DATE DUE

JUL 3 1 2007

D1171490

Air and Surface Patient Transport

Principles and Practice

Air and Surface Patient Transport
Principles and Practice

Third Edition

Edited by

RENEÉ SEMONIN HOLLERAN
RN, PhD, CEN, CCRN, CFRN
Chief Flight Nurse
Emergency Clinical Specialist
University Air Care
University of Cincinnati
Cincinnati, Ohio

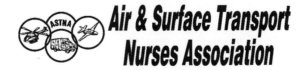

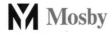

An Affiliate of Elsevier Science
St. Louis   London   Philadelphia   Sydney   Toronto

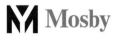

An Affiliate of Elsevier Science

11830 Westline Industrial Drive
St. Louis, Missouri 63146

NOTICE

Nursing is an ever-changing field. Standard safety precautions must be followed, but as new research and clinical experience broaden our knowledge, changes in treatment and drug therapy may become necessary or appropriate. Readers are advised to check the most current product information provided by the manufacturer of each drug to be administered to verify the recommended dose, the method and duration of administration, and contraindications. It is the responsibility of the licensed prescriber, relying on experience and knowledge of the patient, to determine dosages and the best treatment for each individual patient. Neither the publisher nor the editor assumes any liability for any injury and/or damage to persons or property arising from this publication.

Previous editions copyrighted 1991, 1996.

Air and surface patient transport: principles and practice/edited by Renee Semonin Holleran.–3rd ed.
      p.cm.
   Previous editions published under title: Flight nursing.
   Includes bibliographical references and index.
   ISBN 0-323-01701-0 (hardcover)
     1. Aviatiion nursing. 2. Transport of sick and wounded. 3. Airplane ambulances.
   I. Holleran, Reneé Semonin. II. Flight nursing.

   RC1097 .F55 2002   2002029920
   616.9'8021--dc21

Vice President and Publishing Director, Nursing: Sally Schrefer
Executive Editor: Susan R. Epstein
Developmental Editor: Linda Stagg
Publishing Services Manager: John Rogers
Senior Project Manager: Beth Hayes
Designer: Kathi Gosche
Cover Designer: Jennifer Brockett

KI/QWF

Printed in the United States of America

Last digit is the print number: 9 8 7 6 5 4 3 2 1

CONTRIBUTORS TO THE FIRST EDITION

WILLA ADELSTEIN, RN, MSN
Clinical Nurse Specialist, Neurosurgery
University Hospital & Clinics
Columbia, Missouri

LORRAINE ASTON-LINQUIST, RN, BS, CCRN
Flight Nurse, Staff for Life
St. Anthony Hospital Systems
Denver, Colorado

ALLISON L. BOLIN, RN, CEN, CCRN
Charge Nurse, Emergency Department
Community Hospital-Santa Cruz
Santa Cruz, California

DEBBIE BOWMAN, RN, BSN
Flight Nurse
State of Oklahoma Teaching Hospitals
Oklahoma City, Oklahoma

CYNTHIA SALE BRISTOL, RN, BSN, CEN
Flight Nurse, LifeSaver
Carraway Methodist Medical Center
Birmingham, Alabama

JEFFREY H. BROADY
Pilot, Mayo Aeromed
Denver, Colorado

CAPTAIN JAMES T. CANTRELL, R–EMT-P
Little Rock Fire Department
Little Rock, Arkansas

DEBORAH A. CHARLSON, RN, BSN
Trauma Coordinator
Washoe Medical Center
Reno, Nevada

TOM CHURCH, RN
Senior Division Director
Care Team, Health Care Service
Fort Worth, Texas

EDDI COHEN, RN, BS, MICN, CCRN, CFRN
Chief Flight Nurse
AIRescue International
Van Nuys, California
Consultant
EMS Network International
Santa Monica,
California.

ROSE CORDER, RN, BSN, EMT-P
Assistant Nurse Manager
Hermann Hospital Life Flight
Houston, Texas

NANCY COWLES, RN, BSN
Former Flight Nurse, Flight for Life
Penrose-St. Francis Healthcare Systems
Colorado Springs, Colorado

JANET C. CUNNINGHAM, RN, MS
Pediatric Transport Nurse
Children's Emergency Transport Service
The Children's Hospital
Denver, Colorado

RHYS V. DAPAR, MD
Resident, Emergency Medicine
Harbor-UCLA Medical Center
Torrance, California

ANNE F. DARGA, RN, MS, CCRN
Former Flight Nurse Specialist
University of Michigan Hospitals, Ann Arbor
Clinical Nurse Specialist
Cardiology Division, Northern Michigan Hospital
Petoskey, Michigan

TOM DAVIS III
Pilot, Flight for Life
St. Anthony Hospital Systems
Denver, Colorado

CLYDE DEBELL
Mechanic, Flight for Life
St. Anthony Hospital Systems
Denver, Colorado

SUSAN DOUGLAS, RN, TNS, EMT
Life Flight
Georgia Baptist Medical Center
Atlanta, Georgia

**J. SUSAN DOUGLASS, RN, CERTIFIED
   NEPHROLOGY NURSE**
Educational Coordinator, Dialysis Unit
University of Michigan Medical Center
Ann Arbor, Michigan

GARY DROTAR
Pilot, Mayo Aeromed
Denver, Colorado

LYNN E. EASTES, RN, MS
Trauma Coordinator/Case Manager
Oregon Health Sciences University
Portland, Oregon

NANCY GRABOWSKI ELLIOTT, RN, BSN, MBA
National Board Member
Board of Directors, National Flight Nurses
Association
Seattle, Washington

KIM EVERT, RN, BS, CCRN
Former Flight Nurse, Flight for Life
Penrose-St. Francis Healthcare Systems
Colorado Springs, Colorado

REBECCA J. YORI FEAGAN, RN, MS, CCRN
Unit Administrator, Surgical ICU
University of Colorado Health Sciences Center
Denver, Colorado

**VANCE FEREBEE, RN, BSN, CEN, TNS,
ADVANCED EMT**
Life Flight
Georgia Baptist Medical Center
Atlanta, Georgia

MARY M. FREITAG-HAGNEY, RN, MSN
Nursing Manager, CVICU
St. Anthony Hospital Systems
Denver, Colorado

SANDRA GATES, RN, BSN
Nurse Manager
Hermann Hospital Life Flight
Houston, Texas

MARY BUSER GILLS, MS, RNC, NNP
Clinical Director
Children's Transport Service
The Children's Hospital
Denver, Colorado

MAGGIE GRIMES, RN, BSN, EMT-P
Clinical Specialist
Hermann Hospital Life Flight
Houston, Texas

WALT HINTON, RN, MS
Deputy Commander, Sheriff Air Medics
San Bernandino Sheriff's Department
Rialto, California

FORREST HOLDEN, MD
Emergency Medicine Consultants
Phoenix, Arizona

**RENEÉ SEMONIN HOLLERAN, RN PHD, CEN, CCRN,
   CFRN**
Chief Flight Nurse/Emergency Clinical Nurse
   Specialist
University Air Care
University of Cincinnati Medical Center
Cincinnati, Ohio

BUTCH IGNACIO, RN, BSN, TNS, EMT
Life Flight
Georgia Baptist Medical Center
Atlanta, Georgia

JOHN JORDAN, RN, BSN
Chief Flight Nurse
Mayo One, Mayo Foundation
St. Mary's Hospital
Rochester, Minnesota

EVA M. KLINE, RN, BSN
Cardiovascular Research Coordinator
Division of Cardiology
University of Michigan Hospitals
Ann Arbor, Michigan

HEATHER LIGHTFOOT, RN, CEN
Flight Nurse, UTMB Life Flight
University of Texas Medical Branch
Galveston, Texas

LESLEY LOOS, RN, CEN, CFRN, TNS
Flight Nurse, Staff for Life
University Hospital & Clinics
Columbia, Missouri

KATHLEEN MAYER, RN, BSN
Flight Nurse, Flight for Life
St. Anthony Hospital Systems
Denver, Colorado

TERRY McCRARY, RN, CCRN, TNS, EMT
Life Flight
Georgia Baptist Medical Center
Atlanta, Georgia

KEVIN MERIGIAN, MD
Medical Toxicology Consultants
Cincinnati, Ohio

MARY E. MITCHELL, RN, BSN, TNS, NREMT
Life Flight
Georgia Baptist Medical Center
Atlanta, Georgia

PAMELA C. MOORE, RN
Director, Pediatric Life Flight
Primary Children's Medical Center
Salt Lake City, Utah

BETTYE MORRIS, RN, TNS, EMT
Chief Flight Nurse, Life Flight
Georgia Baptist Medical Center
Atlanta, Georgia

DAVE NATHAN, BS, EMT-P
Firefighter-Paramedic
Birmingham Fire and Rescue Service
Assistant Chief Communications Technician
LifeSaver, Carraway Methodist Medical Center
Birmingham, Alabama

SHIRLEY NEVILLE, RN, BHS, CCRN, CFRN,
   CEN, TNS
Flight Nurse, Staff for Life
University Hospital & Clinics
Columbia, Missouri

CYNTHIA NEWTON, RN, TNS, EMT
Life Flight
Georgia Baptist Medical Center
Atlanta, Georgia

MARY ANN NIEHAUS, RN, MSN, CEN, REMT-P
Flight Nurse, University Air Care
University of Cincinnati Medical Center
Cincinnati, Ohio

EDWARD OTTEN, MD
Associate Professor
Director, Prehospital Care
University of Cincinnati Medical Center
Cincinnati, Ohio

PATRICIA A. RAILSBACK, RN, BSN,
   CCRN, CEN
Nursing Manager
Boston MedFlight
Boston, Massachusetts

BOB RUELL
Flight for Life
St. Anthony Hospital Systems
Denver, Colorado

SUSAN RUELL, BA, EMT
Dispatcher, Communications Center
St. Anthony Hospital Systems
Denver, Colorado

PATRICIA M. SCOTT, EMT
Formerly Mayo AeroMed
Denver, Colorado

GAIL D. SKINNER, RN, BSN
Perinatal Flight Nurse
Samaritan AirEvac
Phoenix, Arizona

DANIEL STORER, MD
Associate Professor
Medical Director, University Air Care
University of Cincinnati Medical Center
Cincinnati, Ohio

MARK SWICORD, RN, RNS, CEN, EMT
Life Flight
Georgia Baptist Medical Center
Atlanta, Georgia

KENDRA TJELMELAND, RN, BSN, CCRN
Research/QA Coordinator
Samaritan AirEvac
Phoenix, Arizona

NANCY TUNE, RN-C, BSN
Reengineering Specialist
Critical Care Educator
Boone Hospital Center
Columbia, Missouri

LORRAINE M. VUKICH, RN, MS, ARNP
Director, Trauma & Flight Services
University Medical Center
Jacksonville, Florida

RUSSELL R. WAGGONER, RN, BSN, CEN, EMT-P, IC
Flight Nurse Specialist
University of Michigan Medical Center
Ann Arbor, Michigan

CHRISTINE M. ZALAR, MA
Partner
Fitch & Associates, Inc.
Platte City, Missouri

Contributors to the Second Edition

Willa Adelstein, RN, MSN
Clinical Nurse Specialist, Neurosurgery
University Hospital & Clinics
Columbia, Missouri

Tony Bright, BS
Communications Supervisor
Administrative Assistant
University Air Care
University of Cincinnati Medical Center
Cincinnati, Ohio

Kevin Broford
Line Pilot/Safety Committee Member
PHI Aeromedical Services
University Air Care
Cincinnati, Ohio

Sally Brush, RN, CCRN
Chief Flight Nurse
IHC Life Flight
Intermountain Health Care
Salt Lake City, Utah

Eddi Cohen, RN, BS, MICN, CCRN, CFRN
Chief Flight Nurse
AIRescue International
Van Nuys, California
Consultant
EMS Network International
Santa Monica, California

Tom Culwell, RN, BSN, CEN, CCRN, CFRN, EMT-P
Regional Chief Flight Nurse
Critical Air Medicine
San Antonio, Texas

Janet C. Cunningham, RN, MS
Pediatric Transport Nurse
Children's Emergency Transport Service
The Children's Hospital
Denver, Colorado

Lynn E. Eastes, RN, MS
Trauma Coordinator/Case Manager
Oregon Health Sciences University
Portland, Oregon

Mike Englebert
Lead Pilot
PHI Aeromedical Services
University Air Care
Cincinnati, Ohio

Cheryl J. Erler, RN, MS
Associate Professor
Purdue University
School of Nursing
West Lafayette, Indiana

Ilona Francis, MS, RNC, NNP
Neonatal Nurse Practitioner
Children's Transport Service
The Children's Hospital
Denver, Colorado

Mary Buser Gills, MS, RNC, NNP
Clinical Director
Children's Transport Service
The Children's Hospital
Denver, Colorado

ix

JEANETTE GOLTERMANN, RN, MBA, CFRN
Flight Nurse
Loyola Life Star
Maywood, Illinois

SUE HAGER, RN
Flight Nurse
Survival Flight
University of Michigan Medical Center
Ann Arbor, Michigan

KAREN JOHNSON, RN
Flight Nurse
Samaritan Air Evac
Phoenix, Arizona

LESLEY LOOS, RN, CEN, CFRN, TNS
Flight Nurse, Staff for Life
University Hospital & Clinics
Columbia, Missouri

LAURA LOWE, RN, CCRN, EMT
Flight Nurse, Staff for Life
University Hospital & Clinics
Columbia, Missouri

NEMA MCELVEEN, RN, CCRN
Flight Nurse
Lifestar, Inc.
Savannah, Georgia

HEATHER MCLELLAN, RN, BN, CFRN
Medical Operations Manager
STARS
Calgary, Alberta

SHIRLEY NEVILLE, RN, BHS, CCRN, CFRN, CEN, TNS
Flight Nurse, Staff for Life
University Hospital & Clinics
Columbia, Missouri

MICHELLE NORTH
Director of Safety
Rocky Mountain Helicopters
Sacramento, California

EILEEN PATTON, RN, BHS, CCRN, CEN, TNS, EMT-P
Assistant Manager, Staff for Life
University Hospital & Clinics
Columbia, Missouri

NANCY P. VON ROTZ, RN, MSN
Flight Nurse
University Air Care
University of Cincinnati Medical Center
Cincinnati, Ohio

NANCY PROSSER, RN, BSN, CEN
Flight Nurse
University Air Care
University of Cincinnati Medical Center
Cincinnati, Ohio

MICHAEL ROUSE, RN, BSN, CFRN
Flight Nurse
University Air Care
University of Cincinnati Medical Center
Cincinnati, Ohio

LEEANN RUNYAN, RN, CCRN
Flight Nurse, Staff for Life
University Hospital & Clinics
Columbia, Missouri

MICHAEL SNYDER
Flight Nurse
Survival Flight
University of Michigan Medical Center
Ann Arbor, Michigan

MICHAEL SPADAFORA, MD
Assistant Professor of Emergency Medicine
Director, Hyperbaric Medicine
University of Cincinnati
Center for Emergency Care
Cincinnati, Ohio

FRANK THOMAS, MD
Medical Director
IHC Life Flight
Intermountain Health Care
Salt Lake City, Utah

RICHARD S. TOBIASZ, RN, BS, CEN, CCRN, CFRN, EMT-P
Chief Flight Nurse
Flight for Life
Northern Illinois Medical Center
McHenry, Illinois

NANCY TUNE, RN-C, BSN
Reengineering Specialist
Critical Care Educator
Boone Hospital Center
Columbia, Missouri

RUSSELL R. WAGGONER, RN, BSN, CEN, EMT-P, IC
Flight Nurse Specialist
University of Michigan Medical Center
Ann Arbor, Michigan

CHRISTOPHER WAGNER, RN, CEN, CCRN, EMT-P
Flight Nurse
Survival Flight
University of Michigan Medical Center
Ann Arbor, Michigan

JANET WILLIAMS, RN, MSN, CCRN
Flight Nurse
University Air Care
University of Cincinnati Medical Center
Cincinnati, Ohio

JUDY WILSON, RNC, BSN
Maternal Transport Coordinator
Barnes Hospital
BJC Health Systems
St. Louis, Missouri

CHERYL WRAA, RN, BSN, CFRN
Flight Nurse, Clinical Resource Nurse
Life Flight
University of California, Davis Medical Center
Sacramento, California

DONNA YORK, RN, MS, CFRN
Chief Flight Nurse/Nurse Manager
Stanford Life Flight/Medical Transport Program
Stanford Health Services
San Francisco, California

LINDA YOUNG, RN, MNA
Manager CQI/Research
Samaritan AirEvac
Phoenix, Arizona

CHRISTINE M. ZALAR, MA
Partner
Fitch & Associates, Inc.
Platte City, Missouri

CONTRIBUTORS TO THE THIRD EDITION

REBECCA BAUTE, RN, BSN, CMTE
Clinical Director, Transport
Cincinnati Children's Hospital Medical Center
Cincinnati, Ohio

TONY BRIGHT, BS
Senior Administrative Assistant
University Air Care
Cincinnati, Ohio

THOMAS J. CAHILL, RCP, RRT, EMT-P
Manager Respiratory Care
Shriners Hospital for Children–Cincinnati
Cincinnati, Ohio

DONNA YORK CLARK, RN, MS, CCRN
Director, DHART
Dartmoth-Hitchcock Medical Center
Lebanon, New Hampshire
Air and Surface Transport Nurses Association
Immediate Past President

EDDI COHEN, RN, BS, MICN, CCRN, MRCNA
Director of Training
Airescue International
Van Nuys, California
Medical Director/Clinical Consultant
Mobile Medical Systems International
Sydney, Australia

SCOTT DEBOER, RN, MSN, CFRN
Flight Nurse Educator, UCAN
University of Chicago Hospitals
Founder, Peds-R-Us Medical Education
Dyer, Indiana

EILEEN FRAZER, RN
Executive Director
Commission on Accreditation of Medical
Transport Systems (CAMTS)
Anderson, South Carolina

ANGELA K. GOLDEN, RN, MNED, MS, FNP-C, CNS/CFRN
Family Nurse Practitioner
Verde Valley Medical Center
Emergency Department
Cottonwood, Arizona
Family Nurse Practitioner
White Mountain Regional Medical
Center
Emergency Department
Springerville, Arizona
Assistant Clinical Professor
Northern Arizona University
Flagstaff, Arizona

JONATHAN D. GRYNIUK, FP-C, CCEMT-P, NREMT-P, RRT
Flight Paramedic
National Flight Paramedics Association Board
of Directors
Albany Med FLIGHT/Life Net
Rocky Mountain Helicopters
Albany, New York

MARGARET WATSON HOPKINS, RN, MN, CFRN
Clinical Nurse, Post Anesthesia Care Unit
University of California, Davis, Medical Center
Sacramento, California

SALLY HOULISTON, RCPN, BN, CFN, CRITICAL CARE CERTIFICATE
Flight Nurse, Pacific Air Ambulance
Chairperson, New Zealand Flight Nurses
Association (NZNO)
Auckland, New Zealand

JILL JOHNSON, RN, BSN, BA, CEN, CCRN, CFRN
Flight Nurse
AirLife Denver
Englewood, Colorado
2002 President
Air and Surface Transport Nurses Association

ZEB KORAN, RN, MSN, CEN, TNS
Executive Director
Board of Certification for Emergency Nursing
   (BCEN)
Des Plaines, Illinois

BETTY KOVACH, RN, BSN, CCRN, EMT-P
Chief Flight Nurse, Metro Life Flight
MetroHealth Medical Center
Cleveland, Ohio

ANN LYSTRUP, RN, BSN, CCRN, CEN, CFRN
Flight Nurse
University of Utah AIRMED
Salt Lake City, Utah

GERI MALONE, BSN
President
Flight Nurses Australia 2000-2002
Adelaide, South Australia

CHRISTOPHER MANACCI, RN, CCRN, CFRN
Flight Nurse Specialist, Metro Life Flight
MetroHealth Medical Center
Clinical Faculty
Case Western Reserve University
Cleveland, Ohio

CHARLENE MANCUSO, RN, BSN, MPA, CEN
Operations Director
Division of Burns, Trauma, Critical Care and Metro
   Life Flight
MetroHealth Medical Center
Cleveland, Ohio

HEATHER MCLELLAN, RN, BN, CFRN
QI/Educational Developmental Coordinator
Alberta STARS
Calgary, Alberta
Canada

CAROL PATTERSON, RN, BSN, CCRN
Flight Nurse CN IV
University Air Care
Cincinnati, Ohio

MICHAEL ROUSE, RN, MSN, CRNA
Nurse Anesthetist
University Hospital
Flight Nurse CN-IV
University Air Care
Cincinnati, Ohio

LESLIE C. SWEET, BSN, RN
Ventricular Assist Device Coordinator
Washington Heart, Washington Hospital Center
Washington, D.C.

DENISE TREADWELL, CRNP, MSN, CEN, CFRN
Director of Medical Services
MEDjet International, Inc.
Cabin Services Supervisor
BBJ Charters, Inc.
Birmingham, Alabama

NANCY FLINT VON ROTZ, RN, BSN, MSN, FNP, CCRN
Flight Nurse
University Air Care
Cincinnati, Ohio

CHRISTOPHER WAGNER, RN PARAMEDIC
Flight Nurse Specialist
University of Michigan Medical Center, Survival Flight
Ann Arbor, Michigan

ALLEN C. WOLFE, JR., RN, BSN, TNATC
Clinical Specialist—MedSTAR Transport Program
The Washington Hospital Center
Washington, DC

CHERYL WRAA, RN, MSN
Trauma Program Coordinator
University of California, Davis Medical Center
Sacramento, California

REVIEWERS FOR THE THIRD EDITION

DONNA YORK CLARK, RN, MS, CCRN
Director, DHART
Dartmoth-Hitchcock Medical Center
Lebanon, New Hampshire

SCOTT DEBOER, RN, MSN, CFRN
Flight Nurse Educator, UCAN
University of Chicago Hospitals
Founder, Peds-R-Us Medical Education
Dyer, Indiana

JILL JOHNSON, RN, BSN, BA, CEN, CCRN, CFRN
Flight Nurse
AirLife Denver
Englewood, Colorado
2002 President
Air and Transport Nurses Association

JACQUELINE STOCKING, RN, MSN, CEN, CFRN, FP-C, EMT-P/LP
Director of Clinical Education and Outreach
Critical Air Medicine
Austin, TX

The third edition of this text is dedicated first to my "families." My husband Michael, my children Erin and Sara, and my mom, where the Semonin comes from. My other family is the nurses, communication specialists, mechanics, and pilots with whom I have had the privilege to work for more than 17 years at University Air Care in Cincinnati, Ohio.

Finally, the third edition of this text is for all who provide patient transport and particularly for those who have made the ultimate sacrifice—the loss of their lives doing what they loved, as have Sandy Sigman, Tim Hynes, and Don Green. And to Pam, who inspired us all.

Thank you and please be safe!

Reneé Semonin Holleran RN, PhD, CEN, CCRN, CFRN

FOREWORD

This marks the third generation of a textbook originally intended to serve the needs of the National Flight Nurses Association (NFNA) and a small cadre of other professionals interested in the care of patients during transport. Just as the NFNA has grown to be the Air and Surface Transport Nurses Association (ASTNA) in an effort to include and address issues for all nurses involved in patient transport, *Principles and Practice* has grown.

In this edition, *Air and Surface Patient Transport: Principles and Practice,* the original themes have been expanded to meet the educational and resource needs of all health-care providers dedicated to expert care delivery in transport.

ASTNA is so appreciative for the unending dedication Reneé Semonin Holleran has given to this effort. Truly, without her passion and expertise, this text would not be a reality.

The ASTNA Board of Directors is thankful for the commitment of those members who have authored chapters—we thank you for your time and expertise. We are also grateful to the National Flight Paramedic Association and the Association of Respiratory Care—Transport Section for their contributions to this work. Once again, we have proven greater success can be accomplished when we work together!

In closing, a wish for all involved in the care of patients in transport—may you learn something every day, may you always have great team members, and may safety dictate your decisions!

Donna York Clark RN, MS, CFRN
President
Air and Surface Transport Nurses Association
October, 2000-2001

PREFACE

The National Flight Nurses Association (now the Air and Surface Transport Nurses Association) recognized the need for a comprehensive textbook that contained information pertinent to the practice of flight nursing. The first edition of this book was published in 1991 and edited by Genell Lee, RN, MSN, CEN. The second edition, edited by myself, expanded to include more clinical information, psychosocial needs of the patient and family, and the first description of the roles of those who participate in patient transport.

The first thing you will notice about the third edition of this text is the name change. Patient transport is a collaborative, dynamic process. *Air and Surface Patient Transport: Principles and Practice* attempts to represent the nurses, paramedics, physicians, respiratory therapists, pilots, mechanics, and communication specialists who all play key roles in patient transport. In addition, the focus of the text has broadened to include both air and ground patient transport.

The text is divided into nine units, which include:

- History and the Current Role of Ground and Air Transport Nurses
- General Principles of Practice
- Patient Care Principles
- Trauma
- Medical Problems
- Environmental Emergencies
- Selected Patient Populations
- Patient Care Issues
- Management

Each section contains an updated, collaborative focus on patient transport. However, as some of you may have already found, the more things change, the more they remain the same.

Clinical chapters still list basic competencies and provide a case study that may be used for discussion. Some of the case studies are new. Others are classic teaching tools and have remained the same.

An Appendix has been added that contains descriptions of international patient transport. It also makes available the mission and goals of other transport associations.

Many changes and challenges have arisen in patient transport. Certification, accreditation, legal and ethical issues, and the needs of the family represent only a small number of these.

Transport cannot be done in a vacuum. It is collaborative, and many times it is controlled by forces over which we have little influence. The broader focused we are, better prepared we are, and the more open we are to change, the better care we will provide to those we serve.

ACKNOWLEDGMENTS

The third edition of this book would not have been possible without the work of those who wrote and edited the first and second editions of *Flight Nursing: Principles and Practice.* Genell Lee had the vision and courage to edit the first edition of the text. Cheryl Wraa, Jeanette Goltermann, and Mike Rouse were instrumental in the production of the second edition.

I would like to thank those from the other disciplines who are key in patient transport for their hard work on this third edition. If we do not continue to take pleasure in what makes us the same, we will never become what our patients need.

I would also like to thank all of the editors who have helped me, especially Emily, Laurie, Lisa, and Shari.

INTRODUCTION TO THE FIRST EDITION

In 1980 a steering committee of four flight nurses met to consider the development of a national organization for flight nurses. The members of the steering committee were Jean Mason, RN, of LifeFlight, Hermann Hospital, Houston, Texas; Marcia Katz, RN, of LifeFlight, St. Joseph's Hospital, Omaha, Nebraska; Sally Nielson, RN, of Aircare, University of Iowa Hospital, Iowa City, Iowa; and Pat Noonan, RN, of Aircare, West Jefferson General Hospital, Marerro, Louisiana. After a year of developing bylaws, the organization was founded in 1981. Jean Mason was elected the first President of the National Flight Nurses Association.

The initial goals established by the organization were:

1. To promote the delivery of quality care to patients
2. To develop minimum training standards for flight nurses
3. To develop minimum standards of care for flight nurses
4. To share flight nursing knowledge
5. To provide hospitals considering emergency air service programs with assistance in developing appropriate programs
6. To promote continuing education for all flight crews
7. To promote quality assurance
8. To develop and promote optimum working conditions for all flight nurses

During the first year, the *Flight Nurse Newsletter,* edited by John Jordan, was started. Rose Corder developed the NFNA philosophy and Bill Swanson designed the NFNA Logo.

The NFNA will celebrate its 10-year anniversary in 1991. The textbook *Flight Nursing: Principles and Practice* is a culmination of 5 years of effort on the part of members of NFNA. Its intent is to advance the goals and objectives of the National Flight Nurses Association. This book is dedicated to the efforts and accomplishments of flight nurses past, present, and future.

Genell Lee, RN, MSN, CEN
Editor-In-Chief

INTRODUCTION TO THE THIRD EDITION

Critical care patient transport involves moving patients from various locations to definitive care. The patient may require transport directly from the scene of illness or injury, the emergency department, or a critical care unit. The patient could be moved by air or ground. Care during transport may be provided by a variety of specially qualified teams.

Critical care transport requires a broad knowledge base and expansive clinical experience. Critical care transport teams work collaboratively with a number of other health-care providers, including nurses, physicians, and prehospital care providers. Depending on the type of patient transport, the transport team may be composed of nurses, paramedics, physicians, or respiratory therapists. The transport team also includes a medical director, program management, pilots, drivers, mechanics, and communication specialists.

The role of the critical care transport team is multifaceted and often depends on where the transport team works. The responsibilities of the critical care transport team include clinical practice, patient advocacy and education, research, and management. Because of these varied functions, this practice requires that members of the critical care transport continue their education, practice skill competencies, and be active in their professional organizations.

In the third edition of this text, a decision was made to include as many of the components of patient transport as possible. The text was lengthened to encompass the broader concept of patient transport. Included now are the most common types of transport team members, preparation for practice, certification, research, and accreditation. As indicated, new information has been incorporated so that the most up-to-date information is available for practice. The world of patient transport continues to change, and we as professionals strive to not only keep up with it, but to shape these changes in order to provide safe and competent patient transport.

Reneé Semonin Holleran
RN, PhD, CEN, CCRN, CFRN

THE AIR AND SURFACE TRANSPORT NURSES ASSOCIATION ORGANIZATIONAL PHILOSOPHY

In 1981 the organization known as the National Flight Nurses Association (NFNA) was founded. The initial goals were:

1. To promote the delivery of quality care to patients
2. To develop minimum training standards for flight nurses
3. To develop minimum standards of care for flight nurses
4. To share flight nursing knowledge
5. To provide hospitals considering emergency air service programs with assistance in developing appropriate programs
6. To promote continuing education for all flight crews
7. To promote quality assurance
8. To develop and promote optimum work conditions for all flight nurses

In 1997 NFNA recognized that flight and ground nurses shared a common role. It was decided to change the name of the organization to the Air and Surface Transport Nurses Association. Although the organization has evolved over the years and grown, we still hold on to the core beliefs and philosophy.

Its bylaws and mission as a membership organization of professional nurses who practice transport nursing define the Air and Surface Transport Nurses Association (ASTNA).

Transport nursing is a unique and expanded role for a nursing professional, encompassing the air and surface transport of critically ill and injured patients. This role is characterized by expanded nursing practice based on the ever-growing body of transport nursing knowledge and ASTNA standards of care.

ASTNA is the dominant and leading body representing transport nurses as the voice of clinical care in the transport field with regard to patient and provider advocacy. Its leadership shall be representative of those professional nurses meeting membership criteria.

The activities of ASTNA are performed in a manner that exemplifies a service ethic and orientation toward the membership. ASTNA activities are focused on supporting, serving, and facilitating communication among professional nurses who practice or are actively involved in the support education or management of transport nurses.

MISSION STATEMENT

The Air and Surface Transport Nurses Association is a nonprofit member organization whose mission is to *advance the practice of transport nursing and enhance the quality of patient care.*

GOALS

1. Provide clear and decisive leadership for the unique and distinct specialty of transport nursing

2. Facilitate opportunities for communication and collaboration among transport nurses
3. Provide representation and liaison in forums that relate to the practice of transport nursing
4. Support and promote scientific research that enhances transport nursing knowledge and patient care
5. Promote continuing education specific to the advancement of transport nursing
6. Serve as an information resource about transport nursing and the various modes of transport care delivery systems

CONTENTS

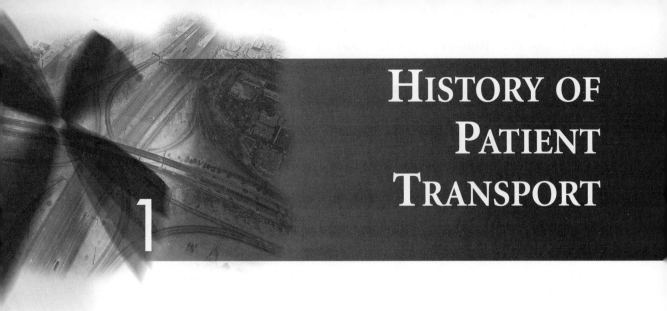

PATIENT TRANSPORT

The history of patient transport can be traced back to before the invention of the wheel, when patients were carried or dragged to care. Ambulance systems were first established in the 1400s to transport war casualties. These ambulances assumed many forms, from a horse-pulled stretcher to wagons developed specifically for patient transport.

During the Civil War the United States Army developed an organized ambulance system for transport of the wounded. Plans were also developed for effective evacuation and treatment of casualties from the battlefield. At this time, trains and steamboats were used to transport patients in addition to conventional ambulance transport.[4,6,11]

In the eighteenth century an intense interest in resuscitation began. The first organized effort to deal with resuscitation was started by a group of wealthy men in 1767 in Amsterdam. They were known as the Society for the Recovery of Drowned Persons. One of the suggestions made by the group was that persons who required resuscitation should be taken to receiving houses (hospitals), where trained individuals could resuscitate them.[5] The need to identify a method of civilian-based transport thus became an important issue.

In 1865 the first hospital-based ambulance service was started at Cincinnati Commercial Hospital in Cincinnati, Ohio (Figure 1-1).

The first electric ambulance was used in 1899 at the Michael Reese Hospital in Chicago. In 1905 a bulletproof ambulance was introduced for military use on the battlefield. During World War I, buses were converted into mobile surgical units to treat the wounded. The Model T Ford was also placed into action during World War I to transport patients.

Despite an old claim that balloons were once used to transport the injured from the battlefield, patient air medical transport was not used until 1915.[10] The French were successful in using planes to evacuate patients during World War I, which led to the French development of ambulance aircraft.

During World War I the United States successfully completed air ambulance transports using old JN-4 aircraft that they converted into air ambulances. The JN-4 aircraft were large, old, and costly to maintain. As they started to break down, the military decided not to invest in the maintenance of the aircraft. The military was interested in a smaller, less-costly aircraft for patient transport.

Igor Sirkorsky developed the first helicopter, and the military subsequently became very interested in its use. The U.S. Army commissioned

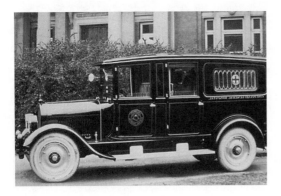

FIGURE 1-1   Early ambulance dispatched from Cincinnati Hospital to transport patients.

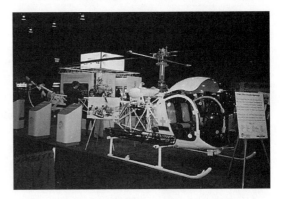

FIGURE 1-2   Helicopter used to transport patients during the Korean War.

Sirkorsky to produce several helicopters for general military use. They found that a helicopter was successful at getting into small areas, and thus the military used it to drop off special units in remote areas.

The first patient helicopter rescue took place in April 1944 in the jungles of Burma. When a helicopter dropped off a military group, a wounded soldier was loaded on to be taken back to a field hospital. This was the beginning of patient transport by helicopter in the military.

Approximately 20,000 wounded men were transported by helicopter during the Korean War. A special helicopter unit was formed and attached to the mobile army surgical hospital (MASH) (Figure 1-2).

During the Vietnam War the care and transport of the ill and injured continued to mature. Approximately 200,000 injured were transported by helicopter during this conflict. Medics were placed on ships to triage and provide care from the battlefield to the field hospital.[3]

In the late 1960s the Scottish Air Ambulance System began patient transports from surrounding islands to the mainland. This was the first civilian air transport system to be placed in service. In 1972 St. Anthony's Hospital in Denver, Colorado, and Lind Loma Hospital in California started the first hospital-based helicopter programs (Figure 1-3).

During the 1980s hospital-based programs were opened at an amazing pace. By 1987 there were 150

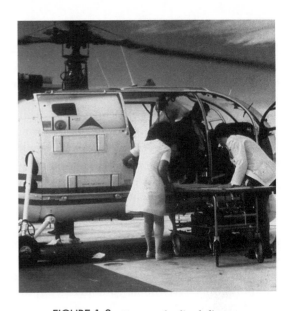

FIGURE 1-3   Nurses unloading helicopter.

programs. Beginning the next century, there are over 400 air medical transport programs worldwide (Figure 1-4).

As ground and air transport of the ill and injured progressed, the care they required before and during transport also advanced. It was not until the twentieth century that reliable methods of resuscitation were developed, studied, and used consistently outside the hospital. In the 1960s the work of Safar and Elam, mouth-to-mouth-resuscitation or the "kiss of

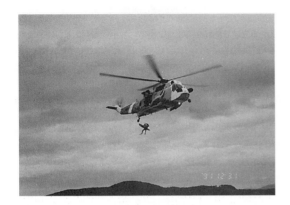

FIGURE 1-4   Norwegian air medical helicopter.

life," was combined with that of Kouwenhoven, who demonstrated the benefits of cardiac massage. Cardiopulmonary resuscitation was then taken from within the walls of the hospital to the field through the pioneering work of Emergency Medical Systems in Los Angeles, California, Warren, Ohio, and Miami, Florida, in the late 1960s and 1970s.[5,6,7]

The initial equipment used in hospital resuscitation was large and nontransportable, and it operated only on AC power. The advent of battery-operated portable monitors and defibrillators greatly improved the care of the critically ill or injured patient during transport. The safety of equipment was improved so that it could be used in any type of transport vehicle without interfering with vehicle operations. Today the monitors used during transport offer multiple functions, such as continuous rhythm monitoring, invasive monitoring, defibrillation, and external pacing.[8]

A Mobile Coronary Care Unit, staffed with both nurses and physicians, was started in Belfast, Ireland, in 1966. In 1968 similar units went into service in Great Britain, the United States, and Australia. The value of trained personnel who could provide critical care outside the hospital continued to grow into the systems that exist throughout the world today.[5]

THE HISTORY OF NURSING IN CRITICAL CARE TRANSPORT

The word *nursing* is derived from the Latin word *nutrire*, to nourish.[1] Florence Nightingale is consid-

ered the founder of modern nursing practice and was one of the original nurses practicing in the "field."[1] In 1854 Florence Nightingale was put in charge of the Female Nursing Establishment of the English General Hospitals in Turkey during the Crimean War. Within 6 months the death rate in the military hospitals went from 47% to 2.2% under her leadership. She went to the front lines where she visited and cared for the ill and injured until she became ill with Crimean fever and was sent back to England. Her work during the Crimean War laid the foundation of prehospital nursing practice.

The U.S. Civil War furnished nurses with an opportunity to demonstrate their skills and administer care to ill and injured soldiers. Nurses served in volunteer corps during the Civil War, offering care to both the Union and Confederate Armies.

Clara Barton emerged as the symbol of nursing's philosophy to meet the health needs of all humans, regardless of race, creed, or color. She was an outspoken opponent of slavery, and she gave care on the battlefield to Northerners, Southerners, blacks, and whites.[4] She went on to establish the American Red Cross in 1882. Many transport nurses today are MAT (Mobile Assist Teams) nurses, who play an integral role in delivering care to victims of disasters.

In the twentieth century, nurses have been active participants in World War I, World War II, the Korean and Vietnam Wars, and more recently, the Gulf War. Nurses, physicians, and corpsman, working only miles from the battlefront, have staffed hospitals known as Mobile Army Surgical Hospitals (MASH) and Medical Unit Self-contained Transportable (MUST). The war experiences of the twentieth century have shown that field stabilization and rapid transport can decrease mortality and morbidity rates. Nurses have played a significant role in the delivery of this care in the field, particularly through flight nursing.

The origin of flight nursing can be traced to Laureate M. Schimmoler, who formed the Emergency Flight Corps in 1933. Ms. Schimmoler influenced the military to open its first flight nurse training program in 1942 at the 349th Air Evacuation Group, Bowman Field, Louisville, Kentucky. The training program lasted 6 weeks and included flight physiology. The "Bees" was the insignia for these nurses (Figure 1-5) A description of its meaning is included.

To become a flight nurse a nurse had to send an application to the Army Nurse Corps and work 6 months at an Army Air Force Hospital. After completion of flight school one could submit a request to the Commanding General of the Army Air Force for the designation "Flight Nurse." Many nurses desired to enter the program because flight nursing represented the elite of the corps (Box 1-1).

On February 18, 1943, the first class of flight nurses graduated from the specialized course of medical training at Bowman Field in Louisville, Kentucky. General David Grant, one of the driving forces behind this new field of military nursing, officiated at the ceremony. Realizing that no one had thought of an insignia for this new group of nurses, he pinned his own flight surgeon's wings on the honor graduate, Geraldine Dishroon. The first to receive the wings, she was designated the first flight nurse (Box 1-2).

During World War II fixed-wing aircraft transported 1.5 million patients with educated flight nurses in attendance.[4,9] During World War II more than 1600 nurses were decorated for meritorious service and bravery under fire. By the end of World War II, 201 nurses were dead, and 16 were missing.

After World War II flight nurse training was conducted by the Air Force. Flight nurses were activated for service during both the Korean and Vietnam Wars.

During the Korean and Vietnam Wars the value of helicopter transport of the injured was recognized. Many of the physicians, nurses, and corpsmen who spent time in these wars felt that there was also a role for helicopter transport in the civilian care of those who were injured or needed to be transported to another care facility.[6]

In 1972 St. Anthony's Hospital in Denver established a civilian-based flight program staffed by nurses with critical care experience. Herman Hospital in Houston, Texas, established a flight

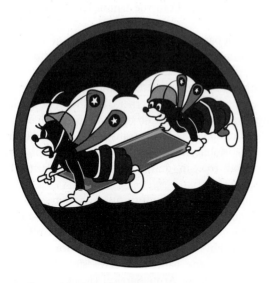

FIGURE 1-5 **Bees insignia.** The insignia of the U.S. Army Air Force's School of Air Evacuation was a dark blue disc with two honeybees, whose bodies were or (gold) and sable (black) with argent (white) wings bearing stars, carrying a brown litter all in front of an argent cloud. Blue and gold are the Air Corps colors. The honeybees, helmeted and wearing red cross armbands, are indicative of the industry displayed by the personnel of the organization. The litter is symbolic of evacuation of the sick and wounded, the cloud indicative of the area in which the mission is carried out. The insignia was designed by Mrs. Don Rider of Buechel, Kentucky, who was greatly impressed by the work of the air evacuation personnel during the flood in Louisville in 1942.

BOX 1-1	"The Song of the Army Nurse Corps"

We march along with faith undaunted beside our
    gallant fighting men;
Whenever they are sick or wounded, we nurse them
    back to health again;
As long as healing hands are wanted, You'll find the
    nurses of the Corps;
On ship, or plane, on transport train, at home or on a
    far off shore;
With loyal heart we do our part, for the Army and the
    Army Nurse Corps.

Copyrighted 1944 by MCA Music; Lou Singen, Composer; Hy Zaret, Lyrics.

BOX 1-2	**Flight Nurses's Creed**

I will summon every resource to prevent the triumph of death over life.

I will stand guard over the medicines and equipment entrusted to my care and ensure their proper use.

I will be untiring in the performance of my duties, and I will remember that upon my disposition and spirit will in large measure depend the morale of my patients.

I will be faithful to my training and to the wisdom handed down to me by those who have gone before me.

I have taken a nurse's oath reverent in man's mind because of the spirit and work of its creator, Florence Nightingale. She, I remember, was called the "lady with the lamp."

It is now my privilege to lift this lamp of hope and faith and courage in my profession to heights not known by her in her time, Together with the help of the flight surgeons and surgical technicians, I, can set the very skies ablaze with life and promise for the sick, injured and wounded who are my sacred charges.

. . .This I will do, I will not falter, in war or in peace.

David N.W. Grant

Major General, U.S.A.

Air Surgeon

program in 1976 and added a physician to the flight team.

During the 1980s there was a boom in the development of hospital-based programs. At one point there were more than 220 programs. The primary crew member has generally been a registered nurse with either emergency or critical care nursing experience. Other members of the flight team include paramedics, other registered nurses, physicians, and respiratory therapists (Figure 1-6). Some flight programs continue to offer specialized flight teams, such as for maternal or neonatal care.

The practice of flight nursing evolved from the role of nursing care in the field and continues to develop based on the type of patients who require transport today. As we begin a new century, we must not forget our roots. Flight nursing is a dynamic component of transport and the key to safe, competent patient care.

THE HISTORY OF THE PARAMEDIC IN CRITICAL CARE TRANSPORT

The lineage of the paramedic can be traced back to the early volunteer ambulance squads organized to provide aid during World War I. These early squads provided little more than transportation of the injured soldier, with squad members having only rudimentary first aid training.

World War II introduced the corpsman, who provided battlefield care to the wounded soldier. In the Korean conflict the corpsman evolved into the field medic, whose rapid care and interventions included packaging the patient for helicopter evacuation.

During the Vietnam War the medics were placed on board the helicopters to provide rapid transport and immediate care.[2,13]

In 1966 significant advancements in civilian emergency medicine occurred in the United States. As a result of the number of traffic deaths in the United States, the U.S. Congress passed the Highway Safety Act, which provided the impetus for the emergence of a nationwide system for prehospital emergency medical services (EMS).[2,13]

In 1969 the federal Department of Transportation developed the first training course for EMTs, and plans were immediately underway to further develop an advanced life support provider, the Emergency Medical Technician-Paramedic (EMT-P).[2] These EMT and paramedic providers were trained in a variety of skills to provide initial stabilization of the acutely ill or injured and to continue this care during transport to a medical facility. The paramedic profession gained official recognition as a health-care occupation in 1975, when the American Medical Association accepted and approved the EMT-P role.[13] Since these early beginnings, EMS has

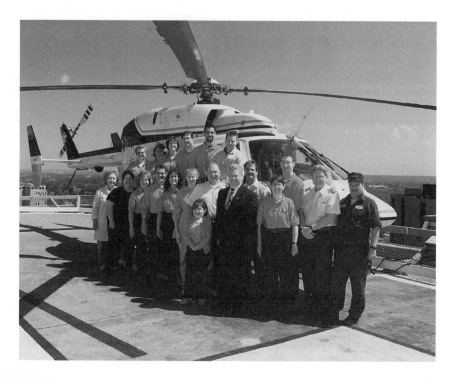

FIGURE 1-6 University Air Care air medical transport crew (Courtesy University Hospital, Cincinnati, Ohio).

evolved to incorporate the use of paramedics within most ambulance systems, including the majority of air medical transport programs.[12]

SUMMARY

Patient transport has existed since patients required movement from the battlefield to areas of safety so care could be rendered. Transport nursing originated through the work of nursing pioneers such as Florence Nightingale and Clara Barton, who became integral to patient care during the battles fought in the nineteenth century. As principles of flight and transport nursing were incorporated into civilian care, hospital-based transport programs were started and staffed by nurses.

Paramedics have been involved in patient transport since the beginning of the century. Their role in critical care transport has continued to expand to critical care paramedics and flight paramedics.

It is important to be familiar with and take pride in where we have come from as we forge into the future. No one profession can provide patient care during the transport process alone.

REFERENCES

1. Bader GB, Terhorst M, Heilman P, DePalma JA: Characteristics of flight nursing practice, Air Med J 14(4):214-218, 1995.
2. Browne B, Jacobs L, Pollack C: *Emergency care and transportation of the sick and injured,* ed 7, Sudbury, Mass, 1999, Jones and Bartlett.
3. Carter G: The evolution of air transport systems: a pictorial review, *J Emerg Med* 6:499-504, 1986.
4. Donahue P: *Nursing: the finest art,* ed 2, St Louis, 1996, Mosby.
5. Eisenberg M, Pantridge J, Cobb L, Geddes J: The revolution and evolution of cardiac care, *Arch Intern Med* 12(26):1-15, 1996.

6. Hackel A: History of medical transport systems. In McClosky K, Orr R, editors: *Pediatric transport medicine,* St Louis, 1995, Mosby.

7. Holleran RS: *Prehospital nursing: a collaborative approach,* St Louis, 1994, Mosby.

8. Holleran RS: Transport monitors: how to choose one for your program, *AirMed* 5(3):43-46, 1999.

9. Lee G: History of flight nursing, *J Emerg Nurs* 13(4):212, 1987.

10. McNab A: Air medical transport: "hot air" and a French lesson, *J Air Med Trans* 11(8):15-16, 1992.

11. Porter R: *The greatest benefit to mankind: a medical history of humanity,* New York, 1999, Knopf.

12. Rau W: 2000 annual transport statistics, *AirMed* 6(4):17-20, 2000.

13. Sanders M: *Mosby's paramedic textbook,* St Louis, 1994, Mosby.

PREPARATION FOR PRACTICE

2

The goals of critical care patient transport[1] are to maintain adequate tissue oxygenation, replace lost fluids and blood, immobilize injured body parts, provide comfort, and deliver early, definitive care, such as the administration of selected therapies. Some examples are the administration of fibrinolytics for acute myocardial infarction or stroke management, methylprednisolone for spinal cord injury, or cerebral resuscitative drugs. The education, skills, and experience needed to provide this care both before and during transport must be diverse and comprehensive.

The Commission on Accreditation of Medical Transport Systems (CAMTS)[4] has standardized the topics that should be covered in a generalized preparation for transport. These topics, which are summarized in Box 2-1, are all considered essential to the initial training of the critical care transport team. Each program should also decide the amount and location of the clinical components, based on their transport profiles.

There are numerous ways to provide a comprehensive orientation. Using adult learning principles, an educational program can be designed that uses self-directed learning packets, traditional lecture with discussion, or case scenario teaching, to name a few techniques.[2,3]

In addition to the didactic information, a practical component of skills training will be needed. This should include various inpatient and prehos-pital care clinical experiences, as well as an invasive skills lab.[4,5]

After the initial education and training is complete, the new transport team member needs to complete an internship or preceptorship. This provides further role definition, recognition of the need for additional education or training, and an opportunity to "put into practice" all the previous learning. Although evaluation is an ongoing process, a final evaluation during the orientation process assists new transport team members in evaluating their experience and the need for any further education.

COMPETENCY-BASED EDUCATION

One of the educational formats that has integrated adult learning principles is competency-based education (CBE). This type of education focuses on the learner's strengths, needs, and learning styles to facilitate mastery of the competencies identified by the transport program.

The components of a CBE program include a skills inventory, which the learner completes and uses to plan the learning experience. A transport program based on role responsibilities creates these inventory lists. Each learner uses a competency checklist to identify learning needs. These competencies are built on the information that transport team members must possess in order to function in their

BOX 2-1 | **CAMTS Initial Training Program Requirements**

Didactic Component
–Advance airway management
–Altitude physiology/stressors of flight
–Anatomy, physiology, and assessment for adult, pediatric, and neonatal patients
–Aviation Ambulance orientation/safety and procedures as appropriate
–Cardiac emergencies and advanced cardiac critical can
–Disaster and triage
–EMS radio communications
–Environmental emergencies
–Hazardious materials recognition and response
–Hemodynamic monitoring, pacemakers, automatic implantable defibrillator (AICD), intra-aortic balloon pump, central lines, pulmonary artery and arterial catheters, ventricular assist devices, and extracorporeal membrane oxygenation (ECMO)
–High risk obstetric emergencies (bleeding, medical, trauma)
–Infection control
–Mechanical ventilation and respiratory physiology for adult, pediatric, and neonatal patients
–Metabolic/endocrine emergencies
–Multi-trauma (chest, abdomen, facial)
–Neonatal emergencies (respiratory distress, surgical, cardiac)
–Oxygen therapy in the medical transport environment—Mechanical ventilation and respiratory physiology for adult, pediatric, and neonatal patients
–Pediatric medical emergencies
–Pediatric trauma
–Pharmacology
–Quality Management
–Respiratory emergencies
–Scene management/rescue/extrication
–Stress recognition and management
–Survival training
–Thermal, chemical, and electrical burns
–Toxicology

Clinical Component
–Critical care
–Emergency care
–Invasive procedures or mannerquin equivalent for practicing invasive procedures
–Neonatal intensive care
–Obstetrics
–Pediatric critical care
–Prehospital care
–Tracheal intubations

BOX 2-2	CAMTS
	Continuing Education Requirements

Didactic continuing education must include the following:

–Aviation—safety issues (if involved in rotorwing or fixed wing operations)

–Altitude physiology/stressors of flight (if involved in both rotorwing and fixed wing operations)

–Critical care courses

–Emergency care courses

–Hazardous materials recognition and response

–Infection control

–State EMS rules and regulations regarding ground and air transport

–Stress recognition and management

–Survival training

Clinical and laboratory continuing education should be developed and documented on an annual basis and must include the following:

–Critical care (adult, pediatric, neontatal)

–Emergency/trauma care

–Invasive procedure labs

–Labor and delivery

–Prehospital experience

–Skills maintenance program documented to comply with number of skills required in a set period of time according to policy of the medical transport service (i.e., endotracheal incubations, chest tubes).

   a. Basic Life Support (BLS)—documented evidence of current BLS certification according to the American Heart Association (AHA)

   b. Advanced Cardiac Life Support (ACLS)—documented evidence of current ACLS according to the AHA.

   c. Advanced Trauma Life Support (ATLS)—according to the American College of Surgeons, ATLS audit, Flight Nurse Advanced Trauma Course (FNATC), or Trauma Nurse Specialist (TNS).

   d. Pediatric Advanced Life Support (PALS)—or Advanced Pediatric Life Support (APLS) according to the AHA and ACEP, or equivalent education.

   e. Neonatal Resuscitation Program (NRP)—documented evidence of current NRP according to the AHA and AAP.

   f. Nursing certifications (such as CEN, CCRN, CFRN, RNC) are encouraged, and if required in position descriptions, certifications must be current.

---

role, as well specific skills that are needed. Once these skills are developed they are used both for the novice (or initial training) and as a continuing checklist for the expert (continuing-education documentation).

Specific behavioral objectives are also needed, which relate to the interpersonal, technical, and critical thinking skills identified in the specific job description and area of clinical responsibilities. These objectives are then used to determine that the initial orientation has been completed. They can also be used for ongoing performance evaluations within the transport program.

The final component of the CBE is the self-learning packages. They are educational resources that allow familiarization with policies, procedures, processes, and knowledge required to perform the transport role.

CBE was originally designed for nursing education, where only one person at a time was being oriented. It is to be used with a preceptor and clinical practice experience. Many transport programs have found this system to be a great addition to their initial orientation. They have used the components of skills inventory lists, competency checklists, and behavioral objectives to design an orientation program for each individual class of transport team members in initial training. The use of self-learning packages has been effective for certain areas, especially repetitive didactic information that is covered annually, such as infection control and altitude physiology.

CONTINUING EDUCATION

CAMTS[1] describes specific components of transport education and skills that should be covered annually (Box 2-2). In addition, individual transport members should recognize their own educational needs independent of any requirements. This is part of the process of becoming an expert in the art and science of critical care transport.

Continuing education in the transport program has a fixed portion of training, including OSHA, local, and state requirements, as well as accreditation standards. The transport team has a professional responsibility to maintain and continue to gain knowledge in the profession. Other sources of continuing education include current books related to transport, online continuing education, and professional journals.[5]

SUMMARY

Critical care transport requires experience, advanced skills, and additional education so that the transport team is able to function autonomously and in collaboration with all the others who may be involved in the transport process. Critical care transport involves the ability to work in a variety of clinical situations. It involves dedication to one's chosen profession and an ability to care for others in diverse and sometimes difficult situations.

REFERENCES

1. Commission on Accreditation of Medical Transport Systems: *Accreditation standards*, ed 5, Anderson, SC, 2002, Author.
2. Miller M, Babcock D: *Critical thinking applied to nursing*, St Louis, 1996, Mosby.
3. Miller P, Epifianio P: Development of a prehospital nursing curriculum in Maryland, *J Emerg Nurs* 19(3):206, 1993.
4. Rottman SJ et al: On-line medical control versus protocol based prehospital care, *Ann Emerg Med* 30(1):62-68, 1997.
5. Shaner S et al: Flight crew physical fitness: a baseline analysis, *Air Med J* 14(1):30, 1995.

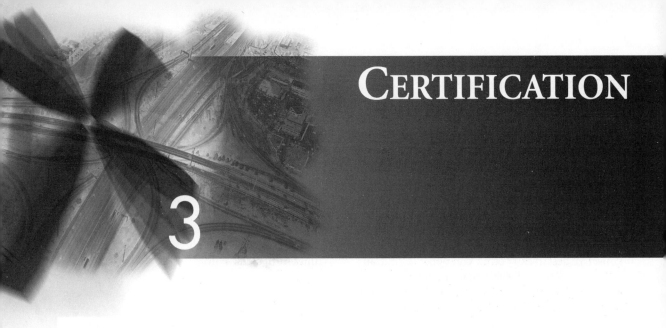

CERTIFICATION

NURSING

Certification in nursing first began in the 1940s. Since that time, the number of certifications has greatly increased. Today more than 40 different certifications exist in nursing.[1,2,3] The National Council's Learning Extension (NCLEX) test is a general, entry-level exam for nursing, whereas a certification exam measures the nurse's knowledge in one specific area of nursing and measures it at a more advanced level than the NCLEX. For example, a nurse specializing in oncology may seek certification as an oncology nurse (OCN), an intensive care or coronary care nurse may seek certification in critical care (CCRN), a nurse practicing in the emergency department may become a certified emergency nurse (CEN), or a flight nurse seeking certification in that specialty would choose to become a certified flight registered nurse (CFRN).

In 1999 the Nursing Credentialing Research Coalition (NCRC), a coalition made up of approximately 20 organizations that certify nurses, conducted a large study on certification. More than 350,000 certified nurses received surveys, and more than 19,500 of them responded. Their responses indicated that certified nurses feel more confident in their skills, experience greater satisfaction from nursing, and feel more competent.[2]

Research conducted by the Board of Certification for Emergency Nursing (BCEN) identified that nurses become certified for financial benefits (pay differentials), potential job opportunities, and personal satisfaction. Other studies have identified that nurses who seek certification have higher self-esteem and value professional growth.

Each certification has various requirements to sit for the examination. Some of these requirements include a number of years of clinical practice experience in the area for which they are testing, specific procedure experience, and an unrestricted nursing license.[6,7]

The length of time that a nurse is certified varies among nursing specialties. Recertification also varies. Because of the growing trend to question whether continuing education provides a measurement of competency, various other methods than continuing education are now being developed for recertification. Some certifications require a written exam as the only method of recertification, whereas others may require a certain number of hours working in the specialty or completion of specific learning modules.[1,3]

Variations also exist in the methods of test administration. Certifications in nursing are considered "high-stakes" certification. This means that the exam must be administered in a very controlled environment and that the exam must be secured at all times. It also means that feedback regarding the answers to questions cannot be given. At the present time, most certification exams are administered in one of two formats—computer based or paper and pencil.

The first certification exams were offered by paper and pencil, and some certifying organizations continue to provide testing by this method. With paper-and-pencil administration, test sites may be more readily available, as they are less expensive than computer-based testing sites. However, because a paper-and-pencil tests are more tedious to process, and because administration of the exams is usually in settings that are not dedicated to test administration (for example, a classroom on a college campus), the frequency of testing is generally less frequent than computerized testing. Registration for paper-and-pencil testing may require more-rigorous deadlines for paper processing than computer-based testing. Applications may need to be received by a specific date, and test scores are generally mailed 6 weeks after taking the examination.

With computer-based examinations, the applicant must schedule a time before taking the exam, but the exam may be offered more frequently than paper-and-pencil tests. For example, the CFRN exam was offered two times per year with paper and pencil, but the computer-based version is now offered 5 days per week (except holidays), two times per day, 50 weeks of the year.

Certification exams are administered at a testing center that has contracted with the certifying organization. Computer-based exams do not require computer experience, and most certifying exams provide a tutorial before taking the exam.

The applicant is given an allotted time to take the exam. With computer-based exams, the applicant can review questions, change answers, and skip questions to return to them later. The exam is composed of a set number of questions.

Most organizations will also have a number of pretest questions in the exam. These are questions that are not counted into the final score. They are new questions that are being tried to see if they are statistically good questions to be used in the future. Many certifications that use computer-based testing will also provide applicants with their scores before they leave the testing facility.

Preparation for taking a certification exam not only includes clinical experience and a general review of information that may be contained on the test, but also knowledge of the type of test being offered (paper and pencil or computer based); the location of testing sites; and the types of identification that may be required to sit for the exam. All this information is usually provided by the certifying organization before the applicant takes the exam. It may be in the application brochure, with more specifics provided in a handbook that is received after registering for the exam.[1,5]

With the vast overlap of knowledge among nursing specialties, nurses sometimes feel unsure which certification they should obtain. A point to consider is what knowledge is required by the specialty one practices in. For example, the transport nurse may choose to take the CEN, CCRN, or CFRN. However, the CFRN addresses issues specific to flight nursing, such as landing zone and scene safety, as well as aircraft operations.

It is important to be sure that the certification organization is legitimate. Various certification programs offer exams that are not psychometrically sound. To eliminate confusion, it is rapidly becoming the norm for certifying organizations to become accredited.

Certification is an important part of nursing practice and may become even more important in the future. The Citizens Advisory Council (CAC) is asking how the consumer can tell which nurses providing patient care posses current knowledge related to their practice. The CAC's concern is that after nurses receive their license, they are not consistently mandated to demonstrate competency or continuing education. For example, in the state of Illinois, unless an employer creates specific criteria identifying competencies, a registered nurse can practice for years without a single evaluation of professional skills.[1,2,3,5]

However, one potential solution that has been proposed is certification in the nurse's specialty. Certification demonstrates that the nurse has achieved a specific level of knowledge in a particular area of nursing.

Certification holds value for health care in many ways. It demonstrates to the consumer and to the employer that the nurse has achieved a level of knowledge in a specific area of nursing. Certification confirms pride in one's profession and in one's specialty.

FLIGHT PARAMEDIC CERTIFICATION

Although the majority of air medical programs have expanded the flight paramedic's roll into that of a critical care provider, some programs continue to provide basic paramedic-level care in the flight environment. This diversity in flight paramedic practice has clouded the definition of the profession. On one hand are a group of flight paramedics who define the practice as the ability to perform paramedic skills in the air medical environment, whereas the majority of flight paramedics define their practice as that of a critical care provider.[4]

To combat this ambiguity and the lack of a nationally recognized flight paramedic examination, the National Flight Paramedics Association (NFPA) introduced the Certified Flight Paramedic exam (FP-C). The FP-C exam was created on the premise that the majority of flight paramedics function as critical care providers.[6] Therefore the certification process that defines the practice of the flight paramedic is not only based on an understanding of basic paramedic skills and flight physiology but also incorporates an understanding of critical care theory and practice. Specific recommendations for attaining and maintaining basic competencies are outlined in the NFPA position statement, "The role of the certified flight paramedic (FP-C) as a critical care provider and the required education."[4] Box 3-1 contains the NFPA's position regarding the training necessary to pass the FP-C exam.

The title FP-C denotes an air medical professional with a broad expanse of knowledge. The FP-C examination process is not regionally specific. It is understood that regional practice and state laws direct the flight paramedic's ability to perform certain procedures or administer specific medications. However, the NFPA does not believe that this precludes the necessity of the flight paramedic to maintain a basic knowledge of these skills or medications.

The FP-C demonstrates, through written testing, the ability to provide care beyond what may be

---

BOX 3-1   **Position of the NFPA Regarding the Training Necessary to Pass Examination and Perform the Duties of a Certified Flight Paramedic (FP-C)**

The NFPA believes the FP-C should have a *minimum* of 5 years of basic paramedic practice after graduation from a DOT recognized paramedic training program before attempting to master the practice of flight medicine.

The NFPA believes the FP-C should maintain currency in the following certifications:

- Basic Cardiac Life Support
- Advanced Cardiac Life Support
- Basic Trauma Life Support
- Prehospital Trauma Life Support of Advanced Trauma Life Support audit
- Pediatric Advanced Life Support
- Neonatal Resuscitation Program

The NFPA believes initial didactic education for the FP-C should include content suitable to fill, at a *minimum*, the following number of hours in each area:

• History, philosophy, and indications for air medical transport	1 hour
• Industry associations and standards to include the standards of the Commission on Accreditation of Medical Transport Systems (CAMTS)	1 hour
• Air medical outcome research, trauma systems and trauma scoring	1 hour
• Kinematics of trauma and injury patterns	1 hour

| BOX 3-1 | **Position of the NFPA Regarding the Training Necessary to Pass Examination and Perform the Duties of a Certified Flight Paramedic (FP-C)—cont'd** |

- Aircraft: fundamentals, safety and survival   3 hours
- Flight physiology   1 hour
- Stress Management   1 hour
- Advanced airway management techniques   2 hours
- Radiographic interpretation   1 hour
- Management of medical neurological emergencies   1 hour
- Management of the critical cardiac patient to include pacemakers and invasive hemodynamic
  monitoring   8 hours
- Intra-aortic balloon pump theory and transport considerations   8 hours
- 12-lead ECG interpretation   8 hours
- Management of the acute respiratiory patient: to include acid-base balance, ABG interpretation
  capnography and ventilator management   6 hours
- Management of septic shock   1 hour
- Management of toxic exposures   1 hour
- Management of the aortic emergency   1 hour
- Management of hypertensive emergencies   1 hour
- Management of obstetric emergencies   3 hours
- Management and delivery of the full-term or pre-term newborn   16 hours
- Neonatal resuscitation program and pediatric advanced life support are acceptable and
  encouraged alternatives
- Management of the critical pediatric, patient   5 hours
- Management of adult thoracic and abdominal trauma   2 hours
- Management of neurological trauma   1 hour
- Management of the burn patient   1 hour
- Management of pediatric trauma   1 hour
- Management of environmental emergencies   1 hour
- Trauma in pregnancy considerations   1 hour

Wherever appropriate, the above education should include information regarding radiographic findings, pertinent laboratory and bedside testing, and pharmacological interventions.

The NFPA believes the FP-C should have initial and annual training in the indications, contraindications, desired effects, and adverse effects of the following skills. Furthermore the NFPA believes that to insure competency the FP-C should have the opportunity to perform the skills in a laboratory setting:

- Rapid sequence induction intubation
- Pericardiocentesis
- Escharotomy
- Central venous access through subclavian, internal jugular or femoral approach
- Chest tube thoracostomy
- Surgical cricothyroidotomy

The NFPA believes the FP-C should be given clinical exposure to critical care suitable to fill at a *minimum* the following number of hours in each area:

- Labor and delivery   8 hours
- Neonatal intensive care   8 hours
- Pediatric intensive care   16 hours

Continued

| BOX 3-1 | **Position of the NFPA Regarding the Training Necessary to Pass Examination and Perform the Duties of a Certified Flight Paramedic (FP-C)—cont'd** |

- Adult cardiac care   16 hours
  To include postoperative cardiothoracic surgery patients
- Adult intensive care   16 hours
  To include medical and surgical patients

The NFPA believes the FP-C should maintain a *minimum* of 24 hours per year of continuing education in areas pertaining to critical care transport and care.

The NFPA believes the FP-C should maintain a *minimum* of 8 hours per year of patient contact hours in the following patient population areas:
   (This time may be met through actual patient contact time during transports or through clinical time spent in the appropriate intensive care unit or specialty unit)
- Labor and delivery
- Neonatal intensive care
- Pediatric intensive care
- Adult cardiac care
- Adult intensive care
- Emergency/trauma care

The listed curriculum and minimum hours of content should not be considered endpoints for the FP-C. The NFPA recognizes that individual learning styles and variances in transport program cultures and practices may require additional content to meet the needs of the individual FP-C provider.

---

allowed within a specific locale. By adopting this philosophy, successful completion of the FP-C examination should be viewed as the pinnacle achievement in the flight paramedic practice. Successful completion of the FP-C exam denotes the ability of the flight paramedic to practice with equal proficiency and without regional discrimination in both prehospital and interfacility transport.

SUMMARY

Certification holds value for health care and healthcare providers in many ways. Certification in transport nursing and as a flight paramedic demonstrates to the consumer and the employer that nurses and paramedics have achieved a certain level of knowledge in a specific area of transport care. Certification confirms pride in one's profession and in one's specialty.

REFERENCES

1. American Nurses Association: Nursing futures and regulation conference policy options for discussion, *Online J Issues Nurs*, May 1-3, 1997.
2. American Nurses Credentialing Center: Certified nurses report fewer adverse events: survey links certification with improved health care, Press release, February 11, 2000.
3. Barnum BS: Licensure, certification and accreditation, *Online J Issues Nurs*, August 13, 1997.
4. The role of the certified paramedic (FP-C) as a critical care provider and the required education, National Flight Paramedics Association Position Statement, Salt Lake City, Utah, 2000.
5. Gunn IP: Regulation of health care professionals, part 2: validation of continued competence, *CRNA* 10(3):135-141, 1999.
6. Hately T et al: Flight paramedic scope of practice: current level and breadth, *J Emerg Med* 16(5):731-735, 1998.
7. Redd ML: Does certification mean better performance? *Nursing Management* 2:6, 1997.

MEMBERS OF THE TRANSPORT TEAM

4

With the advent of advanced treatment modalities and the delineation of specialties at specific tertiary care centers, the need for available critical care transportation has become a matter of life and death. Critical care transport is a collaborative practice and process. Both the mission and the types of patients that are transported determine team members. However, it has been generally agreed in the United States that the primary members of most critical care transport teams are registered nurses.[7,31]

The team approach has proven effective in providing a holistic approach to patient transport. The goal of the transport team is to provide seamless patient care, maintain or enhance the level of care from the referring facility or agency, and render intervention as appropriate. The following discussion covers some of the members of the transport team.

THE TRANSPORT NURSE (FLIGHT, PREHOSPITAL, SURFACE)

The Emergency Nurses Association (ENA) and the National Flight Nurses Association (NFNA) (now known as the Air and Surface Transport Nurses Association [ASTNA]) released a joint position paper in 1987 that described the role of nursing in the prehospital environment. This paper was updated in 1998 and is soon to be revisited again. Essentially, both organizations believe that nurses who practice in the prehospital care environment need to be appropriately educated to function successfully in that role, and that practice should be regulated by state boards of nursing in the state where the flight nurse practices. Box 4-1 presents a summary of this position paper.

Bader et al[2] conducted a national survey to discover the characteristics of flight nursing practice. Their study found that one third of the flight nurses who participated in the flight programs were prepared at the baccalaureate level (BSN) and had 10 to 15 years of nursing experience. Most flight nurses had either emergency or critical care experience, had completed a trauma course, and were verified in pediatric advanced life support (PALS), in prehospital trauma life support/basic trauma life support (PHTLS/BTLS), and certified in emergency nursing (CEN). If the flight nurses were members of a professional organization, they belonged to NFNA or NFNA and ENA.[2]

Currently four curriculums outline the recommended education and skills needed to practice transport nursing. These are the *Transport Nurse Advanced Trauma Course* (now known as the Transport Advanced Trauma Nursing course [TNATC]) from ASTNA; the *Air Medical Crew National Curriculum* from the U.S. Department of Transportation, the *National Standard Guidelines for Prehospital Nursing* from ENA, and the *1997 Flight Nursing Core Curriculum* developed by the Air and

---

BOX 4-1 | **Summary of the ENA/NFNA Position Statement: The Role of the Nurse in the Prehospital Care Environment**

1. ENA and NFNA qualified practicing nurses in the prehospital environment should not be required to certify as emergency medical or flight medical technicians.
2. ENA and NFNA endorse the need for special educational requirements for nurses practicing in the prehospital environment. Nurses need focused education and subsequent maintenance of specifically identified and recognized prehospital knowledge and skill.
3. ENA and NFNA recognize that EMS personnel possess a specialized body of knowledge and skills. Collaboration and communication are needed.
4. ENA and NFNA support that State Boards of nursing are the regulatory body of the profession of nursing.
5. ENA and NFNA seek recognition of registered nurses by state EMS agencies for their unique role in the prehospital care environment.
6. ENA and NFNA endorse a collaborative role for the delivery of prehospital care.
7. ENA and NFNA support the use of the National Standard Guidelines for Prehospital Nursing Curriculum as developed by ENA and collaborating EMS agencies as a foundation for designing a course to meet the state and local requirements to practice in the prehospital environment. Competency-based testing should also be used. ENA and NFNA also support the utilization of the Flight Nursing Principles and Practice, Air Medical Crew National Standard Curriculum in conjunction with Practice Standards for Flight Nursing as the basis for training and education.

From ENA and NFNA Position Statement: Role of the Registered Nurse in the Prehospital Environment. Adopted 1987 and revised 1998.
Please note this is a summary from the position statement. To obtain the entire document go to http://www.ena.org/services/posistate/data/rolreg/htm

---

BOX 4-2 | **Professionalism Standards**

The flight nurse practices autonomously within the scope of practice defined by each institution.
The flight nurse practices in accordance with their state Nurse Practice Acts, state regulations governing prehospital care, NFNA standards, and policies and procedures set forth by medical direction and their institution.
The flight nurse assumes responsibility and accountability for their actions.
The flight nurse identifies self to patients, significant others, and health-care providers.
The flight nurse participates in the education of the health-care team, clients and their significant others, and the community.

From Hepp H: *National flight nurses standards of flight nursing practice*, St Louis, 1995, Mosby.

Surface Transport Nurses Association. ASTNA has published standards of practice that provide nurses with a framework for transport nursing practice. Box 4-2 contains a description of the professionalism standards for nurses.

Some states have prehospital care courses that act as bridge courses for nurses to meet the requirements for EMT and paramedic certification. An example of this is the Prehospital Nursing Course

(PNC) that has been proposed in Maryland.[20] The PNC contains various modules related to prehospital care, and nurses could challenge all but four of these modules. The modules that each nurse is required to complete are disaster/triage, rescue/extrication, vehicle operation, and orientation/role socialization.

There is no question that transport nurses should be prepared to function in the prehospital care environment, particularly if they are first respon-

---

BOX 4-3	Summary of Skills for Flight Nursing Practice

Airway Management

1. Intubation
   Oral
   Nasotracheal
   Digital/manual
   Intubating laryngotracheal mask
2. Cricothyroidotomy
   Needle
   Surgical
3. End-tidal CO_2 monitoring
4. Pulse oximetry

Ventilation Management

1. Needle decompression
2. Chest tube insertion
3. Open thoracotomy-assisting
4. Pericardiocentesis
5. Ventilator management

Circulation Management

1. Vascular access
   Central line placement
   Venous cannulation
   Arterial cannulation
   Intraosseous line placement
   Seldinger technique
2. Medication administration
   Fluids
   Blood

   Blood products
   Vasoactive drugs
   Experimental and research medications
3. Intraaortic balloon pump management/left
   ventricular assist device
4. Pacing devices
   Internal
   External
5. Vital sign monitors
6. Invasive line monitors
   Blood pressure
   Pulmonary catheters
   Intracranial monitors
7. Urinary catheters
8. Gastric catheters
9. ECG monitors
10. 12-lead ECG monitors
11. Temperature management
12. Wound care
    Control of hemorrhage
    Protection from contamination

Additional Skills

1. Pain management during transport
   Movement
   Motion sickness
2. Emotional care
3. Family care

---

ders. Even if flight nurses are not first responders, they still must be familiar with both the potential hazards of scene work and how to keep themselves and their patients safe.

Bader et al[2] found that flight nursing practice consists of both critical care and emergency nursing skills. The procedures that flight nurses performed included intubation, thoracentesis, cricothyroidotomy, escharotomy, intraosseous insertion, cutdowns, chest tube insertion, central line insertion, obstetrics, and transport of patients with intraaortic balloon pumps in place. The ability to perform the skills necessary to carry out these procedures depends on the mission of the transport team, medical direction, and state boards of nursing.

Learning these technical skills and remaining competent in them can be accomplished through laboratory practice and supervision of patient care. Many critical care transport programs require that a specific number of procedures be completed in a designated period of time. Box 4-3 contains a summary of some of the procedures performed by critical care transport nurses.

Critical-thinking skills constitute one of the most important interventions transport nurses bring to air medical transport. Critical care transport nurses constantly question, analyze, and evaluate the entire transport process. Critical thinking involves the use of knowledge and skills to explore practice situations.[21] Critical-thinking skills include the nurse's ability to be autonomous and organized and to view practice situations in an in-depth, comprehensive way to better understand what is happening to the air medical patient.[21] This unique competence was identified in Bader et al,[2] who stated that flight nurses were held accountable for these complex skills. "These complex skills included decisions regarding the administration and titration of medications, initiating therapeutic treatment based on physical assessment findings, communicating and documenting significant findings and performing follow-up activities."[2]

Transport nursing requires experience, education, and continuous evaluation of competence. Transport nurses must be physically and mentally fit to meet the demands of patient care during transport.[27] Although there are some general characteristics of transport nursing, overall, the responsibilities of the nurse depend on the type of service provided, the crew partner, the type of vehicle in which the crew functions, and state regulations, including state boards of nursing. Box 4-4 summarizes general educational preparation for critical transport nursing practice.[26]

PARAMEDICS

Today specially trained skills that had previously been reserved for the hospital setting have now found their way into the paramedic's skill set. Most notably, after appropriate education, paramedics have demonstrated their abilities to perform advanced procedures that have historically been areas of practice for physicians, nurses, or respiratory therapists. Rapid sequence induction (RSI), 12-lead ECG interpretation, and administration of fibrinolytics are a few of the advanced practice skills successfully and appropriately performed by the trained paramedic.[3,17,22,23]

Paramedics performing these skills were once viewed as advanced practice paramedics in that they performed skills outside those taught within the Department of Transportation's EMS curriculum. The paramedics of today are not only responsible for prehospital patient care, but can also frequently be found transporting patients between medical facilities or working as allied health-care providers within the hospital setting.[32] This broadened scope of responsibility has given rise to subspecialty groups of paramedics—the critical care paramedic and the flight paramedic (Figure 4-1).

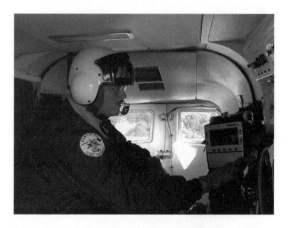

FIGURE 4-1 **Flight medic.**

BOX 4-4	**Summary of Educational Requirements for the Transport Nurse**

Registered nurse (some programs require multiple licensure when providing care across the state line)
Advanced cardiac life support (ACLS)
Pediatric advanced life support (PALS)
Emergency nursing pediatric course (ENPC)
Prehospital care orientation course (determined by state EMS agency)
or
Prehospital registered nurse course
or
EMT/EMT-P certification

Certification in a nursing specialty
Certified emergency nurse (CEN)
Certified critical care nurse (CCRN)
Certified flight registered nurse (CFRN)
Trauma course
Basic trauma life support (BTLS)
Prehospital trauma life support (PHTLS)
Advanced trauma life support (ATLS)
Transport Nurse Advanced Trauma Course (TNATC)
Trauma nursing core course (TNCC)

CRITICAL CARE PARAMEDIC

The resource-scarce health-care environment of the 1990s spurred an increase in the number of patients requiring critical care transport and thus an increase in the need for competent critical care–trained transport providers. Born of this need was the concept of the critical care paramedic (CCP or CC=EMTP), who could complete transports that previously would have required supplementation with hospital staff. CCPs receive training beyond that of "street" paramedics, which prepares them to appropriately assess and manage the patient who has already received significant medical interventions, including the use of advanced pharmacological agents and the insertion of hemodynamic monitoring and assist devices.[28] Use of this new health-care provider has demonstrated promising results with no deterioration of the patient's condition during transport.[10]

Concerns have been raised regarding the ability of the CCP to use the critical-thinking skills that are often necessary in the management of the critical care patient. However, the development of critical-thinking skills can be successfully instilled in the paramedic through an effective scenario-based approach to education and training.[14] Furthermore, no education is complete without the opportunity to apply newly learned skills in a clinical setting under direct observation of another skilled practitioner. Although a variety of CCP training programs offer a clinical practice component, there has been no universal requirement for inclusion of clinical training.[5,11]

Other concerns regarding the CCP have centered on the paramedic's ability to truly identify the critical nature of the patient's condition and ensure that appropriate resources are available during transport. Education and training, again, are the cornerstones to decrease this concern. Paramedics have demonstrated their ability to correctly identify and plan for the transport of the critical care patient after receiving appropriate education.[15]

The CCP is generally partnered with either a critical care transport nurse or respiratory therapist. This type of partnership assures quality patient care.

Although a variety of commercial educational courses offer to train and graduate "critical care paramedics," it is important to note that the use of the title CCP is not currently governed by any private, state, or federal agencies. There is currently no agreement on the content or length of CCP training programs.[19]

FLIGHT PARAMEDIC

The flight paramedic has played a pivotal role in the development of air medical transport. In 1970 the Maryland State Police instituted the first statewide EMS helicopter service. This multifaceted air transport, air rescue, and police program was staffed by EMT-P/police officers and has remained in continuous operation to this day.[9,13]

In 1986 flight paramedics united to form the National Flight Paramedics Association (NFPA). The NFPA was formed to represent the global interests of flight paramedics within the air medical industry with an emphasis on safety and education. In 1990 the NFPA furthered its goals to promote quality within the industry by serving as a founding member of the Commission on Accreditation of Air Medical Services (CAAMS), now known as the Commission on Accreditation of Medical Transport Systems (CAMTS).

Although the concept of the critical care paramedic is fairly new, the ability of the paramedic to function in this advanced capacity is not. The majority of air medical transport programs have used the flight paramedic in a critical care provider capacity since the early beginnings of air medical transport. Due to the complex nature of the patients transported by air medical programs, it quickly became necessary to expand the role of flight paramedics beyond that of their ground counterparts. Additional responsibilities such as surgical airway management, use of anesthetic agents to facilitate intubation, and the use of portable ventilators became necessary to optimize the care of the critically ill and injured patients during air transport. A host of other skills followed, as flight paramedics proved their ability to grasp and maintain competency in skills previously afforded to physicians and advanced practice nurses. These skills commonly include pericardiocentesis, chest tube insertion, escharotomy, and insertion of central venous access devices.

With advances in medical care came the need to maintain care of increasingly complex patients. This required providing a critical care-like setting during transport. Invasive hemodynamic monitoring, administration of blood products, initiation and titration of vasoactive and sedative medications, and analysis of a variety of laboratory data through portable devices became an integral part of air medical transport.[12] Today it is not uncommon to find flight paramedics trained in monitoring and managing patient populations from the adult cardiac patients with an intraaortic balloon pump or a left ventricular assist device to the preterm infant undergoing extracorporeal membrane oxygenation.[1,6,16]

RESPIRATORY THERAPIST

Respiratory therapists (RT) typically work in hospitals, where they perform assessments, diagnostics, intensive critical care procedures, and patient interventions for all patient populations, including the neonate and the elderly. They also function as a vital part of a hospital's lifesaving response team.

A degree in respiratory care requires education in physics (gas laws), biology, pharmacology, chemistry, and microbiology. A respiratory therapist possesses a skill base of more than 100 clinical interventions, including arterial line insertion, chest tube insertion, intubation, surgical airways, and medication administration (inhalation and parenteral). Clinical training includes the use of high-technology medical equipment, such as mechanical ventilation, intraaortic balloon pump, and pulmonary artery catheter monitoring.

This repertoire of education, skills, and clinical training make the respiratory therapist an excellent critical care transport team member who is easily cross trained. Teams with an RN/RT configuration contend that airway management is the first priority in prehospital and transport medicine and have found that specialists in airway maintenance and mechanical ventilation are extremely valuable.

PHYSICIANS

Traditionally, the training of a physician differs from the other transport team members. Physician training includes 4 years of premedical school, 4 years of medical school, a residency program that varies from 3 to 5 years, and a possible fellowship, which also varies in length from 2 to 3 years. Much of a physician's training centers on an understanding of basic science and differential diagnosis of disease processes. The physician team member can make a significant contribution to the care of the critically ill or injured patient who requires transport. Because of their training, physicians can be of great assistance in delineating the causes and, therefore, the required treatment of a medical condition.

A physician involved in a critical care transport program can function in one of three roles: (1) as a transport crew member, (2) for control of medical direction, or (3) as the physician medical director.

THE TRANSPORT CREW MEMBER

Six percent of the flight programs in existence today routinely use a physician as a crew member.[5,7] Only a small number of these physicians are full-time employees of the hospital or the transport program; many are in residency programs.

The need for or benefit of having a physician as a transport team member has been and continues to be a highly debated subject.[5,7,25] The level of expertise of physicians varies from that of an intern, who is in training, to that of a well-experienced, well-seasoned, board-certified physician specialist.[5,7] The selection of physician experience depends on the specific program. Unlike the flight nurse certification examination (CFRN), flight physicians have no available certification test. However, the Commission on Accreditation of Medical Transports Systems (CAMTS) does provide educational and clinical recommendations for physicians involved in critical care transport (Box 4-5).[7]

As a transport team member, the physician is often, but not necessarily, delegated as the final medical authority. Further, because a physician is routinely on board a transport vehicle, it may be less

---

BOX 4-5	**CAMTS Recommendations for Medical Directors**

Medical director shall demonstrate currency in the following or equivalent experiences as appropriate to the mission
    statement and scope of care of the medical transport service:
ACLS
ATLS
Neonatal Resuscitation Program
PALS or APLS
Patient care capabilities and limitations (i.e., assessment and invasive procedures during transport)
Infection control
Stress recognition and management
Altitude physiology
Ground ambulance rules/regulations/driver safety course
Appropriate utilization of air medical/ground interfacility services
Emergency medical services
Hazardous materials recognition and response
Medical director is involved in quality management program
Actively involved in administrative decisions, hiring, firing, training, and continuing education of personnel
Actively involved in care of critically ill and/or injured patients
Actively involved in orienting physicians providing online medical direction
Sets appropriate criteria for use of red lights and sirens for ground transport vehicles

---

necessary to have medical protocols, or standing orders, in existence.

MEDICAL DIRECTION

In programs where physicians are not used as transport team members, control of medical direction of the transport team is often provided by assigning a physician online responsibility for the actions of the transport team. This medical direction physician has the responsibility of overseeing that appropriate medical backup is available for the nonphysician flight team.[24]

Proper medical direction occurs when the physician does one of the following: (1) makes inquiry on the patient's medical condition from the referring institution and relays that information to the transport team, or (2) provides online advice to the transport team.

The overall goal of medical direction is to ensure that the appropriate mode of transport (i.e., helicopter vs. fixed wing vs. ground), proper team (i.e., adult vs. neonatal vs. pediatric), and equipment (i.e., ALS, BLS, specialized) are provided to meet the patient's medical requirements.

THE PHYSICIAN MEDICAL DIRECTOR

The physician medical director has several roles as a team member of the medical flight crew. Specifically, these roles include the following: (1) establishing medical protocols, (2) ensuring adequate training, and (3) providing medical support and advice for problems that may arise during the delivery of medical care by the transport team personnel.

ESTABLISHING MEDICAL PROTOCOLS

For the transport service that does not routinely use physicians as transport team members, the medical director is responsible for establishing medical protocols that enable transport nurses to initiate care and treatment outside their hospital-based nursing practice. These protocols enable the transport team members to engage in the diagnosis, treatment, and initiation of special procedures that, in the past, have been designated as the responsibility of a physician. This is not to say that the transport medical physician director is responsible for writing these protocols, but rather that the transport medical physician is ultimately responsible for the content and accuracy of these protocols. When confusion in treatment results, the team members, in conjunction with the medical director, should develop new policies and protocols that govern future medical care.

ENSURING ADEQUATE TRAINING

The medical director must develop training that ensures the transport team members meet an expected level of medical care. This training can occur prospectively, such as in the introduction courses to critical care transport, which include training on altitude physiology, medical protocols, and medical procedures. In addition to the initial training, the medical director must provide continuous training and updating of the transport team members regarding new innovations in patient care. Often this education occurs during staff meetings where new information can be presented.

Finally, a retrospective analysis of patient care should occur in the weekly or monthly staff meetings. At this time, patient charts are reviewed and reinforcement of current policies and procedures is made. In addition, particular problems that may have arisen from these policies and procedures are presented. The discussion that ensues allows all transport team members an opportunity to develop the best-possible method for patient care in the future.

MEDICAL SUPPORT

The physician must serve as the sounding board and provide medical support to the transport crew members. This may be done pretransport so the physician can provide the transport crew members with valuable information regarding the patient's status and with possible diagnostic or therapeutic suggestions. This support can also be provided during the transport, when the transport team recognizes that additional medical input may be beneficial in diagnosing or providing care to the patient.

Most counsel is done posttransport. In these situations, the transport team may wish to discuss the possible diagnostic and therapeutic options related to the patient's condition. Such interactions are beneficial because the transport crew members gain additional insight, and the medical director

recognizes any need for additional transport team training.

CONFLICT WITH THE PHYSICIAN

Conflict can arise among transport team members, particularly when a nurse, paramedic, or respiratory therapist and a physician disagree about patient treatment. Most often, such conflict is a result of a difference in perspectives. When such conflicts occur, the team member and the physician should work together to resolve the issue. Physicians must attempt to understand transport team members' concerns as they relate to the delivery of patient care. Likewise, the transport team member must recognize that the physician may have a different perspective of the issue as it relates to patient treatment. The best patient care results from a collaborative effort between the team member and the physician.

Physicians may participate in the transport process in a number of ways. They may be crew members, provide online medical direction, or serve as a medical director. Critical care transport team members and physicians in collaboration provide patients with the highest quality of care. Box 4-6 contains the position statement of the Air Medical Physicians Association (AMPA), entitled Medical Direction and Medical Control of Air Medical Services (2002). This statement provides a description of the responsibilities and authority of the medical director, qualifications of the medical director, obligations of the air medical service to the medical director, and a discussion of medical control.

COMMUNICATION SPECIALISTS

Communication is the first step in the transport process. The communication specialist is responsible for obtaining patient information; initiating the transport; transport following; and notification of appropriate personnel before, during, and after the transport process. In addition, many communication centers serve as contact areas for transport team members and their friends and family, as well as other hospital personnel. The transport team must always remember that the communication specialist is the "voice" of the transport team. The communication

BOX 4-6 | **Medical Direction and Medical Control of Air Medical Services Position Statement of The Air Medical Physician Association Approved by the AMPA Board of Trustees Revised April, 2002**

Medical Direction

The Air Medical Physician Association believes that all air medical services require the active involvement and participation of a physician Medical Director(s), who shall be responsible for supervising, evaluating, and ensuring the quality of medical care provided by the air medical transport team.

At all times, Medical Direction must be consistent with the following priorities. Safety of the crew, patient, and vehicle must always be the first priority. The second priority is the provision of appropriate patient care. Finally, after addressing safety and patient care, medical direction should be committed to the appropriate utilization of medical transport resources and cost-effective patient transport.

Responsibility and Authority of the Medical Director

The Medical Director of an air medical service shall:

1. Have the final authority over all patient care and clinical aspects of the air medical service.
2. Oversee and ensure that:
   a. Medical personnel have adequate training and qualifications to deliver appropriate medical care.
   b. Appropriate medical equipment and supplies are available.
   c. Appropriate vehicle selection is made for transport.
   d. Patients are transported to appropriate destinations.
3. Have the responsibility and authority to develop and implement medical care policies and procedures and clinical standards commensurate with the scope of care of the air medical service in accordance with applicable laws and regulations.
4. Participate in the determination of the qualifications, hiring, training, continuing education, and competency evaluation of all air medical service medical personnel.
5. Have the authority to restrict the patient care activities of any medical crew member who does not meet the specified training program or whose performance is inconsistent with established policies, procedures, patient care protocols, or clinical standards of care.
6. Establish criteria to ensure that patients are transported to appropriate destinations.
7. Be involved in any/all air medical service administrative decisions that may affect patient care.
8. Be actively involved in the air medical service continuous quality improvement (CQI) program.
9. Serve as a liaison to the medical community served by the air medical service.
10. Coordinate the orientation and training of any physicians providing on- or off-line medical control for the air medical service with regard to the program policies, procedures, patient care protocols, and clinical standards.
11. Helps resolve disputes regarding medical direction/control and patient care issues.

Qualifications of the Medical Director

The Medical Director of an air medical service shall:

1. Be licensed and authorized to practice in the jurisdiction(s) which serves as a base for the air medical service.
2. Be actively involved in the care of critically ill and/or injured patients.
3. Have the educational experience and exhibit expertise in those areas of medicine commensurate with the scope of care of the air medical service or utilize consultant specialty physicians as indicated.
4. Be experienced and knowledgeable in aspects of air and ground patient transport commensurate with the scope of care of the air medical service. These areas shall include, but are not limited to:
   a. Program safety.
   b. In-flight patient care capabilities and limitations.
   c. Flight physiology and the clinical stresses of flight.
   d. Appropriate utilization of air medical services.

Continued

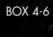 **BOX 4-6** | **Medical Direction and Medical Control of Air Medical Services**
Position Statement of The Air Medical Physician Association
Approved by the AMPA Board of Trustees Revised April, 2002—cont'd

---

    e. Biomedical equipment appropriate to the transport environment.
    f. Infection control.
    g. Stress recognition and management.
    h. Hazardous materials recognition and response.
    i. Any applicable statutory laws, rules, or regulations that may impact patient care.

Obligations of the Air Medical Service

The qualifications, responsibilities, and authority of the Medical Director should be specified in a written agreement between the physician and the air medical service. The air medical service must empower their Medical Director with the authority and necessary resources commensurate with the responsibilities identified, which should include:

1. A job description detailing the Medical Director's authority, responsibility, and expectations.
2. Compensation for professional services.
3. Indemnification for actions and duties as Medical Director of the air medical service.
4. Personnel support, equipment, and supplies.

Medical Control

The Air Medical Physician Association believes that all air medical transports require physician medical control and that the responsibility for ensuring appropriate medical control rests with the Medical Director(s) of the air medical service.

The Medical Director has the final authority over all patient care aspects of the air medical service, which includes medical control for all transports. The Medical Director may, however, delegate the responsibility and authority for medical control to other qualified individuals.

The Medical Director is responsible for selecting, orienting, and ensuring the competency of any medical control physician. Orientation activities shall include review of the policies, procedures, patient care protocols, and in-flight patient care capabilities and limitations of the air medical service.

Appropriate medical control must take into consideration the medical care requirements of the individual patient and a thorough knowledge of the scope of care that can be provided by the medical transport team. The scope of care for each air medical service is based upon the patient care capabilities of the transport personnel, available medical equipment, formulary, and the capabilities and limitations of their transport vehicles.

Medical control physicians must have the experience and knowledge to ensure that appropriate medical control and medical care is rendered and consistent with the scope of practice and the mission of the air medical service. If the experience of the medical control physician in a particular clinical area is insufficient to ensure appropriate care, the medical control physician should seek suitable and timely consultation.

Method of Medical Control

Medical control may be accomplished in one of three ways: on-line, off-line, and visually. On-line medical control represents direct real-time voice communication between the medical control physician and the transport team. During off-line medical control there is no direct contact between the transport team and the medical control physician. Patient interventions follow written medical protocols or standing orders provided by the Medical Director, medical control physician, referring physician, or receiving physician. Visual medical control occurs when a medical control physician is physically present during the transport.

BOX 4-6	Medical Direction and Medical Control of Air Medical Services Position Statement of The Air Medical Physician Association Approved by the AMPA Board of Trustees Revised April, 2002—cont'd

Responsibility and Authority for Medical Control

Interhospital Patient Transfers

While medical control for interfacility transfers may be assumed by the transferring physician, receiving physician, or the Medical Director (or designee) of the air medical service, AMPA believes that medical control should remain the responsibility of the Air Medical Director or his/her designee. Any variation from this standard should be specified in a patient transfer agreement or at the time of request for air medical transport.

Prehospital Patient Transfers

While medical control for prehospital transfers may be assumed by the receiving physician, EMS base station, or air medical service Medical Director (or designee), AMPA believes that medical control should remain the responsibility of the Air Medical Director or his/her designee.

---

specialist must be treated as a team member and included in decision making and stress management.

Communication specialists play a major role in the transport process and are integral members of the transport team.

FLIGHT TEAM AND PILOT INTERACTION

Flight team and pilot interactions play a critical role in the performance of air medical teams. Team- and organization-level factors may enhance or impede the ability of well-trained individuals to work together effectively and efficiently. Each crew member's position must be clearly stated and defined. This establishes structure and determines the flow of communication.

The pilot-in-command (PIC) is the person responsible for the safety of the aircraft, crew, and passengers. The pilot is accountable for nonmedical aspects of the flight and has final authority in all flight-related issues. Flight crew members assist in flight-related duties as outlined by the PIC. Flight team members offer assistance in a variety of flight duties. Some of their contributions include air or ground traffic sightings, hazard and obstacle sightings, obstacle avoidance procedures (landing zones), securing cargo (medical equipment), briefing passengers, monitoring radios, and computation of weight and balance requirements.

It is the responsibility of the PIC to create an atmosphere in which crew participation can flourish. The PIC must help maintain a balanced, predictable environment while responding to changing situations. This implies that shifts of balance will occur and that each crew member should understand that they have the responsibility to participate fully and professionally in every flight.

If the PIC has not succeeded in establishing a comfortable atmosphere of open participation, the flight team will not verbally communicate any concerns or discomforts. It is imperative that the PIC establishes clear leadership and command authority and appropriately applies the use of authority based on the current situation. The pilot must command respect, but at the same time create an atmosphere conducive to crew participation.

When time permits, the pilot may also assist the flight team by helping load and unload patients. In addition, the pilot can transport needed medical equipment to the flight team and relay medical information to the receiving hospital.

The flight team and the pilot's association can have either a positive or negative effect on risk management. Flight team members are in a valuable position to observe the pilot and assist in making safe decisions. For example, if a pilot expresses concern about the weather, this may be an indication that the pilot does not feel entirely comfortable with all aspects of the flight. An appropriate response from the flight team would be to open an objective discussion of alternatives. An inappropriate response would be to indicate displeasure. Accidents have occurred when the pilot, after exhibiting concerns, was met with a negative response or just silence, signifying the flight crew's desire to continue the flight.

The bond between established crew members and the air medical staff could become quite strong. There are eight goals for a successful relationship between the pilot and flight nurse. These are as follows:

1. Communicate positively.
2. Direct assistance as needed.
3. Announce decisions clearly.
4. Offer assistance.
5. Acknowledge the actions of others.
6. Be specific.
7. Know and understand the team's aviation roles and responsibilities.
8. Be vigilant in understanding the interaction between the crew members, the machine, and the environment.

PROGRAM DIRECTOR

In most critical care transport programs, the program director is responsible for coordinating the activities of

---

BOX 4-7   CAMTS Management Recommendations

Commitment to medical transport service
Well-defined line of authority
   Organizational chart
   All personnel understand chain of command
   Disciplinary policies
Encourages ongoing communications between patient
   care personnel, communications personnel, pilots,
   mechanics, and ground personnel
Marketing activities
Oriented to FARs that are pertinent to air medical
   program and regulations pertaining to ground
   ambulance services

---

all systems that are a part of the transport service. The program director may be a registered nurse, physician, pilot, paramedic, or hospital administrator.[29] CAMTS has recommendations on the qualifications of the program administrator, which are listed in Box 4-7.[7]

The major responsibilities of the program director include formulating administrative policies, directing continuous quality improvement activities, managing vehicle contracts and vendors, maintaining the communications system, preparing and monitoring components of the budget, participating in strategic planning and marketing, serving as a resource for problem solving, and serving as community liaison.[18]

The Association of Air Medical Services (AAMS) offers a Medical Transport Leadership Institute whose mission is to enhance the management of medical transportation services. This is a 2-year program that offers courses in human resource management, leadership and administration, financial operations, program development, and asset management.[18] Program directors, medical crew supervisors, operators, lead pilots, and other leadership personnel in critical care transport are provided with a framework to strengthen and/or develop their leadership and administrative skills.

Each critical care transport program dictates the role of the program director. It is important for the transport team to know and understand the director's role in the program, as well as the program's organizational chart and how the transport team functions in the program.

SUMMARY

To accomplish a patient transport, multiple resources need to be involved. The mission of the transport service defines the roles of all the disciplines involved. Unlike other patient care situations in health care, patient transport is very dependent on organized, professional components that must work together smoothly so that patients can be transported both safely and competently.

REFERENCES

1. Albany Med Flight-life Net New York: *Interhospital transfers*, retrieved December 14, 2000 from: http://www.lifeflight-mia.homepage.com.

2. Bader GB, Terhorst M, Heilman P, DePalma JA: Characteristics of flight nursing practice, *Air Med J* 14(4):214-218, 1995.

3. Banerjee S, Rhoden WE: Fast-tracking of myocardial infarction by paramedics, *J Royal Col Phys London* 32(1):36-38, 1998.

4. Baxt W, Moody P: The impact of a physician as part of the aeromedical pre-hospital team in patients with blunt trauma, *JAMA* 257(23):3246-3250, 1987.

5. Baxt W, Moody P, Ireland HC: Hospital-based rotorcraft aeromedical emergency care services and transport: a multicenter study, *Ann Emerg Med* 14(9):859, 1985.

6. British Columbia Ambulance Service: *Paramedic qualifications: infant transport team (EMA III/ITT)*, retrieved November 7, 2000 from: http://www.hlth.gov.bc.ca/bcas/bcasqual.html.

7. Commission on Accreditation of Medical Transport Systems: *Accreditation standards*, ed 5, Anderson, SC, 2002, Author.

8. *Critical care transport program (CCEMTP)*, Baltimore, Md: University of Maryland Baltimore Campus, retrieved November 7, 2000 from: http://ehs.umbc.edu/CE/CCEMT-P/CCEMTP.html.

9. Crowley RA et al: An economical and proved helicopter program for transporting the emergency critically ill and injured patient in Maryland, *J Trauma* 13:1029-1038, 1973.

10. Domier R et al: The development and evaluation of a paramedic-staffed mobile intensive care unit for interfacility patient transport, *Prehospital Disaster Med* 11(1):37-43, 1996.

11. EMS Educators Association of Texas: *WECM: course index*, retrieved November 7, 2000 from: http://www.onr.com/user/jjarvis/wecm.htm.

12. Hatley T et al: Flight paramedic scope of practice: current level of breadth, *J Emerg Med* 16(5):731-735, 1998.

13. Holmes E: *A brief history of aeromedical helicopters, soundings*, retrieved November 28, 2000 from: http://users.exis.net/-eholmes/soun-index.html.

14. Janing J: Assessment of a scenario-based approach to facilitating critical thinking among paramedic students, *Prehospital Disaster Med* 12(3):215-221, 1997.

15. Lee A et al: Interhospital transfers: decision-making in critical care areas, *Crit Care Med* 24(4):618-622, 1996.

16. Life Flight Medical Transport-Miami Children's Hospital: *LifeFlight info page*, retrieved December 14, 2000 from: http://www.lifeflight-mia.homepage.com.

17. McDonald CC, Bailey B: Out-of-hospital use of neuromuscular blocking agents in the United States, *Prehosp Emerg Care* 2(1):29-32, 1998.

18. Medical Transport Leadership Institute: *Association of air medical services*, http://www.aams.org, (Accessed July 19, 2002).

19. Michigan Society of Medicine EMS: *Ad-hoc committee on critical care transport, Instructors/coordinators*, retrieved November 7, 2000 from: http://www.emgint.org/cct/draft.htm.

20. Miller P, Epifianio P: Development of a prehospital nursing curriculum in Maryland, *J Emerg Nurs* 19(3):206, 1993.

21. Miller M, Babcock D: *Critical thinking applied to nursing*, St Louis, 1996, Mosby.

22. Murphy-Macabobby M et al: Neuromuscular blockade in aeromedical airway management, *Ann Emerg Med* 21(6):664-668, 1992.

23. Pace SA, Fuller FP: Out-of-hospital succinylcholine assisted endotracheal intubation by paramedics, *Ann Emerg Med* 35(6):568-572, 2000. http://www.hlth.gov.bc.ca/bcas/bcasqual.html.

24. Pons S, Notterman DA: Roles of the medical program directors. In McClosky K, Orr R, editors: *Pediatric transport medicine*, St Louis, 1995, Mosby.

25. Rhee K, Burney RE: Is a flight physician needed for helicopter emergency services? *Ann Emerg Med* 15(2):174, 1986.

26. Semonin Holleran R: *Prehospital nursing: a collaborative approach*, St Louis, 1994, Mosby.

27. Shaner S et al: Flight crew physical fitness: a baseline analysis, *Air Med J* 14(1):30, 1995.

28. Shoestring Graphics and Printing: *Critical care paramedic protocols*, retrieved November 2000 from: http://www.ssfx.com/CP2020/medtech/procedures/-protocols/htm.

29. Telelz D, Balazs K, Young L: Prehospital transport-air medicine. In McClosky K, Orr R, editors: *Pediatric transport medicine*, St Louis, 1995, Mosby.

30. Weaver WD et al: Prehospital-initiated vs. hospital-initiated thrombolytic therapy, The myocardial infarction and intervention trial, *JAMA* 27(6):426, 1993.

31. Wilson P: Safe patient transport: nurses make a difference, *Nursing Times* 94(26):66-67, 1998.

32. Zempsky WT, Haskell G: Paramedics as allied health care providers in the pediatric emergency department, *Ped Emerg Care* 14(5):329-331, 1998.

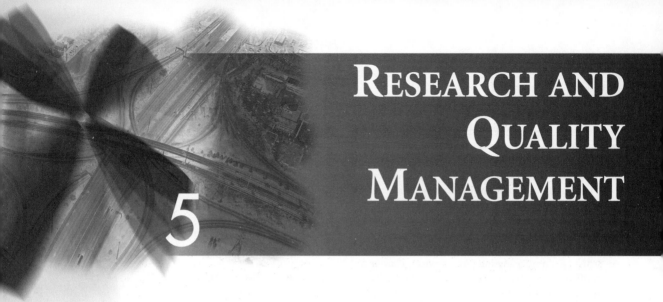

RESEARCH AND QUALITY MANAGEMENT

5

RESEARCH

The art and science of critical care transport has received limited evaluation since its inception. Performing clinical research is time consuming and, unfortunately, does not always receive the support that it should as an important part of the transport process. However, as resources change and challenges increase, the need to identify, describe, and evaluate the value of critical care transport has attained an even greater significance. Research provides a method to identify and describe the art and science of critical care transport and to evaluate and improve the care provided to critically ill or injured patients who must be moved.

CLINICAL RESEARCH

Clinical practice offers a rich source of research ideas. Examples include clinical observations, treatment protocols, new procedures, repeat of previous studies, and identification of gaps in medical or nursing literature.[6] Panacek and Thompson[6] point out that clinical research questions generally fit into one of the following categories.

1. An evaluation of the accuracy or usefulness of a diagnostic test
2. An evaluation of the effectiveness of a new or competing therapy or device

3. An evaluation of the etiology of a clinical condition
4. A description of the natural course or outcome of a medical condition
5. An analysis of clinical decision making or cost effectiveness
6. Description of current practice, emerging trends, or a new observation that is not previously described

There are multiple terms used in research, and it is important to have a basic understanding of these terms so that when each step of the research process is initiated, the researcher has an idea about its components. Box 5-1 contains a definition of these terms.[7]

Once a research question has been identified, a review of the literature should be performed for all the information related to the research topic. Literature reviews have been made much easier with the advent of the Internet. Databases that were once only accessible in libraries are now only one click away from anyone's home desk. Articles pertinent to the topic should be carefully reviewed. Davis, Thompson, and Panacek[3] recommend that each article or paper be evaluated by using the following questions.

1. What are the actual results of the study?
2. Are the results of the study valid?
3. Will the results of the study impact clinical care and/or project design?

BOX 5-1	Definition of Terms

Population - all subjects of interest to the researcher for the study

Sample - the small portion of the population selected for participation in the study

Sampling - the process used for selecting a sample from the population

Simple random sampling - a process in which a sample is selected randomly from the population, with each subject having a known and calculable probability of being chosen

Stratified random sampling - a process in which a population is divided into subgroups and a predetermined portion of the sample is randomly drawn from each subgroup

Systematic random sample - a process in which a sample is drawn by systematically selecting every *n*th subject from a list of all subjects in the population. The starting point in the population must be selected randomly

Cluster sampling - a process in which the sample is selected by randomly choosing smaller and smaller subgroups from the main population

Convenience sampling - a process in which a sample is drawn from conveniently available subjects

Snowball sampling - a process in which the first subjects are drawn by convenience, and these subjects then recruit people they know to participate, and they recruit people they know, etc.

Quota sampling - a process in which the subjects are selected by convenience until the specified number of subjects for a specific subgroup is reached. At this point, subjects are no longer selected for that subgroup but recruitment continues for subgroups that have not yet reached their quota of subjects

Purposive sampling - a process in which subjects are selected by investigator to meet a specific purpose

Judgmental sampling - another name for purposive sample

Internal validity - the degree to which the changes or differences in the dependent variable (the outcome) can be attributed to the independent variable (intervention or group differences). This is related to the degree to which extraneous variables are controlled

History - where natural changes in the outcome variable is attributed to the intervention instead

Maturation - where changes in the dependent variable are a result of normal changes over time

Instrumentation - where changes in the dependent variable are the result of the measurement plan rather than the intervention

Loss of subjects - changes in the dependent variable are a result of differential loss of subjects from the intervention groups

Assignment of subjects - where changes in the dependent variable are a result of preexisting differences in the subjects prior to implementation of the intervention

Blocking - assigning subjects to control and experimental groups based on an extraneous variables. Blocking helps to ensure that one group will not get the preponderance of subjects with a specific value on a variable of interest

External validity - the degree to which the results can be applied to others outside the sample used for the study

Hawthorne effect - subjects respond in a different manner just because they are involved in a study

Biophysiologic measures - measures of biological function obtained through use of technology, such as electrocardiogram or hemodynamic monitoring

Self-report - the variables of interest are measured by asking the subject to report on the perception of the value for the variable

Psychological scale - usually a number of self-report items combined in a questionnaire designed to evaluate the subject on a particular psychological trait, such as self-esteem

Observation - the activity of interest is observed, described, and possibly recorded via audio- or videotape

Validity - how well the tool measures what it is supposed to measure

Face validity - the instrument looks like it is measuring what it should be measuring

Criterion-related validity - the results from the tool of interest are compared to those of another criterion that relates to the variable to be measured

Concurrent validity - criterion-related validity where the measures are obtained at the same time

Continued

BOX 5-1   Definition of Term—cont'd

Predictive validity - criterion-related validity where measurement using one instrument is used to predict the value from another instrument at a future point in time

Content validity - is concerned with whether the questions asked, or observations made actually address all of the variables of interest

Construct validity - a form of validity where the researcher is not as concerned with the values obtained by the instrument but with the abstract match between the true value and the obtained value

Reliability - the degree of consistency with which an instrument measures the variable it is designed to measure

Stability - determination of the degree of change in a measure across time

Determination of stability - is only appropriate when the value for the variable of interest is expected to remain the same over the time period examined

Interrater reliability - the degree to which two or more evaluators agree on the measurement obtained

Internal consistency - the degree to which items on a questionnaire or psychological scale are consistent with each other

---

The research design is the general plan of the study. There are multiple designs that may be used. However, a common mistake made by beginning researchers is the "lack of fit" between the research question and the design of the study. An example would be using a quantitative design (seeking to make predictions) when a qualitative design (an in-depth exploration of the research question) would have better described the research problem. Box 5-2 lists several types of designs.

Once the study has been designed, an institutional review board (IRB) should review it. The purpose of the IRB is to ensure that the patient's rights are protected and to appraise the validity and methodology of the research proposal.[2]

When a patient is to be involved in research, informed consent must be obtained. One of the roles of the IRB is to ensure that the researchers have honored the tenets of informed consent, which include proof that the patient showed decision-making ability, that the patient was not coerced, and that the research has been thoroughly explained.[2]

Research in the prehospital environment can make obtaining timely, informed consent very difficult. Exceptions have been made for life-threatening situations. However, researchers need to be sure that the criteria for these exceptions have been included

BOX 5-2   Examples of Research Designs

True experimental
Quasi-experimental
    Cohort study
    Group sequential
    Cross-sectional study
Nonexperimental
    Case-control
    Historical
    Surveys, questionnaires
    Case series
    Case reports

---

in the research proposal. This is another important role played by the IRB.

After the research design has been ascertained, the sample defined and selected, and the data collected, the data needs to be analyzed and the results interpreted. The research design determines the type of statistics that are used to analyze the data. Descriptive statistics summarize the data and allow the researcher to describe what occurred in the sample. Inferential statistics are numbers that allow the determination of differences between two or more samples.[8] Box 5-3 contains some examples of both descriptive and inferential statistics.

One of the major problems for clinical researchers is in interpretation of the data. As has

BOX 5-3	**Examples of Statistics**

Frequency distribution
Median
Mean
Mode
Chi-square
Correlation analysis
Analysis of variance
Regression analysis
Factor analysis

From Thompson C et al: Basics of research (Part 6): quantitative data analysis, *Air Med J* 15(2):73, 1996.

been said on numerous occasions, numbers can be used to say many things. When interpreting clinical data, there may be statistical significance, but little or no clinical significance. It is also important that the conclusions drawn from the data can be supported.[8]

The final component of clinical research is presentation of the data. Professional associations and journals afford a great opportunity to present findings and link studies and conclusions.

Research in the transport environment can present some unique challenges, including coordination of study protocols with other departments and institutions, an uncontrolled environment, the need for urgent acute-care delivery, and the complications of obtaining or assuring informed consent.[5] Panacek[5] identified several "pearls" for performing clinical research. These include

1. Build group support for clinical research within your transport program.
2. Structure research projects so they are viewed as a benefit rather than a hindrance to patient care.
3. Give adequate time and support to plan the project.
4. The crew leadership must be committed to the project.
5. Clearly define the roles and responsibilities of each member of the research team. This is best done in writing.

6. Be willing to modify the study protocol when necessary in response to problems.
7. Provide frequent positive feedback to *all* who are involved in the project.
8. Consider pilot testing the protocol before full implementation.
9. Make the entire process as user friendly as possible.
10. Follow the KISS principle (keep it simple stupid).

QUALITY MANAGEMENT

Patient transport has become a familiar part of the American health-care system. As health care faces dwindling financial resources, ongoing financial justification and proof of its positive effect on patient outcomes are imperative for patient transport services. For many transport programs, quality management (QM) is often viewed as a time-consuming activity with little measurable impact on actual patient care and outcomes. This section provides an overview of the QM process for transport and flight nursing and provides several practical methods for evaluating patient transport and improving systems of care.

DEFINITION OF TERMS: QUALITY ASSURANCE VERSUS CONTINUOUS QUALITY IMPROVEMENT

A veritable alphabet soup of quality terms has glutted the health-care market. For the sake of clarity, it is important to define the terminology that will be used in this text. *Quality assurance* (QA) implies a traditional approach to evaluation. It includes such activities as monitoring of indicators and comparison of results to a predetermined threshold or standards. Unfortunately, health-care providers sometimes perceive traditional QA negatively because it is associated with the perception that people are doing a bad job or not complying with certain standards. As an alternative to traditional QA, continuous quality improvement (CQI), total quality management (TQM), and many derivations of these terms have deluged the health-care arena over the past decade. These terms are often used interchangeably and essentially embrace the same concepts. They are radically different from traditional QA, but not all individuals who use these terms appreciate the differences.

CQI and QA differ in four major categories: motivation, leadership, methodologic differences, and organization. The motivations for pursuing QA and CQI are radically different. Traditionally, health-care providers have been motivated to perform QA activities mainly to meet externally mandated requirements (regulatory, Joint Commission for the Accreditation of Healthcare Organizations, etc.). In the CQI environment, health-care providers pursue CQI activities as a way to please their customers. This is the era of choice in health care, and patients are informed consumers with discriminating taste in health-care facilities. Although patient choice may not be much of an issue in the emergency setting of transport, patients and their families have certain expectations of health-care providers, regardless of the setting.

The leadership component of CQI versus QA also differs dramatically. In the QA environment, quality initiatives are typically the responsibility of a middle manager, or "QA coordinator." The entire responsibility for quality is relegated to this individual. In the CQI environment, primary accountability for quality rests with lead tier management. The lead tier must be committed to the CQI initiative in both word and deed.

Perhaps the greatest difference between CQI and QA is the methodology used. QA has often depended on retrospective audits, indicators, and less-rigorous QA studies. Decisions are often based on unfounded or spurious data and opinions. In the CQI environment, there is a much greater reliance on statistics and hard facts, not feelings and assumptions. Additionally, CQI uses a standardized problem-solving formula that, if followed carefully, yields a more predictable result than traditional problem-solving techniques.

Finally, the organizational culture of a CQI environment is fundamentally different. In the CQI environment, all processes and plans are centered on the customer (patients and families). Good customer service is a core value of the individuals who work in a CQI environment. Also, employees are empowered to meet the needs of the customer by implementing changes and decisions without being encumbered by bureaucratic rules and regulations.

QUALITY MANAGEMENT MODEL FOR AIR MEDICAL TRANSPORT

Despite their inherent limitations, some traditional QA activities still have merit in air medical transport. Programs might be inclined to discard QA methods completely and adopt CQI exclusively. This approach is not recommended. An integration of the two methods is the most effective way to evaluate and improve care. This model suggests the integration of QA and CQI in an overall QM strategy in which select QA activities serve as a stimulus for multidisciplinary CQI teams. With the significant differences between traditional QA and CQI now elucidated, this chapter will use the term *quality management,* or *QM,* to imply a blending of the best aspects of traditional QA and CQI/TQM.

ASSIGNING ACCOUNTABILITY: THE STAFF-BASED APPROACH TO QUALITY MANAGEMENT

The managers of the air medical program hold the ultimate accountability for the results of quality activities. However, air medical personnel (AMP) involvement in the QM program from its inception through the process of monitoring, data collection, and change is the only way to achieve buy in at the provider level. Managers can delegate much of the monitoring, evaluation, and multidisciplinary team activities to a committee of AMP or to one individual, such as a QM coordinator, but top-down support and involvement are hallmarks of effective QM. Top-down support is demonstrated by financial support for individuals assigned QM responsibilities to receive specialized training and by allowing paid time away from flight duty to complete QM activities and projects. Some air medical services have elected to hire QM coordinators who are assigned most of this workload. Whether the QM coordinator is a full-time staff nurse or an individual who flies part time, it is important that one individual be accountable for overseeing the process. Failure to assign accountability will result in disorganization and lack of direction for the QM program.

The success or failure of an air medical QM program is also related to the degree to which the AMP have been involved in its development, implementation, and ongoing maintenance. If a QM program is conceived and implemented with little or no involvement on the part of those who deliver the care, the staff may perceive the program negatively. If, on the other hand, the AMP are given the opportunity to contribute to the development of the QM program, the personal investment on the part of the staff will improve the chance for greater program success.

THE QUALITY MANAGEMENT COMMITTEE

Development of a QM committee is one way to ensure staff involvement in the air medical QM process. The QM committee approach promotes "ownership" of the QM program on the part of the flight nurses. Also, participation on the multidisciplinary air medical QM committee may be used as a part of the program's clinical advancement system. Committee membership may be made by application, appointment, or election. Whatever the approach, the flight nurse member must be committed to the goals of the committee. Establishment of bylaws for the QM committee that address its structure, reporting mechanisms, voting privileges, attendance requirements, and so on will aid in making the committee more "official" and will serve to heighten the members' sense of commitment to the aims of the committee.

QUALITY MANAGEMENT PROGRAM ORGANIZATIONAL STRATEGIES

The most effective QM program is well organized and multifaceted. Programs that depend too heavily on one monitoring method risk missing opportunities for improvement. However, managing multiple simultaneous studies of indicators and multidisciplinary teams can be overwhelming.

The written QA plan is an effective organizational tool to manage the air medical QM effort. The written plan serves as an infrastructure for all quality efforts and ensures that monitoring and evaluation are systematic and organized.

Table 5-1 displays a generic air medical written QM plan. The development of such a plan is straightforward; however, some essential components must be included.

First, the content of the monitoring plan is based on the air medical service's scope of service, which delineates the types of patients transported and how they are transported. For instance, a flight program that transports 80% scene patients will have a different scope of care than a neonatal transport program. A statement that clearly summarizes the essence of the care provided by the particular air medical service and by its flight nurses could read something like this: "LifeFlight provides for the rapid assessment, diagnosis, and treatment of critically or injured patients of all ages from the scene of an accident or from intraagency transports." With this statement as the framework, QM personnel can begin to develop standards; identify high-risk, high-volume aspects of care; and develop ways to monitor them.

IDENTIFYING IMPORTANT ASPECTS

Important aspects of care are high-risk, problem-prone, high-volume areas of air medical transport with the greatest impact on patient outcome, cost, and efficient functioning of the program. Nursing responsibilities, such as physical assessment, documentation, medication administration, timely response for requests for service, and invasive procedures, are examples of important aspects of flight nursing care. Several examples are shown in Table 5-1.

INDICATOR DEVELOPMENT

Indicators are well-delineated, objective measures of compliance with a particular standard. Two

TABLE 5-1 Generic Air Medical QA and Improvement Plan (1996)

Indicator(s)*	Rate Based (RB) or Sentinel Event (SE)	Goal Benchmark Threshold	Collection Schedule/Method	Collection Responsibility	Date of Next Review
Aspect: Timely and Appropriate Care of the Pediatric Patient					
Pediatric IV fluid rates Maintenance flow rates based on patient weight	RB	95%	Quarterly review of sample (5% or 30 cases) of pediatric patients transported	Pediatric represen-tative	Quarter 2, 1996
Fluid boluses appropriate for patient age/ weight	RB	95%	Same	QM committee	Quarter 2, 1996
Fluid bolus effect documented	RB	95%	Same	QM committee	Quarter 2, 1996
Aspect: Appropriate and Timely Airway Management					
Intubation of pediatric patient Airway size appropriate for weight/age	RB	95%	Quarterly review of all pediatric intubations	Pediatric representative, QM committee	Quarter 3, 1996
Documentation of placement confirmed in nursing notes	RB	95%	Semiannual review of documentation of all intubations	QM committee	Quarter 3, 1996
Intubation (all patients) Tube confirmed in trachea on arrival at receiving facility	SE	100%	All intubation reported to be esophageal reviewed by medical director/team member involved	QM coordinator/ medical director	Quarter 3, 1996
Documentation of all intubation attempts and reasons attempts not successful	RB	95%	Retrospective quarterly review $N =$ all intubations or attempted intubations	QM committee	Quarter 3, 1996

*From Samaritan Air Evac, Phoenix, Ariz, 1996.

indicators dealing with patient physical assessments after intubation might be as follows:

1. Bilateral breath sounds will be documented on all patients postintubation.
2. Esophageal intubations will be recognized and corrected.

THRESHOLDS AND BENCHMARKS

The final step in developing a written QM plan is to establish the level at which lack of compliance with the given standard or indicator of quality will be unacceptable and will require intervention. This level, usually expressed as a percentage, is known as the threshold. Some experts prefer the use of the term *benchmark* to imply an externally determined level of performance.

In the past, national associations have published some thresholds. However, there has been little research done to support their use or effectiveness. Whether this will change in the future remains to be seen. However, this does not preclude a transport program from identifying its own thresholds and benchmarks.

When there is no national data available with which to validate a certain level of performance, how does one realistically assign thresholds? First, thresholds must be attainable and pragmatic. There is no sense establishing thresholds so high that they can never be met. Likewise, in high-risk areas in which failure to meet the threshold 100% of the time could result in deleterious outcome for a patient—for example, esophageal intubations—the threshold should be set at 100%.

ESTABLISHING PRIORITIES FOR MONITORING, EVALUATION, AND MULTIDISCIPLINARY TEAMS

The written plan outlines all general categories of care to be monitored in a given year, how often these aspects of care are to be monitored, and the method to be used. The actual implementation of these activities can be a daunting task. A prioritization tool is needed to determine which activities should be undertaken first.

The decision matrix is a simple but valuable way to prioritize the QM efforts. It is usually most effective if completed as a group by the QM committee or a similar planning structure. The following case study describes the use of the decision matrix.

The Transport XYZ QM committee meets the first week of January to determine "quality initiatives" for the coming year. During this meeting, they hold a brainstorming session to identify all possible clinical and operational nursing, paramedic, respiratory, administration, pilots, and communications. As a result of brainstorming, they target 10 potential opportunities for improvement. These include interfacility AMP bedside time, intubation success rate, documentation of contact with medical control, team composition for maternal transports, improved documentation of chest pain management during cardiac transport, fetal monitor interpretation, refueling turnaround time, transport following compliance, referring hospital satisfaction, and fluid management in the pediatric patient. To decide which of these issues they will address first during the coming year, the QM committee uses a decision matrix (Table 5-2). After completion of the decision matrix, the five highest-ranking issues were (1) team composition for maternal transports, (2) AMP bedside time for interfacility transports, (3) intubation success rate, (4) flight-following compliance, and (5) documentation of contact with medical control. This exercise determines where the QA committee should focus the greatest efforts.

UTILIZATION APPROPRIATENESS

The comprehensive QM plan for patient transport monitors indicators as appropriate and uses this monitoring activity as a stimulus for multidisciplinary team development. Another facet of the comprehensive QM program is the evaluation of appropriateness of the transport. Appropriate use of transportation is as important to the greater quality picture as indicator monitoring and multidisciplinary teams. Yet this important component is often overlooked by many transport services.

What constitutes a medically appropriate transport remains controversial and has not yet been

TABLE 5-2 **Sample Decision Matrix**							
Process Chosen for Improvement	**Patient Outcomes**	**Patient Satisfaction**	**Personnel Satisfaction**	**Safety**	**Cost Savings**	**Customer Satisfaction**	**Total**
Interfacility AMP bedside times	3	3	2	1	3	4	14
Team composition— maternal transports	4	2	4	2	4	4	20
Chest pain management	4	3	1	1	1	3	13
Fetal monitor interpretation	4	2	1	1	1	3	12
Refueling turnaround time	2	2	3	4	4	4	12
Flight-following compliance	2	2	4	4	2	2	16
Referring hospital satisfaction	1	3	4	1	1	4	14
Pediatric fluid management	4	3	2	1	1	3	14
Contact with medical control	4	3	4	2	1	4	18
Intubation success rate	4	4	3	2	1	4	14

Rating: 4 = High/significant improvements will occur if changes made to the process, 3 = moderate improvements will occur if changes made to the process, 2 = low/minimal improvements will occur if changes made to the process, 1 = changes in the process will not affect this area.

scientifically proven. Several professional organizations have proposed utilization appropriateness criteria.[2,3] It is incumbent on the transport program to develop a mechanism to screen medical appropriateness both prospectively and retrospectively. In the development of a method to evaluate the appropriateness of the air or ground transport, several general considerations should be kept in mind. First, does the patient's condition dictate an optimal scene or interhospital transport time? Second, what are the distances covered, the local geography, and traffic conditions that might preclude ground transportation alternatives? Third, what is the availability of appropriate transportation and personnel? Next, what are the prevailing weather conditions that might interfere with air or ground transport? Finally, what is the cost of air transport as opposed to ground transportation?[2]

With these factors as a framework, the transport program can develop criteria for an appropriate versus an inappropriate air medical transport.

LEGAL CONSIDERATIONS FOR QUALITY MANAGEMENT

One of the most underacknowledged considerations in the development of a QM program is the legal issues that surround the quality evaluation process. Laws protecting QM activities and personnel involved in data collection from the threat of subpoena and liability vary significantly from state to state. In fact, in some states, the confidentially of QM documentation is being challenged. This section examines the importance of state discoverability, immunity, and admissibility laws to the QM program and the protection of the QM program and its employees from litigation issues. The legal terminology of QM activities must be defined for the ramifications of state legislation on the QM process to be understood.

Discovery is a term used to describe the acquisition of information and evidence before a trial by oral or written deposition or other means. Admissible evidence is that which is allowed as evidence in court. State laws governing rules of procedure and evidence vary significantly. Information that is not discoverable, however, does not automatically preclude its admissibility by means other than discovery. For example, if a plaintiff's attorney stumbles on undiscoverable QM data stored in sloppy personnel files or carelessly placed in patient records, certain states will allow this information to be admitted.

A *subpoena* is a directive of the court requiring a witness to appear before the court. A subpoena can also force a witness to produce any written evidence that may be pertinent to the case. The difference between subpoena and discoverability becomes problematic because they are two separate legal processes. State laws that prevent discoverability may not necessarily prevent subpoenability. These issues are further confused by the often unclear and ambiguous language used in these laws, which often leave interpretation to the courts.

State laws defining the protection of QM data and QM activities from discoverability, subpoena, and admissibility have a considerable impact on the planning, design, and implementation of the QM plan in the transport services. These laws have bearing on the protection of the health-care providers being monitored and the protection of data obtained from QM monitoring activities from being used against the transport service in court. Without protective legislation, persons in the transport program whose activity initiates QM activities are placing themselves and their employees at risk. Transport programs that implement QM plans with inadequate knowledge of the peer-review statutes in their state are placing the service at risk. The scope and nature of the protection for QM activities vary dramatically from state to state. The transport pro-

gram should request help from an attorney to determine the rules within their state.

Once the transport program has adequate knowledge of the state's discoverability and peer-review statutes, several additional precautions may be taken to ensure protection under the laws, such as the following.

1. Written memoranda regarding adverse patient outcomes, medication errors, and reasons for transport delay (whether valid or otherwise) should not be circulated through the transport service for review.
2. Written documentation of such incidents should never be kept in the employee's personnel file, which may be discoverable and admissible in court.
3. Data derived from all QM studies should be kept in the QM system. It is also helpful to title all QM data, reports, and summaries with "Transport XYZ Quality Management Program: Confidential." If the actual number of the peer-review protective statute and its wording are known, the transport program can stamp it on all documents relating to QM. Explicit discussion of sensitive patient care information should not occur in the open forum of the transport service's weekly or monthly chart review. This practice, though it does have certain educational merit, is essentially placing all of the crew members who attend the forum and hear about the incident at risk for subpoena; these crew members, on hearing the details of the incident, can theoretically be subpoenaed to testify in court about the details of the incident.
4. Any memoranda or other written materials, such as incident reports or other sensitive appropriateness-of-care issues, should not make references to the source of the data.

Laws affecting QM activities are diverse and often ambiguous. Statutes in many states have gone unchallenged. Because of the laws' complexities, it is imperative that program administrators obtain legal assistance in tackling these issues.

SUMMARY

Research provides a way of identifying, describing, and communicating what patient transport is all about. This type of research can be particularly challenging because of the environment in which we practice. However, without research, we may find the future of patient transport difficult to predict and to justify to those we serve.

The evaluation and documentation of quality care in the transport environment remain one of the greatest challenges a program must face. This section has proposed a framework for this evaluation process that is both practical and comprehensive. As health care moves into the 21st century, these tools will be invaluable for sustaining the viability of air medical transport.

REFERENCES

1. American Academy of Pediatric Committee on Hospital Care: Guidelines for air and ground transportation of pediatric patients, *Pediatrics* 78(5):943, 1986.
2. Davis E, Panacek E, Thompson C: Basics of research (Part 5): ethics and human rights, *Air Med J* 15(1): 34, 1996.
3. Davis E, Thompson C, Panacek E: Basics of research (Part 2): reviewing the literature, *Air Med J* 14(2):101, 1995.
4. Falcone RE: Indication for air medical transport: practical applications. In Rodenberg H, Blumen IJ, editors: *Air medical physician handbook,* Salt Lake City, Utah, 1994, Air Medical Physicians Association.
5. Panacek E: Basics of research (Part 9): practical aspects of performing clinical research, *Air Med J* 16(1):19, 1997.
6. Panacek E, Thompson C: Basics of research (Part 1): why conduct clinical research and how to get started, *Air Med J* 14(1):33, 1995.
7. Thompson C, Panacek E, Davis E: Basics of research (Part 4): research study design, *Air Med J* 14(4): 222, 1995.
8. Thompson C, et al: Basics of research (Part 6): quantitative data analysis, *Air Med J* 15(2):73, 1996.

TRANSPORT PHYSIOLOGY

6

1. Identify and define gas laws pertinent to the transport environment.
2. Provide appropriate interventions to prevent the adverse effects of barometric pressure changes during patient transport.
3. Identify the specific management of the stresses that may occur during transport.

Patient transport requires an understanding of physiologic stresses that may occur. Understanding the concepts of physiology transport is crucial because they are the basis for the special skills used by the transport team in transporting patients by fixed-wing or rotor aircraft.

This chapter on transport physiology includes a discussion about the gas laws and their potential effect on patients and the transport team. It also includes information about the physiologic stresses of transport and their effects on the patient and team during transport.

THE GAS LAWS

To provide optimal patient care in the air medical environment, personnel must possess in-depth knowledge of altitude physiology. Altitude physiology exemplifies the concepts of the gas laws, the pri-

mary concern of which is to describe the relationships among the interdependent variables of temperature, pressure, volume, and mass of gases. Before the gas laws are addressed, those factors influencing the behavior of gases need to be considered. The four basic variables that affect gas volumetric relationships are temperature, pressure, volume, and the relative mass of a gas or the number of molecules. These variables—T, P, V, and n—are defined as follows[4]:

1. Temperature (T), when expressed in degrees Kelvin (K), indicates the level of energy of a gas sample and is referred to as *absolute temperature*, converted from temperature centigrade (Celsius [°C]) or Fahrenheit (°F).
2. Pressure (P), defined as absolute or total exerted pressure, is conventionally expressed in atmospheres (torr) or as a given column of mercury in

millimeters (mm Hg) or of water balancing the pressure in centimeters (cm H_2O).

3. Volume (V) is expressed in cubic units, such as cubic meters (m^3), cubic centimeters (cc), or in liters (L).
4. Relative mass of a gas or number of molecules (n) or ions is expressed in gram molecules (the molecular weight of the substance in grams).

Gas laws govern the body's physiologic response to barometric pressure changes by these four variables. When the transport team is taking care of the patient being transported by air, these changes become particularly important on ascent and descent.

BOYLE'S LAW

Boyle's law, which originated from experiments conducted by Robert Boyle in the 1660s, states: "When the temperature remains constant, the volume of a given mass of gas varies inversely as its pressure . . . ." This law applies to all gases and may be expressed as follows[31]:

$$\frac{V_1}{V_2} = \frac{P_2}{P_1} \text{ or } P_1V_1 = P_2V_2$$

where

V_1 = The initial volume

V_2 = The final volume

P_1 = The initial pressure

P_2 = The final pressure

Thus at a constant temperature, the volume of a gas is inversely proportional to the pressure. The gas in a balloon, for example, expands as the balloon ascends.

DALTON'S LAW (LAW OF PARTIAL PRESSURE)

Dalton's law relates to the pressure of a mixture of gases and states: "The total pressure of a gas mixture is the sum of the individual or partial pressures of all the gases in the mixture. . . ."

$$P = P_1 + P_2 + P_3 + P_4 \text{ (and so on)}$$

P is the total pressure of the gas mixture, and P_1, P_2, and P_3 are partial pressures of each gas in the mixture.

The partial pressure of each gas in the mixture is derived from the following equation[31]:

$$P_1 = F_1 \times P$$

where

P_1 = The partial pressure of gas 1

F_1 = The fractional concentration of gas 1 in the mixture

P = The total pressure of the gas mixture[31]

Stated another way, gases in a mixture exert pressure equivalent to the pressure each would exert if present alone in the volume of the total mixture. This means that each gas present in a mixture exerts a partial pressure equal to the fractional concentration (by volume) multiplied by the total pressure.[4]

A mathematical illustration of Dalton's law is shown in the following example, in which the partial pressure of oxygen (P_{O_2}) at sea level is calculated:

$$P_{O_2} = 20.95 \, (21\%) \times 760 \text{ mm Hg} = 159.6$$

Barometric, or atmospheric, pressure is the pressure exerted against an object or a person by the atmosphere (Table 6-1). At sea level this pressure is 15 psi. Increasing altitude results in decreased barometric pressure. Barometric pressure multiplied by the concentration of a gas is equal to the partial pressure of the gas.[22]

$$\text{Barometric pressure} \times \text{Gas concentration} = \text{Gas partial pressure}$$

$$760 \text{ mm Hg} \times 21\% \, O_2{}^* = 159.6 \text{ mm Hg } P_{O_2}$$

---

*Note: Oxygen concentration remains at 21%, regardless of altitude. However, oxygen availability decreases with altitude because the oxygen molecules are farther apart, potentially resulting in hypoxia.

TABLE 6-1	**Dry Atmospheric Composition**	
Gas	Pressure (torr)	Percent (%)
Nitrogen	593.408	78.08
Oxygen	159.22	20.95
Argon	7.144	0.94
Carbon dioxide	0.288	0.03
Hydrogen	0.076	0.01
Neon	0.013	0.0018
Helium	0.003	0.00015

CHARLES' LAW

An additional development in the early formulation of the laws of ideal gases came from the French physicist Jacques Charles, who concluded that, "When pressure is constant, the volume of a gas is very nearly proportional to its absolute temperature." This is expressed as follows[31]:

$$\frac{V_1}{T_1} = \frac{V_2}{T_2}$$

where

V_1 = The initial volume

V_2 = The final volume

T_1 = The initial absolute temperature

T_2 = The final absolute temperature

Thus the volume is directly proportional to the temperature when it is expressed on an absolute scale where all other factors remain constant (where P and n are constant).[4] Consequently, if a mass of gas is kept under a constant pressure as the absolute temperature of the gas is increased or decreased, the volume will increase or decrease accordingly.[7]

The motion of the molecules in a gas is directly related to temperature. A decrease in the temperature of a gas causes the molecules to move more slowly, whereas an increase in the temperature causes a faster motion. The relationship demonstrates that when a greater force is exerted, the volume expands. An example of this would be

achieved by putting a can of shaving cream into a fire and then watching Charles' law at work; however, carrying out this experiment is not recommended.

GAY-LUSSAC'S LAW

Gay-Lussac's law is often combined with Charles' law because it, too, deals with a directly proportional relationship between pressure and temperature. Gay-Lussac's law expresses the same relationship but is stated as follows:

$$\frac{P_1}{T_1} = \frac{P_2}{T_2}$$

where V and n are constant. Thus the pressure of a gas when volume is maintained constant is directly proportional to the absolute temperature for a constant amount of gas.[4] For example, the pressure in an oxygen tank decreases as the temperature decreases.

HENRY'S LAW

Henry's law deals with the solubility of gases in liquids and states: "The quantity of gas dissolved in 1 cm^3 (1 ml) of a liquid is proportional to the partial pressure of the gas in contact with the liquid. . . ." The absolute amount of any gas dissolved in liquid under conditions of equilibrium is dependent on the solubility of the gas in the liquid and the temperature, in addition to the partial pressure of the gas.[31] A simpler interpretation is that the weight of a gas dissolved in a liquid is directly proportional to the weight of the gas above the liquid.[7] An ideal example would be when a can of soda (i.e., a carbonated soft drink) is opened immediately after it has been dropped. The soda was bottled with an equilibrium established between the soda and the gas in the can. When the can is opened, the pressure of the gas above the soda is drastically reduced, releasing the gas within the soda as bubbles. A further example of this law is decompression sickness. When a scuba diver ascends too rapidly from a deep dive, nitrogen bubbles can form in the blood, causing one form of decompression sickness.

Graham's Law (Law of Gaseous Diffusion)

Graham's law states that the rate of diffusion of a gas through a liquid medium is directly related to the solubility of the gas and inversely proportional to the square root of its density or gram molecular weight.[8] This means that gases will go from a higher pressure or concentration to a region of lower pressure or concentration.* Examples would be simple diffusion or gas exchange at the cellular level.

STRESSES OF TRANSPORT

Multiple stresses have been identified that may be caused by transport. According to the U.S. Air Force,[29] which has done the most research on the subject of stresses related to flight, eight classical stresses of flight exist. These stresses are as follows:

- Decreased partial pressure of oxygen
- Barometric pressure changes
- Thermal changes
- Decreased humidity
- Noise
- Vibration
- Fatigue
- Gravitational forces

Additional stresses related to transport include the following:

- Spatial disorientation
- Flicker vertigo
- Fuel vapors

Decreased Partial Pressure of Oxygen

An understanding of the terms *hypoxia, hypoxemia,* and *hypercapnia* is essential for establishing a foundation on which to build knowledge about the effects of decreased partial pressure of oxygen.

Hypoxia is a general term that describes the state of oxygen deficiency in the tissues. It refers to a decrease in tissue oxygen or an oxygen supply inadequate to meet tissue needs.[1,2,16,34] Hypoxia disrupts the intracellular oxidative process and impairs cellular function.[23]

There are many things that may interfere with a blood cell's ability to carry oxygen to the body. Anemia, altitude, alcohol, medications, carbon monoxide poisoning, and heavy smoking can all decrease the blood's ability to absorb and transport oxygen.

Hypoxemia refers to a decrease in arterial blood oxygen tension. A normal Pa_{O_2} does not guarantee adequate tissue oxygenation; conversely, a low Pa_{O_2} may not indicate tissue hypoxia and may be clinically acceptable.[1]

Hypercapnia refers to an increased amount of carbon dioxide in the blood.[27]

Hypoxia

Four stages of hypoxia need to be considered when examining its effects on human pathophysiology. The four stages are divided by altitude. The first stage is the **indifferent stage.** The physiologic zone for this stage starts at sea level and extends to 10,000 feet. In this stage the body reacts to the lessened availability of oxygen in the air with a slight increase in heart rate and ventilation. Night-vision loss occurs at 5000 feet. The second stage is the **compensatory stage,** which occurs from 10,000 to 15,000 feet. This is the stage in which the body attempts to protect itself against hypoxia. An increase in blood pressure, heart rate, and depth and rate of respiration occurs. This stage is when efficiency and performance of tasks requiring mental alertness become impaired. The third stage is the **disturbance stage,** which occurs between 15,000 and 20,000 feet. This stage is characterized by dizziness, sleepiness, tunnel vision, and cyanosis. Thinking becomes slowed, and muscle coordination decreases. The **critical stage** is the fourth stage of hypoxia. This stage occurs between 20,000 and 30,000 feet and features marked mental confusion and incapacitation followed by unconsciousness, usually within a few minutes.[23,26]

---

*Note: Carbon dioxide is 19 times as diffusible as oxygen. Hence the uptake of carbon dioxide occurs 19 times faster than the uptake of oxygen.

Types.   On the basis of the physiologic effects elicited on the body, hypoxia can be divided into four different types: hypoxic hypoxia, hypemic hypoxia, stagnant hypoxia, and histotoxic hypoxia.

Hypoxic hypoxia is a deficiency in alveolar oxygen exchange. A reduction in P_{O_2} in inspired air, or the effective gas exchange area of the lung may cause oxygen deficiency. The result is an inadequate oxygen supply to the arterial blood, which in turn decreases the amount of oxygen available to the tissues.[3,23] Decreased barometric pressure at high altitudes causes a reduction in the alveolar partial pressure of oxygen (Pa_{O_2}). The blood oxygen saturation, which is 98% at sea level, is reduced to 87% at 10,000 feet and 60% at 22,000 feet. This reduction in the amount of oxygen in the blood decreases the availability of the oxygen to the tissues, causing an impairment of body functions.[5] Hypoxic hypoxia is also referred to as *altitude hypoxia* because its primary cause is exposure to low barometric pressure. Hypoxic hypoxia interferes with gas exchange in two phases of respiration: ventilation and diffusion. During the ventilation phase, a reduction in Pa_{O_2} may occur. Specific causes include breathing air at reduced barometric pressure, strangulation/respiratory arrest/laryngospasm, severe asthma, breath-holding, hypoventilation, breathing gas mixtures with insufficient P_{O_2}, and malfunctioning oxygen equipment at altitude. Causes of reduction in the gas exchange area include pneumonia, drowning, atelectasis, emphysema (chronic obstructive pulmonary disease), pneumothorax, pulmonary embolism, congenital heart defects, and physiologic shunting. Some causes of diffusion barriers are pneumonia and drowning.[23]

Hypemic hypoxia is a reduction in the oxygen-carrying capacity of the blood. If the number of red blood cells per unit volume of blood is reduced, as from various types of anemia or from a loss of blood, the oxygen-carrying capacity and thus the oxygen content of the blood are reduced.[6] Even with normal ventilation and diffusion, cellular hypoxia can occur if the rate of delivery of oxygen does not satisfy metabolic requirements.[2,23,34] Hypemic hypoxia interferes with the transportation phase of respiration, causing a reduction in oxygen-carrying capacity. Specific causes of hypemic hypoxia include anemias, hemorrhage, hemoglobin abnormalities, use of drugs (e.g., sulfanilamides, nitrites), and intake of chemicals (e.g., cyanide, carbon monoxide).[23] Carbon monoxide is significant to air medical crews because it is present in the exhaust fumes of both conventional and jet-engine aircraft. It is also present in cigarette smoke. Carbon monoxide binds with hemoglobin 200 times more readily than does oxygen, and it displaces oxygen to form carboxyhemoglobin.[23]

Stagnant hypoxia occurs when conditions exist that result in reduced total cardiac output, pooling of the blood within certain regions of the body, a decreased blood flow to the tissues, or restriction of blood flow.[6,23] Stagnant hypoxia interferes with the transportation phase of respiration by reducing systemic blood flow. Specific causes include heart failure, shock, continuous positive-pressure breathing, acceleration (*g* forces), and pulmonary embolism. A reduction in regional or local blood flow may be caused by extremes of environmental temperatures, postural changes (prolonged sitting, bed rest, or weightlessness), tourniquets (restrictive clothing, straps), hyperventilation, embolism by clots or gas bubbles, and cerebral vascular accidents.[23]

Histotoxic hypoxia (tissue poisoning) occurs when metabolic disorders or poisoning of the cytochrome oxidase enzyme system results in a cell's inability to use molecular oxygen.[23] Histotoxic hypoxia interferes with the utilization phase of respiration because of metabolic poisoning or dysfunction. Specific causes include respiratory enzyme poisoning or degradation and the intake of carbon monoxide, cyanide, or alcohol.[23] Carbon monoxide can cause both hypemic and histotoxic hypoxia.

Effective Performance Time and Time of Useful Consciousness.   Two terms are frequently used synonymously but are not interchangeable: *Effective performance time (EPT)* denotes the amount of time an individual is able to perform useful flying duties in an environment of inadequate oxygen[20]; *time of useful consciousness (TUC)* refers to the elapsed time from the point of exposure to an oxygen-deficient environment to the point at which deliberate function is lost.[6,29] EPT more accurately refers to critical (functional) performance than does TUC. With the loss of effective performance in flight, an individual is no longer capable of taking the proper corrective or protective action.[23] Thus for air medical personnel the emphasis is on prevention. Table 6-2 illustrates the average TUC.

In addition to altitude, factors that influence TUC are rate of ascent and the physical fitness, physical activity, temperature, individual tolerance, and self-imposed stresses, such as smoking, intake of alcohol and medication, and fatigue of the individual.[6] Another factor that dramatically reduces both EPT and TUC is rapid decompression, which occurs when a quick loss of cabin pressure occurs in a pressurized aircraft at high altitudes. On decompression at altitudes above 10,058 meters (33,000 feet), an immediate reversal of oxygen flow in the alveoli takes place, caused by a higher Po_2 within the pulmonary capillaries. This depletes the blood's oxygen reserve and reduces the EPT at rest by up to 50%. Exercise also reduces the EPT considerably.[23]

Causes.   Hypoxia has the three following causes:

1. High altitude
2. Hypoventilation
3. Pathologic condition of the lung

Characteristics.   The onset of hypoxia may be gradual or insidious. Intellectual impairment occurs,

demonstrated by slowed thinking, faulty memory of events, lessened immediate recall, delayed reaction time, and a tendency to fixate.

Early Signs and Symptoms.   The individual symptoms of hypoxia can be identified in subjects under safe and controlled conditions in an altitude chamber. Once recognized, these symptoms do not vary dramatically in similar time exposures or among subjects. Hypoxia can be classified by objective signs (those perceived by an observer) or subjective symptoms (those perceived by the subject).[23] Signs and symptoms that appear on both lists in Box 6-1 may be seen by observers and recognized by the hypoxic subject when they occur.[6,10,22] Cyanosis has been determined to be an unreliable sign of hypoxia because the oxygen saturation must be below 75% in persons with normal hemoglobin before it is detectable.[32]

Treatment.   The treatment for hypoxia is to administer 100% oxygen. The type of hypoxia needs to be determined so that treatment can be administered accordingly. The following are required steps for transport team members:

TABLE 6-2   **Average Time of Useful Consciousness for Nonpressurized Aircraft**

Altitude (in ft)	Time
18,000 and lower	30 min
25,000	3-5 min
30,000	90 sec
35,000	30-60 sec
40,000 and higher	15 sec or less

BOX 6-1   **Signs and Symptoms of Hypoxia**

Objective signs	Subjective symptoms
Confusion	Confusion
Tachycardia	Headache
Tachypnea	Stupor
Seizures	Insomnia
Dyspnea	Change in judgment or
Hypertension	personality
Bradycardia	Dizziness
Arrhythmias	Blurred vision
Restlessness	Tunnel vision
Slouching	Hot and cold flashes
Unconsciousness	Tingling
Hypotension (late)	Numbness
Cyanosis (late)	Nausea
Euphoria	Euphoria
Belligerence	Anger

1. **Administer supplemental oxygen under pressure.** Providing adequate supplemental oxygen is the prime consideration in the treatment of hypoxia. Consideration must be given to the altitude and cause of the oxygen deficiency. Equipment malfunction or altitude exposure above 12,192 meters (40,000 feet) cannot be corrected without the addition of positive pressure.* The physiologic requirements for breathing are as follows:

Normal	Positive pressure*
Inspiration—active	Inspiration—passive
Expiration—passive	Expiration—active

The proper method of positive pressure breathing* is as follows:

Inhale slowly → Pause → Exhale forcibly → Pause

2. **Monitor breathing.** After a hypoxic episode, the resulting hyperventilation must be controlled to achieve complete recovery. Maintaining a breathing rate of 12 to 16 breaths per minute or slightly lower will aid recovery.

3. **Monitor equipment.** The most frequently reported causes of hypoxia are lack of oxygen discipline and equipment malfunction. A conscientious preflight check of equipment and frequent in-flight monitoring will reduce this hazard. Inspection of oxygen equipment when hypoxia is suspected may detect its cause. Ground-transport team members must also conduct the same careful inspection of their equipment before and after transport to prevent any problems with their oxygen-delivery system during transport. Correction of a malfunction should bring immediate relief of the hypoxic condition. If treatment for hypoxia does not remedy the situation, oxygen contamination should be suspected. Use of an alternative oxygen source, such as the emergency oxygen cylinder or portable assembly, should be considered. Descent should be initiated as soon as possible,

and the contents of the oxygen system should be analyzed.

4. **Descend.** Increasing the ambient oxygen pressure by descending to lower altitudes, particularly below 3048 meters (10,000 feet), is also beneficial. Descent to a lower altitude compensates for malfunctioning oxygen equipment that may have caused the hypoxia.[23]

The primary treatment of hypoxia for any patient being transported is prevention. It is important for the transport team to remember that the patient is already compromised and that stresses related to transport increase the risk of the patient experiencing hypoxia unless the transport team continuously monitors the patient and accurately anticipates the oxygen needs of the patient during transport.

HYPERVENTILATION

Hyperventilation at altitude is an important consideration for air medical personnel and also for the air medical patient. Hyperventilation is of concern because it produces changes in cellular respiration. Although unrelated in cause, the symptoms of hyperventilation and hypoxia are similar and often result in confusion and inappropriate corrective procedures. Despite increased knowledge, training, and improved life-support equipment, both hypoxia and hyperventilation are hazards in flying and diving operations.[23] Hyperventilation, an abnormal increase in the rate and depth of breathing that upsets the chemical balance of the blood,[27] is commonly caused by psychologic stress (e.g., fear, anxiety, apprehensiveness, and anger) and environmental stress (e.g., hypoxia, pressure breathing, vibration, and heat). Certain drugs such as salicylates and female sex hormones also cause or enhance hyperventilation, and any condition that creates metabolic acidosis results in hyperventilation at high altitudes.[6,23] Table 6-3 compares the signs and symptoms of hyperventilation with those of hypoxia.

Treatment. At high altitudes, hyperventilation and hypoxia are treated the same way because of similarities in the signs and symptoms. The following steps describe the treatment:

---

*Positive-pressure breathing is the opposite of normal breathing.

TABLE 6-3	Comparison of the Signs and Symptoms of Hyperventilation and Hypoxia	
Signs/symptoms	**Hyperventilation**	**Hypoxia**
Onset of symptoms	Gradual	Rapid (altitude-dependent, may also be gradual)
Muscle activity	Spasmodic	Flaccid
Appearance	Pale	Cyanotic
Tetany	Present	Absent
Breathlessness	X*	X
Dizziness	X	X
Dullness and drowsiness	X	X
Euphoria	X	X
Fatigue	X	X
Headache	X	X
Poor judgment	X	X
Lightheadedness	X	X
Faulty memory	X	X
Muscle incoordination	X	X
Numbness	X	X
Deteriorated performance	X	X
Increased respiratory rate	X	X
Delayed reaction time	X	X
Tingling	X	X
Unconsciousness	X	X
Blurred vision	X	X

From Sheffield PJ, Heimbach RD: Respiratory physiology. In DeHart RI, editor: *Fundamentals of aerospace medicine*, Philadelphia, 1985, Lea & Febiger.
*X means that the sign or symptom can occur in either condition.

1. Administer 100% oxygen.
2. Begin positive-pressure breathing, which is the same as supplemental oxygen under pressure.
3. Regulate breathing and watch for hyperventilation.
4. Check equipment.
5. Descend.

The treatment for hyperventilation in the air medical patient is administration of oxygen. If this is successfully accomplished, the amount of oxygen in the blood will increase. Oxygen transfers from air to blood 20 times slower than carbon dioxide, and carbon dioxide transfers 20 times faster from blood to air than oxygen, which explains why the amount of carbon dioxide in the blood is directly associated with ventilation. When a patient is hyperventilating from anxiety, the act of putting a mask on his or her face to administer oxygen will probably heighten the anxiety and increase tidal volume. Tidal volume must be reduced.[6] More favorable responses can be obtained by talking to patients to distract them, identifying causes of hyperventilation, and suggesting specific exercises to reduce respiratory rate. Following are several helpful exercises:

1. The patient should count to 10 slowly while exhaling.
2. The patient should inhale and exhale only 10 times per minute.
3. Using a watch with a second hand, the patient should set a respiratory rate between 10 and 12 breaths per minute.
4. The air medical team member can provide counter pressure by suggesting isometric or active–passive exercises[5] that cause the patient to hold his or her breath, reducing the respiratory rate.

BAROMETRIC PRESSURE

Boyle's law states that at a constant temperature, the volume of a gas is inversely proportional to the pressure. On ascent, gases expand; on descent, gases contract. Therefore trapped or partially trapped gases within certain body cavities (e.g., the gastrointestinal [GI] tract, lungs, skull, middle ear, sinuses, and teeth) expand in direct proportion to the decrease in pressure.[2,6,16,34]

MIDDLE EAR

The middle ear cavity is an air-filled space connected to the nasopharynx by the eustachian tube. The eustachian tube has a slitlike orifice at the throat end that allows air to vent outward more easily than inward. During ascent, air in the middle ear cavity expands but will normally vent into the throat through the eustachian tube when a pressure differential of approximately 15 mm Hg has been reached. A mild fullness is usually detected but disappears as equalization occurs. This constitutes the passive process.[6] On descent, however, a different situation exists. The eustachian tube remains closed unless actively opened by muscle action or high positive pressure in the nasopharynx. If the eustachian tube opens, any existing pressure differential is immediately equalized. If the tube does not open regularly during descent, a pressure differential may develop. If this pressure differential reaches 80 to 90 mm Hg, the small muscles of the soft palate cannot overcome it, and either reascent or a maneuver that is not physiologic is necessary to open the tube.[10] On descent, equalization of pressure in the middle ear can be accomplished by performing the Valsalva maneuver, yawning, swallowing, moving the lower jaw, controlling administration of vasoconstrictors, or using a Politzer bag or bag-valve mask. These procedures are examples of the active process.

It is not recommended that gum-chewing be used as a method of pressure equalization because it causes swallowing of air, thereby causing gastric distention and discomfort.

Barotitis Media.   Barotitis media, frequently referred to as an *ear block,* results from failure of the middle ear space to ventilate when going from low to high atmospheric pressure (i.e., on descent).[11] Pressure in the middle ear becomes increasingly negative, and a partial vacuum is created. As the pressure differential increases, the tympanic membrane is depressed inward and becomes inflamed, and petechial hemorrhages develop. Blood and tissue fluids are drawn into the middle ear cavity, and if equalization with ambient pressure does not take place, perforation of the tympanic membrane occurs. Severe pain, tinnitus, and possibly vertigo and nausea can accompany acute barotitis.[6] Priority is placed on patient briefing before flight and adequate instructions for air medical crews. The ears should be cleared on descent by using the methods previously described. Patients who are sleeping should be awakened before descent so they can clear their ears in the normal manner.

Patients suffering from colds or upper respiratory tract infections must be closely monitored during both ascent and descent for swollen eustachian tubes, a condition that interferes with normal equalization procedures.[6] Air medical crew members with upper respiratory tract infections should not fly.

If an ear block occurs, mild vasoconstrictors should be administered early, and the plane should reascend to a higher altitude until symptoms lessen or the patient's ear block clears. If patients experience ear pain during ascent, which rarely occurs, air medical personnel should not have them execute a Valsalva maneuver because that would only aggravate the problem; instead, personnel should have them swallow or move their jaw muscles or administer to them a mild vasoconstrictor.[6] Either the Politzer bag or a source of compressed air may be used. A patient's nose should be sprayed well with a decongestant solution to attain maximum shrinkage of the mucosa. For the Politzer bag method, the olive tip is placed in one nostril, the nose is compressed between the air medical crew member's fingers, and the patient is then instructed to say "kick, kick, kick" while the bag is squeezed, thereby increasing the pressure in the nasopharyngeal cavity to the point at which the eustachian tube will be opened and the middle ear space ventilated.[11]

In review, the treatment is as follows:

1. Patient performs Valsalva maneuver.
2. Crew member administers vasoconstrictor spray.
3. Crew member administers Politzer bag or bag-valve mask.
4. Aircraft reascends.

Delayed Ear Block.   A delayed ear block, which occurs after the flight is terminated, results from breathing 100% oxygen during flight. As the ears clear during descent, 100% oxygen is forced into the middle ear cavity.[6] In addition, the absorption of oxygen by the middle ear and mastoid mucosa also contributes to the relatively negative pressure in those cavities. The patient may be symptom-free immediately after flight, but if the oxygen in the middle ear is not replaced with air, the surrounding tissues absorb it, creating a negative pressure within the cavity. **Delayed barotitis media** occurs when oxygen absorption is the primary factor in the development of a pressure differential.[11] This causes a tightness or "stopped-up" sensation in the ears and slight to possibly severe pain. To prevent delayed ear problems, the patient should perform the Valsalva maneuver periodically after the flight.[6] However, if a flight is completed in the late-evening hours or during the night and the individual retires a short time later, a significant pressure differential may develop during sleep because of the combined effects of oxygen absorption and infrequent swallowing.[10] Patients who are maintained on 100% oxygen during flight are especially susceptible to this problem.[6]

Flight crew members who continue to suffer ear pain after flight can treat it with decongestants and analgesics. If their symptoms persist, flying at high altitudes should be avoided until the symptoms subside. If the team member has suffered a ruptured tympanic membrane, it may take several days to weeks before it heals, and they should not fly until cleared. [3]

BAROSINUSITIS (SINUS BLOCK)
The sinuses usually present little problem when subjected to changes in barometric pressure. Because there is a free flow of air between the sinus cavities and the exterior, the sinuses automatically equalize with ambient pressure when the air in them expands or contracts.[6]

Barosinusitis is an acute or chronic inflammation of one or more of the paranasal sinuses produced by the development of a pressure difference, usually negative, between the air in the sinus cavity and that of the surrounding atmosphere.[10] Common causes of barosinusitis are colds and upper respiratory tract infections. Patients with such problems should be closely monitored during ascent and descent.[6] The symptoms of barosinusitis are usually proportional to its severity and may vary from a mild feeling of fullness in or around the involved sinus to excruciating pain. Pain can develop suddenly and be incapacitating.[11] Another symptom is possible persistent local tenderness. The immediate treatment for barosinusitis is to reascend until the pressure within the sinus equals the cabin pressure, administer vasoconstrictors to reduce swelling, and descend as gradually as possible to afford every opportunity for pressure equalization.[6]

BARODONTALGIA
Barodontalgia, or aerodontalgia, is a toothache that is caused by exposure to changing barometric pressures during actual or simulated flight.[11] The precise cause of barodontalgia has not been determined; however, exposure to reduced atmospheric pressure is obviously a significant factor. This exposure is evidently a precipitating factor, with disease of the pulp the primary cause. Pressure changes do not elicit pain in teeth with normal pulps, regardless of whether a tooth is intact, carious, or restored.[11]

Some pathologic conditions may cause no symptoms at ground level but be adversely affected by a change in barometric pressure. It is common for barodontalgia to occur during ascent, with descent bringing relief.[6] Moderate to severe pain that usually develops during ascent and is well localized generally indicates direct barodontalgia. The patient or crew member is frequently able to identify the involved tooth. This condition can usually be prevented by high-quality dental care with an emphasis on slow, careful treatment of cavities and the routine use of a cavity varnish. Indirect barodontalgia is a dull, poorly defined pain that involves the posterior maxillary teeth and develops during descent.[11] If patients complain of tooth pain during descent, especially that involving the upper posterior teeth, they may have barosinusitis and should be treated accordingly.[6]

A crew member who undergoes dental treatment involving deep restorations should be restricted from flying for 48 to 72 hours after treatment to allow time for the dental pulp to stabilize.[11]

GASTROINTESTINAL CHANGES

Gas contained within body cavities is saturated with water vapor, the partial pressure of which is related to body temperature. In determining the mechanical effect of gas expansion, one must account for the non-compressibility of water vapor, which causes wet gases to expand to a greater extent than dry gases.[13] The stomach and intestines normally contain a variable amount of gas at a pressure that is equivalent to the surrounding barometric pressure. On ascending to high altitudes, however, the gases in the GI tract expand. Unless the gases are expelled by belching or the passing of flatus, they may produce pain and discomfort, make breathing more difficult, and possibly lead to hyperventilation or syncope.[6] Severe pain may cause a vasovagal reaction consisting of hypotension, tachycardia, and fainting. Abdominal massage and physical activity may promote the passage of gas. If this is unsuccessful, a descent should be initiated to an altitude at which comfort is achieved.[13] Fortunately, severe gas-expansion problems generally do not occur below flight level 250.* Because the possibility of decompression does exist, however, certain precautionary measures should be taken to reduce the chances of GI gas-expansion difficulties. Such measures include avoiding hasty and heavy meals before flight, such as gas-forming foods, carbonated beverages, and foods that are not easily digested.[6] Normally, the average GI tract has approximately 1 L of gas present at any one time. Wet gas expands to approximately 1½ times its original volume at 9000 feet. Table 6-4 illustrates gas expansion in the GI tract at various altitudes.

One useful example is a pediatric patient with abdominal distention. Gas expansion in the abdominal cavity, if untreated, can increase to such a volume as to raise the diaphragm. With diaphragmatic crowding, lung volume and expansion are decreased. If this distention is large enough, the great blood vessels in the area will be compressed, altering the blood supply to vital organs.[6]

Patients with ileus (bowel obstruction) or recent abdominal surgery should have a gastric tube placed before transport. The gastric tube should not be clamped but should be vented for ambient air or low intermittent suction during transport. After abdominal surgery, pockets of air may remain in the abdominal cavity. For this reason, it is generally recommended that patients not be transported by air until 24 to 48 hours after the surgery. Patients who have undergone colostomy should be advised to carry extra bags because of more-frequent bowel movements resulting from gas expansion.[22] Colostomy bags should be empty and properly vented before air medical transport. Penetrating wounds allow ambient air to travel along the wound tract. According to Boyle's law, penetrating wounds to the eyes, neck, thorax, abdomen, and lower extremities can cause the introduction of emboli, in addition to irreparable damage to nerves and surrounding tissues.

THERMAL CHANGES

An increase in altitude results in a decrease in ambient temperature. As a consequence, cabin

---

Flight level is defined as true altitude, or the actual height above sea level in feet divided by 100, and can be expressed as *FL*. For example, 25,000 feet = FL 250.

TABLE 6-4 **Gas Expansion of 1 Liter in Volume in Gastrointestinal Tract at Various Altitudes**	
Altitude (in feet)	**Amount (times) increased**
Sea level	No increase
9000	1.5
16,500	2
25,000	3
34,000	5
39,000	7
43,000	9

temperature fluctuates considerably depending on the temperature outside the aircraft.[6] The ratio of altitude to temperature is fairly constant from sea level to approximately 35,000 feet. Temperature decreases by 1° C for every 100-m (330 feet) increase in altitude. From FL 350 to FL 990, the temperature fluctuates plus or minus 3° to 5° C. The temperature remains relatively isothermic at approximately –50° C from FL 350 to FL 990.[29] Vibration and thermal change, depending on whether the change is to greater heat or more cold, can have either an antagonistic or a synergistic effect. The body's primary response to heat exposure is vasodilation and activation of cooling mechanisms. Exposure to cold and vibration stimulate vasoconstriction and decreased perspiration.[3] Exposure to whole-body vibration appears to interfere with humans' normal cooling responses in a hot environment by reducing blood flow and decreasing perspiration.[24] Turbulence can be produced by high and low temperature changes in the air. Turbulence increases stress during flight by promoting fatigue and increasing one's susceptibility to motion sickness and disorientation.[24]

The transport team must also keep in mind that some medications can also interfere with the patient's ability to maintain a constant body temperature. Sedatives, analgesics, some psychoactive agents, and neuromuscular blocking agents are only a few examples of the medications that can place the patient at risk for problems with body temperature regulation.

Both hyperthermia and hypothermia increase the body's oxygen requirement. Hyperthermia increases the metabolic rate, and hypothermia increases energy needs as a result of shivering, thereby increasing the body's oxygen consumption.[5] Air medical crews can facilitate maintenance of adequate body temperature by having access to blankets, warm clothing, and warm liquids.[6] An additional way to facilitate thermoregulatory control in the air medical patient is through the use of a first-aid thermal blanket, which is sometimes called a *space blanket*.

DECREASED HUMIDITY

Humidity is the concentration of water vapor in the air; as air cools it loses its ability to hold moisture.

Because temperature is inversely proportional to altitude, an increase in altitude produces a decrease in temperature and, therefore, a decrease in the amount of humidity. The fresh-air supply is drawn into the aircraft cabin from a very dry atmosphere.[5] Before takeoff, small amounts of moisture are present in the cabin air from clothing and other items on board that retain moisture, in addition to expired air from crew members, patients, and other passengers. As the aircraft altitude increases, the air exhausted overboard carries away trapped moisture. Eventually, all the original moisture is lost. The only moisture that remains is supplied by crew members, patients, other passengers on board, and the fresh-air system.[5] For example, on a typical flight of a military jet aircraft known as a C-141 Starlifter, which is a high-speed, high-altitude, long-range aircraft used for troops, cargo, and air medical transport, less than 5% relative humidity remains after 2 hours of flying time. Relative humidity decreases to less than 1% after 4 hours.[5] Propeller-type aircraft are not as dry inside because they do not fly as high; the lowest relative humidity levels reached on typical propeller aircraft flights range from 10% to 25%.[6] Patients and air crew members may become significantly dehydrated because of the decreased humidity at high altitudes. The ventilation systems on aircraft draw off what little moisture there is and contribute further to the decrease in the percentage of humidity. For a healthy person, low humidity results in nothing more than chapped lips, scratchy or slightly sore throat, and hoarseness. Steps that the medical crew member can take to minimize problems caused by decreased humidity include mouth care, use of lip balm, and adequate fluid intake.[5] Patients who receive in-flight oxygen therapy are twice as susceptible to dehydration because oxygen itself is a drying agent. Humidified oxygen should be used on extended patient transports. The transport team must be certain that when humidifiers are used, they are changed often to prevent contamination.

Patients who are unconscious or unable to close their eyelids must be provided with eye care. The administration of artificial tears and the taping shut of lids prevents corneal drying. Before transport, compromised patients predisposed by age, diet, or preexisting medical or surgical complications require special consideration with respect to decreased humidity.

Transport team members should also maintain adequate fluid intake to prevent dehydration. Water or other appropriate liquids need to be available during both air and ground transport.

NOISE

Sound is any undulatory motion in an elastic medium (gaseous, liquid, or solid) capable of producing the sensation of hearing. Normally, the medium is air.[18] Sound waves are variations in air pressure above and below the ambient pressure.[21,31] Sound is described in terms of its intensity, spectrum, and time history. The intensity of a sound wave is the magnitude by which the pressure varies above and below the ambient level. It is measured by a logarithmic scale that expresses the ratio of sound pressure to a reference pressure in decibels (dB), which are the units used to describe levels of acoustic pressure, power, and intensity.[29,30] The spectrum of a sound represents the qualities present distributed across frequency. The frequency of periodic motion (e.g., sound and vibrations) is the number of complete cycles of motion taking place in a unit of time, usually 1 second. The international standard unit of frequency is the hertz (Hz), which is 1 cycle per second.[27] Pressure-time histories describe variations in the sound pressure of a signal as a function of time. The frequency content is not quantified in pressure–time histories of signals, so analytic techniques must be applied to the signal to obtain frequency or spectrum characteristics.[30]

Theoretically, sound waves in open air spread spherically in all directions from an ideal source. As a result of this spherical dispersion, the sound pressure is reduced to half its original value as the distance is doubled, which is a 6-dB reduction in sound pressure level.[27] Hence a number of factors are involved in the creation of sound. In relation to the definition of sound, it is usually easier to think of sound as comprising intensity, which is commonly thought of as merely loudness, in decibels; frequency, in cycles per second and pitch; and duration.

Thus noise, which is dependent on sound, can more easily be defined. Noise may be defined subjectively as a sound that is unpleasant, distracting, unwarranted, or in some other way undesirable.[21] The human hearing mechanism has a wide range and is fairly tolerant, but at times in an aircraft this tolerance is exceeded, with the following potential effects:

- Communications in the form of speech and other auditory signals inside the aircraft or air-to-air or air-to-ground may be degraded.
- The sense of hearing may be temporarily or permanently damaged.
- Noise, acting as a stress, may interfere with patient care and safe transport.
- Noise may induce varying levels of fatigue.[21]

The A-level of a decibel (dBA) is a unit of noise measurement that correlates most closely with the way a human ear accommodates sound or noise. The dBA is a single measurement that incorporates both amplitude and the selective frequency response features that most closely parallel those of the human ear. When ambient noise levels exceed 80 to 85 dBA, a person must usually shout to be heard.[6] Essentially, unprotected exposure to noise can produce one or more of the following three undesirable auditory effects: interference with effective communication, temporary threshold shifts (auditory fatigue), or permanent threshold shifts (sensorineural hearing loss).[6] Auditory fatigue incurred by noise is frequently accompanied by a feeling of "fullness," high-pitched ringing, buzzing, or a roaring sound in the ears (tinnitus). Tinnitus usually subsides within a few minutes after cessation of the noise exposure; however, for some individuals the tinnitus may continue for several hours.[5] Most of the truly significant forms of undesirable response to acoustic noise, such as nausea, disorientation, and excessive general fatigue, are associated with only very intense noise, which air medical personnel rarely encounter during normal airlift operations.[6] Other hazards of exposure are loss of appetite and interest, diaphoresis, salivation, nausea or vomiting, headache, fatigue, and general discomfort.

Noise in the transport environment also impairs the ability of the transport team to perform patient assessment before and during transport. Aircraft noise, sirens, and traffic and crowd noise can interfere with the evaluation of breath sounds, auscultation of blood pressure, or even obtaining patient information.

Transport team members will need to rely on monitoring devices to measure patient blood pressure and monitor oxygen saturation, tube placement, and overall perfusion. Visible signs of distress or discomfort such as increased respiratory rate, changes in skin color, and grimacing may provide additional information about a patient's condition and comfort in a noisy transport environment.

Table 6-5 provides an example of the number of decibels resulting from certain sources. Whenever it is not feasible to control the noise at a desirable level, ear protection devices that attenuate the noise on its way from the surrounding air to the tympanic membrane must be worn, whether in an aircraft or ground transport vehicles. Such devices include helmets, earplugs, and earmuffs. Because effectiveness can vary considerably depending on a device's basic performance and personal fit, all transport team personnel should be carefully instructed regarding quality and size selection and techniques for use.[31] Earplugs are inert devices, and headsets and earmuffs are occluding devices. Earplugs must fit tightly to offer the maximum allowable attenuation; the

only requirement for using airtight earplugs during flight operations is that the plugs be removed before descent. Pressure changes resulting from decreased altitude tend to pull the plugs inward toward the tympanic membrane.[5] Transport team members should have their hearing evaluated on a yearly basis.

A patient's hearing, particularly that of an unconscious patient, needs to be protected during transport. Therefore, a headset or earmuffs should be placed on all patients.

VIBRATION

Vibration is the motion of objects relative to a reference position (usually the object at rest) and is described relative to its effect on human beings in terms of frequency, intensity (amplitude), direction (with regard to anatomic axes of the human body), and duration of exposure.[31] Most vehicles contain two principal sources of vibration: The first originates within the vehicle—specifically, the power source—and the second comes from the environment, which encompasses the terrain over which the land vehicle travels, the turbulence of the air through which the aircraft flies, or the status of the sea in which the ship sails.[27] Thus both air and ground vehicles cause vibration.

Helicopter vibration occurs with broadly similar intensity in all three axes of motion. Large differences in the amplitudes of specific harmonics in different modes of light may exist, but the overall amplitude of vibration tends to increase with airspeed and with the loading of the aircraft. Vibration is usually worse during transition to the hover position.[27]

In fixed-wing aircraft, any vibration coming from the power source is usually at a higher frequency than it is in helicopters. The main source of vibration encountered in fixed-wing aircraft is the atmospheric turbulence through which the aircraft flies. In consequence, the most severe vibration usually occurs during storm-cloud penetration or during high-speed, low-level flight. The response of the aircraft as a whole to atmospheric turbulence is determined by the aerodynamic loading on the wings. An aircraft with a large wing area relative to its weight undergoes greater amplitude low-frequency excursions from level flight as a result of turbulence.[27]

TABLE 6-5 **Number of Decibels in Relation to Source**	
Decibels	**Source**
60	Normal conversation at 1 meter
80	Garbage disposal
88	Propeller aircraft flyover at 1000 feet
90	Noisy factory
	Cockpit of light aircraft
103	Jet flyover at 1000 feet
117	Jet on runway in preparation for takeoff
110-130	Construction site during pile-driving

From Glaister DH: The effects of long-duration acceleration. In Ernsting J, King P, editors: *Aviation medicine*, ed 2, London, 1988, Butterworth.

Resonance frequencies of body structures produce a more pronounced effect than nonresonant frequencies.[4] It has been firmly established that vibration between 1 and 12 Hz causes performance decrement in the cockpit. For example, low-frequency vibration can induce motion sickness, fatigue, shortness of breath, and abdominal and chest pain.[17] Research has established that a human's sensitivity to external vibration is highest between 0.5 and 20 Hz because the human system absorbs most of the vibratory energy applied within this range, with maximal amplification between 5 and 11 Hz. Posture can greatly affect tolerance in test subjects, and wide variability occurs among and in individuals depending on other factors such as fatigue, physical conditioning, and perceived risk.[7]

When the human body is in direct contact with a source of vibration, mechanical energy is transferred, some of which is degraded into heat within those tissues that have dampening properties. The response to whole-body vibration is an increase in muscle activity to maintain posture and possibly to reduce the resonant amplification of body structures. This is reflected in an increase in metabolic rate under vibration and a redistribution of blood flow with peripheral vasoconstriction. The increase in metabolic rate during vibrations is comparable with that seen in gentle exercise. Respiration is increased to achieve the necessary increase in elimination of carbon dioxide (CO_2).[27] Disturbances in dynamic visual acuity, speech, and fine-muscle coordination result from vibration exposure.[5] The effects of vibration on the body can be reduced by attention to the source of vibration, modification of the transmission pathway, or alteration of the dynamic properties of the body.[27]

Vibrations can also interfere with transport equipment such as cardiac and blood pressure monitors. The equipment should be secured in the transport vehicle in a manner least conducive to vibrations.

Aircraft manufacturers have eliminated severe vibrations by improving designs and materials; however, some vibrations still occur as a result of engine operation, flap and landing gear extension and retraction, and general aircraft movement. To minimize reactions to vibrations in either air or ground transport vehicles, transport crew members should properly secure patients, encourage and assist them with position changes, and provide adequate padding and skin care.[6]

FATIGUE

All of the many operational stresses of transport may induce fatigue to some degree. Fatigue is an inherent stress of transport duties. Erratic schedules, hypoxic environments, noise and vibration, and imperfect environmental systems eventually take their toll; therefore, in transport, fatigue is always a potential threat to safety.[20]

Fatigue is the end product of all the physiologic and psychologic stresses of flight associated with exposure to altitude.[6,30] Fatigue can also result from self-imposed stressors whether the transport is by air or ground. Box 6-2 shows self-imposed stresses that can have disastrous results.

BOX 6-2   Factors Affecting Tolerance: DEATH

Factors affecting tolerance to the stresses of flight can be summarized by the acronym *DEATH.*

D = Drugs. Use of over-the-counter drugs and antihistamines, misuse of prescription drugs, and use of stimulants such as caffeine can cause insomnia, tremors, indigestion, and nervousness.

E = Exhaustion (fatigue). Exhaustion can lead to judgment errors, limited response, falling asleep on the job, narrowed attention, and change in circadian rhythm.

A = Alcohol. Use of alcohol can cause histotoxic hypoxia, affect efficiency of cells to use oxygen, interfere with metabolic activity, and result in a hangover.

T = Tobacco. Besides exposing the body to nicotine, tar, and carcinogens, smoking 2 packs of cigarettes per day results in 8% to 10% of the body's hemoglobin being saturated with carbon monoxide.

H = Hypoglycemia (diet). Poor dietary intake can cause nausea, judgment errors, headache, and dizziness.

G Force

To examine force as a stress of flight, an understanding of mass, speed, velocity, and acceleration is helpful to clarify the concepts of exerted forces.

Speed is the rate of movement of a body without regard to the direction of travel.

Velocity is the rate (magnitude) of change of distance and direction of travel of an object and is, therefore, a vector quantity. The velocity of a body changes if its speed or direction of travel changes. Velocity is expressed as the rate of change of distance in a specified direction.

Acceleration is the rate of change of velocity of an object, and like velocity, it is a vector quantity.[10]

Weight is the force exerted by the mass of an accelerating body.[10]

Mass is a measure of the inertia of an object (e.g., its resistance to being accelerated).[9]

Newton's three laws of motion define the relationship between motion and force.[10]

Newton's First Law of Motion. Unless it is acted on by a force, a body at rest will remain at rest and a body in motion will move at a constant speed in a straight line.

Newton's Second Law of Motion. When a force is applied to a body, the body accelerates, and the acceleration is directly proportional to the force applied and inversely proportional to the mass of the body.

Newton's Third Law of Motion. For every action there is an equal and opposite reaction.

Two types of acceleration must be considered—linear and radial acceleration. Linear acceleration is produced by a change of speed without a change in direction. In conventional aviation, prolonged linear accelerations seldom reach a magnitude that could produce significant changes in human performance because most aircraft do not exert sufficient thrust to produce extended changes in linear velocity. However, significant linear accelerations that last 2 to 4 seconds are produced during catapult-assisted takeoffs, arrested landings, and when reheat is engaged in certain high-performance aircraft. Large prolonged linear accelerations occur during the launching of spacecraft and during their slowing on reentry into the Earth's atmosphere. Radial acceleration is produced by a change of direction without a change of speed. Such accelerations occur when the line of flight is changed. Aircraft maneuvers are, by far, the most common source of prolonged acceleration in flight. Accelerations on the order of 6 to 9 g or more can be maintained for many seconds by circular flight in agile military aircraft.[10]

When the main interest is the effect of acceleration on human beings, the direction in which an acceleration or inertial force acts is described by the use of a three-axis coordinate system (X, Y, and Z), in which the vertical (Z) axis is parallel to the long axis of the body. Considerable confusion can result if a clear distinction is not made between the applied acceleration and the resultant inertial force because these, by definition, always act in diametrically opposite directions.[10]

AIRCRAFT MOTION

Because space is three-dimensional, linear motions in space are described by reference to three linear axes, and angular motions by three angular axes. In aviation it is customary to speak of the longitudinal (fore-aft), lateral (right-left), and vertical (up-down) linear axes and the roll, pitch, and yaw angular axes.[9]

Linear Axes	Angular Axes
Longitudinal axis (fore-aft)	Axis of roll
Lateral axis (right-left)	Axis of pitch
Vertical axis (up-down)	Axis of yaw

The relationship of this three-axis system to its action on human beings is illustrated in Table 6-6.

Long-Duration Positive Acceleration. The crews of agile aircraft are frequently exposed to sustained positive accelerations ($+g_z$) by changes in the direction of flight—either in turns or recovery from dives. Exposure to positive acceleration usually causes deterioration of vision before causing any disturbance of consciousness. For example, exposure to $+4.5$ g_z typically produces complete loss of vision, or "blackout," while hearing and mental

TABLE 6-6 Three-Axis Coordinate System for Describing Action on Humans Regarding Direction of Acceleration and Inertial Forces			
Direction of acceleration	Direction of resultant inertial forces	Physiologic and vernacular descriptors	Standard terminology
Headward	Head-to-foot	Positive g Eyeballs down	$+g_z$
Footward	Foot-to-head	Negative g Eyeballs up	$-g_z$
Forward	Chest-to-back	Transverse A-P-G Supine g Eyeballs in	$+g_x$
Backward	Back-to-chest	Transverse P-A-G Prone g Eyeballs out	$-g_x$
To the right	Right-to-left	Left lateral g Eyeballs left	$+g_y$
To the left	Left-to-right	Right lateral g Eyeballs right	$-g_y$

activity remain unaffected. Exposure to a positive acceleration stress somewhat greater than that required to produce blackout results in unconsciousness. At moderate levels of acceleration (5 to 6 g), blackout precedes loss of consciousness, but at higher accelerations, unconsciousness occurs before any visual symptoms occur.[10]

Long-Duration Negative Acceleration. Flight conditions that cause negative accelerations ($-g_z$) are outside loops and spins and simple inverted flight and recovery from such maneuvers. Tolerance for negative acceleration is much lower than that for positive acceleration, and the symptoms produced by even $-2\ g_z$ are unpleasant and alarming. Furthermore, low levels of negative acceleration produce serious decrements in performance.[10]

Long-Duration Transverse Acceleration. Accelerations of long duration acting at right angles to the long axis of the body ($+g_x$) rarely occur in present-day conventional flight. They are usually confined to catapult launches, rocket- and jet-assisted takeoffs, and carrier landings, although forces in excess of $-2\ g_x$ may build up during flat spins. However, the forces in these maneuvers are small relative to human beings' tolerance and do not cause problems.[10]

The definitions of the effects of g forces given here are applicable to high-performance aircraft, mostly fighter-type, and in the event of emergency situations. The longitudinal axis is the most important in air medical transports. However, the effects of g forces are usually encountered only with forces greater than 1.5 g. In terms of practical application for civilian air medical transports, the effects of g force are limited and, in most cases, negligible.

CABIN PRESSURIZATION

The pressure environment surrounding the Earth can be divided into the four following zones: the physiologic zone, the physiologically deficient zone, the space-equivalent zone, and space. These zones are characterized according to their physiologic effects, as follows:

Physiologic zone: from sea level to altitudes up to 10,000 feet

Physiologically deficient zone: altitudes from 10,000 to 50,000 feet

Space-equivalent zone: altitudes from 50,000 to 250,000 feet

Space: altitudes beyond 250,000 feet

In the physiologic zone, human beings are well adapted. Although middle ear or sinus problems may be experienced during ascent or descent in this zone, most physiologic problems occur outside this zone and when proper protective equipment is not used. In the physiologically deficient zone, protective oxygen equipment is mandatory because the decrease in barometric pressure results in oxygen deficiency, causing altitude hypoxia.[14] Additional problems may result from trapped and evolved gases. Travel in the space-equivalent and space zones requires either a sealed cabin or a full-pressure suit.

In general, the most effective way to prevent physiologic problems is to provide an aircraft pressurization system so the occupants of the aircraft are never exposed to pressures outside the physiologic zone. In those cases in which ascent above the physiologic zone is required, protective oxygen equipment must be provided.[14] Aircraft pressurization consists of increased barometric pressure within crew and passenger compartments. This reduces the cabin altitude, creating near-the-Earth atmospheric conditions within the aircraft.[6] Commercial passenger aircraft normally pressurize to the equivalent of 5000 to 8000 feet, with the aircraft ascending a bit over 40,000 feet (FL 400).[12] The conventional method, used in virtually all current aircraft, is to draw air from outside the aircraft, compress it, and deliver it into the cabin. The desired pressure is maintained within the cabin by controlling the flow of compressed gas out of the cabin and to the atmosphere. The continuous flow of air ventilates the compartment, and in most aircraft this flow of air also controls the thermal environment within the cabin.[17]

The difference between the absolute pressure within an aircraft and that of the atmosphere immediately outside an aircraft is called the *cabin differential pressure*. Differential pressure is frequently controlled so that it varies with aircraft altitude.[17] The two principal aircraft pressurization systems— isobaric and isobaric-differential—are described as follows[14]:

Isobaric system. Isobaric control maintains a constant cabin pressure while the ambient barometric pressure decreases. Many military and civilian aircraft are equipped with isobaric pressurization systems. This pressurization increases the comfort and mobility of the passengers, negates the requirement for the routine use of oxygen equipment, and minimizes fatigue.

Isobaric-differential system. Tactical military aircraft are not equipped with isobaric pressurization systems because the added weight would severely limit the range of the aircraft and the large pressure differential would increase the danger of a rapid decompression during combat situations. Instead, these aircraft are equipped with an isobaric-differential cabin pressurization system. The isobaric function controls cabin pressure until a preset pressure differential is reached. With continued ascent, the preset differential is maintained. Thus the apparent cabin altitude progressively increases as the aircraft ascends.

In air medical transports, cabin pressurization is especially important. Not only does it protect the occupants from the physiologic hazards of altitude, but also it provides more effective control of cabin temperature and ventilation, promotes greater mobility and comfort, and reduces fatigue. Cabin pressurization does not eliminate all problems, however. Cabin pressure can be lost as a result of structural failure, such as a window or a door blowing out, or through a mechanical malfunction of pressurization equipment.[6]

DECOMPRESSION

A loss of cabin pressure is referred to as *decompression*. Aircraft decompression can be slow and gradual, taking place over a period of several minutes, or it can be sudden, occurring within a matter of seconds.[6,29] The risk of injury resulting from decompression increases in proportion to the ratio of the area of the defect to the volume of the cabin and to the ratio of cabin pressure before and immediately after the decompression.[15] The following factors control the rate of decompression[14,17]:

- Volume of the pressurized cabin—the larger the cabin, the slower the rate of decompression if all other factors are constant.

- Size of the opening—the larger the opening, the faster the rate of decompression. The most important factor is the ratio between the volume of the cabin and a cross-sectional area of the opening.
- Pressure differential—the initial pressure gradient between the initial cabin pressure and the initial ambient pressure directly influences the rate and severity of decompression. The greater the differential, the more severe the decompression.
- Pressure ratio—time is directly related to the pressure ratio between the cabin and ambient pressures. The greater the ratio, the longer the decompression.
- Flight pressure altitude—the altitude at which decompression occurs relates directly to the physiologic problems that occur after the incident.

Box 6-3 illustrates the physical characteristics of decompression.

The physiologic effects of rapid decompression are hypothermia, gas expansion, hypoxia, and decompression sickness. Hypoxia is by far the most important hazard of cabin decompression of an aircraft flying at high altitudes.[17] The rapid reduction of ambient pressure produces a corresponding drop in the P_{O_2} and reduces the alveolar oxygen tension. A twofold to threefold performance decrement occurs, regardless of altitude. The reduced tolerance for hypoxia after decompression is caused by (1) a reversal in the direction of oxygen flow in the lungs, (2) diminished respiratory activity at the time of decompression, and (3) decreased cardiac activity at the time of decompression.[14,17]

Crew members and passengers must take measures to protect themselves from the potential physiologic hazards caused by loss of cabin pressure. Because hypoxia is the most immediate hazard, all occupants must breathe 100% oxygen. Air medical personnel must first ensure that they are breathing 100% oxygen before attempting to assist their patients. Patients who already have oxygen deficiencies, such as patients with coronary disease, anemia, or pneumonia, must be closely monitored after

---

BOX 6-3   Physical Characteristics of Decompression

Slow Decompression

Onset is insidious and gradual and can occur without detection. Signs and symptoms are the same as for hypoxia. Decompression can be determined by checking the cabin altimeter.

Rapid Decompression

Onset is immediate, in 1 to 3 seconds, and is accompanied by noise, flying debris, and fog.

Noise

When two different air masses collide, a sound is heard that ranges from a *swish* to an explosion.

Flying debris

On decompression, rapidly rushing air from a pressurized cabin causes the velocity of airflow through the cabin to increase rapidly as the air approaches the opening. Loose objects, such as maps, charts, and unsecured medical equipment, can be extracted through the orifice. Dust and dirt hamper vision for a short period of time.

Fog

During rapid decompression, both temperature and pressure suddenly decrease. This decrease reduces the capacity of air to contain water vapor, causing fog. The dissipation rate of fog is fairly rapid in fighter aircraft but considerably slower in larger, multiplace aircraft.

Modified from Chase NB, Kreutzman RJ: Army aviation medicine. In DeHart RL, editor: *Fundamentals of aerospace medicine,* Philadelphia, 1985, Lea & Febiger; Heimbach RD, Sheffield PJ: Decompression sickness and pulmonary overpressure accidents. In DeHart RL, editor: *Fundamentals of aerospace medicine,* Philadelphia, 1985, Lea & Febiger.

decompression. After the prevention or correction of hypoxia, descent is made to an altitude below 10,000 feet if possible.[6]

DECOMPRESSION SICKNESS

The first human case of decompression sickness was reported in 1841 by M. Triger, a French mining engineer who noticed symptoms of pain and muscle cramps in coal miners who had been working in an air-pressurized mine shaft.[13] Because tunnel workers were first to have the syndrome now known as *decompression sickness*, early terminology describing this disorder was related to that occupation; hence the names *caisson disease* and *compressed-air illness*.[13]

There is a distinct difference between compressed-air illness and subatmospheric decompression sickness, although they share the same colloquial nomenclature for the common manifestations. Classically, the main manifestations are limb pain ("the bends"), respiratory disturbances ("the chokes"), skin irritation ("the creeps"), various disturbances of the central nervous system ("the staggers"), and cardiovascular collapse (syncope). These symptoms of subatmospheric decompression sickness virtually always subside or disappear during descent to ground level. Rarely, however, does recovery occur after recompression to ground level, and in some cases the severity of the symptoms may increase, accompanied by a generalized deterioration in the individual's condition, which is known as *postdescent collapse*.[14]

Although the finer points of the pathologic processes underlying some of the manifestations of altitude decompression sickness remain unknown, the basic mechanism is supersaturation of the tissues with nitrogen.[13,17] Because the partial pressure of nitrogen in the inspired air falls with ascent to higher altitudes, nitrogen is carried by the blood from the tissues to the lungs, where it exits the body in the expired gas. In addition, because the solubility of nitrogen in the blood is relatively low and some tissues contain large amounts of nitrogen, the rate of fall of the absolute pressure of the body tissues, which is associated with the ascent in altitude, is greater than the rate of fall of the partial pressure of nitrogen in the tissues. These tissues therefore become supersaturated with nitrogen. Under cer-

tain circumstances, supersaturation gives rise to the formation of bubbles of gas, the main constituent of which is initially nitrogen, in specific tissues of the body. Gas exchange is the governing mechanism in the formation of the bubbles, and these bubbles subsequently grow in size through the diffusion of nitrogen and other gases such as oxygen and carbon dioxide from surrounding tissues.

The driving pressure for bubble formation in a fluid is the difference between the partial pressure of the gas dissolved in the fluid and the absolute hydrostatic pressure.[14] Henry's law can be applied as follows: The amount of a gas that will dissolve in a solution and remain in that solution is directly proportional to the pressure of the gas over the solution. Nitrogen is metabolically inert. At sea level, the amount of nitrogen dissolved in the body tissues and fluid is in equilibrium with the ambient pressure. At a higher altitudes, nitrogen evolves in a manner similar to the formation of bubbles in a carbonated beverage when the bottle cap is removed. Decompression sickness is not usually encountered below a pressure altitude of FL 250.[6] The clinical manifestations of decompression sickness are shown in Box 6-4.

In a small number of cases, circulatory collapse or postdecompression collapse may occur. The clinical symptoms vary. Typically, the patient becomes anxious, develops a frontal headache, and feels sick. Facial pallor, coldness, and sweaty extremities may occur, and peripheral cyanosis almost always occurs. General or focal signs of neurologic involvement such as weakness of the limbs, apraxia, scotomata, and convulsions may occur. Arterial blood pressure is generally well maintained until late in the development of the illness. Finally, in the worst cases, coma supervenes. Recovery can occur at any stage, but in the past it has been very rare once coma has developed.[14,16,30]

In addition to supersaturation of the tissues with nitrogen, other factors that influence susceptibility are the rate of ascent, altitude, time of exposure, reexposure to high altitude, body fat, age (if greater than 40 years), exercise before and after flight, presence of infection, and alcohol ingestion.[13,17,18,33]

The primary treatment of decompression sickness arising at high altitudes is recompression to ground

| BOX 6-4 | **Clinical Manifestations of Decompression Sickness** |

Skin
Paresthesia (numbness or tingling sensation)
Mottled or diffuse rash of short duration
Itching
Cold or warm sensations

Joints
"Bends" pain (mild to severe) in muscles and joints, caused by nitrogen bubbles in the joint space
Pain is mild at onset, becomes deep and penetrating, and eventually becomes severe
Pain usually affects (in order) knee, shoulder, elbow, wrist or hand, and ankle or foot
Pain increases with motion

Lungs
"Chokes" (rare in both diving and aviation)
Deep, sharp pain under sternum
Dry cough
Inability to take a normal breath
Attempted deep breath causes coughing (frequently paroxysmal)
Condition progresses to collapse if exposure to altitude is maintained
"False chokes" (caused by breathing cold, dry oxygen, which dries the throat and causes irritation and a nonproductive cough)

Brain
Visual disturbances
Headache
Spotty motor or sensory loss, or both
Unilateral paresthesia
Confusion
Paresis
Seizures

---

level as rapidly as possible. Breathing 100% oxygen also relieves the tissue hypoxia produced by the reduction of local blood flow. The actual management of a case of serious decompression sickness depends on geographic location and the availability of a suitable hyperbaric chamber. Therefore the order of preference of available treatment is as follows[15,18]:

1. Immediate hyperbaric compression with or without intermittent oxygen breathing should be administered.

2. Where no chamber facility exists, air medical personnel should treat circulatory collapse and arrange for early transfer to a hyperbaric chamber where this facility is available at a reasonable time or distance (less than 6 hours' travel time). Surface transport is preferable; flight to a suitable chamber should be at an altitude below 1000 feet if possible, and not higher than 3000 feet.

3. Air medical crew members should administer full supportive treatment for circulatory collapse if there is no possibility of transfer within a reasonable time to a hyperbaric chamber.

ADDITIONAL STRESSES OF TRANSPORT

SPATIAL DISORIENTATION
Spatial disorientation is described as an individual's inaccurate perception of their position, attitude, and motion in relation to the center of the Earth.[34]

When persons are experiencing spatial disorientation, they cannot correctly interpret or process the information they are being given by their senses. Spatial disorientation is primarily experienced during air transport.

During flight, three systems are involved in maintaining equilibrium. These are the visual, vestibular, and proprioceptive systems. These systems combine to allow the appropriate interpretation of input. However, the visual system plays the most important role.

Spatial disorientation can cause the following visual illusions[34]:

- Cloud formations being confused with the horizon or ground
- Water or desert appearing to be farther away than they are
- During night flight, the perception that another aircraft is moving away when it is actually getting closer

These visual illusions can cause significant motion sickness, which may render pilots or transport team members incapable of performing their duties or providing patient care. Spatial disorientation can also lead to misinterpretation of a landing area and result in a crash.

To prevent spatial disorientation, transport team members should use proper scanning techniques, never stare at lights, get adequate rest and nutrition, and provide conscious patients with a tactile reference during transport.

FLICKER VERTIGO

Flicker vertigo can occur when transport team members and patients are exposed to lights that flicker at a rate of 4 to 20 cycles per second.[34] Flicker vertigo can cause nausea and vomiting. In severe cases, it can cause seizures and unconsciousness.

Flicker vertigo commonly occurs when sunlight flickers through the rotor blades of a helicopter or an airplane propeller. It has also been triggered by light from rotating beacons against an overcast sky.

Transport team members or patients with a history of seizures are at risk for flicker vertigo. Wearing a hat with a bill and sunglasses can prevent flicker vertigo. Adequate rest and stress management may also decrease the risk.

FUEL VAPORS

Both ground and air transport can expose transport crew members and patients to fuel vapors. Jet fuel, diesel fuel, and gasoline are a few examples of what may be used in transport vehicles. Exposure to fuel vapors can cause altered mental status, nausea, and eye inflammation.[34]

Fuel vapors may be an indication of a problem in the transport vehicle and, when detected, should be immediately reported by the transport team. Adequate ventilation can help decrease the effects of exposure.

SUMMARY

To become an effective health-care provider in the transport environment, each transport team member must be thoroughly familiar with the effects of the stresses of transport on the human body. Implementation of correct interventions is an essential responsibility of each team member to minimize the effects of the stresses of transport.

TRANSPORT PHYSIOLOGY CASE STUDY #1

An industrial hydraulic press trapped a 29-year-old man at the substernal level and compressed him to an anterior-posterior diameter of approximately 10 inches, with positive loss of consciousness for approximately 2 minutes. On arrival at the local emergency department, his blood pressure was 80 systolic, and he remained awake and oriented. He was taken immediately to the operating room (OR) for exploratory laparotomy. He had a minor splenic laceration, a grade V laceration to the right lobe of the liver, and a hematoma of the transverse colon. During the operation, he received 22 units of packed red blood cells (PRBCs). He was transferred by fixed-wing aircraft to a level 1 trauma center 310 nautical miles away. He was transferred directly from the referring OR to the receiving OR. In flight he continued to be hemodynamically unstable and hypothermic. Before departure he had received 5 L of intravenous (IV) fluid, 22 units of PRBCs, 4 units of fresh frozen plasma, 10 units of platelets, and 800 ml of Hespan. IV access was triple lumen left (L) subclavian, L antecubital, and right (R) antecubital IV tubes and L radial arterial line. Before departure, the patient was given Norcuron 10 mg and fentanyl 150 μg and orally intubated with an 8.5 endotracheal tube (ETT). A gastric tube and urinary catheter were placed before arrival at the initial OR. The patient's weight was 220 lbs. Vital signs on arrival of the flight team (RN/RN) were blood pressure, 80/P; heart rate, 80; on vent 100% oxygen, O_2 saturation, 92%.

En route, the patient's abdominal distention continued, in addition to the serosanguineous drainage from his abdominal dressing. The fixed-wing flight time was 1 hour. Because of his continuing hemodynamic instability, rotor-wing transport was accomplished from the airport to the receiving hospital. His IV total during transport was 8 units of PRBCs, 1 unit of fresh frozen plasma, 6 units of platelets, and 1500 ml of crystalloid. His total urine output during transport was 1200 ml. He was maintained on Norcuron, Pavulon, and fentanyl IV for transport.

The rotor-wing transport time was 10 minutes. He was placed on the vent TV 850, control of 22, Fio_2 (fractional inspired oxygen concentration) 100%, and positive end-expiratory pressure of 5 cm. He was taken directly to the OR at the trauma center. On repeat exploratory laparotomy, his splenic laceration was managed conservatively. His gallbladder appeared necrotic and was removed, a G tube with a J extension was placed, and multiple drains and packing were placed around the liver. The cervico-thoraco-lumbar spine was negative for injury, and chest x-rays showed pulmonary edema and no pneumothorax. He was transferred to the trauma–burn intensive care unit, hemodynamically stable.

The second postoperative day, he was trached because of pulmonary edema and failure to wean. A large pleural effusion was noted on chest x-rays, and 1500 ml was evacuated after a right-chest-tube insertion. He remained in the intensive care unit for 14 days before being transferred to a general surgery floor. He developed sepsis, and the infection persisted despite treatment with multiple antibiotics.

He was discharged 33 days later with a percutaneously inserted central catheter line for home IV antibiotics, one drain in place for irrigation with antibiotics, and wet-to-dry packing of the abdominal wound.

Discussion
Assessment: On arrival of the flight team to the referring OR, the man was orally intubated with an 8.5 ETT, 27 cm at the lip line and was receiving vent 75% oxygen, TV 650, rate 12. The patient's weight was 220 lb/100 kg. He had the following lines: L radial art line, L triple-lumen subclavian, normal saline (NS) with blood tubing all ports, 16-gauge angiocath R and L antecubital (also NS with blood tubing). His abdomen was distended, with continuously oozing serosanguineous drainage; petechiae were seen from the nipple line up; his bilateral upper and lower extremities were mottled and cool to touch; the femoral pulses were diminished and the pedal pulses were absent; the refill capacity was longer than 5 seconds; and his heart rate was 100 to 110 without ectopy. Also seen were positive fogging of the endotracheal tube and bilateral chest rise symmetrical with ventilation. The R base diminished; in terms of the breath sounds, R > L, rhonchi were bilateral throughout, and the end-tidal CO_2 detector was of the "C" category. Neurologically, previously on neuromuscular blockade, the bilateral pupils were 3 mm, and the patient showed an equal listener response and was awake, talking, and oriented before arrival at the initial OR at the referring hospital. Foley was intact, draining clear amber urine, gastric placed L naris on flight team arrival, positive placement.

Intervention: The ETT was pulled back to 24 cm at the lip, and the ETT cuff was inflated with 8 ml NS; oxygen was increased to 100%, TV to 850 ml, positive end-expiratory pressure to 7, and rate to 20. Diagnostic checks were performed on the transport ventilator for 20 minutes while the patient was being prepared for transport. The

C-collar was applied, and the patient was long-boarded (padded board), secured (body first, head second), and wrapped in a survival blanket on top of spread and bath blankets. Warmed saline IV tubes and a port-a-warm mattress (neonatal) were provided for the axilla, groin, and upper torso. PRBCs were provided during transport.

In-flight: During flight, the gastric tube was open to ambient air, and the abdominal dressing continued to be reinforced as a result of increasing drainage and distention. The abdomen was packed and temporarily closed without drains. The O_2 saturation increased from 90% to 100%. The heart rate continued to increase 110 to 120, and the blood pressure stabilized before takeoff at 110/P to 138/P; became unstable at altitude, decreasing to 70/P; then responded well to continued fluid resuscitation. His IV total during transport was 8 units of PRBCs, 1 unit of fresh frozen plasma, 6 units of platelets, and 1500 ml of crystalloid. His total urine output during transport was 1200 ml. He was maintained on Norcuron, Pavulon, and fentanyl IV during transport. Because of his condition, rotor-wing transport was arranged before landing at the airport 15 nautical miles from the receiving facility. He was flown directly to the receiving facility and taken directly to the OR, where the trauma team was already scrubbed and awaiting his arrival.

Patient outcome was as described previously.

Altitude considerations

Prevent hypoxia by administering 100% oxygen, adequate TV, and positive end-expiratory pressure, if required. Prevent hypemic and stagnant hypoxia, and observe signs and symptoms (subjective). O_2 saturations only give part of the picture regarding oxygenation.

Keep the gastric tube open to ambient air. Barosinusitis and barotitis media are difficult to assess in the paralyzed and comatose patient. All air-filled cuffs and balloons should be replaced with normal saline. Watch for increasing distention in the GI tract or along penetrating-wound tracts, including incision lines. Remember to apply Boyle's law.

The man was initially hypothermic, with increased metabolic needs and acidosis. Decreased perfusion from hypotension and hypothermia caused further decompensation of his health state.

The transport team should provide humidified oxygen or an in-line humidifier. Crew members should administer sterile lubrication for eyes if the patient has neuromuscular blockade or is comatose. Ensure that he has adequate fluid intake. Strict intake and output and best evidence of fluid resuscitation are necessary.

Noise contributes to fatigue and discomfort. A possible option is to make use of hearing protection (even for a patient who is sedated, neuromuscularly blocked, or comatose) and crew, both in rotor-wing and fixed-wing aircraft.

Transport team members must ensure proper securing of the patient for safety and to decrease vibration. As a precautionary measure to protect the cervico-thoraco-lumbar spine, use a padded board, if possible, before transport. Boarded patients pick up all vibrations. Vibration leads to increased fatigue, skin breakdown, and patient discomfort.

Fatigue is the result of all other stresses. Consider the factors affecting tolerance and self-imposed stresses.

TRANSPORT PHYSIOLOGY CASE STUDY # 2

A 70-year-old man with a history of a nonembolic stroke was being transported by rotor-wing aircraft for treatment of sepsis. His vital signs were blood pressure 84/59; pulse rate 120 (sinus tachycardia); respiratory rate (intubated on transport ventilator) 14; and rectal temperature, 97°F.

He has been prepared for transport in a BK 117. When the pilot begins to turn the rotors, the flight nurse notices that the patient's eyes are blinking rapidly and he begins to experience a generalized tonic-clonic seizure. The monitor shows ventricular fibrillation, but a pulse can be palpated.

The flight nurse asks the pilot to stop the engines so that the team may obtain resuscitation assistance from the referring hospital personnel. As the rotors slow down, the patient's seizure activity *ceases. After a quick evaluation and administration of 2 mg of lorazepam, the transport team prepares to leave again. Once again, with the turning of the rotors, the patient experiences the same symptoms.*

This time, the flight nurse covers the patient's eyes with a towel and the seizure activity ceases. The team keeps the patient's eyes covered throughout the transport without further seizure activity.

Discussion
Even though flicker vertigo is not a common condition, sunlight flickering through rotor blades can trigger seizure activity in persons with seizure disorders or neurologic disorders that may place a patient at risk for seizures. This patient had had a recent stroke. Other clues that made the flight nurse consider flicker vertigo as the cause of this man's seizures are as follows:

- *The patient care platform positioned the patient's face in front of a window*
- *It was a sunny day.*
- *The activity ceased when the rotor blades stopped and started again with start-up.*

REFERENCES

1. Alspach JA, editor: *Core curriculum for critical care nursing,* ed 5, Philadelphia, 1998, WB Saunders.
2. Blumen IJ, Rinnert KJ: Altitude physiology and the stresses of flight, *Air Med J* 14(2):87-100, 1995.
3. Browne L, Bodenstedt R, Campbell P, Nehrenz G: The nine stresses of flight, *J Emerg Nurs* 13(4):232-234, 1987.
4. Burton GG, Helmholz HF: Gas laws and certain indispensable conversions. In Burton GG, Hodgkin JE, editors: *Respiratory care: a guide to clinical practice,* ed 2, Philadelphia, 1984, JB Lippincott.
5. Chase NB, Kreutzman RJ: Army aviation medicine. In DeHart RL, editor: *Fundamentals of aerospace medicine,* Philadelphia, 1985, Lea & Febiger.
6. Department of the Air Force: Aeromedical evacuation, U.S. Air Force Pamphlet No 164-2, 1983.
7. deTreville RT: Occupational medical support to the aviation industry. In DeHart RL, editor: *Fundamentals of aerospace medicine,* Philadelphia, 1985, Lea & Febiger.
8. Egan DF, Spearman CB, Sheldon RL: Gases, the atmosphere and the gas laws. In *Egan's fundamentals of respiratory therapy,* ed 4, St Louis, 1982, Mosby.
9. Gillingham KK, Wolfe JW: Spatial orientation in flight. In DeHart RL, editor: *Fundamentals of aerospace medicine,* Philadelphia, 1985, Lea & Febiger.
10. Glaister DH: The effects of long-duration acceleration. In Ernsting J, King P, editors: *Aviation medicine,* ed 2, London, 1988, Butterworth.
11. Hanna HH, Yarington CT: Otolaryngology in aerospace medicine. In DeHart RL, editor: *Fundamentals of aerospace medicine,* Philadelphia, 1985, Lea & Febiger.
12. Hawkins FH: The aircraft cabin and its human payload. In Orlady HW, editor: *Human factors in aviation,* ed 2, England, 1993, Aveberry Technical.
13. Heimbach RD, Sheffield PJ: Decompression sickness and pulmonary overpressure accidents. In DeHart RL, editor: *Fundamentals of aerospace medicine,* Philadelphia, 1985, Lea & Febiger.
14. Heimbach RD, Sheffield PJ: Protection in the pressure environment: cabin pressurization and oxygen equipment. In DeHart RL, editor: *Fundamentals of aerospace medicine,* Philadelphia, 1985, Lea & Febiger.
15. Kizer K: Diving medicine. In Auerbach P, editor, ed 4: *Wilderness medicine,* St Louis, 2001, Mosby.
16. Krupa D, editor: *Flight nursing core curriculum,* Park Ridge, Ill, 1997, National Flight Nurses Association.
17. Macmillan AJ: Decompression sickness. In Ernsting J, King P, editors: *Aviation medicine,* ed 2, London, 1988, Butterworth.
18. Macmillan AJ: The pressure cabin. In Ernsting J, King P, editors: *Aviation medicine,* ed 2, London, 1988, Butterworth.
19. Neubauer JC, Dixon JP, Herndon CM: Fatal pulmonary decompression sickness: a case report, *Aviat Space Environ Med* 59(12):1181-1184, 1988.
20. Raymann RB: Air crew health care maintenance. In DeHart RL, editor: *Fundamentals of aerospace medicine,* Philadelphia, 1985, Lea & Febiger.
21. Rood GM: Noise and communication. In Ernsting J, King P, editors: *Aviation medicine,* ed 2, London, 1988, Butterworth.
22. Sharp GR: The Earth's atmosphere. In *Aviation medicine,* London, 1978, Trimed Books.
23. Sheffield PJ, Heimbach RD: Respiratory physiology. In DeHart RL, editor: *Fundamentals of aerospace medicine,* Philadelphia, 1985, Lea & Febiger.

24. Spaul WA, Spear RC, Greenleaf JE: Thermoregulatory response to heat and vibration in men, *Aviat Space Environ Med* 57(11):1082-1087, 1986.

25. Spoor DH: The passenger and the patient in flight. In DeHart RL, editor: *Fundamentals of aerospace medicine,* Philadelphia, 1985, Lea & Febiger.

26. Sredl D: *Airborne patient care management: a multidisciplinary approach,* St Louis, 1983, Medical Research Associated Publications.

27. Stoot JR: Vibration. In Ernsting J, King P, editors: *Aviation medicine,* ed 2, London, 1988, Butterworth.

28. Thomas CL, editor: *Taber's cyclopedic medical dictionary,* ed 15, Philadelphia, 1985, FA Davis.

29. United States Air Force School of Aerospace Medicine: Flight nurse handouts, June 1995.

30. von Gierke HE, Nixon CW: Vibration, noise and communication. In DeHart RL, editor: *Fundamentals of aerospace medicine,* Philadelphia, 1985, Lea & Febiger.

31. Welch BE: The biosphere. In DeHart RL, editor: *Fundamentals of aerospace medicine,* Philadelphia, 1985, Lea & Febiger.

32. Wilson LM, Price SA: Respiratory pathophysiology. In *Pathophysiology: clinical concepts of disease processes,* ed 2, New York, 1986, McGraw-Hill.

33. Wirjosemito SA, Touhey JE, Workman WT: Type II altitude decompression sickness (DCS): U.S. Air Force experience with 133 cases, *Aviat Space Environ Med* 60(3):256-262, 1989.

34. Wraa C III, editor: *Transport nursing advanced trauma course,* Denver, 2001, Air and Surface Transport Nurses Association.

EXTRICATION AND SCENE MANAGEMENT

7

1. Perform an initial scene evaluation and identify potential safety hazards.
2. Dress appropriately for exposure to hazardous materials.
3. Decontaminate a patient who has been exposed to a toxic substance.
4. Identify whom to call when hazardous materials have been spilled.
5. Preserve evidence from a police scene.

Extrication and scene management are important concepts for the transport team to have a thorough understanding of. Extrication, scene management, and hazardous material management exercises should be included in annual training for all transport personnel. The training officer of the local fire department or rescue team is an excellent resource for either joint agency training or training that is exclusively applicable to transport personnel.

Air medical personnel are frequent participants in patient care in prehospital settings. Often the rescue helicopter has been preceded by rescue personnel who have already freed trapped victims and secured them to backboards or triaged and decontaminated those exposed to hazardous substances. However, when extrication is prolonged or if the helicopter is a first-responder, air medical crews need to use their scene management and extrication skills.

Most citizens and unskilled rescuers immediately rush to the victims. However, doing so can result in direct injury or exposure and contamination to both rescuers and victims, and it may delay the extrication and patient transport. Placing a contaminated patient in a transport vehicle will result in that vehicle being taken out of service for decontamination.

RESCUE MANAGEMENT

The following are rescue management guidelines:

1. Evaluate the situation for potential safety hazards.
2. Secure the accident scene.
3. Wear personal protective equipment (PPE) appropriate to the hazards on the scene (i.e., gloves, goggles, or self-contained breathing apparatus [SCBA]).[7]

4. Gain access to the patient.
5. Provide life-sustaining care to the patient.
6. Disentangle the patient from the vehicle.
7. Prepare the patient for removal from the accident scene (e.g., place cervical collar).
8. Remove the patient.
9. Prepare the patient for transport to the hospital.
10. Provide the patient with treatment en route.

Scene evaluation begins with the communications center obtaining information about possible problems and circumstances the rescuers will confront. The communication specialist should continue to seek information that might aid the rescuers throughout the incident, such as time of day, weather conditions, location, terrain, and number of victims. Information about fire, spilled fuel, toxic chemicals, overturned or entangled vehicles, and downed electrical lines should also be related to the communication specialist.

The general rule is never to compromise the rescuers to aid victims. The utility company should secure downed electrical lines; the fire department will hose down spilled fuel and contain hazardous materials. The rescuer should read placards on heavy trucks or read the manifest in the truck cab to determine the presence of any toxic or radioactive materials.

Scene security is usually provided by law enforcement personnel. Onlookers and the media should be kept well back from the operation. The rescue team should enlist the assistance of responsible adults to walk 100 yards in opposite directions from the scene and divert traffic.[4]

Proper placement of the helicopter is essential so that it does not create a second incident or hazard to personnel on the scene. The pilot retains the ultimate responsibility for landing the helicopter safely. Chapter 10 discusses scene landing recommendations.

The rescue team should enter vehicles through the car doors or by breaking out the glass and crawling through. The transport team should not enter a vehicle unless trained or directed by a trained individual. Although one side of a vehicle may be crushed beyond recognition, the opposite-side car door may be operable. If the vehicle is lying on its side and access is gained by opening the top-side car door, the rescue crew should be prepared for the car to shift. In the most serious crashes, the roof of the vehicle may need to be cut open.

Once inside the vehicle, the rescue team must perform a rapid triage of the occupants. Initial emergency treatment before extrication is extremely limited. Usually the initial-entry rescuer brings in a rigid cervical collar, a pocket face mask, and trauma dressings. The objectives are to (1) establish and maintain an airway with cervical spine precautions by using either the chin-lift maneuver or the jaw-thrust maneuver, (2) provide artificial ventilation (but not oxygenation because the presence of an inadvertent spark can ignite fuel-saturated clothing), (3) control external hemorrhage, and (4) provide cardiopulmonary resuscitation (CPR). CPR is not effective unless the patient is supine and on a firm surface.

The basic principle of extrication is that the rescuers should remove the vehicle from the victim rather than the other way around. If the vehicle is on its side, the extrication is performed through the roof. If the vehicle is on its wheels or roof, extrication is conducted through the doors. Rescue personnel inside an upright vehicle should first unlock the doors and use interior handles while their partners use exterior handles to open the doors.

Once the doors are open, victims can be secured to short backboards that will provide spinal column immobilization. There may be further obstacles to extrication. Typically, a victim's thorax becomes wedged between the forward-displaced seat and the rearward-displaced steering wheel/column, or a victim's feet and legs become trapped under the downward-displaced dashboard and the accelerator or brake pedal.

The victim must be completely immobilized if the seat has been torn from the mechanical track. When the seat tracks snap, there are usually a series of physically jarring pops that could substantially compromise an injured victim.

Pulling the steering wheel usually disentangles the victim's legs and feet because it concurrently lifts the dashboard up and forward.

If the vehicle is resting on its side, extrication can be achieved by cutting an upside-down U in the roof. The vehicle should be stabilized in the side position, the occupants should be warned of the very loud noise about to begin, and a heavy aluminized blanket should cover the occupants for their safety. After the three-sided U-shaped cut of the roof is made, the metal flap should be folded down to provide a smooth edge to move the victims across on their way out.

Extrication and Scene Management

Another hazard that rescuers must be aware of is air bags. Newer cars are now equipped with these safety devices. Studies have documented the effectiveness of air bags in decreasing serious injuries to drivers and passengers.[1,5] However, air bags can also cause injuries such as facial abrasions and lacerations and contusions to the chest and upper extremities.[1,5]

Undeployed air bags may be a potential hazard to the rescuer and can cause injuries similar to those reported in accidents in which the air bag has deployed. If the air bag has not been deployed, the rescuer should observe the following precaution[1,5,7]:

1. Disconnect or cut both battery cables.
2. Avoid placing personnel or objects in front of the air bag deployment path.
3. Do not mechanically displace or cut through the steering column until the system has been deactivated.
4. Do not cut or drill into the air bag module.
5. Do not apply heat in the area of the steering wheel hub.
6. Be aware of other air bags within the vehicle.

AIRCRAFT CRASH

The crash of even a light aircraft requires the response of a variety of emergency service units including fire, rescue, emergency medical service (EMS), and law enforcement. For the response to be quick and effective, it is vital that the person reporting a crash provide as much information about the incident as possible.

The following information should be obtained by communication center personnel and relayed to responders:

1. The time of the crash.
2. The type of aircraft (e.g., small passenger plane, commuter aircraft, large commercial jet, military transport plane, military fighter aircraft, or helicopter).
3. The number of engines, if known.
4. Whether the wreckage is on fire.
5. Whether a parachute was observed.
6. The number of occupants of the aircraft, if known.
7. Identification numbers and markings of the aircraft; military aircraft are marked "U.S. Air Force," "U.S. Navy," and so forth. Commercial aircraft show the name of the carrier. Private aircraft may have a combination of letters and numbers that constitute the identification number.
8. The status (e.g., on fire, damaged, or collapsed) of any structures struck by the aircraft or its components.
9. The status of people in those structures, if known.
10. Vehicles that were struck by the aircraft or parts of it and the status of any persons inside the vehicles, if known.
11. Structures that appear to be endangered by encroaching fire, spilled fuel, military ordnance, and so on.

If the transport team arrives at the crash site before emergency service units, crew members must proceed with caution. Survivors of the crash or persons who have been ejected or who have parachuted from the aircraft may be lying on the roadway leading to the crash site. If the aircraft is military, crew members must avoid both the front and rear ends of any externally mounted tanks or pods because these may be containers for missiles or rockets. The crew must be careful not to disturb any armament thrown clear of the aircraft; it may explode if improperly handled. No one should move body parts or components of the aircraft unless it must be done to care for injured persons. When emergency service units arrive on the scene, the transport team reports to the officer-in-charge, reporting everything known about the incident and the locations of any injured persons who have been assisted.

BUS CRASH

STOPPING THE ENGINE

Buses equipped with diesel engines do not need electrical power to keep running once they have been started. If possible, the rescuers should stop the engine by using the emergency stop button located on the driver's left-hand side switch panel. If the engine does not stop by operating this button, a crew member should discharge CO_2 into the engine air intake located at the left rear corner of the coach, discharging the agent inward and toward the front of the coach. Dry chemical should not be used.

ENTERING THE COACH

The rescuers should enter the coach through the front door if possible. Door unlocking and unlatching mechanisms can be found under the right-side wheel well, behind the front medallion, or to the left of the driver's seat, depending on the make and model of the bus. If the rescuers cannot enter through the front door, they can enter the bus through the windshield by removing the rubber locking strip from around the pane and then removing the pane. To enter the restroom (if the bus is equipped with one), the rescuers should open the small flap at the right rear window and lift the latch bar to open the window. Once inside the coach, the transport team should plan to remove victims confined to stretchers through the side windows.

THE AIR SUSPENSION SYSTEM

The transport team must remember the warning not to place their heads or extremities under any portion of the coach until it is securely blocked. The air suspension system bellows may deflate without warning, in which case the body of the coach may drop suddenly to within inches of the roadway.

ELECTRICAL EMERGENCIES

High voltages are common on roadside utility poles. Wood poles are sometimes used to support conductors of as much as 500,000 volts. Energized downed lines may or may not arc and burn. There is no assurance that a dead line at the scene of a vehicle accident will not become energized again unless it is cut or otherwise disconnected from the system by a representative of the power company. When an interruption of current flow is sensed in most power distribution systems, automatic devices restore the flow two or three times over a period of minutes.

The dispatcher should advise the power company of the exact location of the accident and the number of the power pole. The rescue team member designated to control bystanders should order spectators and nonessential personnel to leave the danger zone. Depending on the distances between poles, the danger zone may be as large as 600 feet by 1500 feet. Any rescuer should stop the approach immediately if a tingling sensation is felt in the legs and lower torso. This sensation signals energized ground, and that current is entering through one foot, passing through the lower body, and leaving through the other foot. This current flow is possible because of the condition known as *ground gradient*. This means the voltage is greatest at the point of contact with the ground and then diminishes as the distance from the point of contact increases.

If a tingling sensation is felt, the proper procedure is to bend one leg at the knee and grasp the foot of that leg with one hand, turn around, and hop to a safe place on one foot. By moving in this manner, the body will not be completing a circuit between sections of ground energized with different voltages. The rescuer should then stand by in a safe place until a representative of the power company can cut the lines or otherwise disconnect them from the power distribution system. The crew member controlling access to the scene must discourage ambulatory accident victims from leaving their vehicles until conductors that are either touching or surrounding the wreckage can be de-energized.

ENERGIZED CHAIN-LINK FENCE

A lethal current can be conducted through a chain-link fence for some distance. If required to work near or climb a chain-link fence that may be energized by a downed conductor, a crew member should not approach the fence with arms extended and fingers pointing forward. If contact is made with an energized fence, the current will cause the person's fingers to curl around the fence mesh and hold the person in place.

The proper approach to the fence is with arms extended and the backs of hands facing forward. If the fence is energized, the current will cause the person to be repelled backward.

HAZARDOUS MATERIALS EMERGENCIES

Emergencies involving hazardous materials occur in all areas of the United States, and transport teams are likely to be involved in the care of those who have been injured. When a hazardous material can be identified from a number or by name, emergency service personnel may obtain advice about managing the emergency from agencies that assist in the management of hazardous materials (Box 7-1). Agencies such as the Chemical Transportation Emergency Center (CHEMTREC) and the U.S. Department of Transportation can offer specific information.

However, not every transport vehicle is marked with a placard that identifies the specific materials on board. Many have placards that identify only the category of material being carried. CHEMTREC should be called for advice if a placard with a four-digit number that identifies the material is noted (Figure 7-1).

Suggested procedures for transport teams responding to the scene of a hazardous material transport emergency are as follows:

1. Land an aircraft upwind of the scene.
2. Keep out of low areas where heavier-than-air vapors can accumulate. Wear full PPE and a self-contained breathing apparatus if working in the hazard area. The use of special protective clothing (such as an acid suit) and a

BOX 7-1 | **Agencies That Assist in Hazardous Materials and Potential Rescue Incidents**

Federal agencies

Environmental Protection Agency (EPA)
Department of Transportation (DOT)
National Response Center (NRC)
United States Coast Guard (USCG)
Centers for Disease Control and Prevention (CDC)
Federal Aviation Administration (FAA)
United States Armed Forces (Army, Navy, Air Force, Marines)
U.S. Department of Energy (DOE)

Regional and state agencies

State EPA
State health departments
National Guard
State police
State emergency management agencies

Local agencies

Emergency management
Fire service (HAZMAT units)
Poison control and information center
Law enforcement agencies
Public utilities
Sewage and treatment facilities

Commercial agencies

American Petroleum Institute
Association of American Railroads (AAR) and Hazardous Materials Systems
Chemical Manufacturers Association
HELP (Union Carbide's emergency response system for company shipments)
Chevron (provides assistance with Chevron products)
Railway industry
Local industry
Local contractors
Local carriers and transporters

From Sanders MJ: *Mosby's paramedic textbook*, St Louis, 1994, Mosby.
HAZMAT, Hazardous material.

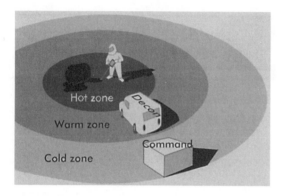

FIGURE 7-1   **Safety zones for hazardous materials incident.** (From Sanders MJ: *Mosby's paramedic textbook*, St Louis, 1994, Mosby.)

positive-pressure breathing apparatus is recommended.

3. If the vehicle is on fire, be aware that some corrosive materials react violently with water. Attempt to extinguish a small fire with dry chemical or CO_2. Extinguish a large fire with water spray, fog, or foam. Fight the fire from the maximum distance that hose streams will allow. Stay away from the ends of tank vehicles. Cool down uninvolved containers exposed to heat. Contain large amounts of spilled materials with dikes for later pick-up by personnel qualified in decontamination procedures.

In the event that someone has had contact with a dangerous substance, these procedures should be followed by personnel trained in decontamination:

1. Move the person to a safe place in fresh air.
2. Support respiration if the person is breathing with difficulty. Administer oxygen if it is available.
3. Initiate pulmonary resuscitation efforts if the person is not breathing.
4. Initiate CPR efforts if the person's breathing or heartbeat has stopped.
5. If skin surfaces (or eyes) have been in contact with a dangerous substance, begin flushing immediately with plenty of running water. The person may also be washed with water and a mild detergent.[7]
6. Strip away contaminated clothing and shoes while flushing with water.

7. Continue to flush the exposed skin surfaces (or eyes) until reasonably certain all traces of the dangerous substance have been removed.
8. Isolate contaminated clothing and shoes.
9. Decontamination procedures must meet Occupational Safety and Health Administration (OSHA) requirements 29 CFR 1910.120.

DECONTAMINATION

The following steps have been recommended for use when a person needs to be decontaminated after exposure to a hazardous material[7]:

1. There should be an entry point established for the "dirty" victims and rescuers to remove their clothing.
2. Surface decontamination should be performed by using plenty of water unless the contaminant requires another decontaminant.
3. PPE should be removed and stored.
4. Other clothing may have to be removed, depending on the level of contamination.
5. Contaminated personnel and victims should be washed at least twice. Water with or without a mild detergent may be used.
6. The victims and personnel should be medically evaluated.
7. Injured individuals should be transported for definitive care.
8. The decontamination site must be cleaned up and contaminated materials disposed of.
9. All equipment that has been used should be decontaminated and cleaned.
10. Contaminated clothing should never be taken home and cleaned.

EXPLOSIVE MATERIALS EMERGENCIES

There has been an increase in the number of injuries and deaths caused by explosives. Between 1980 and 1990 there were 12,261 bombings in the United States. Pipe bombs caused the majority of injuries. The injuries that resulted include both blast and thermal injuries.[3,6] Three classes of explosives are discussed in the following paragraphs.

Class A explosives are the most hazardous types of explosives. They include dynamite, desensitized nitroglycerine, lead azide, mercury, fulminate, black powder, blasting caps, detonators, detonating primers, and certain smokeless propellants.

Class B explosives have a high flammability hazard and include most propellant materials.

Class C explosives include manufactured materials that contain limited quantities of Class A or Class B explosives as one of their components, such as detonating cord, explosive rivets, and fireworks. Class C explosives will not normally detonate under fire conditions.

A vehicle involved in an accident or fire with a placard indicating the presence of Class A or Class B explosives or blasting agents is a potential danger. It is important to stop traffic in all directions, clear the area of nonessential personnel for 2500 feet in all directions, and deny access to all persons not essential to firefighting or the rescue operation.

RADIOACTIVE MATERIAL EMERGENCIES

The degree of hazard will vary greatly depending on the type and quantity of the radioactive material. External radiation can result from exposure to unshielded radioactive material. Internal radiation contamination can result from inhalation, ingestion, or skin absorption. Runoff from fire control or dilution activities can cause water pollution and thus spread the probability of contamination. Although some radioactive materials may burn normally, they do not ignite rapidly.

If only the yellow, black, and white *RADIOACTIVE MATERIAL* placard is visible and the material being carried cannot otherwise be identified, people not essential to the firefighting or rescue operation should be kept at least 150 feet upwind of the area; greater distances may be advised by the radiation authority. A rescuer must enter the spill area only to save a life and, when entry is necessary, should stay only the shortest possible time. The rescuer must wear full PPE and a positive-pressure breathing apparatus. Persons and equipment exposed to the radioactive material must then be detained until the radiation authority arrives or other instructions are received.

If the vehicle is on fire, damaged containers should not be moved; undamaged containers may be moved if it is possible to do so safely. The crew should attempt to extinguish any small fire with dry chemical, CO_2, water fog, or foam.

It is important to be sure that the victim has been appropriately decontaminated before being placed in any transport vehicle. If the victim is not appropriately decontaminated, he or she can contaminate both the team and the transport vehicle if they are not protected. If the transport vehicle is contaminated, it will need to be taken out of service and decontaminated according to decontamination codes and guidelines.[7]

LIQUIFIED PETROLEUM GAS LEAK—NO FIRE

Quick action is necessary when a leak develops in an liquefied petroleum (LP) gas transport vehicle or a large LP-gas storage vessel. A large leak can produce a significant vapor cloud, and the heavier-than-air gas can easily ignite. Vapor releases are usually invisible, and not all LP gas is odorized.

As emergency service units arrive, firefighters will set up large-diameter hose lines and take positions from which they can apply water to the sides of the tank. The officer in charge will establish a danger zone around the leaking container that should extend for at least 2000 feet from each end of the vessel and for at least 1000 feet from each side. Police officers will evacuate the danger zone and deny access to all nonessential personnel until the emergency is over. If a transport team is the first to arrive, a member should first request that police close access roads and then alert the gas company, electric company, and telephone company.

When hose lines are in position, the firefighters will disperse the gas by directing water spray across the vapor path. The crew should remain behind the protective spray so that they will be protected if the vapors ignite unexpectedly. No one should enter the vapor cloud. The gas company or plant operating personnel will stop the flow of gas, if possible.

As utility company personnel arrive, the gas company representative will shut off the gas supply. The power company representative will shut off electricity to the surrounding buildings. The telephone company representative should disconnect the telephone service to buildings. A ringing telephone can trigger an explosion of flammable vapors.

REACTION VESSEL EMERGENCIES

Reaction vessels are steel kettles in which chemicals and other products are combined during a manufacturing process. Essentially "mixing bowls," these vessels can range in capacity from a few hundred to several thousand gallons. Some are simple, open, stainless steel vats with hinged lids; others are thick-walled vessels that can be sealed, pressurized, and heated. Large reaction vessels have manholes several feet in diameter, and others have elliptical openings as small as 12×16 inches. Mixing vessels have agitators, or "beaters," similar to those provided with a kitchen mixer. The edges of the beaters usually come to within a few inches of the vessel wall, and the rescue of a worker behind the beaters (in relation to the manhole) can be a difficult task.

A worker may be injured when he or she fails to follow the established shutdown procedure, enters the vessel, and comes into contact with a hazardous material or a moving beater. A worker may fall and be injured while working inside the vessel. If there is any doubt about the quality of the air within the structure, rescuers should wear self-contained breathing units and a full set of protective clothing.

The rescuer should consult with the plant safety engineer or manager at the vessel location. If a knowledgeable person is not present (as in a multiple-injury situation), look for the **Confined Space Entry Permit** that should be displayed near the entrance to the vessel. From the permit the rescuer should be able to determine the following:

1. Any requirement for special protective clothing
2. The frequency with which the atmosphere should be analyzed for oxygen concentration
3. The frequency with which the atmosphere should be checked for explosive vapors
4. The threshold limit value of any toxic material present
5. The explosive limits of any flammable materials
6. What chemicals were in the vessel before shutdown
7. Any requirement for using nonsparking tools
8. The frequency with which radiation levels should be checked
9. Any requirement to use safety harnesses
10. Any requirement for standby personnel
11. The type of respiratory protection required
12. Any requirement for lifelines

Plant personnel should close feed valves and charging chutes. A rescuer or other responsible person should be assigned to guard the valves and chutes to ensure that they are not inadvertently opened during the rescue operation.

Plant personnel will de-energize the agitator power drive by opening the main disconnect switch and installing a lockout device. The padlock key should be secured until the rescue operation is over.

A rescuer should never be satisfied with someone's assertion that the agitator is "shut off." If there is any doubt that the agitator is inoperative, the rescuer should have plant personnel remove drive belts or chains (or otherwise immobilize) pulleys or flywheels.

CONSTRUCTION SITE EMERGENCIES

If a transport team member is near a piece of construction equipment when aiding a sick or injured operator and the engine of the machine is still running, the team member should not touch any of the operating levers, pedals, or other controls but should ask another operator to shut the engine down. If the injured operator can communicate, the transport team member should ask how to shut the machine down.

If another operator is not available and the sick or injured operator cannot provide instructions in the shutdown procedure and if the equipment is gasoline-powered, the medical team member should turn the key or master switch to the "off" position. If this does not stop the engine, the cable can be disconnected from the negative terminal of the battery. If the equipment is diesel-powered and has a level-type throttle control, pushing the lever all the way forward past the idle position and then turning the key or throwing the master switch to the "off" position will disrupt the electrical circuit to the engine.

RAILROAD INCIDENTS

GRADE-CROSSING ACCIDENT

In the event of an accident at a railroad crossing, the communication specialist should contact the railroad dispatcher with a request to stop all trains that are headed for the crossing.

STOPPING THE TRAIN

The engineer of a train that is traveling at 60 mph has approximately 1 second to determine whether a collision is imminent and activate the emergency-braking system. The train will travel a distance of 7920 feet (1½ miles). After the engineer applies the emergency brake, a train will continue for two thirds of a mile before stopping—even when traveling at only 30 mph.

To stop a train before it reaches a grade crossing, a person should be designated to go down the tracks to a point 1½ to 2 miles from the grade crossing and swing a lighted flare slowly back and forth horizontally at right angles to the track. This is the stop signal that is used by all railroads. The locomotive engineer should acknowledge the signal with two whistle blasts and then stop the train. The engineer might either misinterpret or disregard other signs and not stop the train. A flare can be waved day or night; if a flare is not available, a flashlight, battery-powered hand light, or lantern can be waved at night and a flag or other brightly colored object during daylight.

When responding to a derailment, the transport team should quickly assess the situation, report initial observations to the communication specialist, and request that the railroad dispatcher be notified of the incident. The railroad dispatcher will arrange to halt rail traffic; to dispatch railroad police, rescue, and clean-up crews; and to notify railroad officials.

If the derailed train can be approached safely, the train conductor should be in or near the caboose. The conductor is in charge of the train and will have documents to show whether the train is carrying hazardous materials.

To reach the caboose when passing close to the wreckage, the rescuers should not go under any derailed cars that are piled high. A precariously perched car can come plunging down without warning.

If the conductor and other train members are incapacitated, the crew member can look in the documentation drawer in the caboose for information about the train cargo. There should be car movement waybills and a "consist." Waybills are documents that describe the cargo and identify the shipper and receiver. The consist is a car-by-car listing of the contents of each rail car.

When searching for injured crew members in the locomotive, the crew will observe that there are forward and rear cabin doors. If access cannot be achieved by opening these doors inward, a rescuer can come in through the sliding cabin windows. The entire cabin area including nose section, boiler room, and electrical power transmission areas should be searched for injured persons.

Electric locomotives operate from an overhead electricity system that carries 11,000 V alternating current. It is important to disconnect that overhead power by pressing the **Pantograph Down** button in the locomotive control cab.

Steam generators are powered by diesel fuel. Fuel shutoff controls are located on each side of the car body under a cover plate marked *Fuel Shut Off*. The rescuer should lift the plate and pull the ring straight out 2 inches; the generator will stop running within 1 to 2 minutes.

Searching the train for injured passengers requires sliding open the side or end car doors, or entering through an emergency window. The crew should check the entire car, including the toilet and baggage areas.

Side-entry doors on passenger cars may be locked and will require tools to open. Side doors that slide in the car body panels have electric locks. The conductor and crew members have a skeleton key necessary to open this type of door latch. Access through dual-paned emergency exit windows is accomplished by shattering the outer tempered glass with a heavy, sharp, pointed tool; removing the inner window's rubber molding; and using a pry bar to remove the inner Lexan window.

UNDERGROUND EMERGENCIES

MINE EMERGENCY

In the event of a response to a mine emergency, the medical team should report directly to the mine office for instructions and follow those instructions explicitly.

CAVE EMERGENCY

PREEMERGENCY ACTIVITIES

The medical team should identify cave-rescue specialists, speleologists, and local cavers in the area; catalog their qualifications; and establish procedures for contacting them at the time of a cave emergency.

Rescue equipment and medical supplies should be streamlined. Suggested equipment for cave rescue includes the following[2]:

1. 24 hours of light for a helmet-mounted light
2. Helmet with a chin strap and headlight attachment
3. Warm clothes and gloves that are waterproof and allow mobility
4. Lug-soled boots that are light and drain water
5. Specialized caving rope
6. A litter that can fit through tight spaces
7. Wetsuits when water is expected in the cave
8. Harnesses and rings resistant to chemicals and water
9. Equipment to divert water from the victim and rescue crew
10. Warm food and drink.

The medical crew should participate in cross-training programs so agency rescue personnel can become familiar with cave-rescue techniques, and the administrator should develop a continuing education program so rescue personnel can practice rescue techniques in real cave settings.

CARE FOR AN INJURED PERSON DURING CAVE RESCUE

Caring for victims in a cave presents the medical crew with difficult challenges. Care must be provided in the dark and in muddy conditions. The transport team must be properly trained and experienced before they attempt any cave rescue.

The rescuer should carefully remove the victim from water or water spray, conduct a primary survey for life-threatening problems, and provide basic life support as necessary. The rescuer should remove the victim from drafts, if possible, and if not, should shield the victim using equipment or personnel. Heat loss to the ground can be prevented by placing a ground cover, blanket, articles of clothing, or rope under the victim. Heat loss to the surrounding air can be prevented by replacing the victim's wet clothes with dry clothing that is brought in or worn by the rescuers.

TRENCH COLLAPSE

Workers and emergency service personnel can be buried under tons of earth when unsupported trench walls collapse. Sheeting and shoring a trench are labor-intensive but absolutely necessary if a rescue operation is to be carried out safely. The steps to be followed in case of a trench collapse are as follows:

1. Determine who is in charge.
2. Assess the immediate injury problem.
3. Determine how many people are buried.
4. Determine where people are buried.
5. Assess on-the-scene capabilities of emergency medical services.
6. Request additional resources, if needed.

Hazard-control measures that can be taken include the following:

1. See that rescuers are protected.
2. Control traffic movement.
3. Control spectator movement.
4. Make the trench lip safe.

5. Ventilate the trench.
6. Position a safety observer.
7. Make the trench safe.
8. If the trench cannot be made safe, dig to the angle of repose.

Once access to the trapped victims has been achieved, the rescuers can dig them out by hand and remove the mechanisms of entrapment. First, a rescuer should uncover each victim's head and chest and initiate emergency care measures. When all the victims have been assessed and the ABCs have been treated (airway, breathing, circulation), the rescuers can work to free them completely. Then, as each victim is freed, he or she should be secured to a backboard before being removed from the trench.

WELL EMERGENCIES

Deep wells have shafts that may penetrate the earth for several hundred feet. Depending on the diameter of the shaft, a person who falls into a deep well may become wedged only a few feet from the surface or may go all the way to the bottom. In most cases, rescue (or recovery) is possible only when a parallel shaft is drilled and a horizontal tunnel dug, through which rescuers can pass from the shaft to the well.

Many conditions add to the danger of well emergencies. In shallow wells, the atmosphere may be oxygen deficient. Heavier-than-air toxic gases may be present at the bottom of the well. Methane gas may present the threat of an explosion. Water in the well may cause the victim to drown. Unstable shaft walls may collapse during a rescue operation.

All of these conditions warrant special precautions. To guard against possible shaft-wall collapse, the rescuer should place ground pads (sheets of 4- × 8-foot plywood) around the shaft opening. The pads will distribute the weight of the rescuers and equipment and minimize the possibility of a cave-in. The possibility of an oxygen-deficient atmosphere must be anticipated if the victim at the bottom of the shaft is unconscious or incoherent. The rescuer should ventilate the well by having fresh air blown down the shaft. To reach the victim, the rescuer should put on a safety harness that is secured to a lifeline or a harness that is formed with the end of a lifeline.

The victim, when reached, should be secured in a harness attached to a lifeline or in a harness formed with the end of another lifeline. Rescuers at ground level should hoist the victim from the well before the rescuer in the well climbs out. If it is not possible for the rescuer to climb out, the ground-level rescuers should hoist the rescuer from the shaft with their lifelines.

Rescuers who set up lights to illuminate the shaft of a wet well must be sure the lights are tightly secured. If a lamp falls into the well during the rescue operation it could electrocute victims and rescuers.

POLICE-RELATED SITUATIONS

Police officials expect the cooperation of other emergency personnel when there is a police emergency.

BOMB THREAT

In the event of a bomb threat, the transport team should report the location and give an accurate description of the object to the command post or control point; this information should then be relayed immediately to the police, fire departments, and rescue units. The information should be relayed by telephone even if a two-way radio is available because radio transmission energy can cause detonation of an electric blasting cap. The object should never be touched or otherwise disturbed. Doors and windows should be opened to minimize primary damage from the blast and secondary damage from fragmentation.

FIREARM EMERGENCY

A weapon found at the scene of an emergency must be left in the exact position in which it was discovered. Rescuers should assume the weapon is loaded and in operating order even if it appears otherwise. Law enforcement officers should be called.

If the weapon must be moved for any reason before police officers arrive, a medical crew member may assume responsibility for moving and safeguarding the weapon or should delegate the responsibility to a trustworthy person. Only one person should handle the weapon until it can be turned over to the police officers. If a camera is available, a photograph can be taken of the weapon in place, with reference points, such as doors, windows, furniture, and so on, that will help investigators accurately place the weapon included in the picture. A photograph that shows only the weapon will be useless. The crew member should pick the weapon up with the grips held between the fingers. Although this seems inconsistent with the policy of preserving fingerprints, it is the safe way to handle a handgun. Recognizable fingerprints cannot usually be recovered from checked grips. The crew member should not attempt to clear or unload the weapon. The number of live and expended rounds in a revolver, their position in the cylinder, and the status of the round under the hammer all may be important to investigators. When carrying the weapon, the person should keep the barrel pointed in a safe direction, preferably skyward.

EVIDENCE PRESERVATION

Many investigations have been seriously hindered because emergency service personnel inadvertently disturbed or destroyed articles of evidence at the scene of a crime. Investigators look at everything, and even something that seems of little importance may be a valuable piece of evidence to a police officer.

CRIME SCENE EVIDENCE
The transport team must keep unauthorized persons from the crime scene and not touch, kick, or otherwise move anything unless it is necessary during the rescue or during efforts to care for victims. Mental notes of possible clues such as the position of a weapon, overturned furniture, or pooled blood will be helpful. As soon as rescue or emergency care activities are complete, observations can be shared with the investigating officers.

VEHICLE CRASH SCENE EVIDENCE
Among the items of significance to accident investigators are tire marks, runoff from radiators and crankcases, blood, broken glass, vehicle trim, motor parts, and even clods of dirt turned up by a vehicle's wheels. To assist police investigators at the scene of a vehicle accident, the transport team should first rope off the crash site so physical evidence can be preserved in place and then keep spectators from picking up or moving pieces of debris.

POLICE OFFICER
If responding to assist a wounded or injured officer, the transport team should report to the senior police officer. No one should approach the wounded or injured officer until the police officer–in-charge indicates it is safe to do so. If it will be unsafe to carry out assessment and initial care efforts on the spot, the officer should be moved to a safe place in such a manner that injuries will not be compounded.

SUMMARY

Although the transport team may not be directly involved in extrication or rescue activities, crew members should be prepared to help the rescue effort and not endanger themselves so that they are unable to help the injured after they are rescued. Scene management of various incidences should be a component of all transport teams.

Air and ground transport teams can offer additional medical care and rapid transport to those injured in all types of incidents. *Only transport teams that have had appropriate training, carry the correct equipment, and have experience performing rescues should be the rescuers.* Without the proper equipment and training, the rescue crew may find themselves needing to be rescued.

REFERENCES

1. Antosia RE, Partridge RA, Virk AS: Air bag safety, *Ann Emerg Med* 25(6):794-798, 1995.
2. Cooper DC, LaValla PH, Stoffel RC: Search and rescue. In Auerbach P, editor: *Wilderness medicine*, St Louis, 2001, Mosby.
3. Karmy-Jones R, Kissinger D, Golocovsky M, Jordan M, et al: Bomb-related injuries, *Mil Med* 159(7):536-539, 1994.

4. Kramer A, Evans J: Ambulance operations and special response situations. In Holleran RS, editor: *Prehospital nursing: a collaborative approach*, St Louis, 1994, Mosby.

5. Kuner EH, Schlickewei W, Oltmanns D: [Protective air bags in traffic accidents: change in the injury pattern and reduction in the severity of injuries], *Unfallchirurgie* 21(2):92-99, 1995.

6. Mellor SG: The relationship of blast loading to death and injury from explosion, *World J Surg* 16(5):893-898, 1992.

7. Sanders MJ: *Mosby's paramedic textbook*, St Louis, 1994, Mosby.

DISASTER MANAGEMENT

8

COMPETENCIES

1. Delineate disaster criteria on the basis of location, number of victims, and resources available.
2. Identify the safety issues that should be considered by the transport team when responding to a disaster.
3. Perform disaster triage using a designated system of patient identification.

Disasters represent a serious challenge to helicopter emergency medical services and transport teams, including the sudden and sometimes unplanned experience of working with agencies that do not routinely work together. Disasters are often a result of a complex series of events that lead to a constantly changing environment and situation. Managing them demands plans that are adaptive in the face of a frequently chaotic and often emotionally overwhelming situation. By their nature, disasters are unpredictable, unexpected, and certainly unwanted events. Yet responding to a disaster is an aspect of any emergency service, and both air and ground transport teams may be asked to participate in an operation that must be addressed and carefully planned for before a disaster strikes.

Medical disaster management refers to the medical treatment, prioritization, and disposition/transportation of large numbers of victims during natural and man-made catastrophes. However, disasters are often described in limiting numeric terms, such as *mass casualty* or *multicasualty*, which generally refer to victim statistics only.

The development of disaster-management principles starts with the operational definition of *disaster* and its related levels of intensity. A particular level of intensity or impact on one community may not be the same from one agency to another. For ground emergency medical service (EMS) agencies, a disaster may vary depending on the location of the incident, resources available, number of victims and their acuity levels, and environmental factors. The use of helicopter emergency medical service (HEMS) responders will be affected by weather, the number of victims and their acuity levels, the type of ground EMS providers (advanced life support [ALS] versus basic life support [BLS]), the distance from hospitals, and geography.

The levels of intensity and impact are best illustrated by comparing the response capabilities of rural areas with those of a large urban community. A disaster for one may merely be a busy day for another. Accordingly, the term *disaster* is often vague and can vary from one locality to another. Often the definition of a disaster is influenced by the extent of media interest, numbers of victims, and the spectacular nature of the event. Assuming large numbers of people are involved, if all injuries are relatively minor, the use of the term *disaster* becomes questionable. In such cases the favored term has become *near disaster*. However, the issue is not what to call the event but whether the local EMS disaster plan was activated. Because of this, there is a more accurate *operational* definition of a disaster. The operational definition is used to aid the decision whether to activate the plan when responders are initially confronted with a possible disaster. Thus the operational definition of a disaster is not determined by what type of incident has occurred but rather by the understanding that a disaster is any event that overwhelms the existing personnel, facilities, equipment, and capabilities of responding agencies or institutions.[1-4] The development of disaster-management principles starts with an understanding of the operational definition and its related levels of intensity.

Interestingly, the Association of Air Medical Services (AAMS) Air Medical Crew National Standard Curriculum cites the definitions of disasters using the Association of Standard Testing Management (ASTM) standard F30.03.07.[1] These disaster levels, labeled *Level I Emergency Response (Extended Medical Incident)*, *Level II Emergency Response (Major Medical Incident)*, and *Level III Emergency Response (Disaster)*. Level I incidents can be handled by local resources and facilities. Level II incidents involve large numbers of victims and require multijurisdictional mutual medical aid. Level III incidents result in many casualties, overwhelm local and multijurisdictional resources, and require assistance from state or federal resources, or both.

For emergency planners, an additional variation on these definitions can be used. Rather than the use of Levels II, III, and I, which essentially refer to the number of victims, apply definitions that make use of language that is more common. This definition format refers to disasters as *simple* versus *compound* and expands on the concept of multijurisdictional aid. A simple disaster occurs when a community's

physical integrity is not disrupted, roads and communities remain intact, and local resources are enough to manage the incident. These disasters tend to be short-lived and may cover a limited area but could involve overlapping boundaries and jurisdictions. A compound disaster disrupts both the structure and function of a community and requires the assistance of outside agencies, usually state and federal, to manage the incident. Classically, this event has multiple or widespread incident sites that may overlap multiple jurisdictions and boundaries and often involves mass casualties and fatalities. Operations, including rescue and recovery, may last several days, weeks, or in extreme cases, months.

It is to this environment of overwhelming numbers of victims and an emotionally charged atmosphere that HEMS providers are asked to respond. Whether the incident is a 5-victim traffic accident or a jetliner crash (Figure 8-1), air medical crews must be prepared to interact with local public service agencies and private EMS providers. HEMS transport units must be an integral part of the disaster plan, not just an afterthought. Air medical crew members must train extensively for their roles and responsibilities in the disaster plan. They must know how they are activated to respond and who their command officials are, understand their role in the Incident Command System (ICS), and have the ability to function in a prehospital care environment.

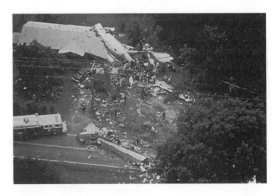

FIGURE 8-1 **Aerial view of the site of USAir 1016 crash in Charlotte, NC, July 2, 1994.** (Courtesy Medcenter Air, Charlotte, NC.)

HEMS organizations must continually update, train, and adjust plans as necessary on the basis of the experiences of others who have responded to multicasualty and mass-casualty incidents. Lessons learned by HEMS operators provide valuable information about what went right, what problems were encountered, what component(s) of their plan failed, and what in their training and their plan has been changed because of this understanding.

This chapter reviews the principles of disaster management, triage, incident command, and postincident debriefing. Focus is on the expected roles and responsibilities of air medical crews in disaster operations, regardless of the size and impact of the disaster. Even though the focus is on HEMS, the principles are applicable to ground transport services that may also be called to participate in disaster management.

DISASTER MANAGEMENT

The primary concern for HEMS disaster-management planners is not the number of victims but rather the development and implementation of a well-researched and well-prepared disaster plan. The development of a disaster plan starts with an evaluation process known as the *preplan*. The preplan is an honest and unbiased evaluation of the existing resources and capabilities of a particular organization. Community emergency planners, in general, should look at resource issues as they apply to all prehospital care providers (in the public and private sectors), public service agencies (fire, police), local and state agencies, and finally, local and regional health care facilities. All area HEMS organizations must be identified by type of service (mission profiles), including training and expertise in scene work, level of on-board medical expertise, number and types of aircraft, availability (hours of operation), flight times to different localities, aircraft capabilities for ground and air communication, and emergency dispatch numbers.

Those responsible for developing a HEMS operational disaster plan must take into consideration the normal mission profile of their service, the training and experience in prehospital care opera-

tions of their medical flight teams, the normal level of emergency medical and other equipment carried, their communication capabilities, and safety-related issues such as protective clothing for flight crews. Deliberation must be given to operating in hazardous environments with uneven terrain, sharp-edged debris, hazardous materials, poor lighting, inclement or hazardous weather conditions, and confined space or structurally impaired areas. Therefore scrutiny must be given to the part of the preplan assessment that looks at the availability of protective clothing, light sources, crew training for operations in and around hazardous materials, confined space, and hazardous environments.

Personnel at Medcenter Air of Charlotte, North Carolina, learned a lesson in scene safety in the postincident critique of the July 1994 USAir jetliner crash.[5] Arriving in the early stages of the incident, the flight team functioned in a first-responder role, which is not normally part of Medcenter Air's mission profile. The air medical crews initially worked in and among the wreckage without wearing the standard type of personal protection gear normally worn by fire and prehospital care personnel. They thereby exposed themselves to increased risks of injury. Other hazards that result from inexperience include arriving at the disaster site wearing unsafe footwear, such as high-top sneakers. This can result in penetrating foot injuries to flight crews as they walk around and over sharp debris that can penetrate the soles of the shoe. Other injuries include strains, sprains, and fractures of the lower extremities. The same hazard issues apply to not wearing leather work gloves and helmets. The most tragic lesson of this type occurred following the April 1995 terrorist bombing in Oklahoma City, Oklahoma. A local nurse voluntarily responded to the scene and was killed by falling debris. She had responded wearing only a pair of jeans, a shirt, and sneakers.

Other scene safety issues relate to the security, control, and location of landing zones but, most crucially, to control and safety when loading and unloading victims from the aircraft. In the atmosphere of heightened activity and emotions at a large disaster scene, the loading and unloading of victims often becomes chaotic. Nevertheless, scene safety measures must be strictly followed. In disasters, EMS pilots will have to deal with additional environmental, communication, and geographic issues not normally encountered as part of a routine scene call. As with the USAir incident, predesignated sites may not always work, and alternative-landing zones may need to be used when otherwise indicated (Figure 8-2). This may mean that initial landing zones may be assessed as suboptimal, and aircraft may need to be relocated after touching down at a scene.

Multiple aircraft may be involved in a disaster response or incident. Responding aircraft include those belonging to the military, public service agencies, other HEMS operators, and the media. Preplanning should include a look at organized plans by these groups to work, communicate, and coordinate efforts to avoid any other unfortunate incidents such as midair accidents or collisions. Add the mix of multiple HEMS operations, fire or police aircraft, and a swarm of media helicopters, and it makes for a very crowded sky. In previous large-scale incidents, the Federal Aviation Administration (FAA) has restricted airspace above and around an ongoing incident to prevent such occurrences and to control the presence of unauthorized aircraft. However, this is not always the case in the early stages of a disaster event.

Another issue to explore during the preplan phase is the need to provide large inventories of medical supplies and be prepared to resupply for protracted disaster incidents. Typically, EMS and HEMS aircraft medical supplies are rapidly exhausted early on in the incident. HEMS providers, with local authorities and hospitals, should evaluate their systems' ability to bring disaster packs or additional caches of medical equipment to the incident site or prearranged localities. This transporting of medical supplies and, possibly, hospital-based medical response teams should be included in the mission profile of HEMS disaster operations. Other secondary uses for HEMS aircraft may include performing aerial scene surveillance to assist local authorities.

Further essential elements in the preplan phase include the vital issues of activation and dispatch of resources and, ultimately, of communications. A strong community disaster plan is one that includes timely activation of all required resources, including notification of those anticipated for response and alerting of local and regional HEMS providers. The longer the delay in activation of resources, the greater the delay in rescuing, treating, and transporting victims when a disaster occurs. The best example of being well prepared for emergency response was the 1989 crash of a DC-10 in Sioux City, Iowa. Emergency responders were given at least a 30-minute warning of the impending crash. Ground ambulances, fire and police units, military rescue, and HEMS were all activated in advance and were in place when the airliner arrived and crashed on airport property. Essentially the disaster came to them, for all resources were able to respond immediately. Obviously, this was an extraordinary case with an extraordinary outcome. This prewarning alarm of the impending disaster, which resulted in the early activation of resources, aided in the overall coordination of rescue efforts and ensured an instantaneous response to the event. If, however, there is no warning of the event, it is imperative that there be no delays in activating and notifying needed agencies and resources, including hospitals and HEMS providers. Imagine what the response and outcome would have been if the Sioux City crash had occurred without any warning whatsoever. This is the reality of most disaster responses.

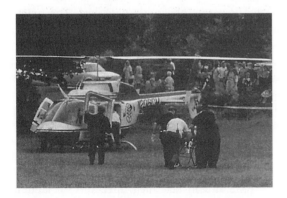

FIGURE 8-2   **The loading of a USAir 1016 crash victim at the established landing zone.** (Courtesy Medcenter Air, Charlotte, NC.)

The communications capabilities of HEMS providers are equally as crucial as the issues of early notification, activation, and response. As part of the preplan, helicopter and ground vehicle radio capabilities must be evaluated for ground-to-air and ground-to-ground compatibility with those of fire, EMS, and police ground units, particularly when multiple frequencies and agencies are involved.

A comprehensive preplan looks at internal issues, but also the interface and coordination required with all other responding agencies, including nontraditional ones. Hospital, prehospital, fire, and law enforcement are just some of the agencies to be assessed when developing a well-rounded and flexible HEMS disaster-response plan. Once the preplan is completed, it becomes the working foundation for the development of the operations and disaster plan itself.

THE DISASTER-RESPONSE PLAN

Once the preplan is completed, the response plan is developed and put into action through instructional and practical training, with yearly continuing education and practice. Most public service agencies use a system known as the *Incident Command System (ICS)*. Initially developed for use during multijurisdictional wildfires occurring in Southern California, it allowed fire agencies to develop ongoing letters of agreement and plans to jointly manage catastrophic brush fires while recognizing the need for a lead agency and command structure. Later the ICS was expanded to cover any large-scale event requiring multiple units or agencies, either fire rescue or EMS. Included in the ICS are operational roles for fire, law enforcement, and EMS. The ICS is a management system that allows multijurisdictional agencies to work harmoniously under joint management and control.

Under the ICS, one *Incident Commander (IC)* is responsible for all aspects of the operation. The IC is usually the highest-ranking fire or law enforcement officer on the scene (depending on the incident). The highest-ranking officer may initially be a fire captain or paramedic, but this job is delegated to the highest-ranking official as that person arrives on the scene, usually a battalion chief or higher-ranking

officer. The IC is not directly involved with medical operations but rather with the operation as a whole, including search-and-rescue efforts, fire suppression, hazardous materials containment (if necessary), logistics, medical aid, and transportation. The IC delegates others to control each of the separate efforts; for example, the IC would assign the highest-ranking medical person (usually a senior-level paramedic) to medical operations (*medical control*). This chapter deals exclusively with the medical operation branch under the ICS.

The medical division functions under the operations sector of the ICS. A medical division/branch supervisor or medical control officer (different areas use different titles) coordinates all medical transportation, hospital communications, supply, and medical air operations as they relate to transport of victims, and, in some cases, extrication where medical care is needed.[7] The *medical control officer* serves as the resource and coordinator for division leaders/supervisors (also known as subsector or branch).

The medical control officer is responsible for delegating supervisory responsibilities to personnel who are in charge of triage, treatment areas, transportation (ambulance loading and staging), and communications. The *communications supervisor* is responsible for communications with base hospitals or medical control and maintains logs of victim destination. Each branch supervisor has line responsibility and involvement with direct victim care and related issues as previously described. The *ambulance control officer* or *transportation supervisor* works closely with the *air operations supervisor* when requesting HEMS response. The medical control officer also coordinates supply needs and resupply issues, working with branch supervisors as needed. The medical control officer communicates directly with the IC. No other subordinates report to this level of command. All EMS operational requests and considerations are passed through the medical control officer.

HEMS aircraft take their directions for landing from the air operations supervisor. They will guide in aircraft, establish air-to-ground communications, and secure the landing zone. In smaller operations, someone other than EMS or fire personnel can perform this task. It is imperative that someone with a direct line of communication with incoming aircraft has responsibility for this task. Normally, landing zones are kept at a distance from the incident site to minimize rotor wash and maintain control and security. The transportation officer is responsible for dispatching ground vehicles to transport air medical crews if their presence is desired anywhere other than at the landing zone itself.

Depending on local operational plans, air medical crews may either be required to remain with their aircraft and accept victims brought to them for evacuation or asked to report to medical control for further directions. Medical control may request air medical crews to assist in stabilizing victims before air evacuation. Timely air evacuation is a priority once airways are secured. Other procedures may be accomplished in flight, depending on aircraft and crew configuration. In either case, air medical crews should not self-dispatch to victim care areas, get involved with rescue efforts, or provide direction on where victims will be transported unless this is part of the local organizational plan.

Once air medical crews are physically separated from their aircraft, a situation may develop in which ambulances arrive at the landing zone ready to transport victims and then find that the only person there is the pilot. This situation has occurred in small and large events across the nation.

Decisions regarding which hospital a victim will be transported to and by what means (ground or air) are made by the transportation supervisor. This individual receives information on patient destinations by the medical control supervisor, who coordinates efforts with local receiving hospitals. It is this coordinated effort that prevents "relocating the disaster" to area hospitals and reduces the chances of unintentionally overloading one or more of the facilities.

The ICS provides for a coordinated effort among all responding agencies and is only as effective as those who implement and work within it. The primary role of HEMS is that of transportation to and from the scene. Under ICS, added responsibilities of transporting supplies or equipment and additional

medical personnel may occur. In rare cases, HEMS aircraft may be used for search-and-rescue operations or scene surveillance once the primary task of victim transport is completed.

COMMON PROBLEMS IN DISASTER MANAGEMENT

In past years, EMS and HEMS agencies have responded to disasters small and large, simple and compound, and those involving the complicated issues of terrorist events. A pattern of consistent problems, which I have dubbed the "Five Cs," has emerged as endemic to all disaster events. Disaster planners should use these consistent problems as a guide in anticipating and developing disaster operational plans for HEMS organizations. Understanding what problems continually develop during disaster operations allows planners to mitigate the situation by developing flexible operational disaster plans that take into consideration the variables of such events. The Five Cs of disaster management are problems with *Communications, Control* and command, *Congestion, Collection* of resources, and *Coordination* of triage and transportation.[4]

COMMUNICATIONS

Communication problems occur because of nonfunctioning or marginally functioning communications hardware, inappropriate use or lack of radio frequencies, incompatible frequencies, insufficient numbers of radios and cellular phones, or poor verbal and alternative communications skills by field and hospital personnel. "Ten codes," or coded radio language, should be avoided when dealing with interagency communications, particularly when those agencies normally do not use coded language. Simple language is used to accurately convey a picture of the incident and its victims, the additional resources being requested, and information being passed on. As previously discussed, good communication from the scene is important. Dispatch centers need immediate information and accurate descriptions of the incident and, in addition, need to know what resources are needed or anticipated. They must be advised whether the disaster is impending (as an inbound crippled jetliner) or is occurring. Historically in disasters occurring in the United States, communication delays of up to 20 minutes have hindered activation of disaster plans and the timely response of resources, equipment, and personnel. Communication is the foundation on which all of management and operations is built. Without a well-thought-out plan that anticipates communication needs and all contingencies, overall operational plans will fail.

For example, the flight team from Medcenter Air, Carolinas Medical Center, Charlotte, North Carolina, experienced communication difficulties during a HEMS disaster response. Their postcritique of Medcenter Air's response to the commercial airliner crash of USAir Flight 1016 revealed communication problems that developed immediately on arrival at the scene. The landing zone was located a half mile from the incident site. Ironically this site had been selected in a previous drill simulating aircraft crashes at the local airport. However, once the flight team was away from the aircraft, they had no way of staying in communication with the pilot, dispatch center, or medical control officer at the hospital. In addition, after arriving at the crash site, members of the medical flight crew became separated and were unable to communicate with each other. Drawing from this experience, Medcenter Air evaluated the use of alternate communication devices such as hand-held radios and cellular phones.[5]

CONTROL AND COMMAND

Control and command are only as effective as those persons assigned to leadership positions and those responsible for following their orders. If the command position is not recognized or acknowledged by all involved, then the commander or leader becomes ineffective. This is particularly true when there is a jurisdictional conflict among responding agencies and disputes or conflicts of operational plans develop among the respective organizational heads. Command decisions and plans may fail when there is inappropriate assignment of personnel to job tasks, not taking into consideration the skill, experience, and routine roles of the particular indi-

vidual or organization. However, even appropriate implementation of the ICS does not guarantee that problems will not develop in the end.

CONGESTION

An expectation in any disaster is pedestrian and vehicular congestion, whether it is at the scene or at the hospital. Civilian, media, fire, rescue, and law enforcement vehicles can cause traffic obstructions. Additional impediments are caused by onlookers, the media, law enforcement, victims, and rescuers (fire and EMS) alike. This congestion becomes a management problem for the control of ambulance movement and the transport of victims from one area to another, including HEMS landing zones. If a rotorcraft lands too close to an incident, rotor wash can cause havoc and unintentional injuries from flying debris. If the landing zone is too far from the incident, coordinated and timely patient transport from the incident site to waiting aircraft is hampered.

COLLECTION OF RESOURCES

Resources, both personnel and equipment, may create problems either because they are limited or are overabundant. Anticipated resources may or may not appear quickly at the scene. Unrequested responders, volunteers (bystander rescuers), or unauthorized responders may appear at the scene or the hospital. Overstaffing or an excess of available resources complicates the issues of congestion, command, and coordination. The greatest error in judgment is to rely on resources that are not yet on the scene, rather than on those that are already available. Those in command must not allow extra personnel to remain in the area when they are not needed for effective operations. These resources can be used later on for relief, particularly in long-term operations.

COORDINATION OF TRIAGE AND TRANSPORTATION

The process of triage is only effective if those who are the triageurs coordinate their activities and actions. Transportation of victims from the scene to area hospitals and the means of transporting them must not occur because of independent decisions and actions by field personnel. The tendency to transport all victims or "relocate the disaster" to one local facility (unless only one exists) must be avoided. Victims need to be dispersed among existing facilities, taking into consideration transportation times, distance from scene, and the capabilities of the facilities, including whether they have trauma and pediatric centers.[6]

From the moment resources arrive on the scene, communication must be established with local hospitals to determine their patient care capacity and capabilities. Once those capacities are established, victims should be dispersed among all available facilities; their destination should be established on the basis of acuity levels, hospital capabilities, and distance/transportation times from the scene. In compound disasters, the hospital themselves may become unusable or diminished in their capabilities. In some cases, hospitals have required emergency evacuations of patients and personnel because of structural failure or danger, thus turning them into additional disaster incident sites. All responding field personnel (EMS, HEMS, fire, law enforcement) must be trained in similar triage techniques.[7]

As part of the preplan, area hospitals capable of receiving helicopter transports should have been previously identified. However, air medical crews should not assume that the closest hospital with a helipad or landing zone will automatically receive victims by air. These facilities are inundated with victims arriving by ambulances or private vehicles because of their close proximity to the incident. Helicopter transport may often take victims to facilities farther from the scene to avoid overwhelming the closest hospitals. Victims benefit both from shortened transport times to these remote health care facilities and from the fact that these centers are less likely to be overwhelmed with victims arriving by ambulance. Thus the staff at these facilities can give more attention to the limited numbers of victims they receive, assuming they have the ability to provide advanced medical care.

TRIAGE

Triage comes from the French verb *trier*, which means "to sort." In medical terms, *triage* is the process of prioritizing medical care, treatment, and transportation of a number of patients. Its purpose is to sort large numbers of victims, maximize limited resources, and do the most good for those best able to survive. Triage should be based solely on the chances for survival and not necessarily the severity of the injury. The process of triage is instituted when existing resources are overwhelmed and medical personnel are unable to render complete care to all of the victims. In other words, the process of triage is to assess the victim's clinical condition as it relates to other victims, assign priority of field treatment, and determine the disposition of that victim.

Triage is used to avoid making decisions that involve the performance of heroic life-saving procedures on those victims who have obvious lethal injuries and are therefore deemed nonviable. This is contrary to routine EMS response, where extraordinary care is rendered to the dead and near-dead as a matter of course.

A number of triage systems have been developed over the years. Air medical crews should familiarize themselves with the system used in their response area. Historically, patient categorization by triage was carried out on the basis of specific injury types and an assumed diagnosis of injuries—for example, giving priority to a victim with a tension pneumothorax over one with a fractured femur. The process of triage has turned away from the traditional injury/diagnostic approach to the more realistic response to injury and clinical presentation approach, or assessing the patient's hemodynamic status in response to the injury. This approach, called *START (Simple Triage and Rapid Treatment)*, has been gaining popularity since its development in the early 1980s.[6]

START is a way to categorize victims by evaluating three clinical parameters: level of consciousness, respirations, and perfusion. It does not take into consideration the traditional trauma triage criteria of injury type or mechanism of injury. START is a primary triage system and not meant for use in secondary or more advanced triage. Its focus is on initial triage efforts during the early phases of a multicasualty or mass casualty incident. It separates higher-priority victims from lower-priority victims and quickly and efficiently maximizes the efforts of limited resources. Secondary triage would take into consideration the types of injures and hemodynamic status of the victim by using more advanced assessment techniques. START is useful in hospital settings, especially when the hospital staff is confronted with a sudden onslaught of victims that overloads the facility's capabilities. It usually involves situations in which emergency departments are flooded with ambulatory victims who arrive at hospitals by means other than EMS vehicles and who have not had primary triage. This has been the experience of hospitals affected by compound disasters such as earthquakes, tornadoes, and massive explosions.

Triage is conducted on the basis of the victim's potential for survival without the immediate availability of heroic, time-consuming, and extraordinary medical management. Triage by means of START assesses the victim's clinical condition as it relates to other victims, assigns priority for field treatment, and determines the disposition of that victim. The terms used most often for triage classifications are *immediate care* (sometimes designated by the color red), *delayed care* (designated by the color yellow), *minor* or *ambulatory care* (designated by the color green), and *dead* (designated by the color black). My preference is the use of both simple descriptive language and color keys in triaging.

Some prehospital care systems use numeric categorizations when triaging, traditionally rating victims from 1 to 5 or 0 to 3. Because numbers can be hard to remember and offer no "free association" to memory when the rescuer is under stress, the numeric system has fallen out of favor in lieu of the previously discussed classifications. Therefore the START approach categorizes the victim into one of two primary classifications: immediate and delayed.

A victim classified as *immediate care* is one who is considered clinically salvable but who requires advanced intervention within 1 hour to survive. This category does not include the dead or near-dead. A victim categorized as *delayed care* is one who does not fall into the classification of immediate care. This includes victims with significant severe injuries whose lives are not threatened and whose condition would not deteriorate within 1 hour if otherwise untreated.

The delayed care classification includes those victims with minor injuries (or ambulatory victims) and those with critical injuries who would require extraordinary efforts for survival. If these victims are still alive after all victims classified as immediate care have been treated and transported, then these victims are given attention and care. Under normal circumstances, victims such as these would be considered the most urgent. However, in disaster operations (events in which resources are overwhelmed), victims such as these would require efforts that exceed the capabilities of those on the scene and would draw resources away from those who are more viable. Thus the essence of what triage accomplishes is the efficient use of limited resources to maximize outcomes for the greater good.

To implement the START system, the triageur assesses the victim's level of consciousness, respirations, and perfusion. START is based on the assumption that the triageur is in an overwhelming situation with limited equipment and resources and thus uses his or her eyes, ears, and senses of touch and smell to assess the victim. Ancillary equipment such as stethoscopes, blood pressure cuffs, and so on may not be available, and the triageur is forced into the "basics." Triage is completed in 15 to 30 seconds and is performed rapidly and succinctly.

Except for those who fall into the category secondary to mortal/lethal and nonviable injuries, victims classified as *delayed care* must have presentations in level of consciousness, respirations, and perfusion that fall within normal parameters. This triage decision is made regardless of injury type and mechanism of injury.

A victim categorized as *immediate care* is one whose level of consciousness, respiration, or perfusion (at least one of the three) is not within normal parameters. In assessing victims, it is important to note that the level of consciousness is not measured by the Glasgow Coma Scale but rather is determined on the basis of a simplified approach of assessing mental activity and consciousness by the victim's ability to follow simple commands. If the victim does not appear awake, alert, and oriented, the level of consciousness is considered "abnormal." However, there is one pitfall with START: that of *the moribund, nonviable victim.* This victim would obviously present as "abnormal" in all three areas and thus technically is classified as *immediate care.* However, this victim is not classified as *immediate care* because of the extent of injuries and the probability that the victim cannot be saved. To prevent this problem, the triageur should assess pupillary signs on any unconscious, nonresponsive victim to determine whether lethal brain injuries exist. If present, the victim is excluded from immediate care and designated as a *delayed-care patient.*

In the assessment of respiration status, the issue again is presentation within normal parameters. The triageur would assess the victim for obvious tachypnea, use of accessory muscles, audible adventitious sounds with or without the use of a stethoscope, or respiratory distress. If any of these signs are present, the victim is categorized as *immediate care.* This does not include the abnormal respiratory status of a moribund victim with agonal respirations, who is assigned to *delayed care* rather than *immediate care.*

Finally, the triageur would assess perfusion. The assessment of perfusion is a controversial issue. The original START formula called for assessing perfusion by looking only at capillary refill, assuming a blood pressure reading is not feasible. Capillary refill has questionable validity when assessing perfusion. However, given the disaster situation and lack of time, equipment, and alternative assessment abilities, capillary refill is used as an assessment tool under the START system. Optimally, assess capillary refill by evaluating the mucous membranes of the lower lip rather than distal areas such as fingers and toes.

A capillary refill of more than 2 seconds is outside normal parameters; therefore assign the victim to *immediate care.* However, this does not preclude the triageur from using other assessment techniques such as skin vitals and quality of carotid pulses, as long as the entire triage process does not exceed 30 seconds per victim.

There is one exception to the rules of START. *Any patient with penetrating trunk trauma is automatically an immediate-care patient regardless of the presence of three normal assessment parameters.* The rationale behind this exception is that the nature of penetrating trauma, particularly high-velocity missiles, tends to cause victims to appear well compensated until they suddenly and rapidly deteriorate.

Finally, in addition to familiarizing themselves with and practicing their region's triage system, air medical crews must also acquaint themselves with the triage tags used by local EMS systems. Some triage tags are miniature medical records, and others are simply a "filing" system that displays a victim's triage category. Regardless of the systems used, air medical crews will be expected to know how these tags and systems are utilized. There are three major reasons why triage is beneficial in a disaster response[2]:

1. Triage singles out those who need rapid medical care to save life, or, if appropriate, limb.
2. By singling out the minor injuries, triage reduces the urgent burden on medical facilities and organizations. On average, only 10% to 15% of disaster casualties are serious enough to require overnight hospitalization.
3. By providing for the equitable and rational distribution of casualties among the available hospitals, triage reduces the burden on each to a manageable level, often even to "nondisaster" levels.

POSTDISASTER PLANNING

No disaster plan is complete without a postdisaster management or recovery plan. In the past, the short-term and long-term psychologic effects of a disaster on rescuers were ignored or minimized. Fortunately, because of the efforts of such people as Jeffrey Mitchell, PhD, who developed the Critical Incident Stress Debriefing System (CISD) for psychologic recovery and intervention, management personnel are now more aware of the effects of posttraumatic stress (PTS) and critical incidents on rescuers and victims alike.[7-8]

HEMS providers are also potential victims of critical incidents such as disasters and, particularly, death or serious injuries of colleagues involved in aviation accidents. Postincident debriefing is crucial for all members of the HEMS/EMS teams, including medical crews, pilots, dispatchers, and support personnel to ensure psychologic survival and optimum recovery.[8]

TERRORISM AND DISASTERS

Terrorism is a reality that has struck the United States too many times in the past few years. Whether it is the bombings at the World Trade Center in 1993, the Alfred P. Murrah Federal Building in 1995, and Atlanta's Centennial Olympic Park in 1996; the World Trade Center and Pentagon assaults in 2001; product tampering; or workplace violence and its multiple shootings, acts of terrorism and their aftermath must be addressed.

Particularly worrisome is that terrorists, be they international or homegrown, are also more willing to use NBC (nuclear, biologic, chemical) weapons and explosive devices. Therefore, in 1996, the "Defense Against Weapons of Mass Destruction Act" (Nunn-Lugar-Domenici Legislation) was passed by the U.S. government. This bill highlighted the lack of preparedness by most first-responders and provided the necessary funding and authority to train U.S. cities to respond to acts of terrorism in a manner that protected themselves and the public they serve.[4]

Impetuous for this bill was the growing evidence showing an alarming lack of centralized and readily available stores of antidote and personal protective equipment (PPE) against chemical attacks for EMS, fire, and police personnel. The Gulf War had exposed problems in preparing for large-scale chemical warfare, and the 1995 subway Sarin attack in Tokyo resulted in 135 injured first-responders. More than 80% of victims were "walking wounded" who were brought to area hospitals by other than emergency vehicles, resulting in contamination of hospitals and their personnel.

This legislation resulted in the development of mandatory NBC training programs aimed at the Responder Awareness Level, Operations Level, HAZMAT/Technician Level, IC Level, EMS/Technician Level, and Hospital Provider Level. Depending on

the level, courses range from 8 hours to multiple days and are built on the "train the trainer" concept.

The NBC 'Delta' (uniqueness) plan builds or adds to the responders'/providers' existing disaster plans and training in mass-casualty incidents (MCIs), HAZMAT, and other types of emergency responses. Established in 1996, the Domestic Preparedness Program was designed to assist state, local, and federal emergency responders/providers in preparing for NBC incidents. Conducted as a partnership among federal agencies, this program was developed by the Departments of Defense and Energy, Federal Bureau of Investigation (FBI), Federal Emergency Management Agency (FEMA), Public Health Service, and the Environmental Protection Agency (EPA).

Traditional EMS disaster planning and training do not include planning for responding to issues unique to a terrorist-generated MCI. Conventional command protocols and triage may not work and may even endanger EMS personnel.

The potential for danger and personal injury is a reality faced by rescuers around the world. Look at the Los Angeles and the Cincinnati riots and the injury and danger faced by responding fire and EMS personnel as a timely lesson. At the Murrah Building bombing, fears of a secondary explosive device designed to kill and maim emergency responders was of real concern.

Therefore besides training in NBC situations, disaster planning for incidents related to terrorism must include a coordinated effort and plan to include prehospital care providers, fire, police, hospitals, local health services, and other law enforcement agencies. Unfortunately, terrorism from NBC weapons is an all-too-real threat to the public and responding providers.

SUMMARY

Disaster drills must continually test and challenge local EMS, fire, and law enforcement agencies; hospitals; and HEMS providers. HEMS have proved to be invaluable, when used wisely, in lessening the overloading of local hospitals with disaster victims and providing valuable scene support.

Air medical crews, pilots, and dispatchers must be trained and updated in their responsibilities during disaster operations to perform maximally and efficiently. EMS systems must include HEMS operations as part of a systemwide approach to disaster management. However, it is the responsibility of those HEMS providers to be well versed in triage, scene operations, prehospital medical care, and the ICS to function more effectively.

REFERENCES

1. *Air Medical Crew National Standard Curriculum,* Pasadena, 1988, U.S. Department of Transportation, Samaritan Air Evac and ASHBEAMS.

2. Auf der Heide E: *Disaster response: principles of preparation and coordination,* St Louis, 1989, Mosby.

3. Cohen E: *Disasters! an emergency care workbook,* San Diego, 1983, Idea Inc.

4. Cohen E: Terrorism and EMS, a U.S. perspective, *Rescue Pacific Magazine,* Winter 1999.

5. Vaughan DM, Pierce R: Medcenter Air Carolinas Medical Center, Charlotte, NC.

6. Groth S, et al: Simple triage and rapid treatment: the START system, Hoag Memorial Hospital, Newport Beach, Calif, 1984.

7. LeSage S, et al: *Fire service field guide: a pocket reference for firefighters and command officers,* Los Angeles, 1995, InforMed.

8. Mitchell JT: Stress. Development and functions of a critical incident stress debriefing team. *J Emerg Med Serv JEMS* 13(12):42-46, 1988.

COMMUNICATIONS

9

1. Demonstrate knowledge about communications systems and their use in patient transport.
2. Use appropriate communication skills before, during, and after transport.
3. Use appropriate communication equipment to provide safe and competent patient transport.

Communication encompasses more than use of a radio or telephone; it is a total system that ensures the smooth operation of routine daily patient transports while guaranteeing optimal patient care and transport team safety (Figure 9-1). No one perfect communications system exists for all transport programs. The communications system must meet the present and future needs of the program it serves.

COMMUNICATION CENTERS

PLANNING

Planning for the needs of the communications system should be an integral part of every program's overall strategic planning effort. Each administration must decide very early how highly it values a communications system. Some administrators see it as a costly, non–revenue-producing entity, whereas others understand not only the intangible value of a first-rate communications center, but the potential it has for saving the lives of an air medical crew. Death benefits, potential liability damages, and legal costs far exceed the cost of installing an elaborate communications center.

The most recent Communications Survey[8] found that more than 90% of the transport programs operated a separate communication center line for patient transport. Ninety-nine percent of the centers had phone lines dedicated to receiving transport requests. Some of these phone lines also serve to provide communication during disasters. These findings help to illustrate that in planning communication centers, the overall role of communication needs to be considered. Therefore the following question must be answered: "Is the communication center also responsible for other aspects of communication, including disaster management, diversion protocols, and other incidents that may require open lines within the hospital or in the communities in which the transport program is based?"

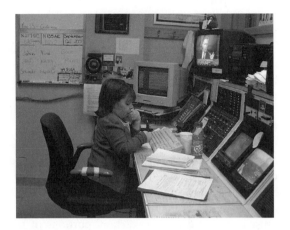

FIGURE 9-1 **Communications Center, University Air Care, Cincinnati, Ohio.** (Courtesy Rose DeJarnette and John Robinson.)

MANAGEMENT
STYLE
Management style plays a critical role in the success of a communications center. With the proactive management style, problems and issues that are likely to occur are addressed before they actually happen, present conditions are continually evaluated, and unanticipated problems are dealt with in a timely, definitive manner.

The reactive management style is not strong on planning and evaluation. With this style, sometimes known as "management by crisis," problems are dealt with only after they occur. In communications centers that operate under this style, little things keep going wrong, details are overlooked, and morale falls until finally an acute crisis occurs and everyone involved looks around, wondering what happened. In the final step in this sequence, a scapegoat is selected, and the problem is fixed in a reactive fashion. Repeated patchwork repairs to any system ultimately result in system degradation and failure.

SUPPORT
Administrative support must be available to the communications specialist (CS) around the clock. The CS must always have someone to turn to who can make a decision about unusual events or circumstances not covered in the policy and procedures manual.

Similarly, in programs in which medical direction is required, the CS must have a physician available to communicate with the crew if the normal medical protocol fails for any reason.

COMMUNICATIONS
A major aspect of any communications program is the physical environment of the communications center.[6] Following are some major considerations in the planning process for a communications center.

LOCATION
Whether it is located in a hospital, at an airfield, or within a separate facility, the communications center should be in an area with little pedestrian traffic. Physical inaccessibility and program policy discourage casual visitors.

SEISMIC STABILITY
In some areas of the United States, the structural and functional integrity of the facility in the face of a major seismic disturbance is a very real concern and should be discussed with the facility's architect. It should not be taken for granted that seismic stability is part of the design of the facility.

SECURITY
The level of security needed for a given communications center will vary considerably, depending on its location. A steel door with a deadbolt lock should be considered a minimum level of security. Numerous high-technology security systems may be acquired; the level of security attained will ultimately be a function of the budget.

Security does not end with a locked door. Additional security issues are fire alarm and fire suppression systems. Although the communications center may meet current local fire codes, one must remember that most fire codes are minimums for protection, not maximums. It is permissible to adopt stricter safeguards than those required by the code. For more detailed information, one should contact the local or state fire marshal.

EMERGENCY ELECTRICAL POWER

Each communications center should have its own emergency power supply. Although an independent source of electrical energy is preferable, it is common for hospital-based communication centers to receive emergency power from the hospital's emergency generator.

An electrical generator of sufficient capacity for a given communications center should be located nearby. This generator may be powered by diesel fuel, gasoline, or natural gas, depending on which type of fuel is most economical in a given locale. Consideration should also be given to the use of alternative energy sources abundant in the region, such as sunlight, wind, or hydroelectric power. The technology for these alternative energy sources is available, and it is possible to calculate economies for the program when these energy sources are used.

Emergency power must also be instantly available for remote transmitter/receiver sites.

WIRING ACCESS

Each communications center includes enough wiring and cables to stretch the length of several football fields. These wires, which are vital to the operation of the system, should be readily accessible, and the function of each wire should be readily identifiable. This may be accomplished either by running all wiring underneath a raised floor or by terminating all wiring into a utility room behind the wall where the console is located.

LIGHTING

Whether the communications operations center has the appearance of an office or resembles a combat information center on a ship is a matter of preference. The bottom line is that the CS is able to clearly see everything that must be done. It is necessary to have emergency lighting that comes on the instant that power is lost, even if this is only for a short duration.

HEATING, VENTILATION, AND AIR-CONDITIONING

Heating, ventilation, and air-conditioning systems should be engineered with local geographic weather conditions in mind.[4] These systems not only keep personnel comfortable, but also help prevent equipment from malfunctioning.

If smoking is permitted in the communications center, an air-filtration system is useful because the byproducts of any type of smoke can be harmful to electronic equipment.

CONSOLE LAYOUT AND DESIGN

Once a custom console is built and installed, it is costly to alter; therefore consoles should be designed carefully, with use of full-scale plans and even cardboard mock-ups. In addition, a console should be designed to be ergonomically functional. The CS must be able to see and reach all portions of the console without twisting, craning, stretching, or squinting. The seat for a console must roll, swivel, tilt, and be comfortable while providing good lumbar support.

ACOUSTIC INSULATION

The amount of insulation required to render the communications center oblivious to the external environment will vary with the location of the center. Enough insulation should be used to deaden the noise from an aircraft engine 100 yards away at ground level. A communications center located deep within a building or above or below ground level will probably not be as sensitive to external street or airfield noise.

RESTROOM FACILITIES

Each communications center should be equipped with full restroom facilities, including a toilet, sink, and shower. Depending on the schedule and program volume, the CS may not have the time to go elsewhere to use restroom facilities and certainly should not have to leave the communications center during a tour of duty.

LOUNGE AREAS

It is useful to have a room adjacent to the operations room of the communications center that the CS may use during slack periods or periods of inclement weather when flights are not being made. This room may contain a couch, chair, coffee table, television, and videocassette player. The CS should not be in this room while a transport is underway. Whether such a lounge area is available in a given program depends both on policy and space constraints.

The lounge might also contain the kitchen area or dormitory area, or both.

DORMITORIES

The existence of a dormitory depends on program policy, shift schedules, program volume, and the number of personnel on duty. Sleeping while on duty is a controversial topic, and its appropriateness for specific types of personnel must be evaluated by each individual program.

KITCHEN EQUIPMENT

It is necessary to have a small kitchen and pantry area in communications centers in which the CS cannot obtain nutrition because they are not able to leave the communication center. This area should include a small refrigerator and freezer, a small microwave oven, a coffee maker, and cabinet and counter space.

STORAGE

A secure storage area should be provided for communications center supplies, backup equipment, and archives. This space should not be shared with other departments. Some communication centers are also used to store disaster supplies because of their central location.

DECORATION

The decor of the communications center should be pleasant, easy to maintain, and in keeping with the character of the organization. It is an excellent idea for the personnel who work in a given area to have input into its decor.

ALTERNATIVE SITES/BACKUP EQUIPMENT

A worst-case scenario should be prepared by every air medical program, along with a plan of action to deal with such a scenario should it ever occur. Each communications center should be able to continue operations at an alternative site with backup equipment if for any reason the primary communications center becomes inoperable.

Plans should also be made for rapidly repairing or replacing any piece of essential equipment in the communications center.

EQUIPMENT

Selection of equipment for a communications center should be based on the mission of the transport program, present and anticipated needs, functions, durability, reliability, expendability, serviceability, and, last but not least, cost.

To make a decision about a given piece of equipment, a program should prioritize these factors, add any others that are applicable, and then determine the most cost-effective choice. The most costly item is not always the best item. However, it is also worth noting that you get what you pay for.

TELEPHONES

Emergency telephone lines should not go through a switchboard; instead they should be dedicated central office lines, so that if the switchboard fails, the communications center will still have telephone communications. The number of incoming local and wide area telephone service lines should be based on the size of the service area and the projected volume of calls. Phone lines can be added relatively quickly when needed.

All calls made with use of emergency phone lines should be recorded, as should any outgoing call pertaining to requests for assistance or notifications.

Telephones today are available with a wide variety of features that may prove useful in a given operation. These features include speed-dialing, memory banks of phone numbers, call queuing, hands-free operation, automatic redial, and so on.

RADIOS

Radios are the key hardware elements in an air medical communications system. The radio frequencies on which a program operates are assigned by the Federal Communications Commission (FCC) on the basis of recommendations by the state chapter of Associated Public Safety Communications Officers,

---

BOX 9-1	**Radio Bands**

VHF high-band FM (148-174 MHz): The radio signal in this band follows a straight line.

VHF low-band FM (30-50 MHz): The radio signal in this band follows the curvature of the Earth and has the greatest range.

VHF AM (118-136 MHz): This band is typically used for aviation-related communications.

UHF (403-941 MHz): These ultra-high frequencies have limited range and are most often used between ground units and base stations. They can be used for air-to-ground and ground-to-air communications for relatively short distances that will fluctuate with the terrain.

800 MHz: Digital communication controlled by computers. Allows multiple agencies to communicate with each other. Higher frequency, less noise, and greater penetration outside of buildings.

AM, Amplitude modulation; *FM,* frequency modulation; MHz, megahertz; *VHF,* very high frequency; *UHF,* ultra-high frequency.

---

to which it has delegated responsibility for frequency coordination. It is the FCC that issues licenses and assigns call letters. A program's assigned frequencies may be found in several radio bands (Box 9-1).

Included in the ultra-high frequency (UHF) spectrum are the so-called MED channels. MED channels are a set of 10 paired frequencies set aside by the FCC for the exclusive use of emergency medical service (EMS) units. The channels from MED 9 to MED 10 are frequency allocation channels used in metropolitan regions where UHF traffic is high. To use such a channel, an EMS unit calls the frequency allocation center, usually located in a fire department or ambulance service communications center, and requests assignment to a channel for the purpose of speaking with a specific hospital. The unit is then assigned an open channel or is told to stand by until one is available (Box 9-2).

Some programs will have their own private very high frequency (VHF) assigned to them. Others may choose to use one of the existing UHFs allocated for EMS use nationwide. The same rules and principles apply to use of any of them.

There are several basic types of radio systems, as follows[3,6]:

1. Simplex system: The simplex system has the ability to transmit in one direction at a time by using a single frequency.
2. Full duplex system: The full duplex system has the ability to transmit and receive simulta-

BOX 9-2	**MED Channel Frequencies**

463.000/468.000 MHz ("MED-ONE")
463.025/468.025 MHz ("MED-TWO")
463.050/468.050 MHz ("MED-THREE")
463.075/486.075 MHz ("MED-FOUR")
463.100/468.100 MHz ("MED-SIX")
463.150/468.150 MHz ("MED-SEVEN")
463.175/468.175 MHz ("MED-EIGHT")
462.950/467.950 MHz ("MED-NINE")
462.975/467.975 MHz ("MED-TEN")

neously by using two frequencies (typically UHF).

3. Half duplex system: The half duplex system has the ability to transmit or receive in one direction at a time by using two frequencies (typically UHF high-band).
4. Multiplex system: The multiplex system has the ability to transmit from two or more sources over the same frequency.

A repeater system is a type of half duplex system that involves a base station "repeater" at an elevated site remote from the communications center. This system is particularly useful in regions with mountainous terrain. A repeater system receives a signal on one frequency and instantly retransmits it on a second frequency to the other radios in the system, extending the communications center's range. The process is reversed when the repeater receives signals coming into the base station.

PHONE-RADIO OR RADIO-PHONE PATCH

With a phone-radio or radio-phone patch, special circuits in the radio console permit a radio and telephone to be linked together, one direction at a time, so that the medical crew can speak to a person who is not in the communications center and vice versa. This capability is useful for programs that require voice contact with a medical control physician and for occasions when a member of the medical crew needs to speak with the receiving physician. These optional circuits can be included when the radio console is purchased, or they can be added at a later date.

Programs that use a phone-radio or radio-phone patch have found that radio-like procedures must be used because transmissions are simplex. At times, this presents problems when patched through to persons who may not understand the system. Cellular telephones have supplanted this feature in many programs.

SQUELCH CONTROL

Nearly all radios have squelch control, which is accessed by turning the knob until static is heard and then turning it in the opposite direction just past the point where the static ends. It is best to make this adjustment before using the radio.

CONTINUOUS TONE CONTROLLED SUBAUDIBLE SQUELCH

Continuous tone controlled subaudible squelch circuits act as a filter to other users of the radio's frequency. Only users of radios with the same tone-control frequency setting will normally hear each other. This feature may be disabled when the tone of a transmitting radio is unknown or different or the radio operator wishes to monitor the entire frequency. *Private line* and *channel guard* are proprietary names for continuous tone controlled subaudible squelch.

PAGERS

Most programs have a need for transport crews to carry personal pagers. The communications center should have its own paging encoder rather than use pagers that are accessed by dialing a telephone number. Telephone pagers have a lag time of up to several minutes, depending on the volume of pager calls in a given region. Direct encoding will both speed crew response time and result in long-term savings. A variety of pagers are available that can beep, buzz, vibrate, speak, or even display alphanumeric messages.

Recent introduction of two-way paging with use of satellite communications allows voiceless pages to be sent and an acknowledgment to be received with use of data terminals; this technology will no doubt change much of our existing radio communications and paging systems.

An extremely detailed needs assessment should be undertaken by qualified technical personnel before the implementation of any radio system. It is ill-advised for a program to purchase a system identical to that of another program on the basis of their satisfaction with it.

HEADSETS, MICROPHONES, AND FOOT SWITCHES

The use of headsets rather than microphones should be considered in busy communications centers. When used in conjunction with a foot switch, a headset leaves the CS's hands free, which is particularly desirable in operations in which only one CS is on duty.

When microphones are used, they should be of the type that filters out background noises. A microphone placed on a bracket or gooseneck fixture attached to the console is preferable because it leaves the desktop space clear. When a headset microphone is used, it should be fairly close to the lips; proximity to the lips will vary because of the varying speech characteristics of different people.

LOGGING RECORDERS

All business-related telephone calls and all radio transmissions should be recorded. A program may elect to use an audiocassette logging system, digital audiocassette, VHS audiotape, or a reel-to-reel logging system.

Cassette systems are more suitable for low-volume, low-traffic operations. Cassette loggers typically limit the program to three recorded channels, with a fourth channel allocated for injection of the time signal. Most programs will need a greater capacity than this.

Traditional reel-to-reel loggers are expensive; however, VHS and digital technology have reduced the cost and size of past generations of reel-to-reel recorders. The tapes for the reel-to-reel system are also expensive, but they are reusable. Currently available technology permits the contents of a 24-hour tape to be compressed and stored on a cassette for future reference. A program might elect to store several days of recording on reels, but this is costly and creates a storage problem.

If the program's budget permits, a dual logger should be purchased. A dual logger provides the redundancy needed in a communications center and permits playback of older tapes while still recording in real-time.

SHORT-TERM PLAYBACK DEVICES

Short-term playback devices, through the use of either a continuous loop of recording tape or digital technology, record the last several minutes of telephone or radio traffic for review by the CS when needed. This device enables the CS to double-check any recent conversation at the touch of a button.

COMPUTERS AND PERIPHERALS

Computers are an integral part of the well-equipped communications center. What a computer can do for a program is limited primarily by imagination and budget.

Needs should be assessed before any computer system is purchased. First, it should be decided what the program wishes the computer system to do; second, it is necessary to find the appropriate software; and finally, a computer system should be selected that has the speed and power to accomplish the task.

A wide variety of software is available to aid in communications before, during, and after transport. Computer-aided dispatch programs can allow the CS and other transport team members to input data about the transport and the patient and keep track of data regarding medical procedures, trans-

port times, delays, and downtimes. In addition, there is software available now that provides revenue management.[7]

The communication center must also have access to the Internet. This allows communication outside of the program. Internet access also allows the program to keep up to date on information pertinent to transport.

MOBILE DATA TERMINALS

Mobile data terminals are small computer terminals that are attached to a radio and have the ability to send data to and receive data from the base station or another mobile data terminal. These systems vary in complexity and require a dedicated radio frequency for their use.

WEATHER RADAR

All pilots have access to Federal Aviation Administration (FAA) Flight Service weather information. While the FAA generally does an excellent job, its reports may not be as up-to-the-minute as desired at a given point in time.

Weather radar display systems are available through several commercial services. These systems may be connected to the National Weather Service radar site in the region by telephone line or computer modem. All weather radar display systems provide displays and printouts of excellent quality. The Internet also has many sites that offer real-time radar and weather for no cost. The display should be installed in a place where the pilots have access to it. If the pilot needs an update while airborne, the CS should also have access to it. This may not be a problem if the aircraft has its own weather radar. If a program has a computer-driven system, the CS can access the weather report from the communications center. An alternative to the phone-line system is to place a remote monitor in the communications center.[3]

CELLULAR TELEPHONES

Cellular telephones have proved to be invaluable both in air and ground transport communication. Cellular telephones have the distinct advantage of providing a medical crew direct access to medical direction or to a receiving facility without going through the troublesome radiophone patch procedure. Cellular telephone technology continues to progress. Some cellular telephones can also be used as communication devices similar to portable radios.

Today, many transport team members carry cellular telephones. It is important for transport team members to use these phones appropriately. FCC regulations (Code of Regulations # 47, Parts 20-39, Section 22.925; October 1, 1996) state that the use of cellular telephones in an aircraft when the craft is airborne is not permitted. The use of a cellular telephone during flight could result in suspension of service or a fine, or both.[1]

FAX MACHINES
A fax machine is an almost indispensable tool in a communications center today because it enables any needed or requested documentation or information to be sent or received at low cost. For example, if a page has been omitted from a transferred patient's chart and this is not discovered until the patient is en route, a simple telephone call to request that the page be faxed can correct this problem in short order. Fax machines today are multifunctional and may also operate scanners and copiers.

UNINTERRUPTIBLE POWER SUPPLY
An uninterruptible power supply is a device that provides steady electrical current to sensitive electronic equipment when there is a power drop-off or surge and serves as a battery backup for a finite

period of time until power is restored. It is essential to have an uninterruptible power supply when computers are used for important tasks. These devices can support an operation for periods ranging from a few minutes to several hours. Support for longer periods of time costs more money.

CLOSED-CIRCUIT TELEVISION
It may be desirable for the CS to have access to video scanning of the helipad or hangar ramp. Such scanning serves as a security system and enables the CS who does not have direct visual contact with the program's parked aircraft to see what is occurring. Television monitors are available that may serve as a computer screen or as a video monitor by pressing a button, thus reducing the cost to the program.

CLOCKS
Each communications center should have several clocks, which may be analog, digital, or a mix of both types. At least one good-quality, battery-operated clock should be available to provide backup during power failures. Air medical crew members should familiarize themselves with the military time system used in aviation. Programs that operate in more than one time zone may wish to keep parallel sets of clocks in operation to avoid confusion in calculating arrival times (Box 9-3).

STATUS BOARD
Every communication center must have a status board that displays, for each aircraft and ground vehicle, their assigned aircraft (N) numbers, the crew

BOX 9-3	24-Hour Clock								
A.M.									
	1:00	0100	4:00	0400	7:00	0700	10:00	1000	
	2:00	0200	5:00	0500	8:00	0800	11:00	1100	
	3:00	0300	6:00	0600	9:00	0900	Noon	1200	
P.M.									
	1:00	1300	4:00	1600	7:00	1900	10:00	2200	
	2:00	1400	5:00	1700	8:00	2000	11:00	2300	
	3:00	1500	6:00	1800	9:00	2100	Midnight	2400	(0000)

on board, and its current status. Any type of board, from a chalkboard to an elaborate electronic device, may be used.

MAPS

An aviation sectional map or maps of the program's normal area of operations should be mounted on a wall in the communications center. A compass radial overlay with a center string attached should be affixed to the map, centered over the base of operations. A heavy, dark line radiating from the base operations should be drawn on the map and marked off in 10-mile increments. This map enables the CS to rapidly obtain a heading and distance to a given point.

There should also be a street map of the metropolitan area around the base of rotary-wing operations as they are called on to precede directly to the scene. This map should be modified, as previously mentioned.

Topographic maps that show variation in terrain contour and various other maps that may be obtained from state or county highway departments will prove useful in the communications center.

Mapping software is available that allows the CS to point and click on selected response sites, displaying coordinates for navigational purposes. The software can also create driving maps for ground transport teams.

ROLODEX

A Rolodex may serve as the primary reference device in an office. It is inexpensive, consumes no energy, and is 100% reliable in operation. Computerized communications centers should have one on hand as part of their backup inventory. Rolodexes are available in several different sizes and configurations.

CARDEX

A Cardex is a book similar to a Rolodex in that it has a separate card for each hospital in the service area. Information included in a Cardex should be updated and dated, and each card should include landing zone information and all telephone numbers. Even though many communication centers are

now computerized, a written back-up system is imperative if there is a power failure or data loss.

REFERENCE MATERIAL

There is no limit to the amount of useful reference material that should be available in the communications center. Available reference materials should include telephone books, aviation material, medical information, hazardous materials data, and anything else thought to be useful by a particular program.

SERVICE CONTRACTS

A service contract should be purchased for all equipment selected for inclusion in a communications center. Service contracts will usually result in long-term savings and more efficient operations because of decreased downtime of equipment. Before any purchase is made, it should be determined whether a vendor is able to support the operation with a loaner piece of equipment if the program does not have backup equipment.

The Commission on Accreditation of Medical Transport Systems[2] lists the components that a communication center must contain. Box 9-4 lists these components.

POLICIES AND PROCEDURES

A detailed policy and procedures manual is necessary for any organization that wishes to function in a systematic, effective manner. The communications center manual must be a part of the program's overall policy and procedures manual. When the communications center manual is written, it should be carefully integrated with existing policies and procedures to minimize potential conflicting instructions to the CS.

The manual must cover all aspects of operation that have anything to do with communications. Each segment of the manual should be extremely detailed so that if a question arises about a specific item, it can be resolved by referring to the manual.

A typical communications center manual would include the sections shown in Box 9-5 and any additional sections that would be appropriate for a particular program.

| BOX 9-4 | **Components of a Communication Center** |

At least one dedicated phone line
A system for recording all incoming and outgoing telephone and radio transmissions, which should be stored for 30 days, with time recording and playback capabilities
Capability to notify the transport team and online medical direction for a request and during transport
Back-up emergency power when power outages occur
A status board to follow transport vehicles and show who is on the transport crews, weather status, and so on
Local aircraft service area maps and navigation charts
Road maps available for ground transport
Communication Policy and Procedures manual

From Commission on Accreditation of Medical Transport Systems: *Accreditation standards*, ed 5, Anderson, SC, 2002, The Commission.

| BOX 9-5 | **Typical Communications Center Manual** |

A. Mission statement: A succinct statement of the program's objectives and how they will be accomplished
B. Table of organization: A graphic depiction of how the program's components are related
C. Table of contents: A detailed listing of the contents of each page in the manual
D. Air medical communications specialist: A detailed listing of job descriptions, schedules, training programs, job requirements, and anything else pertaining to the CS
E. Documentation: Detailed instructions on the use of all forms used by the communications center, whether paper or computerized
F. Equipment: Step-by-step instructions on how to use and troubleshoot potential problems for each piece of equipment used by the communications center; the manufacturer's list of instructions may be inserted as is, or, if they are difficult to understand, they may be rewritten and inserted in simplified form.
G. Operational procedures: Detailed instructions on every known aspect of a program's operation as it pertains to communications (typically the largest section of the manual)
H. Quality assurance plan: Components include but are not limited to an in-depth review of CS performance,* routine preventive maintenance schedules for equipment, and critique sessions held soon after any event in which a communications problem played a role
I. Index: A complete alphabetical listing of the manual's contents

*Performance evaluation of the CS must be based on written objectives and guidelines, which should be derived from the policy and procedures manual. Areas of evaluation include completeness of documentation, audio review, and procedural accuracy review.
CS, Communications specialist.

THE COMMUNICATIONS SPECIALIST

The complexities of organizing a communications system pale with respect to its operation. Beyond dealing with electronic hardware and computer software, the program is faced with one of the most challenging of tasks—dealing with people.

Human beings are both the strongest and weakest points in a system. People represent a broad spectrum of personalities and egos, and no two individuals are quite the same.

ROLES AND RESPONSIBILITIES

The CS is designated to coordinate requests for aircraft and ground response. The title assigned to the person with the CS function varies from program to program. The only limitation is that the FAA uses the term *dispatcher* to designate a person who has a decision-making role regarding whether or not an aircraft takes off. Unless this is the case with a program, another title should be used.

The CS is responsible for coordinating intraagency and interagency communications pertaining to any phase of a transport, from a request to hospital admission. The role of the CS is to serve as a facilitator for the smooth integration of all the resources at the program's disposal, with the dual objectives of program safety and excellent patient care.

The CS must perform a variety of tasks. These include the following[2]:

- Listening intently
- Accurately repeating what was said
- Reading maps (including using computer mapping software)
- Spelling
- Using medical, aviation, and EMS terms
- Setting, evaluating, and resetting priorities

SELECTION

Applicants for CS positions should be screened as thoroughly as applicants for transport team positions. Just as all persons who desire to be part of a transport team are not suited for the work, all persons who desire to be a CS may not be suited to the type of stress inherent in the job.

The decision about whom to hire as a CS must be determined by each individual program. Certain minimum educational requirements must be met in any case, but some controversy has arisen about background requirements. Areas of controversy include the following:

1. Should the CS have medical field experience? If so, at what level and how much?
2. Should the CS have communications center experience? If so, what type(s) of experience are acceptable, and how much experience is necessary?

Neither medical field experience nor communications center experience alone qualifies a person to be a CS; neither does being a friend or relative of someone employed by the program.

The Commission on Accreditation of Medical Transport Systems[2] recommends that the CS have emergency medical technician certification or its equivalent, knowledge of or experience with medical terminology, and knowledge of EMS.

TRAINING

Regardless of the background of the CS applicant, the person must be trained as a CS. A curriculum that may be used as a foundation for a program's own curriculum is included in *The AAMS Manual for Air Medical Communications Operations.*[1] Training must be an ongoing process to ensure currency and proficiency. During training, the CS should be given a variety of situations, be allowed to make decisions, and discuss why decisions were made. Just as many use their "transports from Hell" to teach others, the "communication situations from Hell" presented and discussed with new CSs may assist them in their future work.

TESTING

The CS should be tested periodically on all elements of the position. The CS has the responsibility of knowing everything about the program and being able to use that information at a moment's notice with a high degree of accuracy. In terms of communications procedures, less than 100% accuracy is unacceptable.

DRESS CODE

The attire that is considered proper for communications personnel is a matter of preference for each program. Consideration should be given to whether anything is gained by the additional expense of uniforms or if civilian attire in certain color combinations is acceptable.

COMMUNICATING

RADIOS

LANGUAGE

To effectively communicate within a program, standardized terminology should be used so that meanings are not lost or misinterpreted.

In general, it is preferable to communicate in plain language instead of using various codes; this precludes errors caused by misunderstanding of a garbled coded transmission. Because of the broad area over which an air medical program operates, it would be extremely difficult to know codes for each of the many jurisdictions in the program's service area.

SPEAKING

When initiating a radio transmission, a transport team member should begin with the name or call sign of the unit being called, followed by the member's own name or call sign. When older radio systems and poorly maintained new systems are used, it may be advantageous, when keying the microphone, for the speaker to pause for a second before speaking to allow the radio to reach its maximum output level. This helps prevent the frequent problem of incomplete messages being received. Another cause of this problem is speaking before keying the microphone.

The speaker should talk at a normal level; yelling into the microphone distorts the transmission. The speaker should know what he or she is going to say before keying the microphone; speak clearly and concisely without irrelevant comments; attempt to control the voice level and intonation even when under stress; try to avoid transmissions that reflect disgust, irritation, or sarcasm; and avoid the use of profanity at all times. Radio transmissions are a measure of a program's professionalism, and both the media and a large population of citizens with scanners hear every word that is said on the radio.

It is important that transport team members know how to properly operate the two-directional radio-intercom switch commonly found on headset cords in aircraft or ground vehicle. Many transport team members have been embarrassed when personal conversations or comments less than socially acceptable were broadcast over a wide area. This is less of a problem in programs that operate pressurized aircraft, in which transport team members may not be using a headset system.

Intracrew communications are also very important. The pilot should keep the medical crew informed of any developments in a clear, complete message that leaves no doubt about what is happening. The following two anecdotes illustrate this point. Although the incidents are somewhat humorous now, the crews involved did not think so at the time. In the first incident, the crew received a badly scrawled note from the pilot, pushed through an opening behind his seat, just as the helicopter began an unexpected banking turn. The note read, "I can't talk." The crew members looked at each other, each thinking that the pilot had experienced a cerebrovascular accident. They were about to become upset when the aircraft resumed straight and level flight. The pilot came on the intercom and explained that he could not talk on the medical radio, that he had spoken to approach control, and that he was returning to base for another aircraft. A more complete written message or advance warning on the intercom could have prevented a tense few moments for the crew.

In the second incident, the pilot of an outbound aircraft observed a transmission chip light blink on. In accordance with company policy, he immediately began a descent in preparation for landing. He told the crew, "We're going down." The crew went into a not-so-happy mode, prepared themselves for a hard landing, and then began a vigorous discussion over the use of the one pillow on board. A normal landing was made, the mechanic arrived and corrected the problem, and the aircraft returned to its base. Once again, a more complete explanation would have prevented these tense moments.

During a flight the pilot of an airport-based aircraft will communicate with each of the following, in addition to the CS: ground control, airport tower departure control, air route traffic control center, approach control, airport tower, and ground control again.

Hospital-based rotorcraft may or may not be near an airport but will be in communication with the appropriate segments of the air traffic control system and the program's own communications center. In either case, only the pilots should communicate with air traffic control. Aircraft on scene flights will also speak with units already on the scene.

The medical crew should be aware that there are certain times when they should refrain from speaking to the pilot unless absolutely imperative. These times are as follows[5]:

1. During takeoff
2. During landing
3. During instrument approaches
4. In dense air traffic areas

Air crews in programs with multiple aircraft should also be aware that nonessential interaircraft conversations may make it difficult for the CS to carry on a telephone conversation or to receive an essential transmission from another unit.

If a crew member asks the CS to make a telephone call, a minute or so should be allowed to pass before transmitting again to avoid interrupting the call.

If either party is having difficulty making a word understood, then that person should spell it using the phonetic alphabet (see Box 9-6).

TELEPHONES

Often a requesting party's first impression of a program is created by the CS who answers the telephone. A courteous manner combined with comprehensive knowledge of the program will help give the caller the impression that the program is staffed by competent, professional personnel.

MEDICAL DIRECTION

Programs that operate with nurses or paramedics are included under medical direction regulations that vary from state to state. Whether communicating with their medical direction physician by radio, radiophone patch, or cellular telephone, the medical crew should follow the medical reporting format used in their region. All reports should be to-the-point. Any treatment order received should be acknowledged by repeating the order verbatim.

FACE-TO-FACE

Of particular importance to the success of a program are interpersonal communications among all program personnel. An understanding of the problems and stress inherent to each position tends to foster patience. Cross-orientation sessions between transport team members and communications

---

BOX 9-6	**Phonetic Alphabet and Numbers**[3]

Phonetic Alphabet

A – Alpha
B – Bravo
C – Charlie
D – Delta
E – Echo
F – Foxtrot
G – Gulf
H – Hotel
I – India
J – Juliet
K – Kilo
L – Lima
M – Mike
N – November
O – Oscar
P – Papa
Q – Quebec
R – Romeo
S – Sierra
T – Tango
U – Uniform
V – Victor
W – Whiskey
X – X-ray
Y – Yankee
Z – Zulu

Phonetic Numbers

1 – WUN
2 – TOO
3 – TREE
4 – FOW-ER
5 – FIFE
6 – SIX
7 – SEV-EN
8 – AIT
9 – NIN-ER
0 – ZEE-RO

From *Federal Aviation Administration*, http://www.faa.gov. Accessed June, 2002.

---

personnel are useful in creating this understanding. Anyone who works in a program is going to have an occasional bad day, and colleagues must be able to deal with this circumspectly.

Successful working relationships frequently lead to personal friendships. Social events within programs also tend to relieve stress and improve working relationships.[5]

ON PAPER

In this litigious age, everything that occurs must be documented. "If it is not written down, then it did not happen" is a concept pursued by attorneys who specialize in the field of malpractice.

All forms used by the program should be filled out assiduously. If something does not apply, a line should be drawn through the space, or the letters *NA* should be inserted.

When forms to be used in the program are created, an attempt should be made to minimize the number of times that any one piece of information must be written. If the originals do not have separate destinations, forms should be consolidated. Communications forms should have the same flow as those used by the medical crew to make it easier for the medical crew member to write down what the CS says.

A 6-month supply of most forms should be adequate as long as a new supply is ordered before they are used up. All forms should be evaluated periodically to determine whether they are still functional.

All written communications from administration should be placed in a file folder or in loose-leaf books in reverse chronological order for easy reference. If appropriate, they may be placed in the policy and procedures manual.

Some programs have found that the use of an electronic means of communication such as e-mail or a Web site has increased their ability to communicate new policies and procedures and social information.

WITH THE MEDIA

Local news media usually have a high level of interest in the activities of an air medical program. The CS must be able to politely—but firmly—deal with their calls when they interfere with operations. The CS must be aware of program policy with respect to giving out information and should refer the caller to the appropriate person if this is dictated by policy.

Establishing a good rapport with the local media is essential. Many people have strong negative feelings about certain aspects of the news media. A decision may be reached within a program to notify the media of the types of events in which they usually express interest, time permitting. The flight operation always comes first.

EMERGENCY PROCEDURES

The operational procedures section of the policy and procedures manual should include a subsection dealing with procedures to be followed in the event of any unscheduled event that affects the use of the aircraft or directly involves the aircraft.

MASS-CASUALTY INCIDENTS

Most transport programs are undoubtedly a part of any mass-casualty incident plan developed in the program's service area. Copies of the program's roles in these situations should be immediately accessible to the CS.

UNSCHEDULED EVENTS

Detailed contingency plans must exist for various emergencies involving the program's aircraft and ground vehicles. These plans must be immediately accessible to the CS.

DRILLS

The CS should participate in practice exercises, both scheduled and unscheduled, relating to various emergencies that might occur. These practice exercises reinforce the CS's knowledge of the procedures and test the procedures for weak spots.

CRITICAL-INCIDENT STRESS MANAGEMENT

Each program should have a critical-incident stress-management plan in place in the event of the loss of an aircraft and its crew. It is imperative that the CS on duty at the time be included in this plan. The CS will experience all the same feelings of grief and loss as the other program members, and more. The CS may believe that he or she could have done something more or failed to do something and, thus, take on unwarranted feelings of guilt. Unless counseled immediately, this CS will be lost to the program at some point in the future.

AIRCRAFT RADIOS

Each medical crew member should be familiar with the operation of the radios used in the program's aircraft. In some aircraft there may be more than one radio, thus permitting the medical crew to communicate with someone on the ground while the pilot is talking to someone else.

Other aircraft will have one radio and two control heads, one for the pilot and the other for the medical crew. The medical crew member should check with the pilot before using the radio to be certain that the pilot has no need of it at the time.

PORTABLE UNITS

A program may elect to provide medical crew members with portable handheld radios for use on the ground outside the aircraft. These radios are particularly useful for programs that do emergency scene flights, and they are also useful during transfer flights for alerting the pilot to the imminent return of the crew with the patient.

SUMMARY

The communications center of a transport program is the foundation of a successful venture. Planning and implementation of a communications center must be organized, logical, and cost-effective. The program's mission, philosophy, and resources must be continually evaluated to ensure the quality of its communications.

REFERENCES

1. Association of Air Medical Services: *Manual for air medical communications operations*, Pasadena, Calif, 1989, AAMS.
2. Commission on Accreditation of Medical Transport Systems: *Accreditation standards*, ed 5, Anderson, SC, 2002, Author.
3. *Federal Aviation Administration*, http://www.faa.gov. Accessed June, 2002.
4. Hawsey KO, Lee A: "This is a drill": Overdue aircraft drill for a postaccident/incident plan, *Air Med J* 20(5):15-17, 2001.
5. Herron S: Communications. In McCloskey K, Orr R, editors: *Pediatric transport medicine*, St Louis, 1995, Mosby.
6. Illman P: *Pilot's communication handbook*, ed 5, New York, 1998, McGraw-Hill.
7. Quinlan BJ: 21st century telecom, *Air Ambulance* 3(4):18-20, 1999.
8. Rau W: 2000 Communications survey, *Air Med J* 6(2):22-26, 2000.
9. Rogers LC, Fiege A: Missing/overdue aircraft: are you prepared? *Air Med J* 5(2):24-26, 1999.
10. Yocum K: A new look at hiring communication specialists, *Air Med J* 5(2):132-34, 1999.

Safety and Survival

10

1. Identify safety issues related to air and surface transport.
2. Perform a safety checklist before and after patient transport.
3. Perform safety procedures during transport.
4. Identify the components of the postaccident incident (PAIP).
5. Perform basic survival skills including signaling and fire and shelter building.

The majority of the chapters in this book contain information written to help the practitioner who performs in the air medical setting to provide care for critically ill or injured patients. The information in this chapter is written for the practitioners themselves, who face unique and challenging hazards in the transport environment. Nurses, paramedics, physicians, respiratory therapists, and pilots are responsible for the care and transport of patients, but these professionals also share a greater responsibility: to function as safety advocates. Transport team members must recognize that their actions affect not only their own safety but also the safety of others. With that knowledge in mind, transport team members must develop a safety-consciousness that guides their actions. A safety-consciousness is developed as a result of training, repetition, and complete familiarity with equipment and procedures. It is only after

developing a safety-consciousness that transport team members are ready to assume the responsibility of maintaining a secure and protected environment for the patients they transport, other team members, ancillary staff, public service personnel, bystanders, and all other persons who interact with the transport service.

Like other skills, safety requires time, work, and desire. The role of safety advocate is the most important responsibility of any transport team member because failure to provide the safest environment possible will at some point significantly undermine the ability of transport team members to perform the diverse responsibilities required for patient care.

DEFINITION OF SAFETY

Every transport program (air or ground) must provide a safe work environment. The Occupational

Safety and Health Act that was passed in 1970 makes it mandatory that the workplace preserve human resources by reducing workplace illnesses and injuries. Unfortunately, not all human endeavors are totally free of risk. Many work environments present significant risk to those who work in them. However, steps can be taken to assess and prioritize the risk, safety plans can be implemented to address known risk, and an ongoing monitoring program can evaluate the effectiveness of efforts to reduce the risks to an acceptable degree. Over time the work environment will change, which requires flexibility in the safety plan. New information may dictate new approaches to old problems. What must never change is the commitment of the people involved to continually work toward keeping risk at or below an acceptable level.

All persons directly involved in daily transport operations must also define within themselves their personal degree of acceptable risk because, if individuals have serious doubts regarding their personal safety, the stress created by those concerns will ultimately interfere with their job performance.

SAFETY PROGRAM

Each transport program must develop a safety program that is comprehensive and includes a number of components including:

- A safety officer
- Communication tools: e-mail, bulletin board, website, and so on
- A reporting process to identify safety issues and corrective action
- Annual safety training
- Safety evaluations
- Hearing conservation
- Scene safety training

A strong commitment to safety must begin early in the development of any transport program.

The Commission on Accreditation of Medical Transport Systems (CAMTS) requires that each transport program establish a safety committee.[7] The safety committee is composed of various members of the transport program, representing pilots, drivers, mechanics, communication specialists, and medical personnel, in addition to administrative staff. The committee should establish a hazard-reporting system in which potential hazards in the work environment are reported to the committee and are then channeled for further discussion and resolution by the committee.

The recommendations and actions of the safety committee need to be linked to the transport program's performance improvement (PI) or quality management (QM) programs.[13] An action cycle should be initiated and completed and information appropriately communicated and incorporated into the program's policies, procedures, and operations.

Safety problems are discussed at safety meetings, appropriate action is decided on, and responsibilities to complete the action are assigned. Safety information is reviewed frequently, changes are made as required, and new information is disseminated during regularly scheduled safety meetings at which all members of the program are present.

Statewide and regional safety councils are made up of local programs that work together to address common safety concerns.[21,23,28] The safety forum allows member programs an opportunity to exchange program policy information on topics such as weather guidelines, communication procedures, and ongoing training. Agreements to provide mutual transport following for member programs are also addressed by state or regional safety committees. One objective of regional or state safety committees should be the elimination of any negative influence caused by competition between programs that operate in the same area.

A successful, comprehensive safety program evaluates training, equipment, policies, and procedures and is strengthened by commitment, teamwork, and open communication by all members of the air medical program.

AIR MEDICAL ACCIDENT RATES

The first hospital air medical program was established in 1972. In the following years the air medical industry underwent tremendous growth. With the growth in the industry came the realization that air medical helicopters had an accident rate far greater than that of helicopters engaged in general aviation. From 1980 through 1985 the air medical helicopter industry had an estimated accident rate of 12.34 accidents per 100,000 patients (1.1 patient transport = 1 flight hour). The accident rate for a comparable non-emergency medical service population, such as nonscheduled turbine-powered air taxi helicopter operators, was 6.9 for the same time period.[30] The emergency medical service (EMS) accident rate was almost double the rate for air taxi operators. In 1982, the worst year on record, the air medical helicopter accident rate climbed to nearly 16 accidents per 100,000 patients transported compared with the non-EMS air taxi rate of 4.51.[24] In addition, the fatal accident rate among EMS helicopters (5.4) was more than three times that of helicopter air taxis (1.6) for the same period (1980 through 1985).[30,34] These alarming statistics led those involved in air medical transport to take a serious look at what was causing these accidents.

In 1988 the National Transportation Safety Board (NTSB) released the results of an investigation of 59 EMS accidents that occurred between 1978 and 1986. The study concluded that weather-related accidents were the most common and most serious type of accident experienced by EMS helicopters. In 1999, 2000, and 2001 Frazer[14-16] published a review of 121 EMS air medical accidents. Again weather-related accidents were found to be the most common type of accident. In comparison with the 1980s, the 1990s saw a 10% increase in weather-related accidents. Fog was the common denominator in these weather-related incidents.[15]

In 1990 the CAMTS was established. One of CAMTS's standards is a recommendation for weather minimums.[7] It seems that weather, particularly fog—which can impair pilot visualization—continues to be a cause of helicopter crashes. Flight programs need to establish weather minimums based on the terrain in which they operate and then adhere to them. Each program must have a policy that allows any crew member to refuse or abort a flight if they feel uncomfort-

able. Unfortunately it seems we have yet to learn from our past.

AIR AND SURFACE TRANSPORT NURSES ASSOCIATION POSITION PAPER

The Air and Surface Transport Nurses Association (ASTNA; formerly the National Flight Nurses Association [NFNA]) is a professional nursing organization with a membership that includes flight nurses from throughout the United States and Canada, and it is involved in establishing professional practice standards for flight nursing. The NFNA[31] (ASTNA) published a position paper in 1988 in which the organization endorsed many of the recommendations of the NTSB study published earlier the same year. The NFNA (ASTNA) stated that "available knowledge and technology which could significantly enhance [a] flight nurse's safety in the air medical helicopter environment is not consistently applied and utilized in all air medical transport programs."[31] The NFNA (ASTNA) proposed several corrective measures. The proposals dealt with (1) crew scheduling and rest periods, (2) the right of flight nurses to refuse to participate in a flight as a result of concerns for personal safety, (3) the need for programs to develop written protocols for the use of physical and pharmacologic restraints when combative or potentially combative patients are being transported, (4) the need for programs to critically evaluate hot-loading and unloading polices and procedures and to ensure personnel assigned to hot-load or unload do so only after proper training, and (5) the adoption of measures to maximize safety and reduce the potential of serious injury to flight nurses by use of helicopter design changes such as energy-attenuating seats, addition of shoulder harnesses to lap belts at each position in the aircraft, and development and installation of crash-resistant fuel systems in aircraft as soon as possible.

The final position statement dealt with specific in-flight duties to be performed by flight nurses to ensure a safe aviation environment. Identified flight nurse responsibilities included (1) equipment securement during flight, (2) use of seat belts and shoulder harnesses, (3) proper patient securement within the aircraft, (4) judicious use of night lighting, and (5) isolation of the pilot and controls from potential patient movement.

The NFNA (ASTNA) also stated that flight nurses should be active in working with pilots in developing initial and recurrent safety briefings, premission briefings, and postmission debriefings and that flight nurses should be trained in position-reporting procedures, communication terminology, landing-zone safety, helicopter emergency fuel and system shutdown, radio communications, and other aspects of crew member emergency training.

In 1998 *Improving Flight Nurse Safety in the Air Medical Helicopter Environment* was revised.[31] The revised position paper reinforces the positions of the first paper with the addition of the following recommendations:

1. Flight nurses interact more with the pilot in command by participating in recurrent safety, permission, and postmission briefings; by being taught how to report aircraft position; and by undergoing crew member emergency training.
2. Appropriate personal protective gear including helmets, flame-resistant flight uniforms, and protective footwear should be used.
3. Stress-management programs should be used to enhance flight nursing performance.
4. Back-up aircraft that are similar to the primary aircraft in the flight program should be used.

PERSONAL SAFETY

Personal safety is not only as the phrase indicates. As a part of a transport team, one is responsible for other team members, the patient, and any others that are involved in the transport process. Limmer[24] offers *10 Commandments* to help ensure survival in the prehospital environment. These include the need to remain observant; listen to one's "gut" feelings; stay safe in traffic (both air and ground); practice legal survival (provide quality care, document that care, and treat people well); make an informed decision about the use of additional safety gear such as body armor; remain wary of all weapons; know and practice safety tactics; communicate and work

as a team; deal with stress; and realize that safety and survival are a mindset.

FITNESS STANDARDS

The transport environment is physically challenging and requires that medical crew members maintain a high personal level of physical and emotional fitness. Requirements of each program vary, and no industrywide formal guidelines exist.[37] However, a common-sense approach would seem to dictate some minimal fitness requirements.

Minimum physical requirements of any person wishing to work in the transport environment should include the ability to wear installed seat belts and the ability to work within the confined space limitations of an individual transport vehicle. Transport team members must also have no preexisting conditions that would interfere with their flexibility, strength, or cardiovascular fitness. Transport team members must not have any condition that would cause altered mental or neurologic function.

PREGNANCY

Many women of childbearing age work in the transport setting. For those contemplating pregnancy, there is no existing industry standard regarding pregnancy employment policies.[11] The effects of high altitude, high noise levels, vibrations, and increased risk for injury in mishaps have been identified as risks to the fetus and may adversely affect maternal health.[25] Further studies are warranted to assess the environmental and physical effects of air and surface medical stressors on the health of the mother and unborn child.

PERSONAL PROTECTIVE EQUIPMENT

The NTSB study of 1988 recommended that air medical personnel who routinely fly EMS helicopter missions wear protective clothing and equipment to reduce the chance of injury or death in survivable accidents.[18] The ASTNA position paper also endorses the use of protective equipment. Protective equipment consists of helmets, fire-resistant uniforms, and boots with steel toes and shanks.

HELMETS

In the military the use of flight helmets has been shown to protect significantly against head injuries.[9] Despite the obvious advantages afforded to the military by flight helmets, acceptance in civilian air medical programs has not been widespread. Reasons cited for not wearing helmets included high cost, uncertain benefit, and negative public relations.[22] However, a survey performed to determine the public's perception of helmet usage found that patients and family members positively viewed the use of helmets by air medical personnel.[35]

Factors air medical personnel should evaluate when selecting a helmet include choosing a knowledgeable vendor who is familiar with custom-fitting helmets. The helmet should be lightweight and should match the center of gravity of the unhelmeted head. Some manufacturers use customized liners that are molded to the individual's head size and fit into the hard outer shell of the helmet, which reduces the cost of a complete helmet for each team member. The helmet's liner must absorb energy and fit comfortably, and the chinstrap should hold the helmet firmly in place.

FIRE-RESISTANT CLOTHING

The goal of fire-resistant clothing is to minimize skin exposure to the intense thermal energy from a postaccident fire. The uniform should be made of a flame-resistant, heat-resistant material, such as Nomex, that is designed to withstand high temperatures for a brief period, usually less than 20 seconds, to enable the wearer to evacuate a burning aircraft.[19] The fabric may reduce the risk or severity of tissue damage but will not prevent thermal injury to the skin.

The fire-resistant suit should be worn in combination with cotton, silk, or wool/cotton undergarments that include both briefs and a T-shirt or long underwear.[18] When exposed to flames, synthetic materials such as polyester or polypropylene melt and become embedded into the skin; therefore they should not be worn under the suit. The uniform should also fit to allow 0.25 inch of air space between the suit and undergarments. Although not specifically recommended by the 1988 NTSB safety

study, Nomex gloves can be useful in protecting the hands and should be considered by persons who wear fire-resistant uniforms.

PROTECTIVE FOOTWEAR

Footwear is an important consideration for transport team members, especially for programs that respond to scene work. Boots protect the foot from punctures, lacerations, and thermal injuries and provide stability to the ankle on rough or unlevel ground.

The boot should be constructed of leather that extends several inches above the ankle. The sole should be thick and oil-resistant, and the boot should have steel toes and shanks. The boot should also have adequate ventilation to prevent moisture from being trapped. When boots are worn in combination with fire-resistant flight suits, the pant legs should be tucked inside the boot.

HEARING PROTECTION

Noise is a hazard faced daily by flight crews in the air medical industry. Long-term exposure to high noise levels is associated with hearing loss, and often the hearing loss goes unnoticed by the person involved,[32] although sound emission is different for each aircraft, the average sound level is between 90 and 100 dB. The Occupational Safety and Health Administration (OSHA) currently require employers to provide hearing-conservation programs for employees exposed to time-weighted average sound levels of 85 dB or greater. Hearing protectors, such as earplugs or earmuffs, should be worn during high decibel exposures such as hot loading and unloading or when extreme noise levels exist at scenes. Earplugs are smaller and less expensive, but noise protection varies with fit. Earmuffs offer more uniform protection but are more expensive, are not easily carried or stored, and are less comfortable than earplugs.

GROUND VEHICLE SAFETY

Unlike air medical accidents, which have to be reported and are investigated by the NTSB, ground vehicle crashes are generally monitored on a state or local level. It is difficult to know how many accidents occur each year, but periodic reports that are published in the EMS literature point out that they do occur and there are fatalities and serious injuries. Elling[12] reviewed ambulance accident data reported to the police in New York state over a 48-month period. He found that there was an increased risk of having an accident on wet roads, although the majority of accidents occurred on dry roads; the majority of accidents occurred when the ambulance was making turns or when they were broadsided at an intersection; and locations where traffic signaling devices exist presented the greatest risk for an ambulance accident to occur. He also found that few medical personnel were appropriately restrained in the transport vehicle.

Each state, county, or local government may set guidelines for the use of lights and sirens. Generally that decision is left to the transport team, but the safety of all involved needs to be considered. It is also recommended that ambulance service vehicles should not exceed posted speed limits when proceeding through an intersection.

Appropriate safety equipment should be used by the ground transport service. Equipment should be stowed and secured. In addition, the transport team must be restrained when the vehicle is in motion when not attending to the patient. Even then, their time out of restraint needs to be limited to decrease their risk of injury.[12]

TRANSPORT PREPARATION

Safe performance of duties in the transport environment begins with education and training. Classroom instruction should include topics such as transport physiology, safety, communications, stress management, survival training, and legal aspects of patient transport. When possible, opportunities to practice classroom instruction in the actual environment should be done, such as an exercise in the wilderness to practice survival skills. Safe performance in the transport environment requires a foundation of knowledge, gained through training and experience, which ultimately builds confidence in the ability to perform safely and effectively. Safety

should be the number-one priority for both air and ground transport. Even though this section focuses specifically on air medical transport, the basic concepts of safety presented here are applicable to either air or surface transport environments.

AIRCRAFT SAFETY

An introduction to flight safety should begin with an orientation to the characteristics of the particular aircraft in use at the air medical program. Individual aircraft characteristics exist, but only general information will be discussed here.

The wind created by the rotor blades, referred to as *rotor wash,* can exceed 50 mph. In a hover and on the ground during the warm-up or cooldown stage, a rotor wash of approximately 25 mph can occur. This wind becomes a hazard in the form of flying dust, litter, loose clothing, and anything that is not tied down. Personnel should be aware of this and take proper precautions, such as wearing protective glasses to prevent injuries to the eyes. Hats, scarves, blankets, sheets, towels, mattress pads, and loose papers must be secured to prevent them from being blown away. More importantly, objects that are kept secure will be prevented from being pulled into the air intake of the helicopter, damaging the engine, and possibly leading to engine failure.

Rotor wash also increases the risk of wind-chill to skin. A 25-mph rotor wash with an air temperature of 10° F creates a wind-chill of 30° F, which can damage exposed skin in minutes. Flight crew members must consider this hazard when flying in cold weather and must take steps to protect the patient accordingly.

The most obvious hazards of a helicopter are the main rotor and tail rotor blades. These blades turn at approximately 400 rpm, with rotor tips spinning at approximately 500 mph. At full speed the main rotor blades create a disk that can be seen above the cabin; however, at lower–rotor velocity speeds, such as the warm-up and cool-down stages, the blades can "flap" or "sail" with wind gusts. This may allow the blades to drop below shoulder level. The crouch position is advised for anyone approaching or departing an aircraft while the blades are turning.

When a helicopter lands on uneven ground or on a slope, the rotor disk will come closer to the ground on the uphill side. The aircraft should be approached and departed on the downhill side in the crouched position with constant attention paid to the terrain and the rotor blades at all times. At scenes a safety person should be designated to ensure that those loading the aircraft do not inadvertently walk under the tail rotor area. When loading or unloading patients and equipment, the flight crew must take measures to ensure that nothing is carried above the head.

The tail rotor is potentially more hazardous than the main rotor. At greater than 2000 rpm it is nearly invisible. Efforts to reduce tail rotor risk to EMS workers include conduction of routine training sessions with first-responders, provision of high-visibility tail-rotor lighting on EMS aircraft, use of a helicopter with a fenestron, or installation of high skids under the aircraft to raise the height of the rotor.[10] Flight crew members must always approach the aircraft from the front in full view of the pilot. Those working around the aircraft, such as EMS personnel, must be instructed to remain back from the aircraft after it lands and to approach only after being signaled by the pilot. The safe approach zone is in front of the helicopter and from the sides within the pilot's vision, never from the rear.

The engine exhaust area is another hazardous area that should be avoided. The exhaust coming from the engine is approximately 400° C. The metal pipes in the system should be avoided.

DAILY PREFLIGHT PROCEDURES

Daily preflight procedures should include an aircraft check to ensure all essential equipment is present, functioning, and properly stored. A daily (or more often, such as at each shift change) preflight briefing should be held during which the pilot, flight team, and communications specialist discuss forecasted weather and any other potential problems that might be encountered during the shift. Opportunities for the crew to conduct postflight briefings should occur, when necessary, to address any safety concern and allow for corrective action.

A daily briefing should also be a part of ground transport services. Procedures should include a vehicle check to ensure all essential equipment is present and functioning. If there have been any problems, this is a good time to brief the team and develop an action plan to solve the problem. Posttransport briefings may also be beneficial.

HELIPAD SAFETY

Safety should be a primary focus in design of a hospital helipad. The air medical hospital's helipad should be well planned and designed according to FAA regulations. Considerations include approach and departure routes; the location of the helipad relative to patient care areas; the size of the helipad; and the provision of emergency exits, fire protection equipment, and lighting.[27] In addition, provisions for snow removal and cleaning must be made.

The helipad should be inaccessible to unauthorized persons, and a member of the flight crew should accompany anyone wanting to see the helicopter. All flight crew members should be trained in fire safety and should know the location of fire alarm boxes and extinguishers. Smoking should be prohibited around or near the aircraft. Figure 10-1 illustrates a marked rooftop helipad.

IN-FLIGHT SAFETY
SECUREMENT OF EQUIPMENT AND PATIENTS

In-flight safety is an important responsibility of flight nurses. Responsibility begins with the use of seat belts and shoulder harnesses during all phases of flight. At times patient needs will require that the shoulder restraint or lap belt be removed; however, the removal should be done only in level flight and only after the need is communicated to the pilot. The safety restraints should then be reapplied as soon as possible.

Flight nurses must develop the habit of always securing equipment such as monitors, intravenous equipment controllers, and equipment and medication boxes to prevent these objects from becoming projectiles and inflicting injuries to the patient or crew (Figure 10-2). The flight team must securely restrain patients during flight to prevent injury, and

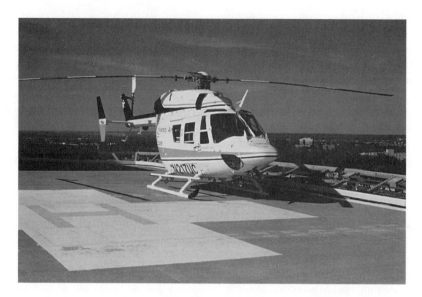

FIGURE 10-1   A marked hospital rooftop helipad.

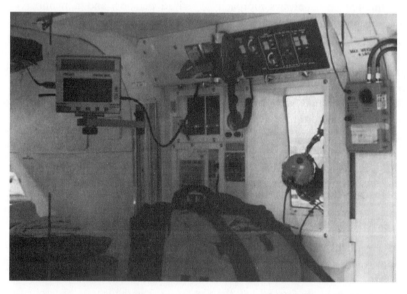

FIGURE 10-2   An example of methods that may be used to ensure that equipment is appropriately secured.

they must ensure that the patient is isolated from the pilot and the controls. Flight team members have special responsibilities when securing pediatric patients during flight. Infants and small children must not be held during transport. The pediatric patient should be restrained snugly in an infant carrier or car seat that conforms to applicable federal motor-vehicle safety standards, and the carrier or car seat should then be restrained to the aircraft stretcher in a rear-facing position. Pediatric immobilization devices are available for those patients who require spinal immobilization.

Combative patients should be evaluated for the use of physical or chemical restraints. Physical restraints should be applied before takeoff. The use of physical or chemical restraints should be guided by program policies that are periodically reviewed and updated.

OTHER IN-FLIGHT DUTIES

The transport team is also responsible for assisting the pilot in command with in-flight duties such as scanning for other aircraft, maintaining a "sterile cockpit" during critical phases of flight, and observing for hazards on approach at scenes or at other unfamiliar landing areas. Other aircraft should be scanned for as an ongoing process, especially when there is no patient aboard. When other air traffic or obstacles are spotted, the flight team should report their position by the clock method. The nose of the aircraft is in the 12 o'clock position, and the tail is in the 6 o'clock position. To ensure that no obstacle goes unnoticed by the pilot, flight team members should report any obstacle or air traffic even though the pilot may have seen it. Aircraft reporting is helpful to pilots, particularly in areas of congested air traffic. One effective technique for scanning is the front-to-side method.[33] This method involves the flight team member starting with a fixed point in the center of the front windshield, slowly adjusting his or her vision leftward, returning to the center, refocusing, and then moving the eyes to the right. There are other scanning techniques, and selection of one is a matter of preference, but the technique should involve some series of fixations to be successful. When the head is in motion, vision is blurred, and the mind will not register targets as easily.[33]

Observance of a sterile cockpit is a regulation of the FAA (FAR 135.100) that prohibits nonessential communications between the medical crew and pilot during critical phases of flight. The critical phases of flight include all ground operations that involve taxi, takeoff, and landing and all other flight operations except cruise flight.

When approaching unfamiliar landing areas or landing at scenes, flight team members should be attentive to the radio conversations between the pilot

and the on-scene personnel. The flight team should understand the landing-zone description and look for additional hazards not mentioned in the landing-zone briefing. Hazards to look for include wires, trees, vehicles, loose articles, and persons.

IN-FLIGHT EMERGENCIES

An in-flight emergency is often considered only when an accident is reported or has occurred. Training in emergency in-flight procedures should be part of an overall safety program, and proficiency should be demonstrated yearly. Training and retraining will ensure that safety procedures are automatic. During an actual emergency, flight team members are responsible for (1) confirming with the pilot that an actual emergency exists and assisting as necessary, (2) shutting off the main oxygen supply, and (3) preparing patients by placing them flat and tightening the stretcher straps.[4] As the final step in preparation, the flight team members should get into the survival position by placing the arms across the chest, forming an X with the forearms, and grasping the shoulder harness, while placing the knees together and the feet approximately 6 inches apart.

FIRE EMERGENCIES

The successful prevention of serious injury or death from an in-flight fire requires quick action. Smoke can quickly fill the cabin of an EMS helicopter. The heat and smoke can incapacitate the crew, with disastrous consequences. Fire extinguishers should be located within easy reach of the crew. On larger aircraft in which the medical crew is separated from the pilot, a fire extinguisher should be located in each compartment. If the fire is electrical, caused by medical equipment plugged into the aircraft power supply, the crew should unplug the equipment, turn off the inverter, turn off the oxygen source, and close the windows and vents to prevent accelerating the fire. If the smoke and heat become excessive, the crew should open windows or doors with discretion, fight the fire aggressively with the fire extinguisher, and prepare for an emergency landing as soon as possible.[26]

EMERGENCY EGRESS

The actions of the flight crew members immediately after an emergency landing may directly influence their survival. Disorientation and panic threaten survival.[4] Crew members must make a quick survey to reestablish orientation and assess the condition of the aircraft, other crew members, and the patient. In night conditions or in smoke-filled cabins, orientation can be maintained by use of the hand-over-hand method, wherein an old reference point is kept with one hand while a new one is selected with the other. After a forced landing the main danger is fire. If the pilot has become incapacitated, the fuel switch and master battery switch should be turned off. The position of these switches varies with the aircraft, and the flight team must be familiar with the procedure for their specific aircraft. After the aircraft has come to a complete stop, the aircraft should be exited by normal means first, jettison doors only if necessary, and forcible means if required.[26] Crew members should meet at a predesignated position a safe distance from the aircraft. After the threat of fire has passed, they should return to the aircraft and assist any persons who were injured during the emergency.

FORCED WATER LANDING

Flight crew members of air medical programs that frequently fly over large bodies of water need to be familiar with emergency egress procedures in the event of a forced water landing. Personal flotation devices should be worn by all flight crew members when missions require flight over water. If the pilot announces an in-flight emergency, the same procedure as outlined in the preceding paragraph should be followed. After a helicopter has made contact with the water, it will usually capsize because helicopters are top heavy as a result of the weight of the engines and transmission. It is important that no attempt be made to exit the aircraft until the blades have completely stopped. Flight crew members should establish a fixed reference point with one hand while finding a new one with the other, jettison the aircraft door after releasing the seat restraints, and maintain a fixed reference orientation with the hands, which is crucial in finding the

exits. Air bubbles always travel to the surface, and observing them may help crew members establish orientation; however, poor lighting conditions may prevent adequate visualization of bubbles. Crew members should gently use their arms to push themselves out of the aircraft and avoid kicking to prevent injury to crew members following behind. During surface ascent they should exhale slowly to prevent serious lung damage should they attempt to hold their breath.[36]

Some air medical programs practice emergency egress procedures with an egress simulator.[17,36,38] Wright et al[38] found that egress training can improve the ability of flight crew members to quickly evacuate an aircraft in a forced-landing situation, and a training program that focuses on in-flight emergencies can increase the flight crew's confidence to deal with these emergencies.

POSTACCIDENT DUTIES

After safely exiting a disabled aircraft, flight team members should meet at a predesignated safe distance from the aircraft until the danger of fire is eliminated. Measures to stabilize the patient and injured crew members should be taken. They should then try to ensure that chances for rescue are optimized.[19]

All EMS aircraft are required by the FAA to carry an emergency locator transmitter (ELT). These transmitters are designed to emit a radio signal when activated that will be received by satellites and relayed to rescue personnel. The radio signal does not pinpoint the position of the aircraft but gives rescuers a general area in which to begin a search. The ELT is activated by an impact exceeding 4 g (4 times the force of gravity) and broadcasts on the universal distress channel 121.5. Flight team members should know the location of the ELT and ensure that it has been activated. If an impact does not automatically activate the ELT, it can be activated manually by use of the directions on the front.

After the ELT is checked, the crew's situation needs to be evaluated, and survival priorities must be established. The environment in which the forced landing occurred will largely determine these priorities. Immediate goals are to secure a shelter and build a fire. The crew should stay with the aircraft unless a road or building is in sight. After the crew members secure shelter and build a fire, their next priority should be signaling. For a more detailed discussion refer to Survival Principles in this chapter.

DOWNED AIRCRAFT OR MISSING GROUND VEHICLE PROCEDURE

The practice of flight or ground transport following, in which a communication specialist keeps abreast of the progress of the transport by periodic scheduled communications with the pilot or driver, should be a standard operating procedure in all transport programs. Where distances between the transport vehicle and base are too great, the pilot or driver should make contact with other programs along the flight or transport path or with airports or hospitals and ask them to notify the base with transport status reports. Because cellular telephones can be used without consequence while performing ground transport, the surface transport team can generally provide position reports by calling when other modes of communication fail. Policies and procedures must be in place to aid the communication specialist in the event of an overdue transport vehicle.

The postaccident incident policy[7,29] should be a graduated response that outlines the responsibilities of the communication specialist in situations such as the following: (1) an unscheduled landing, which covers any precautionary landing; (2) a missing or overdue aircraft, such as an aircraft that is 15 minutes overdue; (3) aircraft emergency protocol, such as a serious emergency in which the crew is in jeopardy and needs immediate assistance; (4) aircraft postaccident protocol, such as notification that an aircraft accident has occurred; and (5) ground vehicle accident or emergencies.

Resources that should be used by the communication specialist in assisting in a missing aircraft location include local EMS agencies, state and local police agencies, other nearby air medical programs, airport facilities along the flight path, and the FAA. Similar resources should be used in locating overdue ground vehicles, with the exception of the FAA. Administrative personnel must also be notified, and an administrative crisis team must be assembled to assist in incident command. Members of the administrative crisis team should be listed in the procedural policy and should have the following duties: notifying next of kin, establishing a family reception center, providing for stress debriefing, coordinating all press releases, and establishing short- and long-term planning. The response to any disaster requires detailed planning and preparation, with the responsibilities of those involved clearly outlined in a procedural policy that is easily located during an emergency. Periodic review of the procedure and program drills can identify problem areas, and proper revisions can be instituted.[23] Figure 10-3 contains an example of a downed-aircraft policy and in the AAMS Postaccident Resource Document is located in the Addendum.

SCENE SAFETY

Air medical assistance at the scene of accidents has become a common occurrence in the prehospital setting. Flight teams must be aware of the potentially dangerous situations of landing at unfamiliar locations. The selection and preparation of the landing zone are often the responsibilities of the local EMS agency in charge at the scene, although the pilot has ultimate decision-making responsibility for landing at the site. If the pilot detects a problem with the site, he or she will relay those concerns to the ground guide, and a new site will be chosen. If the concern can be immediately addressed, such as an emergency vehicle too close to the landing zone, steps to correct the concern can be taken, and the site may be used.

Landing-zone selection and preparation should be part of an ongoing emergency service education program provided by various members of the flight team. The educational program should include discussion of ground and helicopter communication procedures, hazards such as rotor wash and noise, and the need for eye-protection measures. Instructions on hot-loading procedures and an aircraft-specific orientation should also be included.

Predesignated landing zones (PDLZs) are useful in areas of high congestion or in areas in which the terrain prevents a safe landing.[6] PDLZs are selected

Rev: 8/1/2000

AD _B_ MD _SLC_ FNC _BM_ LP _ME_

University Air Care

Subject: **Accident/Incident Plan**

Policy: University Air Care personnel will follow a defined process for timely and appropriate notification of individuals following identification of an actual or perceived emergency.

Purpose: This plan is a professional approach to dealing with any adversity that may have an effect on the program. It is designed to be a concise, workable guide through any accident or incident involving the University Air Care aircraft and personnel.

Procedure: This plan is a sequenced procedural guide that covers any incident or accident that may occur to a University Air Care helicopter. The protocols listed below are addressed in the pages that follow:

1. **Unscheduled landing protocol** - Any unscheduled (precautionary) landing (e.g., mechanical deficiency, inclement weather, or medical emergency).

2. **Missing/overdue aircraft protocol** - The aircraft is overdue 15 minutes after its estimated time of arrival (ETA).

3. **Aircraft emergency protocol** - A serious emergency in which the crew is in jeopardy and needs immediate help.

4. **Aircraft post accident protocol** - Notification that an aircraft accident has occurred.

In the event of an aircraft mishap, *never* transmit the names of the suspected injured or deceased persons over the radio.

Only the Air Care Program Director and his/her representative or the Medical Center Public Relations Department shall release information to the media. *UNDER NO CIRCUMSTANCES* shall any information be released to any member of the news media, Federal Aviation Administration (FAA), or any other persons unless the information is released by the above-stated individuals.

FIGURE 10-3 **Downed aircraft policy accident/incident plan.** (Courtesy University Air Care, Cincinnati, Ohio.)

by local EMS officials, who then consult with the program lead pilot, who schedules an evaluation of the zone. If the zone selection is mutually agreed on, information on the PDLZ is recorded and kept on file in the dispatch center. Potential PDLZs include parks, ball fields, schoolyards, vacant lots, and church or business parking lots. Time of day may be a consideration in the use of a particular PDLZ, and any restrictions should be noted in the dispatch file.

When a request from the community EMS agency is received, the communication specialist can transmit the information to the pilot. Included in the information are the coordinates and a written description of the PDLZ, together with any time restrictions. An advantage of PDLZ identification is faster dispatch of the helicopter, especially if the scene is less than 10 minutes away.[6]

Flight team members must also be aware of the dangers encountered in the prehospital setting and should take precautions to prevent themselves from becoming another victim at the scene. Unless specifically trained, flight nurses should not engage in the extrication or rescue effort. The extrication effort should proceed uninterrupted by the flight team, unless airway measures are required and only if the procedure can be done without the rescuer being put in jeopardy. While the extrication of a victim continues, the flight team should prepare the equipment and plan as rapid a departure as possible.

Response to the scene of a violent crime requires special caution. The prehospital setting is becoming more dangerous to emergency care providers. No longer is crime contained to the larger inner cities; it is becoming common in rural areas as well.[3] Flight teams can protect themselves by consulting with law enforcement personnel to ensure the scene is safe. When caring for a victim of a violent crime, flight nurses must try to disturb the scene no more than necessary to preserve evidence.

SURVIVAL PRINCIPLES

Preparation and education are the best means of dealing with the uncertainty and fear associated with survival. Good physical and mental health are essential components of survival.[1,2] Air medical aircraft should be equipped with a complete survival kit, and all crew members should be instructed in its use. The periodic checking of survival equipment and review of emergency protocols and procedures are essential parts of pretransport duties.

Each transport program should conduct annual survival and safety skills reviews. These should include a review of the weather conditions and how to prepare for those in which the program operates and a review of safety procedures such as emergency egress (Figure 10-4).

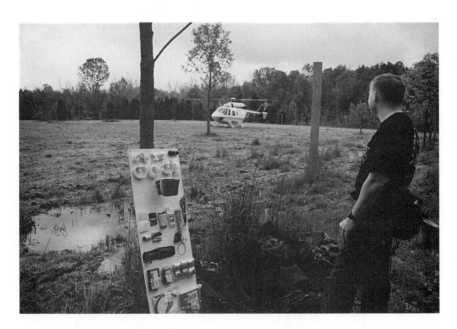

FIGURE 10-4   **Air care survival day.**

Psychological Preparation

By understanding and dealing with the potential for loss of life or serious injury, the flight nurse can build coping mechanisms that will help in the event of an aircraft emergency or postcrash scenario. Fear, anxiety, anger, and denial can be experienced during the preimpact phase of the emergency. A sound safety program, survival education, and experience will help prepare for a situation that requires survival skills.

Leadership is vital when danger is imminent so that panic and denial can be prevented. To alleviate panic, flight crew members should keep busy with tasks or help others. By providing support, comfort, rest, and medical attention to those injured, flight crew members will help all the survivors psychologically.

Those directly or indirectly involved in the incident or accident should be offered counseling after rescue by a qualified mental health professionals experienced in critical-incident debriefing.

Clothing

In cold-weather environments, measures should be taken to protect all parts of the body because a person's clothing may be the only shelter from the environment and protection against hypothermia. Clothing should protect the wearer against the environment and be comfortable and practical. Tight-fitting clothing, which may restrict movement and circulation during physical exercise, should be avoided. Clothing must be layered for best effect and have proper ventilation to ensure adequate heat regulation.

Warm-weather clothing should protect against the sun. Long-sleeve shirts and pants together with head and eye protection diminish water loss and exposure. Preplanning for a mission in desert terrain should recognize the potential for significant variations in temperature from day to night.

Priorities

Knowledge of the rule of threes when priorities are set will greatly increase the chances of survival in the outdoors. This rule states that the average person can survive 3 minutes without oxygen, 3 hours without shelter in extreme conditions, 3 days without water, and 3 weeks without food.[2,19] Medical concerns and safety are more important in an accident, but once these are addressed, the rule of threes should guide priorities. With this rule in mind, the flight crew's immediate concerns after an accident should be creating or seeking shelter, building a fire, and making appropriate fire signals.[2]

Shelter

The ability to create a shelter is vital and cannot be overemphasized. Shelter provides protection from extremes in environmental temperatures. Warmth and dryness are best achieved when the shelter is kept small and simple. The aircraft and natural shelters require little physical energy and are the easiest to prepare. When formulating a plan for building a shelter, the flight crew should consider the following points: (1) the shelter should be kept as close to the aircraft as possible; (2) the area should be checked for future danger, such as dry stream beds that could flood quickly, avalanche chutes, and steep terrain; and (3) the three basic parts of any shelter are the roof, floor, and walls; if not enough material is available to build a complete shelter, the sequence of priorities is a roof, floor (insulated if possible), windward side, and leeward side. Figure 10-5 illustrates some general-purpose shelters.

The aircraft provides excellent shelter. If the fuselage of an aircraft is used for shelter, the flight crew should ensure that is supported and will not roll or tilt on the terrain or during adverse weather conditions. Any holes inside the aircraft should be patched with sheets, tarps, or space blankets. All windows or exposed metal should be insulated to prevent heat loss. The flight crew should avoid sleeping on or placing the injured on exposed metal or ground.

The flight crew can strip the aircraft of its resources and materials and improvise to meet the survival goal. Following is a partial list of uses for aircraft parts:

1. Battery: signal lights, communications, and fire starter
2. Cowling: signal panels, water collection, fire pit, windbreaker, and shelter

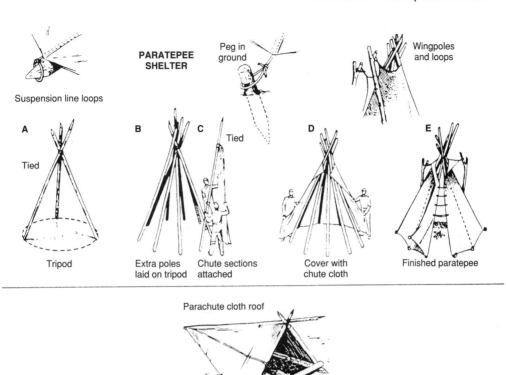

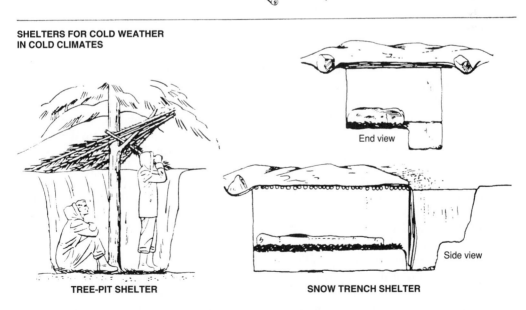

FIGURE 10-5   **General-purpose shelters.** (From Department of the Air Force: *Survival-training education*, AFM 64-3, Washington, DC, 1969, US Government Printing Office.)

3. Doors: shelter, windbreaker, signal panel
4. Fuselage: shelter
5. Engine oil or fuel: fire starter, signal fire
6. Nose spinner: bucket, water collection, tool for snow
7. Seats: insulation, sleeping cushions, fire material, signal material
8. Tires: black smoke signal
9. Vertical stabilizer: shelter supports, signal panel
10. Wings: windbreaks, shelter supports, overhead shade, water collection for dew and rain

The flight team must first consider the length of time and the amount of energy required to build a shelter. Natural shelter provides an alternative that will protect a flight crew member from the environment. The flight crew must be aware of potential dangers when selecting a natural shelter; for example, dead trees or tree limbs that may fall in a strong wind; rock slides; caves with other inhabitants such as bears, skunks, or cougars; and trees or rocks that may conduct lightning.[19] A formation in the earth made of rock, snow, timber, or sand may provide a place in which crew members can burrow. When constructing a shelter, the flight team member must investigate natural resources to discover ventilation and insulation materials available, such as rocks, tree branches, and snow, to incorporate with materials in the aircraft or survival kit. Trapped air with ventilation is an effective insulator; therefore snow caves are excellent shelters in cold climates. Whether it is a space blanket raised between two trees or an elaborate construction job, the flight crew member should consider the expenditure of energy to build it. Optimally the shelter should be in sight of the aircraft. The flight crew should keep survival gear in the shelter close to the air medical team members and out of the elements. Diagrams of the steps in shelter building are helpful when they can be applied to a complete program that incorporates aircraft configuration, terrain, climate, and survival equipment available to the flight nurse.

FIRE-BUILDING

A fire provides warmth, light, and a sense of security. If adequate clothing and shelter are available, a fire may not be needed. When the need is recognized, the crew member should prepare materials and start the fire before dark, considering the placement of the shelter and direction of reflected heat. Once the location of the fire has been chosen, the fire should be contained with some type of boundary. The crew member should gather enough combustible material such as tinder, kindling (small pieces), and large pieces of wood to last through the night. Using the available fire-starting equipment, the crew member should first build the fire with small combustible material and then add larger pieces of wood. Once the fire has evolved, kindling can be added to the tinder. The flight crew should be prepared to use the fire as a signaling tool. Oil or greenery can be added to create effective smoke that can be seen by aerial search-and-rescue aircraft. There are many methods of fire building and many materials to use (Figure 10-6). Crew members should be instructed about what fuel is available in the service area and how to use the fire starter available in the aircraft survival pack.

SIGNALING

Once the basic needs of the flight team have been met, signaling becomes the next priority. The chance of being rescued increases with enhanced visibility. However, signaling must be accomplished without the crew members being further endangered.

The aircraft radio and ELT discussed in the section on Postaccident Duties are the most effective rescue aids. When the aircraft radio is not operational, alternative signaling methods must be used. Smoke is the most effective means by day to signal search-and-rescue aircraft. Signaling should be one purpose of the survival fire. Other signaling methods are as follows:

1. Smoke: Addition of oil, rubber, or plastic to the fire creates black smoke; addition of green leaves, grass, or water creates white smoke. The flight crew member should pick the color of smoke that will provide the most contrast with the environment.

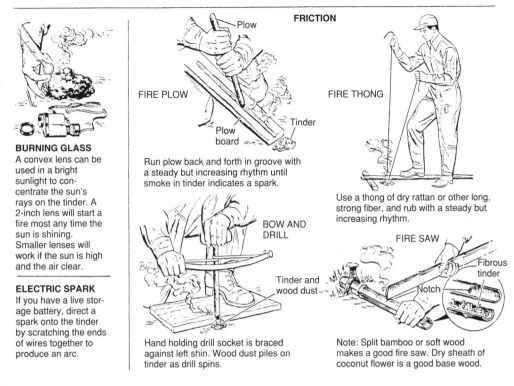

FIGURE 10-6   **Fire-making without matches.** (From Department of the Air Force: *Survival-training education*, AFM 64-3, Washington, DC, 1969, US Government Printing Office.)

2. Signal mirror: Reflections off shiny metal objects, cans, or foil can be seen on overcast days. The crew member should practice using a signal mirror by flashing the mirror in the direction of the aircraft when heard, even if it cannot be seen.

3. Flares or flashlight: The flight crew member can signal with a flashlight at night. Flares can be used if they are available in the aircraft.

4. Clothing: Orange parkas, sheets, or other items with bright colors that provide a contrast with the colors of the surrounding nature are useful signals.

5. Whistle: A plastic police whistle will provide ground search-and-rescue units with easy signaling communication on the ground. Whistles can be used in adverse weather or at night for guidance.[1]

6. Dyes or signal panels: Depending on terrain, the flight crew member can clear an area and lay signal panels in a geometric pattern. Dyes are effective in water and on snow. Fine dyes should be used downwind because they will penetrate clothing and food.

In winter environments, the signal fire should be made on top of a platform. In desert environments, a can with sand and oil can provide a smoke device that will continue to burn for a long time.

WATER

Hydration maintenance is crucial in the survival setting. Available intravenous fluids provide electrolyte solutions and some glucose for energy. Air medical crew members should conserve all available water stores by rationing. Crew members must boil water or use water-purification tablets to prevent bacterial gastrointestinal infection; vomiting and diarrhea cause large amounts of water loss.

In snow environments, snow should be melted before ingestion to prevent body heat loss. If water is kept in a container, the expansion of the container and its possible rupture if it freezes must be considered; it is better to keep water in a shallow open container for future use. Available water mixed with hot chocolate or instant soup and heated provides a hot meal and liquid.

FOOD

The need for food is a low priority during a survival situation of fewer than 4 to 5 days. It is vital that the air medical crew recognize depleted energy stores. The psychologic effects of depleted energy stores include personality changes, depression, and diminished problem-solving capabilities.

SPECIFIC ENVIRONMENTAL CONSIDERATIONS

When flying over water, all flight team members should wear personal flotation devices. Flight team members may consider wearing survival gear and signal devices in a vest system. All personnel should be knowledgeable about the use of these devices. The ability to swim should be mandatory, and open-sea survival should be part of the training received by all flight team members who frequently operate over large bodies of water.

Both rotor and fixed-wing aircraft should provide seat cushions that can be used as flotation devices. The program safety officer should investigate the availability of open-water survival gear and make specific equipment available when appropriate.

Jettisoning of doors, evacuation of the aircraft, and other emergency procedures should be directed by the pilot. Any available time before the aircraft sinks should be spent on evacuation and gathering of open-sea survival equipment. The crew must be prepared for the aircraft to flip over once it hits the water. Engine weight on rotor aircraft will turn the aircraft upside-down.

Once in the water, the flight team can minimize heat loss by using the heat escape–lessening posture (HELP). Team members can achieve this position by bringing the knees up to the chest and putting the arms across the chest. They must use a flotation device with the heat escape–lessening posture to stay afloat. The surviving flight team members should huddle together to decrease heat loss. The flight team should protect against salt and sun exposure by covering any exposed skin surface. Protection against exposure, care of the raft, and signaling are the primary objectives in open-water survival.

SURVIVAL IN THE DESERT

By following basic survival principles with education about heat illness and exposure, the flight team will be better able to survive in desert terrain. Water collection, insect precautions, snakebite treatment procedures, and shelter construction to protect flight team members from the sun are major topics to be covered in a complete desert terrain survival education program. Long-sleeve shirts and long pants should be worn, and complete head, neck, and eye protection is vital.

INTERNATIONAL SURVIVAL CONCERNS

Because flight nurses cross international boundaries, international survival concerns need to be addressed. Air medical team members should be aware of climates and terrain that will be flown over and at the final destination of the mission. Recognition of the need for additional survival equipment and food stores should be part of a complete preflight check. Preparation for customs, ports of entry, and passport checks is just the beginning for fixed-wing and rotor aircraft involved in international flights.

In Canada and Mexico complete flight plans are required for entrance into and departure from the country. The ELT and the emergency frequency 121.5 are used in Canada. However, in some countries search-and-rescue efforts are limited, and in many others they are nonexistent.

SURVIVAL EQUIPMENT

Survival equipment should be standard on every air medical aircraft. Specific service area, climate, type of aircraft, and time of year are considerations when survival gear is assembled. The survival gear should

BOX 10-1	**Basic Survival Kits**

Personal survival kit

Waterproof matches
Small flashlight
Sunglasses
Pocketknife
Compass
Parachute cord

Aircraft survival kit

Waterproof matches
Candle, dry tinder
Space blanket, tarps, tents, plastic poncho
Nylon cord, rope, duct tape
Mirror, signal flares, plastic whistle, flashlight
Canned smoke
Compass, knife, sunglasses, sunscreen
Water-purification tablets, insect repellant
Foodstuffs, appropriate additional clothing
Cooking kit, drinking cup, toilet paper
Sleeping bag, snowshoes, inflatable raft
Fishing kit, ax or saw, aluminum foil

be assembled and stored in a manner that affords easy access. Box 10-1 lists items to be included in basic survival kits.

REFERENCES

1. Air Training Command: *Air Force manual of search and rescue survival*, Washington, DC, 1962, Department of the Air Force.

2. Arnold M: Winter survival tactics, *Hosp Aviat* 5(10):14, 1986.

3. Benson K: Violence, trauma, and EMS, *J Emerg Services* 26(4):40, 1994.

4. Bush C: Emergency egress scenarios, *J Air Med Transport* 10(10):35, 1991.

5. Collett HM: Air medical accident rates: a historical look back at causes, *J Air Med Transport* 10(2):14, 1991.

6. Collins MH: Pre-designated landing zones, *Hosp Aviat* 7(6):6, 1988.

7. Commission on Accreditation of Medical Transport Systems: *Accreditation standards,* ed 5, Anderson, SC, 2001, Author.

8. Cooper LT: An administrator's perspective on managing safety, *J Air Med Transport* 10(3):15, 1991.

9. Crowley JS, Licina JR, Bruckart JE: Flight helmets: How they work and why you should wear one, *J Air Med Transport* 11(8):19, 1992.

10. Dolan J: Keep safe from tail rotor strikes, *J Air Med Transport* 9(2):9, 1990.

11. Drew K: Should a pregnant flight nurse be allowed to fly? *J Air Med Transport* 10(7):11, 1991.

12. Elling R: Dispelling myths on ambulance accidents, *J Emerg Serv* 7:1, 1989.

13. Frazer R: Operational quality assurance: a new concept defined, *J Air Med Transport* 10(3):19, 1991.

14. Frazer R: Air medical accidents: a 20 year search for information, *Air Med J* 8(5):33, 1999.

15. Frazer R: Weather accidents and the air medical industry, *Air Med J* 6(6):49, 2000.

16. Frazer R: Air medical accidents involving collision with objects, *Air Med J* 20(3):13, 2001.

17. Green B: Egress simulator, *Hosp Aviat* 8(7):28, 1989.

18. Hawkins M: Personal protective equipment in helicopter EMS, *Air Med J* 13(4):1123, 1994.

19. Holleran RS: Prehospital safety. In Holleran RS, editor: *Prehospital nursing: a collaborative approach,* St Louis, 1994, Mosby.

20. Homer S: Development of an air medical outreach program: practical applications, *Top Emerg Med* 16(4):45, 1994.

21. Jones K: Regional air medical safety committees, *J Air Med Transport* 9(9):44, 1990.

22. Kruppa RM: Air medical safety, a follow-up survey, *J Air Med Transport* 8(10):10, 1991.

23. Lillie J, Larsen B: Safety in the '90s, *J Air Med Transport* 10(2):16, 1991.

24. Limmer D: 10 commandments for EMS survival, *J Emerg Med Serv JEMS* 25(8):24, 2000.

25. Mason KT: Letter, *Air Med J* 13(6):242, 1994.

26. Mayberry RT: Medical air crew roles and responsibilities during aircraft emergencies, *Aero Med J* 3(4):16, 1988.

27. Militello PR, Ramzy AI: Safety by design, *J Air Med Transport* 9(8):15, 1990.

28. Moon T, Broome R: Air medical safety program, *Top Emerg Med* 16(4):31, 1994.

29. Mrochek P, Sorenson P: Missing aircraft: if disaster strikes, is your program prepared? *Air Med Transport* 8(12):17, 1989.

30. National Transportation Safety Board: Safety study commercial emergency medical service helicopter

operations, National Technical Information Service, NTSB/SS 1988, US Department of Commerce.

31. National Flight Nurses Association: *Improving flight nurse safety in the air medical helicopter environment*, Park Ridge, Ill, July 1998, NFNA.

32. Nordberg M: Listen up, *Emerg Med Serv* 22(4):35, 1993.

33. PHI Training Department: *Aeromedical crew member training manual*, Lafayette, La, 1994.

34. Preston N: 1991 Air medical helicopter accident rates, *J Air Med Transport* 11(2):14, 1992.

35. Ryan T, Studebaker B, Brennan G: Patient impression of the use of helmets by HEMS personnel, *J Air Med Transport* 11(10):65, 1992 (abstract).

36. Stinson WF: Forced water landing: a practice in survival, *J Air Med Transport* 9(1):23, 1990.

37. Wraa CE, O'Malley JO: Flight nurse physical requirements, *J Air Med Transport* 11(10):17, 1992.

38. Wright AE, Campos JA, Gorder T: The effect of an in-flight emergency training program on crew confidence, *Air Med J* 13(4):127, 1994.

11

PATIENT ASSESSMENT AND PREPARATION FOR TRANSPORT

1. Obtain initial, focused, and comprehensive subjective and objective data through history-taking, physical examination, review of records, pertinent laboratory values and radiographic/diagnostic studies, and communication with other health care providers, including prehospital and referring personnel.
2. Recognize and anticipate critical signs and symptoms related to the patient's illness or injury.
3. Perform critical patient interventions as indicated by the patient's illness or injury.
4. Prepare the patient for transport by ground or rotor or fixed-wing aircraft.
5. Identify and prepare for issues related to international transport.

The first half of this chapter presents an overview of patient assessment and preparation for transport, including identification of the indications for transport; communication; consent for transport; all the factors involved in performing a patient assessment; and steps that must be taken to prepare the patient for transport. The second half of this chapter discusses all issues pertinent to fixed-wing transport, including international transport.

The transport process begins with identification of the need to transfer a patient. In many cases this step has been initiated by members of the referring agency, such as prehospital care providers or health care providers in the transferring hospital.

Communication about the need for transport and the care the patient has received and will require from the transport team is an integral part of preparing the patient for transport. This communication begins before the transport team arrives, continues during transport, and concludes with patient follow-up information to the referring agency.

Performing a patient assessment provides the transport team with an opportunity to identify patient problems and what interventions are needed before transport. Patient assessment also allows the transport team to anticipate and prepare for events that may occur during transport.

Patient assessment and preparation for transport is composed of multiple elements, including primary and secondary assessment, performance of critical interventions, and dealing with specific problems such as pain management.

The transport environment may not always be conducive to performing all of the components of patient assessment and preparation. However, the transport team must be familiar with all of these components of patient assessment and preparation so that they can perform the appropriate interventions required for a safe and successful patient transport.

INDICATIONS FOR PATIENT TRANSPORT

Currently no universal agreement exists on what is an indication for transport. Numerous research studies have identified reasons to transport patients,* and national organizations have suggested indications for air medical transport, particularly rotor-wing transport.[1,3,32] In general the need to move or transfer a patient is based on the severity of the patient's illness or injury, time, distance, terrain, weather, need for nursing and medical expertise or diagnostic procedures not available at the referring health facility, and a request by the patient's family that the patient be transferred to another facility.[26]

TRAUMA PATIENTS

Numerous guidelines for air medical transport of trauma patients are available. The reason that air medical transport of trauma patients is commonly accepted is probably related to the history of helicopters, which were first used to transport injured patients from the battlefield and were subsequently used to transport trauma patients in the civilian population (*see* Chapter 1 for the history of air medical transport). In 1992 the National Association of Emergency Medical Services Physicians published extensive guidelines for air medical transport use.[44] Some indications for the use of air medical transport identified in these guidelines are listed in Appendix G. Scoring systems have also been used to determine

indications for patient transport. Some examples of these scoring systems are the trauma revised trauma score, the CRAMS score, the trauma triage rule, the Glasgow coma score, a Glasgow motor score (GMR) greater than 5, and the vehicular trauma checklist.

The American College of Surgeons (ACS)[3] continues to include recommendations for the transfer of injured patients in both their Advanced Trauma Life Support Course and their Resources for the Optimal Care of the Injured Patient. In addition, the ACS recommends that the trauma patient should no longer be transferred to the closest hospital, but to the closest appropriate hospital, preferably a verified trauma center (ACS, 1997). Some of the recommendations of the ACS are listed in Box 11-1.

PATIENTS WITH CARDIOVASCULAR AND MEDICAL EMERGENCIES

Even though most of the research related to the indications for transport involves trauma patients, some indications have been recognized for the patient with a cardiovascular emergency. These include the need for cardiac critical care that is not available at the referring facility, cardiac catheterization, treatment for cardiogenic shock that may include insertion of a balloon pump, mechanical assistance devices, experimental medications, and an organ transplant.[12,14,27] Research and case reports have demonstrated that patients with cardiovascular emergencies tolerate the transport process fairly and have benefited from it.[27]

Loos, Runyan, and Pelch[40] developed a Medical Classification Criteria Tool (MCCT) modeled on trauma classification tools to assist in determining the severity of illness and what resources may be needed to appropriately transport these patients. The advantages of using this tool included enhancement of communication between the referring and receiving facility and advanced notification of the severity of the patient's illness so that the receiving facility can be appropriately prepared. This tool could also be used to monitor the appropriateness of medical transfers. Box 11-2 details the Medical Classification Criteria Tool.

PREGNANT WOMEN AND NEONATES

Other patients who may require transfer and transport include pregnant women and neonatal patients. Indications for the transport of pregnant

---

* References 1, 4, 23, 26, 37, and 40.

<table>
<tr><td>BOX 11-1</td><td>ACS Indications for Transfer of the Injured Patient</td></tr>
</table>

Central Nervous System
- Penetrating injury or depressed skull fracture
- GCS >14 or deteriorating GCS
- Spinal cord injury

Chest
- Widened mediastinum
- Pulmonary contusion
- Patients who may require prolonged ventilation

Pelvis/Abdomen
- Unstable pelvic ring fracture
- Open pelvic fracture

Extremity
- Severe open fractures
- Traumatic amputation with potential for reimplantation
- Ischemic injury

Multisystem Trauma
- Injury to more than two body regions
- Major burns associated with multiple trauma
- Multiple proximal long bone fractures

Comorbid Factors
- Age >55 years
- Pediatric patients
- Cardiovascular disease
- Pulmonary disease
- Pregnancy

Secondary Deterioration
- Mechanical ventilation required
- Sepsis
- Multiple-organ system failure

ACS, American College of Surgeons; *GCS,* Glasgow coma score.

---

women include placenta previa, fetal distress, maternal trauma, prenatal complications, and perimortem delivery. Indications for the transport of neonates include the age and weight of the infant and neonatal illness and injury that cannot be appropriately cared for at the referring facility.[4,42]

APPROPRIATE PATIENT TRANSFER

In 1986 the Consolidated Omnibus Reconciliation Act (COBRA) was implemented. This legislation furnishes guidelines, regulations, and penalties that govern patient transfer and transport. The implications of this law and its recent revisions are discussed in Chapter 32.

When transporting an ill or injured patient, transport services should provide (1) a transport team with the experience necessary to perform an initial assessment and stabilize the patient before and during transport; (2) staff who are capable of using the equipment and technology necessary to deliver care during transport to specific groups of patients, such as the critically ill or injured; and (3) the ability to demonstrate that the transport will make a difference in patient outcome.[1-4,13,15,16]

The American College of Emergency Physicians has developed guidelines for appropriate transfer and transport of ill or injured patients. These guidelines are summarized in Box 11-3. In addition, the American College of Critical Care Medicine has proposed its own recommendations for the transport of critically ill or injured patients. Box 11-4 contains a summary of these guidelines, which address both interhospital and intrahospital transport of patients. Box 11-5 provides recommendations from the Air Medical Physician Association (AMPA) for air medical transport in acute coronary syndromes.

Finally, in 1995 the Emergency Nurses Association (ENA) developed a document (revised in 1998) that provides guidelines for the transport of ill or injured children. Unlike the documents previously mentioned, this document specifically addresses the needs of the ill or injured child. These guidelines are available from the ENA.

MAKING THE DECISION TO TRANSPORT

Several factors must be considered by referring personnel when they are deciding whether to transport a patient. The first factor to be considered is the appropriateness of transport, which was previously discussed. Identification of a suitable receiving facility is a second factor that must be considered. When choosing a receiving facility, referring personnel

---

BOX 11-2	Medical Classification Criteria Tool

Staff for Life Helicopter Service University of Missouri Hospital and Clinics

Code blue: Cardiopulmonary arrest (nontraumatic source)

Class I: Life-threatening illness and/or unstable vital signs

    A. Unstable airway

        Acute respiratory distress (i.e., acute pulmonary edema, unconscious patient, patient requires recent intubation)

    B. Patient requires ventilatory support (oxygen saturation <80% via pulse oximetry)

    C. Circulatory instability

        Clinical signs and symptoms of shock

        Symptomatic hypotension <90 mm Hg systolic

        Symptomatic hypertension >200 mm Hg systolic or >110 diastolic

        Unstable/symptomatic cardiac rhythms

        Uncontrolled chest pain

        S/P arrest

        Therapies to include but not limited to:

        • Transvenous pacer

        • Intraaortic balloon pump

        • External pacer

        • Vasopressor administration

    D. GCS <8 (i.e., acute mental status changes, status epilepticus)

Class II: Potentially life-threatening illness, but vital signs currently stable

    A. Controlled pulmonary disease

    B. Controlled/decreasing chest pain

    C. Controlled acute cardiac dysrhythmias

    D. S/P new-onset seizures

    E. Vascular disorders

    F. Thrombolytic therapy

    G. Previously Class I patient who has been stabilized with treatment

    H. GCS = 9-12

Class III: No obvious life-threatening illness and vital signs stable

From Loos L, Runyan L, Pelch D: Development of prehospital medical classification criteria, *Air Med J* 17(1):14, 1998.

---

must look at the resources available at the receiving facility, such as specialized care staff, equipment, and expertise. The location of the receiving facility is also an important consideration.

Another factor that should be considered when deciding whether to transport a patient involves the existence of written policies and agreements among the receiving and referring agencies. The identification of centers that are capable of providing certain types of services and generating triage guidelines could save precious time.

COMMUNICATION

Communication is probably one of the most important components in the preparation of the patient for transport. Communications center operations are discussed in Chapter 9. This discussion will focus on the communication process among personnel at the referring and receiving agencies (either a health care facility or an emergency medical services [EMS] agency).

Communication should begin before the transport team arrives. Written policies, procedures, and

---

BOX 11-3	**American College of Emergency Physicians Guidelines for Transfer and Transport of Injured or Ill Patients**

1. The health and well-being of the patient must be the overriding concerns when any patient transport is considered.
2. The patient should be evaluated before transfer.
3. The referring personnel should stabilize the patient (to the extent possible) before transport.
4. The patient and patient's family should be informed about the reasons for and the risks of transport.
5. The patient should be transferred to a facility that is appropriate to the medical needs of the patient and that has adequate space and available personnel.
6. The receiving facility must agree to accept the patient.
7. Economic reasons should not be the basis for transferring a patient to a receiving facility or refusing to admit a patient at a receiving facility.
8. Information about the patient's condition and initial care must be communicated to the receiving facility.
9. The patient should be transferred in a vehicle that is staffed by quality personnel and that contains the equipment necessary to provide appropriate treatment for the patient who is being transferred.
10. When possible, written protocols and transfer agreements should be in place.

From American College of Emergency Physicians: Principles of appropriate transfer, *Ann Emerg Med* 3:337, 1990.

BOX 11-4	**Summary of American College of Critical Care Medicine Guidelines for the Transport of the Critically Ill or Injured Patient**

1. The benefits of transferring the patient should outweigh the risks.
2. The practitioner needs to be aware of the legal implications of patient transfer and transport.
3. Before the patient is transported, physicians and nurses at the referring and receiving facilities should be in contact, a decision should be made about the mode of transportation to be used, and a copy of all medical records relevant to the patient's care should be secured.
4. Accompanying transport personnel should include a minimum of two patient care providers and a vehicle operator. At least one care provider should be a registered nurse.
5. The equipment (including monitors) and medications necessary to manage the patient's airway, breathing, and circulation should be available. Communication equipment used during transport should also be available.
6. Continuous monitoring should take place during transport. At a minimum, ECG monitoring and monitoring of vital signs are required. Patients with specific problems may require additional monitoring, such as capnography and invasive monitoring.

Modified from the Guidelines Committee of the American College of Critical Care Medicine Society of Critical Care Medicine and the Transfer Guidelines Task Force of the American Association of Critical Care Nurses: *Guidelines for the transport of the critically ill patient*, 1997.

---

triage guidelines should be in place at the referring agency. These documents should address the type of patient who should be transferred and by what mode of transportation, the care that is required before transport, and the steps that need to be taken by the referring agency to prepare for the arrival of the transport vehicle. For example, if a helicopter will be transporting the patient, where will it land, who will meet it, and who will monitor it while the team prepares the patient for transport?

When initial contact has been made by the referring agency, information that should be provided for the transport team includes the patient's chief complaint, the indications for transport, interventions and their effects, and the patient's current condition. The reason why the patient needs transfer should be

BOX 11-5   Appropriateness of Air Medical Transport in Acute Coronary Syndromes

Position Statement of The Air Medical Physician Association
Approved by the AMPA Board of Trustees November 10, 2001

Background

Acute coronary syndromes and common reasons to utilize air medical transport. Regionalization of cardiac care to highly specialized centers, increasing use of invasive and time sensitive therapies, and efforts to minimize both the absolute time to therapy and the dangerous out of hospital time are significant drivers in improving cardiac care and for increasing the utilization of air medical transport.

AMPA Position Statement

AMPA supports the use of air medical transport for adult patients with acute coronary syndromes requiring or potentially requiring urgent/time-sensitive intervention not available at the sending facility.

As outlined by the American Heart Association, acute coronary syndromes represents the spectrum of clinical disease presenting with syndromes ranging from unstable angina to Q-wave and non-Q-wave myocardial infarctions.

It is AMPA's position that the determination for the need for urgent/time-sensitive interventions is made by a physician, as documented on a written Certification of Medical Necessity.

Furthermore, AMPA acknowledges that scene air medical transport of acute coronary syndromes occurs routinely and supports that the medical necessity is determined by the requesting authorized provider based on regional policy and their best medical judgment at the time of the request for transport. AMPA supports that a receiving physician or the transport program medical director may complete the Certificate of Medical Necessity on scene transports.

AMPA does not support the use of discharge ICD-9 codes or other methodologies that retrospectively determine medical appropriateness of acute coronary syndromes as this may adversely restrict access to appropriate care and may contradict the intent of EMTALA regulations. AMPA also believes that retrospective determination of medical appropriateness also negates the regional, environmental, level of prehospital care, and situational issues that are important factors at the time of transport in determining medical appropriateness for air medical transport in acute and potentially acute coronary syndromes.

clearly identified and documented. Some transport programs require signed documentation before they will transfer the patient because of recent reimbursement issues, particularly from Medicare.

It is important to relay the patient's problem, age, and location so the most suitable transport team can be sent to provide care for the patient. For example, some areas of the United States have transport teams specifically designed to provide care for pregnant women, children, and critical care patients. The equipment required by the patient's illness or injury might influence the clinical skills that may be needed during transport (e.g., an intraaortic balloon pump requires personnel who are trained in its use in the transport environment).

Once the transport team arrives, they can obtain any information about the patient directly from the staff at the referring agency. When the transport team members arrive at the scene, they should identify the person in charge and offer assistance.

During the initial assessment and preparation of the patient for transport, transport team members will communicate with referring individuals. The communication process is composed of both verbal and nonverbal behaviors, and one's attitude is an important intervention. Thus the transport team should always involve those who have been caring for the patient.

Any laboratory results and radiographic and diagnostic study results should be copied and sent with the patient. Technology continues to make some paperwork easier to transfer. For example, radiographic and diagnostic study results may be transmitted by means of telemedicine before the patient leaves the receiving facility. If the patient has any valuables, they must be accounted for. Sometimes it is easier to leave valuables with a family member, but this may not be possible.

Recording a list of what was brought with the patient and to whom it was given on arrival at the receiving facility may prevent problems. Clothing or other valuables are sometimes considered evidence and should be treated as such on the basis of evidence protocols.

CONSENT

Patients must consent to treatment. However, it is not always possible to obtain written or verbal consent for transport and for emergency treatment directly from the patient or family. Consent for transport is usually implied. Implied consent is considered to be given only in an emergency situation, when the patient is incapacitated and is in a life-threatening situation.[15]

Even though the patient's consent is implied, the transport team should always explain to the patient and available family members all procedures and the transport process. If family members are available, they may be able to provide consent for treatment. If consent forms are part of the transport documentation, the transport team should ensure that they are transported with the patient.

A TWENTY-FIRST CENTURY PATIENT TRANSPORT CHALLENGE

Over the past few years the closing of hospitals, the decrease in nursing and other health care providers, and the lack of funds to provide health care have created a unique crisis that has grave implications to patient transport.[56] Many facilities that in the past accepted patients without question have now adopted diversion policies. This means a decrease in available beds, longer waits for transfer, refusal of some patients, and diversion. The American College of Emergency Physicians has developed Guidelines for Ambulance Diversion.[10] Box 11-6 contains a summary of these guidelines.

Transport programs need to ensure that the patient has a receiving facility. Diversion notification should also include all services that provide patient transport to prevent any undue delay in patient transfer and transport.

PERFORMING A PATIENT ASSESSMENT

Primary and secondary assessment, identification of patient problems, and initiation of critical interventions provide a framework for preparing a patient for transport. Each of these tasks must be performed in an organized, rapid, and complete manner. It is important to note that patient assessment is a continuous process that occurs before, during, and after transport.

ASSESSMENT OF THE PATIENT IN THE PREHOSPITAL CARE ENVIRONMENT

Assessment of the patient in the prehospital care environment can be an intense challenge. The location of the patient (e.g., trapped in a vehicle) (Figure 11-1), the limited availability of personnel and

---

BOX 11-6   Guidelines for Ambulance Diversion

- Identify situations in which a hospital's resources are not available (critical care beds, nursing staff) and temporary diversion is required.
- EMS systems and hospital personnel must be notified of such occurrences, and the notification must occur through a lead EMS agency or designated communication coordination center.
- The hospital's diversion status must be regularly reviewed.
- Policies and resources need to be in place to provide for the safe, appropriate, and timely care of patients who continue to enter the EMS system during the period of diversion.
- The EMS system and other appropriate personnel should be notified when the diversion status has changed.
- Explore solutions that address the causes of diversion and implement policies that minimize the need for diversions.
- Continuously review polices and guidelines governing diversion.

Modified from Brennan J: *Guidelines for ambulance diversion,* American College of Emergency Physicians, Irving, Tex, 1999, American College of Emergency Physicians.
EMS, Emergency medical service.

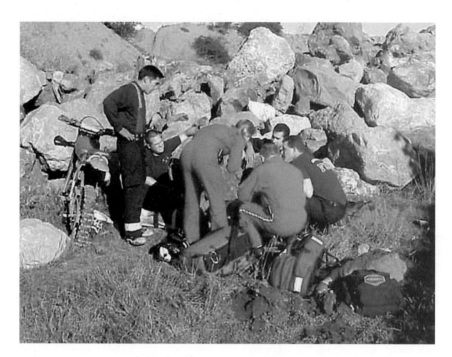

FIGURE 11-1   **It is difficult to perform primary and secondary assessments depending on patient location.** (Courtesy, Stanford Life Flight.)

equipment, and the nature of the illness or injury the patient has sustained present potential barriers to performing prehospital patient assessment.

The environment in which the patient is located poses additional barriers to assessment. Noise, a lack of light and space, vehicle movement and the speed at which the vehicle is moving, and outside weather can make normal assessment maneuvers such as auscultation difficult to perform.

The type of vehicle used to transport the patient may also pose a barrier to patient assessment. Assessing patients in ground, helicopter, or fixed-wing vehicles can be troublesome. Even though equipment is now more portable, some pieces of equipment are still susceptible to movement and vibrations that could affect their reliability when they are used for patient assessment. Noise hampers patient assessment no matter what mode of transport may be used.

SCENE ASSESSMENT

Assessment of the patient before he or she reaches the hospital begins with assessment of the scene,

whether the transport team will be responding directly to the patient or to another facility. The transport team should assess the surrounding environment for hazards. Box 11-7 contains a summary of some of the hazards that may be encountered.

On arrival at the referring facility, the transport team should survey the resources that are available to assist in preparing the patient for transport. Equipment and supplies necessary for patient stabilization may be limited, and thus it may be necessary for the team to bring additional equipment.

The principles of patient assessment used by the transport team are no different than those used when patients are assessed within the walls of a hospital. However, the prehospital environment dictates that the assessment be organized, direct, and rapid. Adaptation and flexibility are necessary when patient assessment is performed outside the hospital. Tight spaces, lack of light, noise, and equipment that may or may not be functioning can present challenges to patient assessment in the prehospital care environment.

BOX 11-7 | Potential Environmental Hazards

Hazards at the Scene

Wires
Uneven ground
Vehicles
Accident itself
People
Signs
Light poles
Water
Loose debris

Hazards at the Referring Facility

Buildings
Wires
People

HISTORY

Patient assessment begins with obtaining a history as the primary assessment is being performed. The history of the illness or injury provides a guide for performing critical interventions, preparing the patient for transport, and ongoing assessment during transport and also alerts the transport team to problems that may develop during transport. For example, the situation of a patient who has suffered multiple rib fractures who will be flown will alert the transport team to the potential for the development of a tension pneumothorax.

Generally the transport team is given some information while en route to the patient. However, experience has demonstrated that the situation on arrival may be quite different than that described beforehand.

GENERAL PRINCIPLES OF HISTORY GATHERING

According to Henry and Stapleton,[32] "history is the patient's story of significant events related to and surrounding the present problem." Some general principles should be followed when gathering information related to the patient's illness or injury. One of these principles is that the patient's chief complaint or problem should be identified. If the patient is unable to provide this information, the transport team may obtain it from others at the scene (prehospital care providers, police, or bystanders), referring personnel (nurses or physicians), or any persons who may be with the patient. A survey of the scene by the transport team can also provide valuable information about what may have happened. If the patient is unconscious, the transport team should look for medic alert jewelry, syringes, medications, pill bottles, or information in the patient's wallet or purse.

A common mnemonic used to collect general history information is AMPLE:

A   Allergies, alcohol, or substance abuse

M   Medications including immunizations, particularly when obtaining a pediatric history

P   Past medical history including illnesses, injuries

L   Last meal or intake

E   Events leading to the emergency. Everything that has been done before the arrival of the transport team

If the patient's chief complaint or problem is related to pain, the PQRST method will be of use when collecting information on history. PQRST[29,32,37] represents the following:

P   Provoking factors: What caused or causes the pain? Does anything relieve the pain or make it worse? What was the patient doing when the pain began?

Q   Quality of the pain: Some of the words used to describe the pain may provide the nurse with clues to the origin of the pain. For example, patients who describe chest pain often use words such as "burning" or "crushing."

R   Region and radiation: The patient should be asked to point to the area where he or she feels pain. Pain patterns can provide the transport team with clues to the cause of the patient's pain and may help guide the management of the patient's pain.

S   Severity: Numbering, such as from 1 to 10, can be used to describe the severity of the pain.

T   Time: The patient should be asked to describe the temporal nature of the pain, such as how long it has been present and when or at what time of day it began

The transport team may find it difficult to obtain a history in the prehospital care environment because of obstacles such as the patient's inability to communicate because of illness or injury, the lack of witnesses to a particular event, and the absence of family members or significant others at the scene of the illness or injury.

When possible, and particularly when the patient is being transported from a referring facility, as much information as possible should be collected and communicated with the receiving facility. At other times, particularly when patients are transported directly from the scene, this may not be possible. The transport team should keep in mind that history provides key information. History will also alert the nurse to problems that may develop during transport.

TRAUMA HISTORY

History gathering is different for the trauma patient than it is for the patient with a medical illness. The mechanism of injury generally triggers the trauma history. The transport team must find out in what manner, when, where, and how the patient was injured. A complete description of the event is often limited. However, a general idea of the mechanism of injury will provide clues regarding additional injuries and complications that may occur during transport. Box 11-8 describes predictable injuries that may occur as a result of motor vehicle crashes, an example of taking a trauma history.[23,26,32]

In recent years instant photographs, video recorders, and digital camera have been used to provide information about the mechanism of injury. Dickinson, Krett, and O'Connor[19] reported that when photography was used to provide details related to a motor vehicle crash, receiving physicians altered their perceptions about the patient's injuries in 46% of the cases. In addition, the receiving physician upgraded the severity of the motor vehicle crash after viewing the photographs in 22 of 26 cases (85%).

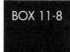

BOX 11-8   **Predictable Injuries Resulting From Motor Vehicle Crashes**

Unrestrained Driver
Head injuries
Facial injuries
Fractured larynx
Fractured sternum
Cardiac contusion
Lacerated liver or spleen
Lacerated great vessels
Fractured patella and femur
Fractured clavicle

Restrained Driver
Caused by a lap restraint
Pelvic injuries
Spleen, liver, and pancreas injuries
Caused by a shoulder restraint
Cervical fractures
Rupture of mitral valve or diaphragm

Modified from McSwai N, Frame S, Salomone J: *Basic and advanced prehospital trauma life support,* ed 5, St Louis, 2003, Mosby.

When obtaining the history of a trauma patient, the transport team should also gather information that describes the scene of the crash. Did the accident involve multiple victims? Are all of the victims accounted for? If the on-scene patients are unable to provide information about additional patients, the presence of schoolbooks, clothing, or toys may suggest that additional victims are present.[13]

HISTORY RELATED TO MEDICAL ILLNESS

A patient's medical history begins with the chief complaint or current problem. The PQRST mnemonic previously described can be of assistance when obtaining a medical history. The transport team should obtain history related to the present illness, including related signs and symptoms. Significant medical history and risk factors for a particular disease process (such as smoking and chronic obstructive pulmonary disease) can provide additional pieces of meaningful information.

Information about current medications should be provided. Drug interactions or the effects of not taking a scheduled medication may cause additional problems during transport.

Information about care initiated before the arrival of the transport team must be gathered. These data[29,32] should include initial physical findings, initial treatments and results, vital sign trends, medications given, laboratory results, radiographic/diagnostic study findings, ECG interpretation, intravenous infusions given, intake and output, and status of family notification.

DIVERSITY ASSESSMENT

Even though the focus of patient care during the transport process is generally on critical needs, their age, class, culture, ethnicity, sex, nationality, race, religion, and sexual orientation will influence their response to illness and injury. The transport team must take into consideration these factors when providing care and respect and, when possible, adapt their care to include the impact of their diversity on their response to their illness, injuries, and the need to be transported.[22]

It is impossible to be aware and knowledgeable about the diversity of patients. However, not ignoring that there are multiple factors that influence a patient's response to illness and injury can make the

transport process a little less stressful for the patient, their family, and the transport team.

In 1997 the Emergency Nurses Association developed a Diversity Practice Model that can assist in approaching patient diversity.[22] The components of this model are summarized in Table 11-1. The use of this model may offer some added patient care information and help us recognize what makes us different and the same.

PRIMARY ASSESSMENT AND CRITICAL INTERVENTIONS

Primary assessment is based on assessment of the patient's airway, breathing, circulation, neurologic disability, and exposure. During the primary assessment, as patient problems are identified, critical interventions are initiated. The basic steps remain the same whether at a scene or an interfacility transport.

AIRWAY

The patient's airway is assessed to determine whether it is patent, maintainable, or not maintainable. For any patient who is suspected of having a traumatic injury, cervical spine precautions are used while the airway is evaluated. Assessment of the patient's level of consciousness, in concert with assessment of the airway status, provides the transport team with an

TABLE 11-1   The Diversity Practice Model

A	Assumption	What do we assume or take for granted about this individual or the community that they come from?
B	Beliefs or behaviors	How does my belief system affect the care I provide for this patient?
		Are my beliefs mirrored in the way I behave toward the patient? For example, a patient who may not have bathed for a long period of time may be viewed as homeless.
C	Communication	How does the patient communicate? Do they speak English? If not, is there a translator available? Can the patient hear, see? Has the patient suffered an injury such as a stroke that impairs their ability to communicate or understand?
D	Diversity or identification of how the patient differs	Some diversity is visible, such as skin color, age, or ethnic background. Some is invisible, such as sexual orientation or class.
E	Education Ethics	Education involves learning about the patient's diversity. Ethical decisions are influenced by one's diversity.

Emergency Nurses Association Diversity Task Force: *Approaching diversity: an interactive journey.* Des Plaines, Ill, 1997, Author.

BOX 11-9	Summary of Primary Airway Assessment

- Airway: patent, maintainable, nonmaintainable
- Level of consciousness
- Skin appearance: ashen, pale, gray, cyanotic, or mottled
- Preferred posture to maintain airway
- Airway clearance
- Sounds of obstruction

BOX 11-10	Summary of Primary Breathing Assessment

- Rate and depth of respirations
- Cyanosis
- Position of the trachea
- Presence of obvious injury or deformity
- Work of breathing
- Use of accessory muscles
- Flaring of nostrils
- Presence of breath sounds bilaterally
- Presence of adventitious breath sounds
- Asymmetric chest movements
- Palpation of crepitus

impression of the effectiveness of the patient's current airway status (Box 11-9).

If an airway problem is identified, the appropriate intervention should be started. The decision to use a particular intervention will depend on the nature of the patient's problem and the potential for complications during transport. Airway interventions are addressed in Chapter 12. Supplemental oxygen should be given to all patients before transport. Specific equipment such as a pulse oximeter or CO_2 detector will help provide continuous airway evaluation during transport. The indications and the procedures for use of these devices are included in Chapter 12.

Pharmacologic Adjuncts for Airway Management. Specific pharmacologic agents have been found to be useful in prehospital airway management. These agents include those that provide sedation and amnesia and neuromuscular blocking agents that facilitate intubation. An in-depth discussion of the use of these medications is provided in Chapter 12.

It is important for transport team members to remember when these medications are used, particularly if the patient received neuromuscular blocking agents—then they are totally dependent on the transport team. Measures to ensure patient safety and comfort, including keeping the patient warm and providing sedation and analgesia, must be provided by the team during transport.

BREATHING

The assessment of ventilation begins with noting whether the patient is breathing; if the patient is

breathing, the work of ventilation should begin. If the patient is apneic or in severe respiratory distress, immediate interventions are indicated. If the patient is having any difficulty with ventilation, the transport team must identify the problem and proceed with the appropriate interventions. Emergent interventions may include decompression with a needle or insertion of a chest tube (Box 11-10). Ventilation interventions are discussed in Chapters 12 and 16.

CIRCULATION

Palpation of both the peripheral and the central pulse provides information about the patient's circulatory status. The quality, location, and rate of the patient's pulses should be noted. The temperature of the patient's skin can be assessed along with the pulses. Observation of the level of consciousness will help evaluate the patient's perfusion (Box 11-11).

Active bleeding should be quickly controlled with interventions such as direct pressure. The transport team should observe the patient for indications of circulatory compromise. Skin color, diaphoresis, and capillary refill are appraised during circulatory assessment.

Intravenous access is obtained for administration of fluid, blood, and medications. Depending on the patient's location and the accessibility of veins, peripheral, central, or intraosseous access may be used. Fluid resuscitation must be guided by the patient's response.

BOX 11-11	**Summary of Primary Circulation Assessment**

- Pulse rate and quality
- Skin appearance—color
- Peripheral pulses
- Skin temperature
- Level of consciousness
- Urinary output
- Blood pressure
- Cardiac monitor
- Invasive monitor

DISABILITY: NEUROLOGIC ASSESSMENT

Neurologic assessment includes assessment of the level of consciousness; the size, shape, and response of the pupil; and motor sensory function. The following simple method may be used to evaluate the patient's level of consciousness; it is called the AVPU method:

A Alert
V Responds to verbal stimuli
P Responds to painful stimuli
U Unresponsive

Both the Glasgow and Pediatric Glasgow Coma Scales provide assessment of the patient's level of consciousness and motor function.[37]

If the patient has an altered mental status, the transport team needs to determine whether the patient has ingested any toxic substances such as alcohol or other drugs or may be hypoxic because of illness or injury. A patient with an altered mental status may pose a safety problem during transport. Use of chemical paralysis, sedation, or physical restraints may be required to ensure safe transport.

EXPOSURE

As much of the patient's body as possible should be exposed for examination, keeping in mind the effects of the environment on the patient. Discovering hidden problems before the patient is loaded for transport allows the transport team to intervene and prevent potentially disastrous complications. Although exposure for examination has been emphasized most

BOX 11-12	**Summary of Exposure Assessment**

- Appropriate tube placement: endotracheal tubes, nasotracheal tubes, chest tubes, nasogastric or orogastric tubes, and urinary catheters
- Intravenous access: peripheral, central, and intraosseous
- Identification of injury; active bleeding; indication of a serious illness such as presence of purpura

frequently in the care of the trauma patient, it is just as important in the primary assessment of the patient with a medical illness.

Team members should always look under dressings or clothing, which may "hide" complications or potential problems. Intravenous access can be wrongly assumed underneath a bulky cover. Clothing can also hide bleeding that occurs as a result of thrombolytic therapy (Box 11-12).

Once patient assessment has been completed, the patient needs to be kept warm. Hypothermia can cause cardiac arrhythmias, increased stress response, and hypoxia. Medications such as neuromuscular blocking agents interfere with the patient's ability to maintain a stable body temperature.

Preventing hypothermia should be considered a critical intervention, and methods to decrease the risk of heat loss initiated during the primary assessment should be initiated by the transport team. These include the following[31]:

- Covering the patient with blankets or an insulated layer
- Limiting exposure when examinations are required
- Keeping the patient away from metal during transport or anything that may draw heat away from the patient
- Shielding the patient from wind rotor wash
- Using oxygen and intravenous fluids

EQUIPMENT ASSESSMENT

Even though the concept of equipment assessment has not been routinely included in previous descriptions of primary assessment, it is an important process that must be performed. Before the patient is transported, the transport team should ensure that the patient is wearing an appropriately sized cervical collar, that the chest tube drainage system is functioning, and that the patient is correctly restrained. This assessment of equipment will help prevent problems during transport that could potentially leave the patient at risk for further injury.

SECONDARY ASSESSMENT

Whether a secondary assessment can be performed depends on the patient's condition and the amount of time needed for transport. Lack of space in the transport vehicle, lack of light, and noise may interfere with the transport team's ability to perform a secondary assessment during transport.

Secondary assessment involves evaluating the patient from head to toe.[6] Patient data are collected by means of inspection, palpation, and auscultation during secondary assessment. Whether the patient has suffered an injury or is critically ill, the evaluator should observe, touch, and listen to the patient.

Secondary assessment begins with an evaluation of the patient's general appearance. The transport team should observe the surrounding environment and evaluate its effects on the patient. Is the patient aware of the environment? Is there appropriate interaction between the patient and the environment?

Additional systems that should be assessed include the integumentary (color, presence of wounds, tem-

---

BOX 11-13   Summary of Secondary Assessment

Skin
- Presence of petechia, purpura, abrasions, bruises, scars, birthmarks
- Rashes
- Abnormal skin turgor
- Signs of abuse and neglect

Head and Neck
- Presence of lacerations, contusions, raccoon eyes, Battle's sign, or drainage from the nose, mouth, and ears
- In the infant, examination of the anterior fontanelle
- Gross visual examination
- Abnormal extraocular movements
- Position of the trachea
- Neck veins
- Swallowing difficulties
- Nuchal rigidity
- Presence of lymphadenopathy or neck masses

Eyes, Ears, Nose
- Lack of tearing
- Sunken eyes
- Color of the sclera
- Drainage
- Gross assessment of hearing

Mouth and Throat
- Mucous membranes
- Breath odor
- Injuries to teeth

- Drooling
- Drainage

Thorax, Lungs, Cardiovascular System
- Breath sounds
- Heart sounds

Abdomen
- Shape and size
- Bowel sounds
- Tenderness
- Firmness
- Masses (e.g., suprapubic mass)
- Femoral pulses
- Pelvic tenderness
- Color of drainage from nasogastric or orogastric tube

Genitourinary
- Blood at meatus
- Rectal bleeding
- Color of urine in catheter

Extremities and Back
- Gross motor and sensory function
- Peripheral pulses
- Lack of use of an extremity
- Deformity, angulation
- Wounds, abrasions
- Equipment is appropriately applied (e.g., traction splints)
- Vertebral column, flank, buttock

perature); head and neck (deformities, crepitus, pain); eyes, ears, and nose (drainage); thorax and lungs (chest movement and heart and breath sounds); abdomen; genitourinary; and extremities and back (Box 11-13).

PAIN ASSESSMENT

Determination of the amount of pain the patient is experiencing as a result of illness or injury is an important component of patient assessment. Physiologic indicators of pain include uncontrolled respi... tension, hyper-... diaphoresis. ...ing, protective ...cusing.*

...the pain the ...fectiveness of ...ng transport.

...d to identify ...that was not ...as patients ...trauma cen-...field and for ...interfacility ...monly been ...ems include ...Scale Score, ...'s Trauma ...e regarding ...be used for

...aration for ...ut patient preparation are contained in the clinical care sections of this book. The patient is prepared for transport on the basis of information obtained from the primary and secondary assessment, the type of vehicle the patient will be transported in, the amount of time the transport will take, and the problems that may develop in relation to the patient's illness or injury during transport. Patient preparation includes anticipatory planning; preparing for potential patient problems makes patient care easier and safer.

Over the past 20 years, technology has markedly improved transport equipment. Continenza and Hill[16] recommend that the equipment meet the following criteria:

- It should be useful in the transport setting.
- It should be lightweight, portable, and perhaps fulfill several functions (Figure 11-2).
- It should be easy to clean and maintain.
- It should have a battery life or power source that will last the length of the transport.
- It should have the ability to be used both inside and outside the transport vehicle.
- It should be able to withstand the stresses of transport, such as movement, altitude changes, being dropped, water or fluid contamination, weather changes, and use by multiple persons.

Box 11-14 contains a generic list of equipment that may be used during transport. The types of patients cared for dictate the amount and type of equipment carried by each service.

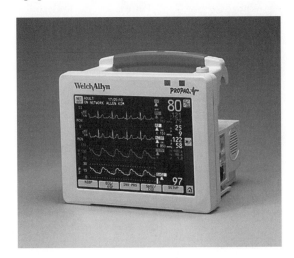

FIGURE 11-2 **An example of a multifunctional monitor.** (Courtesy of Welch Allyn Monitoring, Beaverton, Oregon.)

*References 6, 7, 38, 43, 50, and 53.

BOX 11-14	**Equipment for Transport**

A comprehensive list of equipment that needs to be stocked by transport services consists of a core set of supplies. The following equipment list serves as a guide, but it must be upgraded for special patient considerations and streamlined in the event of cost constraints.

1. Airway equipment
   Resuscitation bags (infant, child, adult)
   All sizes of masks for bag-valve-mask ventilation
   Nonrebreather masks
     Pediatric
     Adult
   Nasal cannula
   Oral and NP airways
   Nebulizer setup
   Portable suction unit
   Tonsil suction
   Suction catheters in the following sizes: 5/6, 8, 10, 14 and 18 Fr
   Magill forceps (pediatric and adult)
   Laryngoscope handles (pediatric and adult)
   Laryngoscope blades in the following sizes:
     Miller 0, 1, 2, and 3
     MAC 2, 3, and 4
   Spare laryngoscope batteries and bulbs
   Endotracheal tubes

Uncuffed		Cuffed		Endotrol
2.5	4.0	5.5	7.0	7.0
3.0	4.5	6.0	7.5	8.0
3.5	5.0	6.5	8.0	

   Stylets
   Benzoin, adhesive tape, and tracheostomy tape
   End-tidal CO_2 monitor
   PEEP valve
   Pulse oximeter
   Ventilator and filter and spirometer
   Cricothyrotomy tray
   Tracheostomy tubes
   Needle cricothyrotomy setup
   Gastric tubes in sizes 5 to 18
   Catheter tip syringe
   Surgilube
2. Cardiothoracic equipment
   Cardiac monitor and supplies, including extra batteries

Defibrillator and supplies, including adult and pediatric paddles
Defibrillator pads
Multipurpose pads (defibrillator/pacer)
External pacer and supplies
Transvenous pulse generator and cable
Noninvasive blood pressure monitor
Manual blood pressure equipment (pediatric, adult, and obese)
Doppler
Pressure monitor and transducer and tubing kit
MAST pants (depends on state regulations)
Thoracotomy tray and drainage system
Chest tubes in sizes 12 Fr to 36 Fr
Chest tube dressing
Needle decompression supplies
Pericardiocentesis setup
Multiple adapters (Sims, connectors, small and large Y)

3. Intravenous access equipment
   Intravenous solutions based on local protocols
   Blood tubing
   Minidrip tubing
   Extension tubing
   Intravenous needles (24 to 14 ga)
   Butterfly needles (27 to 19 ga)
   Intraosseous needles (15 and 18 ga)
   Rapid-infusion catheters
   Triple lumen catheter set-up
   Syringes of multiple sizes
   Intravenous start packs
   Razors
   Arm boards
   Laboratory blood tubes
   Stopcocks
   Pressure bag
   Intravenous controllers or pumps and setup
   Blood products and blood cooler
4. Medications
   ACLS medications
   Antianginal agents
   Antiarrhythmics
   Anticonvulsants
   Antiemetics
   Antihistamines
   Antihypertensives
   Diuretics

BOX 11-14	Equipment for Transport—cont'd

4. Medications—cont'd
   Local anesthetics
   Narcotics
   Nasal decongestant
   Neuromuscular blocking agents
   Steroids
   Tocolytics
   Vasopressor agents
5. Miscellaneous
   Oxygen
   Stethoscope
   Standard Precautions equipment
   Infectious waste management receptacles
   Sharp object safety boxes
   Instruments
      Bandage scissors
      Trauma scissors
      Hemostats
      Ring-cutter
   Tape
   Betadine solution
   Dressing supplies (4 × 4s, elastic, bandages, cravats)
   Eye shields
   Burn cable and electrodes
   Cervical collars
   Cervical immobilization device
   Pediatric transport board
   Car seat
   Isolette
   Obstetrics delivery tray
   Bubble bag

Stockinette cap
Stuffed toys
Pediatric dosage calculation references
Soft or leather restraints
Linen, blankets, towels
Flashlight
Cellular telephone
Two-way radio
Thermometer
Camera: instant, digital, video recorder
Documents
Directions and map to receiving facilities
Additional equipment specific to a particular type of service may include the following:
Ambulance
   Immobilization devices (because space and weight are less of a consideration in an ambulance than in a helicopter or fixed-wing aircraft)
   Backboard
   Traction splint
   Vacuum splints
Helicopter
   Ear protection for the patient and crew
   Survival bag stocked with necessary equipment in the event of an emergency landing
Fixed-wing aircraft
   Certain bulk supplies (because of extended transport times)
   Intravenous solutions, medication
   Food and drink for the crew
   Patient "comfort kit" (e.g., bedpan, urinal, urinary catheter)

ACLS, Advanced cardiac life support; *Fr*, French; *ga*, gauge; *NP*, nasopharyngeal airway; *PEEP*, positive end-expiratory pressure

AIRWAY MANAGEMENT

Patient preparation begins with assessment and management of the patient's airway. The location of the patient may limit the type of airway management the team will be able to provide. For example, if a patient is trapped in a vehicle, the team may have limited access for airway management.

Factors that may influence the decision about how to manage the airway include the nature of the patient's illness or injury, the amount of time the transport will take, the room available in the transport vehicle, and the positioning of the crew in the transport vehicle.

If intubation has already been performed, tube placement and security should be evaluated. An unsecured endotracheal tube may inadvertently come out during transport. In addition, movement of the endotracheal tube can cause mucosal damage, induce gagging and coughing, and increase the patient's intracranial or intraocular pressure.[60]

Oxygen should be administered to the patient. When available, additional monitoring equipment such as a pulse oximeter, CO_2 monitor, or apnea monitor should be used for continuous airway evaluation. These monitoring devices are discussed further in Chapter 12.

VENTILATION MANAGEMENT

A rapid, focused assessment of the patient's ventilatory status should be performed as the patient is being prepared for transport. If a chest radiograph has been obtained before arrival, it should be viewed to determine whether any pathosis exists. Breath sounds should be auscultated before the patient is placed in the transport vehicle because of noise interference.

If pneumothorax is suspected or is present on the chest radiograph, appropriate interventions should be initiated. If a chest tube or tubes are already in place, the nurse should check to see whether they are functioning. The drainage system may need to be changed so that it will continue to function during transport.

If a portable ventilator is to be used, the patient's tidal volume, respiratory rate, and FiO_2 must be calculated before the patient is connected to the ventilator. Patients who are dependent on a ventilator may need to spend some time connected to the transport ventilator so it can be ascertained that they are able to tolerate the change.[15] Ventilator use is discussed in Chapter 12.

CIRCULATION MANAGEMENT

Initial care related to circulation management is directed at controlling any active bleeding. Bleeding can be controlled with direct pressure by applying gauze pads and elastic tape or bandages. Air splints and MAST (military antishock trousers) pants have also been used to help control bleeding. However, the source and cause of the bleeding should be carefully evaluated before transport. Once the patient is "packaged," sheets and blankets can easily hide bleeding.

Intravenous access must be ensured. Whether one or two lines are inserted depends on individual protocols. However, having access to the intravenous line is important for fluid replacement, blood administration, and medication administration.

When medications are being infused, intravenous monitors may be used to ensure the appropriate delivery of medication. Medication concentrations and dosages should always be checked before a change is made in the equipment being used. Some transport nurses have found that it is easier to prepare medications with their own equipment and then make any changes in concentration and dosage, particularly when their own equipment requires specific types of tubing.

Urinary catheters must be appropriately placed and affixed so that they are not pulled out with patient movement. It is recommended that the catheter bag be emptied before the patient leaves the referring facility. The amount of urine emptied from the bag and its color should be recorded.

If invasive lines such as pulmonary or arterial catheters are in place, the transport team will need to check the patency and functioning of these lines. In some cases, transport monitors that offer specific readings during transport may not be available. The lines must be appropriately secured so that their functioning is not impaired. If a transport monitor is available, readings should be taken and recorded before, during, and after transport.

GASTRIC DECOMPRESSION

A gastric tube should be inserted to prevent the potential for aspiration and to provide gastric decompression during transport.[3] This procedure is not generally performed when a patient is transported directly from a scene, but it should be considered, particularly when the patient has undergone bag-valve-mask ventilation.

As with the urinary catheter, the gastric decompression tube must be appropriately placed and secured to prevent it from being pulled out. If the tube is not going to be placed on suction during transport, it should be capped so that it does not spill. When possible, the patient's stomach should be drained before the tube is plugged. The amount of the drainage and its color should be recorded.

When patients are being treated for extensive gastrointestinal (GI) bleeding, such as that seen in the patient with liver disease, a specific type of gastric tube, such as the Sengstaken-Blakemore tube, may be in place. Traction must be maintained so that the tube will continue to function properly. When this tube is present, the patient may be at risk for aspiration, asphyxia, gastric rupture, and erosion of the esophageal wall.[38] When this patient is transported, the airway should be secured by intubation, and the transport team must be prepared to intervene if any complications occur and to provide continued traction on the tube.

WOUND CARE AND SPLINTING

Wounds and splinting devices should be surveyed quickly, before the patient is moved. Hidden wounds may cause the patient discomfort and place the patient at risk for bleeding and long-term complications. Improperly placed splints or lack of splinting when indicated may also cause problems.

Several types of splints and splint devices are available to be used for the patient being transported. The transport team must be familiar with the type of equipment that is being used. Placement of the splint, potential complications of the device, and when it should be removed are some examples of the kind of information needed. The neurovascular status of the extremity to which the splint is applied should be assessed and documented. Orthopedic and vascular emergencies are discussed in Chapter 18. Wound care is provided for patient comfort and protection. Dressing the wound will help control bleeding and keep it free of debris. If there is concern about additional bleeding or neurovascular compromise, the wound should be dressed in such a manner that continuous assessment is possible during transport. Any wet dressings are replaced with dry sterile dressings to prevent heat loss during transport.

It is important to keep in mind the need for infection control when tending to the wounds of the patient being prepared for transport. Many patients being transported may have infected wounds that can put at risk the transport team and anyone else who may need to be transported in the vehicle.

SAFETY

An entire chapter in this textbook (Chapter 10) has been devoted to safety issues. In this section we will examine the safety measures that must be taken into consideration by the transport team when preparing the patient for transport. If the patient is combative, neuromuscular blocking agents and sedation may be indicated to ensure the safety of both the patient and the transport team.

A policy based on guidelines issued by the Food and Drug Administration should be in place regarding the use of restraints. These guidelines include the need to clearly document the necessity of the use of restraints during transport, follow local and state laws regarding the use of patient restraints, closely monitor the patient in restraints, carefully apply the restraining device(s) and adjust them properly so that they maintain body alignment and are not uncomfortable, and consider restraints to be a temporary solution.

When transporting a child, the child's size, weight, and state laws necessitate that restraint systems appropriate for a child be used. Devices that may be used include care beds, car seats, and transport boards. Any equipment that is used during transport needs to meet both federal and state standards.

PAIN MANAGEMENT

Pain management in the prehospital care environment is frequently not given priority consideration.[42] Several factors influence the use or lack of use of pain medications in the field, including the location of the patient, the nature of the patient's illness or injury, the possible masking of symptoms, and the effect of pain medications on the patient's vital signs. Movement, noise, changes in temperature, and fear may be contributing factors that cause or increase the patient's pain during preparation and transport.

Certain patient problems, such as chest pain related to myocardial infarction, have been dealt with outside of the hospital without any difficulty. However, pain management for trauma or other disease states continues to cause controversy.[53]

In 1992 the United States Department of Health and Human Services published its *Clinical Practice Guidelines for Acute Pain Management: Operative or Medical Procedures and Trauma.* The need for appropriate pain management is emphasized in these guidelines. Even though the prehospital management of pain is not directly addressed, these guidelines can easily be applied to the transport process.

The guidelines point out the following[53]:

The presence of a condition that could eventually result in cardiovascular, hemodynamic, neurologic, or pulmonary instability (e.g., femur fracture, pneumothorax, skull fracture) is not an absolute contraindication to systemic analgesia, although careful titration and monitoring must be provided.

The transport team should perform a brief assessment related to the patient's pain. The PQRST mnemonic previously described will help provide the nurse with a baseline description of the patient's pain. If the patient received medication before the team's arrival, information about the medication used and its effect on the patient should be included in the pain assessment.

Pain medications used for analgesia in the prehospital care environment need to be rapid in onset, short in duration, easy to administer, and easy to store.[50] The intravenous route is the quickest method of administration and has a rapid onset. However, intravenous access may not always be available. The transport team needs to be familiar with specific medications that can be used during transport to provide analgesia and sedation. This knowledge must include appropriate medications dosage, possible drug interactions, adverse reactions, and management of these adverse reactions.

Another important point to keep in mind regarding pain management during transport is that many patients have received neuromuscular blocking agents for safe transport, management of specific problems, or both. The transport team should pay particular attention to these patients' needs for sedation and pain management because they are unable to let the flight team know when they are anxious or in pain.

Additional methods that may be used by the transport team to help the patient manage pain during transport include the following:

- Distracting the patient: for example, if the patient is alert enough to look out the window, he or she

should be allowed to do so; a security object such as a stuffed toy may be of help to a child
- Talking to the patient
- Keeping the patient warm
- Placing the patient in a comfortable position when possible
- Describing everything that is going to occur
- Allowing a family member to accompany the patient
- Using therapeutic touch

PATIENT PREPARATION: THE FAMILY

Any time a family member is ill or injured, a crisis is created in the family. The need to transfer the patient to a distant facility produces additional stress.

At times the transport team will not have the opportunity to interact with the patient's family. Family members may not be present at the scene of the illness or injury, or they themselves may be injured. When family members are present, the team may be able to obtain a pertinent patient history from them.

The transport team should ensure that information is provided to the family before, during, and after transport of the patient. Policies and procedures that address when a family member may accompany an injured or ill family member should be in place. A discussion about family needs, how to care for the family, and when transport of a family member is appropriate is contained in Chapter 34.

DOCUMENTATION

Copies of any relevant documentation from the referring agency or EMS care providers should accompany the patient. If pictures of the scene of the accident are available, the transport team should bring them as well.

Copies of lab results, radiographic and diagnostic studies, and documentation by other health care providers should also accompany the patient. Consent forms, reasons for transport, and any other pertinent papers should be placed in the transport vehicle so that the team will not forget them when the patient arrives at the receiving facility. Remember to maintain patient confidentially when transporting or reviewing patient records.

Documentation by the transport team should reflect the reason the patient was transported; the interventions performed before, during, and after transport; and how the transport was completed. Strong and Thompson[51] found that the top 10 decisions made and documented during transport regarded fluid administration, immobilization, ventilation, oxygen administration, safety management, monitor use, intubation decisions, intravenous access, how to load the patient (hot vs. cold), and the use of neuromuscular blockade.

It also important to document not only what was done, but how the decision was made to perform the specific intervention. For example, why was the decision made to perform Rapid Sequence Induction (RSI) to secure the patient's airway? If medications are administered for pain or arrhythmia management, did they have an effect on the patient and what was that effect?

The patient's chart is not only used to document interventions and their indications, but it is also used for continuous quality improvement and reimbursement of services. Documentation is an integral part of patient care. It is important that it be clear, complete, and readable.

What is documented and who does the documentation is determined by the transport service and the specific standards. Nurses and paramedics have standards that describe their practice and provide guidelines for documentation (e.g., Air and Surface Transport Nurses Association [ASTNA]—formerly called the National Flight Nurses Association [NFNA]).

PATIENT ASSESSMENT DURING TRANSPORT

The nature of the patient's illness or injuries and the initial interventions performed will influence the assessment and management needed during air medical transport. Each of the clinical chapters in this textbook addresses the specific care required during transport as a result of the patient's illness or injury. Some general principles of assessment and management during transport include the following:

- Transport team members should position themselves in the aircraft so that they can effectively manage the patient's airway, breathing, and circulation (ABCs).
- Airway equipment, including suction equipment, should be easily accessible.
- All intravenous, central, or intraosseous lines should be accessible and functioning.
- All tubes and drainage systems should be functioning and secured to decrease the risk of dislodgement.
- If there is any question about cervical spine injury, the cervical spine should be immobilized for transport.
- A combative patient should be properly restrained—both physically and chemically—if indicated. If chemical restraint is chosen, the transport team needs to ensure that the patient receives adequate analgesia, sedation, and environmental control during the transport.
- All monitors should be placed within the transport team's field of vision.
- When indicated, wounds and injured limbs should remain exposed for inspection.

SUMMARY

Assessment and preparation are the foundation of patient transport. Primary and secondary assessments provide initial information about the patient's current and potential problems. On the basis of these assessments, the transport team initiates appropriate interventions. Box 11-15 lists some of these interventions.[41]

Patient preparation includes not only obvious care, but also anticipation of what may occur. In the prehospital care environment, resources are limited and anticipatory planning, safety, and prevention are key care interventions.

FIXED-WING PATIENT TRANSPORT

When transporting patients in fixed-wing aircraft, the transport team must pay critical attention to preflight preparation because of long periods of time typically spent on the ground and in flight. Fixed-wing aircraft transports usually entail lengthy periods of patient

---

BOX 11-15 | **Patient Care Interventions**

- Airway management
- Electrolyte and acid base management
- Drug management
- Neurologic management
- Respiratory management
- Physical comfort promotion
- Thermoregulation
- Tissue perfusion
- Psychologic comfort promotion
- Crisis management
- Risk management
- Lifespan care
- Information management

From McCloskey J, Bulechek G: *Nursing interventions classification,* St Louis, 1996, Mosby.

---

care; thus it is imperative that the detailed preflight information be obtained so that air medical personnel can make appropriate preparations for the transport. The aircraft should not depart to pick up the patient until all preflight preparations are complete. In addition to preparing for the medical aspects of the flight, the logistics and itinerary must be worked out, and any other preflight information required by the pilots must be obtained. The transport team and pilot(s) should collaborate in gathering this preflight information and in coordinating the entire flight to ensure appropriate quality patient care.

In this section of the chapter, issues encountered by care providers in the fixed-wing transport environment will be discussed. The following topics will be covered: preflight preparation, federal aviation regulations, preparing for patient transport, patient "packaging," in-flight factors influencing patient care, air medical personnel resources, in-flight codes, and safety and emergency procedures. In addition, issues related to international transports and escort flights will be highlighted.

PREFLIGHT PREPARATION

Preplanning by air medical personnel and the pilot is necessary if the patient transport is to go smoothly. Fixed-wing aircraft flight times are usu-

ally much longer than rotor-wing aircraft flight times and may vary greatly from service to service. Fixed-wing aircraft flight times may be as brief as 40 minutes within the state or as long as 3 to 6 hours within a particular region or across the country. In addition, transport distances may range from 150 to 500 miles for a propellor or turbopropellor aircraft to more than 500 miles for a jet. Once the patient transfer has been agreed on by a receiving physician and facility, the transport team should begin by obtaining information such as physicians' names, telephone numbers, and an accurate account of the patient's diagnosis and condition. This information will, it is hoped, ensure that the skills of the air medical personnel and the medical equipment available during transport are appropriate for the anticipated medical needs of the patient. In addition, logistic information such as patient and luggage weights, the number of family members who will ride along and their weights, and the "do not resuscitate" (DNR) status of the patient must also be obtained.

Preflight preparation also entails coordination of information with the pilot(s). Issues to be discussed should include location of airports, refueling and restroom stops, weight and balance issues, in-flight times to and from airports, ground ambulance times to referring and receiving facilities, ground unit resources, nutritional and fluid requirements, and disposal of wastes. The transport team must take into account in-flight and ground times when calculating the amount of intravenous (IV) fluids, medications, medical supplies, and oxygen that will be needed and when checking to ensure that medical equipment is fully charged.[33-36]

FEDERAL AVIATION REGULATIONS

Air medical services must actively participate in the daily aviation operations dictated by the Federal Aviation Administration (FAA) or national and international regulations specific to the operations of the air medical service in the country of residence, as applicable, to provide safety for all patients and care providers in the air transport environment. The fixed-wing air taxi certificate holder must comply with the appropriate Federal Aviation Regulations (FARs). These regulations pertain to air traffic control, airports, visual and instrument flight rules, and aircraft operations.[11] The majority of air medical services must comply with the appropriate FARs, depending on who possesses the air taxi certificate.

FAR Part 91 pertains to general operating and flight rules for aircraft flying in U.S. airspace. FAR Part 135 provides specific rules for air taxi operators and commercial operators. Most air medical services are regulated under Part 135 of the FARs because of the nature of transporting "passengers" or "persons" for compensation or hire.[11] Currently, more than half of the fixed-wing transport programs in operation possess their own FAR Part 135 certificate.[20] A brief explanation of weather minimums, weight and balance, the term *lifeguard,* and ambient temperatures as they relate to FARs will give the transport team an understanding of how they can assist the pilot in complying with FARs and ultimately with safety.[56]

WEATHER MINIMUMS—VISUAL AND INSTRUMENT FLIGHT RULES

The FARs define explicit weather minimums and rules that must be in effect for an aircraft to operate within consistent safety standards. Under FAR Part 135, air medical services operate under either Visual Flight Rules (VFRs) or Instrument Flight Rules (IFRs).[56] The pilot of a fixed-wing aircraft must comply with the appropriate rules that define flying limitations in adverse weather conditions.

VFRs govern the procedures for conducting flight under visual conditions as interpreted by the pilot. Flight visibility is defined by the distance forward into the visible horizon, and the ceiling (vertical boundary) is the height above the ground or water to the base of the lowest (broken) layer of clouds.[14,56] FAR Part 91.155 addresses the basic VFR weather minimums that are maintained for the corresponding altitude and class airspace for all aircraft.[56]

IFRs govern the procedures for conducting instrument flight when weather conditions do not meet the minimum requirements for flight under VFRs.[14,56] IFRs indicate that the pilot intends to navigate by instrumentation for at least a portion of the flight. Most programs that operate with fixed-wing aircraft have the capability to operate under IFRs. However, IFRs pose other limitations, such as the need to land at approved airports when instrument approaches are used; complying with restrictions for takeoff, approach, and landing minimums; and having plans in place in case of the need to use approved alternate airports.

WEIGHT AND BALANCE

It is important to meet weight and balance requirements for rotor-wing and fixed-wing aircraft as specified in the airplane or rotorcraft flight manual. The manual contains aircraft performance data regarding maximum certified gross weights, center-of-gravity limits, and runway lengths that fixed-wing aircraft will use for takeoff. Because fixed-wing airplanes (depending on the model) have fewer weight restrictions and more cabin space than rotor-wing aircraft,[48] family members and other persons frequently accompany patients on fixed-wing aircraft transports.

According to FAR Part 91.605, the pilot must ensure that the aircraft is loaded within weight and balance limits at all times.[11] Because the gross weight of the aircraft is predetermined by the airplane flight manual, the pilot is responsible for determining the daily operational weight, which is the weight of the aircraft, fuel, pilot(s), air medical personnel, and equipment. These calculations must be completed before taking off on a medical transport. Therefore, when in contact with the referring facility, air medical personnel should attempt to obtain the weights of patients and persons who will ride along. The pilot(s) can benefit from early notification of a patient's weight, especially for the patient who weighs more than 300 pounds. The pilot has final authority for weight limitations and may decide that family members or other persons may not accompany the patient. In addition, the pilot may decide to decrease fuel loads, rearrange the seating of passengers, unload unnecessary equipment, leave behind unnecessary passengers and air medical personnel, or depart from an airport with a longer runway.

A second important weight and balance requirement is that aircraft be loaded within the center-of-gravity range or limitations.[11] Once the maximum weight has been determined, the weight distribution, or where the weight is placed in an aircraft, is critical for aerodynamic performance and safety while the aircraft is in flight.[14,55] The weight must be properly loaded fore and aft of the center of gravity, according to the manufacturer's airplane flight manual.

LIFEGUARD STATUS

Air ambulance services may declare *lifeguard* status for priority flights in the air traffic control system. Lifeguard affords the airplane priority when taking off or landing and should be used with extreme discretion. It is only "intended for those missions of an urgent medical nature" (i.e., when a patient is deteriorating or is in full arrest) when a patient is on board or for the "portion of the flight requiring expeditious handling."[48] Lifeguard status is filed with a flight service station. Although landing and departing time differences are minimal at small airports, lifeguard status often achieves a tremendous time advantage at metropolitan and international airports. An air medical aircraft that is on lifeguard status may be allowed to take off or land ahead of multiple commercial and private aircraft, but this causes delays for these aircraft or extends their holding pattern time, costing thousands of dollars. Therefore an air medical service must reserve lifeguard status for those times when it is absolutely necessary.

AMBIENT TEMPERATURES

Several aircraft temperature considerations should be addressed before a flight commences because temperature can present potential problems in the air medical environment. The first consideration is the amount of time the aircraft will spend on the ground because air conditioning or heating cannot be left on for more than a few minutes during this time unless an auxiliary power unit is used. Unfortunately, auxiliary power units are usually not available at smaller airports, where most fixed-wing transports originate.

A second temperature consideration is evident at higher altitudes, at which the ambient temperature decreases. As the altitude increases, temperature decreases to the tropopause, which is the location at which the temperature reaches its lowest point and remains constant. The fuselage circumference of most air medical aircraft tends to be relatively small, and insulation of the walls is such that the walls and floor will feel cool.[33] The cumulative effect of all of these factors is often a cooler environment in a fixed-wing aircraft.

A third temperature consideration is encountered when descending into tropical or humid climates. On descent, windows will become fogged and other types of condensation will occur inside the aircraft.

PREPARING FOR PATIENT TRANSPORT

TRANSFERRING AND ACCEPTING PHYSICIAN AND FACILITY

The transport team must ensure that an appropriate referral is arranged for the fixed-wing transport. Because additional time is usually available to preplan for an interfacility fixed-wing transport, the names of both the referring and the accepting physician should be documented for the transfer.

In 1985 Congress enacted the Consolidated Omnibus Budget Reconciliation Act (COBRA), which was amended in July and November 1990. COBRA protects indigent, uninsured patients from being denied access to emergency care by hospitals or from being transferred inappropriately between hospitals on the basis of the patient's inability to pay.[52] This legislation requires that the referring hospital assume liability for the adequacy of stabilization before transport. COBRA also requires documentation before the transfer that the receiving hospital has been verified and that a receiving physician is willing to accept the patient. If a transfer is required for a patient who is not yet stabilized, COBRA states that various conditions are to be met, including the following[52]:

(1) The physician certifies in writing that, in his/her professional opinion, the benefits of the transfer outweigh the risks; (2) the transferring hospital treats the patient within its capacity, which minimizes the risks to the patient; (3) the receiving facility agrees to accept the patient and has available space and qualified personnel to provide appropriate medical treatment; (4) the transferring hospital sends to the receiving facility all medical records (copies) available at the time of transfer; and (5) the transfer is effected through qualified personnel and transportation equipment.

The transport team must often validate transfer information from the communications center. It is important that this information be validated because these patients are transferred from towns, cities, and states in which air medical personnel are not necessarily familiar with the hospitals and physicians involved in the transfer.

Oxygen Requirements

Determination of in-flight and ground ambulance times from the referring to the receiving facility assists the flight nurse in calculating the amount of oxygen that will be required to meet the needs of the patient. The transport team must ensure sufficient oxygen to deliver 1.0 FiO_2 or to operate a ventilator, if needed, for 1 to 1.3 times the entire length of the patient transport.[11,47] In some patient transports, more time is spent on the ground than in flight. Time spent on the ground may be 90 minutes or longer. Therefore all fixed-wing aircraft should carry a portable back-up oxygen tank in case the main system fails or the ground ambulance has no oxygen available. Some foreign countries do not carry oxygen in their ambulances (Table 11-2).

Patient Medical Equipment Requirements

Air medical services are improving fixed-wing aircraft standards by providing dedicated aircraft with custom medical configurations, which allows services to permanently secure ventilators, heart moni-

TABLE 11-2   Calculating Oxygen Cylinder Time

$$Time = \frac{Pcylinder \times CF}{V}$$

Cylinder	CF
D Cylinder	0.16
Jumbo D Cylinder	0.25
E Cylinder	0.28
G Cylinder	2.41
H Cylinder	3.14

From Oakes D: *Clinical practitioner's pocket guide to respiratory care,* Philadelphia, 1998, Health Educator Publications.
CF, Conversion factor; *Pcylinder,* total pressure in cylinder is 500; *V,* flow rate in liters per minute.

tors, and other patient medical equipment. Equipment that is required may be chosen on the basis of the mission and the scope of care provided by the air medical service. For example, a service whose mission is critical care for children and adults should have appropriate transport equipment readily available. This may include a heart and hemodynamic monitor, a noninvasive blood pressure (BP) monitor, a pulse generator, IV pumps, a pulse oximeter, an on-board suction device, a transport ventilator, an isolette, and a transport intraaortic balloon pump.

Medical equipment that requires battery power should also have auxiliary power capabilities that can use the aircraft's invertor. The transport team should always ensure that the invertor power source on the aircraft and ground ambulance work properly in case batteries should fail. Because many ground ambulances outside the United States do not have invertors, the transport team should have spare batteries available.

For example, a critically ill patient in severe cardiogenic shock with severely depressed left ventricular function can be successfully transported by fixed-wing aircraft. Wedge-Stecher[58] reviewed a case report of a patient who required not only intraaortic balloon pump therapy but also a left ventricular assistance device to take over the left ventricular workload. The patient was transported with all these devices, which gave him his only chance of survival until he was able to receive a heart transplant at a tertiary center. The patient was discharged from the hospital 1 month after the flight. The team coordinator ensured that the proper equipment for the transfer, including the IV pumps and the intraaortic balloon pump, was available and fully charged and that extra batteries were available.

A portable suction unit should also be included in the standard equipment for fixed-wing transports. This unit provides the team with back-up equipment should the main suction system fail in the fixed-wing aircraft. The portable suction unit is also valuable during transport once the patient is removed from the aircraft at isolated or foreign airports.

Finally, transport services must comply with their state licensure requirements for air medical aircraft, which include specifications about medical equipment that must be placed on the aircraft. Because these requirements vary from state to state, some aircraft may be required to carry additional equipment according to state regulations.

PATIENT CARE SUPPLIES AND MEDICATIONS

The aircraft must be stocked with adequate medical supplies and medications to provide the nursing care required by the patient. In addition to the required air ambulance equipment, extra supplies may be tailored to the anticipated needs of the patient. For example, if a patient requires breathing treatments while in flight, additional nebulizer setups and extra or multivial doses of the medication may be stocked. Also, because an intubated patient may require frequent suctioning, additional saline bullets and sterile suction catheters should be stocked on the aircraft.

BEDDING AND LINENS

Because fixed-wing flights involve longer periods of patient care, comfort becomes a major issue. The traditional fixed-wing aircraft stretcher pads are hard, thin, narrow, and have limited flexibility. The transport team can plan ahead and attempt to use bedding, egg crates, or blankets on top of the stretcher to provide

extra padding and create a softer surface. If an air mattress is to be used, air must be able to be released to prevent the mattress from rupturing in flight as a result of gas expansion at higher altitudes.

In addition, the transport nurse may stock extra pillows for use in supporting the head, neck, back, and knees, positioning between knees and elbows and elevating extremities and feet. On longer flights, the team must pay greater attention to the patient's position. Patients, especially those who are comatose or paralyzed, may need to be turned to prevent skin breakdowns. The patient may be placed on a "turn" or "draw sheet" so that air medical personnel can reposition the patient more easily in flight. Passive range-of-motion exercises will also decrease the risk of blood pooling and additional skin injury from immobility.

The transport team should also pay attention to their own immobility on long flights. Stretching exercises and increased fluid intake can help prevent circulatory problems.

NUTRITION AND FLUID REQUIREMENTS

Adequate nutrition and fluids should be provided for all persons on board the aircraft. Depending on the transport time and the time of day, food may be catered for the patient, family, pilots, and air medical personnel. The team must choose the proper food or provide the specialized diet (e.g., a low-fat or diabetic diet) required by the patient. Proper storage of the food and fluids is necessary. In addition, there should be an adequate stock of fluids, such as juice, and plenty of water for the entire length of the transport. Because of the longer in-flight times, higher altitudes, and stresses of flight, the nurse should provide sources for replenishing energy and preventing dehydration for all persons on board the aircraft. Emphasis should be placed on taking care of oneself in addition to the patient and other passengers during the transport.

DISPOSING OF CONTAMINATED WASTES

All air medical personnel must comply with Occupational Safety and Health Administration (OSHA) regulations regarding occupational exposure to bloodborne pathogens.[54] The air medical service must have an exposure-control plan. Policies, procedures, and equipment must be provided in the plan to comply with these regulations and protect employees from infectious diseases. Air medical personnel must follow infection control policies by observing standard precautions and stocking extra personal protective equipment, supplies, and cleaning agents for these long flights. Depending on the flight distance and in-flight patient care times, the team must plan for the containment and disposal of contaminated needles, dressings, empty IV fluid bags, and human wastes according to OSHA regulations. A urinary catheter makes it easy to dispose of urine. The team must also plan for providing care and properly disposing of wastes should the patient have a bowel movement. Multiple large red isolation bags may be used to dispose of wipes, bedpans, and urinals.

Air medical personnel, pilots, and family members should plan to use restroom facilities before departure and during fuel stops. Some fixed-wing aircraft have toilet facilities on board, but most do not.

REQUIRED GROUND AMBULANCE CAPABILITIES

For fixed-wing transports, the transport team can never assume that a particular ground ambulance unit will be available. The team must investigate the capabilities and resources of the ambulance that arrives at the airport. If the patient requires various kinds of medical equipment, invertor power should be available on the ambulance to power the equipment. The transport team should also assess the resources of the ambulance service to determine whether it can provide the appropriate basic life-support or advanced life-support services. In some countries, no resources may be available in the ambulance, in which case *all* medical equipment, medications, and oxygen required for the patient must be provided by the flight team.

PATIENT "PACKAGING" FOR TRANSPORT

PREPARATION

Preparation of a patient for a fixed-wing transport usually requires a thorough assessment, stabilization, and preparation process because of lengthy patient care times. In rare cases the transport team may swoop and scoop the patient, primarily as a result of the patient's condition or when the patient is brought to the transport team at an airport. Most of the time, the team will perform a rapid assessment at the referring facility and initiate patient care. A preflight plan helps minimize the amount of time spent on the ground before departure.

LOADING CONSIDERATIONS

After ground transport to the aircraft, air medical personnel must plan to transfer the patient into the aircraft and secure the medical equipment. Because most aircraft doors are relatively narrow, the team must make the "patient package" as slender as possible.[45,48] Once on the aircraft, equipment must be secured according to FAA regulations and placed in a position that will permit continuous assessments while allowing the tubes and catheters to remain patent and accessible.

Numerous companies provide equipment for loading a patient into fixed-wing aircraft. Because there has been an increase in fixed-wing transports, these companies have developed and marketed stands, lifts, slides, and sleds to assist with loading and unloading patients through narrow fixed-wing aircraft doors. These loading devices have significantly eased the loading procedure, but more importantly, they assist with preventing work-related injuries for the pilot and air medical personnel.

IMMOBILIZATION EQUIPMENT

Immobilization devices present unique challenges for loading a patient through a fixed-wing aircraft door and positioning the patient in the aircraft. Some aircraft doors are too narrow to accommodate standard backboards for loading patients into aircraft. For this reason, tapered backboards are suggested. The team must also prepare for patients who have other immobilization devices, such as a traction splint, in place. Loading the patient on the aircraft may be difficult because of the length of the splint. In addition, positioning the patient can present challenges.

Bulky dressings, splints, and the need to maintain a position of comfort for an injured extremity may make it difficult to transfer the patient smoothly through the aircraft door. In addition, the patient will need to be positioned in the aircraft so that the extremity can be supported, while maintaining optimal positioning and allowing access for nursing care.

IN-FLIGHT FACTORS INFLUENCING PATIENT CARE

LIMITED SPACE

The fixed-wing transport team must consider several issues that may not be factors in rotor-wing aircraft transport. Space may vary greatly from one aircraft to another. Propellor and turbopropellor aircraft tend to be more spacious than the jet models, which can be extremely important when patients require large advanced life-support equipment or immobilization devices or when family members desire to accompany the patient.

AIR-CONDITIONER AND HEATER

In-flight climate-control systems may not meet most caregivers' expectations. The thin walls and floor of the fuselage do not allow much space for thermal insulation. Therefore the air-conditioning may not adequately cool the airplane to the desired temperature on extremely hot summer days, and in the winter, some aircraft cabins may still feel cool when heaters are performing at maximum capacity.

DIVERSIONS

Because fixed-wing transport times are often longer than for other types of patient transport, the potential for diversion of the flight is increased. Diversion can be prompted by mechanical problems, weather, or even a significant deterioration in the patient's status. Plans must be in place before transport to address diversion so that patient care is not jeopardized.

AIR MEDICAL PERSONNEL RESOURCES

One of the most critical factors for fixed-wing transports is the teams' knowledge of available resources and how these resources can be accessed.

The transport team must be familiar with medical control policies and procedures. Medical control may be extremely helpful to those involved with political situations, a patient whose condition is deteriorating, cardiac arrests that occur during the flight, interstate transports, and flights outside of the United States. The transport team must ensure that the air medical service has policies and procedures in place and must know how to contact the medical control to deal with these situations. In addition, the transport team must be able to use the resources of the communications center to contact the program director, clinical supervisor, or medical director as needed to assist with patient decisions and coordination of the patient transfer in emergency situations.[14]

MEDICAL CONTROL

Most air medical services receive medical control services from the medical director and the designated medical control physicians. As discussed earlier in this chapter, most fixed-wing aircraft flights are interfacility transports. Therefore a physician referral has been made to transfer the patient to an accepting physician and facility. Before departing from the referring facility, a nurse may initiate patching to a medical control physician by telephone to discuss a patient's medical condition and request further orders as needed. Once the team is in the ground ambulance or in flight, the opportunities for medical patching may be limited for some air medical services.

COMMUNICATION

The transport team should be familiar with all of the capabilities and aircraft communications of the communications center. The team should also become familiar with the various nonaviation radio frequencies for contacting the communications center and ground EMS agencies. In addition, air medical services should be encouraged to provide flite telephones on the aircraft to initiate medical patching during the flight if the patient's condition deteriorates. It is legal to use flite telephones during flight, whereas it is illegal to use cellular telephones when airborne. Flite telephones are licensed and regulated by the Federal Communications Commission. When a flite telephone is available, the transport team can contact medical control during in-flight medical emergencies.

IN-FLIGHT CODES

The transport team faces unique challenges and must use decision-making skills when a patient goes into cardiopulmonary arrest during a fixed-wing aircraft transport. The air medical personnel should be apprised of the patient's current code status. In addition, before transport, the patient and family members accompanying the patient should be made aware of the risks of air medical transport and the potential for diversions should the patient's condition deteriorate.

The team must address four essential issues if a patient has a full cardiopulmonary arrest during the fixed-wing aircraft transport. The team must consider the following: the (1) service's policies and procedures for in-flight codes; (2) decision to return, divert, or continue to proceed to the destination; (3) availability of resuscitation equipment and medications; and (4) endurance of the air medical personnel. After all of these issues have been weighed and deliberated, the team shall make the final decision in conjunction with medical control.

First, air medical personnel need to be well versed in the air medical service's policies and procedures for full codes on a fixed-wing aircraft transport. Every state has specific laws dealing with terminating resuscitation efforts in the prehospital arena. The program should have policies and procedures in place that relate to patients in full cardiopulmonary arrest and the actions that are required by air medical personnel in consultation with the service's medical control.

In addition, legal aspects of interstate and international transport may complicate the decision to terminate resuscitation en route or before reaching the destination. Therefore some air medical services have a policy that a patient cannot be pronounced dead until the aircraft has landed, especially if the transport takes place outside the United States.[29,30]

Second, if the patient deteriorates into a full code during any portion of the transport, the air medical personnel must weigh distance and time factors to decide literally in which direction to transport. This decision may be based on the distance and time it would take to return to the referring facility or to the closest appropriate facility, on the availability of ground ambulances, and on overall patient status. The question for the air medical personnel will be whether to divert the aircraft or continue to the final destination after weighing all these factors.

The third essential issue relates to the service's available resuscitation equipment and medications. This may include oxygen, endotracheal tubes, advanced cardiac life-support medications, fluids, and the battery power on life-support equipment. Given the limited supplies available on fixed-wing aircraft, the transport team may be required to make a decision based on the air medical team exhausting all of the resuscitation equipment.

Finally the endurance of the air medical personnel on the transport should be considered, especially for transports that also require ground times in excess of 90 minutes. The air medical personnel may be required to contact medical control and recommend ceasing resuscitation efforts if the patient does not respond to medical therapy on an extremely long flight.

"Do Not Resuscitate" Orders

Fixed-wing aircraft transport services may provide "Do Not Resuscitate" (DNR) transports at the family's request and not because of medical necessity. These flights are prescheduled with an air medical service, but again, the transport team should be familiar with DNR policies and procedures. Because various states have different definitions for DNR patients, services that conduct these types of flights should provide policies and procedures for air medical personnel.

SAFETY AND EMERGENCY PROCEDURES

Safety is the number one priority for any patient transport. In the fixed-wing aircraft transport environment, the transport team should receive initial and annual ongoing education regarding fixed-wing aircraft operations, regulations, and unscheduled aircraft emergencies. According to FAR 91.505 and 135.331, all flight crew members should receive emergency training for each aircraft type and model.[55] Because air medical personnel are considered passengers and not "flight crew," an air medical service may not provide all the crew member emergency training requirements. All air medical personnel should receive safety education in potential in-flight emergencies and procedures appropriate for each kind and model of aircraft flown. This will allow the air medical personnel to understand and assist the pilot with various procedures. According to Wright et al,[59] education regarding in-flight emergencies increases the confidence of air medical personnel and pilots and affects their ability to deal effectively with these emergencies before and after the emergency. At a minimum, education should be provided for dealing with the following emergencies: (1) fire during the flight, (2) electrical failure; (3) hydraulic failure; (4) slow or rapid decompression; (5) water ditching, if flying over water; (6) rapid egress procedures; and (7) survival procedures and available equipment. For further review of emergency procedures and survival, see Chapter 10.

INTERNATIONAL TRANSPORT ISSUES

AIR MEDICAL SERVICE INTERNATIONAL TRANSPORTS

The discussion of air medical transport no longer focuses only on domestic transports. International transports continue to increase for patients who require medical transport from one country to another. Although similarities exist between domestic and international air medical transports, there are many unique differences. This section will focus on some of the issues and obstacles that may be encountered with international transports, such as preflight preparation and logistics, documentation, language barriers, patient locations, ground ambulance times and resources, pilot and air medical personnel duty times, and medical equipment and supplies.[33-36]

PREFLIGHT PREPARATION AND LOGISTICS

Preflight preparation becomes extremely critical for international air medical transports. As with fixed-wing transports, extensive plans for the logistics must be completed by the entire team with the realization that the flights will often be much longer than other air medical transports. Additional preflight plans must include Customs, Immigrations, international weather briefings, landing permits, refueling stops, ground handling, oxygen requirements, catering arrangements, medical equipment needs, and rest requirements.[32] Inadequate preparations or failure to notify the appropriate authorities will only frustrate the air medical team and create enormous delays. In addition, meticulous attention should be given to obtaining as much accurate patient information as possible to prepare for the medical needs of the patient.[26,27,32] Because international transports of critically ill and injured patients may not be accomplished on some commercial airliners, some air medical services conduct routine international transports. These programs have dedicated jets that are medically configured. To prepare for the worst-case scenario, these aircraft have redundant medical equipment and systems. These jets also offer lavatory facilities and auxiliary power units for maintaining a comfortable cabin environment and charging medical equipment during ground times of the transport.[26] Many aviation companies are able to assist an air medical service in preparing for an international transport.

DOCUMENTATION

Air medical personnel and pilots should always have the appropriate documentation for customs and immigration requirements on their person. This documentation may include passports, driver's licenses, voter registrations, visas, and immunization records.[33-36] International guideline charts are available to explain requirements for different countries.[33-36] The State Department can advise on the specific customs and immigration requirements for a country.

The Centers for Disease Control and the World Health Organization publish guidelines for required and recommended immunizations for each country. The patient and all companying passengers should also have the required customs and immigration papers. The transport company will be held responsible for any fines or citations incurred resulting from the lack of these required documents.

When planning for the flight, the appropriate documentation must also be verified for the patient and any passengers. Frequently the pilot(s) will organize this information when filing the flight plan and making arrangements with customs.

LANGUAGE BARRIERS

When attempting to obtain an accurate patient diagnosis and discover the patient's medical condition and care needs, air medical personnel may deal with language barriers from the referring facility, physician(s), and family members that may require the use of a translator. Many long-distance telephone companies now offer translators fluent in multiple languages.[33] In addition, insurance companies that coordinate these international flights have resources available for translating patient information.

It is imperative that the medical director or clinical supervisor and the flight nurse involved with the flight use the necessary resources to obtain patient information that is as accurate as possible, even if this delays the transport.[32] This will ensure that the skills of the air medical personnel and the available medical equipment are appropriate for the anticipated medical needs of the patient. In some cases, when transporting an American citizen back to the United States, the transport team may be able to obtain medical information by speaking directly with the patient or family members.

The air medical personnel must also plan for language barriers when arriving at the patient location and during the flight. It may be necessary to request an interpreter at the referring hospital or clinic to translate the medical terms, current treatment, and patient care needs.[33] In addition, the air medical personnel on the flight will benefit from learning specific medical terms and words related to caring for the patient during the flight—for example, terms related to current chest pain status and restroom needs.

PATIENT LOCATION

International air medical transports may involve patients who are located not only in hospitals but also in clinics, private homes, trailers, hotels, physicians' offices, cruise ships or docks, and other locations that may never before have been encountered. It may not be possible to predict how stable the patient will be on one's arrival; therefore the flight nurse must prepare for the worst-case scenario. Patients arriving at the airport by taxi may have had minimal care. The air medical personnel, being the only providers of advanced life support, will have to initiate medical care.

Transport times should allow for a visit to the patient by the medical team at the referring facility. This time should involve a patient evaluation, obtaining medical records, and completing final arrangements. Each team member must always practice professional courtesy and obtain permission before entering the patient care area, examining the patient, and reviewing medical records. The transport team must keep in mind that medical care and local customs may influence their approach to the patient and the referring facility.

GROUND TRANSPORT TIMES

Preflight planning must include an accurate calculation of the distance and ground times between the patient's location and the airport. Information such as traffic and road conditions may also be sought.[33-36] This information is extremely important for calculating oxygen requirements for ventilatory patients, battery life of equipment, and necessary supplies for the patient during transport.

GROUND AMBULANCE RESOURCES

Whether the patient is transported to the airport or the team is transported to the patient, the resources of the ground unit may be very limited. The ambulance vehicle may be a private car, a taxicab, a suburban vehicle, a Volkswagen camper, a pickup truck with a camper shell, or an ambulance unit.[27] Some ambulances may be stripped to an empty unit with no oxygen source or suction equipment. Others may be elaborately stocked with supplies and medical equipment. In addition, the skills of the ambulance personnel accompanying the team and patient may vary widely, from a driver with no medical knowledge to emergency medical personnel, nurses, or physicians with varying degrees of skills.

Finally one must consider the safety issues of the ground transport to and from the airplane. Road conditions, driving skills and compliance with traffic laws, and the inability to secure equipment are a few of the concerns that may be faced during the ground transport. All of these issues contribute additional stresses to the international transport of patients.

Pilot and Air Medical Personnel Duty Times

Duty and rest times must be considered for each international transport for the pilot(s) and air medical personnel. This is already addressed for the pilot(s) because they must comply with FAR Part 135.267 flight time limitations and rest requirements.[55] Therefore during the preflight preparation, rest requirements must be calculated into the plan and arrangements made for relief pilots to assume flight duties at appropriate fuel stops or at the destination.

When making preflight preparations, air medical personnel should determine the length of the flight and patient care times and use judgment in scheduling adequate team breaks. Depending on the duty times of the flight and medical crew members, an overnight stay may be necessary to comply with crew rest and FAA requirements. This may involve the acquisition of lodging for each team member. Many times these arrangements are easily facilitated by employing a handling agent in the country to which the patient is transferred; this agent can assist with hotel arrangements, aircraft refueling, catering, and so on.

Rest for air medical personnel may be accomplished during the flight, with "members of the team sleeping in a rotation where the transport nurse or physician is always awake with the patient."[33] For extremely long transports, the air medical service may send a relief team of air medical personnel to a scheduled fuel stop to assume patient care.

Medical Equipment and Supplies

Just as with preflight preparations for any fixed-wing aircraft transport, it is imperative that the transport team ensures that plans are complete for international transports. The transport nurse must be meticulous in planning and arranging for adequate oxygen, medical equipment, batteries, supplies, bedding and linens, nutrition and fluids, and disposal of contaminated wastes. It is important to remember that there is a greater potential for unexpected delays for these transports because of customs coordination, ambulance delays, and refueling stops. In addition, international transports may be of longer duration than other transports and to destinations with no stock of medical supplies or supplies incompatible with that of the air medical personnel. Therefore air medical personnel should stock enough medical supplies and medications for twice the predicted time of transport.[33-36]

Many countries require special permits or have adopted specific requirements for the transport of certain medications. These should be identified before the team's arrival to prevent any delays or confiscation of the medications needed to care for the patient. Medications should be kept in kits or medical packs and never carried in the team members' personal luggage.

Finally the compatibility of medical equipment with foreign electrical current may need to be considered. The team may need to obtain several types of foreign adapters to convert the current so that monitors and suction units can be properly charged.

ESCORT AND MEDICAL ASSIST TRANSPORTS ON COMMERCIAL AIRLINERS

One more form of patient transport, called an *escort flight* or *medical assist transport,* should be discussed. Escorts may be either domestic or international transports. These transports are referred to as *commercial escorts.* A commercial escort is defined as the escort of a stable patient on a contracted aircraft or a commercial airliner with the airliner's approval with only one attendant who may be a emergency medical technician (EMT), emergency medical technician–paramedic (EMT-P), registered nurse (RN), or medical doctor (MD).[14] These flights may involve transporting a patient at the basic life-support level who requires medical assistance, a critically ill or injured patient, or one who requires advanced life support or extensive nursing care.[33]

With regard to preflight preparation and logistics for this type of transport, the flight nurse should ensure that all arrangements are complete and plan to address several unique obstacles. These issues include not only commercial air carrier regulations, documentation, airline oxygen requirements, oxygen adapters, and electrical power, but also privacy and nonstop flights. Because transporting a patient on a commercial airliner requires coordination that is not under the control of the air medical service, these arrangements may take several days to an entire week to complete.

COMMERCIAL AIR CARRIER REGULATIONS

Regulations for transporting a patient on an airliner vary, depending on the patient's designated level and condition. Many commercial air carriers will allow a stable patient who requires limited care to sit in the first-class or business-class section for transport.[33] On the other hand, transferring a critically ill patient may require the purchase of multiple seats (6 to 12) in the business-class section or in the rear coach compartment of the airplane so the litter can be secured. Many airliners have a dedicated patient litter that rests above the folded passenger seats and is bolted to the seat tracks. Special arrangements should be made with each commercial airliner because each carrier has a different patient litter, loading and securing procedures, and quantity of medical oxygen available. The transport team should plan for the logistics of these escorts to ensure that the transport is completed smoothly.

In addition, provisions must be made for transporting medical equipment and supplies in such a way that they are readily available for the patient and yet secured according to the FARs. The equipment also should be organized in such a manner that it can be easily transferred and checked by customs and immigration authorities.

DOCUMENTATION

The air medical personnel must organize all of the paperwork necessary for the entire transport, including the airline tickets, passports, itinerary, and customs documents. This documentation for the air medical personnel, patient, and family members must be readily available for customs and immigration authorities. Air medical personnel should always keep this paperwork on their person.

AIRLINE OXYGEN REQUIREMENTS

Each air carrier has a different procedure for obtaining oxygen and securing the O_2 tanks. The oxygen tanks routinely provided by most airliners deliver only 2 to 4 L per minute. Therefore, arrangements must be made to have extra oxygen tanks available for patients who require 100% O_2 or a ventilator. A minimum of 24 hours' notice is necessary, but it may frequently take several days to make such arrangements.[33-36] Several airliners do not have the capacity to carry and secure larger oxygen tanks.

OXYGEN ADAPTERS

Particular attention should be given to the oxygen adapters and regulators available on each airliner. Most of this equipment is not compatible with air medical transport ventilator fittings. In addition, oxygen flow meters are often irregular. For instance, in some airliners, the O_2 outlet has three prongs.

ELECTRICAL POWER AND ADAPTERS

The commercial air carrier's electrical power sources must be assessed and coordinated to power the medical equipment. A power source may be needed for transport ventilators, heart monitors, intravenous pumps, and suction equipment. As previously mentioned, the appropriate adapters must be obtained to convert the current in these foreign airplanes.

PRIVACY

Most commercial airliners have various rules pertaining to patients in critical condition. Their presence may offend or upset other paying passengers. Some airlines provide privacy for the patient by installing temporary curtains, but most of the time they are inadequate. Therefore it may be necessary to bring additional sheets and clothespins to provide adequate privacy for the patient.

Nonstop Flight

Every attempt should be made to make reservations on a nonstop flight for the patient transport.[33-36] This eliminates the frustrations of making additional arrangements to get on and off of the airplane, to transfer the patient, and to provide documentation for customs and immigrations officials. In addition, plans must be made to organize all of the medical equipment, patient and family belongings, and luggage of air medical personnel for each transfer.

SUMMARY

Although many general principles of practice and patient care are identical in the rotor-wing aircraft and fixed-wing aircraft and ground transport environments, differences do exist. First, one must focus on learning the safety and emergency procedures to be used in the fixed-wing aircraft. Second, because air medical transport on fixed-wing aircraft requires longer patient care times than other types of transport, the transport team must be meticulous in preplanning for the entire flight, coordinating resources, and providing care for all persons on board. Fixed-wing transport, both national and international, offers unique challenges to patient transport; to ensure safe and competent care, team members need to be appropriately selected and educated.

REFERENCES

1. American College of Emergency Physicians: Principles of appropriate transfer, *Ann Emerg Med* 3:337, 1990.
2. American College of Surgeons Committee on Trauma: Interhospital transfer. In *Resources for optimal care of the injured patient*, Chicago, 1999, American College of Surgeons Committee on Trauma.
3. American College of Surgeons: *Advanced trauma life support program for doctors*, Chicago, 1997, ACS.
4. Aoki B, McClosky K: *Evaluation, stabilization, and transport of the critically ill child*, St Louis, 1992, Mosby.
5. Association of Air Medical Services: Recommended minimum quality standards for rotor-wing and fixed-wing standards, Pasadena, CA, 1992, Author.
6. Barson W, Jastremski M, Syverud S: *Emergency drug therapy*, Philadelphia, 1991, WB Saunders.
7. Benevilli W, Thomas S, Brown D, Wedel S: Safety of fentanyl during transport of trauma patients, *Air Med J* 14(3):156, 1995.
8. Bennet-Jacobs B, Baker P: *Trauma nursing core course*, Park Ridge, Ill, 1995, Emergency Nurses Association.
9. Benson J: *FDA safety alert: potential hazards with restraint devices*, Rockville, Md, 1992, Food and Drug Administration.
10. Brennan JA: *Guidelines for ambulance diversion. American College of Emergency Physicians*, Irving, Tex, 1999, American College of Emergency Physicians.
11. Brink LW, et al: Air transport, transport medicine, *Pediatr Clin North Am* 40(2):452, 1993.
12. Burney R, et al: Evaluation of hospital based aeromedical programs using therapeutic intervention scoring, *Aviat Space Environ Med* 6:563, 1990.
13. Campbell J: *Basic trauma life support*, ed 4, Upper Saddle River, NJ, 2000, Brady/Prentice Hall Health.
14. Commission on Accreditation of Medical Transport Systems (CAMTS): *Standards*. Anderson, SC, 2002, CAMTS.
15. Cohn H: Legal issues. In Neff J, Kidd P, editors: *Trauma nursing: the art and science*, St Louis, 1993, Mosby.
16. Continenza K, Hill J: Transport of the critical child. In Blumer J, editor: *Pediatric intensive care*, St Louis, 1990, Mosby.
17. Crippen D: Critical care transportation medicine: new concepts in pretransport stabilization of the critically ill patient, *Am J Emerg Med* 11:551, 1990.
18. DeJarnette R, editor: *Flight nurse advanced trauma course*, Park Ridge, Ill, 1994, National Flight Nurses Association.
19. Dickinson E, Krett R, O'Connor R: The impact of prehospital instant photography of motor crashes on physician perception and patient management in the emergency department, *Prehosp Disaster Med* 7(suppl 1), 1992.
20. Newberry L: Directory of Air Medical Services, *Air Med J* 20(6):41, 2001.
21. Emergency Nurses Association: *Sheehy's emergency nursing: principles and practice*, ed 4, St Louis, 1998, Mosby.
22. Emergency Nurses Association Diversity Task Force: *Approaching diversity: an interactive journey*. Des Plaines, Ill, 1997, Author.
23. Emerman C, Shade B, Kubincanek J: Comparative performance of the Best trauma triage rule, *Am J Emerg Med* 10(4):294, 1992.

24. Federal Aviation Administration: *Code of federal regulations: title 14, aeronautics and space, parts 91 and 135,* 1996, U.S. Department of Transportation.

25. Flight Safety International Inc: *Lear Jet 20 Series, pilot training manual,* 1986.

26. Forgey WW: *Wilderness medical practice guidelines for wilderness emergency care,* Guilford, CT, 2001, the Globe Pequot Press.

27. Gabram S, Piancentini L, Jacobs L: The risk of aeromedical transport for the cardiac patient, *Emerg Care Q* 2:72, 1990.

28. Haley C, Baker P, Eckles N: *Emergency nursing pediatric course,* Park Ridge, Ill, 1998, Emergency Nurses Association.

29. Hart M: Patient assessment, preparation and care. In U.S. Department of Transportation: *Air medical crew national standard curriculum,* 1988, U.S. Department of Transportation.

30. Hart M, et al: Air transport of the pediatric trauma patient, *Emerg Care Q* 3:21, 1986.

31. Hatfield ML, Lang A, Han ZQ, Proksch M: The effect of helicopter transport on adult patients' body temperature, *Air Med J* 18(3):103, 1999.

32. Henry M, Stapleton E: *EMT prehospital care,* Philadelphia, 1992, WB Saunders.

33. Holdefer WF, Diethelm AG, Tolbert FT: International air medical transport, part I: methods and logistics, *J Air Med Transport* 9(7):6, 1990.

34. Holdefer WF, et al: International air medical transport, part II: results and discussion, *J Air Med Transport* 9(8):8, 1990.

35. Holdefer WF, Treadwell D, Tolbert JT: International air medical transport, program profile, *Int Air Amb* 7:36, 1998.

36. Holdefer WF, Treadwell D, Moore S, Kay M, et al: International air medical transport ventilator dependent patients, *Int Air Amb* 9:22, 1999.

37. Kidd P: Assessment of the trauma patient. In Neff J, Kidd P, editors: *Trauma nursing: the art and science,* St Louis, 1993, Mosby.

38. Kitt S, et al: *Emergency nursing,* Philadelphia, 1995, WB Saunders.

39. Lee G: *Quick emergency care reference,* St Louis, 1992, Mosby.

40. Loos L, Runyan L, Pelch D: Development of prehospital medical classification criteria, *Air Med J* 17(1):13, 1998.

41. McCloskey J, Bulechek G: *Nursing interventions classification,* St Louis, 1996, Mosby.

42. McCloskey K, Orr R, editors: *Textbook of pediatric transport medicine,* St Louis, 1995, Mosby.

43. Mirski M, et al: Sedation for the critically ill neurologic patient, *Crit Care Med* 23(12):2038, 1995.

44. National Association of Emergency Medical Services Physicians: Air medical dispatch: guidelines for scene response, *Prehosp Disaster Med* 7:75, 1992.

45. National Flight Nurses Association: *Practice standards for flight nursing,* St Louis, 1995, Mosby.

46. Neff JA, Kidd PS, editors: *Trauma nursing: the art and science,* St Louis, 1993, Mosby.

47. Oakes D: *Clinical practitioner's pocket guide to respiratory care,* Philadelphia, 1998, Health Educator Publications, Inc.

48. Schneider C, et al: Evaluation of ground ambulance, rotor-wing and fixed-wing aircraft services, *Crit Care Clin* 8(3):543, 1992.

49. Sheehy SB, Jimmerson CL: *Manual of clinical trauma care: the first hour,* ed 2, St Louis, 1994, Mosby.

50. Stewart R: Analgesia in the field, *Prehosp Disaster Med* 4(1):31, 1989.

51. Strong C, Thompson CB: Documentation of decision-making during air transport, *Air Med J* 19(3):77, 2000.

52. United States Code: Consolidation Omnibus Budget Reconciliation Act (COBRA) of 1985 (42USC139dd), as amended by the Omnibus Budget Reconciliation Acts (OBRA) of 1987, 1989, and 1990.

53. U.S. Department of Health and Human Services: *Acute pain management: operative or medical procedures,* Washington DC, 1992, USDHHS.

54. U.S. Department of Labor, Occupational Safety and Health Administration: *Occupational exposure to bloodborne pathogens,* 29 CFR part 1910.1030, Washington DC, 1991, OSHA.

55. U.S. Department of Transportation Regulations: *Code of federal regulations and aeronautical information manual,* Newcastle, Wash, 1996, Aviation Supplies and Academics.

56. U.S. Department of Transportation: *Pilot's handbook of aeromedical knowledge,* Washington DC, 1984, USDOT.

57. Velianoff G: Overcrowding and diversion in the emergency department, *Nurs Clin North Am* 37(1): 59, 2002.

58. Wedige-Stecher T: Fixed-wing transport of a patient requiring IABP and left ventricular assist device, *J Air Med Transport* 9(2):6, 1990.

59. Wright A, et al: The effect of an in-flight emergency training program on crew confidence, *Air Med J* 13(4):127, 1994.

60. Zecca A, et al: Endotracheal tube stabilization in the air medical setting, *J Air Med Transport* 3:7, 1991.

AIRWAY AND VENTILATION MANAGEMENT

12

Airway management is the first priority of patient care and often accounts for one of the most difficult clinical dilemmas encountered by transport personnel. The most common error in airway management is failure to anticipate the need for active intervention in patients at high risk for airway obstruction or respiratory insufficiency.[5] Patients with a decreased level of consciousness, cardiopulmonary disease, head and neck injuries, and major traumatic injuries require quick, decisive airway management, based on a sound knowledge of physiologic and anatomic principles, to prevent life-threatening complications during transport.

Many skills and much equipment are required for control of the airway, but none is more important than the clinical judgment required to recognize that interventions are indicated. In addition to judgment skills, the competent transport team member must also possess the technical skill to per-form an intervention when it is indicated. Judgment skills are developed through experience and practice. Technical performance is improved through advanced instruction and practice. Transport team members must be familiar with alternative airway options and their risks and benefits when deciding on a particular airway management technique.

Any vehicle used for patient transport may be an unfavorable environment for airway management. Noise, vibrations, sudden movements, inadequate lighting, lack of assistive personnel, limited access to the patient, and the inability to position the patient for better airway management are only a few of the reasons that airway management can be made difficult in the transport environment.[12,32,62] Failure of transport personnel to properly secure the airway before transport can lead to further respiratory decompensation, which can hasten systemic failure or produce an unmanageable transport in which safety may be compromised. Safety must never become a secondary consideration for the transport. Therefore it is essential that the airway be fully controlled before critical care transport, even at the expense of additional time being spent at the scene or referring institution.

This chapter describes assessment parameters, airway interventions, and methods of evaluating the patient's airway and ventilation during transport. Therapies to restore breathing and circulation are discussed in later chapters.

PATHOPHYSIOLOGY

INDICATIONS FOR INTUBATION

There are multiple indications to initiate airway management including apnea, airway obstruction, airway protection, and respiratory failure. There may also be times when the decision is made to intubate when there is not an obvious reason, but there is the anticipation of a problem during transport. For example, the size of the transport vehicle may dictate that the patient has a secure airway before transport. The transport team should never ignore the competence that experience brings them. It is also important to note that even though intubation is a life-saving procedure, it is not without the potential for the development of serious complications. These include soft tissue injuries to the mouth, dental injury, vocal cord injury, tracheal or bronchial disruption, right mainstem intubation, aspiration, the development of a pneumothorax, esophageal intubation, and cardiac dysrhythmias. There are also complications that can occur with the use of neuromuscular blocking agents, anxiolytics, and sedative-hypnotics that are used to facilitate intubation.[68]

Over the past 20 years, a great deal of research has been done related to airway management in the prehospital environment.[1,12,32,62,68] The National Emergency Airway Management Course[68] recommends an approach to airway management that uses a clinical critical thinking approach. Algorithms are used to make airway management decisions. Figures 12-1 through 12-5 contain the universal emergency airway algorithm; main emergency airway management algorithm; crash airway algorithm; difficult airway algorithm; and the failed-airway algorithm. The different airway interventions that are presented in these algorithms are discussed throughout this chapter. These algorithms also provide a framework to develop quality management and research programs related to airway management in the transport environment.

SELECTED PATHOPHYSIOLOGY RELATED TO AIRWAY MANAGEMENT

Apnea can be the result of cardiac or traumatic arrest and is easily recognized and quickly treated. Upper airway obstruction in the trauma patient is usually caused by the tongue or teeth or by blood. In the nontrauma patient excessive secretions or an edematous epiglottis may obstruct the upper airway. Airway protection must be considered for the patient with actual or potential emesis and active bleeding.

A closed head injury produces increased intracranial pressure (ICP) as a result of cerebral edema. Hypoxia and hypercapnia cause cerebral blood vessels to dilate, increasing blood flow and volume, which further escalate the ICP. The resulting brain swelling compromises oxygen and glucose delivery to neurons. Intubation can help assure airway protection and adequate oxygenation during transport.[40]

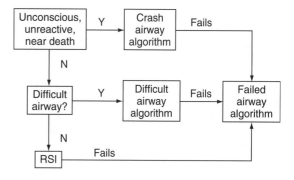

FIGURE 12-1   **Universal emergency airway algorithm.** (Reprinted from Walls, Luten, Murphy, Schneider, editors: *Manual of emergency airway management, a companion manual for the National Airway Management Course*, www.theairwaysite.com, Philadelphia, 2000, Lippincott Williams and Wilkins.)

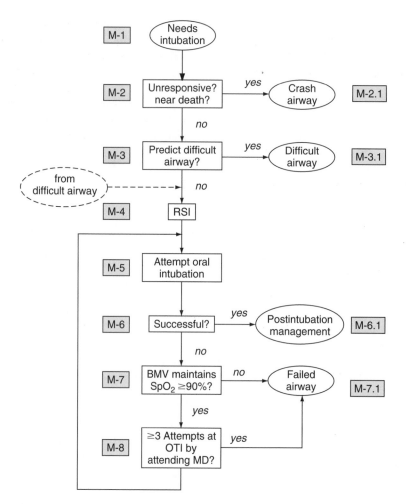

FIGURE 12-2   Main emergency airway management algorithm. (Reprinted from Walls, Luten, Murphy, Schneider, editors: *Manual of emergency airway management, a companion manual for the National Airway Management Course,* www.theairwaysite.com, Philadelphia, 2000, Lippincott Williams and Wilkins.)

Respiratory insufficiency may be traumatic or non-traumatic in origin and involves disease of the lower airways, where actual gas exchange takes place. Traumatic respiratory insufficiency may result, for example, from a flail segment or pulmonary contusion. Nontraumatic conditions that cause respiratory distress include pulmonary emboli, congestive heart failure, adult respiratory distress syndrome, and status asthmaticus.

Impending or potential airway compromise may be the most difficult situation to ascertain.

Consideration must be given to the history of illness or injury, therapies used to treat the patient before the transport teams' arrival, the patient's response to the therapies, and transport time to the receiving agency. A situation in which a patient has sustained burn trauma with an inhalation injury and circumferential burns of the neck and chest should leave the transport team with little doubt of the need for airway control. However, the transport team frequently finds themselves in situations in which the potential for airway compromise is not as

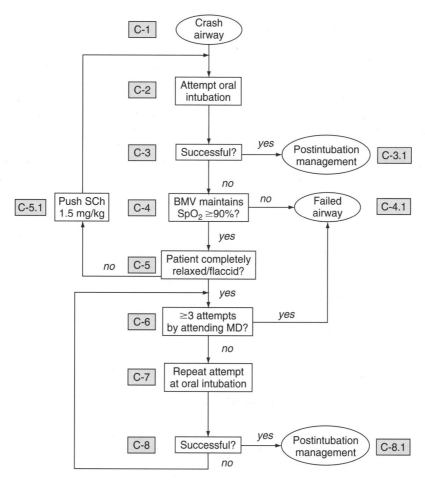

FIGURE 12-3   Crash airway algorithm. (Reprinted from Walls, Luten, Murphy, Schneider, editors: *Manual of emergency airway management, a companion manual for the National Airway Management Course,* www.theairwaysite.com, Philadelphia, 2000, Lippincott Williams and Wilkins.)

obvious. Under these circumstances the transport team must rely on subjective and objective assessment parameters and past experience to guide their judgment.

ASSESSMENT

Assessment of the airway is a two-part process. The primary survey is quick and crude; the secondary survey is slower and refined. The primary survey begins by assessment of airway patency. If a problem is discovered, the assessment stops, and immediate action is taken to establish airway patency. During the secondary survey the transport team must determine whether airway patency and an appropriate level of oxygenation can be maintained throughout transport. If in doubt, the transport team must initiate appropriate interventions.

Initially, the transport team assesses the patient by looking, listening, and feeling for spontaneous respirations. The mouth is opened and observed for

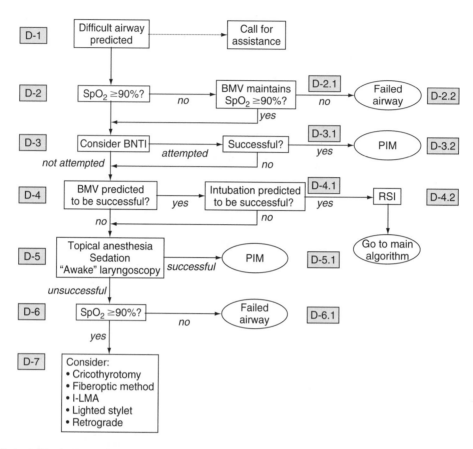

FIGURE 12-4   **Difficult airway algorithm.** (Reprinted from Walls, Luten, Murphy, Schneider, editors: *Manual of emergency airway management, a companion manual for the National Airway Management Course,* www.theairwaysite.com, Philadelphia, 2000, Lippincott Williams and Wilkins.)

obvious injuries and the presence of blood, teeth, the tongue, or foreign bodies obstructing the upper airway. An altered level of consciousness may indicate hypoxia. The patient in the compensatory stage of shock may also have an increase in the rate, rhythm, and depth of respiration; pale, moist skin; and tachypnea and tachycardia caused by a stimulation of the sympathetic nervous system. Pallor, rather than cyanosis, is an indicator of shock for both adult and pediatric patients because sympathetic nerve stimulation causes blood to shunt from minor to major organs; the skin is considered a minor organ. Major organs are the heart and brain, and the body will strive to maintain their oxygena-

tion. The patient's general appearance may also provide assessment data. The use of accessory muscles, nasal flaring, and the position the patient assumes should all be noted. The hypoxic patient may attempt to sit upright and appear anxious and apprehensive and subjectively report shortness of breath.

The neck should be observed for obvious injuries that may produce an expanding hematoma, edema subcutaneous emphysema. The position of the trachea and presence of jugular vein distention should also be noted.

The purpose of auscultation is to identify the presence of absent, decreased, or adventitious

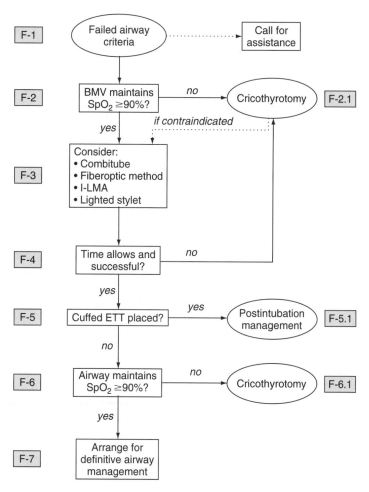

FIGURE 12-5   **Failed airway algorithm.** (Reprinted from Walls, Luten, Murphy, Schneider, editors: *Manual of emergency airway management, a companion manual for the National Airway Management Course,* www.theairwaysite.com, Philadelphia, 2000, Lippincott Williams and Wilkins.)

breath sounds. Absent or decreased breath sounds may be present with a pneumothorax or hemothorax. Adventitious breath sounds will be auscultated if there is obstruction of upper or lower airway structures.

The chest wall should be palpated for tenderness, crepitus, subcutaneous air, and symmetry of movement. Percussion is not a practical tool in the field at a noisy scene. However, in a quiet environment percussion, like palpation, can provide excellent information about the status of the underlying thoracic structures. The normal lung sound is resonant,

a hemothorax is dull, and a tension pneumothorax is hyperresonant.

The history of mechanism of injury or progression of illness may also provide subjective and objective data and assist the transport team when determining a course of action.

Pediatric patients should be assessed in the same manner as adults. However, children do not have the chronic diseases of adulthood and therefore compensate more efficiently. To the untrained or unsuspecting eye, the child who appears in mild respiratory distress may be severely ill. (See Chapter 31 for discussion of the pediatric patient.) It is essential to recognize that bradypnea and bradycardia are critical signs of impending respiratory failure in the pediatric patient. Primary cardiac arrest in children is rare. Cardiac arrest is usually caused by respiratory failure, and interventions to support respirations will also sustain the cardiac system. Therefore early and aggressive airway management for children is mandatory.

The child with respiratory insufficiency may demonstrate general signs and symptoms of fatigue, restlessness, irritability, and confusion and may cling to his or her parents with anxiety and apprehension. A weak cry is also typical. Observation may also reveal nasal flaring and substernal, supraclavicular, or intercostal retractions. Skin color is an excellent indicator of oxygenation in children; skin that is pale, with a capillary refill time of greater than 2 seconds, mottled, or cyanotic represents distress in the nontrauma patient. In the pediatric trauma patient cyanosis may not be seen as a result of hypovolemia. Cyanosis is the result of desaturated hemoglobin. Active bleeding will deplete the system of hemoglobin, and cyanosis will not be observed. A fever may be present if the respiratory distress or failure is the result of an infectious process.

Auscultation may reveal expiratory grunting or wheezing and inspiratory strider. Upper airway problems usually involve a barking cough or strider, whereas wheezing and grunting breath sounds are associated with lower airway disease or obstruction. Diminished breath sounds may be present even in the face of a nontraumatic event.

Examination of the traumatized child may yield findings similar to those previously discussed. However, palpation, percussion, and a high index of suspicion are necessary for a thorough examination. The chest wall and mediastinal structures are more mobile in children than in adults. Children can withstand severe blunt chest trauma without sustaining rib fractures, but the heart and lungs may be severely contused. Likewise, the child with a tension pneumothorax may have a shift of the mediastinal structures much faster than an adult would. Interventions for the child with chest trauma are

discussed later. It is crucial for the transport team to recognize that any sign or symptom of respiratory compromise warrants aggressive airway management in children.[16]

INTERVENTION

BASIC LIFE SUPPORT AIRWAY INTERVENTIONS

In the patient with a history of trauma, all airway interventions must be performed with protection of the cervical spine. The airway should be opened, all blood or emesis suctioned, and foreign bodies removed. The tongue may be displaced from the oropharynx through placement of an airway adjunct or by use of a modified jaw thrust. If the patient's mandible is not intact, the tongue can be protracted directly by traction with a towel clip, suture, or clamp. When properly positioned, an oropharyngeal airway rests in the lower posterior pharynx. For an adult it is inserted backward until it reaches the posterior wall of the pharynx and then is rotated into the proper position. This method of insertion is contraindicated for the pediatric patient because rotation of the rigid plastic device may cause dental or soft palate injuries. Instead, the oropharyngeal airway should be inserted with a tongue depressor.

With either method of insertion, proper position must be confirmed by assessment of airflow and efficacy of ventilation. An incorrectly placed oropharyngeal airway may worsen airflow or create an airway obstruction where none existed, created by the tongue being pushed posteriorly against the pharyngeal wall or the epiglottis being pushed against the laryngeal opening. The use of an oropharyngeal airway may induce vomiting in a conscious patient; therefore it should be used only in unconscious patients (Figure 12-6).

Nasopharyngeal airways may be used in patients with marginal stupor or coma who need assistance in maintaining an open airway. However, nasopharyngeal airways should be avoided for any patient with suspected head or facial trauma. Like that of the oral airway, the nasal airway's tip lies in the posterior pharynx behind the tongue. Selection of the

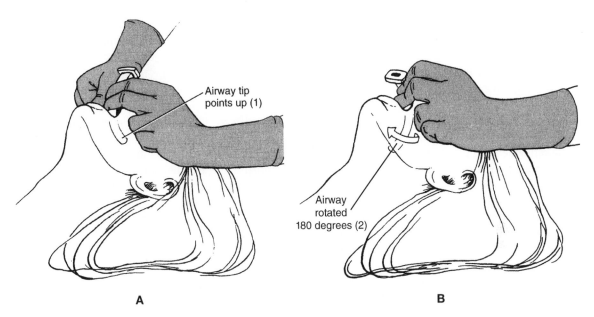

A   **B**

FIGURE 12-6   **Insertion of an oropharyngeal airway.** (From Lynn-McHale D, Carlson K, editors: *AACN procedure manual for critical care* [ed 4], Philadelphia, 2001, WB Saunders.)

appropriate size of nasal airway is important because traumatic insertion may cause severe epistaxis or adenoid bleeding, especially in children. Lubricant use facilitates its insertion. The airway is inserted with the beveled edge along the nasal septum. When the left nostril is used, the nasopharyngeal airway must be inserted upside down to maintain the beveled edge against the septum and then rotated once the airway tip is in the posterior pharynx. If significant resistance is met, the other nostril should be tried. The appropriate size for both the oral and nasal airways are obtained by comparison of the length of the airway device to the distance from the nares or mouth to the angle of the mandible (Figure 12-7).

Ventilatory assistance must be initiated immediately for the apneic patient and for the patient with severe hypoventilation. In preparation for intubation respirations can be assisted with a bag-valve mask device. Supplemental oxygen can be delivered through this device. The bag-valve mask with a reservoir can deliver a FiO$_2$ of 90% to 100% at flow rates of 10 to 15 L/min. So that emesis can be immediately identified, all masks should be transparent,

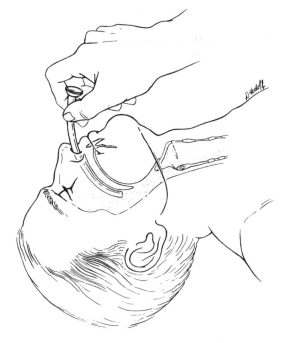

FIGURE 12-7   **Correct placement of nasopharyngeal airway.** (From Proehl J: *Emergency nursing procedures*, ed 2, Philadelphia, 1999, WB Saunders.)

the airway should be promptly suctioned, and assisted ventilations should be resumed.

ESOPHAGEAL INTUBATION

The technique of esophageal intubation began during the late 1960s and has been in use primarily in the prehospital setting since that time. Criticisms of the earlier esophageal obturator airways (EOAs) led to refinements in the esophageal airway that are frequently encountered by the critical care transport team today in areas in which medical personnel are not trained in endotracheal intubation techniques or when attempts at endotracheal intubation are unsuccessful. Contraindications to the use of the esophageal airway follow: (1) age less than 16 years or height under 5 feet, (2) presence of a gag reflex, (3) conscious or semiconscious patient, (4) known or suspected esophageal disease or injury, and (5) known or suspected caustic ingestion. The presence of maxillofacial injuries is considered to be a relative contraindication to the use of esophageal airways.[27,46,52]

The original EOA developed in 1968 is a two-part device—a mask and tube. The tube is approximately 37 cm long, open at the top, and blind at the bottom. An inflatable cuff lies above the blind end. Several holes are near the top portion of the tube, and when the tube is inserted, these holes lie in the oropharynx. The tube attaches to the mask through an opening at the lower end of the mask. A tightly sealed face mask and the cuffed end of the blunt tube theoretically prevent air from escaping through the mouth and into the stomach. If the chest does not rise, the tube should be removed immediately because it may have passed into the trachea. If placement is correct, air is forced into the tube from an external source and enters the trachea because the distal inflatable obturator cuff effectively seals off the esophagus. Achievement of a tight seal on the face mask and ventilation of the patient requires two people. With removal of the EOA, vomiting will occur. Therefore, before the EOA is removed, the patient must be tracheally intubated for airway protection.

A later modification of the EOA, the esophageal gastric tube airway (EGTA), is essentially an EOA with a lumen that allows passage of a 16-gauge gastric tube for removal of gastric contents and relief of gastric distention. However, the EGTA also requires two people for optimal ventilatory assistance. There are several disadvantages to the EOA and EGTA. First, the airway may be completely obstructed with both devices if the trachea is inadvertently intubated.[72] Second, during transport it is difficult for a tight face mask seal to be obtained and for adequate ventilation to be maintained, and esophageal and gastric ruptures have been reported.[8] Because of the problems previously discussed, the use of the EOA has fallen out of favor, although the concept of the EOA has not.

The pharyngeotracheal lumen airway (PTLA)[1] (Figure 12-8) is a further modification of the esophageal airway device and was quickly followed by the esophageal tracheal combitube[27,15] (Figure 12-9). Both devices are double tubes inserted the same way as described for the EOA. The double-tube system allows for either tracheal or esophageal intubation without ventilatory compromise. Both devices also incorporate double-balloon systems that serve as airway seals. The distal balloon, which holds 12 to 20 ml of air, seals the esophagus and prevents gastric regurgitation or, in the event of tracheal intubation, aspiration. The proximal balloon is inflated with 85 to 140 ml of air and is designed to be positioned between the base of the tongue and the soft palate so that the mouth and nasopharynx will be sealed off and the escape of air through the mouth will be prevented. The pharyngeal balloon may also tamponade oral bleeding and prevent aspiration of blood into the trachea. Both devices require only one person to manage them.[15,41] The PTLA is a definite improvement over the EOA or EGTA but still has some significant disadvantages. The oropharyngeal balloon does not prevent aspiration of teeth or other oral debris, and the oropharyngeal balloon can migrate out of the mouth anteriorly, partially dislodging the airway. Also, endotracheal intubation around the PTLA is difficult because of the residual air in the oral balloon.[68]

Neiman[41] compared blood gas measurements achieved between the PTLA and traditional

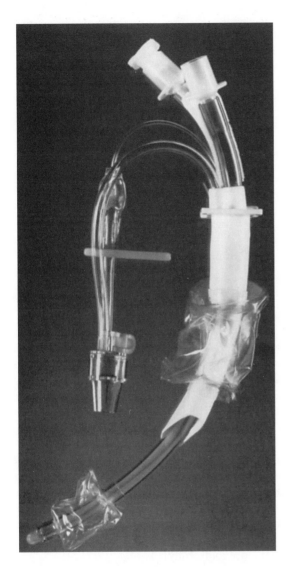

FIGURE 12-8   Pharyngeotracheal lumen airway.
(Courtesy Respironics, Inc, Monroeville, Penn.)

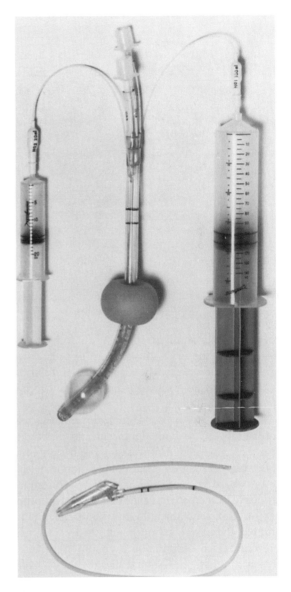

FIGURE 12-9   Esophageal tracheal combitube. (Courtesy Sheridan Catheter Corp., Argyle, NY.)

endotracheal tube (ETT). Frass et al[15] conducted a similar comparison using the esophageal tracheal combitube. Both devices have demonstrated adequate oxygenation. However, endotracheal intubation provides the best method of protecting the patient's airway and assuring adequate oxygenation during transport. Figure 12-10 illustrates insertion of the combitube.

TRACHEAL INTUBATION

Intubation of the trachea involves the passage of an ETT through the nose (nasotracheal) or mouth (orotracheal) into the trachea. Tracheal intubation provides protection against aspiration, allows for controlled and precise ventilation, and provides a

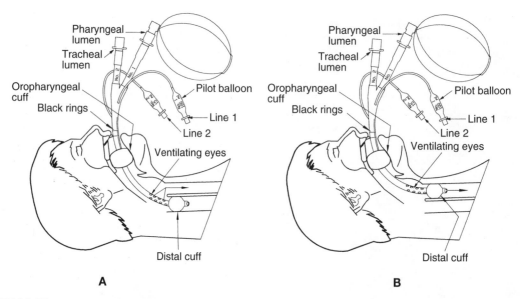

FIGURE 12-10   **Insertion of the combitube.** (From Proehl J: *Emergency nursing procedures*, ed 2, Philadelphia, 1999, WB Saunders.)

method of drug administration. In addition, intubation protects the airway in situations of progressive airway closure caused by epiglottitis, inhalation burns, soft tissue trauma or infections, and other obstructive conditions.

Complications of oral and nasal endotracheal intubation can be both significant and disastrous (see Box 12-1.).[68,9] Unsuccessful intubation or a missed inadvertent esophageal intubation may lead to prolonged hypoxia resulting in long-term injury or death. If the patient cannot be intubated, other means of oxygenation and ventilation must be substituted. Pulse oximetry during intubation can help prevent oxygen desaturation during multiple intubation attempts and should always be available. Intubation predisposes the patient to a number of harmful physiologic responses, including laryngospasm, bronchospasm caused by airway irritability or aspirated secretions, hypertension, and dysrhythmias unrelated to hypoxia.[68] In addition, the process of intubation increases the patient's ICP.[40] An unrecognized right mainstem bronchus intubation is a complication that may lead to inadequate ventilation and left lung atelectasis.

The ability to perform advanced airway maneuvers must begin with knowledge of normal anatomy. Knowledge of the anatomic structures is especially important when structures are only partially visible or are displaced as a result of injury. Familiarity with the anatomic differences between the adult and child is equally important.

THE LARYNX

Endotracheal intubation entails manipulation of the anatomy to allow passage of an ETT through the larynx either blindly or through direct visualization with a laryngoscope. An understanding of the relationship of the cartilages of the larynx and their relative positions will help to perform intubation faster and more confidently.

The larynx, or voice box, is an intricate arrangement of nine cartilages, three single and six paired, connected by membranes and ligaments and moved by nine muscles. From above it attaches to the hyoid bone and opens into the laryngopharynx, and on the inside it is continuous with the trachea. In an adult it extends from the level of the fourth to the sixth cervical vertebrae.

The three single cartilages form the basic boxlike structure of the larynx and provide the major external landmarks. The thyroid cartilage, commonly known as the Adam's apple, is formed by the fusion

BOX 12-1 Complications of Intubation

Early Complications Occurring During the Intubation Procedure

1. Neck
Cervical strain: subluxation/dislocation, fracture, and neurologic injury

2. Mouth
Soft tissue injury resulting in abrasion and hemorrhage involving lips, tongue, buccal mucosa, and pharynx
Temporomandibular joint subluxation/dislocation
Dental injury

3. Airway/respiratory
Arytenoid: dislocation and avulsion
Vocal cord: spasm, avulsion, and laceration
Pyriform sinus perforation resulting in pneumothorax and pneumomediastinum
Tracheal and bronchial rupture
Right main stem bronchus intubation, with atelectasis and respiratory compromise
Bronchospasm

4. Gastrointestinal
Esophageal: intubation and perforation
Vomiting and aspiration

5. Cardiovascular
Hypertension, tachycardia, bradycardia, and dysrhythmias
Cardiac arrest and interruption of CPR

Late Complications Occurring After Tube Is in Place

1. Airway/respiratory
Tube obstruction: secretions, blood, and kinking
Accidental extubation and endobronchial intubation
Vocal cords: ulceration
Trachea: ulceration, ischemic necrosis, and paralysis
Pneumothorax and pneumomediastinum
Aspiration and atelectasis
Cough resulting in increased intrathoracic, intracranial, and intraocular pressures

2. Gastrointestinal
Esophageal intubation
Tracheoesophageal fistula

3. Cardiovascular
Tracheoinnominate artery fistula

4. Infections
Sinusitis, pneumonia, tracheobronchitis, mediastinitis, and abscess

5. Tube dislodgment

From Walls R, editor: *Emergency airway management*, Phildelphia,2000, Lippincott Williams and Wilkins; Dauphinee K: Orotracheal intubation; nasotracheal intubation, *Emerg Med Clin North Am* 6(4): 7110, 1988.

of two curving cartilage plates and is typically larger in men than in women because of the growth-stimulating influence of male sex hormones during puberty. The ring-shaped cricoid cartilage is sand-wiched between the thyroid cartilage above the first tracheal ring. Because the cricoid cartilage is a complete ring, the tracheal diameter does not narrow during cricoid pressure.[6] The cricoid cartilage is

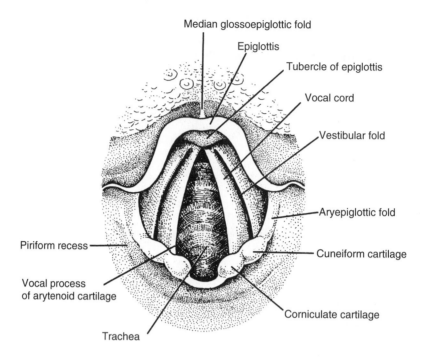

Median glossoepiglottic fold

Epiglottis

Tubercle of epiglottis

Vocal cord

Vestibular fold

Aryepiglottic fold

Cuneiform cartilage

Corniculate cartilage

Trachea

Vocal process
of arytenoid cartilage

Piriform recess

FIGURE 12-11   Laryngoscopic view of the airway. (From Rosen P et al: *Emergency medicine: concepts and clinical practice*, vol 1, ed 3, St Louis, 1992, Mosby.)

connected to the thyroid cartilage by the cricothyroid membrane and is the desired location for a cricothyrotomy.[68] The upper free edge of the cricothyroid membrane forms the vocal cords. Because of the attachment of the vocal cords to the cricoid ring, downward pressure on the cricoid ring helps to bring the vocal cords into view when they are hidden behind the tongue (the Sellick maneuver).[6] The third single cartilage is the epiglottis, a spoon-shaped structure that prevents anything other than air from entering the tracheal inlet. The epiglottis is a major visual landmark during intubation (Figures 12-11 and 12-12).

The most important paired cartilages of the larynx are the arytenoids. The arytenoids are pyramid-shaped and anchor the vocal cords in the larynx. The vocal cords look pearly white because of their avascular nature. At rest the vocal cords lie partially separated or abducted. Excessive secretions or aspiration stimulates the airway and activates the defense reflexes. Laryngospasm, or spasmodic clo-

sure of the vocal cords, is the most severe form of airway closure and can totally prevent ventilation and the passage of an ETT.[73] If a tube is forced through the cords with excessive pressure, an arytenoid can actually be dislocated and permanent hoarseness can result.[73] The remaining two pairs of cartilages, the cuneiform and corniculate, form the posterior wall of the larynx. Committing these structures to memory will assist the transport team in quickly identifying the glottic opening, and when the opening is obscured from view, the ETT can be steered into position with the structures in view as reference points.

OROTRACHEAL INTUBATION

Orotracheal intubation is the most common method of airway management for all age groups. In children orotracheal intubation is used almost exclusively.[68,13] It is a safe procedure that involves psychomotor skills that are easily mastered. There are few, if any, true contraindications to

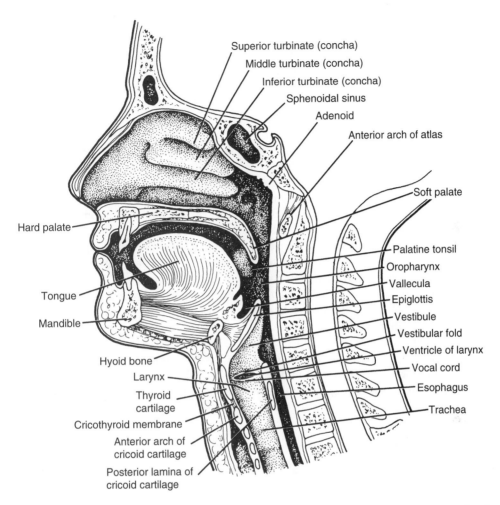

FIGURE 12-12   Sagittal view of the airway. (From Rosen P et al: *Emergency medicine: concepts and clinical practice*, vol 1, ed 3, St Louis, 1992, Mosby.)

orotracheal intubation in the emergency setting. However, during circumstances in which major facial and neck trauma prevents recognition of landmarks or during isolated mandibular trauma in which the temporomandibular joint may be immobile, the orotracheal route becomes much more difficult and may necessitate a surgical airway. Other conditions that might dictate a surgical airway include circumstances in which there is significant bleeding in the oral pharynx or supraglottic area and in patients with epiglottitis in whom

landmarks are obscured or passage of a tube is impossible.[68,51] Again, these conditions are considered relative, not absolute, contraindications. Another relative contraindication for oral intubation is the patient with a suspected unstable cervical spine injury. Oral intubation may be acceptable if strict in-line cervical spine immobilization is maintained.[34,47] Trauma to the teeth, soft tissues of the mouth, posterior pharynx, or vocal cords caused by improper use of the laryngoscope blade are complications of oral intubation.

In the adult the narrowest portion of the airway is the glottic opening, the space between the true vocal cords. In children the narrowest portion is at the cricoid cartilage below the vocal cords. In the child it is possible to see the tube pass through the vocal cords but to be unable to pass the tube through the cricoid ring. If this situation occurs, a smaller tube should be chosen; an ETT should never be forced down a child's airway.

The choice of blade, straight or curved, is left to the personal preference of the intubator, although the straight blade is recommended in obese patients and in patients with short, muscular necks. In these persons the airway is located more forward, and curved blades often do not provide an adequate view.[47] Patients with receding chins also tend to have an anterior larynx, which may make intubation more difficult with a curved blade.[12] The adult-size blade is a no. 3 or 4. Steps for orotracheal intubation are included in Box 12-2. Selection of the appropriate size tube is an important consideration in patient intubation. In general, the largest tube possible should be selected. This will minimize airway resistance, assist in suctioning, and minimize the need for excessive inflation of the tube

cuff, which can cause mucosal damage. The cuff pressure should be at minimal occluding volume. At pressures greater than 25 mm Hg, mucosal ischemia starts to occur. A persistent air leak in the balloon is often caused by a faulty valve at the pilot balloon.

To correct this condition without reintubating, the transport team member should attach a stopcock to the balloon, reinflate the balloon, and close the stopcock.[51] The average adult female airway can accommodate a 7 to 8 mm tube (the size refers to the inside diameter of the tube), and the average male airway, an 8 to 9 mm tube. The pilot balloon should be tested for leaks before insertion.

Preoxygenation is an important step that is frequently terminated prematurely. The procedure requires a tight seal on the face mask and use of a bag-valve mask device with reservoir to deliver the highest FiO_2 for 3 to 5 minutes. If done correctly, preoxygenation will supersaturate the patient and allow for as much as 5 to 8 minutes of apnea. Another method of preoxygenation involves placing a high flow mask on a breathing patient. Pulse oximetry should be available to aid in oxygen desaturation detection. If CPR is being performed, it

---

BOX 12-2   Steps for Orotracheal Intubation

1. Position the patient. Nontrauma patient: Flex the neck forward and extend the head backward, creating a "sniffing" position. Trauma patient: Maintain in-line traction.
2. Preoxygenate the patient.
3. Hold the laryngoscope in the left hand, and open the patient's mouth with the right hand.
4. Insert the blade into the right side of the mouth, sweep the tongue to the left, and advance to the appropriate landmarks. The Miller (straight) blade tip goes beyond the epiglottis; the MacIntosh (curved) blade tip enters the vallecula.
5. Pull the laryngoscope blade at a 45-degree angle; avoid twisting the laryngoscope handle. Visualize the epiglottis and vocal cords. Apply cricoid pressure.
6. Insert the ETT from the right corner of the mouth, and watch the tube pass through the vocal cords. Use the largest tube possible. Remove the stylet.
7. Inflate the tube cuff with 5 to 10 ml of air or to minimal occluding volume. (Minimal occluding volume is determined by placing the hand over the mouth and noting cessation of air leak with ventilation.) Capillary flow pressure in the tracheal mucosa is approximately 25 mm Hg, so cuff pressure should be less than that.
8. Confirm tube placement by auscultating bilateral breath sounds over the chest and axilla and by noting a lack of gurgling over the epigastrium. Observe for symmetry of chest wall motion. For a child observe the cardiac monitor for the maintenance of an appropriate pulse rate and improvement in the patient's color.
9. Secure the tube in place.

should not be interrupted for more than 15 seconds for any single intubation attempt,[1] but unforeseen obstacles frequently prolong the procedure. With proper preoxygenation, the transport team has more than adequate time for intubation to occur in a very deliberate, nonhurried, and controlled environment rather than in a state of panic.

The Sellick maneuver (digital pressure over the cricoid cartilage exerted posteriorly) can assist with intubation in two ways and is useful in both oral and nasal intubation. It improves visualization of the glottic opening by pressing the larynx downward and perhaps into the field of view. Cricoid pressure forces the cricoid ring against the vertebral column and effectively seals the esophagus, preventing the aspiration of passively regurgitated gastric contents or swallowed blood. In general, gastric emptying ceases when a person sustains significant trauma, and a patient is considered to have a full stomach if he or she has eaten within 6 hours of sustaining trauma or receiving anesthesia.[6] If the patient actively vomits, the assistant should immediately release the cricoid pressure and actively suction the patient's airway. Cricoid pressure may occasionally prevent the passage of a tube if the posterior pressure is too great or if the pressure is over the thyroid cartilage and not the cricoid ring. This is especially true in the pediatric patient because of the child's pliable airway structures. If difficulty is encountered, the assistant should release part or all of the pressure.

BURP is an additional maneuver to improve visualization of the glottis during difficult intubations. The BURP method (Backward, Upward, Rightward, Pressure) involves pressure on the thyroid cartilage. At present, there is little in the literature about its use in the transport environment.[29]

Insertion of the tube through the relaxed cords should continue until the cuff is just past the cords. To ensure the tip of the tube is above the carina, the tube is placed so that the teeth are approximately at the 21-cm mark on the tube for women and at the 23-cm mark for men.[68] With completion of the intubation, the laryngoscope is gently withdrawn, the cuff is inflated with 5 to 10 ml of air, and placement of the tube is confirmed. Tube placement confirmation begins with auscultation of breath sounds in the right and left chest areas and over the stomach. A number of adjuncts are available to assist in confirmation of tube placement and are discussed later in this chapter.

Once intubated and oxygenated, previously hypoxic patients may have an increased level of consciousness and may become combative. In a patient's confusion their first priority is extubation. Soft restraints and a bite block may be in order. An oral airway may be used as a bite block to prevent the patient from biting down on the ETT. The bite block should be secured in place separately from the ETT. If the bite block and the ETT are secured together, the patient may inadvertently extubate him or herself by lodging the tongue behind the oral airway and pushing it and the ETT out.

NASOTRACHEAL INTUBATION

Nasotracheal intubation is often referred to as a blind procedure because the larynx is not visualized as in the orotracheal method. For successful performance of the blind method of tracheal intubation, the patient must have spontaneous respirations, although the use of a lighted stylet in an apneic patient can facilitate the nasotracheal route. In addition to the patient having spontaneous respirations, the nasotracheal method also requires a relatively quiet environment, which could make it a difficult procedure at a noisy scene. In general, the nasotracheal technique requires more time than the orotracheal technique[45,68] but also offers many advantages over the orotracheal technique (Box 12-3).

Nasotracheal intubation is a relatively easy procedure that is usually well tolerated by patients. The technique is especially useful in dyspneic patients because they have breath sounds that are easily heard and their glottis tends to remain open. For trauma patients the procedure can be performed with no movement of the cervical spine and can be performed on a patient who is sitting. Therefore the nasotracheal method can be a useful procedure in the trauma patient who needs airway management but who is still trapped upright in a vehicle. Also, the patient cannot bite the tube, and the tube is easily secured in place so mouth care is easily provided.

BOX 12-3 | **Advantages of Nasotracheal Intubation Versus the Orotracheal Technique**

1. Tube is more easily secured and hence is less likely to be dislodged.
2. More comfort during awake intubation and on the patient awakening.
3. Easier insertion in a patient with impaired neck or jaw motion.
4. No danger of the patient biting the tube.
5. Facilitates surgery to the oral cavity.
6. Favored in patients in whom laryngoscopy is difficult or contraindicated.
7. Useful in patients in whom neuromuscular blockade is hazardous.

Modified from Walls R et al: *Manual of emergency airway management*, Philadelphia, 2000, Lippincott Williams and Wilkins.

A disadvantage of blind nasal intubation is that any upper airway bleeding induced by this technique can obscure visualization during subsequent attempts at direct laryngoscopy should the blind technique fail.

The only absolute contraindication to the standard blind nasotracheal technique of intubation is apnea or near apnea. Other contraindications to nasotracheal intubation are considered relative, and they include (1) a suspected basilar skull fracture (may risk cranial intubation) or other closed head injury; (2) acute epiglottitis; (3) severe nasal or maxillofacial fractures; (4) upper airway foreign body, abscess, or tumor; and (5) anticoagulation therapy or other blood-clotting abnormalities causing epistaxis. There are disadvantages that are not contraindications to the procedure that should be noted. Nasotracheal intubation puts the patient at risk for the development of meningitis or encephalitis. Special consideration must also be given to the patient for whom bacteremia would be detrimental, such as the immunocompromised patient or the patient with a cardiac valve abnormality or prosthesis.

The most common complication of nasotracheal intubation is hemorrhage. Traumatic intubation may cause epistaxis through abrasion of the nasal mucosa or rupture of a nasal polyp. Bleeding can be minimized by use of a tube 1 mm smaller than would be used orally. Use of a vasoconstrictive agent to the nasal mucosa, such as topical phenylephrine, lubrication of the tube well, and avoidance of excessive pressure will also help prevent excessive bleeding. In the awake patient it is also advisable to provide nasopharyngeal anesthesia with lidocaine or Cetacaine, and aqueous lidocaine gel may be used to lubricate the tube.[45,68] In children the relatively large size of the tonsils and adenoidal tissue may produce severe bleeding if ruptured. Perforation and dissection of the posterior pharyngeal wall have also been reported.[9] Steps for nasotracheal intubation are included in Box 12-4.

The proper head position in the patient being nasotracheally intubated is the sniffing position with a bit less extension than when an oral intubation is performed. Extreme extension creates a more acute angle for the tube to pass through the larynx and makes the procedure more difficult. However, if cervical spine injury is suspected, the head and neck must be maintained in the neutral position. The beveled edge of the tube should be introduced against the nasal septum of the nostril chosen. The tube is advanced through the nose and into the pharynx with continuous forward pressure and gentle rotation. If the nasal passage appears to be obstructed, the other nostril may be used, or the tube may be substituted with a smaller one. The tube must never be forced. The intubator must listen and feel for air movement through the tube as the tube enters the pharynx and advances toward the glottis. Cricoid pressure may also be helpful. As the tube approaches the glottis, breath sounds will be heard maximally. On inspiration the tube is advanced through the cords. Tube position is then verified as described earlier.

Several devices are available to aid placement of the nasotracheal tube. The Endotrol tube is

BOX 12-4	**Steps for Nasotracheal Intubation**

1. Assess nasal patency. Alternately occlude each naris, listen to air passage, and ask the patient or family members about past medical problems.
2. Anesthetize the nasal passage with lidocaine and a vasoconstrictor such as phenylephrine. Cetacaine to the posterior pharynx may also be used.
3. Position the patient. Nontrauma patient: may sit upright or assume a sniffing position with a bit less extension than for oral intubation. Trauma patient: maintain in-line traction.
4. Provide supplemental oxygen.
5. Lubricate the tube liberally.
6. Introduce the tube perpendicular to the floor for the supine patient or to the bed for the upright patient.
7. Point the bevel of the tube toward the nasal septum. (If the left naris is used, the tube is inserted backward.)
8. Gently pass the tube and listen to breath sounds through the end of the tube as it is advanced. Occlusion of the opposite naris may make the breath sounds louder.
9. Just proximal to the glottis, the breath sounds become maximal. Take care not to touch the cords prematurely so as not to induce laryngospasm and cough.
10. Quickly advance the tube on inspiration into the trachea. An assistant should apply the Sellick maneuver (cricoid pressure) to help align the glottic opening.
11. Confirm the tube position by auscultating breath sounds and observing symmetric chest wall motion, and ensure that the patient is unable to speak.
12. Secure the tube in place.

specifically designed for nasotracheal intubation and for use in patients with an anterior larynx. The Endotrol tube has a ring on the upper portion that directs the tip anteriorly when traction is applied to the ring. Should cord spasm develop, a topical anesthetic may be sprayed onto the cords through the tube. Another device used to aid placement of the nasotracheal tube is the airway whistle or BAAM (Beck Airway Airflow Monitor). The whistle is attached to the standard 15-mm endotracheal connector and amplifies the patient's breathing as the tube is being advanced through the posterior nasopharynx. As the tube is advanced further, the sound increases in intensity. Deviation from the airflow tract will result in a decrease or loss of the whistle sound, indicating a need for tube redirection. Once intubation is complete, the airway whistle is removed. An air medical program evaluated the BAAM airway whistle and found that it was easy to use even in the noisy in-flight environment and had the added advantage of protecting the intubator against contact with blood, vomitus, and sputum during the intubation procedure.[30] A technique for using the BAAM airway whistle combined with the controllable-tip ETT during blind oral intubation and digital intubation has also been described.[7]

LIGHTED STYLET

An optional method of endotracheal intubation is the use of the lighted stylet. Referred to as the transillumination method, it uses a rigid wire stylet with a light bulb at the distal end and is powered by a small battery source in the proximal end. The technique relies on the transillumination of the neck tissue to guide the placement of the ETT. The lighted stylet was originally designed to aid in the blind nasotracheal method of intubation; however, design modifications have now been made to allow use in both orotracheal or nasotracheal methods.[68] The brighter transilluminated glow from the trachea is easily distinguished from the dull or absent glow should the esophagus be intubated. Medical personnel can also use the lighted stylet to accurately position the ETT of an intubated patient by adjusting the stylet so that the transilluminated glow is at the level of the sternal notch. The tube is then slid to align proximally with a point that will also align the light with the distal tip of the ETT (Box 12-5).[30]

BOX 12-5 | **Steps for Using the Lighted Stylet**

1. Position the patient. Nontrauma patient: Flex the neck forward and extend the head backward, creating the sniffing position. Trauma patient: Maintain in-line traction.
2. Preoxygenate the patient.
3. The lighted stylet should be checked to ensure its light is bright enough by directly looking at the light. If the light is not uncomfortable to the eyes, it should be discarded and a new one used.
4. The lubricated stylet is inserted into a transparent ETT, and the light is positioned at the tip of the ETT, but not beyond.
5. The distal end of the ETT is then bent at a slightly greater than 90° angle.
6. The intubator kneels or stands on either side of the patient at the level of the shoulders, facing the patient.
7. For the oral technique lift the tongue or the tongue and jaw, pulling the epiglottis anteriorly and clearing the supraglottic area for introduction of the tube stylet. Slide the tube down along the tongue, and lift the glottis in a "soup ladle" motion. For the nasal technique use the lighted stylet with a directional tip tube such as the Endotrol tube. The tube stylet is inserted with the beveled edge against the septum after applying a topical anesthetic and phenylephrine.
8. As the tube stylet is advanced, observe for the transilluminated glow in the midline. If the tip is off midline, a dim glow will be observed. If the glow is extremely dim or cannot be seen, the epiglottis has not been elevated and is probably covering the glottic opening. Correct by lifting forward on the jaw, tongue, or both.
9. When a bright midline glow is observed, the tube stylet is advanced until the glow is located at the sternal notch.
10. Carefully remove the stylet without dislodging the tube. Secure the tube.
11. Confirm proper tube placement in the usual manner.

Verdile[64] described the advantages of the transillumination method in prehospital care as follows: (1) rapidity of intubation, an average of 20 seconds; (2) ability to intubate without manipulation of the head and neck; and (3) low incidence of complications. Vollmer et al[66] published similar results.

DIGITAL INTUBATION

Digital intubation, or tactile orotracheal intubation, was the original method of intubation beginning in the mid-1700s.[26] With the invention of the laryngoscope the technique became obsolete. Although not the method of choice, digital intubation can be helpful when other conventional methods have failed. The technique is useful in comatose patients with head and neck trauma, in obese patients or those with short, muscular necks, and in patients with severe bleeding or excessive secretions that prevent direct visualization by laryngoscopy. The digital technique may also be useful in cramped spaces, such as ground or air ambulances in which space is limited, or in situations in which equipment such as a laryngoscope or suction apparatus is lacking or has failed.[56,68]

Digital intubation requires that the patient be completely unconscious and that the mouth can be opened widely without fear of the patient biting. In an air medical program this technique has been used with remarkable success in children and neonates, despite their small mouth openings.[17] It relies on the ability of the intubator to guide the tip of the tube through the glottic opening using the middle and index fingers of the nondominant hand (Box 12-6).

LARYNGEAL MASK AIRWAY (LMA)

The laryngeal mask airway offers another method of airway management in the transport environment. A British anesthesiologist named Archie Brain designed the LMA. The device is designed to surround and cover the supraglottic area. The LMA consists of an airway tube, a mask, and a mask inflation tube (Figure 12-13). There are two rubber bars that cross the tube opening at the mask end to prevent the herniation of the epiglottis into the LMA tube.[68] Figure 12-14 illustrates insertion of the LMA.

BOX 12-6	**Steps for Digital Oral Intubation**

1. Position the patient. Nontrauma patient: Flex the neck forward and extend the head backward, creating a sniffing position. Trauma patient: Maintain in-line traction.
2. Preoxygenate the patient.
3. Select the appropriate size ETT in the usual manner. Insert an intubation stylet and bend the tube stylet in an open J configuration. Lubricate the tube.
4. Kneels or stand on either side of the patient at the level of the shoulders, facing the patient.
5. With gloved hands insert the fingers of the nondominant hand along the patient's tongue, pull the tongue forward, and "walk" the fingers down to palpate the epiglottis with the middle finger. If the epiglottis is not palpated, pull forward on the tongue.
6. The tube stylet is then slid along the left side of the mouth, with the medial aspect of the middle finger and the volar aspect of the index finger used to guide the tube tip in the direction of the epiglottis. Keep the index finger above the tube and the tube tip in contact with the middle finger.
7. Hold the tube against the epiglottis with the index finger, and slip the tube distally toward the glottic opening.
8. As the tube enters the glottic opening, resistance will increase. At this point hold the tube firmly and withdraw the stylet slightly. Advance the tube through the cords and then completely remove the stylet.
9. Confirm proper tube placement in the usual manner.

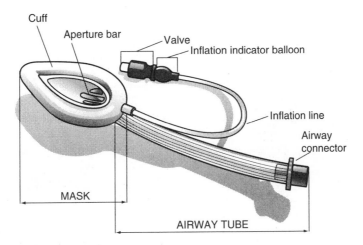

FIGURE 12-13   **Laryngeal tracheal mask.** (Courtesy of LMA North America, Inc.)

There is also a LMA device that allows for the insertion of an endotracheal tube once the LMA is in place. It is known as the intubating laryngeal mask (ILM).[37] One available device is called the LMA-Fastrach. It is designed to allow the insertion of an endotracheal tube that comes with the device to be inserted through the LMA-Fastrach. With use of a stabilizing rod, the LMA-Fastrach is then removed, and the endotracheal tube remains in place.[68]

Advantages of the use of the LMA or ILM in the transport environment include: minimal skill and training are required for their use; the devices can be inserted with minimal manipulation of the patient's head and neck; the insertion can occur either in front of or behind the patient which may make it particularly useful for the patient who is entrapped and if laryngoscopy is contraindicated or impossible, the patient can be intubated through the device.[35,37,68] Another advantage this device may

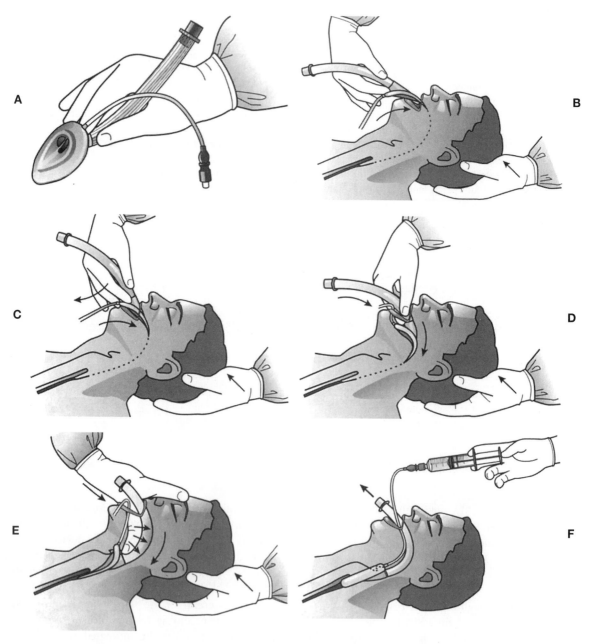

FIGURE 12-14   **Insertion of the laryngeal mask airway.** (Courtesy of LMA North America, Inc.)

offer for airway management in the transport environment is that it is available in pediatric sizes while many airway rescue devices are not.

The major disadvantage of the use of LMA in the transport environment is that the patient must be deeply sedated or unconsciousness to insert the device. Other contraindications to the use of the LMA that the transport team must consider include the risk of aspiration, poor pulmonary compliance, laryngeal problems, and local pharyngeal abnormality.

The major indication for the use of the LMA or the intubating LMA in the transport environment is as a temporizing measure when there is a failed-airway situation. However, because the majority of patients who require intubation in the transport environment may have full stomachs, the transport team must always consider the risk of aspiration because the LMA does not protect the tracheobronchial tree from gastrointestinal contents. Figure 12-15 illustrates insertion of the intubating LMA (ILMA), and Figure 12-16 illustrates insertion of the endotracheal tube through the ILMA.

PEDIATRIC MANAGEMENT

Successful management of the pediatric airway begins with the knowledge that anatomic differences in children require adaptations to the techniques described earlier for proper care to be provided. Fortunately, the differences slowly diminish as a child ages. Not only does the clinician have to be familiar with anatomic differences but also the child's fear or apprehension can complicate treatment efforts. Even the routine act of supplemental oxygenation with a nasal cannula or mask can become a challenge in an awake child because of the child's fear of having something in his or her nose or wrapped around his or her face. The child should be prepared by being talked to and comforted as much as possible. This step is important to the child and to the adult.

The indications for intubation are the same for the pediatric patient as for the adult. Complications are also similar in both populations. The most common complications of orotracheal intubation for all age groups include dental trauma and esophageal

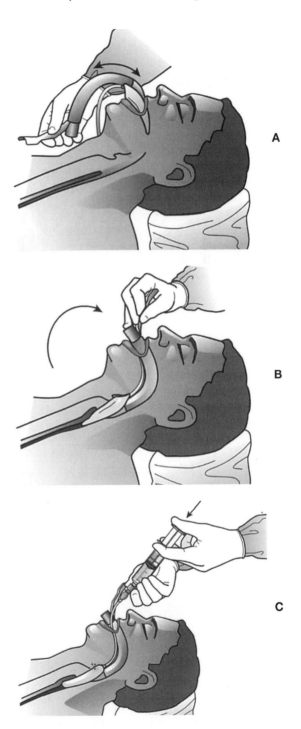

FIGURE 12-15   **Insertion of the intubating laryngeal mask airway (ILMA).** (Courtesy of LMA North America, Inc.)

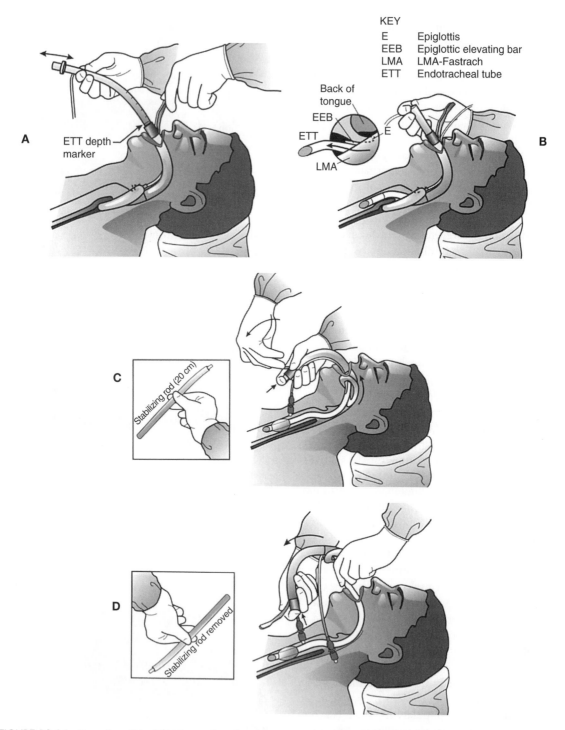

FIGURE 12-16 **Insertion of the LMA-Fastrach endotracheal tube and removal of the LMA-Fastrach.** (Courtesy of LMA North America, Inc.)

and right mainstem bronchus intubations that go unrecognized. The most common cause of unsuccessful pediatric intubation is operator inexperience.[13,68] Although the complications appear to be many and severe, benefits of orotracheal intubation far outweigh the disadvantages. Orotracheal intubation is considered the gold standard of airway control and is a skill the should be mastered by all transport personnel who are responsible for advanced airway management.

There are anatomic differences in the upper and lower airways of the infant who is 1 year or younger, the child who is 1 to 8 years old, and the older child or adolescent who is 8 to 16 years old. As the child approaches 8 years of age, the larynx closely resembles that of the adult in structure and position. However, the overall size remains less than that of the adult. An infant's head is much larger in proportion to the rest of the body and results in a natural sniffing position. In infants and some young children the sniffing position is too pronounced, and the flight nurse may need to place a towel under the infant's shoulders to raise the rest of the body and straighten the airway, thereby improving airflow. The infant is also an obligate nose breather, and secretions or edema in this area can cause airway compromise. Infants and small children also have tongues that are large in relation to the size of their oropharynges, which makes the tongue, as it is in the adult, the most common cause of airway obstruction. The relatively small size of children's mouths also makes intubation more difficult. Because of the small size of the pediatric airway, minimal edema can create a life-threatening obstruction. An infant's airway, normally 4 mm in diameter, will decrease to 2 mm with 1 mm of circumferential edema caused by secretions or trauma caused by intubation. By comparison, the adult airway, normally 8 mm in diameter, will decrease to 6 mm with 1 mm of circumferential edema. The result is only a 25% decrease in diameter as compared with a 50% decrease in the infant with an equal amount of swelling.[23] The vocal cords of a young child are more pliable than those of the adult and are easier to damage, resulting in potential obstruction. Additionally, the larynx is more anterior in the young child, which leads to more frequent intubation of the esophagus.

Lungs can easily be overdistended and barotrauma induced by overzealous rescue attempts. Ventilation should be limited to the amount of air needed to cause the chest to rise. Excessive volumes exacerbate gastric distention and increase the risk of pneumothorax.[68] When possible, a self-inflating bag-valve ventilation system should be used, optimally with a pop-off valve. Resuscitation bags are available for neonates (delivering volumes of 500 to 600 ml) and adults (delivering volumes of 1.0 to 1.5 L). An oxygen reservoir should be used to enhance the oxygen concentration.[68] Initial respiratory rates used for controlled ventilation should approximate normal spontaneous respiratory rates based on age.[13,50,68]

The proper ETT size can be determined in several ways. It can be approximated by the size of the child's little finger or nares. A more precise method to ensure proper ETT size is as follows:

$$\text{Newborn: Preterm} = 3.0$$

$$\text{Full-term} = 3.5$$

Then:

$$\frac{\text{Age (years)} + 16}{4} = \text{Internal diameter of ETT (mm)}$$

ETT depth (cm) in orally intubated children (or adults), tube measured at lip line = Tube size × 3

Pediatric tubes are cuffless, which prevents subglottic stenosis and ulceration, and they range in size from 2.5 to 6.5 mm. Cuffless tubes are recommended in children younger than 8 years of age[14] because the cricoid cartilage is the narrowest portion of the trachea, and if the proper size tube is used, it serves as a physiologic cuff. A tube that is too large will not pass through the cricoid cartilage. A tube that is too small will not provide total airway protection.

The anatomic differences between the pediatric and adult airways are illustrated in Figure 12-1. The anatomic differences can be summarized as follows[50,68]:

1. A child's larynx lies more cephalad than an adult's.

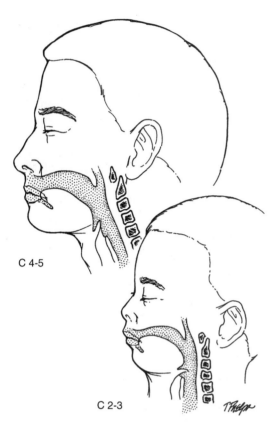

C 4-5

C 2-3

FIGURE 12-17   **Comparative anatomy of the adult and infant airways.** (From Nichols DG et al, editors: *Golden hour— the handbook of advanced pediatric life support,* ed 2, St Louis, 1996, Mosby.)

2. A child's epiglottis is at an angle of 45 degrees to the anterior pharyngeal wall, whereas an adult's lies parallel to the base of the tongue.
3. A child's epiglottis is large, stiff, and U-shaped, whereas an adult's is flattened and more flexible.
4. The larger tongue of infants and children and the position of the hyoid bone depress the epiglottis.
5. The cricoid ring is the narrowest portion of a child's airway.

The use of a Miller (straight) blade permits easier cord visualization. A straight blade is inserted beyond the epiglottis, which is lifted up along with the tongue and jaw. If the blade is inserted too far

and landmarks are not easily recognized, the blade should be gently backed out, and the glottic opening will often "pop" into view. Inability to recognize the epiglottis increases the likelihood of tracheal intubation. Pediatric Miller blades range in size from 0 to 2. The 0 blade is used for the premature and small newborn, and the Miller 1 is used for the larger newborn to age 2 years. A Miller 2 or the MacIntosh 2 is used in children older than 2 years. For the child older than 12 years, the MacIntosh 3 is frequently used.[13]

During intubation, it is beneficial to assign an assistant the task of observing the cardiac monitor for heart rate. In young infants the cardiac output is very rate dependent, and bradycardia is universally associated with hypotension.[13] A heart rate of less than 100 beats/min in a neonate, less than 80 beats/min in an infant, and less than 60 beats/min in a child constitutes bradycardia. Should this be observed, the intubation attempt is aborted, and oxygenation by bag-valve mask is initiated. Atropine should be administered to all children and adolescents receiving succinylcholine to block vagal stimulation.

Tube placement is confirmed by auscultation with observation, palpation, and the use of an endotracheal tube confirmation device such as an end-tidal CO_2 detector. Breath sounds are transmitted readily, although the child's thorax and abdomen make it hard to judge tube placement. Therefore along with auscultation the transport team should observe the symmetric rise and fall of the chest wall, monitor for maintenance of heart rate, and check the patient's color for improvement. The chest wall should also be palpated for symmetry of movement.

ETT depth is generally three times the inside diameter of the tube size. This rule of thumb applies to premature infants and to adults when the appropriate size tube for the patient's age is in place.[13] Once placed, the tube should be well secured with tape and tincture of benzoin. The use of tracheostomy tape should be avoided because it may kink the tube or reduce the tube's diameter if secured too tightly. Because the tube is cuffless and the child's trachea is so short, movement of the child's head may lead to a mainstem intubation or to extubation. As with the adult, assessment of tube placement should occur after each patient transfer—for example, after the child is loaded into the aircraft before liftoff.

A part of airway management for children is the placement of a gastric tube. A child's stomach is relatively larger than an adult's and may contain food and a significant amount of air. Children tend to swallow air when crying (aerophagia). If full, the stomach may impinge on the diaphragm and decrease vital capacity. If a postintubation chest radiograph is available, the tip of the ETT should be at the T2 to T3 vertebral level or at the level of the lower edge of the medial aspect of the clavicle.

INVASIVE AIRWAY MANAGEMENT

Invasive airway management offers additional methods to manage a difficult or failed airway. The likelihood is good, particularly for the transport team who frequently care for trauma victims, that at some time these skills will be needed. Because of the relatively infrequent opportunity to gain experience, there can be reluctance to attempt the procedure when the clinical situation clearly dictates the need for an invasive airway. Reluctance to perform the procedure and the delay that results can add additional urgency to a situation that necessitates swift action. Transport team members must be knowledgeable in the techniques of invasive airway management: needle cricothyrotomy and surgical cricothyrotomy.

Cricothyroidotomy is a procedure used to gain airway control that requires a surgical incision through the cricothyroid space. A needle cricothyrotomy (also called transtracheal jet ventilation and percutaneous transtracheal jet ventilation) is a method of airway control that uses a needle through the cricothyroid space and therefore requires less surgical skill than a cricothyroidotomy. Needle cricothyrotomy is generally accepted as the preferred surgical airway maneuver in children 10 years and older. Palpation and identification of landmarks of the neck may be difficult in children, and identification of the cricothyroid membrane may be especially difficult in infants. An additional compli-

cating factor is that the laryngeal prominence does not develop until late childhood and adolescence. The procedure is a technically difficult one in children and is generally not recommended in children less than 10 years of age.[68] The goal is to avoid damage to the cricoid cartilage, which in children is the only circumferential structure supporting the larynx and upper trachea (Figure 12-18).

Indications for the establishment of a surgical airway include (1) the inability to gain airway access by other means (the failed airway) and (2) complete upper airway obstruction. Airway inaccessibility during orotracheal or nasotracheal intubation may be the result of trauma, which can cause abnormal anatomy or profuse bleeding and thereby obscure visualization of the glottic opening. Upper airway obstruction may be the result of a foreign body, mass lesion, or edema. Edema can be caused by infection, caustic ingestion, allergic reaction, or an inhalation injury. There are also a number of contraindications to surgical airway maneuver. However, these are considered relative contraindications and include (1) the inability to locate the correct landmarks for puncture, (2) gross infection over the puncture site, (3) primary laryngeal injury, and (4) a patient younger than 10 years of age.

NEEDLE CRICOTHYROTOMY

Needle cricothyrotomy involves the insertion of an over-the-needle cannula through the cricothyroid membrane into the trachea. Steps for this procedure are included in Box 12-7. The use of a kink-resistant catheter, 10-, 14- or 16-gauge cannula, is recommended. The needle is removed, and the cannula is left in place. Commercially available cannulas are designed with side holes in addition to the distal port and incorporate a flange that aids securement of the catheter. The additional holes decrease pressure-related mucosal damage. The cannula must then be connected to an oxygen-delivery device capable of delivering short bursts of oxygen from a high-pressure source of 50 psi. This method of ventilation is known as translaryngeal jet ventilation, and it provides emergency oxygenation but not ventilation if there is an upper airway obstruction.[58] The ventilatory rate should be from 12 to 20 breaths

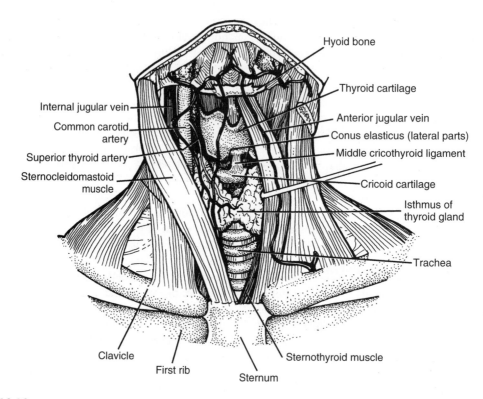

FIGURE 12-18 **Anterior aspect of the neck with relative anatomic structures.** (From Rosen P et al: *Emergency medicine: concepts and clinical practice*, vol 1, ed 2, St Louis, 1988, Mosby)

BOX 12-7   Steps for Needle Cricothyrotomy

1. Stabilize the patient's head in a neutral position.
2. Identify the cricothyroid membrane and prepare the skin.
3. Stabilize the cricoid and thyroid cartilages with the nondominant hand.
4. Insert a 12- or 14-gauge over-the-needle intravenous catheter into the membrane at a 45-degree angle caudally (toward the feet). On passage into the trachea, the needle is removed, and the cannula is advanced caudally.
5. The hub of the needle is connected, preferably to a jet ventilator capable of delivering oxygen at a pressure of 50 psi. Otherwise, the connector is removed from a 3.0-mm ETT and attached to the intravenous catheter. It is then connected to a bag-valve mask. This method is temporary until other means of airway securement can be achieved.

---

per minute with an insufflation time of about 1 to 2 seconds.

Frequently described is an alternative method to the use of the jet ventilator in which the connector from a no. 3 ETT is connected to the cannula, which is then connected to a resuscitation bag. This tech-

nique meets oxygen requirements. However, ventilation cannot be achieved, and respiratory acidosis quickly results.[58] The respiratory acidosis that results generally limits ventilation in this manner to approximately 30 minutes. The use of a resuscitation bag is at best a temporary measure, whereas jet

BOX 12-8 **Steps for Surgical Cricothyrotomy**

1. Stabilize the patient's head in a neutral position.
2. Identify the cricothyroid membrane and prepare the skin.
3. Stabilize the cricoid and thyroid cartilages with the nondominant hand.
4. Make a vertical incision 5 to 7 cm through the skin.
5. Identify the cricoid membrane, and insert the tracheal hook. Use the tracheal hook, now in the nondominant hand, to stabilize the thyroid. Apply upward traction (45-degree angle) on the inferior margin of the thyroid cartilage.
6. Use the tip of a no. 11 blade to create a horizontal incision through the cricoid membrane. Avoid insertion of the blade too deeply and injury of the posterior wall of the trachea or the esophagus.
7. Insert a Trousseau dilator and spread vertically to enlarge the diameter of the cricoid space. Mayo scissors may be used to help enlarge the space in the transverse direction.
8. Remove the tracheal hook.
9. Place a cuffed ETT or tracheostomy tube through the dilator.
10. Remove the dilator. Secure the tube, and verify proper position in the usual manner.

ventilation is considered a true-positive pressure-ventilation technique. Another advantage of jet ventilation is that aspiration of airway secretions is prevented as the high airway pressures escape proximally through the open glottis. Normally, air flows passively from the lungs, up through the larynx, and out the mouth. With upper airway obstruction, normal airflow is not possible, and provision for exhalation must be made or barotrauma will occur. A Y connector can be placed onto the cannula after its insertion.

SURGICAL CRICOTHYROTOMY

Surgical cricothyrotomy is an invasive procedure that should be governed by protocols. Steps for surgical cricothyrotomy are detailed in Box 12-8. Under circumstances in which the anatomy of the neck is distorted, the trachea can be identified by slow advancement of a needle connected to a syringe through the skin and attempted aspiration of air. Once air has been aspirated, signaling entrance into the trachea, the needle and syringe should be left in place and cut down over the needle. If the incision is too small, identification of the structures will be more difficult. A vertical incision over the midline is recommended for minimization of bleeding. The nondominant hand should be used for grasping and stabilization of the larynx until the tracheostomy hook can be inserted. If a tracheostomy hook is not available, one can be made by removal of the

cannula from a 16- or 14-gauge catheter and bending of the needle into a hook about 0.25 inches above the tip with a hemostat. After the skin incision has been made and the cricoid membrane identified, the membrane should be incised, and the tracheostomy hook should be inserted through the membrane and used to stabilize the inferior border of the trachea. The diameter of the cricothyroid space is enlarged by insertion and spreading of a Trousseau dilator. Once the dilator is in place, the hook is removed to prevent puncture of the balloon of the tracheostomy tube. A cuffed 6.0-mm ETT or a Shiley tracheostomy tube is placed through the dilator, and the dilator is then removed. The balloon is inflated, and the tube is checked for correct position in the usual manner.

RAPID FOUR-STEP CRICOTHYROTOMY TECHNIQUE

The Rapid Four-Step Cricothyrotomy Technique was developed for use in the prehospital environment. This technique relies on palpation rather than direct visualization of the cricothyroid membrane, thus decreasing the need for suction and additional light (Figure 12-19). The steps for this procedure include[5]:

1. Palpation (Figure 12-19A). The person performing the procedure should position him or herself at the patient's left shoulder and

palpate the cricoid membrane using the index finger of the left hand, allowing the thumb and middle finger to palpate and stabilize the trachea.

2. Incision (Figure 12-19B). Using the right hand, a no. 20 scalpel is used to make a horizontal incision into the inferior aspect of the cricothyroid membrane. The scalpel is pushed through the membrane at a 60-degree angle to create a 2.5-cm horizontal incision. The scalpel is NOT removed but held in place.

3. Traction (Figure 12-19C). A tracheal hook is held perpendicular to the longitudinal axis of the patient. Using the left hand, the tracheal hook is placed flush against the caudal surface of the scalpel blade and slid down along the trachea. The tip of the hook is rotated 90 degrees in the inferior direction, and ventral/caudal traction is applied to the superior margin of the cricoid cartilage. The scalpel is then removed, and traction is maintained on the trachea by placing the left hand on the patient's sternum.

4. Intubation (Figure 12-19D). This step is very similar to orotracheal intubation. A cuffed endotracheal tube or tracheostomy tube is placed with the right hand. Tube placement is confirmed and the hook is removed. If an endotracheal tube is used, the beveled side initially should be facing the cephalad during insertion to decrease advancement of the tube superior to the vocal cords.

CRICOTHYROTOMY: SELDINGER TECHNIQUE

The development of the Seldinger technique for insertion of catheters and other tubes has also provided an additional method of performing a cricothyrotomy. Commercial kits are available that contain all the components needed to perform this procedure. Steps include:

1. Position the patient and identify appropriate landmarks.

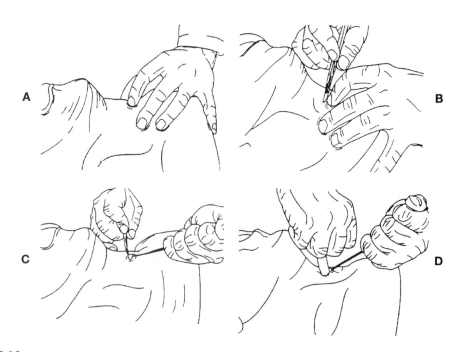

FIGURE 12-19   **Four-step cricothyrotomy. A,** Palpation. **B,** Incision. **C,** Traction. **D,** Intubation. (From Brofeldt BT, Osborn ML, Sakles JC, Panacek EA: Evaluation of the rapid four-step cricothyrotomy technique: an interim report, *Air Med J* 17[3]:127, 1998.)

2. Insert a small locator needle into the cricothyroid membrane. Aspirate air to confirm needle placement into the trachea.

3. Pass a soft-tipped wire through the needle, and thread it into the trachea. Keep control of the wire at all times to prevent wire aspiration.

4. Using a no. 11 blade cut a small incision adjacent to the needle to facilitate passage of the airway device.

5. Place the airway tube with its internal dilator over the wire through the tissue into the trachea. If resistance is met, extend or deepen the skin incision. A gentle screwing motion may also facilitate passage.

6. Confirm tube placement.[18, 68]

PHARMACOLOGY OF ADVANCED AIRWAY MANAGEMENT

The use of sedation and neuromuscular blocking agents to facilitate advanced airway management before and during transport has helped to prevent complications such as aspiration, airway trauma, and failed intubation.[31,32,39,70,71] The use of sedation and neuromuscular blocking agents to facilitate advanced airway management is now used by all types of transport teams and team members including nurses, paramedics, and physicians.*

RAPID-SEQUENCE INDUCTION

Rapid-sequence induction refers to a specific method of inducing general anesthesia while securing active airway control.[33,68] The procedure calls for preoxygenation of the patient with 100% oxygen and cautious avoidance, when possible, of positive-pressure ventilation, which results in gastric distention. Cricoid pressure and medication for sedation and analgesia, followed by a neuromuscular blocking agent (NMBA), are then used to facilitate intubation. If the situation warrants, neuromuscular blockade may be maintained by administration of a longer-acting NMBA. Before the use of NMBAs a brief neurologic assessment should be performed. It is important that this assessment be performed and documented.

NEUROMUSCULAR BLOCKING AGENTS

The use of NMBAs to achieve intubation and to facilitate ventilation has proved effective in the emergency department and the prehospital, and it enhances the safety of patients transported by air or ground. However, these medications are not without serious adverse effects and must be used appropriately and only by those who have been educated in their use and possess advanced airway management skills.

All NMBAs work at the level of the neuromuscular end plate, disrupting neurotransmitter (acetylcholine) function and preventing effective contraction of skeletal muscle (Figure 12-20). These agents do not produce analgesia, anesthesia, or amnesia, and reports of patients with total recall and pain perception who were paralyzed without sufficient anesthesia during operations and procedures exist.[43,22,63] Therefore it is essential to sedate the patient before and during extended periods of paralysis. Clinically, neuromuscular blockade may result in hyperkalemia, regurgitation, and aspiration of gastric contents, and it is also associated with a risk of globe rupture in patients with ocular trauma.

NMBAs can be classified in three ways: type of block produced (depolarizing versus nondepolarizing), duration of action (ultra short, short, intermediate, or long), and structure (acetylcholine-like, benzylisoquinolinium compound, or aminosteroid compound).[39,54]

SUCCINYLCHOLINE

Succinylcholine is the only ultra short-acting NMBA and the only depolarizing agent in common clinical use.[1,10,32] Despite having more adverse effects than nondepolarizing agents, succinylcholine remains the agent of choice for rapid-sequence induction because of the rapid onset of paralysis (30 to 60 seconds) and the short duration of action (4 to 6 minutes). If the transport team is unable to intubate a patient who receives succinylcholine, the patient can be bag-valve mask–supported for the relatively

---

*References 1, 22, 32, 36, 39, 43, 60, 63.

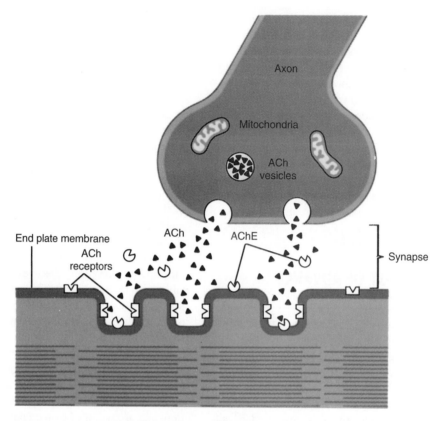

FIGURE 12-20   **Disruption of acetylcholine function by neuromuscular blocking agents.** (From Clark JB, Queener SF, Karb VB: *Pharmacologic basis of nursing practice*, ed 4, St Louis, 1993, Mosby.)

short time until spontaneous respirations return. A nondepolarizing agent given for rapid-sequence induction has the disadvantage of longer onset of action (2 to 5 minutes) and a longer duration (12 to 40 minutes) before return of spontaneous respirations.[1,10,32] Nondepolarizing agents such as vecuronium will work almost as rapidly if given in higher doses. However, the patient will be unable to assist with respirations for 30 minutes or more.

Succinylcholine is associated with several potential complications including the following: hyperkalemia; increases in intracranial, intraocular, and intragastric pressure; cardiac dysrhythmias; and pseudocholinesterase deficiency.[33,39,54] The hyperkalemia associated with succinylcholine, which can approach or exceed life-threatening levels, is of greater consequence in patients who have had burn or massive muscle trauma 2 to 3 days previously, and patients may continue to be at risk for 2 to 3 months.[33,39] Bradydysrhythmia is a complication that frequently is associated with succinylcholine use, especially in young children, but may also occur in adults. Pretreatment with atropine 0.02 mg/kg is advised in children to prevent bradycardia and pretreatment with lidocaine 1.5 mg/kg in patients with suspected head injury has been shown to attenuate the rise in ICP associated with endotracheal intubation.[68] In patients who have sustained significant skeletal fractures, the fasciculations (irregular muscle contractions produced by depolarization of the muscle membrane before complete cessation of muscle activity) caused by succinylcholine can cause additional injury at the fracture site. Administration of a defasciculation dose of a nondepolarizing agent can prevent this complication.[33,68] Succinylcholine will also cause the release of a small amount of histamine into the systemic circulation and can result in bronchospasm, which can be a concern but not a contraindication in patients with chronic obstructive pulmonary disease or asthma.[33]

The are two absolute contraindications to the use of succinylcholine. One is its use in situations in which a cricothyrotomy would be difficult or impossible. Examples include (1) children younger than 10 years, (2) patients with massive neck swelling or trauma in which landmarks are obscured, or (3) cases in which ventilation and intubation would be difficult, such as epiglottis or upper airway obstruction. The second absolute contraindication is its use by individuals who do not possess a thorough knowledge about the pharmacology of neuromuscular blocking agents, and they do not possess advanced airway management skills or an alternative plan if they should encounter a failed intubation.

NONDEPOLARIZING AGENTS

Nondepolarizing agents are used to extend the time of neuromuscular blockade after intubation. Pancuronium was the first nondepolarizing NMBA to be used, beginning in the 1960s, and was used exclusively until the mid-1980s when the newer agents atracurium and vecuronium were marketed. In the 1990s mivacurium and rocuronium were introduced.[57] The new nondepolarizing agents were developed to produce onset of paralysis more rapidly but have duration of activity shorter than that of pancuronium, and they prevent tachycardia and increased peripheral vascular resistance, which occur with the use of pancuronium. All of the new agents produce fewer cardiovascular effects and have a fairly predictable recovery profile.

Nondepolarizing agents as a rule have a slower onset of action and maintain neuromuscular blockade longer than succinylcholine. The onset of action of these medications may be increased with a higher dose of the drug, but there is a greater risk of triggering cardiovascular side effects such as tachycardia and prolonging the duration of paralysis.

Indications for the use of neuromuscular blocking agents in the critical care transport environment include: facilitation of intubation, ventilation control, safety (management of an agitated patient), and improvement in oxygenation and treatment of pathologic muscle rigidity. Table 12-1 lists some of the NMBAs used in critical care transport.

There are medications, disease processes, and physiologic conditions that may interfere with the effectiveness of neuromuscular blocking agents. Neurologic diseases such as myasthenia gravis can prolong paralysis. Hyper and hypothermia both may have an impact on the pharmacology of selected neuromuscular blocking agents. Electrolyte imbalances such a hypermagnesia may also prolong paralysis. Table 12-2 contains some of the medications that may affect neuromuscular blocking agents. The transport team must be very comfortable with the medications that they may administer and the management of potential adverse reactions that may occur.

After the introduction of these agents in critical care units, case reports began to describe prolonged weakness and muscle atrophy in patients who received NMBAs for 24 to 48 hours or longer. The drugs most often implicated were pancuronium and vecuronium, and patients at greatest risk were those with kidney or liver dysfunction.[54] This side effect of NMBAs has been shown to be prevented by monitoring of the degree of blockade with a peripheral nerve stimulator, thereby avoiding overdosage, which has been implicated as a cause of prolonged weakness.[42]

A peripheral nerve stimulator is a device that delivers an electric current to one of several peripheral nerves (the ulnar nerve is the most widely used) through pregelled electrodes placed over the skin. The muscle response to nerve stimulation is then observed. The muscle response to nerve stimulation is also dependent on the type of test. There are three test modes of stimulation, but the "train of four" (TOF) is the best and most common method of peripheral nerve stimulator monitoring to assess the level of neuromuscular blockage.[41] TOF stimulation involves initiation of four electrical stimuli during a 2-second period (2 Hz). An unparalyzed patient will

TABLE 12-1 NMBAs

NMBAs	Intravenous dosage (mg/kg)	Onset (min)	Duration (min)	Comments
Depolarizing				
Succinylcholine	Adult dose: 1.0-1.5 Pediatric dose: 1.5-2.0	1.5-2.0	4-6	Pretreat with atropine in children and adolescents; many adverse effects
Nondepolarizing				
Pancuronium	00.04-0.01	3-5	60-100	Stimulate heart rate and cardiac output; no histamine release
Atracurium	0.4-0.5	2-3	20-45	Metabolism independent of kidney or liver function; histamine release
Rocuronium	0.5-1.0	1-2	20-40	Shortest onset of all nondepolarizing NMBAs; no histamine release
Vecuronium	0.1	2-3	20-40	Minimal cardiovascular effects; no histamine release
Mivacurium	0.15-0.25	2-3	12-20	Shortest duration of all nondepolarizing NMBAs; histamine release

TABLE 12-2 Medications That May Affect NMBAs

Medications	Effects
Aminoglycosides	Prolonged duration of relaxation
Lidocaine	Prolonged duration of relaxation
Local anesthetics	Prolonged duration of relaxation
Beta blockers	Prolonged relaxation
Magnesium	Prolonged relaxation
Procainamide	Prolonged relaxation
Quinidine	Prolonged relaxation
Potassium depleting medications	Prolonged relaxation
Lithium	Prolonged relaxation
Digoxin	Prolonged relaxation
Corticosteroids	Prolonged relaxation

have no fatigue and will have four equal twitches when tested at this frequency. As paralysis increases, the number of twitches will decrease because of fatigue at the neuromuscular junction. Blockade is quantified by a count of the number of thumb adductions or twitches. Four twitches correlate with approximately 75% receptor blockade; three twitches, 80%; two twitches, 85%; and one twitch, 90%. When all four twitches are absent, 100%, or total neuromuscular blockade, is assumed to be present.[41] The frequency of TOF monitoring is recommended every 4 hours during active titration and every 8 hours during maintenance infusion.[14,53] It is important to note that thus far all reports of prolonged weakness have been in intensive care unit patients receiving long-term administration of these agents. Monitoring with a peripheral nerve stimulator has not yet been identified as beneficial in patients receiving short-term neuromuscular blockade.

TABLE 12-3 **Drugs Used to Reverse NMBAs**	
Drug	**Dosage**
First-line drug combination	
Neostigmine	0.05 mg/kg (not to exceed 5 mg) and atropine 0.015 mg/kg
Given by slow intravenous push	
Repeat dose not recommended	
Second-line drug combination	
Pyridostigmine	0.2 mg/kg and atropine 0.015 mg/kg
Given by slow intravenous push	
Repeat dose not recommended	
Or	
Edrophonium	0.5 mg/kg and atropine 0.007 mg/kg
May repeat 10 min after initial dose	
(mixed thoroughly in same syringe)	

Data from Nissen D, ed: *2001 Mosby's GenRx*, ed 11, St Louis, 2001 Mosby.

REVERSAL OF NEUROMUSCULAR BLOCKADE

On rare occasions prolonged paralysis after the administration of NMBAs presents a problem in patient evaluation or treatment, and the need to reverse the agent arises. Pharmacologic reversal of these agents is possible. However, in most situations it is safer and easier to allow normal drug metabolism and excretion to clear the neuromuscular agent.[61] Succinylcholine has no known reversal agent. The patient's respirations must be supported during the duration of action time (4 to 6 minutes), after which the drug will undergo normal metabolism and muscle action will return.

Reversal of the nondepolarizing agents involves administration of drugs that inhibit acetylcholinesterase. This allows the local concentration of acetylcholine molecules to rise. The reversal agents include neostigmine, pyridostigmine, and edrophonium (Table 12-3).[48,54] The administration of these anticholinesterase-inhibiting drugs causes a strong parasympathetic response consisting of cardiovascular effects, bronchoconstriction, and increased glandular secretions. The cardiovascular effects are of greatest concern and include bradycardia, heart block, and cardiac arrest.[48] These effects can be countered by administration of anticholinergic agents such as atropine or glycopyrrolate, given in conjunction with anticholinesterase inhibitors.

MONITORING AIRWAY MANAGEMENT AND VENTILATION DURING TRANSPORT

Evaluation of airway interventions occurs under less than optimal conditions during transport. Transport vehicles may be noisy and dimly lit. Traditional auscultation is extremely difficult, and poor vehicle lighting may interfere with the normal visual cues of assessment.[21,24] Parameters used for evaluation include the level of consciousness, stability of vital signs, observation of the patient's color, and symmetric rise and fall of the chest wall. Several pieces of equipment may assist with evaluation and provide objective data.

END-TIDAL CO_2 DETECTION

The disposable end-tidal CO_2 detector Easy Cap (Figure 12-21) assists proper ETT placement by incorporating a nontoxic, chemically treated indicator that changes color in the presence of carbon dioxide.[70] The device can reliably function for up to 2 hours and is not affected by environmental temperature extremes. With early use of the Easy Cap it was thought that patients in cardiopulmonary arrest might not have

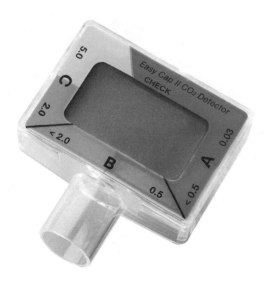

FIGURE 12-21   **Easy Cap end-tidal CO_2 detector.**
(Courtesy Nellcor Puritan Bennett, Inc, Pleasanton, Calif.)

enough perfusion to generate a color change in the device. Recent investigations have concluded that when used during cardiopulmonary resuscitation in patients with low end-tidal carbon dioxide levels, the device should produce a detectable color change.[28] Hayden et al[19] found in a study of 566 prehospital intubations of patients in cardiac arrest that a color change occurred in 95.6%, with only 1 false-positive result. In addition to verifying endotracheal placement after intubation, the Easy Cap device can also be used to monitor tube placement while in flight.[4,44] If the indicator becomes contaminated with pulmonary secretions or comes in contact with medications administered through the ETT, the indicator will no longer function. The device may be removed from the ETT after administration of medications given through the ETT for at least six breaths, or until fluids are no longer visible, and then replaced with no loss of function. Pedi-Cap (Figure 12-22), a new, smaller

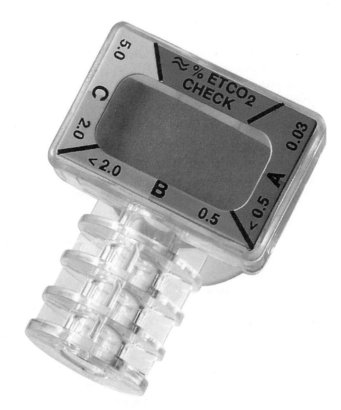

FIGURE 12-22   **Pedi-Cap pediatric end-tidal CO_2 detector.** (Courtesy Nellcor, Puritan, Bennett, Inc, Pleasanton, Calif.)

detector, is now available and is designed for neonates and children who weigh up to 15 kg. It provides 2 hours of continuous service. The adult model is not recommended in patients who weigh less than 15 kg.

CAPNOGRAPHY

Capnography is the measurement of end-tidal CO_2 volumes with each breath by use of infrared light absorption by placement of a sensor between the breathing circuit and the ETT. The instrument works by emitting an infrared light beam through a sensor located immediately distal to the ETT. As carbon dioxide is exhaled, the CO_2 molecules absorb the infrared light. The instrument then measures how much light was absorbed, thereby determining the concentration of CO_2.[44,59] The data are then displayed in digital or waveform or both. Figure 12-23 shows two such instruments. The graphic waveform, called a capnogram, displays levels of CO_2 over time. Capnometry refers to the numeric display. Normal end-tidal CO_2 volume is a close indicator of the arterial pressure of carbon dioxide, and the difference between these two parameters, known as the CO_2 gradient ($P\{a- ET\}CO_2$) has been reported to be less than 6 mm Hg in normal patients.[20]

Capnography technology has been in use during the last decade in the operating room for assessment of the respiratory status of patients during surgery, for detection of hyperventilation or hypoventilation, and for detection of equipment problems. The value of capnography to the transport team is its ability to confirm proper ETT placement, to indicate situations in which the ETT has become displaced, and to detect disruption of the ventilator circuit. Monitors that provide continuous waveforms can also assist the transport team in evaluating the clinical status of the patient as well. However, as with any piece of equipment, caution should be exercised when capnography is used to ensure the clinical picture matches the readings. Carbon dioxide present in the exhaled gas indicates that alveolar ventilation has transpired but does not necessarily mean that the ETT is in the trachea. A tube positioned in the pharynx will also provide normal readings.

Continuous capnography has been used during blind nasotracheal intubation in spontaneously breathing patients. The posterior displacement of the tip of the tube to the larynx was recognized promptly by the use of continuous capnography. Likewise, when the tube was repositioned for entry into the trachea, the capnograph monitor displayed the presence of CO_2.[59]

Recent advances in technology have allowed smaller, more durable instruments for prehospital use. Even though there is currently no national standard that dictates the use of capnography during critical care transport, many transport programs do use some type of monitoring during transport.[20,44,59]

PULSE OXIMETRY

In the emergency department or critical care unit, health-care providers rely on arterial blood gases or, more specifically, the partial pressure of oxygen tension (PaO_2) drawn on an intermittent basis to guide therapy. Pulse oximetry provides a reliable and continuous evaluation of oxygenation.

Oxygen in the blood is dissolved in the plasma or is bound to hemoglobin. The oxygen dissolved in the plasma is referred to as the partial pressure of oxygen (PO_2). The normal value of oxygen dissolved in the arterial blood (PaO_2) is measured in millimeters of mercury or torr. In children and adults this value ranges from 80 to 100, with higher values expected in the pediatric population. The PO_2 accounts for 1% to 2% of the total oxygen content.[20]

The portion of oxygen bound to hemoglobin is referred to as oxygen saturation (SO_2). In arterial blood the normal value of oxygen saturation (SaO_2) ranges from 95% to 97.5%. The SO_2 accounts for 98% or more of the total oxygen content.

The relationship between the PaO_2 and SaO_2 is displayed in Figure 12-24, the oxyhemoglobin dissociation curve. If one value is known, the other can be estimated. It is important to note that the relationship is not a linear one. The upper portion of the curve demonstrates a compensatory mechanism of the body; in a normal healthy adult, more oxygen

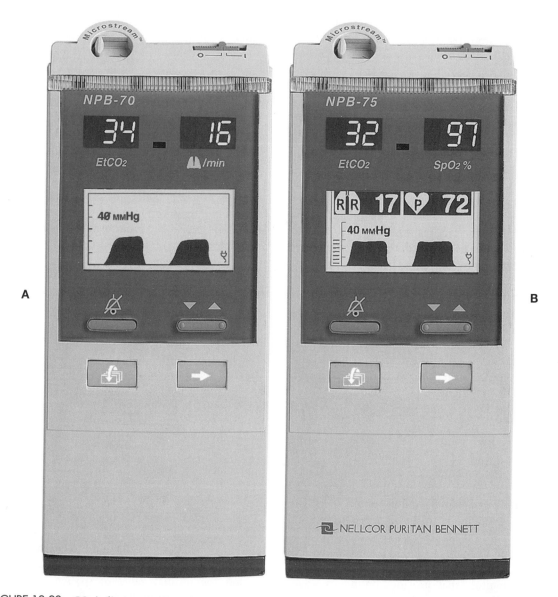

FIGURE 12-23 CO_2 **indicators. A,** NPB-70 handheld capnograph; **B,** NPB-75 combination handheld capnograph and pulse oximeter. (Courtesy Nellcor Puritan Bennett, Inc., Pleasanton, Calif.)

than necessary is carried. A drop in the PaO_2 from 100 to 80 mm Hg shows a minimal change in the SaO_2. The steep portion of the curve demonstrates a rapid decline in SaO_2 with small decreases in PaO_2. When the SaO_2 falls below 90%, there is a rapid decline in the oxygen content.

Pulse oximetry continuously monitors the SaO_2 value. A sensor device is placed across a pulsating arteriolar bed, such as the toe, nose, or finger. Figure 12-25 illustrates two types of pulse oximeters. The sensor houses a light source and photo detector device. The pulse oximeter processes the light

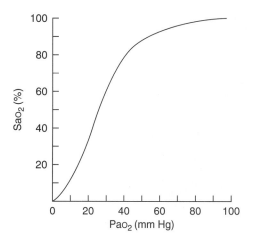

FIGURE 12-24 **Oxyhemoglobin dissociation curve.**

absorption to determine SaO_2 values. The successful use of an oximetry device is dependent on proper placement of the sensor device. It should be positioned such that the light source and photo detector are in direct alignment. The patient's skin at the placement site should be clean and dry. The ability to obtain a pulse at the site of placement is also important. The accuracy of pulse oximetry may be affected by clinical conditions such as hypotension or hypothermia, or during vasopressor therapy secondary to vasoconstriction.

The accuracy and efficacy of pulse oximetry in the critical care transport environment have also been established. The value of this device to the transport team lies in its ability to act as an early warning system. A low SaO_2 is detected much earlier than by clinical observation, permitting expeditious and aggressive interventions. Continuous pulse oximetry monitoring improves the recognition and management of hypoxemia during emergency endotracheal intubation,[68] and during critical care transport it offers visual reassurance to the team that airway management is having its intended effect. If oxygen saturation measured by pulse oximetry suddenly changes, a repeat airway assessment should be performed to determine the cause, and corrective action should be taken.[61]

Pulse oximetry has also been found to be useful in determination of systolic blood pressure in the air medical setting by application of an appropriate size blood pressure cuff on the same arm as the pulse oximetry probe. The cuff is inflated until the palatial display on the pulse oximeter is obliterated. The manometer reading at the point of obliteration is recorded as the systolic blood pressure.[38,61]

TRANSPORT VENTILATORS

Once the airway is controlled, ventilations can be assisted with either a bag-valve mask device or a ventilator. In recent years, the market has been flooded with transport ventilators. In 1985 Branson et al[4] provided a description and performance evaluation of several models. They recommended that air and ground ambulance ventilators be "compact, lightweight, fuel efficient, flexible, user friendly, durable, and require little maintenance." This statement still reflects the requirements of ventilators. Of these criteria fuel efficiency and flexibility deserve the greatest consideration.[2,26]

Most transport ventilators are oxygen-powered devices. Thus, when selecting one to purchase or deciding which patient should be placed on a ventilator, medical personnel should consider the amount of oxygen on board the aircraft. Figure 12-26 shows two models of transport ventilators.

Flexibility is a must. The majority of ventilators manufactured for the prehospital setting are capable of providing ventilation for both adults and children. Some of the more sophisticated models are capable of providing a wide range of ventilatory modes and therefore are useful in meeting the requirements of patients with routine tidal volume and rate settings. In addition, they can meet the demands of the critically ill patient with special ventilatory needs such as control, assist-control, and synchronized intermittent mandatory ventilation operating modes. Many are PEEP-compensable and use comprehensive alarm systems for continuous system self-checks.

The use of ventilators versus manual ventilation remains controversial, particularly in the initial treatment of patients with obvious chest trauma or in patients who have potential chest injuries. Ventilators, particularly those without a peak inspiratory pressure alarm, eliminate the ability to "feel"

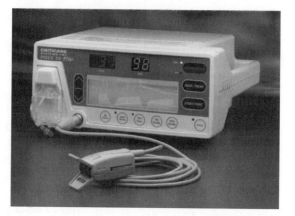

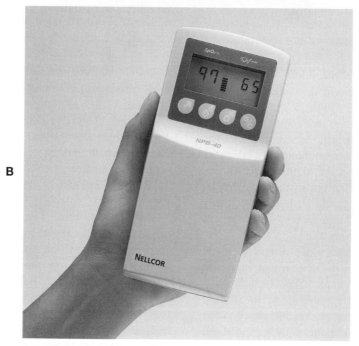

FIGURE 12-25   **Pulse oximeters. A,** Poet TE Plus combination capnograph and pulse oximeter. **B,** N40 portable pulse oximeter.
(**A** Courtesy of Criticare Systems Inc, Milwaukee, Wis. Reprinted with permission; **B** Reprinted by permission of Nellcor Puritan Bennett, Inc.)

lung compliance, which can indicate a pneumothorax is developing or can signal an obstruction in or displacement of the ETT.

The primary use for mechanical ventilation during transport is to maintain alveolar ventilation by causing airflow in and out of the lungs via changing airway pressures. Mechanical ventilators deliver a specific and reliable concentration of oxygen,

decrease the work of breathing for critically ill patients, and avoid the prolonged use of bag-valve device ventilation during transport.[23]

Consistent ventilation is one of the major uses of mechanical ventilators during transport. Because of the nature of the transport environment, the rate and tidal volume delivered by a bag-valve device will vary as a result of movement, interruptions (loading and

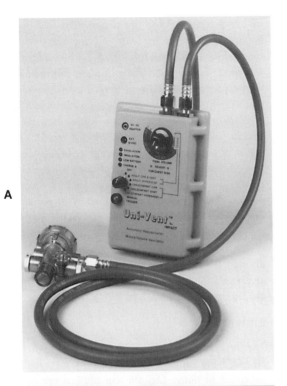

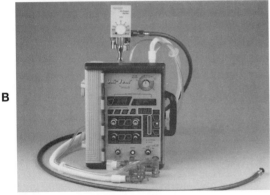

FIGURE 12-26 **Transport ventilators. A,** Uni-Vent Model 706 automatic resuscitator. **B,** Uni-Vent Model 750 transport ventilator. (Courtesy Impact Medical Co, West Caldwell, NJ.)

unloading the patient), and operator variations.[11] These changes in oxygenation and acid-base balance may be detrimental to a patient, particularly on long transports, and result in significant impacts such as alteration in cerebral blood flow or pulmonary shunting.[11]

Transport ventilators have the additional benefit of allowing both members of the critical care transport team to continue patient care unencumbered by the need to manually ventilate the patient after initial ventilator setup. A sensible policy may be that a transport ventilator not to be used for patients with potential chest injuries, such as from trauma scenes, and to use transport ventilators for patients with head injuries or for other critical care transports.

Mechanical ventilation is not without the potential for causing complications and injury. Complications related to mechanical ventilation include infection and adverse hemodynamic changes. Injury to lung parenchyma can result from volutrauma and acute lung injury.

When using a transport ventilator, a transport team should calculate tidal volumes at 6 to 10 ml/kg and then check them using a spirometer, especially in children to prevent the risk of barotrauma.[11]

Many transport ventilators today provide a variety of settings and modes so that the patient may maintain similar ventilation as to what they were receiving in the critical care unit. However, a ventilator should not be used unless the critical care transport team is familiar with its mechanics and the physiologic consequences of its use.

ESOPHAGEAL INTUBATION DETECTION

Assessment of ETT placement is a routine maneuver after intubation. The potentially catastrophic consequences of an undetected esophageal intubation stress the importance of the ability to recognize and correct the situation should it occur. Observations such as chest movement, breath sounds, epigastric auscultation and observation, reservoir bag compliance, and tube condensation are some of the more commonly prescribed methods of tube position assessment. However, each of these methods at times may prove inaccurate.[68]

A tool for detection of esophageal intubation is commercially available. The detector consists of a 60-ml syringe fitted with a standard 15-mm ETT adaptor on the end of the syringe. After intubation, the device is connected to the ETT, and the plunger is pulled back. Because of the rigid support provided by the cartilaginous rings, when the plunger of the syringe is pulled back, air will be aspirated without resistance if the ETT is placed in the trachea. If resistance or negative pressure is encountered when the plunger is pulled back, the esophagus has been intubated. The esophagus readily collapses when a negative pressure is applied because, unlike the trachea, it has no cartilaginous support. The syringe aspiration technique of verifying ETT position was found to be accurate in both the emergency department and the prehospital setting.[25]

A further modification of the plunger device incorporates a self-inflating bulb fitted with an ETT adaptor. The bulb is squeezed before it is connected to the ETT. If the bulb self-inflates, tracheal intubation is signaled. If the bulb remains deflated, esophageal intubation is indicated. Studies have concluded that prior bag-mask ventilation or esophageal ventilation does not interfere with the reliability of the self-inflating bulb in detecting esophageal intubation.[67] The self-inflating bulb has also been shown to be useful in correct identification of placement of the esophageal tracheal combitube.[69]

SUMMARY

Assessment and management of the patient's airway is the primary role of the transport team. When and how to perform basic and advanced airway management is critical in the transport environment. Good clinical judgment, skill, and familiarity with the pharmacology of airway management are required so that patients receive competent care and complications are prevented that can occur in the care of the critically ill or injured patient.

Airway Management and Ventilation Case Study

The transport team of a major regional trauma center was called by the local fire and EMS service of a small town 40 miles away for a motorcycle accident involving two people. In 5 minutes the BK-117 with a flight nurse and paramedic were en route for the 20-minute flight. The accident happened near the center of the small community within 2 blocks of the fire department who was holding their monthly staff meeting when they received the call. Upon landing, the transport team was immediately met by the incident commander who told them that there were 2 non-helmeted motorcyclists who were traveling an estimated 30 mph through an intersection when they were struck, T-bone fashion, by a pickup truck. The driver of the pickup was only slightly injured and refused treatment. The flight team was further told that a middle-aged male was the operator of the motorcycle and riding with him was a 20-year-old male recognized by EMS providers. They reported the young passenger had Down syndrome and many times had required transport for a seizure disorder. The team was first directed to the middle-aged male. The initial assessment revealed the following information:

AIRWAY

The patient was awake, confused, and combative. He was lying supine on a backboard with a cervical collar in place. Oxygen was applied per nonrebreather mask, but he was attempting to remove it. There was no blood, vomitus, or other foreign material obstructing the airway.

BREATHING

Respiratory rate was 28 breaths per minute with bilateral equal chest expansion noted. The chest was palpated and found to have no subcutaneous air or crepitus.

CIRCULATION

Skin was pale, warm, and dry with 2+ radial pulses bilaterally. Capillary refill was 3 seconds.

DEFICITS

Movement was noted in all extremities. Pupils were midrange, round, and reactive bilaterally. The patient was screaming and was being physically restrained by numerous EMS personnel. He did not follow commands, and his speech was at times garbled. Upper extremity restraints were in place and secured to the back board. His Glasgow Coma Scale (GCS) was 11 (E3, V3, M5).

EXTREMITIES

No upper extremity fractures were noted; however, he had an obvious open distal tibia-fibula fracture on the right. His pelvis appeared stable.

The transport team discussed their options. There was concern for the patients mental status, and his uncooperative behavior presented a safety risk inflight. They decided to intubate the patient per RSI protocol. An intravenous line was started, the patient was pre-oxygenated and received lidocaine, an induction agent, succinylcholine, and he was successfully intubated on the first attempt. The ETT was secured, and the patient then received a non-depolarizing paralytic agent and a narcotic analgesic. While one team member finished up, the second team member went to evaluate the other victim.

The second victim, a 20-year-old male with Down syndrome was lying supine on the pavement. There was no C-collar in place, and the patient was being manually ventilated by two rescuers with an ambu bag. The EMT in charge reported that the patient was found lying on his side in a head–chest position and was not breathing. His color was blue, and his pulse was slow and bounding. He was turned on his back, and bag-mask ventilations were started. One person was holding the mask, and another was squeezing the ambu bag. Numerous attempts to start an intravenous (IV) line were unsuccessful. The primary exam was as follows.

AIRWAY

The airway was difficult to evaluate. The tongue was large, and it obstructed the view of the mouth. There was no obvious blood, vomitus, or foreign material in the mouth. The flight nurse inserted an oral airway, which immediately improved ventilatory exchange.

BREATHING

The patient had no spontaneous effort. The was no subcutaneous air of crepitus noted. There were notable contusions to the right anterior hemithorax. There seemed adequate chest excursion with manual ventilations.

CIRCULATION

Color was ashen with slow bounding radial pulses bilaterally.

DEFICIT

There was no eye opening and no movement to pain on the left or right side. The pupils were large, round, and minimally reactive. GCS was 3 (E_1, V_1, M_1)

EXTREMITIES

There were numerous abrasions and contusions but no obvious long bone fractures.

The transport team member was joined by the other, who was now finished packaging the first patient. The second patient also needed intubation, but IV access had still not been established. One team member attempted to start an IV while the other took over bag-mask ventilations. Despite multiple attempts, an IV could not be established. The decision was made to attempt oral intubation. A cardiac and pulse oximeter were established. The heart rate was 68, and the pulse oximeter was 92%. The first attempt at intubation was made with a no. 4 Macintosh blade, but the attempt was quickly abandoned because of the large tongue. A second and third attempt was made with a smaller no. 3 curved blade without success. Cricoid pressure using the BURP method was applied throughout each attempt. It was decided the second team member would attempt intubation. He chose to use a straight blade and on each attempt (3) was unsuccessful. He was unable to visualize any structures beyond the tongue. Between attempts, the oximetry reading dropped to the mid 80s. At this time, the flight crew elected to attempt intubation using their rescue device, the intubating laryngeal mask airway (ILMA or Fastrach). A no. 3-size ILMA was inserted into the mouth with the laryngeal surface down and pressed onto the hard palate. The device was advanced over the back of the tongue following the natural curvature of the oropharynx and hypopharynx to where it "seated" over the larynx. The cuff was filled with approximately 20 ml of air. The patient was again ventilated, this time with the ILMA. In a few minutes the saturations improved to 100%. Next, the silicone-tipped armored ETT was lubricated and inserted into the metal tube of the ILMA until the horizontal black line on the ETT was at the proximal entrance to the ILMA. Resistance was felt as the ETT advanced through the distal end of the ILMA. The metal handle was withdrawn slightly, and the ETT advanced without difficulty. The balloon of the ETT was inflated, and position was confirmed with a disposable end-tidal CO_2 detector. The ILMA cuff was then deflated and withdrawn over the ETT. The patient was quickly immobilized on a backboard; rolled towels were used to secure the head in neutral position. Both patients were loaded in the aircraft. While inflight patient number one, the middle-aged man, remained hemodynamically stable with an oxygen saturation of 100%. Patient number two was hypotensive with a blood pressure of 80 and a pulse of 60 to 70. His oxygen saturation remained 98 to 100% with significant improvement in his color from his initial evaluation.

Patient number one's evaluation revealed a cerebral contusion and an open distal tibia-fibula fracture. He was taken to surgery for open reduction and internal fixation of his orthopaedic injury and then admitted to the neurologic unit where he remained for 48 hours. At that time he was extubated and moved to a regular floor. Four days later he was discharged home with full neurologic recovery.

Patient number two was the son of patient one's girlfriend. The older man often gave the younger man rides on his motorcycle. The patient was found to have an atlanto-occipital dislocation and a severe anoxic injury. He too was admitted to the neurologic intensive care unit (ICU) where, consistent with the family's wishes, he was removed from life support 36 hours post-injury and expired.

DISCUSSION

The transport team was faced a number of difficult patient management issues which were successfully negotiated. With a GCS of 11, the motorcycle operator required intubation to facilitate safe transport more so than to treat his neurologic compromise. The patient with Down syndrome displayed the usual airway characteristics of the abnormality. These include a short neck, irregular dentition, and a large tongue, which made the airway difficult to manage. In addition he had a known seizure disorder. The congenital laxity of the ligaments of the neck most likely contributed to the atlanto-occipital dislocation, and had the initial responders been delayed another minute, the patient would not have likely survived to be transported from the scene. The transport crew made several important decisions in caring for this patient. First, a properly sized oral airway is important as first-line management of a difficult airway. Secondly, after each intubation attempt, the patient was re-oxygenated and ventilated. At the same time the situation was re-assessed and the team changed something. In this example, the size and type of laryngoscope blade was changed. Following a failed intubation it is good practice to change something to improve the chances for success on the following attempt. The flight team also recognized that this was a "can't intubate but can oxygenate" situation. Available options in this situation included lighted stylet intubation, retrograde intubation, digital intubation, the intubating laryngeal mask airway, and the esophageal tracheal combitube. The flight team recognized that because of the patient's short neck, a cricothyrotomy would have been extremely difficult and therefore chose to use the intubating laryngeal mask airway (ILMA or Fastrach). This particular design differs from the original LMA in that the ILMA or Fastrach allows for the blind introduction of an ETT through it. The classic LMA does not constitute definitive airway management. The classic LMA does not protect against airway aspiration, ventilation pressures greater than 20 to 25 cm can dislodge the LMA, and the device is difficult to secure during patient transport. Patients must be significantly obtunded to allow insertion of the ILMA or the classic LMA. The combitube may actually be a better rescue device than the classic LMA because it allows for gastric decompression and aspiration of gastric contents by passing a suction catheter through the clear connecting tube into the stomach. In addition, it is more stable and less likely to become dislodged during transport. This case study underscores the importance of good airway skills and proper equipment, combined with sound judgment gained through practice and experience, in managing a difficult airway situation.

REFERENCES

1. Austin P: A literature review of the prehospital use of neuromuscular blocking agents by air medical personnel to facilitate endotracheal intubation, *Air Med J* 19(3):90, 2000.
2. Bell T: Understanding transport ventilators, *Air Med J* 6(6):24, 2000.
3. Birnbaumer DM, Biemann JT: Esophageal airways. In Dailey R et al, editors: *The airway: emergency management*, St Louis, 1992, Mosby.
4. Branson R et al: Ventilators for aeromedical transport, description, and performance evaluations, *Hosp Aviat* 4(11):13, 1985.
5. Brofeldt B et al: Evaluation of the rapid four-step cricothyrotomy technique: an interim report, *Air Med J* 17:128, 1998.
6. Bryant A, Tingen M: The use of cricoid pressure during emergency intubation, *J Emerg Nurs* 25(4):283, 1999.
7. Cook RT, Stene JK, Marcolina B: Use of a Beck Airflow Monitor and controllable-tip endotracheal tube in two cases of nonlaryngoscopic oral intubation, *Am J Emerg Med* 13(2):180, 1995.
8. Crippen D, Oleevy S, Graffis R: Gastric rupture: an esophageal obturator complication, *Ann Emerg Med* 10(2):370, 1981.
9. Dauphinee K: Orotracheal intubation, nasotracheal intubation, *Emerg Med Clinic North Am* 6(4):699, 1988.
10. Dickens MD: Pharmacology of neuromuscular blockade: interactions and implications for concurrent drug therapies, *Crit Care Nursing Q* 18(2):1, 1985.
11. Dockery WK et al: A comparison of manual and mechanical ventilation during pediatric transport, *Crit Care Med* :802, 1999.
12. Duchynski R et al: The quick look airway classification, *Air Med J* 17(4):46, 1998.
13. Feaster WW: Oral endotracheal intubation: pediatric perspective. In Dailey R et al, editors: *The airway: emergency management*, St Louis, 1992, Mosby.
14. Ford EV: Monitoring neuromuscular blockade in the adult ICU, *Am J Crit Care* 4(2):28, 1987.
15. Frass M et al: The esophageal tracheal combitube: preliminary results with a new airway for CPR, *Ann Emerg Med* 16(7):768, 1987.
16. Haley K, Eckles N, Baker P: *Emergency nursing pediatric course*, Des Plaines, Ill, 1998, Emergency Nurses Association.
17. Hancock PJ: Finger intubation, *Air Med J* 13(10):421, 1994 (abstract).
18. Hawkins M: Cricothyrotomy. In Proehl J: *Emergency nursing procedures*, Philadelphia, 1999, WB Saunders.
19. Hayden SR et al: Coloremic end-tidal CO_2 detector for verification of endotracheal tube placement in out-of-hospital cardiac arrest, *Acad Emerg Med* 2:499, 1995.
20. Hicks GH: Blood gas and acid-base management. In Dantzer D et al, editors: *Comprehensive respiratory care*, ed 5, Philadelphia, 1995, WB Saunders.
21. Hightower DP et al: Red cabin lights impair air medical crew performance of color-dependent tasks, *Air Med J* 14(1):75, 1995.
22. Holleran RS: The use of neuromuscular blocking agents in critical care nursing practice, *Crit Care Nursing P* 5:344, 1993.
23. Holleran RS, Rouse M: Mechanical ventilators. In Proehl J, editor: *Emergency nursing procedures*, ed 2, Philadelphia, 1999, WB Saunders.
24. Hunt RC et al: Inability to assess breath sounds during air medical transports by helicopter, *JAMA* 265(15):1982, 1991.
25. Jenkins WA, Verduke VP, Paris PM: The syringe aspiration technique to verify endotracheal tube position, *Am J Emerg Med* 12(4):413, 1994.
26. Johanningman J: Prehospital respiratory care. In Dantzer D et al, editors: *Comprehensive respiratory care*, ed 5, Philadelphia, 1995, WB Saunders.
27. Johnson JC, Atherton GL: The esophageal tracheal combitube: an alternative route to airway management, *J Emerg Med Serv* 16(5):29, 1991.
28. Jones BR, Dorsey MJ: Sensitivity of a disposable end-tidal carbon dioxide detector, *J Clin Monit* 7(3):268, 1991.
29. Knill RL: Difficult laryngoscopy made easy with a "BURP", *Canadian J Anesth* 279, 1993.
30. Krishel S, Jackimcuzk K, Balazs K: Endotracheal tube whistle
31. Li J et al: Complications of emergency intubation with and without paralysis, *Amer J Emerg Med* 17(2):141-143, 1999.
32. Lowe L, Sagehorn K, Madsen R: The effect of a rapid sequence induction protocol on intubation success rates in an air medical program, *Air Med J* 17:101, 1998.
33. Ma OJ et al: Intubation success rates improve for an air medical program after implementing the use neuromuscular blocking agents, *Am J Emerg Med* 16(2):128-131, 1998.
34. Majernick T et al: Cervical spine motion during orotracheal intubation, *Ann Emerg Med* 15(4):417, 1986.
35. Martin S, Ochsner M, Jarman R: The LMA: a viable alternative for securing the airway, *Air Med J* 18(2):89, 1999.
36. McDonald C, Bailey B: Out-of-hospital use of neuromuscular blocking agents in the United States, *Prehosp Emerg Care* 30:29-32, 1998.

37. Minkowitz H: Laryngeal mask airway and esophageal tracheal combitube. In Hagberg C, editor: *Handbook of difficult airway management*, Philadelphia, 2000, Churchill Livingston.

38. Mohler J, Hart SC: Use of a pulse oximeter for determination of systolic blood pressure in a helicopter air ambulance, *Air Med J* 13(11-12):479, 1994.

39. Munford B: Practical pharmacology of neuromuscular blockade, *Air Med J* 4:149, 1998.

40. Ng S: Pathophysiological effects of tracheal intubation. In Linto IP, Vaughan RS, eds: *Difficulties in tracheal intubation,* London, 1997, WB Saunders.

41. Nieman JT et al: The pharyngealtracheal lumen airway: preliminary investigation of a new adjunct, *Ann Emerg Med* 13(8):591, 1984.

42. Parker M et al: Perception of a critically ill patient experiencing therapeutic paralysis in an ICU, *Crit Care Med* 12(1):69, 1984.

43. Pepe PE, Copass MK, Joyce T: Prehospital endotracheal intubation: rationale for training emergency medical personnel, *Ann Emerg Med* 14:1085, 1985.

44. Perez L, Klofas E, Wise L: Oxygenation/ventilation of transported intubated adult patients: a national survey of organization practices, *Air Med J* 19(2):55, 2000.

45. Pointer JE: Nasotracheal intubation. In Dailey R et al, editors: *The airway: emergency management*, St Louis, 1992, Mosby.

46. Pons PT: esophageal obturator airway, *Emerg Med Clin North Am* 6(4):693, 1988.

47. Rhee KJ et al: Oral intubation in the multiply injured patient: the risk of exacerbating spinal cord damage, *Ann Emerg Med* 19(5):511,1990.

48. Roberts DJ, Clinton JE, Ruiz E: Neuromuscular blockage for critical patients in the emergency department, *Ann Emerg Med* 15(2):152, 1986.

49. Rouse MJ, Branson R, Holleran RS: Mechanical ventilation during air medical transport, *J Air Med Transport* 11(10):5, 1992.

50. Sage F, Bingham R: Intubation. In Macnab A, Macrae D, Henning R, editors: *Care of the critically ill child*, London, 1999, Churchill Livingston.

51. Scott J: Oral endotracheal intubation. In Daily R et al, editors: *The airway: emergency management*, St Louis, 1992, Mosby.

52. Shea SR, MacDonald JR, Grouzinski G: Prehospital endotracheal tube airway or esophageal gastric tube airway: a critical comparison, *Ann Emerg Med* 14(2):102, 1985.

53. Silverman D: *Neuromuscular block*, Philadelphia, 1994, JB Lippincott, Co.

54. Simon B: Pharmacologic aids in airway management. In Dailey R et al, editors: *The airway: emergency management*, St Louis, 1992, Mosby.

55. Smith SB et al: Introduction of pulse oximetry in the air medical setting, *J Air Med Transport* 10(11):11, 1991.

56. Stewart R: Digital intubation. In Daily R et al, editors: *The airway: emergency management*, St Louis, 1992, Mosby.

57. Stewart R: Lighted stylet. In Daily R et al: *The airway: emergency management*, St Louis, 1992, Mosby.

58. Stewart R: Manual translaryngeal jet ventilation. In Daily R et al, editors: *The airway: emergency management*, St Louis, 1992, Mosby.

59. Stock MC: Capnography for adults, *Crit Care Clin* 11(1):219, 1995.

60. Syverud S et al: Prehospital use of neuromuscular agents in a helicopter ambulance program, *Ann Emerg Med* 17:236, 1988.

61. Thomas F, Blumen I: Assessing oxygenation in the transport environment, *Air Med J* 18(2):79, 1999.

62. Thompson C et al: Intubation quality assurance thresholds, *Air Med J* 14:55, 1995.

63. Thompson JD, Fish S, Ruiz E: Succinylcholine for endotracheal intubation, *Ann Emer Med* 12:526, 1982.

64. Verdile VP: Digital and transillumination intubation, *Emerg Care Q* 3(3):77, 1987.

65. Vitello-Cicciu JM: Recalled perceptions of patients administered pancuronium bromide, *Focus Crit Care* 11:28, 1984.

66. Vollmer TP et al: Use of a lighted stylet for guided orotracheal intubation in the prehospital setting, *Ann Emerg Med* 14(4):324, 1985.

67. Wafai Y et al: Effectiveness of the self-inflating bulb for verification of proper placement of the esophageal tracheal combitube, *Anesth Analg* 80(1):122, 1995.

68. Walls R: Course Manual National Emergency Airway Management Course, Wesley, MA, 1998, Airway Management Education Center.

69. Walls R, editor: *Emergency airway management*, Philadelphia, 2000, Lippincott Williams and Wilkins.

70. Walter FG, Lowe RA: Airway management. In Hamilton G et al, editors: *Emergency medicine: an approach to clinical problem solving*, Philadelphia, 1991, WB Saunders.

71. Wayne M, Friedland E: Prehospital use of succinylcholine: a 20-year review, *Prehosp Emerg Care* 10:107, 1999.

72. Yancey W et al: Unrecognized tracheal intubation: a complication of the esophageal obturator airway, *Ann Emerg Med* 9(1):18, 1980.

73. Young GP: Clinical airway anatomy. In Daily R et al, editors: *The airway: emergency management*, St Louis, 1992, Mosby.

SHOCK MANAGEMENT

13

COMPETENCIES

1. Describe the pathophysiology of shock.
2. Identify the patient at risk for shock.
3. Initiate critical interventions to manage the patient in shock before and during transport.
4. Identify the supportive care required by the patient who is in shock.
5. Describe the treatment of selected coagulopathies.

Shock has been described as the "rude unhinging of the machinery of life." Shock is the manifestation of cellular insufficiency. No matter what the cause of shock, the common denominator of all shock states is the amount of oxygen consumed by the cells.[8,52,77] Despite the technologies and treatments available today, the mortality from shock remains high. Unfortunately, many patients suffer sepsis, systemic inflammatory response, multiple organ system failure, and death. The mortality and morbidity related to shock is best managed through prevention, early recognition, and rapid transport to definitive care.

Shock is divided into three major phases: a compensatory stage, a progressive stage, and an irreversible stage.[93] Shock can result from alterations in circulating volume, cardiac pump function, and peripheral vascular resistance.[93] It causes myriad physiologic changes in the nervous, respiratory, renal, and gastrointestinal systems.[19]

Alteration in circulating volume, particularly hemorrhage, is one of the most common causes of shock and one that is frequently encountered by transport teams. One complication of hemorrhage is the development of a coagulopathy. Dilutional effects of massive transfusions, continued bleeding, and hypothermia are some of the causes of coagulopathy encountered by transport teams.[7,27,48]

Disseminated Intravascular Coagulation (DIC) is a secondary complication of such disease states as shock from traumatic injury, abruptio placentae, and anaphylaxis.[40,42] It is frequently found in critically ill patients when their transport has been delayed.

This chapter discusses the etiology, pathophysiology, and initial management of shock. It also includes a discussion about coagulopathies because they are common complications related to the management of shock.

| BOX 13-1 | **Etiology of Shock** |

Hemorrhagic: Acute blood loss from an internal or external vascular injury
External: Penetrating trauma, amputation, and open fractures
Internal: Injury (splenic, liver) fractures—particularly pelvic, body tissue injury, bleeding from other internal source such as gastrointestinal (GI) tract, and esophageal varices
Hypovolemia: Fluid loss such as from third spacing, burn injury, vomiting, diarrhea, diabetes mellitus, diabetes insipidus, and diuresis
Neurogenic: Spinal cord injury, alteration in vascular tone from drugs, food, plants, and venom
Anaphylaxis: Allergic reaction to a foreign substance including drugs, food, plants, and venom
Obstructive: Obstruction of blood flow (e.g., from a tension pneumothorax or cardiac tamponade)
Cardiac: Pump failure that may result from a myocardial infarction, valvular malfunction, septal defect, right-sided infarct, or direct injury to the heart such as a myocardial contusion
Sepsis: Infectious agent that compromises the host defense mechanism

---

ETIOLOGY

The multiple causes of shock are summarized in Box 13-1. Even though multiple causes have been described as putting a patient at risk of developing shock, the entire body is affected by shock. Shock treatment is multifaceted.

PATHOPHYSIOLOGY

The research surrounding shock during the past decade has focused on the role of the immune system and the multisystem effect that a clinical insult may trigger. Cellular injury induces an adaptive response. One of these adaptive responses is apoptosis.[10,77] Apoptosis is a molecularly regulated cell death, which can be induced by environmental, physical, or chemical stressors. It is characterized by a sequence of precisely regulated events that culminate in the self-destruction of a cell. This may provide an explanation of why, despite aggressive resuscitation, patients do not get better.[10,77]

As previously stated, shock is the manifestation of cellular metabolic insufficiency. The amount of oxygen available for tissue consumption has been defined as oxygen delivery (DO_2). The body tissues do not extract all the oxygen available to them, which allows the body to maintain some reserve.[93]

The amount of oxygen extracted from tissues for metabolism has been defined as *oxygen consumption* (VO_2). Oxygen consumption is calculated by determining the differences between the amount of oxygen delivered to the tissues and the amount returned to the right side of the heart. Oxygen consumption depends on cardiac output, hemoglobin, Sao_2, and venous oxygen saturation (SVO_2). The normal VO_2 is 180 to 250 ml/min.[84,93]

When blood flow is diminished because of blood or fluid loss or redistribution of the circulating blood flow, the delivery of oxygen to the tissues is diminished. When not enough oxygen is available to meet the needs of the body tissues, an oxygen debt results. Oxygen debt has been described as the difference between tissue oxygen demand and oxygen consumption.[84,77,93]

Shock has been divided into three specific stages. These are the compensatory stage, the progressive stage, and the irreversible stage. No matter what the origin of shock, a decrease in available oxygen triggers cellular responses, which in turn affect all body systems.

CELLULAR RESPONSE

A reduction in the amount of available oxygen causes an alteration in cellular metabolism, resulting in a cascade of significant cellular changes and leading to injury and death if interventions prove ineffective or are too late. Figures 13-1 and 13-2 illustrate the cellular and micropathophysiologic changes that occur during cellular ischemia.[84]

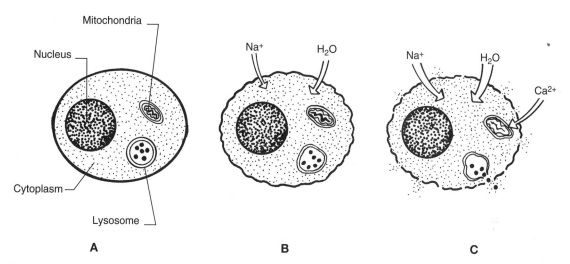

FIGURE 13-1 **A,** Normal cell. **B,** Massive amounts of water and sodium enter the cytoplasm, causing blebs to develop. **C,** Calcium changes in the mitochondria causing destruction; lysosomes rupture, spilling proteolytic enzymes into the cytoplasm; the cell wall loses integrity, and the cell dies. (Modified from Kitt S et al: *Emergency nursing,* Philadelphia, 1995, Saunders.)

BODY SYSTEMS RESPONSE

The lack of available oxygen to the cell initiates a cellular response, as discussed, that results in body system changes. As demonstrated in Figure 13-3, the immune system reacts with the activation of a complement cascade that eventually releases cytokines such as tissue necrosis factor (TNF) and interleukin 1 (IN-1). These cytokines are key in the production of cellular toxins, such as arachidonic acid, thromboxane, and leukotrienes. These substances lead to bronchoconstriction, platelet aggregation, capillary permeability, and vasoconstriction or vasodilation.[83,84]

Figure 13-4 summarizes the other system changes associated with the hypoxia of shock that result in some of the classic signs and symptoms of shock. These include altered mental status, changes in skin color and temperature, and a decrease in or an absence of urinary output.[80,84,93]

Regardless of the source of shock, if it is not quickly recognized, the concomitant changes occurring in blood pressure, flow, and volume and the alterations in oxygen transport causing hypoxia will lead to tissue hypoxia, organ dysfunction, multiple organ failure, and death.[3,20,45,60]

The transport team must always be cognizant of the causes of shock and the subtlety of its signs and symptoms in its early stages. They must also take into account comorbid risk factors that cause additional stress on the patient's body systems and that may increase a patient's risk of becoming compromised even with a moderate illness or injury. Some of these factors include a history of cardiovascular disease, pulmonary disease, or diabetes. Research demonstrates that shock needs to be treated and reversed as soon as possible to prevent additional injury and eventual death.[5,9,73]

STAGES

COMPENSATORY

During the compensatory phase of shock, the body attempts to compensate for the stress that has been caused by a specific illness or injury. One compensatory mechanism is stimulation of the baroreceptors, which causes a decrease in vagal tone and an increase in sympathetic discharge. The results of this mechanism are some of the classic signs and symptoms of shock, including an increase in heart rate, force of myocardial contractility, and venous and

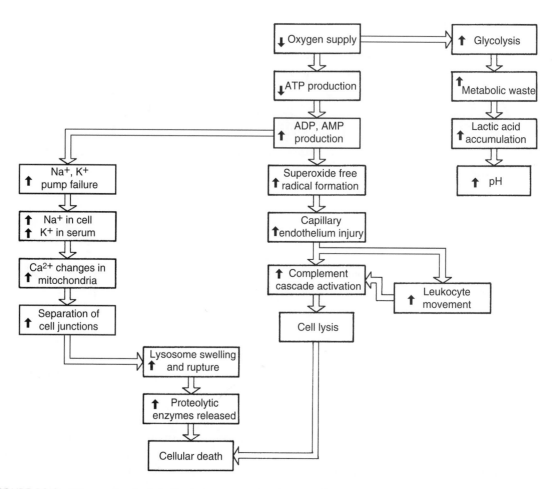

FIGURE 13-2   **Micropathophysiologic changes occurring during cellular ischemia.** *ATP*, Adenosine triphosphate; *ADP*, adenosine diphosphate; *AMP*, adenosine monophosphate; *Na+*, sodium ion; *K+*, potassium ion; *Ca2+*, calcium ion; *pH*, logarithm of the reciprocal of the hydrogen ion concentration. (Modified from Kitt S et al: *Emergency nursing,* Philadelphia, 1995, Saunders.)

arterial vasoconstriction. This stage of shock is generally reversible.

PROGRESSIVE

If the presence of shock goes unrecognized or the cause of it is not managed, the shock cycle will continue to progress. The initial insult that caused shock will continue to activate vicious cycles of compensatory mechanisms that, if not appropriately managed, will lead to death. During this phase, the effects of tissue hypoxia and anaerobic metabolism are experienced.[37] Cytokines such as TNF and the interleukins, especially 1 and 6, initiate the pathophysiologic changes that may eventually lead to multiple organ failure.

IRREVERSIBLE

In the irreversible stage of shock the body becomes refractory to treatment. In the final stages of shock the patient may still be alive, but treatments such as fluid resuscitation, antibiotic administration, and ventilatory management become ineffective (Figure 13-5). The reason this occurs remains unknown.

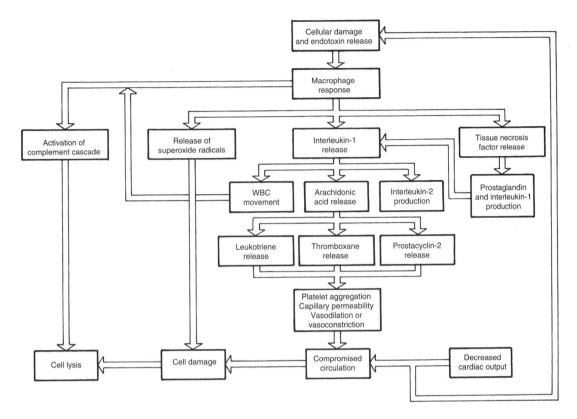

FIGURE 13-3 **Cascading response of the immune system in shock.** (Modified from Kitt S et al: *Emergency nursing,* Philadelphia, 1995, Saunders.)

SYSTEMIC INFLAMMATORY RESPONSE SYNDROME

In 1992 a new description for the shock cascade was proposed. The body's response to a clinical insult that causes shock or systemic inflammatory response syndrome (SIRS) was at first related more directly to septic shock, but as research continues, indications are that SIRS is probably involved in the first phase of shock.[8,15] In recent years research has been focused on the effects of a clinical insult on the immune system and its response, particularly the neutrophils.[14] Moore et al[60] proposed that this model can be easily applied to the management of the trauma patient and that unrecognized and undertreated shock after injury contributes to the occurrence of multiple organ failure and eventual death in the multiply injured patient.

The pathophysiology of shock and current research emphasize the need for the transport team to recognize the risk or presence of shock and act quickly to prevent further injury. This may be through fluid resuscitation, blood administration, use of selected medications such as vasoactive drugs, and rapid transport to definitive care.[76]

MULTIPLE ORGAN DYSFUNCTION SYNDROME

Bone has described multiple organ dysfunction syndrome (MODS) as a clinical syndrome characterized by the development of potentially reversible physiologic dysfunction in two or more organ systems.[34,93] This pathology can be caused by a variety of acute insults including trauma, sepsis, and poison. Research has shown that there is little consensus on what exactly constitutes MODS. However,

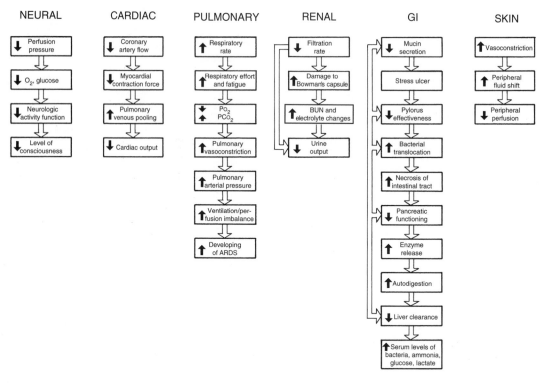

FIGURE 13-4   **Major organ system changes that occur from hypoxia associated with shock.** O_2, Oxygen; Po_2, partial pressure of oxygen; Pco_2, partial pressure of carbon dioxide; *ARDS*, adult respiratory distress syndrome; *BUN*, blood urea nitrogen. (Modified from Kitt S et al: *Emergency nursing*, Philadelphia, 1995, Saunders.)

most experts agree that seven systems are generally included in the definition. These systems are cardiovascular, central nervous, gastrointestinal, hematologic, hepatic, renal, and respiratory systems.

The patient with MODS is generally transported after a referring center can no longer provide care. They may present a unique challenge because they are more likely to have multiple invasive lines, medications, and complex ventilator settings.

PATIENT ASSESSMENT AND SHOCK MANAGEMENT

The management of the patient in shock begins with the recognition that the patient is in shock. Early recognition of shock directly affects the

morbidity or mortality of the patient. Shock can be diagnosed early based on history and clinical signs such as weak and thready pulse, cold and clammy skin, pallor, and mottled skin. Simultaneous goals of therapy include the following.[99]

1. Correction of the initial insult by hemostasis, pericardiocentesis, treatment of arrhythmias, or antibiotics
2. Maintenance of vital organ function such as cardiac output, arterial blood pressure, and urinary output
3. Correction of secondary consequences such as hypovolemia, acidosis, hypoxemia, and DIC
4. Identification and correction of any aggravating factors manifested by evidence or suggested by a history of preexisting disease

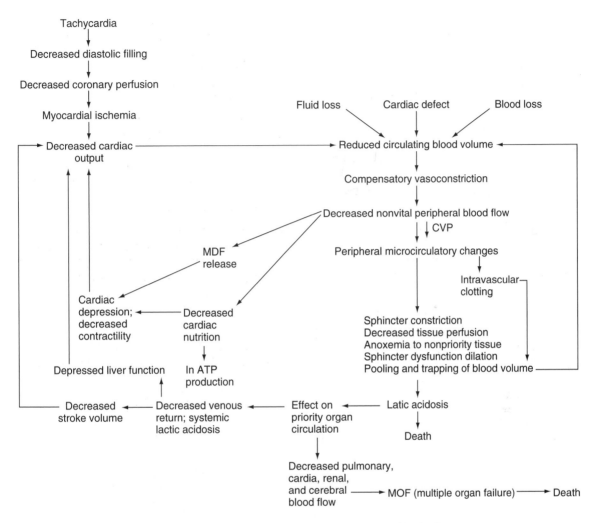

FIGURE 13-5   **Compounding factors in irreversible shock.**

Complete assessments and general therapy are accomplished almost simultaneously and should proceed as shown in Box 13-2.

CORRECTION OF HYPOXIA

The goal of correcting hypoxia during the initial resuscitation of the patient in shock is to correct the oxygen deficit that has occurred. The transport team should place the patient, intubate or perform cricothyrotomy when necessary, and provide mechanical ventilation.[88,96] Respiratory muscle effort is the major site of oxygen expenditure for the resting patient and may place undue metabolic demands on the heart. Assisted ventilation providing maximal analgesia, sedation, and neuromuscular blockade may be necessary for the transport of a critically ill patient.

FLUID RESUSCITATION

Fluid resuscitation has become and continues to be one of the most controversial topics in shock management. Research has questioned some of the

---

BOX 13-2   **Steps in Initial Management of the Patient in Shock**

1. Assess airway patency, administer 100% oxygen, perform advanced airway management as indicated.
2. Assess breathing effectiveness, perform decompression if indicated.
3. Inspect for and control active bleeding.
4. Assess perfusion: peripheral and central pulses, capillary refill, skin temperature, color, jugular veins.
5. Initiate fluid resuscitation, closely monitoring patient during resuscitation.
6. Assess neurologic function: AVPU, GCS, pupillary function, motor and sensory response, immobilize patient if indicated.
7. Assess skin and skeleton; note abnormalities, deformities of skeleton, potential sources of blood, volume loss.
8. Keep patient warm.
9. Apply monitoring devices: cardiac, pulse oximeter, end-tidal.
10. Check invasive lines if in place.
11. Check urinary catheter if in place; monitor output.
12. Review laboratory studies before transport when available.
13. Review radiographic and diagnostic studies when available.

---

previously common methods used to manage the patient in shock in prehospital and transport environments.* Unfortunately, despite continued research, inappropriate fluid resuscitation continues, as do the complications that come with it.[43,44,50,51,90]

The purpose of volume resuscitation is to restore oxygen transport and cellular uptake of needed oxygen, militate against the oxygen debt accumulation, repay a preresuscitation oxygen deficit, and prevent the complications of SIRS and the development of multiple organ failure. The prehospital and transport management of fluid resuscitation must pay careful attention to the long-term consequences of any intervention.[9,11-13,93,94]

Research has shown that hypotension may be a protective mechanism. Unless the source of bleeding can be adequately managed in the prehospital care environment, aggressively resuscitating a patient may do more harm than good. Increasing a shock patient's blood pressure increases the risk of bleeding, may dislodge formed clots, and depending on the resuscitation fluid, dilutes circulating volume and increases clotting time. Crystalloids and colloids do not carry oxygen, which is one of the primary things cells need to survive.[26,30,31,68]

The amount of fluid required by the shock patient—particularly those in hemorrhagic or hypovolemic shock—depends on the amount of intravascular volume depletion. During resuscitation the transport team needs to monitor the patient closely for sufficiency of volume replacement. The patient's blood pressure, pulse rate, level of consciousness, and urinary output (when available) provide parameters that can be monitored during transport. These parameters may also provide the transport team with indications of a fluid overload.[86]

Multiple fluids have been used for resuscitation, including lactated Ringer's, normal saline, hypertonic saline, Hetastarch, and plasmanate. In hemorrhagic shock, blood and blood products are required for resuscitation. However, some transport programs do not carry O negative blood with them. Regardless of which fluids are chosen for resuscitation, the patient needs to be monitored closely for the effectiveness of resuscitation and the potential complications that may occur.

The complications of massive fluid resuscitation include hypothermia, coagulopathy, metabolic derangements such as hypocalcemia and hypokalemia, organ dysfunction, and extravascular fluid shifts. These may lead to the development of adult respiratory distress syndrome (ARDS), sepsis syndrome, acute renal failure, DIC, pneumonia, multiple organ failure, and death.[72,87]

---

*References 11-13, 50, 54, 80, 81, 84, 85, 87-89.

BOX 13-3	**Summary of 1989 MAST Study**

1. PASG application does not increase the length of prehospital time.
2. PASG does increase blood pressure.
3. PASG does not decrease the length of time in the emergency department, operating room, or hospital.
4. When PASG was applied, an overall increased mortality was seen for all patients.
5. Patients with prehospital time greater than 30 minutes and PASG application did not have better survival rates.
6. Patients with thoracic injuries had a greater chance of dying before arrival at the hospital if PASG was applied.
7. Patients with major abdominal injuries did not have an overall better survival rate if PASG was applied.

From Liberman M, Mulder D, Sampalis J: Advanced or basic life support for trauma: meta-analyis and critical review of the literature, *J Trauma* 49(4):584, 2000.
MAST, Military antishock trousers; *PASG*, pneumatic antishock garment

---

PNEUMATIC ANTISHOCK GARMENT

One of the most common methods once used in the management of the injured patient in shock was the application of pneumatic antishock garments (PASGs) or military antishock trousers (MAST). As the original name, *MAST*, suggests, this device was found to be of great use during the Vietnam War. However, little research had been done related to their effectiveness and the potential complications that could occur once they have been applied.[22,75,92]

Mattox et al[55] published a landmark study in 1989 that demonstrated several important points about the use of PASGs (Box 13-3). This study and other animal model studies proved that PASGs did work, but that their application in certain patient populations may actually increase patient morbidity and mortality.[55]

Currently, the Basic Trauma Life Support Course[20] recommends that the indications for the applications of PASG in the prehospital environment include external hemorrhage that can be controlled (PASG possibly being used initially until fluids are replaced), neurogenic shock without evidence of internal injuries, isolated fractures of legs without evidence of other internal injuries, and systolic blood pressure of less than 50 mm Hg (which still remains controversial).[19] Absolute contraindications to the use of PSAG include pulmonary edema, bleeding that cannot be controlled. They must be used with caution in the woman who is pregnant, keeping pressure off the fetus.[20]

BOX 13-4	**Medications Used in the Management of Shock**

Antibiotics and antiinfectives
Vasoactive drugs
Analgesics and sedation medications
Steroids

When PSAG are used during transport, the transport team needs to weigh the advantages over the disadvantages and monitor the patient closely. Continued use of PASG can lead to the development of decubiti and other stasis injuries.[2,24]

PHARMACOLOGIC MANAGEMENT

The pharmacologic management of shock depends on the source of the shock. For example, usually little need exists for pharmacologic agents in traumatic hemorrhagic shock. The primary therapy is administration of fluids, blood, and blood products. However, once the primary therapy has been initiated, pharmacologic management may be indicated if the patient does not improve.

Commonly used medications in the management of shock include inotropic agents, vasopressors, vasodilators, antibiotics, and steroids. Box 13-4 contains a summary of some of the medications that may be used in shock management and indications for their use. Because dosages depend on the age, size, and severity of the patient's condition, the transport team needs to be familiar with the indications, dosages, and side effects of these medications.[46,47]

OTHER INTERVENTIONS

As summarized in Box 13-1, multiple causes of shock exist. When the blood flow is obstructed, as in cardiac tamponade and tension pneumothorax, the patient will exhibit signs and symptoms of shock. Critical interventions in obstructive shock include pericardiocentesis and thoracic decompression. Although some disease states may induce a pericardial tamponade or tension pneumothorax and contribute to obstructive shock, the most common causes of these life-threatening maladies are blunt and penetrating thoracic trauma.[4,20,23]

Pericardiocentesis is indicated for the patient in shock when blunt or penetrating trauma to the chest (particularly the sternum) has occurred, and the patient is hypotensive and has bradycardia, distended neck veins, and muffled heart sounds.[4,20,23]

Needle decompression or chest tube insertion is indicated when the patient is in shock and experiencing severe respiratory distress, hypotension, bradycardia, jugular vein distention, and tracheal deviation. When the patient is intubated, difficulty ventilating this type of patient should alert the flight nurse to the potential of a tension pneumothorax, once again in the patient with a history of blunt and penetrating trauma.[20,23]

Other interventions that may be used in the management of shock are the mechanical devices to assist circulation or increase tissue perfusion. Some of these devices include intraaortic balloon pumps (IAB), left ventricular assist devices (LVAD), and extracorporeal oxygenation devices (ECHMO). The uses of these types of equipment require special skills and significant preparation.[25]

CLINICAL MONITORING

Depending on the time, location, and initiation of interventions, the patient in shock may not have clinical monitoring devices in place. Multiple methods may be used to monitor the patient in shock, including hemodynamic and SVo_2 monitors. Box 13-5 contains a summary of some of these clinical monitors.[17,21,33]

| BOX 13-5 | **Cardiopulmonary and Metabolic Measurements in Shock** |

Arterial pressure
Left ventricular function (pulmonary artery catheter)
Cardiac output
Cardiac index
Mixed venous blood gases
Lactic acidosis
Base deficit
Intramucosal pH

Central venous and pulmonary artery catheter pressures provide an index of the status of absolute and relative blood volume, the need for fluid replacement, and the effects of interventions. Accurate serial measurement of heart rate and rhythm, respiratory rate, cardiac filling pressure, cardiac output, tissue perfusion indices, and end-organ function (mental state and UO) must be done when possible.[37,36,84,85,99]

Regardless of the types of clinical monitor being used, the transport team needs to ensure that they can be used during transport. All ports, intravenous and invasive lines, and monitors need to be secured and accessible as well as protected from the possibility of contamination, particularly when invasive lines are in place.[53] If invasive monitors are being used, the transport team should document an initial reading once equipment has been changed and according to transport protocols or as the patient's condition indicates during transport.[33]

SELECTED SHOCK PATHOPHYSIOLOGY
HEMORRHAGE

Description. Circulation can be compromised in various ways. Failure of circulation occurs either locally or systemically, resulting in shock. Systemic circulation failure is caused by inadequate blood volume or a pump defect. The first of three types of inadequate volume is hemorrhage, or loss of plasma and red cell mass from the vascular system. Hemorrhage is either internal or external: the amount depends on the vessel, the extent of damage, and the ability to form and maintain a clot. The effect of hemorrhage depends on the preexisting state of the cardiovascular, respiratory, renal, and hematologic systems.[6,73]

Normal blood volume is approximately 7% of the ideal adult body weight (approximately 70 ml/kg) and 80 to 90 ml/kg in children.[28] In hemorrhage a graded physiologic response is based on the percentage of blood volume lost acutely. The clinical symptoms progress as blood loss increases.

The blood pressure sometimes does not change until 30% to 40% of the total blood volume is lost. Specific attention should be paid to pulse rate, respiratory rate, skin circulation, pulse pressure, and the patient's mental status.[28]

Intrathoracic and intraabdominal bleeding (cavitary hemorrhage) are well recognized as causes of hypovolemia in trauma. Significant losses from noncavitary causes (pelvic fracture, skin laceration, and multiple long-bone fractures) may result in a 20% to 50% total blood loss, placing the patient into a severe shock state.

An isolated, closed femur fracture can result in up to 2½ L of blood lost in the fracture hematoma. In pelvic fractures, 40% to 50% of the total blood volume may be lost. The mortality rate in pelvic fracture is 6.4% to 15%; however, 42% to 70% of the deaths are attributed to blood loss. These patients require aggressive resuscitation.

Noncavitary blood losses contribute to additional loss of blood in 85.2% of patients with intraabdominal or intrathoracic hemorrhage. Blood losses will occur in 2 to 5 hours after the injury, so air medical crew members should be alert for delayed hypovolemia.

Treatment requires tamponading of the bleeding and supporting and splinting fractures. Fluid management includes administering crystalloid and blood. Knowing that severe blood losses can occur with noncavitary losses is essential for early recognition to ensure proper treatment and prevent wasted time in searching for cavitary hemorrhage.[63-65,67,68]

Indicators.   A history of any of the following factors should lead to suspicion of hemorrhage.

Trauma to the thorax, abdomen, pelvis, or an extremity
Melena or hematochezia
Hematemesis
Hemoptysis or epistaxis
Vaginal bleeding
Surgery

Predisposing Conditions.   The following conditions can predispose to hemorrhage.

Anemia
Hemoglobinopathies
Thrombocytopenia
Liver disease
Any hemorrhagic diathesis, hemophilia, and DIC
Neoplastic disease
Peptic ulcer disease
Alcoholism
Atherosclerosis
Sepsis
Surgery

Causes

Internal Hemorrhage

Pleural cavity hemorrhage: intrathoracic vessel trauma, dissecting aortic aneurysm, ruptured varices, fracture

Peritoneal cavity hemorrhage: liver, spleen, or any artery trauma; abdominal aneurysm; tumor; arteritis; volvulus; strangulated ovarian cyst

Retroperitoneum hemorrhage: tumor, trauma fracture, ectopic pregnancy; soft tissue extremity trauma, fracture, venipuncture; skin trauma, purpura

Bladder hemorrhage: tumor, transurethral prostatectomy

Cavity hemorrhage: complication of surgery

External Hemorrhage

GI tract hemorrhage (associated with hematemesis): inflammatory gastritis, peptic ulcer disease (PUD), esophagitis, and tumor of esophagus, stomach

Endotracheal hemorrhage: esophageal lacerations, foreign body ingestion, abdominal trauma

Vascular hemorrhage: varices, aneurysms, mesenteric occlusion, and hematologic disease

GI tract (associated with hematochezia): ulcerative colitis (inflammatory), shigellosis (infectious), amebiasis, tumor, vascular hemorrhoids, volvulus, mesenteric occlusion; Meckel's diverticulum (congenital)

Respiratory tract hemorrhage: trauma, inflammation, infection, vascular lesions, infarction of lung, bleeding in an abscess, ruptured aortic aneurysm, and bronchiectasis

Vaginal hemorrhage: pregnancy, abortion, abruptio placentae, placenta previa, lacerations from delivery, cervical and endometrial cancer, dysfunctional uterine bleeding

FLUID LOSS

Description.   The second of the three major types of inadequate volume is fluid loss. This occurs in conditions with a reduced blood volume and hemoconcentration because of water loss and unusually high solute loss. The usual modes of fluid loss are vomiting, diarrhea, excessive sweating (fever, heatstroke), excessive urination, and loss from body surface area of denuded skin. (The management of burns and burn shock is discussed in Chapter 19.)

Indicators.   A history of the following would indicate low blood volume due to fluid loss. In addition, hematocrit levels and CVP values are good indicators of fluid loss.

Burns

Diarrhea, vomiting, excessive urination, sweating

Poorly controlled diabetes, lowered insulin usage with polyuria

Exposure to environment for prolonged time with decreased food and water supply

Fever

Ascites

Extensive surgery

Diuretic use or abuse

Predisposing Conditions.   A patient with any of the following conditions could be predisposed to low blood volume caused by fluid loss.

Age: very young or very old

Surgery: GI resections, hyposectomy, and extensive resections

Diabetes mellitus

Adrenal insufficiency

Drugs: diuretic therapy

Hyperthyroidism

Regional enteritis, ulcerative colitis

Liver disease

PUD

Malnutrition, anemia

Peritonitis, pelvic inflammatory disease

Neoplasia

Diabetes insipidus

ABNORMAL PERIPHERAL DISTRIBUTION

Description.   Loss of blood volume can be caused by vasomotor dysfunction with sequestration of blood in the resistance circuit or venous capacitance bed. The absolute blood volume does not change, but an increase in vascular space results in a decrease of effective blood volume and tissue perfusion. Vasomotor dysfunction results in (1) high or normal arterial resistance with expanded venous capacitance (pooling) or (2) low arterial resistance with arteriovenous shunting. This is sometimes referred to as distributive shock.[20]

Sepsis.   Septic shock was a term used to describe the shock state associated with infection. In 1992 septic shock was reclassified and defined as sepsis-induced hypotension despite adequate fluid resuscitation with lactic acidosis, oliguria, and acute alteration in mental status.* *Sepsis* is described as a spectrum of clinical conditions caused by the immune response of a host to a clinical insult such as an injury or illness and characterized by systemic

---

*References 1, 2, 49, 73, 74, 91, 95, 96.

inflammation and coagulation.[34] Each year thousands of people die of sepsis in the United States.[34,39,41]

The body responds to infection through an inflammatory response. Multiple proinflammatory mediators such as tumor necrosis factor (TNF-a); interleukins 1 and 6 and platelet activating factor (PAF) are released. These help the body repair and prevent further injury. The body also releases anti-inflammatory mediators to balance the effects.[34]

In sepsis there is an overwhelming inflammatory response. TNF and interleukins cause tissue and capillary injury. One of these injuries is the activation of the coagulation system and depletion of endogenous anticoagulants. This results in the diffuse microthrombus formation.[34] The primary cause of sepsis and septic shock is an event that interferes with local or systemic host defense mechanisms. These causes may include a primary infection, for example, pneumonia, or an iatrogenic cause such as the presence of a urinary catheter or pulmonary catheter. The increased, indiscriminate use of broad-spectrum antibiotics has lead to a proliferation of antibiotic resistant infective and increased the risk of sepsis. [34]

As with the management of any type of shock, prevention is primary in the treatment of sepsis. The transport team must use meticulous methods to decrease the risk of exposing patients to infection, particularly when transporting patients with invasive lines.

Indicators of sepsis or septic shock include:

- Fever
- Hypothermia
- Obvious source of infection
  - Urinary catheter
  - Central venous access
  - Invasive monitoring
  - Opens
  - Postsurgery
- Risk of infection
  - Penetrating injury
  - Open fractures
- Hyperdynamic state
  - Increased cardiac index

- Decreased vascular resistance
- Hypoxia

Research is directed at identifying ways to stop the devastating cascade that is initiated with sepsis and septic shock, which can lead to multiple organ dysfunction and death. Examples of current research include development of medications to manage the coagulopathy that occurs with sepsis, anti-infective agents that selectively render the invading agent ineffective, and methods to correct impaired oxygen deliver.[34]

Neurogenic Shock. Neurogenic shock is a result of an injury or insult to the reticular activating system and spinal cord. In the presence of major brain stem dysfunction or spinal cord injury, hypotension without tachycardia or cutaneous vasoconstriction may be of neurogenic cause. Vasoactive drugs should not be administered until volume is restored. Many times, if no blood loss has occurred, hypotension may be resolved by placing the patient flat or in a slight Trendelenburg position if no injury to the cervical spine has occurred, as confirmed by medical personnel. Respiratory insufficiency is common, and ventilatory support should be implemented as necessary.[25,28,66]

The treatment of spinal shock includes appropriate immobilization for transport and initiation of pharmacologic management for hypotension. Vasoactive drugs may be needed to maintain peripheral vasoconstriction once any source of bleeding has been ruled out. If the transport team comes in contact with the patient within 8 hours of the injury, methylprednisolone should be started to decrease the effects of inflammation on the spinal cord. The initial dose of methylprednisolone is 30 mg/kg over 15 minutes followed 45 minutes later by a maintenance infusion of 5.4 mg/kg over 23 hours.

The transport team must also ensure that the patient is kept warm because spinal cord injury leaves the patient poikilothermic. In addition the team must be sure no pressure is being exerted on the patient's skin that may cause further injury because the patient is insensitive to it.

Anaphylaxis. Anaphylaxis is an acute systemic allergic reaction as a result of the release of chemical mediators after an antigen-antibody reaction. It is mediated by immunoglobin E (IgE), which rests on the surface of mast cells and basophils in the body, especially along the respiratory and GI tracts. When a reaction occurs, it results in the formation and release of histamine, the kinins, and the slow, reactive substance of anaphylaxis. These cause three major effects: (1) vasodilation, (2) smooth muscle spasm, and (3) increased vascular permeability with edema formation[41,36,84] (Figure 13-6).

Anaphylactoid reactions (not mediated by IgE) have identical signs and symptoms and are caused most often by drugs, such as iodinated radiograph contrast, procaine compounds, and fluorescein. In either reaction the sooner the onset, the more severe the reaction is likely to be.

Patients experience a sense of impending doom; pruritus, especially of the palms and feet; and sudden headache. Adverse reactions may occur quickly and affect all systems.[36,84]

Respiratory: upper airway edema; angioedema of hypopharynx, epiglottis, larynx, and trachea; asthma; stridulous breathing with supraclavicular, suprasternal, and intercostal retractions

Cutaneous: flushing, pruritus, urticaria, and angioedema

Cardiovascular: arrhythmias and electrocardiogram (ECG) abnormalities, probably caused by decreased coronary perfusion and oxygenation; vasodilation and hypotension possibly occurring with or without other symptoms from venous pooling or increased capillary permeability and water loss into the interstitial space

Neurologic: sudden loss of consciousness, seizures, cerebral anoxia secondary to airway obstruction, and decreased blood pressure

Rarely, GI spasm of smooth muscle leading to cramps, diarrhea, sudden and explosive involuntary defecation, and vomiting with potential for aspiration

Genitourinary: incontinence and labor-like pains in female uterus

Death from upper airway obstruction, vomiting and aspiration, bronchospasm, and vascular collapse

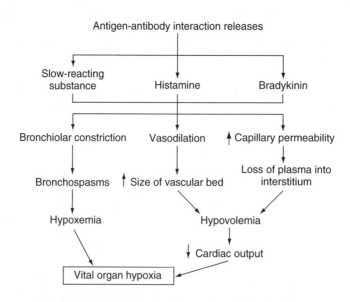

FIGURE 13-6　**Pathophysiology of anaphylactic shock.**

Management. Treatment for patients with anaphylaxis is as follows.

For some stings and bites, compression dressings may be applied to decrease the progress of the toxin. The Sawyer extractor may be used to remove the stinger.

Resuscitation should be initiated, depending on the severity of the reaction. The transport team must keep in mind that airway management may be made more difficult because of swelling. Definitive airway management may need to be performed before transport, depending on the size of the transport vehicle and the length of the transport.

Epinephrine—Administration of 1:1000 epinephrine subcutaneously dilates bronchial smooth muscle, causes vasoconstriction, and decreases vascular permeability.

For severe reactions a 1:10,000 epinephrine solution (5 ml) may be given intravenously and repeated every 5 to 10 minutes.

Antihistamine (Diphenhydramine)—An antihistamine will compete with the binding sites.

Administration of steroids is also needed.

Unexpected anaphylaxis with a rapid clinical course may result in a swift recovery or death. There is little time to act; early recognition is therefore essential.

Obstructive Shock

Description. Circulation can be compromised and the patient become hypotensive and hypoxic because of direct failure of the heart muscle or compression or obstruction of vessels that provide central circulation. The result of this pathophysiologic process may be a pericardial tamponade or tension pneumothorax.[20]

Cardiac tamponade and tension pneumothorax, once recognized, are easily reversible mechanical obstructions to cardiac output. Cardiac tamponade occurs when blood or effusion accumulates in the closed pericardial sac. The heart is unable to fill, the central venous pressure rises, blood pressure and pulse rate decrease, and heart sounds may be muffled (Beck's triad).[36] Needle pericardiocentesis is the treatment of choice.

Tension pneumothorax results in a complete collapse of one or both lungs with compression on mediastinal vessels and organs. Air under tension may be evacuated by needle or chest tube insertion.

Indicators. A history of any of the following may indicate the potential for mechanical obstruction resulting in hypotension and hypoxia.

Chest pain
Dyspnea
Syncope
Trauma to the chest

Signs and symptoms include:

Apprehension
Shortness of breath
Tracheal deviation
Jugular vein distention

Predisposing Conditions. Predisposing conditions include the following.

Blunt or penetrating trauma
Preexisting pulmonary disease, such as chronic obstructive pulmonary disease or asthma
Cardiomyopathy
Bacterial endocarditis

Management should include:

- Decompression of the obstruction by a needle or chest tube for a tension pneumothorax
- Pericardiocentesis
- Transporting the patient at lower altitudes

COAGULOPATHIES

One of the common complications of shock is the development of coagulopathies and DIC, particularly as the result of massive blood loss and fluid resuscitation. In addition, the presence of a preexisting condition, such as hemophilia, or the patient's use of a medication such as coumarin that interferes with coagulation poses further challenges in patient care.

Most patients who are bleeding have normal clotting mechanisms, and when normal measures taken to control bleeding are not effective, a coagulopathy, or bleeding disorder, may be suspected. Diagnosing a specific coagulopathy in the transport environment is difficult or impossible, but an index of suspicion should be raised in certain cases based on the assessment of the patient, the available history, and an evaluation of laboratory findings that may be available. Some patients will have an established history of an inherited coagulopathy, whereas others may be expected to have a bleeding disorder or tendency toward such a disorder based on their current disease process. Confirmation of that suspicion will require more extensive laboratory testing than is available in most community hospitals and is best determined by consultation with a hematologist or an internist in a medical center with experience and facilities to properly evaluate and care for the patient.

A *coagulopathy* is defined as "any disorder of blood coagulation."[35,38,48,97] This is a broad categorization of a variety of disorders that interfere with the body's ability to control hemorrhage. Some coagulopathies are inherited disorders, whereas others are acquired and unrelated to genetic tendencies. Coagulopathies can be either primary disorders or secondary to an underlying disease. Of the 12 clotting factors (Box 13-6), clotting factor may be deficient, or another stage of the clotting cascade may not function normally. Some coagulopathies are life threatening; others are so mild that they go undetected until late in life. Approximately 80,000 deaths in the United States occur each year from bleeding disorders of acquired or congenital origin.[7]

INCIDENCE

Some coagulopathies are hereditary in origin. The famous "bleeders" of history have been victims of hemophilia. Any deficiency of 1 of the 12 clotting factors may cause a clotting disorder, but the most commonly seen hereditary coagulopathies are hemophilia A, hemophilia B, and von Willebrand's disease.

BOX 13-6	**Common Names of Coagulation Factors**
Factor I	Fibrinogen
Factor II	Prothrombin
Factor III	Tissue thromboplastin
Factor IV	Calcium
Factor V	Ac globulin
Factor VII	Proconvertin
Factor VIII	Antihemophilic factor (AHG)
Factor IX	Plasma thromboplastin component (PTC) (Christmas factor)
Factor X	Stuart factor
Factor XI	Plasma thromboplastin antecedent (PTA)
Factor XII	Hageman factor
Factor XIII	Fibrin stabilizing factor

HEREDITARY COAGULOPATHIES
HEMOPHILIA A
Of all the hereditary coagulopathies, hemophilia A, sometimes called "classic hemophilia," is the most common. About 70% to 90% of "hemophiliacs" have hemophilia A. It is seen in 1 to 2 of every 10,000 people in the United States.[63] The gene is found on the X chromosome and is transmitted as a sex-linked recessive trait; therefore nearly all its victims are male. Female carriers (heterozygotes) pass the gene to one half their daughters, who then also become carriers, and to one half their sons, who will have the disease. Males with the disease (hemizygotes) pass the gene to all of their daughters, who become asymptomatic carriers; sons are normal. Of hemophilia patients, 30% have no family history of the disease.

HEMOPHILIA B
Also called "Christmas disease," hemophilia B is similar to hemophilia A. About 9% of those with inherited coagulation defects have this disease. It is 15% as frequent as hemophilia A and is found in approximately 1 of every 100,000 persons in the United States.[63] Like hemophilia A, it is found almost entirely in males as a sex-linked recessive trait.

von Willebrand's Disease

This form of hemophilia occurs in 5 to 10 of every 1,000,000 persons in the United States. It is found in both genders because it is inherited as an autosomal dominant trait.[7,35]

Acquired Disorders

Coagulopathies may also be acquired rather than inherited. Acquired disorders occur much more commonly than inherited ones.[7,35] These bleeding disorders are secondary to another disease process or therapy. Although many varieties exist, the types most likely to confront the transport team are described in the following sections.

Vitamin K Deficiency

Vitamin K must be present in the blood for clotting to occur. It is obtained by the body through the diet and produced by intestinal bacteria. Vitamin K levels may be deficient due to poor diet or sterilization of the gut from antibiotic therapy. Patients at risk include the postoperative patient with oral intake who is on an extended course of antibiotic therapy.

Hepatic Coagulopathy

Liver disease is one of the most common risk factors for the development of coagulopathy. Because 11 of the 12 clotting factors are synthesized in the liver, patients with liver dysfunction, particularly those with severe cirrhosis, are deficient in those factors. In addition, vitamin K deficiency often contributes to the coagulopathy because patients with liver disease are unable to store vitamin K at optimum levels.

Disseminated Intravascular Coagulation

DIC is a complex disease and not uncommon in critically ill or injured patients. It is a secondary response to many diseases, including some infections, malignancies, and obstetric complications.[48] Braunwald[16] stated that sepsis is one of the most common disorders associated with DIC. Box 13-7 lists many of the disease states for which DIC may be a further complication.

Robbins[16,48] stated that 50% of DIC patients are obstetric patients, and 33% have terminal cancers. DIC appears to result from the entrance of

---

BOX 13-7 Diseases That Precipitate DIC

Obstetric
Abruptio placentae
Amniotic fluid embolism
Toxemia of pregnancy
Hydatidiform mole
Retained dead fetus
Septic abortion

Infection
Bacterial: gram-negative or gram-positive septicemia
Rickettsial: Rocky Mountain spotted fever
Viral: varicella, rubella, arboviruses, influenza A
Parasitic: *Plasmodium falciparum* malaria
Fungal: histoplasmosis

Trauma
Trauma with shock
Head injury
Burns
Anoxia
Heatstroke

Malignancy
Metastatic carcinoma: pancreas, lung, breast, stomach, prostate, colon
Acute promyelocytic leukemia

Shock States
Cardiac arrest

Miscellaneous
Aortic aneurysm
Snakebite
Transfusion reactions
Anaphylactic drug reactions
Prostatic surgery
Lung surgery
Extracorporal circulation

---

substances into the blood that cause accelerated clotting, thus the variety of primary diseases (see box) with which it has been associated.

Drug-Induced Coagulopathies

A variety of medications can either enhance or inhibit clotting. Drug-induced coagulopathies may be the most commonly seen cause of abnormal bleeding.[70] However, a few of these medications alone will cause significant problems without accompanying platelet or clotting-factor deficiency.[59]

MASSIVE TRANSFUSIONS

Another cause of bleeding that can be encountered by transport team personnel is the coagulopathy associated with massive transfusions. Massive blood loss, the use of banked blood, which is deficient in clotting factors and platelets, and resuscitation with large amounts of crystalloids and colloids are significant contributing factors to the coagulopathy associated with massive transfusions. Those at risk include patients with major trauma, GI hemorrhage, or obstetric complications.

NORMAL PHYSIOLOGY

Hemostasis, the arrest of bleeding, is an extremely complex process. The normal coagulation process is a balance between uncontrolled bleeding and generalized thrombosis or clotting. The transport team needs some understanding of the coagulative process to be adequately prepared for patients with actual or potential coagulopathies.

At least four components are necessary for normal clotting to take place: (1) blood vessels, (2) platelets, (3) clotting, and (4) fibrinolysis, or clot dissolution.[82] If any one of these components malfunctions or is deficient, a coagulopathy will result. Nearly every conceivable aspect of these four components has been known to malfunction. A few disorders are seen much more frequently than others; the remaining bleeding disorders are rather rare.

Blood vessels are composed of connective and smooth muscle tissue lined with endothelial cells. Vessel walls serve as an important protective barrier to contain and protect the circulating blood. If injured, the vessel constricts at the site of injury through a reflex nervous system response. This decreases blood flow and slows bleeding. In addition, after blunt trauma, blood flowing into the injured tissue creates a hematoma, which decreases blood loss by mechanical pressure, tamponading the ruptured vessel.

The second and third components, platelets and clotting factors, interact to form the clot. Platelets, also known as *thrombocytes*, are actually cell fragments from larger cells called *karyocytes*, which are formed in the bone marrow. When a blood vessel is injured, collagen is exposed in the connective tissue. Collagen is oppositely charged to the circulating platelets, causing platelets to be attracted to the injured site. The platelets adhere to exposed tissue and vessel walls, but they also stick or aggregate to one another, forming a platelet plug. Platelets then rupture as they plug the damaged vessel wall, releasing incomplete thromboplastin, also known as *clotting factor III*. Clotting factor III reacts with calcium, called *factor IV*, and several other blood factors to help form the permanent clot. The platelet plug is adequate to stop minor bleeding at least temporarily, but more severe bleeding also requires the interaction of coagulation factors to form a stable fibrin clot.

Collagen exposed at the injured site activates factor XII, which stimulates other reactions, eventually forming thrombin, enhancing the aggregation of platelets. Thrombin also converts fibrinogen, factor I, which is present in plasma, into fibrin, an insoluble protein of densely intertwined threads that catch erythrocytes and platelets.

After the clot has served its purpose in stopping the hemorrhage, the fibrin clot is dissolved by the fibrinolytic system. This process, known as *fibrinolysis*, begins within 24 hours after clot formation. Plasminogen, a serum globulin found in the clot, is activated by substances in the blood and becomes plasmin, a proteolytic enzyme that digests proteins, including fibrin, fibrinogen, and factors V and VIII. This prevents the permanent thrombosis of the injured blood vessel.

PATHOPHYSIOLOGY

HEREDITARY COAGULOPATHIES
HEMOPHILIA A

The hemophilias are the most common hereditary bleeding disorders, and hemophilia A is the most prevalent of the hemophilias. The deficiency in this disease is factor VIII, also known as *antihemophilic factor*, with severity of symptoms closely related to the level of factor VIII in the blood. Platelet plug formation is normal; however, deficiency of factor VIII impairs the capacity to form a stable fibrin clot. The disease is almost always discovered by age 5, although mild cases may not be recognized until after trauma or surgery as an adult.[82]

Between acute episodes of bleeding, hemophiliacs may be without symptoms unless they are anemic from previous blood loss. Medical attention will be sought for hemarthroses (bleeding into joints), hematuria, and epistaxis. Bleeding can also occur into deep tissues. Mucosal bleeding is unusual, as is GI bleeding, unless peptic ulcer disease is also present. Trauma is often the cause of bleeding, and that bleeding may occur or reoccur 8 hours or even 1 to 3 days after the injury and continue for days or weeks.

Bleeding is particularly dangerous when pressure is exerted on organs, vessels, or nerves. It can be life threatening when it is intracranial, lingual, laryngeal, retropharyngeal, pericardial, pleural, or simply exsanguinating. CNS hemorrhage is the leading cause of death of hemophiliacs and should be taken seriously.[70] CNS bleeding may occur spontaneously unrelated to trauma or a specific lesion.

A long history of severe or poorly controlled hemophilia may leave the patient severely handicapped, with permanent joint damage resulting from hemarthroses, causing fibrous or bony ankylosis. Hemophiliacs may also suffer complications secondary to the treatment process. Multiple blood product transfusions or factor-concentrate infusions can result in liver disease, hepatitis, and HIV.

HEMOPHILIA B

Hemophilia B is very similar to hemophilia A. It is a hereditary disorder with the same genetic pattern, affecting primarily males. Hemophilia B is caused by a deficiency of factor IX activity. This results in prolonged partial thromboplastin (PT) times. Clinical symptoms and bleeding are the same as in hemophilia A, as is the risk to the patient's life.

VON WILLEBRAND'S DISEASE

von Willebrand's disease is a result of two defects: defective platelet adherence and decreased levels of factor VIII. Platelets occur in normal numbers but do not adhere to the subendothelial collagen of the capillary wall to form the platelet plug. Therefore bleeding is prolonged. von Willebrand's disease is usually milder than hemophilia A or B. Bleeding is mostly from skin or mucous membranes rather than deep bleeding into tissue or joints. Easy bruising, epistaxis, dental bleeding, menorrhagia, and GI bleeding are the usual clinical manifestations.[70]

ACQUIRED COAGULOPATHIES

Bleeding disorders that are acquired are seen more often by the transport team than inherited coagulopathies.

VITAMIN K DEFICIENCY

Factors II, VII, IX, and X are vitamin K dependent, requiring the presence of vitamin K to function normally.[59] The body acquires vitamin K from leafy green vegetables in the diet and as a by-product of intestinal bacteria. If these sources are not available to the body, a deficiency will result in 2 to 4 weeks. Hemorrhage from vitamin K deficiency can occur in patients receiving antibiotic therapy for extended periods while taking nothing by mouth because antibiotics may "sterilize" the gut, eliminating the bacterial source of vitamin K. Intestinal malabsorption and liver disease can cause bleeding from vitamin K deficiency. Hemorrhagic disease of the newborn is also a vitamin K deficiency, caused by a lack of vitamin K-producing intestinal flora and the immaturity of the liver.[16]

HEPATIC COAGULOPATHY

Liver disease is a common cause of coagulopathy. It is most often seen in patients with severe hepatic cirrhosis but also occurs with other acute and chronic liver diseases. Any patient with severe liver dysfunction is at risk for hemorrhage. All coagulation factors except VIII are synthesized in the liver by hepatocytes. Therefore patients with liver disease will be deficient in those factors. However, before bleeding occurs, liver disease is usually advanced and easily recognized by other signs of the disease.

Other factors may contribute to bleeding tendencies in the patient with liver disease. A vitamin K deficiency may result from intestinal malabsorption, poor dietary habits, or the anorexia associated with liver disease. Further coagulopathy is often present because of low platelet count and platelet dysfunction. Finally, liver disease results in increased proteolytic activity in the blood, probably because the liver has a decreased ability to remove these proteolytic substances from circulation. The clinical picture is very close to that of DIC, which may also develop.

DISSEMINATED INTRAVASCULAR COAGULATION

DIC has been called the most important coagulopathy in the emergency department.[70] This life-threatening disorder is actually a secondary complication of a broad spectrum of diseases (see Box 13-7). It may have a variety of causes, including the entry of foreign protein into circulation or massive vascular injury, as occurs in crushing trauma. Whatever the cause, the result is that the coagulation and fibrinolytic systems are out of control. Platelets and coagulation factors are consumed by this abnormal clotting. Thrombin formation overwhelms its inhibitor system, further accelerating clotting and activation of fibrinogen. Fibrin is deposited in the microvasculature of many organs, resulting in poor tissue perfusion and eventual focal necrosis of tissue. Organ failure may result. Later the fibrinolytic system loses fibrin and impairs thrombin formation, and clots wash away. In summary, platelets, clotting factors, and fibrinogen are consumed so quickly that the body is unable to replace them and maintain hemostatic levels. This creates a clinical picture of petechiae, peripheral cyanosis, GI bleeding, vaginal bleeding, prolonged bleeding, ecchymosis, hematomas, bleeding from surgical or invasive procedure sites, and signs of organ injury.

DRUG-INDUCED COAGULOPATHIES

Coumarin. The coumarin drugs, primarily dicoumarol and warfarin, are medications frequently prescribed. Coumarin interferes with the action of vitamin K, causing a deficiency with resultant bleeding. Levels of prothrombin and factors VII and X are particularly decreased. Inappropriate dosage levels, the need for dosage adjustment, or intentional overdosage by the patient can be the cause of the coagulopathy.

Heparin. Heparin has several actions, the most important of which is the inactivation of thrombin.

With the inactivation of thrombin, fibrinogen is not converted to fibrin (insoluble protein threads that strengthen clots). Heparin also interferes in the action of factors IX, X, XI, and XII, resulting in bleeding at single or multiple sites.

Other Medications. Aspirin affects platelet function and may cause bleeding. Aspirin blocks an enzyme called *cyclooxygenase*, which results in a decrease in platelet aggregation and decreased vasoconstriction. The clinical manifestations of aspirin-induced platelet dysfunction are minimal unless the patient also has an underlying coagulation defect such as von Willebrand's disease or other platelet or coagulation disorders.[59]

Fibrinolytic therapy is used in the management of acute myocardial infarction, pulmonary embolus, and stroke. A serious complication of this therapy is bleeding.

These medications work by causing clot dissolution by specific mechanisms, such as binding to fibrin and activating plasminogen to form plasmin, which in turn dissolves fibrin clots, fibrinogen, and other clotting factors. Even though some drugs are clot specific, their action mechanisms leave the patient at risk for bleeding from puncture sites, from procedures such as intubation, and into specific places such as the brain or GI tract. Patients with previous histories of medical or surgical problems that can leave them at risk for bleeding are particularly vulnerable.[46,47] Other medications may interfere with platelet and clotting functions, but symptoms are generally mild and easily treated (Box 13-8).[46,47]

MASSIVE TRANSFUSIONS

Patients receiving large quantities of banked blood over a short period of time experience coagulopathies because of a dilutional effect. Banked blood becomes deficient in platelets and factors

BOX 13-8	**Drugs Causing Decreased Platelet Number or Function**

Drug-Induced Thrombocytopenia

Alcohol
Antibiotics (sulfa, rifampin)
Aspirin
Cytotoxic agents
Digitoxin
Diphenylhydantoin
Estrogen
Gold salts
Heparin
Heroin
Nonsteroidal antiinflammatory drugs (NSAIDs)
Para-aminosalicylic acid
Phenylbutazone
Phenytoin
Quinidine, quinine
Streptokinase
Thiazides
Fibrinolytics

Drug-Induced Decreased Platelet Function

Aspirin
Clofibrate
Dextran
Dipyridamole
NSAIDs (indomethacin)
Sulfinpyrazone

V and VII after storage at 4° C for 48 hours or longer. An estimated 10 to 12 units or more of blood given in a 24-hour period will cause coagulopathies if platelets or fresh blood are not also given to increase platelet and clotting-factor levels.[56] The transport team must help prevent this type of coagulopathy from reaching clinically significant proportions.

ASSESSMENT

PHYSICAL ASSESSMENT

As with any other physical assessment, the transport team should first evaluate the airway, breathing, and circulation (the ABCs). Once any necessary interventions have been undertaken to support those

systems, attention can be given to a more detailed physical assessment.

Most bleeding, ecchymosis, and hematoma nearly always result from identifiable local trauma. However, as the transport team continues to assess the patient, certain observations indicate that a coagulopathy may be present. Some of these red flags include the following.[82]

1. Bleeding at multiple sites or in several body systems concurrently
2. "Spontaneous" deep hematomas or hemarthroses
3. Unusually prolonged bleeding after local injury
4. Disproportionately large hemorrhage after a minor insult
5. Late bleeding that follows a period of apparently normal hemostasis after surgery or trauma
6. Inability to find an organic cause for hemorrhage in a specific area or an organ system

The transport team must be careful not to overlook the obvious. Many patients with previously diagnosed coagulopathies wear an identification tag such as the Medic-Alert tag as a necklace or bracelet, others carry a card identifying their specific disorder, and some carry a treatment protocol at all times. This kind of documentation saves valuable time in directing patient assessment and care delivery.

During the assessment, the transport team should examine the skin and mucous membranes for signs of bleeding and note petechiae, purpura, ecchymosis, and hematomas. Oozing from IV sites or hematoma or ecchymosis around those sites may be significant. The patient should be observed for gingival or other mucous membrane bleeding; hematuria or GI bleeding may be part of the pattern indicating coagulopathy. Joint deformities or stiffness may be present from previous hemarthroses. CNS bleeding is a life-threatening occurrence that is easily missed, and headache or other CNS signs should be aggressively pursued. The team should look for signs of liver, renal, or splenic disease or infection.

Any bleeding that is unusual or does not stop with direct pressure as expected should alert the team to suspect a coagulopathy is present.

Identifying a specific coagulopathy based on physical assessment, particularly in the transport environment, is almost impossible. However, characterizing the signs and symptoms of some of the major categories of coagulopathies is useful. Bleeding typical of a coagulation defect, such as the hemophilias, is large-vessel bleeding, often intramuscular, with large, deep hematomas and hemarthrosis. Crippling joint deformities may be present from previous hemarthrosis.

In hemophilia the platelet plug forms normally, but coagulation, which should follow, is defective. Therefore the platelet plug may initially control bleeding. Later, delayed onset of bleeding may occur, or there may be rebleeding after initial control of hemorrhage. In general, coagulation factor deficiencies are less responsive to local pressure than platelet abnormalities. Bleeding in DIC usually occurs at multiple sites, such as an oozing around IV or venipuncture sites or frank bleeding from mucosa. Purpura and ecchymosis may be present. The patient is often in shock.

Platelet defects, as in aspirin-induced bleeding or other types of thrombocytopenia, is manifested as small-vessel bleeding. Spontaneous bleeding occurs into the skin, such as petechiae, purpura, or numerous overlapping ecchymosis. Bleeding may be mucosal. Bleeding after trauma is more immediate than in clotting-factor deficiencies, and it usually stops with local pressure. Bleeding does not reoccur hours or days later, as does the pattern seen in clotting-factor disorders.

History

A thorough history is extremely important in patients with suspected coagulopathies. The patient with a known coagulopathy may be more knowledgeable and expert about needed clinical management than the average nurse or physician. Family history of a coagulopathy may also guide in the assessment; however, this information should be substantiated by accompanying clinical signs and symptoms of the disease.

The patient's medical history may include unusual bleeding from the umbilical stump after birth and bleeding after dental extractions, trauma,

or surgical procedures. A history of hemarthrosis, frequent epistaxis, or menorrhagia is significant. The flight nurse should question the patient about taking anticoagulants or other drugs that affect platelet function. A history of liver disease or other organ system failure is significant, as is evidence of infection or DIC-associated factors.

Laboratory Values

Frequently, laboratory values are included in the patient's medical record received during an interfacility transport. These values should be referred to when the transport team undertakes the initial evaluation of the patient's condition (Box 13-9).

Table 13-1 lists possible diagnoses based on results of the most readily available blood tests that evaluate coagulation and fibrinolysis. A definitive evaluation and diagnosis of the patient will require further laboratory testing at the receiving medical center.

In general the intrinsic pathway is measured by the PTT. The extrinsic pathway is also evaluated by the PT (Figure 13-7).

A platelet count will reveal thrombocytopenia but will not establish that platelet function is normal. Bleeding time, another widely available screening test, is increased in significant thrombocytopenia or platelet dysfunction disorders such as von Willebrand's disease. Fibrinogen concentration does not measure fibrinolysis directly but can suggest it when evaluated in conjunction with the other tests described.

INTERVENTIONS AND TREATMENT

Diagnosis of a specific coagulopathy is difficult or impossible in the transport environment. Emergency interventions appropriate for patients experiencing acute effects of a coagulopathy are primarily supportive.

The first priority is airway management. This may be required if there is evidence of obstruction caused by bleeding or hematomas in the pharyngeal or laryngeal areas. Airway obstruction worsens as bleeding continues into the airway. An enlarging hematoma caused by bleeding into the soft tissues

BOX 13-9	Normal Laboratory Values*

Bleeding time (Surgicutt)	1.5-8 min	
Fibrinogen concentration	195-365 mg/dl	
Hematocrit	Males:	42.0%-54.0%
	Females:	38.0%-46.0%
Hemoglobin	Males:	14.0-17.0 g/dl
	Females:	12.0-15.0 g/dl
Partial thromboplastin time (activated)	25-35 sec	
Prothrombin time	10.9-12.8 sec	
Platelet count		

Males:	6-11 years	235-534	$10^3/\mu l$
	12-16 years	184-485	$10^3/\mu l$
	>16 years	184-370	$10^3/\mu l$
Females	6-11 years	227-539	$10^3/\mu l$
	12-16 years	200-390	$10^3/\mu l$
	>16 year s	196-451	$10^3/\mu l$

*Normal values vary among laboratories depending on reagents used and the method and instrumentation used.

TABLE 13-1	Laboratory Evaluation of Coagulopathies

Abnormal tests	Possible diagnoses
Plat or Plat BT	Idiopathic thrombocytopenic purpura, drug reaction, bone marrow depression
Plat, PT, PTT, Fib	DIC, liver disease
BT	Platelet dysfunction, mild von Willebrand's disease, salicylates, uremia
BT, PTT	von Willebrand's disease
PT	Factor VII deficiency (rare)
PTT	Hemophilia, heparin
PT, PTT	Vitamin K deficiency, coumarin drugs, liver disease, heparin, factor V, X, II, or I deficiency
Fib	Decreased fibrinogen (rare)
Fib, PT, ± PTT	DIC, primary fibrinolysis
All normal	Normal hemostasis, factor XII deficiency, allergic vasculitis, scurvy, dysproteinemia, etc.

BT, Bleeding time; *Fib*, fibrinogen concentration; *Plat*, platelet count; *PT*, prothrombin time; *PTT*, partial thromboplastin time

could completely obstruct the airway. Endotracheal intubation may be necessary to preserve the airway. Nasal intubation should be avoided because of a high likelihood of serious epistaxis. Supplemental oxygen should be delivered to the bleeding patient.

The next priority is to stop ongoing major hemorrhage. Patients who are continuing to hemorrhage should be treated similarly to any bleeding patient that the transport team may encounter. Direct pressure or pressure applied to appropriate pressure points helps control bleeding. Raising the bleeding part above the patient's heart decreases hydrostatic pressure and slows bleeding; however, pressure must be held for a much greater time than for the patient with normal coagulation mechanisms.

Volume replacement of shed blood is important. Fluids should be administered and the patient's response closely monitored. If assessment indicates the need for additional volume replacement, blood products should be considered if available.

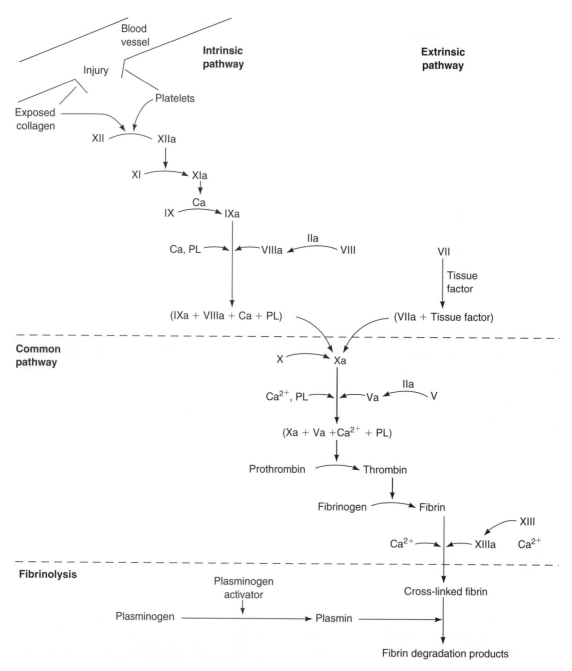

(1) Factors in the intrinsic pathway are present in circulating blood.
(2) The extrinsic pathway depends on the release of thromboplastin from damaged cells.
(3) "a" refers to the activated form of the designated factor.
(4) Ca = calcium. PL = phospholipid.

FIGURE 13-7   Coagulation and fibrinolytic system.

The patient should be protected from additional trauma during loading and unloading from the transport vehicle. The transport team should minimize needle sticks, and prolonged pressure should be applied to venipuncture sites. Intubation, catheterization, and other invasive procedures should be undertaken gently with good technique and only when indicated by the patient's condition.

Medications that depress platelet function should be withheld until medical consultation is available. Anticoagulants should also be withheld, with the exception of heparin in the case of DIC. This is an accepted therapy appropriate in some situations to control the clotting system that is out of hemostatic balance.

Infusion of packed red blood cells, fresh frozen plasma, or platelets may be started at the referring hospital in an attempt to raise clotting factor or platelet levels. This is a useful therapy but is rather inexact when undertaken before complete laboratory evaluation. Only the specifically indicated blood component should be given because of the risk of autoimmunization and the possible transmission of infectious disease.[98]

Fresh frozen plasma can be infused to increase clotting-factor levels in deficient patients. A unit of fresh frozen plasma raises any clotting-factor level 2% to 3% in the average-size adult. Fresh frozen plasma is not recommended if PT and PTT times are less than one and one-half times normal. Fresh frozen plasma is a useful method for correcting warfarin-induced hemorrhage when the seriousness of the patient's condition does not allow time for correction by simply discontinuing warfarin therapy or administering vitamin K.

Platelets can also be infused to correct bleeding caused by low platelet counts (thrombocytopenia) or deficiencies in platelet function. One unit of platelets should raise the platelet count by at least 5000 in the average adult. The decision to infuse platelets depends on clinical parameters in addition to platelet count. Patients who are clinically stable may require platelet counts for less than 10,000 to 20,000/μl. Patients undergoing invasive procedures generally should have a platelet count of 50,000/μl. However, patients with coagulation defects,

hemorrhage, sepsis, or other unstable conditions may require higher platelet counts.

Specific treatment of certain disorders bears comment. Hemophilia A patients should be treated early and aggressively for any bleeding episode. Standard treatment involves infusion of a factor VIII replacement. Cryoprecipitate is a frozen form of factor VIII concentrate. Most patients use factor VIII concentrate supplied in powder form. A single dose corrects minor bleeding, but severe hemorrhage may require continuous infusion for up to several weeks.

Hemophilia B is clinically indistinguishable from hemophilia A but requires treatment with either fresh frozen plasma or a concentrate enriched in the deficient factor IX. von Willebrand's disease is treated similarly to hemophilia A, often with cryoprecipitate.

Vitamin K deficiency should be treated with parenteral replacement. Administration of vitamin K intravenously is in a slow, diluted infusion. An attempt should be made to correct the cause of the deficiency. Emergency treatment of hemorrhage with fresh frozen plasma should correct the clotting defect, at least temporarily.

Emergency treatment for hepatic coagulopathies includes administration of vitamin K. Fresh frozen plasma infusion replaces all known coagulation factors and is safer and more complete therapy than prothrombin complex replacements. For patients with thrombosis, treatment by anticoagulation with heparin can be dangerous because heparin metabolism is unpredictable in cirrhosis, and severe bleeding may result.

DIC is treated by identification and treatment of the underlying cause. Once this is eliminated, DIC will resolve. Any significant bleeding or thrombosis requires immediate treatment. Fresh frozen plasma and cryoprecipitate are recommended to replace clotting factors. Platelet concentrates are given to increase the platelet count.[16] Heparinization is a controversial treatment of the thrombosis seen in DIC. The clotting cascade is out of control in DIC, and clotting factors are rapidly consumed, resulting in uncontrollable hemorrhage. Heparin reduces thrombin generation and prevents the further consumption of clotting factors. The risk is that heparin may cause further bleeding.

SUMMARY

The management of the patient who is in shock or may be suffering from the complications of coagulopathy is based on early recognition, swift and appropriate treatment, and rapid transport. Regardless of the cause, uncontrolled shock leads to fatal derangement. The early diagnosis of shock requires consideration of the history of the precipitating incident, the patient's medical history, and the sometimes-subtle signs exhibited by patients while compensatory mechanisms manage to maintain blood pressure and cardiac output.

An improved understanding of the pathophysiologic signs of shock helps the transport team recognize patients with shock and potential or actual bleeding disorders. Although definitive diagnosis and treatment are generally not possible during transport, early recognition enhances the patient's chances for timely treatment. Supportive measures routinely practiced by transport team will help stabilize the patient in shock until further evaluation and treatment become available at the tertiary receiving facility.

SHOCK AND COAGULOPATHY CASE STUDY

A 23-year-old female, restrained passenger of a motor vehicle was struck on her side of the car by a tractor-trailer. The car was driven into a ditch. On arrival of the transport team, they found a confused and combative patient in the back of an ambulance. The patient was on 100% oxygen by mask, appropriately immobilized, and one intravenous line of normal saline had been established.

Primary survey:
Spontaneous airway
Equal breath sounds
Pale, diaphoretic, cool skin
No palpable peripheral pulses, palpable femoral pulse
Monitor showed heart rate of 157, sinus tachycardia

Combative patient, GCS: 9
  Eye Opening   1
  Verbal   3
  Motor   5

Because of her signs of shock, the patient was intubated using RSI including Amidate, Lidocaine, and Succinylcholine. She was intubated on the first attempt and ventilated with 100% oxygen. Initial color change on the end-tidal CO_2, yellow.

A second line was established because the first line was tenuous. Additional sedation was given with the Amidate, soft restraints were applied, and the patient was secured to the stretcher. During the 10-minute flight, 1500 of fluid was administered. The patient had a palpable pulse of 90 and a heart rate of 140, which decreased briefly to 110. Her ventilations were assisted with 100%, and she occasionally pulled against the restraints. Verbal assurance was given by the team.

On arrival at the trauma center, the patient was hot unloaded and taken to the Shock Resuscitation Unit. Her heart rate increased again to 150, and no blood pressure could be palpated. It was obtained by Doppler at 70 over palpation. A FAST exam was performed on arrival. A large amount of fluid was observed. Within minutes, she was taken directly to the operating room.

Blood and fluid resuscitation in the OR returned a pressure of 90. The patient had sustained a severe splenic injury and as repair began, her blood pressure dropped and she began to bleed profusely. A lacerated inferior vena cava was found.

Despite aggressive resuscitation and repair of the injury, the patient continued to bleed. Unfortunately, she expired approximately 90 minutes after her accident.

This case illustrates the need for early recognition of shock (no palpable peripheral pulses, tachycardia, altered mental status), the initial critical interventions (intubation and oxygenation with 100% oxygen, fluid bolus), and rapid transport to an appropriate center for definitive care. However, it points out that even when all the pieces fall in place, the injury or illness that causes irreversible shock remains a challenge.

REFERENCES

1. Ackerman M: The systemic inflammatory response, sepsis, and multiple organ dysfunction, *Crit Care Nurs Clin North Am* 6:243, 1994.
2. Ali J, Qi W: Fluid and electrolyte deficit with prolonged pneumatic anti-shock garment application, *J Trauma* 38(4):612, 1994.
3. Alspach JG, Williams SM: *Core curriculum for critical care nursing*, ed 3, Philadelphia, 1985, Saunders.
4. American Heart Association: *Textbook of advanced cardiac life support*, Dallas, 2000, Author.
5. Anderson HL III et al: Extracorporeal life support for respiratory failure after multiple trauma, *J Trauma* 37(2):266, 1994.
6. Angelica A, Todaro A: Action stat! Reversing acute dehydration, *Nurs 93* 23(6):33, 1993.
7. Bang N: Diagnosis and management of bleeding disorders. In Grenvik A, editor: *Textbook of critical care*, ed 4, Philadelphia, 2000, Saunders.
8. Barone J, Snyder A: Treatment strategies in shock: use of oxygen transport measures, *Heart Lung* 1:81, 1991.
9. Battistella F, Wisner D: Combined hemorrhagic shock and head injury: effects of hypertonic saline (7.5%) resuscitation, *J Trauma* 31(2):182, 1991.
10. Beere HM, Green DR: Stress management: heat shock protein–70 and the regulation of apoptosis, *Trends in Cell Biology* 11(1):6, 2001.
11. Behrman S et al: Microcirculatory flow changes after initial resuscitation of hemorrhagic shock with 7.5% hypertonic saline/6% dextran, *J Trauma* 31(5):589, 1991.
12. Bickell W et al: Immediate versus delayed fluid resuscitation for hypotensive patients with penetrating torso injuries, *N Engl J Med* 331(17):1105, 1994.
13. Bickell WH et al: Resuscitation of canine hemorrhage hypotension with large volume isotonic crystalloid: impact on lung water, venous admixture, and systemic arterial oxygen saturation, *Am J Emerg Med* 12(1):36, 1994.
14. Biffl WL, Moore EE: Role of the gut in multiple organ failure. In Grenvik A, ed: *Textbook of critical care*, ed 4, Philadelphia, 2000, Saunders.
15. Bone R: Sepsis, sepsis syndrome, and the systemic inflammatory response syndrome (SIRS): Gullivar in Laputa, *JAMA* 273:155, 1995.
16. Braunwald E: *Harrison's principles of internal medicine*, ed 10, New York, 1987, McGraw-Hill.
17. Bridges EJ, Woods SL: Pulmonary artery pressure measurement: state of the art, *Heart Lung* 22(2):99, 1993.
18. Brown KK: Critical interventions in septic shock, *Am J Nurs* 94:21, 1994.
19. Brown KK: Septic shock: how to stop the deadly cascade, *Am J Nurs* 94:20, 1994.
20. Campbell JE: *Basic trauma life support, advanced prehospital care*, ed 4, Upper Saddle River, NJ, 2000, Brady/Prentice Hall Health.
21. Cardona VD et al: *Trauma nursing: from resuscitation through rehabilitation*, ed 2, Philadelphia, 1994, WB Saunders.
22. Cayten CG et al: A study of pneumatic anti-shock garments in severely hypotensive trauma patients, *J Trauma* 34(5):728, 1993.
23. Chameides L, Hazinski MF: *Textbook of pediatric advanced life support*, Dallas, 1997, American Heart Association.
24. Chang FC et al: PSAG: does it help in the management of traumatic shock? *J Trauma* 39(3):453, 1995.
25. Chikanori T et al: Effects of mild Trendelenburg on central hemodynamics and internal jugular vein velocity, cross sectional area flow, *Am J Emerg Med* 13(3):255, 1995.
26. Cohn SM, Farrell TJ: Diasprin cross-linked hemoglobin, resuscitation of hemorrhage: comparison of a blood substitute with hypertonic saline and isotonic saline, *J Trauma* 39(2):210, 1995.
27. Committee on Trauma: *Advanced trauma life support manual*, Chicago, 1997, American College of Surgeons.
28. Committee on Trauma: *A guide to the evaluation and treatment of serious head injuries*, Chicago, 1983, American College of Surgeons.
29. Committee on Trauma: *A guide to the initial therapy of shock*, Chicago, 1983, American College of Surgeons.
30. Cross J et al: Hypertonic saline fluid therapy following surgery: a prospective study, *J Trauma* 30(6):817, 1989.
31. Dabich MA, Wade CE: A review of the efficacy and safety of 7.5% NaCl/6% dextran 70 in experimental animals and humans, *J Trauma* 36(3):323, 1994.
32. Darling GE: Multi-organ failure in critical patients, *Can J Surg* 31(3):172, 1988.
33. Darls EK, Schroeder JS: *Techniques in bedside hemodynamic monitoring*, ed 4, St Louis, Mosby.
34. Dhainaut JF, Thijs L, Park G: Septic shock. London, 2000, WB Saunders Company Limited.
35. Ebb D, Bray G: Bleeding disorders in children. In Ayers S et al, editors: *Textbook of critical care*, Philadelphia, 1995, Saunders.

36. Emergency Nurses Association: *Sheehy's Emergency Nursing: Principles and Practice*, ed 4, St Louis, 1998, Mosby.

37. Epstein CD, Herning RJP: Oxygen transport variables in the identification and treatment of tissue hypoxia, *Heart Lung* 22(4):328, 1993.

38. Ertel W et al: Release of anti-inflammatory mediators after mechanical trauma correlates with severity of injury and clinical outcome, *J Trauma* 39(5):879, 1995.

39. Fisher J: *The plague makers*, New York, 1994, Simon and Schuster.

40. Gaedeke MK: Action stat! Disseminated intravascular coagulation, *Nurs 94* 24(7):53, 1994.

41. Guyton AC: *Textbook of medical physiology*, ed 8, Philadelphia, 1991, Saunders.

42. Hudak C et al: *Critical care nursing*, ed 4, Philadelphia, 1986, Lippincott.

43. Jacobs L: Timing of fluid resuscitation in trauma, *N Engl J Med* 331(17):1153, 1994.

44. Jones S, Nesper T, Alcoulmre E: Prehospital intravenous line placement: a prospective study, *Ann Emerg Med* 10:1039, 1990.

45. Jordan K, editor: *Emergency nursing core curriculum*, ed 5, Philadelphia, 2000, Saunders.

46. Katzung BG: *Basic and clinical pharmacology*, New York, 2001, McGraw-Hill.

47. Keen J: *Critical care and emergency drug reference*, St Louis, 1994, Mosby.

48. Keenan A: Hematologic emergencies. In Kitt S et al, editors: *Emergency nursing*, Philadelphia, 1995, Saunders.

49. Kokiki J: Septic shock: a review and update for the emergency department clinician, *J Emerg Nurs* 19(2):102, 1993.

50. Kowalenkno T et al: Improved outcome with hypotensive resuscitation of uncontrolled hemorrhagic shock in a swine model, *J Trauma* 33(3):349, 1992.

51. Liberman M, Mulder D, Sampalis J: Advanced or basic life support for trauma: meta-analysis and critical review of the literature, *J Trauma* 49(4):584, 2000.

52. Maclean LD: Shock: a century of progress, *Ann Surg* 201(4):407, 1985.

53. Marthay MA, Chatterjee K: Bedside catheterization of the pulmonary artery: risks compared with benefits, *Ann Intern Med* 109(10):826, 1988.

54. Martin R et al: Prospective evaluation of preoperative fluid resuscitation in hypotensive patients with penetrating truncal injury: a preliminary report, *J Trauma* 33(3):354, 1992.

55. Mattox K et al: Prospective MAST study in 911 patients, *J Trauma* 30(8):1104, 1989.

56. May HL: *Emergency medicine*, New York, 1984, Wiley.

57. Mazzoni M et al: The efficiency of iso- and hyperosmotic fluids as volume expanders in fixed-volume and uncontrolled hemorrhage, *Ann Emerg Med* 19(4):350, 1990.

58. McQuillan K: Initial management of traumatic shock. In Cardona V et al, editors: *Trauma nursing*, Philadelphia, 1994, Saunders.

59. Mills J: *Current emergency diagnosis and treatment*, ed 2, Los Altos, Calif, 1985, Lange Medical.

60. Moore E et al: The post-ischemic gut serves as a priming bed for circulating neutrophils that provoke multiple organ failure, *J Trauma* 37:881, 1994.

61. Moore F, Moore E, Peterson V: Inflammatory models of multiple organ failure, *Trauma Q* 12(1):47, 1995.

62. Mountz J et al: The role of programmed cell death as an emerging new concept for the pathogenesis of autoimmune diseases, *Clin Immunol Immunopath* 80(3): S2, 1996.

63. Oman KS: Use of hematocrit changes as an indicator of blood loss in adult trauma patients who receive intravenous fluids, *J Emerg Nurs* 21(5):395, 1995.

64. Owens TS et al: Limiting initial resuscitation of uncontrolled hemorrhage reduces internal bleeding and subsequent volume requirements, *J Trauma* 39(2):200, 1995.

65. Pedowitz RA, Shackford SR: Noncavitary hemorrhage producing shock in trauma patients: incidence and severity, *J Trauma* 29(2):219, 1989.

66. Pettijean ME et al: Thoracic spinal trauma and associated injuries: should early decompression be considered? *J Trauma* 39(2)368, 1995.

67. Price S, Wilson LM: *Pathophysiology: clinical concepts of disease process*, ed 5, St Louis, 1996, Mosby.

68. Querin JJ, Dixon LS: Twelve simple sensible steps to successful blood transfusions, *Nurs 90* 20(10):68, 1990.

69. Rifkind R et al: *Fundamentals of hematology*, ed 3, St Louis, 1986, Mosby.

70. Rosen P: *Emergency medicine concepts and clinical practice*, St Louis, 1992, Mosby.

71. Rottman S, Larmon B, Manix T: Rapid volume infusion in prehospital care, *Prehosp Disas Med* 3:225, 1990.

72. Rueden K, Dunham CM: Sequelae of massive fluid resuscitation in trauma patients, *Crit Care Nurs Clin North Am* 6:463, 1994.

73. Russell S: Hypovolemic shock: is your patient at risk? *Nurs 94* 24(4):34, 1994.

74. Russell S: Septic shock: can you recognize the clues? *Nurs 94* 24(4):40, 1994.

75. Samuels D, Bock H: *Air medical crew national standard curriculum*, Pasadena, Calif, 1988, ASHBEAMS.

76. Sayre MR: What's new in the treatment of hemorrhagic shock, *J Air Med Transport* 10(5):20, 1991.

77. Scalea TM, Boswell SA: Initial management of traumatic shock. In McQuillan KA et al: *Trauma nursing: from resuscitation through rehabilitation*, ed 3, Philadelphia, 2002, Saunders.

78. Schmoker JD et al: Hypertonic fluid resuscitation improves cerebral oxygen delivery and reduces intracranial pressure after hemorrhagic shock, *J Trauma* 31(12):1607, 1991.

79. Schrieber TL, Miller DH, Zola B: Management of myocardial infarction shock: current status, *Am Heart J* 117(2):435, 1989.

80. Schultz SC et al: The efficacy of diaspirin cross-linked hemoglobin solution resuscitation in a model of uncontrolled hemorrhage, *J Trauma* 37(3):408, 1994.

81. Schultz SC et al: Use of base deficit to compare resuscitation with lactated Ringer's solution, Hemaccel, whole blood, and diaspirin cross linked hemoglobin following hemorrhage in rats, *J Trauma* 35(4):619, 1993.

82. Schwartz GR: *Principles and practices of emergency medicine*, ed 2, Philadelphia, 1986, Saunders.

83. Schwartzberg S: Cytokines: experimental and clinical studies, *Trauma Q* 22(1):7, 1995.

84. Selfridge-Thomas J: Shock. In Kitt S et al, editors: *Emergency nursing*, Philadelphia, 1995, Saunders.

85. Shatney CH: Initial resuscitation and assessment of patients with multisystem blunt trauma, *South Med J* 81(4):501, 1988.

86. Shoemaker WC: Diagnosis and treatment of shock and circulatory dysfunction. In Grenvik A, editor: *Textbook of critical care*, ed 4, Philadelphia, 2000, WB Saunders.

87. Sommers M: Rapid fluid resuscitation: how to correct dangerous deficits, *Nurs 90* 20(1):52, 1990.

88. Spearing-Bolgiano C: Administering oxygen therapy: what you need to know, *Nurs 90* 20(6):47, 1990.

89. Stark JL: Interpreting BUN/creatine levels: it's not as simple as you think, *Nurs 94* 24(9):58, 1994.

90. Stern S et al: Effect of blood pressure on hemorrhage volume and survival in a near-fetal hemorrhage model incorporating vascular injury, *Ann Emerg Med* 22(2):155, 1993.

91. Talan D: Recent developments in our understanding of sepsis: evaluation of antiendotoxin antibodies and biological modifiers, *Ann Emerg Med* 22:1871, 1993.

92. Valedi MH: Pneumatic anti-shock garment: associated compartment syndrome in uninjured lower extremities, *J Trauma* 38(4):616, 1995.

93. Vary T, McLean B, Von Rueden K: Shock and multiple organ dysfunction syndrome. In McQuillan K et al, editors: *Trauma nursing: from resuscitation through rehabilitation*, Philadelphia, 2002, Saunders.

94. Vassar MJ et al: Prehospital resuscitation of hypotensive trauma patient with 7.5% NaCl vs 7.5% NaCl with added dextran: a controlled trial, *J Trauma* 34(5):622, 1993.

95. Warren BL et al: Kybersept trial study group, *JAMA* 286(1): 1894, 2001.

96. Wheeler AP, Bernard GR. Treating patients with severe sepsis, *N Engl J Med* 340: 207, 1999.

97. Whitney J: Wound healing. In Cardona V et al, editors: *Trauma nursing*, Philadelphia, 1995, Saunders.

98. Willis JL: Use of blood components, *FDA Drug Bulletin* 19:14, 1989.

99. Wyngaarden JB, Smith LH Jr: *Cecil's textbook of medicine*, ed 18, Philadelphia, 1988, Saunders.

14

GENERAL PRINCIPLES OF TRAUMA MANAGEMENT

COMPETENCIES

1. Demonstrate the ability to perform scene safety and trauma triage.
2. Perform a primary and secondary assessment of the injured patient.
3. Initiate critical interventions for the injured patient before and during transport.

Trauma is the leading cause of death in persons younger than 40 years and the fourth-leading cause of death of persons of all age groups.[21] It is estimated that more than 60 million injuries occur in the United States annually, and 150,000 people die of these injuries.[1] Disability from injury outweighs mortality by three to one.[1] Unpublished results from "U.S. Burden of Disease and Injury Study," done by the U.S. Centers for Disease Control and Harvard University, look at disability-adjusted life years (DALYs). DALYs equal years of healthy life lost to disability plus years of life lost to premature death. The study showed that in 1996, road traffic crashes, homicide, violence, and other unintentional injuries, taken together, accounted for more DALYs for men than did ischemic heart disease. Road traffic crashes alone accounted for an estimated 366,316 DALYs due to injury for both men and women.[24]

Unintentional injuries are a major source of morbidity and mortality. For this reason, injury prevention has become a major public health goal. The U.S. Department of Health and Human Services and Public Health Service have developed the "Healthy People 2010: National Health Promotion and Disease Prevention Objectives" (Box 14-1).[21] More than half of all motor vehicle crashes are the result of improper driving practices or human error, with alcohol being a factor in 50% to 75% of all fatal crashes.[21]

Another often-preventable injury is from a fall. Falls account for approximately half of the deaths that are a result from trauma in the home.[21] The elder population is especially at risk for falls, and homes should be checked for loose rugs, poor lighting, and other preventable conditions.

Bicycle, skateboard, and scooter injuries are a major source of trauma in the pediatric population.

| BOX 14-1 | Objectives for Injury and Violence Prevention, Healthy People 2010 |

1. Reduce hospitalization for nonfatal head injuries.
2. Reduce hospitalization for nonfatal spinal cord injuries.
3. Reduce firearm-related deaths.
4. Reduce the proportion of persons living in homes with firearms that are loaded and unlocked.
5. Reduce nonfatal firearm-related injuries.
6. (Developmental) Extend state-level child fatality review of deaths due to external causes for children aged 14 years and under.
7. Reduce deaths caused by suffocation.
8. Increase the number of states and the District of Columbia with statewide emergency department surveillance systems that collect data on external causes of injury.
9. Increase the number of states and the District of Columbia that collect data on external causes of injury through hospital discharge data systems.
10. Reduce hospital emergency department visits caused by injuries.
11. Reduce deaths caused by unintentional injuries.
12. (Developmental) Reduce nonfatal unintentional injuries.
13. Reduce deaths caused by motor vehicle crashes.
14. Reduce pedestrian deaths on public roads.
15. Reduce nonfatal injuries caused by motor vehicle crashes.
16. Reduce nonfatal pedestrian injuries on public roads.
17. Increase use of safety belts.
18. Increase use of child restraints.
19. Increase the number of states and the District of Columbia that have adopted a graduated driver licensing model law.
20. (Developmental) Increase use of helmets by bicyclists.
21. Increase the number of states and the District of Columbia with laws requiring bicyle helmets for bicycle riders.
22. Reduce residential fire deaths.
23. Increase functioning residential smoke alarms.
24. Reduce deaths from falls.
25. Reduce hip fractures among older adults.
26. Reduce drownings.
27. Reduce hospital emergency department visits for nonfatal dog bite injuries.
28. (Developmental) Increase the proportion of public and private schools that require use of appropriate head, face, eye, and mouth protection for students participating in school-sponsored physical activities.
29. Reduce homicides.
30. Reduce maltreatment and maltreatment fatalities of children.
31. Reduce the rate of physical assault by current or former intimate partners.
32. Reduce the annual rate of rape or attempted rape.
33. Reduce sexual assault other than rape.
34. Reduce physical assaults.
35. Reduce weapon carrying by adolescents on school property.

Modified from U.S. Department of Health and Human Services, Public Health Service: Healthy People 2010 *Understanding and improving health.*

Head injuries cause 67% of bicycle-related deaths and 68% of bicycle-related hospital admissions.[21] Helmets have been shown to be effective in decreasing head injuries in children and should be encouraged.

Costs associated with these trauma injuries are staggering. Approximately 40% of health-care dollars are expended annually because of trauma. In approximately the next 10 minutes, 2 people will be killed, approximately 350 will have a disabling injury, and approximately $7,800,000 will be spent on the unintentionally injured.[1,2,10] Private insurance monies are rapidly exhausted, and reimbursement, according to the federal government prospective payment system (diagnosis-related groups), does not adequately cover expenses incurred.

INJURY DYNAMICS

One of the most important factors that has positively influenced the morbidity and mortality of trauma patients is rapid transport because the time from the accident to initiation of definitive care is the key to patient survivability. The addition of highly trained medical personnel has brought critical care management outside the trauma center to the rural hospital or the scene of the trauma.

The transport of the multiply injured patient requires in-depth knowledge and skills, as well as expert prioritization and organization skills. A thorough understanding of the mechanisms of injury and the kinematics of trauma are essential for any transport team member caring for injured patients. These principles will provide a direction of care.

HISTORY

One of the first steps taken in caring for a multiply injured victim is to elicit a history of events preceding and following the traumatic event. With hospital transfers this is most commonly obtained from other nurses, physicians, and family members. A history obtained at the scene generally involves many additional reporters, including law enforcement, firefighters, and other paramedics.

When responding at the scene of a trauma by helicopter, an aerial view of the situation helps begin the history (Figure 14-1). The flight crew has the

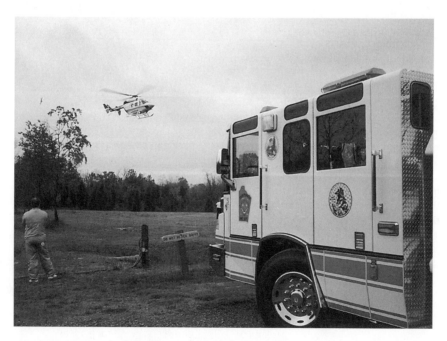

FIGURE 14-1   When approaching a scene from the air, the flight team begins collecting information about the incident.

advantage of evaluating the entire scene, the damage sustained to the vehicles or the buildings, the extent of impact, and the objects flung or blown out of the central area of impact.

At the scene, life-threatening injuries are always top priority, and obtaining a detailed history may be impractical in certain cases. However, the importance of a thorough history is vital to direct the patient's care. Because time is a critical factor for the survivability of the trauma patient, the history should be obtained while gaining access to the patient or while simultaneously performing the primary assessment. If the patient has an altered level of consciousness, the only history obtained may be from the hospital or emergency personnel present, who may not be going to the receiving hospital. It is important to learn to elicit the history while concurrently assessing the patient because you may never get another chance to obtain needed information.

Important information to elicit in the history includes time of incident, mechanism of injury, any alteration in the patient's level of consciousness, and the patient's past medical history and current medications.

A further detailed history may be obtained from the patient during the secondary survey as time and patient condition allow, and this can be routinely performed in the transport vehicle.

MECHANISM OF INJURY

Injuries occur when external forces are applied to the body. The type and amount of injuring force and the tissue response to the force determine the extent of injury.[2] When the body's tissue cannot withstand any additional force, destruction occurs, as evidenced by the common injuries seen in the multiply injured patient: fractures, lacerations, and ruptured internal organs. A complete understanding of a force and the way it is applied is necessary to predict potential injuries and thus adequately care for the injured patient.

Newton's first law of motion states that a body at rest tends to remain at rest, and a body in motion tends to remain in motion until acted on by an outside force. When the body contacts an object, energy is transferred, and damage occurs (Figure 14-2).

Force is a result of energy transference, which can be explained by the laws of physics.

1. Energy can be neither created not destroyed; it can change form.

2. Kinetic energy (KE) = $\dfrac{\text{Mass} \times \text{Velocity}^2}{2}$

3. Force = Mass × Acceleration

Because energy is neither created nor destroyed, it is transferred, and its transference is dependent on the mass of the object times the speed squared over a common denominator of 2. For example, an automobile weighing 3000 pounds is traveling at 40 miles/hr when it strikes a telephone pole.

$$KE = \frac{3000 \times 40^2}{2}$$

The kinetic energy transferred in this impact to both objects is 2,400,000 units.

The same force is applied to destruction of the body. Energy is transferred from the automobile to the human being. Several factors determine the amount of energy the human being absorbs, including the following.

1. The amount of energy absorbed by the objects that initially collide (the telephone pole and the automobile, for example)
2. The amount absorbed by protective factors, such as seat belts, helmets, padded steering wheels, dashboards, and airbags

The forces involved in the impact will cause varying degrees of destruction. The more slowly the force is applied, the less energy transference and the lower the degree of destruction. The extent of injury is also dependent on which body parts receive the impact.[19] For example, the skull can take more force before damage occurs than can the abdomen.

Force can be delivered by compression, acceleration, deceleration, or shearing.[19]

Compression: Direct compression or pressure on a structure is the most common type of force applied. The amount of injury sustained is dependent on the length of time of compression and the area compressed. [19]

Acceleration/deceleration: Acceleration is the increase in the velocity of a moving object. Deceleration is the decrease in velocity of an object.[19] In an automobile crash, the body is thrown forward (acceleration) by the impact and decelerates as it comes in contact with the steering wheel, seatbelt, or dashboard. The internal organs also accelerate and decelerate, causing destruction to the tissues and vasculature.

Shearing: Shearing forces occur when the tissues, organs, or both are pushed ahead. The most common mechanism causing a shearing injury occurs when a pedestrian is run over by a vehicle. As the vehicle grabs a part of the body, the area is pushed forward until it can no longer take the force, and it tears. Degloving routinely occurs from shearing forces.

The viscoelastic properties of tissues in the body help to absorb energy. When the energy delivered is below the limit of injury, the energy will be absorbed and cause no damage. When the forces applied deliver more energy than the body can absorb, strains occur.[19] Strains may be classified as tensile, shearing, or compressive. Table 14-1 displays the characteristics and examples of each type of strain.

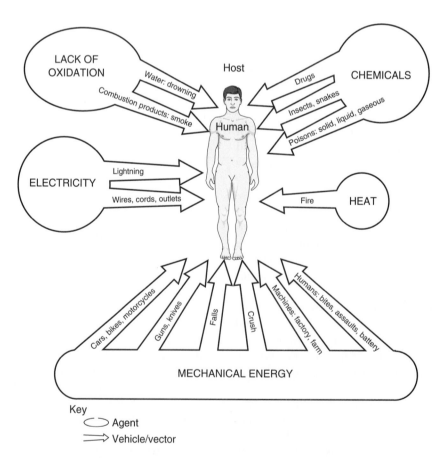

FIGURE 14-2   **Energy forces that can affect the human body.**

TABLE 14-1	**Characteristics of Strains**	
Type	**Reaction**	**Examples**
Tensile	Stretching	Bony fractures, aortic tears
Shearing	Movement of tissue in opposite directions	Brain injuries, lacerations/ avulsions
Compressive	Crushing force	Compartment syndrome, ruptures

KINEMATICS OF TRAUMA

Patterns of injury have been identified by evaluation of the type of trauma that has occurred and the amount of force generated. Although all patients should be evaluated individually, certain injuries are common to certain forces. Prediction of these injuries is referred to as kinematics. Age, preventive measures taken, and velocity are factors in the alteration of injury patterns, and the caregiver should consider them when evaluating a patient.[15]

BLUNT INJURIES
MOTOR VEHICLE CRASHES

Head-on Collisions.   As an automobile collides with another automobile or with any object head-on, energy is transferred to the vehicle. The front of the vehicle routinely stops less than one-half second after impact. The rear of the automobile continues to move forward until all the energy is dispersed. Although the front end of the car is destroyed, it is the rear of the vehicle that causes the destruction by its continued forward movement. The same principle of injury occurs with the body during a head-on collision. The initial impact occurs in the front of the vehicle. The unrestrained driver will hit the steering wheel with the thorax; the head may hit the windshield, and the knees contact the dashboard (Figure 14-3). Predictable initial injuries from initial impact are fractured ribs, pneumothorax, or hemopneumothorax; concussion; skull fractures; patella and femur fractures; dislocated hips; and acetabular fractures. The progression of injury proceeds, as will the automobile, and the person's internal organs will be thrown from the rear forward until all energy is dispersed. Common injuries include ruptured spleens (direct

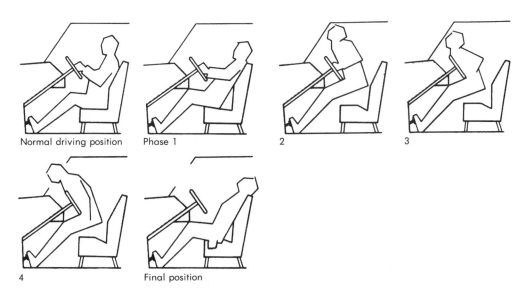

Normal driving position   Phase 1   2   3

4   Final position

FIGURE 14-3   **Phases of movement of the unrestrained occupant during frontal collision.**

compression from the steering wheel), lacerated livers (stretching of hilum until the tensile strength is exceeded), and ruptured thoracic aortas (heart and aorta are forcibly thrown forward, stretched, and then compressed against the ribs).

The restrained driver in a head-on collision has much of the energy absorbed by the seat belt and air bag, if present. The seat belt may impose a load 20 to 50 times as great as the body weight. The only portion of the human body capable of incurring this load is the pelvis. Unless the patient has the belt properly applied securely over the pelvis, direct compression of the abdomen may occur. The first indicator of these injuries is often the presence of abrasions over the abdomen from the belt. Other injuries associated with seat belt use include sternal fractures, breast injuries, and lumbar vertebral body fractures. As seen with abdominal seat belt injuries, abrasions, ecchymosis, or both are important indicators. A study done by C. F. Chandler at the UCLA School of Medicine (1997) showed that in 117 patients who were involved in a motor vehicle crash, 12% of the patients arrived with an abdominal seat belt sign. Of these with a positive sign, 64% had abdominal injury and 36% required operative intervention. In contrast, the patients who did not have an abdominal seat belt sign had significantly fewer abdominal injuries (8.7%). Lap belts should be worn with a diagonal shoulder strap to stop forward movement of the upper body. Diagonal straps worn alone can cause severe neck injuries, including decapitation. Air bags are to cushion forward motion only. They are very effective in the first collision, but because they deflate immediately, they are not effective in multiple-impact collisions. When the air bag deploys, it can produce injury to the patient. The most common injuries seen are abrasions of the arms, chest, and face, which can include injuries caused by the patient's eyeglasses.[19]

Rear-end Collisions.   An automobile hit from behind rapidly accelerates, causing the car to move forward under the patient. Predictable injuries are to the back (T12-L1 is the most common area of injury), legs (femur, tibia/fibula, and ankle fractures), and neck (cervical strain, C21 frac-

ture caused by hyperextension) if the head restraint is not in the proper position. If the automobile undergoes a second collision by striking a car in front of it, the predictable head-on injuries also need to be evaluated.

Side Impact.   An automobile hit on the side will routinely cause lateral injuries to the patient. An unrestrained driver hit on the side will sustain initial injuries to the left clavicle, ribs, femur, and tibia/fibula. Abdominal injuries, such as ruptured spleens, are seen in these crashes, usually because of the fractured lower lateral ribs, but also because of direct compression on the abdomen.[19] Secondary injuries occur when the patient is propelled to the other side of the car, which causes injuries to the opposite side.

Rollovers.   Predictable injuries caused by vehicle rollovers are more difficult to define (Figure 14-4). The unrestrained patient tumbles inside the vehicle, and injury occurs to the areas of the body that are hit. The caregiver should always care for these patients judiciously and realize the potential for multiple-system injuries.

MOTORCYCLE CRASHES

Because motorcycles offer minimal or no initial energy transference, energy is directly absorbed by the rider, and injuries are substantially more severe than with other motor vehicle crashes. The predicted injuries during a motorcycle crash, like those during other motor vehicle crashes, depend on the type of collision that occurs.

Head-on Collisions.   To accurately predict injuries involving the motorcycle rider, it helps to understand the design of a motorcycle (Figure 14-5). The center of gravity is located in front of the driver's seat. As the cycle strikes an object head on, the rear (or lighter portion) tips upward from the weight under the handlebars, which prevent the driver, who is propelled over the handlebars, from total ejection. Associated injuries with this type of crash are fractured femurs, tibias, and fibulas (from the handlebars); chest and abdominal injuries (from direct compression against the handlebars or tire); and head and neck

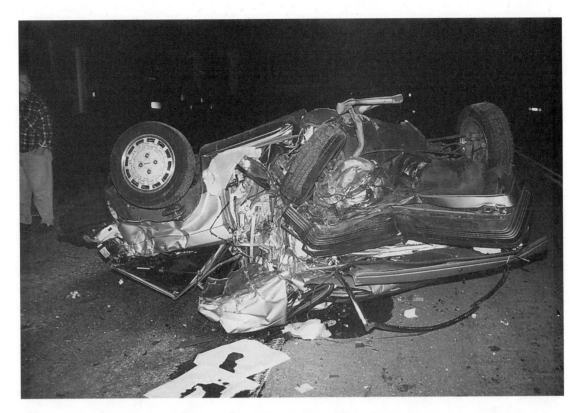

FIGURE 14-4   Rollover motor vehicle crashes.

injuries (from impact with the tire or any object in front of the cycle). Any motorcycle crash can cause the rider to be ejected, but it is most common during head-on collisions. As with ejection from any vehicle, the head acts as the missile. Suspicion of and intervention for major head and cervical spine injuries is imperative with any ejected patient.

Side Impact.   Injuries associated with a side-impact motorcycle crash are related to the body parts crushed between the cycle and the second object. Most commonly seen injuries involve the leg and foot on the impact side. Open fracture of the femur, tibia/fibula, and malleolus are predictable.

Laying Down the Motorcycle.   Motorcycle riders have learned the technique of laying down the bike and sliding off to the side before colliding with another object. The energy transference is a result of sliding away from the bike. Commonly seen are abrasions on the affected side. Fractures may occur if the patient hits the road hard or comes in contact with another object. Preventive clothing, such as leather jackets, pants, and gloves, will absorb more energy than average clothing, and in this type of impact they may prevent abrasions from occurring.

FALLS

Falls from heights greater than 15 to 20 feet are associated with severe injuries. In predicting injuries associated with falls, caregivers should understand the following:

1.   The average roof of a one-story house is approximately 15 feet off the ground; a two-story fall is approximately 30 feet.

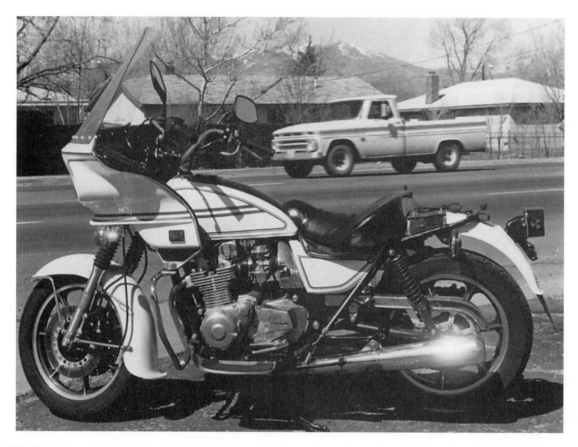

FIGURE 14-5   **Construction of a motorcycle places the center or gravity in front of the driver's seat.** Head-on collision will cause the cycle to up and throw the occupant over the front.

2. With a fall greater than 15 feet, adults will usually land on their feet. Below 15 feet, adults will land as they fell; that is, if the person falls head first, he or she will land on his or her head.
3. Because small children have proportionally larger heads, no matter what the distance, they will tend to fall headfirst.

It is important for the caregiver to estimate the distance fallen. Second, it must be determined what the patient landed on. A soft landing surface, such as dirt or sand, will absorb much more energy than a hard surface, such as concrete.

Three predictable injuries are seen in falls. The forces involved are deceleration and compression.

The first injury, calcaneus fractures, is caused by compression of the feet on impact. Second, as the energy dissipates after impact and the top of the body pushes down toward the point of impact, compression fractures to T12-L1 are seen. Finally, as the body moves forward and the patient puts both arms out to complete the fall, bilateral wrist fractures occur.

PENETRATING TRAUMA

All objects that cause injury from penetration deliver the same two types of force: crushing and stretching.[13] Depending on the velocity of the penetrating object, the wound can be small or massive.

STAB WOUNDS

Stab wounds are considered low velocity and produce their major damage by crushing tissues as the penetrating object enters. An object that is narrow at the beginning and thicker at the end will crush the tissues as it enters and stretch them apart as the thicker part is inserted. The area of injury for stab wounds is typically localized to the area of insertion. The penetrating instrument might remain embedded in the patient or might have been removed; embedded penetrating objects should be stabilized with bandages for transport and not removed (Figure 14-6)

GUNSHOT WOUNDS

Wounding from bullets can have four causes: (1) direct contact by the missile, (2) crushing force in the immediate vicinity of the missile, (3) temporary cavity formation, and (4) collapse of the temporary cavity.[10]

The degree of wounding depends on the amount of energy transferred from the bullet to the body. The type of weapon used, the type of bullet, the distance at which the weapon was fired, and the body part penetrated are key factors in wound severity.

Firearms can be handguns, rifles, and shotguns. Handguns and some rifles are considered medium energy, with assault rifles and hunting rifles being high energy. The greater the amount of gunpowder in the cartridge, the greater the speed of the bullet, and therefore the kinetic energy increases.[19] The degree of deformation by the penetrating missile is influenced by the following factors.

Yaw and tumbling: Yaw is deviation of the bullet up to 90 degrees from a straight path, and tumbling is rotation of the bullet 360 degrees. Both cause increased tissue crush and stretching.

Deformation of a bullet when striking tissue: Certain missiles are constructed of soft lead and flatten on impact. Other bullets have hollow points that cause a "mushrooming" effect on impact; hollow-point bullets are also known as expanding bullets. The increased diameter of these bullets increases tissue destruction.

Fragmentation: Each fragmented portion of the missile causes damage in its path. Increased velocity increases the potential of fragmentation.

Explosive effect: Explosive bullets are intended to cause massive damage with a single shot. The bullet is composed of black powder and lead shot. On impact, detonation of the powder causes explosion and disintegration of the bullet casing, further propelling the lead shot.[19]

The closer to the target the bullet was fired, the greater the amount of kinetic energy transferred to the tissues. For that reason, firing distance is important to ascertain during the history taking.

Cavitation occurs with all penetrating objects. The permanent cavity is formed from the crushed tissue produced by the object. Temporary cavity formation occurs from transfer of kinetic energy from the missile to the tissue. The velocity, size, shape, and ballistic behavior of the missile and the biophysical properties of the tissue determine the extent of the temporary cavity. As a missile strikes tissue, temporary cavitation occurs forward of and lateral to the missile. Relatively elastic tissues, such as lung, bowel wall, and muscle, tolerate the stretch of the temporary cavity much better than the solid, nonelastic organs, such as the liver and spleen.[14] Past literature has estimated temporary cavity formation as large as 30 to 40 times the missile diameter.[5] Studies have indicated that temporary cavitation is usually no more than 10 to 20 times the missile diameter for high-velocity missiles[14,18] (Figure 14-7).

PATHOPHYSIOLOGIC FACTORS

Multiple trauma causes severe stress to the human body and is associated with a flux of hormones and physiologic reactions (Table 14-2). The degree of metabolic and hormonal changes depends on the severity of injury, the effectiveness of resuscitation, and the preinjury condition of the patient. The pathophysiologic analysis of traumatic injuries is discussed in detail in the chapters that individually discuss specific traumas. In general, metabolic response to shock from injury in the early stage differs from that in the late stage (Table 14-3).

In the early stage the body responds to hypoperfusion as a stress to the body. Many of the changes

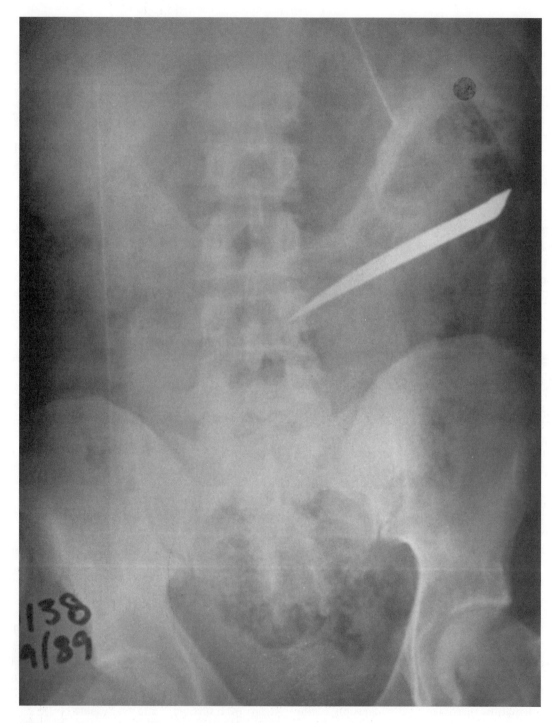

FIGURE 14-6   Knife with the handle broken off embedded in a patient. Object was discovered when the radiograph was taken.

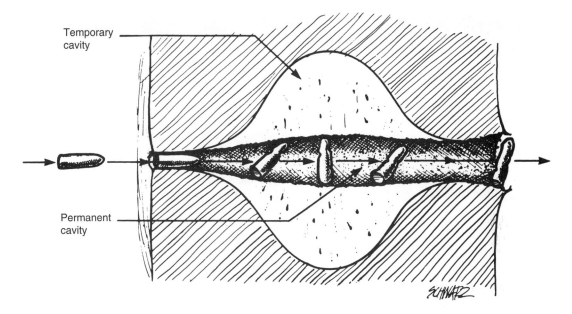

Temporary
cavity

Permanent
cavity

FIGURE 14-7   **Effects of yaw and temporary and permanent cavitation from a missile.** Permanent cavity is caused by necrotic muscle tissue. Temporary cavity is caused by stretching of soft tissue. (From Weiner SL, Barrett J: *Trauma management for civilian and military positions*, Philadelphia, 1986, Saunders.)

are mediated through the sympathetic nervous system that occur rapidly. The overall effect is an increase in systemic vascular resistance. A response is mediated through the renin-angiotensin system that occurs more slowly. The response is again to vasoconstrict and also to increase blood volume via retention.[21]

In the early stage the compensatory mechanisms are beneficial in that the heart and brain receive adequate blood supply, but at the expense of the kidneys and other abdominal organs. If the underlying cause of shock is corrected, then the patient may do well. If it is not, the compensatory mechanisms will not be able to continue to perfuse vital organs well enough, and the mechanisms themselves will be deleterious to the body. The patient will then progress to the late stage.[21]

During the late stage, as shock progresses, blood flow to all body tissues is impaired. The cell's metabolism fails and acidosis and energy deficiency result. Without enough energy the cell functions fail, and lysosomes are damaged, spilling digestive enzymes into the rest of the cell destroying it. As the enzymes come into contact with adjacent cells, these cells also are destroyed, and eventually the cellular death results in organ death. Shock is a dynamic process, and at some point a cycle begins that cannot be stopped, and an irreversible stage of shock develops.

One syndrome is seen after a severe physiologic insult when the patient initially was successfully resuscitated. The syndrome has been termed *multiple organ dysfunction,* and it is thought that the local injury from trauma and hypoperfusion causes a local inflammatory response. The response is probably a result of endothelial injury, platelet activation, the release of inflammatory mediators, and activation of the clotting cascade. This leads to the development of a hyperinflammatory state and a hypermetabolic state, with increases in oxygen consumption and demand. The lung is usually the first organ to fail, with the kidneys, immune system, gastrointestinal tract, and liver following, resulting ultimately in sepsis, cardiovascular collapse, and death. There is evidence that the gastrointestinal tract plays

TABLE 14-2 Major Pathophysiologic Changes in Shock

Change	Effect
Early Stage (Compensatory/Nonprogressive)	
Increased epinephrine and norepinephrine	Increased cardiac output to increase blood flow to tissues
Alpha- and beta-adrenergic receptors stimulated	
Alpha effects: skin and most viscera	Vasoconstriction and decreased blood supply
Beta effects: heart and skeletal muscles	Vasodilation and increased blood supply and heart rate
Renin-angiotensin response	Vasoconstriction and secretion of aldosterone; sodium and water retention, which supports intravascular volume; potassium loss
Increased glucocorticoids and mineralocorticoids	Sodium and water retention to increase intravascular volume; potassium loss
Hypoxemia	Hyperventilation and bronchodilation; provides more oxygen to tissues; may cause respiratory alkalosis
Decreased hydrostatic fluid pressure	Fluid shifts from interstitial space to intravascular space to increase vascular volume
Late Stage (Noncompensatory/Progressive)	
Decreased blood flow to heart	Impaired cardiac pumping ability (decreased cardiac output); blood pressure decreases
Anaerobic metabolism	Acidosis; decreased adenosine triphosphate; failure of cellular sodium-potassium pump (potassium leaves cell; sodium and water enter cell); cellular damage
Arteriolar dilation and venule constriction	Fluid shift from intravascular to interstitial space, reducing blood pressure
Decreased blood flow to kidneys with acute tubular necrosis	Decreased kidney function (oliguria or anuria, retention of nitrogenous waste products and potassium)
Decreased blood flow to pancreas	Production of myocardial depressant factor (MDF)

From Phipps WJ, Sands JK, Marek JF: *Medical-surgical nursing: concepts and clinical practice*, ed 6, St Louis, 1999, Mosby.

a strong role in the initiation and continuation of the syndrome. Patients who are subjected to circulatory shock may sustain mild ischemia to the gut. This may lead to necrosis of the superficial mucosa, with loss of epithelial barrier function. Once the barrier function is lost, bacterial translocation is facilitated. It is thought that this release of bacteria, endotoxin, and other luminal factors may contribute to a systemic inflammatory response.[22]

These factors emphasize the importance of the amount of physiologic stress the patient receives and the need for rapid assessment and transport of the trauma patient to definitive care.

PRIMARY AND SECONDARY ASSESSMENT

When developing a systematic approach for assessing the trauma patient, caregivers must intervene in life-threatening injuries, discover occult injuries, and prioritize care. In the prehospital setting, scene evaluation is very important and includes an assessment of safety. Every transport team member is responsible for recognizing all possible dangers and ensuring that none still exist. No one should become a victim. Caregivers should evaluate the scene and if necessary move the patient to a safe area before

TABLE 14-3   Comparison of Signs and Symptoms in Early and Late Shock by Body System

	Early Shock	Late Shock
Respiratory system	Hyperventilation; ↑ minute volume; ↓ $Paco_2$;* normal Pao_2; bronchodilation	Respirations shallow; breath sounds may suggest congestion; ↑ $Paco_2$; ↓ Pao_2; pulmonary edema; ↓ pulse oximetry
Cardiovascular system	Blood pressure normal to slightly lowered; ↑ diastolic pressure; ↓ pulse pressure; tachycardia; cardiac output normal in hypovolemic shock, slightly decreased in cardiogenic shock, and increased in septic shock; mild vasoconstriction in hypovolemic and cardiogenic shock; vasodilation in septic shock	↓ Blood pressure; ↓ cardiac output; tachycardia continues; vasoconstriction worsens in hypovolemic, cardiogenic, and septic shock
Renal system	Decreased urine output; ↑ urine osmolality; ↓ urine sodium concentration; hypokelemia	Oliguria or complete renal shutdown; hyperkalemia; buildup of waste products
Acid-base balance	Respiratory alkalosis	Metabolic acidosis; respiratory acidosis
Vascular compartment	Fluid shift from interstitial space to intravascular compartment; thirst	Fluid shift from intravascular to interstitial and intracellular spaces, causing edema
Skin	Minimal to no changes in hypovolemic and cardiogenic shock; warm, flushed skin in septic shock	Cool, clammy skin in hypovolemic, cardiogenic, and septic shock; cool, mottled skin in neurogenic and vasogenic shock
Hematological system	Release of red blood cells (RBCs) from bone marrow to increase vascular volume; platelet aggregation	Disseminated intravascular coagulation (DIC); ↓ hematopoiesis leading to ↓ white blood cells, ↓ hemoglobin, ↓ hematocrit, ↓ platelets
Mental-neurological system	Restless; alert; confused	Lethargy; unconsciousness
GI-hepatic system	No obvious changes	Perfusion decreases; bowel sounds possibly diminished; gastric distention; nausea, vomiting

*$Paco_2$, Arterial carbon dioxide pressure; Pao_2, arterial oxygen pressure.
From Phipps WJ, Sants JK, Marek JF: *Medical-surgical nursing: concepts and clinical practice,* ed 6, St Louis, 1999, Mosby.

initiating treatment. The crew is challenged by many factors while attempting to perform a detailed assessment. Three of the most common factors are time, noise level, and the inability to fully disrobe a patient. It is the responsibility of the transport team to evaluate each patient situation individually to determine the best approach for assessment. For example, transporting a patient by helicopter from the scene of the accident may routinely require that you perform the primary assessment on the scene, load the patient, and do the secondary assessment in the aircraft or ground vehicle, thus avoiding delay of definitive care. However, the auscultation of breath sounds and bowel sounds is not possible during a helicopter flight and thus should be performed before liftoff and out of the normal assessment sequence.

Primary Assessment

The focuses of the primary assessment are evaluation of the airway, breathing, and circulation and intervention when life-threatening conditions are identified. The primary assessment should be performed quickly and in the following order of priority: (1) airway and cervical spine stabilization, (2) breathing and ventilation, (3) circulation with hemorrhage control, (4) disability (neurologic status), and (5) exposure (the patient is undressed).

Airway

A secure, patent airway is the first priority. While the airway is being assessed, the patient's cervical spine should not be moved. The patient's airway should be assessed for patency. Basic maneuvers should be instituted, including suctioning and opening of the airway with a chin-lift or jaw-thrust technique. A patient with a head injury or facial fractures risks losing their airway, and the transport team should always be prepared to manage the airway before it occludes. Frequent suctioning is often indicated, and the equipment should be at hand. Endotracheal intubation allows for optimal control of the airway. It is important that the transport team to be able to recognize the indications for airway management and perform the type of intervention (basic or advanced) that is optimal for the situation and clinical condition.

Breathing

The majority of life-threatening injuries are in the chest and affect breathing (Box 14-2). Recognition of these injuries is imperative to effectively manage ventilation. Once a patent airway is established, the caregiver must determine the effectiveness of air exchange. The rise and fall of the chest alone is not sufficient for the caregiver to determine the status of breathing. The caregiver should assess the rate of ventilation, use of accessory muscles, and presence of circumoral cyanosis. If spontaneous breathing is absent, the crew should initiate positive-pressure ventilation through a bag-valve device. For patients who do not require a bag-valve mask, high-flow oxygen through a nonrebreather mask is effective to augment ventilations. All multisystem trauma patients should receive

BOX 14-2	Indicators of Immediate Life-Threatening Chest Injury

1. Open pneumothorax
2. Flail chest
3. Massive hemothorax
4. Tension pneumothorax
5. Cardiac tamponade
6. Penetrating cardiac wounds
7. Air embolus

supplemental oxygen during transport, regardless of whether they are symptomatic.

Circulation

Evaluation of circulation is accomplished by assessing the patient's pulse. A quick palpation of radial pulses may be sufficient for the caregiver to determine effective circulation. If a radial, femoral, or carotid pulse is not palpated, then chest compressions should be initiated. As soon as possible, the patient should be placed on a cardiac monitor.

The crew performing airway, breathing, and cervical spine control at the scene and gaining venous access en route may best treat patients who need immediate surgical intervention. This process allows minimal delay for the patient requiring immediate surgery. The concept that an intravenous line is supportive, rather that restorative, care to the patient is important to remember. Unlike intubation and ventilation of the patient, an intravenous line cannot correct a problem. It only provides supplemental fluid until the underlying condition is corrected. A patient in hypotensive shock may need immediate surgery, and extra time taken, especially at the scene, for lines to be initiated only adds to the delay of definitive care for that patient.

Intravenous lines may be required to administer medications to secure the airway or provide pain management during transport. However, the transport team needs to carefully evaluate whether a delay may occur with multiple intravenous attempts.

Before moving on to the secondary assessment, the caregiver should judiciously check the patient for any uncontrolled hemorrhage. Active bleeding is controlled by direct pressure.

A quick neurologic examination with the components of the Glasgow Coma Scale Score is performed at the first assessment stage. The AVPU scale (A-alert; V-responds to verbal stimulus; P-responds to pain; and U-unresponsive) may also provide a quick assessment of the patient's level of consciousness and assist the transport team in determining if critical interventions, such as airway management, may be required before transport.

SECONDARY ASSESSMENT

The optimal preliminary step in the secondary assessment is for the patient to be completely disrobed. As mentioned earlier, this is often impractical in the prehospital setting. Baring of the chest is essential for evaluation of life-threatening injuries, and exposure of the abdomen is crucial for proper examination, and both should be done in all trauma patients. All restrictive clothing, such as belts or bras, should be removed or cut away. When the patient is exposed for assessment, attention must be given to keeping him or her warm; blankets should cover body areas not being examined at the time.

The secondary assessment proceeds in a systematic fashion from head to toe to reveal all injuries the patient has sustained. During this assessment, the caregiver strictly adheres to assessment of the patient and does not intervene for specific injuries. To avoid missed injuries, the caregiver must develop a routine when performing the secondary assessment. Inspection, auscultation, palpation, and information the patient offers are key to performing this assessment. When proficient, the transport team should be able to perform the secondary assessment in approximately 60 seconds. It is easy to focus on obvious injuries during this assessment, but the challenge is to discover occult injuries that may have an adverse affect on the patient's morbidity or mortality and cause major problems for both the patient and the team during transport.

After completing the secondary assessment, the caregiver can focus on the patient's specific injuries to determine their severity and to intervene when necessary, for example, by splinting an extremity. It is very important to remember during the assessment and transport of the trauma patient the importance of protecting them from becoming hypothermic, which can be very detrimental to the patient. Also, reporting all information regarding the patient to the receiving trauma team is very important, especially if there were any episodes of hypotension or loss of consciousness that the patient may have experienced.

The primary and secondary assessments, along with the treatment of life-threatening injuries, are the most important aspects of trauma care the transport crew can deliver. They direct the priorities of care during transport and for the staff at the receiving hospital and are the cornerstone for optimal outcome of the patient with multiple injuries.

SCORING OF TRAUMA PATIENTS

Numeric scoring for determination of the severity of injuries is common practice. Scoring provides a potential outcome classification for trauma patients, through either single-system injuries, multisystem injuries, or the patient's physiologic condition. A variety of injury-severity scores exist; none of them is 100% accurate, and their questionable reliability should be considered with their use. Two common prehospital scoring systems and accepted retrospective scores are discussed in the following subsections.

PROSPECTIVE SCORING

It has long been a goal of emergency response personnel to develop a numeric score to determine the severity of a patient's injuries at the accident scene. Use of such a score would mean rapid verification of trauma patients and appropriate triage to a trauma center; thus appropriate resources could be used, and morbidity and mortality could be significantly improved. Numerous prehospital scoring indexes have been developed, and two have gained national support.

TRAUMA SCORE

The Trauma Score is a physiologic index that is composed of five categories: systolic blood pressure, respiratory rate, respiratory expansion, capillary refill rate, and score on the Glasgow Coma Scale (Figure 14-8). The score is a number between 1 and 15. Associated with each score is a probability of survival for that score. The lower scores are associated with higher mortality rates. To increase reliability of outcome predictions, the Revised Trauma Score has been developed. The Revised Trauma Score includes the Glasgow Coma Score, systolic blood pressure, and respiratory rate (Table 14-4), but both capillary refill rate and respiratory expansion have been removed because of their subjectivity.[10] The major limitation to the Trauma Score remains the fact that it measures physiologic response; as long as the patient compensates, the score will not accurately reflect his or her condition. The Trauma Score has a sensitivity rate of approximately 80%, and therefore 20% of patients with severe injuries will not be identified with this score.[6]

CRAMS Score

The CRAMS score is also used in the prehospital setting. The CRAMS scale involves assessment of the following areas: circulation, respiration, abdomen and chest, motor, and speech. Each area is graded either 2 (normal), 1 (a deviation form normal), or 0 (absent or none). The highest possible score is 10, which indicates an uninjured patient. The major drawback to the CRAMS score is the need for an actual hands-on assessment for scoring of the abdomen and chest section.[18]

For all prospective scales, only acute injuries should be scored. A person with paraplegia involved in a motor vehicle crash will have only additional injuries scored, not the previous paraplegia.

Retrospective Scoring

Attachment of a numeric score to each diagnosed injury is the concept of retrospective scoring.

Abbreviated Injury Scale

The Abbreviated Injury Scale (AIS), published by the American Association for Automotive Medicine, categorizes injuries into six body regions (head, neck, thorax, abdomen, spine, and extremity and external) and assigns an individual score to each injury (Box 14-3). Scores are integers from 1 to 6, according to severity. The lower the score, the less severe the injury.[11] The AIS method was designed to determine severity of motor vehicle injuries. In the 1985 revision of the AIS, penetrating injuries were addressed in all body regions, but the scale is still considered more sensitive to blunt injuries. The AIS allows determination of individual injury severity but does not take into account multisystem injuries.

BOX 14-3   Abbreviated Injury Scale

0. No injury
1. Minor
2. Moderate
3. Severe
4. Serious
5. Critical
6. Maximum, virtually unsurvivable

TABLE 14-4   Revised Trauma Score Variable Break Points

Glasgow Coma Scale score	Systolic blood pressure (mm Hg)	Respiratory rate (breaths/min)	Coded value
13-15	> 89	10-29	4
9-12	76-89	> 29	3
6-8	50-75	6-9	2
4-5	1-49	1-5	1
3	0	0	0

	Rate	Codes	Score
A. Respiratory rate	10-24	4	
Number of respirations in 15	25-35	3	
seconds: Multiply by 4	>35	2	
	<10	1	
	0	0	A. _____
B. Respiratory effort	Normal	1	
Retroactive: Use of accessory	Retractive	0	
muscles or intercostal retraction			B. _____
C. Systolic blood pressure	≥90	4	
Systolic cuff pressure: Either arm,	70-89	3	
auscultate or palpate	50-69	2	
	>50	1	
No carotid pulse	0	0	C. _____
D. Capillary refill			
Normal: Forehead or lip mucosa			
color refill in 2 seconds	Normal	2	
Delayed: More than 2 seconds			
capillary refill	Delayed	1	
None: No capillary refill	None	0	D. _____
E. Glasgow Coma Scale	Total GSC points	Score	
1. Eye opening			
Spontaneous _____ 4	14-15	5	
To voice _____ 3	11-13	4	
To pain _____ 2	8-10	3	
None _____ 1	5-7	2	
	3-4	1	E. _____
2. Verbal response			
Oriented _____ 5			
Confused _____ 4			
Inappropriate words _____ 3			
Incomprehensible			
sounds _____ 2			
None _____ 1			
3. Motor response			
Obeys commands _____ 6			
Purposeful move-			
ments (pain) _____ 5			
Withdraw (pain) _____ 4			
Flexion (pain) _____ 3			
Extension (pain) _____ 2			
None _____ 1			
Total GCS points (1 + 2 + 3) _____		Trauma Score _____	
	(Total points A + B + C + D + E)		

FIGURE 14-8   **Components of the Trauma Score.**

INJURY SEVERITY SCORE

The Injury Severity Score (ISS) quantifies multisystem injury by use of the AIS scores. The ISS is determined by adding of the squares of the highest AIS scores in the three most severely injured body systems. The ISS is a number between 1 and 75, with 1 being a minor injury and 75 being largely nonsurvivable. A patient who receives a score of 6 in any AIS category is automatically scored as having an ISS of 75. It is widely accepted that any patient with an ISS greater than 15 is a major trauma patient.

TRISS

The TRISS method ties together the Trauma Score, ISS, age, and type of injury to determine the probability of survival for the patient.[6,7]

With the focus on percent of mortality, the injury scoring systems have yet to address the probable morbidity associated with physiologic response and actual injuries.

FIELD TRIAGE

Using triage to determine whether to take a patient to a trauma center is a necessary skill for caregivers in many parts of the United States today. Proper identification of patients who meet trauma center criteria is routinely based on physiologic criteria such as blood pressure lower than 90 mm Hg, anatomic criteria such as two long-bone fractures, and a field triage score such as the Revised or Pediatric Trauma Score.[1] Figure 14-9 displays the standard field triage criteria for delivering a patient to a trauma center.

TRIAGE PATIENT TRANSPORT

Care of the multiply injured patient during transport is aimed at maintaining adequate airway, breathing, and circulation; continued stabilization; and constant monitoring of the patient. The success of the transport depends on the caregiver's ability to anticipate the patient's progression and expect the unexpected (Figure 14-10).

SUMMARY

The members of the transport team provide a critical level of knowledge and expertise of care for the multiply injured patient in the prehospital setting. By understanding the kinematics of trauma, performing a thorough assessment, and delivering care in an organized manner, the transport team will have a positive effect on decreasing the morbidity and mortality of such patients.

MULTIPLE TRAUMA CASE STUDY

The flight team was dispatched to a multiple-victim scene 15 minutes from the hospital. It was reported that two victims were dead and two others were severely injured. The rescue squad performed the initial care practice at the advanced level. On arrival, the flight crew's aerial view of the scene revealed a single car that had been split in half. Rescuers were attending to two victims, and two bodies lying near the wreckage were covered with sheets.

On the basis of the report the flight team received before arrival, they began preparation to transport two victims in the aircraft. Both viable patients had been thrown from the vehicle over the guardrail. Patient 1 was a 15-year-old female whose left leg had been amputated above the knee. Bleeding was controlled with a pressure dressing. She had multiple abrasions and lacerations on her face and chest. Her Glasgow Coma Scale score was 7 (eyes 1; verbal 1; motor 5). She was pale and diaphoretic. She had a palpable femoral pulse of 130 beats/min and a respiratory rate of 8 breaths/minute. Patient 2 was a 16-year-old female who was awake, screaming, and not following any commands. She had multiple abrasions and lacerations to her face, head, and extremities. Her vital signs included a radial pulse of 100 beats/minute and a respiratory rate of 22 breaths/minute. Both were immobilized on backboards with cervical collars and head blocks. Each had one intravenous line in place.

The flight team elected to intubate the first patient because of her low Glasgow Coma Scale score and her advanced level of shock.

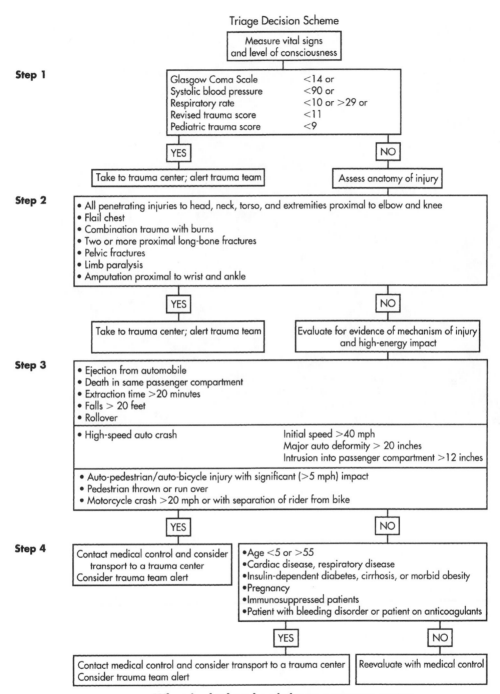

FIGURE 14-9   **Trauma triage decision making.** (From Committee on Trauma, American College of Surgeons: *Resources for optimal care of the injured patient,* 1993, American College of Surgeons.)

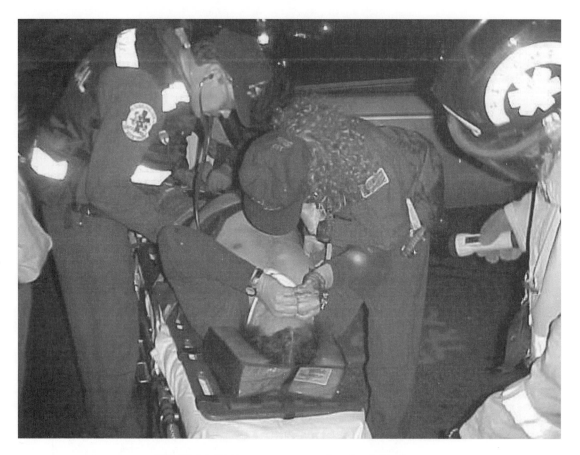

FIGURE 14-10 Transport team performing field triage.

Rapid-sequence induction was initiated, and the patient was intubated without difficulty. During the intubation, a member of the rescue squad placed a second intravenous line. A palpable systolic pressure of 70 mm Hg was ascertained. Both patients were loaded into the aircraft and secured. The second patient was placed on oxygen at high flow per nonrebreather mask. Soft restraints were applied as a precaution.

During the 15-minute transport to the trauma center, the first patient remained hypotensive and tachycardic. No additional neuromuscular blocking agent was administered. The second patient remained stable. Both patients were admitted to the shock resuscitation unit, and a report was given to the resuscitation team.

REFERENCES

1. American College of Surgeons: *Advanced trauma life support student manual,* Chicago, 1997, American College of Surgeons.
2. American College of Surgeons: *Hospital and prehospital resources for optimal care of the injured patient,* appendixes A through J, Chicago, 1993, American College of Surgeons.
3. Amoroso T: Evaluation of the patient with blunt abdominal trauma: an evidence based approach, *Emerg Med Clin North Am* 17(1):63, 1999.
4. Baker SP, O'Neill B, Karpf R: *The injury fact book,* New York, 1992, Oxford.
5. Barach E, Tomlanovich M, Nowak R: Ballistics: a pathophysiologic examination of the wounding mechanisms of firearms: part I, *J Trauma* 26(3):225, 1986.

6. Boyd CR, Tolson MA, Copes WS: Evaluating trauma care: the TRISS method, *J Trauma* 27(4):370, 1987.

7. Champion HR et al: A new characterization of injury severity, *J Trauma* 30(5):539, 1990.

8. Chan L, Bartfield JM, Reilly KM: The significance of out-of-hospital hypotension in blunt trauma patients, *Acad Emerg Med*, 4(8):785, 1997.

9. Chandler CF, Lane JS, Waxman KS: Seatbelt sign following blunt trauma is associated with increased incidence of abdominal injury, *Am Surg* 63(10):885, 1997.

10. Copes W: Major trauma outcome study: letter to MTOS participants, Aug 11, 1988, American College of Surgeons.

11. Copes WS et al: The Injury Severity Score revisited, *J Trauma* 28(1):69, 1988.

12. Daffner RH et al: Patterns of high-speed impact injuries in motor vehicle occupants, *J Trauma*, 28(4):498, 1988.

13. Fackler ML, Bellamy RF, Malinowski JA: The wound profile: illustration of the missile-tissue interaction, *J Trauma* 28(2 suppl):S21, 1988.

14. Fackler ML, Malinowski JA: The wound profile: a visual method quantifying gunshot wound components, *J Trauma* 26(6):522, 1985.

15. Jacobs B, Baker P: *Trauma nursing care course*, Park Ridge, Ill, 1995, Emergency Nurses Association.

16. Janzon B: *High-energy missile trauma: a study of the mechanisms of wounding of muscle tissue*, Goteborg, Sweden, 1983, University of Goteborg.

17. Mackenzie C, Lippert FK: Emergency department management of trauma, *Anesthesiol Clin North Am* 17(1):45, 1999.

18. Mattox K, Moore EE, Feliciano DV, editors: *Trauma*, Norwalk, Conn, 1996, Appleton & Lange.

19. National Association of Emergency Medical Technicians: *Prehospital trauma life support student manual*, ed 3, St Louis, 1994, Mosby.

20. Pepe P, Eckstein M: Reappraising the prehospital care of the patient with major trauma, *Emerg Med Clin North Am* 16(1):1, 1998.

21. Phipps W, Sands J, Marek J, editors: *Medical-surgical nursing concepts & clinical practice*, ed 6, St Louis, 1999, Mosby.

22. Reilly P et al: Reactive oxygen metabolites, *Scientific American*, Chicago, Ill, 1997, American College of Surgeons.

23. Sumchai A, Eliastam M, Werner P: Seatbelt cervical injury in an intersection type vehicular collision, *J Trauma* 28(4):498, 1988.

24. U.S. Centers for Disease Control, Harvard School of Public Health: *U.S. burden of disease and injury study*, Preliminary, unpublished results, 2000, CDC.

25. Watts DD et al: Hypothermic coagulopathy in trauma: effect of varying levels of hypothermia on enzyme speed, platelet function, and fibrinolytic activity, *J Trauma* 44:846, 1998

NEUROLOGIC TRAUMA

15

COMPETENCIES

1. Perform a baseline neurologic assessment and ongoing serial evaluations of the trauma patient.
2. Provide life-sustaining and supportive care with appropriate and aggressive interventions to patients with neurologic trauma to achieve maximum potential for recovery.
3. Use guidelines in the management of the patient with a traumatic brain or spinal cord injury during transport.

Traumatic neurologic emergencies involve disorders of both the central and the peripheral nervous systems. In one way or another the vast majority of these disorders will ultimately affect the respiratory system, and thus airway management will be crucial. However, depending on the patient's condition, specific treatment may be instituted that will lessen the impact of emergencies with which the transport team will have to contend. The ultimate result may be a progression to coma, often in association with increased intracranial pressure (ICP) or a spinal injury. Therefore it is essential that the transport team understand the causes of increased ICP and the neurologic syndromes discussed later in this chapter. Because of the extensive nature of this topic, we have categorized types of neurologic traumatic emergencies and listed by headings the components and management issues as they relate to patient transport.

HEAD INJURIES

Head injury statistics are staggering. Head injuries that result in traumatic brain injury (TBI) are the leading cause of death related to trauma. It has been estimated that both fatal and nonfatal traumatic brain injuries in the United States occur 237 per 100,000 people.[12,28,51] Two thirds of those who sustain head injuries are under the age of 30 years. The cost of care for people who survive neurologic injuries is in the millions of dollars. In general, 10% to 20% of all head injuries are classified as severe and potentially life threatening.[20,39,40,45]

Head injuries are the major cause of death of people involved in motor vehicle crashes.[20] The primary solution to the death and devastation caused by neurologic trauma is prevention.

The outcome for a patient who has sustained a head injury may be determined by the severity of the injury and the time elapsed before the patient receives adequate medical attention; thus there is a need for rapid evaluation, assessment, and transfer of the patient to an appropriate-level care facility by the transport team. The transport team must possess a basic knowledge of the principles of pathophysiology of head injury to apply appropriate diagnostic and therapeutic methods and perform a thorough and ongoing systemic evaluation of the patient.

When trauma to the head occurs, the hair and scalp provide some dampening effect on impact. However, the brunt of the blow is delivered to the skull, which has enough elasticity to be flattened or indented when struck with a blunt object. The maximum depression occurs instantly and is followed within a few milliseconds by several oscillations. A severe blow to the skull actually causes a generalized deformation by flattening in the direction of the impact, with a corresponding widening of the diameter at right angles to the impact line.[4,14]

The skull travels faster under impact than does the brain. Although the unbending skull often contuses the brain at the site of impact, severe brain injuries occur when the brain is hurled against the skull's rough, bony prominence, the crista galli, the major sphenoid wings, or the petrous bones. It is not uncommon for the frontal and temporal poles to be injured. The undersurface of the temporal poles and, less often, the occipital poles are contused or pulped as a result of the unbending skull. Similar damage can also be caused by the edges of the relatively unyielding falx and tentorium. So-called coup lesions develop in opposite areas of the brain on impact.[14,44]

Damage may result from direct injury or may be secondary to compression, tension, or shearing forces caused by the particular injury. In addition, secondary complications result from the head injury. Ischemia and cerebral edema may ensue. There seems to be an immediate increase in ICP on impact; however, there is also a secondary increase several minutes after the injury. The increase in ICP at the time of impact results from acceleration and deceleration of the head and deformation of the skull, the former being more significant than the latter.[3,14,21]

During impact, cerebral spinal fluid may offer some protection to the brain. However, this protective layer is insufficient in the subarachnoid space around the frontal and temporal lobes, the most frequent sites of contusion.[44]

TYPES OF HEAD INJURIES: PATHOLOGIC AND CLINICAL CONSIDERATIONS

Head injury may exist in isolation; however, various combinations of injuries usually occur. Each component contributes in a different degree to the overall severity and outcome of the injury.[25]

SKULL FRACTURE

The skull is composed of three layers: an outer layer, a middle cancellous layer, and an inner layer that is half as thick as the outer layer and contains grooves that have large vessels. Whether a fracture actually occurs in the area of impact depends on the type of injury. The more concentrated and focused the impact tends to be, the greater the likelihood of a fracture.

A vast majority of skull fractures are linear.[19] A linear skull fracture produces a line that usually extends toward the base of the skull. Impact can produce a single linear fracture or multiple fractures, referred to as *linear stellate fractures,* that radiate from the compressed area. Although linear fractures may look benign, they can cause serious complications. One such complication is infection. If the fracture line is open a few millimeters at the time of impact, debris such as hair, dirt, and glass may travel into the cranial vault. Linear fractures may also lead to epidural hematoma if the fracture line crosses a groove in the layer of the skull that houses the middle meningeal artery. Another complication occurs when the dura, which is strongly attached to the skull, tears at the fracture site.

Diastatic and Basilar Skull Fractures. Diastatic fracture involves a separation of bones at a suture line or a marked separation of bone fragments; both are usually visible on skull x-ray films. Facial fracture may also play a role in head injuries. A blow to the lower jaw when the jaw is closed can cause the mandibular condyles to displace upward and backward against the base of the skull, leading to a concussion or a basilar skull fracture. Another type of facial fracture, which may or may not involve the cranium, is an orbital blowout fracture, which usually involves the floor of the orbit and is caused by blunt impact to the orbit and its contents.

Basilar skull fractures can occur when the mandibular condyles perforate into the base of the skull, but they most often result from extension of fractures of the calvaria. Many basilar skull fractures are impossible to see on an x-ray film. Basilar fractures often produce Battle's sign (an oval-shaped bruise over the mastoid) or "raccoon eyes" (ecchymotic areas around the eyes).

Depressed Skull Fracture. The presence of depressed elements of a fracture may warrant specific diagnostic and therapeutic measures. If the depressed fracture is closed, the rationale for surgical correction is to evacuate any local mass if present, repair any dural lacerations to prevent cerebral herniation through the defect, and correct any cosmetic disfigurement caused by the depression. In general, if the depression on the tangential view of the skull is greater than the thickness of the skull, the dura is probably lacerated, and surgery is recommended. Depressions of a lesser degree, unless over the forehead, rarely require surgical exploration.

A compound depressed skull fracture usually requires surgical debridement. If the injury has been caused by a blow to a static head, the patient's level of consciousness is frequently well preserved, and there may be no neurologic deficits. When a blow has been sustained to a moving head, consciousness is impaired.

Skull fractures can be the source of various complications, including intracranial infections, hematomas, and meningeal and brain tissue damage. Approximately 3% of all skull fractures are associated with *pneumocephalus,* which is defined as the presence of air within the cranial vault.[4] Traumatic pneumocephalus may occur if the frontal, ethmoid, or sphenoid sinuses or the mastoid processes are fractured. Air that has entered the skull will locate in the epidural, subdural, subarachnoid, interventricular, or intercerebral space. Pneumocephalus seldom

produces symptoms unless it is under tension and thus produces compression of the underlying brain tissue. The incidence of pneumocephalus and cerebral spinal fluid rhinorrhea with sella turcica fractures is small, but there is a high incidence of infection if this condition is present. There may be associated palsies of the oculi motor, trochlear, trigeminal, or abducens nerves.[33]

In general, temporal bone fractures can cause pneumocephalus if dural tearing occurs in conjunction with injury to the eustachian tube, the middle ear, or the mastoid process. The patient may have sensory neurologic hearing loss, otorrhagia, or cerebral spinal fluid rhinorrhea in the presence of a temporal bone fracture.

Hemorrhage

Subdural Hematoma. Subdural hematoma is a collection of blood between the brain surface and the dura. It may occur as a result of a contusion or laceration of the brain with bleeding into the subdural space, tearing of the veins that bridge the subdural space, or an extension of an intercerebral hematoma through the brain surface into the subdural space. Subdural hematoma might be unassociated with skull fracture.[41]

Subdural hematomas are classified as acute, subacute, or chronic, depending on the time elapsed between the injury and the appearance of signs and symptoms of neurologic dysfunction. As with other types of head injury, the time course of development and the degree and rate of neurologic dysfunction depend on many factors. As a general rule, if dysfunction occurs within 24 hours, the hematoma is acute; if it occurs between 2 and 10 days, it is subacute; and if it occurs after 2 weeks, the hematoma is chronic. This particular classification is partially pathologic. The location of the hematoma and the amount of mass effect play important roles in determining the timing of surgical intervention.

Elderly patients may have larger subdural hematomas with slowly developing symptoms because they have larger potential subdural spaces as a result of cerebral atrophy. In contrast, symptoms may be displayed rapidly, and marked increases in intercranial pressure may develop in a younger patient with a small subdural space.

Subdural hematomas generally occur in children under the age of 2 years. Signs and symptoms include a bulging fontanelle and a large head (because of separation of the sutures) and retinal hemorrhages (because of increased ICP). In the infant patient a shocklike state may also develop because a relatively large blood volume loss may be caused by a subdural hematoma.

Acute subdural hematomas are usually associated with a high morbidity and mortality, reflecting the usually severe nature of the associated injuries and the not-infrequent association of rapidly rising ICP resulting from the mass effect and development of cerebral edema. Two separate related pathophysiologic problems are cerebral contusion and edema and the presence of blood in the subdural space. The computed tomography (CT) scan is very valuable in determining whether surgical intervention may be indicated. If the major problem contributing to the patient's poor neurologic status is the mass effect, then surgical intervention may be necessary. If the major problem is the cerebral injury, then corrective treatment should be directed toward treating increased ICP.

Epidural Hematoma. Epidural hematomas are classified as acute or subacute. An acute epidural hematoma that is arterial in origin generally produces symptoms within a few hours. Subacute epidural hematomas are venous in origin and take a longer time to produce symptoms. These hematomas are associated with linear skull fractures in 90% of patients, but they may also occur as a result of blunt injuries in which there is no evidence of fracture.[4] The classic symptoms displayed by a patient with an epidural hematoma are transient loss of consciousness, recovery with a lucid interval during which the patient's neurologic status returns to normal, and the secondary onset of headache and a decreasing level of consciousness. As a result of the initial injury, the middle meningeal artery may tear, causing traumatic unconsciousness. Spasm and clotting then occur in the middle meningeal artery, and the bleeding stops. During the next several

hours the artery gradually bleeds, and a hematoma is formed, stripping the dura from the inside of the skull. Once a headache with a decreasing level of consciousness becomes obvious, the secondary rise in ICP has already occurred, and distortion of the brain with significant mass effect occurs. Because compensatory mechanisms of the inner cranial space have already been exhausted, the patient's neurologic status rapidly deteriorates. The patient experiences a downhill course, usually with dilatation of the ipsilateral pupil because of third-nerve compression by the herniating temporal structures, progressive unconsciousness with weakness or decerebration of either the contralateral extremities or the ipsilateral extremities, Cheyne-Stokes respirations, and if no treatment is initiated, loss of pupillary reflexes, caloric responses, bradycardia, and death. It is thus extremely important to identify the epidural hematoma in the earliest possible stage, when a headache and drowsiness are the only complaints, and to transfer the patient for immediate neurosurgical intervention.[26] The classic history and clinical progression, however, is only seen in one third of patients with epidural hematomas. Another third are unconscious from the time of injury, and the final third are never unconscious. In children, bradycardia and early papilledema may be the only warning signs.[4,30]

Intracerebral Hematoma. Movement of one section of brain tissue over or against another section causes tears in blood vessels, which leads to contusions or intracerebral hematomas. Most intracerebral hematomas are found in the frontal and temporal lobes, usually very deep, and are associated with necrosis and hemorrhage. The anatomic relationship between these areas and irregularities of the skull have already been discussed. Intracerebral hematomas are readily identified on the CT scan. The clinical picture may vary from no neurologic defect to deep coma.

CLOSED HEAD INJURY

Concussion. The term *concussion* applies to injuries that result in transient alterations of consciousness. There have been reports of deaths when prolonged apnea ensues, but recovery is the rule. No specific neurologic abnormalities are present, although a postconcussive syndrome may follow even minor injuries.

Cerebral Contusion.   Cerebral hemorrhagic contusions frequently occur in patients, particularly adults, after head injury. Of the patients who die as a result of head injury, 75% have contusions at autopsy. Hemorrhagic contusions are infrequently seen in children, but areas of localized decreased density on a CT scan may represent nonhemorrhagic contusions or possibly local ischemia.[22]

Generally, no surgical intervention is recommended for cerebral contusions because brain matter cannot be removed in areas of the brain that control motor, sensory, or visual functioning. If, however, the contusion occurs over the frontal or temporal lobes, with significant edema and shift, it is feasible to remove contused portions of the brain surgically. When a temporal lobe contusion is present and signs of herniation are seen, surgical excision of the temporal lobe may be beneficial. Generally, patients with contusion are treated by controlling elevated ICP medically.[15]

Diffuse Axonal Injury.   Diffuse axonal injury occurs when the delicate axons of the brain are starched and damaged as a result of rapid movement of the brain. Mechanisms of injury associated with the acceleration and deceleration that occurs with high-speed motor vehicle crashes or ejection from a vehicle can cause this type of diffuse brain injury. Because the axons have been damaged, there is interference with neuron transmission, and multiple neurologic deficits occur including deep coma, posturing, and respiratory compromise. This type of head injury is generally severe with a high morbidity and mortality.[12,51]

PENETRATING INJURIES

Gunshot Wounds.   When a person is shot at close range, there may be evidence of smoke on the skin. When the muzzle of the gun is somewhat farther from the scalp but still close, there may be evidence of powder burns. A bullet striking the skull can cause great destruction of the underlying brain tissue.

Although some of the energy of impact may be dissipated by the shattering of bones and soft tissues, the impact on the brain after a bullet penetrates the skull is still great. The bullet's ability to destroy tissues is directly related to its kinetic energy at the moment of impact. The degree of damage to the brain depends primarily on the muzzle velocity of the bullet and the distance between the gun and its target.

A bullet that passes through the head produces a larger defect on the inner table of the skull than that produced on the outer table. High-velocity bullets cause extensive injury to the brain and cranium. The entrance wound is usually smaller than the exit wound, but there may be a great deal of variation in their sizes. Multiple linear fractures that radiate from either the entrance or exit wound are common. Some fractures may be far away from the trajectory of the bullet, particularly in thin bones. The transport team should describe the wounds but not attempt to determine whether they are entrance or exit wounds.

Injuries to the major cerebral arteries, veins, or venous sinuses can occur during any of the bullet's intracranial passages. Cerebral injuries cause an immediate but transitory increase in ICP. The eventual ICP depends on the degree of intracranial bleeding, which may be profuse even in the absence of injury to major vessels. Secondary cerebral edema causes a delayed increase in ICP. Damage to the hemisphere causes loss of autoregulation, falling cerebral blood flow, an increase in cerebral blood volume and ICP, and eventually, brain death.

Intracranial hematomas are frequently associated with penetrating wounds to the brain. If the bullet passes close to or transverses the ventricle, an intraventricular hematoma may result.

Infection is seen often in injuries caused by shell fragments because these fragments are more likely than bullets to carry dirt, hair, and bone fragments into the brain. Infections develop most often from retained bone fragments, improper closure of the scalp and dura, and delay of definitive surgery beyond 48 hours.

TABLE 15-1	**Physiologic Disturbance Correlated With Anatomic Level of Lesion**					
Parameters	Cerebral cortex	Diencephalon (thalamus)		Midbrain	Pons	Medulla
Mental status	Awake, alert, lethargic, obtunded	Light stupor	Deep stupor	Coma	Coma	Coma
Motor response	Appropriate	Focal response to pain	General response to pain	Decerebrate posturing, decorticate posturing	Flaccid	Flaccid
Pupil response	Normal size and reactivity	Small	Small	Midposition	Small	Small
Oculocephalic, oculovestibular reflex	Not testable	Normal response	Normal response	Abnormal	Abnormal	Abnormal*
Respiratory status	Variable	Variable	Cheyne-Stokes	Central neurogenic hyperventilation	Apneustic pattern	Apnea

*May be normal with isolated medullary injury.

Stab Wounds. Whenever the skull has been penetrated, there is a risk of intracranial infection. The injury should be managed to minimize that risk. All patients with penetrating injuries should receive tetanus prophylaxis.

Most stab wounds are caused by assaults with sharp instruments such as knives, scissors, and screwdrivers or when the patient (often a child) falls on a stick or sharp toy. It is best to transport a stab-wound patient with the object immobilized, secured, and left in place.

If the penetrating object has been removed, it may be difficult to determine exactly where penetration of the skull occurred, particularly if entry occurred at the eyelid or sclera. When the patient arrives at the hospital, the area of injury is explored and debrided, as with an open injury.

PHYSICAL ASSESSMENT: HEAD INJURY

Examination of a patient who is unconscious requires integration of information from several systems: mental status, the pupils, other cranial nerves, the motor system, and respiratory function (Table 15-1).

LEVEL OF CONSCIOUSNESS

The best indicator of changes in intracranial pressure, especially from a mass lesion, is a patient's level of consciousness.[28] Consciousness is a mental state in which the person is stimulated by the environment and can react appropriately to it. A useful way of describing the conscious state is to divide it into alert, lethargic, or obtunded stages (Box 15-1).

The **alert** patient readily responds to the examiner, although, depending on the state of the central nervous system (CNS) injury, there may be some confusion, speech disturbance, and motor deficits. The **lethargic** patient appears to be drowsy or asleep but can be aroused easily and can respond reasonably appropriately to the examiner's questions, although if left alone, he or she will slowly return to an apparent sleep state or certainly lack attentiveness. The **obtunded** patient is extremely drowsy, arouses with greater difficulty than a lethargic patient, rarely answers in complete sentences, and certainly does not volunteer information. In fact, during the active questioning period the examiner may have to repeatedly stimulate the patient to gain attention.

BOX 15-1   Stages in Progression From Consciousness to Unconsciousness

---

Conscious State

Alert: Patient responds readily but may have some confusion, speech disturbance, or motor deficit.
Lethargic: Patient appears drowsy or sleepy but can be aroused to respond to questioning.
Obtunded: Patient is extremely drowsy, is difficult to arouse, and rarely answers in complete sentences.

Unconscious State

Stuporous: Patient does not verbalize appropriately or coherently; may moan and groan or utter monosyllables.
Comatose: Patient gives no evidence of awareness.

Deterioration beyond the obtunded level results in the unconscious state. This state may be classified as either stupor or coma.

The **stuporous** patient does not verbalize appropriately or coherently. Two distinct levels of activity can characterize this state. The patient in a lightly stuporous state may moan and groan in response to stimulation or may utter an occasional recognizable monosyllabic word, often a slang or curse word. The patient who is in a light stuporous condition will respond to pain by moving all extremities, unless there is a primary motor system injury, and will appear to crudely localize the site of the pain. However, a patient who is in a deeply stuporous state will not appear to localize and protect against pain. The patient who is in true coma may have decorticate posturing, decerebrate posturing, or flaccid motor response.

In examining the pattern of motor response, it is important to be aware of the possibility of primary motor system injury. For example, a left cortical lesion or a lesion in the left internal capsule may cause a contralateral hemiparesis that even in the awake patient may distort the motor response.

The **comatose** state roughly divides into three levels of reflex motor activity: **decorticate posturing, decerebrate posturing,** and **flaccidity,** to use clinically descriptive terms rather than more precise neurophysiologic descriptions. The patient in a decorticate state is unconscious and gives no evidence of awareness. Painful stimulation causes extensor rigidity in the lower extremities combined with a flexor posture of the upper extremities. Depending on the extent of the underlying damage to the motor system, this posturing may occur spontaneously or after painful stimulation and may be more prominent on one side than the other. Decerebrate posturing is exhibited by extensor rigidity in all four extremities. The patient who is flaccid has no motor response to painful stimulation.

For consciousness to be present, a stimulus must be presented to the CNS and must pass through the brain stem (with the exception of visual stimulation) to the diencephalon. From there the stimulus must reach the cerebral cortex, where it is recorded. The patient must have sufficient cortical function so that the stimulus can excite associations through memory, which will let the patient acknowledge the presence of the stimulus and make use of that stimulus to relate appropriately to the external environment.

For example, when an intracranial mass lesion develops after head trauma and unconsciousness does not initially result, the patient may be expected, as the mass lesion increases, to progress systematically through the various levels and stages just described. The mass lesion may be a hematoma or a significant cerebral edema. A patient with a head injury resulting in a primary upper brain stem lesion might be unconscious and would immediately evidence a comatose state without having ever experienced cortical or diencephalic deterioration. A person who survives a near drowning or delayed cardiopulmonary resuscitation may have severe bilateral cortical injury and may not progress significantly. A person who experiences a spontaneous hemorrhage in the brain stem, particularly in the region of the pons or midbrain, would be expected to become suddenly comatose with no evidence of an orderly progression through the stages noted previously.

EXAMINATION OF THE PUPILS

The pupils are innervated by both the parasympathetic (third-nerve) and the sympathetic systems, with the former causing constriction and the latter causing dilatation. The size of the pupil will depend on the degree to which each system is influencing the pupil at the time of examination. The normal pupil will constrict promptly to light. Examination of the pupils consists of assessment of the relative size of the two pupils and their reactivity to light. Injury to the parasympathetic system will result in pupillary dilatation. Injury to the parasympathetic system may occur within the midbrain at the origin of the parasympathetic contribution to the third nerve, or it may occur outside the brain stem where the third nerve exits and proceeds forward beneath the brain into the region of the cavernous sinus. The sympathetic innervation begins in the posterior hypothalamus, descends the length of the brain stem and cervical cord, and exits in the lower cervical upper thoracic area, where it proceeds up the neck in the cervical sympathetic chain to the base of the skull and then out to the orbit where innervation occurs. Injury to the sympathetic system results in pupillary constriction because of the actions of the unopposed third nerve. The sympathetic system can be injured within the CNS anywhere along its pathway and during its course through the chest and neck. Because of the relatively small size of the structures involved, it is unlikely that lesions within the brain or brain stem will affect either the parasympathetic or the sympathetic systems unilaterally. Therefore, it can be assumed that if bilateral pupil abnormalities are seen, a lesion in the brain or brain stem has affected the nerve supply to the pupils. For example, bilaterally small pupils may very well be caused by a lesion within the brain stem that affects both descending sympathetic tracts. On the other hand, a unilateral affected pupil can be expected to be caused by a lesion of the tracts outside the brain or brain stem (extraaxial). A unilaterally dilated pupil may be caused by compression of the third nerve by a herniating temporal lobe after it has exited the midbrain and as it crosses the floor of the skull. A unilateral small pupil resulting from sympathetic denervation will react more sluggishly to light. Bilaterally dilated and fixed pupils are generally caused by global hypoxia or by bilateral temporal lobe herniation from central cerebral edema with bilateral third-nerve compression. Bilaterally constricted pupils may be caused by central herniation of the posterior hypothalamus at the site of origin of the sympathetic fibers through the tentorial notch or by bilateral involvement within the brain stem, such as from a pontine hemorrhage. Midbrain lesions that affect the parasympathetic bilaterally will yield pupils that are in midposition and are nonreactive to light. It is helpful to examine other cranial nerves because they can reveal the competency of brain stem function.

BRAIN STEM AND CRANIAL NERVES

The integrity of the brain stem can be evaluated by examining certain cranial nerves, especially those related to conjugate gaze. In the patient who is awake, conjugate gaze is controlled by visual input through the complex system that coordinates the function of the extraocular muscles by way of cranial nerves III, IV, and VI. In the patient who is unconscious, however, visual input gives way to vestibular input to control conjugate gaze. This is best evaluated by examining the oculocephalic or oculovestibular reflexes.[38]

The oculocephalic reflex is demonstrated by stimulating the vestibular system through movement of the head in reference to the neck. While the patient lies supine on the ground, stretcher, or bed, the person performing the assessment opens the patient's eyelids. Under normal circumstances the eyes should stare at the sky or ceiling. The nurse then rotates the head briskly but gently to one side or the other. Under normal circumstances the eyes may momentarily remain in their position in the orbits but will immediately track conjugately to the side opposite the direction of the movement so that the eyes will be directed once again toward the sky or ceiling. If conjugate activity cannot be observed, for example, if one eye tracks and the other one does not or if neither eye tracks, this signals an abnormality and suggests a disturbance of the brain stem. This maneuver should never be performed in a patient with a head injury or multiple trauma until the cervical spine has been determined to be without injury.

The oculovestibular reflex is demonstrated by cold caloric stimulation, in which cold saline solution is irrigated into the external auditory canal. In a few seconds the eyes will conjugately deviate to the side of the irrigation and remain in that position from several seconds to several minutes. If this response is not seen, an abnormality is present in the brain stem involving the medial longitudinal fasciculus, the vestibular system, or both. The flight nurse should not perform this maneuver on a patient with head injury until the possibility of a basal skull fracture involving the temporal bone has been excluded.

The midportion of the pons may be evaluated by the presence or absence of the corneal reflex. The corneal reflex can quickly be assessed by lightly touching the cornea with the corner of a soft gauze dressing and observing whether a blink reflex occurs.

MOTOR EXAMINATION

The motor system is best examined in conjunction with an examination of the patient's mental status or level of consciousness. The awake patient can be asked to perform certain motor tasks, such as moving his or her legs or gripping. If the patient is unconscious, motor activity in response to pain is a good way to determine the level of unconsciousness, as previously described.

RESPIRATORY PATTERN

Most patients with significant head injuries will hypoventilate early after the injury. Later the respiratory pattern may vary, depending on the level of the lesion. Patients with decorticate posturing often demonstrate an accompanying Cheyne-Stokes pattern of respiration in which there is a regular crescendo-decrescendo change in the volume of inspiration, with the rate remaining rather regular.

The patient with decerebrate posturing may exhibit central neurogenic hyperventilation. Patients with brain stem lesions may have varying rates and depths of respiration, and an ataxic element is often noted. With lower brain stem lesions, the rate becomes more irregular, more shallow, and less frequent, until medullary lesions result in respiratory paralysis. It is often necessary for the transport team to intubate the patient for respiratory control.

The respiratory patterns of patients in a metabolic coma will be dictated by the cause of the coma. Patients with intrinsic metabolic lesions that lead to conditions such as diabetic ketoacidosis or hepatic coma may demonstrate a driven hyperventilation; patients who have ingested opiates will have a much more shallow respiratory pattern with a decreased frequency, depending on the drug level.

THE GLASGOW COMA SCALE

The Glasgow Coma Scale (GCS), as shown in Table 15-2, is widely used to measure the severity of coma in patients and is therefore an indicator of prognosis. However, eye-opening response may not be accurately assessed in the patient with severe maxillofacial injuries whose airway is being mechanically supported. In addition, in a patient with a contralateral mass lesion, the best motor response may not depict progressing hemiparesis. When examining a patient, it is best to record the GCS results in the narrative record that goes to the receiving health-care providers.

REEXAMINATION

Successful acute management of the comatose patient depends on frequent examination of the patient to determine his or her level of neurologic function and rate of deterioration. The information provided in Table 15-2 can be helpful in this analysis.

When the transport team sees the injured patient for the first time, a baseline neurologic evaluation should be performed. Findings during subsequent examinations will provide the transport team with an understanding of the intracranial injury. When a focal mass lesion such as a hematoma or focal contusion develops in a patient, he or she will steadily

TABLE 15-2 **The Glasgow Coma Scale**

Circle the Appropriate Number and Compute the Total

Best eye-opening response:	_____ **Right**		_____ **Left**	
	Never		1	
	To pain		2	
	To verbal stimuli		3	
	Spontaneously		4	
Best verbal response:				
	No response		1	
	Incomprehensible sounds		2	
	Inappropriate words		3	
	Disoriented and converses		4	
	Oriented and converses		5	
Best motor response:	_____ **Right**		_____ **Left**	
	No response		1	
	Extension abnormal (decerebrate rigidity)		2	
	Flexion abnormal (decorticate rigidity)		3	
	Flexion withdrawal		4	
	Localizes pain		5	
	Obeys commands		6	
	Total:_____ **3-15**			
Neurologic evaluation:	Record on Glasgow Coma Scale sheet.			
	Repeat evaluation frequently. A score of 15 is normal; below 7 indicates coma; 3 signifies brain death.			
	Vital signs:			
	Level of consciousness			
	Glasgow Coma Scale			
	Pupillary size and reactivity			
	Right_____			
	Left_____			
	Focal weakness			
	Present_____			
	Absent_____			

progress in depth of coma through the various levels depicted in Table 15-2. For example, when the initial examination of a patient results in findings compatible with a diencephalic level of coma, the coma will be determined to have deteriorated to a midbrain level if the patient is subsequently found to have decerebrate posturing, midposition pupils, and central neurogenic hyperventilation. If the insult is unilateral, hemiparesis and an ipsilateral dilated pupil will be seen before bilateral motor signs of herniation are seen. If the patient initially shows signs of coma resulting from a primary brain stem injury—a static lesion—a further deterioration in the level will not be demonstrated within the next few hours, other than what would normally be seen with a developing mass lesion. Finally, if the patient does not have a significant head injury but rather on initial examination is found to have a suppressed level of consciousness because of a metabolic disorder, such as drug intoxication, the examinations over time will demonstrate a pattern of what appears to be multilevel involvement, depending on the sensitivity of the system being examined to the drug concentration in the blood.

INTERVENTIONS AND TREATMENT

There has been a concerted effort on the part of the Brain Trauma Foundation, American Association of Neurological Surgeons, and the Congress of Neurological Surgeons to develop guidelines for the management of the patient with a head injury.[6,24] A summary of these guidelines appears in Box 15-2.

Management is based on the severity of the injury, which is usually measured by the patient's

GCS. The following classification using the GCS has been suggested to identify the gravity of the patient's injury[6,24,51]:

- Mild   GCS 14-15
- Moderate   GCS 9-13
- Severe   GCS 3-8

Because the transport team may not always know what is the patient's primary injury (i.e., subdural hematoma or epidural hematoma), managing patients based on their GCS as well as the related physical exam will assist the team in providing the appropriate care to these patients.

| BOX 15-2 | **Summary of the Guidelines for the Management of Severe Head Injury That Affect Patient Transport** |

Initial Resuscitation

Complete and rapid physiological resuscitation is the first priority, and no treatment should be directed toward intracranial hypertension in the absence of indications that deterioration in neurologic status exists. However, when signs of neurologic deterioration are present, aggressive management must be initiated and should include:

- Hyperventilation
- Administration of mannitol

Sedation and neuromuscular blockade must be used in a discretionary manner.

Resuscitation of Blood Pressure and Oxygenation

Mean arterial blood pressure should be maintained at more than 90 mm Hg throughout to keep the patient's cerebral perfusion pressure greater than 70 mm Hg. Patients with a GCS score of less than 9 who cannot maintain their airway or who are hypoxic require a secured airway.

ICP Treatment Threshold

Interpretation and treatment of ICP based on any threshold should be corroborated by frequent clinical examination and monitoring.

Hyperventilation

Avoid hyperventilation during the first 24 hours because reduced blood flow compromises cerebral perfusion.

Use of Mannitol

Administration of mannitol may occur before initiation of ICP monitoring when there are signs of transtentorial herniations or deterioration of neurologic status.

Role of Glococorticoids

Glucocorticoids are not recommended in severe head injury.

Modified from Bullock R, Chestnut RM, Clifton G et al: *Management and prognosis of severe traumatic brain injury,* New York, 2000, Brain Trauma Foundation and American Association of Neurological Surgeons; McQuillan KA, Mitchell PH: Traumatic brain injuries. In McQuillan KA, Von Rueden KT, Hartsock RL, Flynn MB, Whalen E, editors: *Trauma nursing: from resuscitation through rehabilitation,* ed 3, Philadelphia, 2002, Saunders; and Wraa C, editor: *Transport nursing advanced trauma course,* ed 3, Denver, 2001, Air and Surface Transport Nurses Association.

The transport teams' highest priority is establishing an adequate airway and oxygenation. The awake patient should be placed on 100% oxygen. If the patient is unable to maintain the airway or the transport team anticipates the potential for deterioration during transport, the patient should be intubated. Care must be taken to maintain cervical spine immobilization while gaining access to the airway. A gastric tube should be inserted with care to prevent aspiration. Pulse oximetry and end-tidal CO_2 ($ETCO_2$) devices should be used throughout the transport process to monitor the patient's oxygenation and perfusion.[30,37]

Hypotension has been found to contribute to the mortality and morbidity of head-injured patients. The patient's mean arterial pressure should be maintained at more than 90 mm Hg. Fluids and blood products should be administered to maintain blood pressure. Rapid transport for definitive surgical intervention may be the only way that some hemorrhagic hypotension can be managed.

If the patient is restless or agitated, hypoxia should be suspected until a specific cause can be found. Most patients with head injuries have sustained other injuries that will cause pain. Even in the patient who is inattentive or stuporous, hypoxia rather than pain should be considered the cause of restlessness until this is proven otherwise.

The intubated patient who is restless or who resists ventilatory support is increasing his or her ICP, which may be extremely critical. These patients should be subdued with pharmacologically appropriate doses of sedation, analgesia, and neuromuscular blocking agents.[8] Because of the effects of analgesic and sedation agents on the patient's hemodynamic status, the effects of these medications must be closely monitored by the transport team. However, pain can be a powerful stimulus to increasing physiologic metabolism and oxygen consumption, and its effects must be considered on the patient's ICP.

If neuromuscular blocking agents are used, it is important to closely monitor the patient's temperature for the presence of hypothermia, because of the inability of the patient to shiver, or for evidence of malignant hyperthermia, particularly in children.

Seizures that develop during transport should be promptly treated because they produce hypoxia and cause increased ICP. Intravenous administration of benzodiazepines are indicated for initial seizure management. Prophylactic use of antiepileptic medications may also be considered, especially if the patient is receiving neuromuscular blocking agents.[45,52] Unconscious patients or those who have a depressed level of consciousness associated with seizure activities should be intubated for maximal control of the airway. Because having an adequate airway is of paramount importance, the airway should be secured immediately.

In general, hypertension and bradycardia may develop in patients who have increased ICP. Hypotension and tachycardia are not signs of intracranial injury, except in a patient who is herniating. However, small children may become hypovolemic from scalp lacerations associated with head injuries and should be monitored and treated accordingly with volume replacement.

Patients with head injuries may lose their cerebral autoregulation (Figure 15-1). If this is the case, cerebral perfusion is directly related to mean systemic arterial pressure. Thus hypotension may lead to underperfusion, and hypertension may lead to vascular congestion and mass effect. Both extremes should be avoided.

Hyperthermia also increases ICP, and thus normal body temperatures should be maintained with

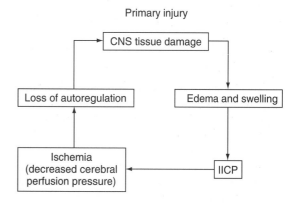

FIGURE 15-1   **Sequence of pathophysiologic events initiated by primary injury.**

the use of acetaminophen suppositories or cooling techniques. Shivering should be controlled because it increases ICP.

Routine hyperventilation is no longer recommended in the initial management of the patient with a traumatic brain injury. It may be indicated with any of the following signs.[6,28,51]

- Unilateral or bilateral pupillary dilation
- Asymmetric pupillary reactivity
- Motor posturing
- Other evidence of deterioration of the neurologic exam

The patient's CO_2 should be maintained between 35 to 45 mm Hg. End-tidal CO_2 monitoring will aid the transport team in the appropriate ventilation of the patient with a traumatic brain injury. The transport team must pay careful attention when manually assisting an intubated head-injured patient. Aggressive bagging can potentially cause additional injury.[6,28]

Mannitol may be used to treat increasing intracranial pressure manifested by deterioration in the patient's neurologic status. Mannitol will decrease the patient's ICP by enhancing cerebral blood flow because it can draw excess fluid into the vascular space and reduce blood viscosity. Mannitol should be administered through an intravenous filter.[6,28]

SPINAL CORD INJURY

The transport team should perform a baseline evaluation of the patient with a spine injury before transfer and should monitor the patient closely for changes in neurologic status during the transfer process. All trauma patients are suspect for spine injury and should be treated accordingly.[40] These patients should be transferred supine on a firm surface with the spine in good alignment.[42] Studies suggest that logrolling of patients with spine injuries is destabilizing at the fracture site and should be avoided if possible. A scoop stretcher may be used to transfer the patient onto the rigid transport stretcher to avoid the torsion effects produced by the logrolling maneuver.[27]

When appropriate and delineated by established guidelines, patients with cervical spine injury may be transported in traction. Proper equipment, such as a spring-loaded scale system, is necessary because use of hanging weights is inappropriate in the transport setting.

ETIOLOGY AND INCIDENCE

The incidence of spinal cord injuries (SCIs) that result in paralysis or debilitating weakness as a consequence of trauma to the spinal cord has been analyzed statistically in many different ways in many different countries. Studies reported in the Head and Spinal Cord Injury System Data Bank show that the occurrence rate is about 30 to 40 new cases per million population per year.

The age distribution of acute SCIs peaks in the 15- to 24-year-old age-group. Frequency decreases in the middle-age group, with a second peak occurring at about the age of 55 years.[12,20] The incidence in women is lower for all age groups. Traffic accidents continue to be the most frequent cause of SCIs in all age groups. Among children, 65% of cases of SCI are caused by traffic accidents. Motorcycles and bicycles cause 10% to 12% of SCIs. Excessive consumption of alcohol is a factor in one third of cases involving accident victims with SCIs.[12,20]

More than half of work-related SCIs are caused by falls, and falls are the primary cause of SCIs in the home, particularly among the elderly, who fall down steps, from chairs, or off ladders.[5]

Approximately 7% of SCIs are caused by accidents that occur during sporting and recreational activities, and these SCIs most commonly occur as a result of diving into shallow water. The increasing number of women involved in sports is reflected in the rise of injuries for that group.[20]

INITIAL ASSESSMENT

Management of spine trauma begins with the realization that the patient may have an unstable spine. Whether at the accident scene or at a local referring hospital, the transport team should conduct a rapid, thorough primary and secondary assessment of the patient with an SCI before he or she is transferred. This assessment will provide a baseline for serial assessments and will reveal additional injuries and commonly associated complications, such as aspiration, neurogenic shock (bradycardia and hypotension), and poikilothermy.[16,34]

AIRWAY

The patient's airway should be checked for patency and cleared of foreign matter or secretions. While maintaining alignment of the spine, the upper airway in a patient with an altered mental status should be opened with use of the modified jaw-thrust maneuver to allow spontaneous or assisted ventilation.[1,12,51]

BREATHING

Breathing may be absent or inadequate in patients with high cervical cord injury (C4 or above), resulting in loss of both diaphragmatic and intercostal phrenic nerve intervention and paralysis of these respiratory muscles. In such cases assisted ventilation with a bag-valve mask and tracheal intubation with oxygen supplementation is indicated.[1,12,51] Rapid-sequence intubation with judicious spine immobilization may be required for airway and ventilation control.[18,35] Whatever method is chosen to manage the patient's airway, the transport team must ensure proper, consistent alignment of the entire spine.

CIRCULATION

As with all critically injured patients, intravenous access is mandatory for patients with SCIs. Intravenous lines may be inserted on the scene or en route, depending on the patient's condition, distance of transfer, and existing protocols. Isotonic solutions such as lactated Ringer's solution or normal saline solution are preferred, with the rate and volume of infusion based on the patient's cardiovascular response. Neurogenic shock may be present in patients with cervical or high thoracic spine injury. Interruption of sympathetic outflow below the level of injury results in loss of autoregulation, a decrease in vascular tone, and inability of the heart to increase its intrinsic rate. With passive vasodilation and a normal or bradycardic state, the patient becomes hypotensive.[52] The transport team should differentiate this shock state from hypovolemia and infuse crystalloids accordingly. In the absence of hypov-

olemia, the patient with an SCI can be considered "normotensive," with a blood pressure of 80 to 90 mm Hg. If the patient is hemodynamically unstable, administration of a vasoactive drug such as dopamine may be indicated. Hypovolemia must be ruled out before vasopressor therapy is begun.[1,51,52]

This sympathetic block or injury-induced sympathectomy produces poikilothermy. In this state the patient loses the ability to vasodilate and sweat in hot environments and the ability to vasoconstrict and shiver in cold environments. Thus the patient's core body temperature will often reflect the environment and must be considered if warming or cooling techniques are withheld.[35,52]

Vasovagal reflex with tracheal suctioning must also be considered for these patients. Preoxygenation is important to prevent vagal stimulation and severe bradycardia, which could lead to cardiac arrest.[35]

SECONDARY ASSESSMENT

Once the primary survey has been completed, critical interventions have been initiated, and the patient has been stabilized, the transport team can perform a secondary assessment, which includes performing a baseline neurologic evaluation; obtaining a history of the incident and of allergies, medications, previous illnesses or injuries, and the time of the patient's last meal; and completely exposing and examining the patient. Data about the mechanism and time of injury are valuable. To help expedite the transfer, this information can be obtained during the head-to-toe assessment.

Examination of the patient with an SCI should be performed with the patient maintained in a neutral position and the entire spine immobilized. A sensory and motor assessment will help the transport team determine the level and extent of injury. Autonomic function such as anal sphincter control can be assessed, and if sacral sparing is present, the injury should be considered incomplete.[1]

The transport team should visually inspect and carefully palpate the cervical spine area to determine the presence of deformity, crepitus, pain, and muscle spasm, which is frequently associated with cervical spine injury.[1] A second team member should maintain cervical spine immobilization while this is being performed.

LOWER SPINE INJURIES

The patient should be asked to wiggle his or her toes. If the patient can move the toes of both feet, he or she should be asked to raise each leg slightly, one at a time. The patient's legs should not be raised if the prior examination revealed no movement or association. If the patient shows any obvious weakness, it must be assumed that he or she has sustained an injury to the spinal cord.

CERVICAL SPINE INJURIES

The patient should be asked to wiggle his or her fingers. If the patient can do so, he or she should be asked to raise each arm one at a time. Again, substantial active movement of the upper extremity should be avoided if evidence exists of obvious fractures of the spine or extremity. The transport team should ask the patient to squeeze his or her fingers with both hands. In addition, the transport team should ascertain the patient's dominant hand and cross over, matching the team member's dominant hand to the patient's dominant hand. The strength of the patient's grasp should be similar. If the patient cannot move his or her fingers and arms or has obvious weakness, it should be assumed that the patient has an SCI in the cervical region.[19]

SENSORY EXAMINATION

The presence of a sensory deficit confirms the suspicion of a cord or nerve-root injury. The transport team should test the patient's ankles and wrists and ask the patient if he or she can feel the touch. In the event that the patient cannot feel the touch in one or more places or reports numbness and/or tingling, it can be assumed that the patient has sustained an SCI.[19]

NEUROLOGIC EXAMINATION OF THE UNCONSCIOUS PATIENT

The condition of an unconscious patient's spinal cord should be checked by pricking the skin lightly on the soles of the feet or ankles with a sharp object. If there is no spinal cord damage, the painful stimulus triggers an involuntary muscle reflex, and the extremities will move, unless the patient is in a profound coma. If the cord is damaged, there may be no such reaction. The lack of response to pinpricks in the upper extremities indicates damage to the spinal cord in the cervical region. Failure of only the lower extremities to respond indicates an SCI in the thoracic or lumbar regions.[19]

The degree of functional loss with sudden spinal cord transection depends on the level of the injury. The higher the injury, the more function lost. Complete sudden cord transection results in complete flaccid paralysis below the level of injury, areflexia (spinal shock) below the level of injury, urinary retention, and occasionally in the male patient, priapism.

Incomplete sudden cord transection results in varying degrees of paralysis and sensory loss below the level of injury, areflexia (below the level of injury), and varying degrees of bladder or bowel paralysis. Box 15-3 may be used as a guide for evaluation of muscle strength and motor function.

INTERVENTIONS AND TREATMENT

The patient with an SCI frequently has association trauma and therefore may have varying degrees of stability.[19] Judicious airway assessment and management is required for the patient with an SCI when there are injuries in the cervical region. In the absence of hypovolemia, intravenous fluids should be monitored closely and maintained at a rate that will prevent pulmonary overload. Within 8 hours of an isolated cervical spine injury, the transport team may initiate steroids if the injury is at L1 or above. Methylprednisone 30 mg/kg bolus over 15 minutes followed by an infusion of 5.4 mg/kg/hr beginning 45 minutes after is the recommended treatment of choice.[12,51] If the patient's potential spine injury has not be appropriately ruled out, the transport team must ensure that they remain immobilized until arrival at the receiving facility. However, particularly in a patient who cannot move and who may undergo a lengthy transport, assessment of the patient's skin for injury from a backboard should take place frequently. New methods of immobilization are being introduced that hopefully will

BOX 15-3	Muscles to be Tested for Evaluation of Motor Strength	
Actions to be Tested	**Muscles**	**Cord Segment**
Abduction of the arm	Deltoid	C5
Flexion of the forearm	Biceps	C5, C6
Extension of the forearm	Triceps	C7
Flexion of digits 2, 3, 4, and 5	Flexor digitorum and profundus	C8
Opposition of metacarpal of thumb	Opponens pollicis	C8, T1
Hip flexion	Iliopsoas	L12
Knee extension	Quadriceps femoris	L34
Dorsiflexion of foot	Deep peroneal	L5
Dorsiflexion of big toe	Extensor hallucis longus	L5
Plantar flexion of foot and big toe	Gastrocnemius flexor	S1

decrease the risk of skin breakdown when a patient must remain immobilized for long transports.[51]

CLASSIFICATION OF CERVICAL SPINE INJURIES BY MECHANISM OF INJURY
FLEXION INJURIES
Anterior subluxation (Box 15-3) is a flexion lesion characterized by disruption of the posterior ligament complex (Figure 15-2). Because the anterior longitudinal ligament remains intact and the disk is not completely disrupted, this lesion is stable at the time of injury and is difficult to see radiographically.[17]

Physicians disagree on whether bilateral interfacetal dislocations result from hyperflexion or a combined flexion and rotary force. Unilateral and bilateral interfacetal dislocations involve soft-tissue injury of the posterior ligament complex, and tomograms frequently reveal an unstable injury with a high incidence of cord damage.[9,17]

The stability of a simple wedge fracture depends on associated posterior ligament disruption. This flexion injury usually results from a compressive force on the anterior portion of the vertebral body with stretching of the posterior ligament complex. These fractures are generally in the mid or lower cervical segments and are considered stable fractures because of maintenance of posterior and anterior ligaments and the integrity of the interfacetal points.[17]

"Teardrop" hyperflexion fracture dislocations are seen as a result of diving or traffic accidents and falls. This type of fracture is extremely unstable because the vertebra is displaced posteriorly as the person strikes an object, and displacement disrupts the apophyseal joint capsule disk below. The anterior margin of the vertebra fractures in a teardrop-shaped fragment, and the fractured vertebra remains displaced posteriorly. Although often severe, the degree of neurologic deficit depends on the severity of hyperflexion compression. Patients who sustain "teardrop" flexion fractures frequently have acute anterior cervical cord syndrome. Immediate quadriplegia, loss of anterior cord senses (pain and temperature), and retention of posterior cord senses (position, motion, and vibration) result.[17]

FLEXION-ROTATION INJURIES
Fractures resulting from flexion-rotation are characterized by the displacement or fracture of one or more vertebrae. Fractured vertebrae may produce a unilateral facet dislocation with corresponding nerve-root compression. Severe distraction forces may cause an anterior displacement of the upper cervical body greater than 50%, which can result in bilateral locked facets and major cord injury, such as quadriplegia.[17]

EXTENSION-ROTATION INJURIES
Pillar fractures, usually caused by motor vehicle accidents and falls, are the most common "combined" injury of the cervical spine. The mechanism of injury

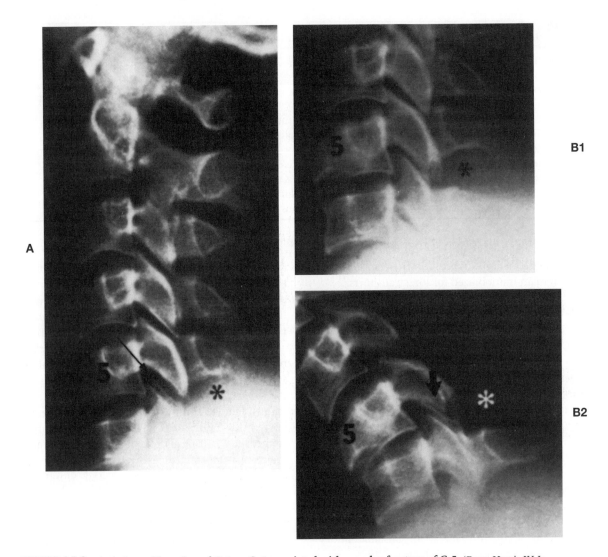

FIGURE 15-2   **Anterior subluxation of C-5 on C-6 associated with a wedge fracture of C-5.** (From Harris JH Jr, Edeiken-Monroe B: *The radiology of acute cervical spine trauma,* Baltimore, 1987, Williams and Wilkins.)

results in force concentrated on the apophyseal joints of the mid and lower cervical segments and resultant vertical fractures of a lateral mass. A distraction of the fracture elements is probably caused by rebound flexion of the head and neck.[17]

VERTICAL COMPRESSION

Compression cervical spine injuries include the "Jefferson" fracture of the atlas and the bursting

fracture of the lower cervical vertebrae. Compression fractures of the cervical spine are uncommon because the injury must occur from force transmitted vertically through the skull and occipital condyles of the spine at the precise moment the spine is straight.[17]

EXTENSION INJURIES

Most hyperextension injuries result from contact with a windshield or other structure in the interior of an automobile. Extension injuries can be of three types. The extension "teardrop" fracture is a rare extension injury that involves the anterior corner of the axis. This type of fracture is usually associated with degenerative arthritis of the cervical spine. The hangman's fracture is an unstable, bilateral fracture of the pedicles of the axis. This fracture is often associated with dislocation of the C-2 or C-3 cord segment and prevertebral soft-tissue swelling.[17] Hyperextension fracture-dislocation injuries are associated with direct force backward or a backward and upward force without an axial loading force. The typical hyperextension-dislocation injury is accompanied by the following triad of signs: (1) midface skeletal or soft-tissue injury; (2) varying degrees of central cord syndrome; and (3) a lateral cervical spine radiograph that appears normal with the exception of diffuse prevertebral soft-tissue swelling[17] (Figure 15-3). This type of extension injury is believed to be responsible for the quadriplegia in the rare patient whose cervical spine films appear normal. The probable mechanism of injury is cord compression between the posterior vertebral body, lamina, and ligamentum flavum during extension.

THORACIC SPINE INJURIES

Injuries to the thoracic and lumbar spine vary in severity from muscle strains and ligamentous strain to fractures of the vertebral body, fractures of the dorsal elements, dislocation of the facets, and complex combination fracture dislocations. The spinal cord and the nerve roots may be injured by an encroachment into the spinal canal. Patients with stable compression fractures may sustain concomitant injury to the spinal cord, and patients with grossly unstable comminuted fractures may escape neurologic injury. In general, however, the more comminuted, displaced, and unstable the spine fracture, the greater the likelihood of severe cord damage.[5]

Direct injuries to the spine and the spinal cord may occur as a result of a direct blow, such as from a falling tree limb or other heavy object, a stab wound, or a gunshot wound. Most injuries are caused by indirect trauma to the vertebral column

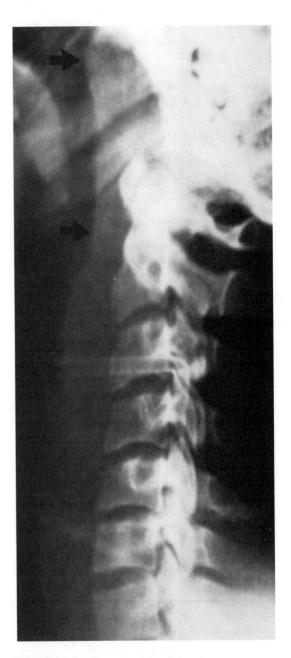

FIGURE 15-3 **Hyperextension dislocation characterized by intact cervical vertebrae and diffuse prevertebral soft tissue swelling** *(arrows)* **extending throughout the cervical region and into the nasopharynx.** (From Harris JH Jr, Edeiken-Monroe B: *The radiology of acute cervical spine trauma,* Baltimore, 1987, Williams and Wilkins.)

resulting from energy generated by forces applied to the head, shoulders, trunk, or pelvis. These forces may contain an axial load as the main force with varying degrees of lateral bending, flexion, extension, or torsion. The thoracic and lumbar spine are most commonly injured by the kinetic energy produced by the person's body traveling through space and a sudden deceleration of the shoulders, upper trunk, or buttocks against an immovable object, with the vector of forces concentrated in an area of the thoracic or the lumbar spine. The most common area is that of the thoracolumbar junction, with specific patterns of vertebral body fractures and dorsal-element dislocation at T11 and T12, rotational-flexion fractures of both body and dorsal elements at T12 to L1, and bursting fractures of the body of L1. Fractures of the midthoracic spine usually occur at the T5 or T6 level.[50]

The most common site of lumbar fractures is L2 or L3. A specific type of flexion-distraction injury occurs when a person is restrained by a seat belt and experiences sudden deceleration, which causes sudden flexion and distraction centered at the midlumbar spine. Patients with these fractures often escape spinal cord cauda equina damage, and the fracture may be overlooked in the presence of head injury or associated small intestinal injuries. Any person who has pain after being in an automobile accident in which he or she wore a seat belt must be examined specifically for the presence of a spinal fracture.

The thoracic spine is protected from injury by the rib cage, the sternum, and the chest wall. These bony structures permit little flexion and extension motion of the upper and midthoracic spine; however, there is a normal rotation motion. The lumbar spine allows for more flexion, extension, and lateral motion because it lacks the above-mentioned supporting structures.[50]

Midthoracic spine injuries are usually caused by acute flexion, rotation, and axial load forces at the midthoracic region, resulting in either a simple compression fracture of the vertebral bodies or a complex fracture dislocation in which the vertebral body and the dorsal elements are fractured.

Most injuries at the thoracolumbar junction are caused by a combination of flexion, rotation, and axial load. An injury that is centered at T11 to T12 frequently causes a dislocation without fracture of the posterior facets and a slice fracture through the upper portion of the T12 vertebral body.

Rotational forces are commonly associated with fracture dislocations of T12 to L1 level. If the injury has more of an axial load than a rotational force, the body of L1 suffers a burst injury. In this type of injury, the posterior elements of the lamina, spinous process, and facet joints may be intact or may also be fractured.

SUMMARY

The management of all neurologic traumatic emergencies includes rapid assessment, airway management with spinal immobilization, and serial examinations throughout the assessment and transfer phases. On completion of the transfer, it is important that the receiving caregivers be provided with a thorough report of events, including the time of the incident, the mechanism of injury or preceding events, care rendered by the referring facility and the transport team, response of the patient to care initiated, the past medical history of patient, and observed changes in the patient's condition. This thorough report will provide the receiving caregivers with information to guide their management and ensure continuity of care for the patient with the best possible chance for a positive outcome.

NEUROLOGIC TRAUMA CASE STUDY

A 22-year-old male unrestrained driver struck the back end of a parked car. He was thrown 25 feet from the vehicle. Because of the mechanism of injury, the local EMS agency called the flight team directly to the scene so that the patient could be transferred to a Level I trauma center.

The flight team found on arrival that the patient was unresponsive with a GCS of 5. He had facial abrasions and swelling with palpable crepitus.

1. *Eye Opening:*   1
2. *Verbal Response:*   1
3. *Motor Response:*   3

He was being ventilated by BVM, and his jaws were clenched. He was successfully intubated using RSI on the first attempt. He had strong peripheral pulses and the monitor showed a sinus tachycardia at a rate of 120. One intravenous line had been established before arrival, and the patient was appropriately immobilized and packaged for transport.

During transport, the patient's blood pressure was measured at 180/128. His heart rate decreased to 48. His right pupil became fixed and dilated.

Discussion

The patient's change in vital signs reflected his increasing intracranial pressure. Based on his blood pressure, pulse rate, and fixed dilated pupil, the flight team initiated hyperventilation at a rate of 26 and administered 50 g of mannitol in route. These acute changes in the patient's neurologic status were clear indications for aggressive management to decrease his ICP.

On arrival at the receiving facility, the patient's blood pressure had decreased to 160/100, and his heart rate had increased to 100. He was taken for emergent CT, which showed a large epidural with mass effect on the left. He was then taken to the operating room for decompression.

REFERENCES

1. *Advanced Trauma Life Support Course for Physicians,* Chicago, 1997, American College of Surgeons Committee on Trauma, ATLS/ACS.
2. Anderson L, Rose W, Edmond S: Analysis of intubations: before and after establishment of a rapid sequence intubation protocol, *Scientific Abstract,* 15th Annual Air Medical Transport Conference, Detroit, Michigan, October 17-21, 1994.
3. Baker S, O'Neill B, Karpf R: *The injury fact book,* Lexington, Mass, 1984, Lexington Books.
4. Becker DP, Gardner S: Intensive management of head injury. In *Neurosurgery,* vol 2, St Louis, 1985, McGraw-Hill.
5. Bohlman HH, Ducker TB, Lucas JT: Spine and spinal cord injuries. In Rothman RH, Simeone FA, editors: *The spine,* vol 2, Philadelphia, 1982, Saunders.
6. Bullock R et al: *Management and prognosis of severe traumatic brain injury,* New York, 2000, Brain Trauma Foundation and American Association of Neurological Surgeons.
7. Chen FH, Fetzer JD: Complete cricotracheal separation and third cervical spinal cord transection following blunt neck trauma: a case report of one survivor, *J Trauma* 35(1):140, 1993.
8. Chestnut RM, Marshall LF: Management of head injury: treatment of abnormal intracranial pressure, *Neurosurg Clin North Am* 2(2):267, 1991.
9. Cooper PR, Chalif DJ: Fractures and dislocations of the upper cervical spine, *Contemp Neurosurg* 5(16):1, 1983.
10. Crutchfield WG: Skeletal traction for dislocation of cervical spine: report of a case, *Southern Surgeon* 2:156, 1933.
11. Davis M, Lucatorto M: Mannitol revisited, *J Neurosci Nurs* 26(3):170, 1994.
12. Emergency Nurses Association: *Trauma nursing core course,* ed. 5, Des Plaines, Ill, 2000, Author.
13. Fessler RD, Diaz FG: The management of cerebral perfusion pressure and intracranial pressure after severe head injury, *Ann Emerg Med* 22(6):998, 1993.
14. Gennarelli T, Thibault L: Biomechanics of head injury. In *Neurosurgery,* vol 2, St Louis, 1985, McGraw-Hill.
15. Gennarelli TA et al: Diffuse axonal injury and traumatic coma in the primate, *Ann Neurol* 12:564, 1982.
16. Geisler FH: Acute management of cervical spinal cord injury, *Trauma Q* 4(3), May 1988.
17. Harris JH Jr: *The radiology of acute cervical spine trauma,* Baltimore, 1987, Williams and Wilkins.
18. Hastings RH, Wood PR: Head extension and laryngeal view during laryngoscopy with cervical spine immobilization maneuvers, *Anesthesiology* 80(4):825, 1994.
19. Hickey J: *The clinical practice of neurological and neurosurgical nursing,* ed 2, Philadelphia, 1985, Lippincott.
20. National Academy of Sciences, National Academy of Engineering and the Institute of Medicine: *Injury in America: a continuing public health problem,* Chicago, 1985, National Academy Press.
21. Jennett B, Teasdale G: *Management of head injuries,* Philadelphia, 1981, Davis.
22. Keller TS, Schneider RC: Craniocerebral trauma. In *Correlative neurosurgery,* ed 3, vol 2, Springfield, Ill, 1982, Charles C Thomas.

23. Krupa D: *Flight nursing core curriculum*. Des Plaines, Ill, 1997, Air and Surface Transport Nurses Association.

24. Littlejohns LR, Bader MK: Guidelines for the management of severe head injury: Clinical application and change in practice, *Critical Care Nurse* 21(6):48, 2001.

25. Manifold S: Craniocerebral trauma: a review of primary and secondary injury and therapeutic modalities, *Focus Crit Care* 13:33, 1986.

26. Marshall LE: Surgical treatment of extracerebral lesions in head injury. In Pitts LH, Wagner FC Jr, editors: *Craniospinal trauma*, New York, 1990, Thieme Medical.

27. McGuire RA et al: Spine instability and logrolling maneuver, *J Trauma* 27:525, 1987.

28. McQuillan KA, Mitchell PH: Traumatic brain injuries. In McQuillan KA et al, editors: *Trauma nursing: from resuscitation through rehabilitation,* ed 3, Philadelphia, 2002, Saunders.

29. Miller JD: Head injury and brain ischemia, *Br J Anesthesiol* 57:120, 1985.

30. Morris M, Kinkade S: The effect of capnometry on manual ventilation technique, *Air Med J* 14(2):79, 1995.

31. Muizelaar JP, Schroder ML: Overview of monitoring of cerebral blood flow and metabolism after severe head injury, *Can J Neurol Sci* 21(2):S6, 1994.

32. Nayduch D, Lee A, Butler D: High-dose methylprednisolone after acute spinal cord injury, *Crit Care Nurse* 14(4):69, 1994.

33. Neave V, Weiss M: Neurological evaluation of a patient with head trauma: coma scales. In *Neurosurgery*, vol 2, St Louis, 1985, McGraw-Hill.

34. Nikas D: Pathophysiology and nursing interventions in acute SCI, *Trauma Q* 4(3), May 1988.

35. Norwood S, Myers MB, Butler TJ: The safety of emergency neuromuscular blockade and orotracheal intubation in the acutely injured trauma patient, *J Am Coll Surg* 179(6):646, 1994.

36. Oman KS: Commentary on methylprednisolone for acute spinal cord injury, *ENA's Nurs Scan Emerg Care* 3(1):11, 1993.

37. Peterson C, Budd R, Balazs K: Comparative evaluation of three end-tidal CO_2 monitors used during air medical transport, *J Air Med Transport* 11(2):7, 1992.

38. Popp A, Bourke R: Pathophysiology of head injury. In *Neurosurgery,* vol 2, St Louis, 1985, McGraw-Hill.

39. Prolo DJ, Hanbery JW: Cervical stabilization-traction board, *J Am Med Assoc* 224(5):615, 1973.

40. Saboe LA et al: Spine trauma and associated injuries, *J Trauma* 31(1):43, 1991.

41. Seeling JM et al: Traumatic acute subdural hematoma: major mortality reduction in comatose patients treated within four hours, *N Engl J Med* 304:1511, 1981.

42. Smith M, Bourn S, Larmm B: Ties that bind-immobilizing the injury spine, *J Emerg Med Serv* 14(4), 1989.

43. Sullivan TE et al: Closed head injury assessment and research methodology, *J Neurosci Nurs* 26(1):24, 1994.

44. Tabaddor K: Nonoperative management of head trauma, *Contemp Neurosurg* 2(26):1, 1980.

45. Temkin NR, Dikem SS, Winn HR: Management of head injury, posttraumatic seizures, *Neurosurg Clin North Am* 2(2):425, 1991.

46. Ward JD: Management of head injury: prehospital care, *Neurosurg Clin North Am* 2(2):251, 1991.

47. Watts C: Trauma to the cervical spine, *Mod Med* 101, 1986.

48. White RJ: Acute evacuation and management of head injury. In Najarian JS, Delaney JP, editors: *Emergency surgery: trauma-shock-sepsis-burns*, St Louis, 1982, Mosby.

49. White RJ, Likavec MJ: Current concepts: the diagnosis and initial management of head injury, *N Engl J Med* 327(21):1507, 1992.

50. Whiteside TE Jr, Shah S: On management of unstable fractures of thoraco-lumbar spine, *Spine* 1:99, 1976.

51. Wraa C, editor: *Transport nursing advanced trauma course,* ed 3, Denver, 2001, Air and Surface Transport Nurses Association.

52. Yablon SA: Posttraumatic seizures, *Arch Physical Med Rehabil* 74(9):983, 1993.

THORACIC TRAUMA

16

COMPETENCIES

1. Perform a patient assessment identifying the indications of a thoracic injury.
2. Identify signs and symptoms of life-threatening thoracic injuries, including a tension pneumothorax, a hemothorax, and a flail chest.
3. Initiate appropriate critical interventions to manage a thoracic injury.

Thoracic injuries present a demanding challenge for patient transport. Approximately 25% of all trauma deaths involve thoracic injuries. Thoracic injury remains second only to central nervous system injury as the leading cause of all trauma deaths.[1] In the pediatric population, with the exception of lung contusions, serious injuries to vital thoracic structures are associated with a mortality rate of more than 50%.[8] An understanding of the severity and mechanism of injury, management concerns of specific thoracic injuries, and special transport considerations aids the transport team in providing care.

Thoracic trauma is classified by either the mechanism of injury or the degree to which the injury is life threatening. Classification of thoracic trauma by mechanism of injury encompasses two categories: blunt and penetrating traumas. Blunt trauma is associated with motor vehicle crashes, compression injuries, falls, and assaults. Penetrating trauma occurs as a result of gunshot wounds, stab wounds, and impalement.

Thoracic injuries may also be categorized as life-threatening or potentially life-threatening conditions. Life-threatening thoracic conditions are airway obstruction, tension pneumothorax, massive hemothorax, open pneumothorax, flail chest, cardiac tamponade, aortic rupture, and myocardial rupture. Potentially life-threatening conditions are myocardial contusion, pulmonary contusion, aortic disruption, tracheobronchial disruption, esophageal rupture, and diaphragmatic disruption. Because many of the thoracic injuries are life threatening, rapid transport to a regional trauma center or tertiary care setting may be indicated.

Special considerations for in-flight care of the patient with thoracic trauma relate to altitude changes and gas expansion. As previously discussed in transport physiology, gases expand with increasing altitude. Because of this, a patient with an untreated pneumothorax or a nonfunctioning chest tube may be at great risk for a tension pneumothorax developing.[25] As part of the anticipatory planning and managing of care during transport, the way changes in altitude may affect a patient with thoracic injuries must be considered.

The greatest threat in the management of a patient with a thoracic injury is hypoxia.[25] After thoracic injury, the contributing causes of hypoxia may be decreased blood volume, failure to ventilate the lungs, ventilation-perfusion mismatches, or pressure changes within the intrapleural space. The ABCs of resuscitation (maintenance of airway, breathing, and circulation) serve as a framework for management of each injury. The ABC framework assists in quick detection of life-threatening injuries and implementation of rapid interventions.

LIFE-THREATENING THORACIC INJURIES

TENSION PNEUMOTHORAX

ETIOLOGIC FACTORS
Both blunt and penetrating thoracic trauma cause tension pneumothorax, or it can occur as a complication of treatment of an open pneumothorax. Air progressively accumulates under pressure, and the flap of the injured lung acts as a one-way valve; air is allowed to enter the pleural space on inspiration but not allowed to escape on expiration.

PATHOPHYSIOLOGIC FACTORS
Ventilation is inadequate because the air entering the pleural space increases the intrapleural pressure with each inspiration. This causes collapse of the ipsilateral lung and a mediastinal shift to the opposite side, leading to compression of the contralateral lung (Figure 16-1). Perfusion becomes inadequate because of decreased venous return to the heart as a result of the increased intrapleural pressure and shift of mediastinal structures.

ASSESSMENT
The mechanism of injury establishes a high index of suspicion. The patient with a tension pneumothorax will exhibit severe respiratory distress, dyspnea, and cyanosis. Agitation and anxiety are common.[13,19] Clinical evidence of shock may be present. Breath sounds will be either decreased or absent over the involved hemithorax. The trachea should

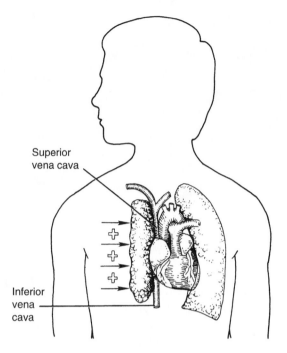

FIGURE 16-1   **Tension pneumothorax.** (From Sheehy SB: *Emergency nursing: principles and practice,* ed 3, St Louis, 1992, Mosby.)

be assessed because a shift to the unaffected side occurs as intrapleural pressure increases. As air passes into the tissues, subcutaneous emphysema can be palpated. Jugular venous distention occurs because of the increased intrapleural pressure. Constant observation of the patient's chest excursion is important during transport because auscultation is next to impossible.

INTERVENTIONS
The immediate lifesaving intervention is rapid decompression of the pleural space. To release the intrapleural pressure, a large-bore needle should be placed into the pleural space, specifically into the second intercostal space, two-finger breadths lateral to the sternal border on the affected side. The needle should then be placed superior to the rib margin to avoid the intercostal artery. The anterior site is used for avoidance of the internal mammary vessels.[5,13,19] If a tension pneumothorax is present, the

air within the pleural space will force the plunger out of the syringe attached to the needle, or a rush of air may be heard.

The needle thoracostomy should be converted to a tube thoracostomy as soon as possible. A single chest tube is acceptable for a pneumothorax, hemothorax, or hemopneumothorax.[16] In addition, intravenous access and fluid resuscitation should be done. Supplemental oxygen using a nonrebreather mask is indicated because hypoxia is a real threat.

EVALUATION

Constant reevaluation of the patient's cardiopulmonary status is warranted. If a chest tube is placed and a persistent air leak occurs, the presence of a tracheobronchial disruption must be considered.

MASSIVE HEMOTHORAX

ETIOLOGIC FACTORS

Massive hemothorax develops as a result of blunt or penetrating injuries of intrathoracic organs or laceration of an intercostal artery. The rapid and massive accumulation of blood and fluid in the pleural space can result in severe hemodynamic compromise.

PATHOPHYSIOLOGIC FACTORS

The compliant lung offers little resistance to a large amount of blood becoming sequestered in the pleural space (Figure 16-2), and hypovolemic shock results. Compression of the ipsilateral lung occurs

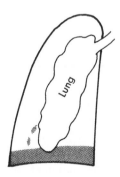

FIGURE 16-2   **Hemothorax.** (From Sheehy SB: *Emergency nursing: principles and practice*, ed 3, St Louis, 1992, Mosby.)

from the accumulation of blood, and a mediastinal shift can occur from compression of the contralateral lung. In this way ventilation-perfusion mismatches happen.

ASSESSMENT

The mechanism of injury is vital to the initial assessment of the patient suspected of having a massive hemothorax. Because of the decrease in blood volume, manifestations of hypovolemic shock will appear. Altered mentation, decrease in blood pressure, increase in heart rate, and signs of peripheral vasoconstriction are common. Breath sounds are decreased or absent over the involved hemothorax, and chest excursion on the affected side is decreased. Unlike the symptoms of cardiac tamponade, the trachea is generally in the midline, and the neck veins are flat.[21]

INTERVENTIONS

Restoration of lost blood volume is of primary importance, and an initial response is to achieve intravenous access with at least two large-bore catheters and to administer crystalloids or colloids. Supplemental oxygen should be administered. Endotracheal intubation may be required. Emergent management involves placement of a tube thoracostomy.

Fluid resuscitation must be carefully monitored. The transport team must also be cognizant that excessive fluid resuscitation, particularly in penetrating thoracic trauma, can be detrimental.

In cases of massive hemothorax, the transport team may consider autotransfusion. The use of autotransfusion in thoracic trauma patients has been greatly debated because of the potential effect of anticoagulants and abdominal contaminants.[3,15] Considerations related to autotransfusion are transport delay during supply setup and space limitation during transport. In situations of prolonged transport times, isolated chest trauma, conflicting religious beliefs, or cross-matching difficulty, autotransfusion may serve as a bridge until definitive care is provided. The need for surgical intervention, a thoracotomy, is based not only on the initial amount of chest tube drainage, hemodynamic status, and fluid resuscitation amounts, but also on the location of chest-wall penetration or the rate of ongoing blood loss (200 ml/hr).[3,17]

EVALUATION
The transport crew members must constantly reassesses the ventilatory status of the patient and monitor the parameters of the patient's response to volume replacement.

OPEN PNEUMOTHORAX
ETIOLOGIC FACTORS
A penetrating object causes an open pneumothorax, or sucking chest wound. Air enters the pleural space through the opening or defect in the chest wall (Figure 16-3).

PATHOPHYSIOLOGIC FACTORS
If the diameter of the chest-wall defect is greater than the diameter of the patient's trachea, air will move through the chest wound rather than through the trachea and airways. The defect in the thoracic wall leads to an equilibration of atmospheric and pleural pressure. The result is loss of the negative intrathoracic pressure, which leads to respiratory insufficiency. Air in the pleural space promotes collapse of the ipsilateral lung and a mediastinal shift to the unaffected side. The mediastinal shift and loss of

normal negative intrathoracic pressure produce decreased venous return to the heart and cardiac insufficiency.

ASSESSMENT
A penetrating injury to the thorax should lead the transport team to closely assess the thorax to determine whether a sucking chest wound is present. The patient will be in respiratory distress, with tachypnea and grunting, and as air enters and leaves the pleural space through the chest-wall defect, a sucking noise may be heard during respiration. Clinical manifestations of shock occur as a result of intermittent obstruction of venous return.[13,19]

INTERVENTIONS
In the prehospital setting the wound should be covered, but not sealed, with an occlusive dressing. A dressing taped on three sides creates a flutter-valve effect; air is prevented from entering the chest on inspiration but is not prevented from leaving the chest on expiration. If an occlusive dressing is used and a defect in the lung exists, a tension pneumothorax may develop because the air is not allowed to escape from the pleural space.

If a tension pneumothorax develops, the occlusive dressing should be immediately removed. The patient may require the placement of a chest tube to treat the underlying lung defect.[5,25] If the patient's ventilation and oxygenation continue to deteriorate, the team should immediately prepare to intubate. Maintenance of intravenous access is also imperative as a route for volume resuscitation and medication administration.

EVALUATION
Evaluation must consist of continuous monitoring of the patient's cardiopulmonary status. Assessment parameters for expanding pneumothoraces are limited during transport because of the background noise levels. Astute evaluation of the patient's chest pain, tachycardia, increasing dyspnea, tracheal deviation, and development of subcutaneous emphysema prompts the flight nurse to begin hemodynamic compromise.[1,25]

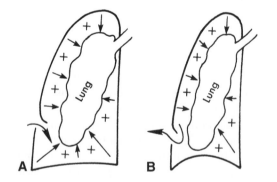

FIGURE 16-3 **Sucking chest wound. A,** Inspiration. **B,** Expiration. (From Sheehy SB: *Emergency nursing: principles and practice,* ed 3, St Louis, 1992, Mosby.)

FLAIL CHEST

ETIOLOGIC FACTORS

A flail chest usually occurs as a result of blunt thoracic trauma. Multiple rib fractures cause separation of a portion of the rib cage and loss of stability of the chest wall. The flail segment usually involves the anterior or lateral chest wall because heavy posterior muscles and the scapula protect the posterior chest wall.

PATHOPHYSIOLOGIC FACTORS

Paradoxical chest movement interferes with the normal "bellows" function of the thoracic cage, causing inadequate gas exchange. The underlying pulmonary contusion causes progressive respiratory insufficiency. The instability of the chest wall and the pain from the fracture sites lead to hypoventilation and subsequent hypoxemia.

ASSESSMENT

Observation of chest excursion is important; however, the paradoxical movement may not be obvious except in cases of severe flail. The flail segment moves in the opposite direction from the rest of the thoracic cage during respiration, moving inward during inspiration and outward during expiration (Figure 16-4). Initially, the flail may not be obvious because of spasms of the muscles in the thoracic wall. The patient is also in respiratory distress, with cyanosis, grunting, and use of accessory muscles, and will report severe chest pain on the involved side.

INTERVENTIONS

For the patient in severe distress, endotracheal intubation will be required to treat hypoxia. The patient should be manually ventilated if the transport ventilator does not have the appropriate settings to recognize the development of a tension pneumothorax. External stabilization techniques include application of gentle pressure over the flail segment with a pillow or a pad or placement of the patient with the injured side down, if their condition allows. And of course, the patient needs intravenous access and supplemental oxygen.

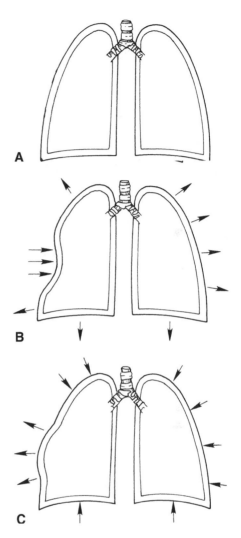

FIGURE 16-4 **Flail chest. A,** Normal lungs. **B,** Flail chest on inspiration. **C,** Flail chest on expiration. (From Sheehy SB: *Emergency nursing: principles and practice,* ed 3, St Louis, 1992, Mosby.)

EVALUATION

Constant reassessment of the patient's cardiopulmonary status is vital to treatment of the patient with a flail chest. Mentation, skin color, and Sao_2 measurements, in addition to vital signs, are parameters to monitor. Pain control cannot be accomplished until the patient's condition is fully evaluated.

ACUTE CARDIAC TAMPONADE
ETIOLOGIC FACTORS
Acute cardiac tamponade occurs when blood accumulates in the pericardial sac (Figure 16-5) as a result of blunt and penetrating cardiac trauma.

PATHOPHYSIOLOGIC FACTORS
The hemodynamic effects of cardiac tamponade depend on how quickly fluid (blood) accumulates in the pericardial sac; rapid accumulation of blood (from 150 to 250 ml) may be fatal because the normal pericardial sac contains 20 to 50 ml of pericardial fluid. If the accumulation is slow, the fibrous pericardium stretches and can accommodate several liters of fluid without hemodynamic consequences. The main hemodynamic consequence is a decrease in diastolic filling because of increased intrapericardial pressure. Once the diastolic filling decreases, stroke volume and cardiac output fall. Central venous pressure increases as a result of increased intrapericardial pressure.

ASSESSMENT
The patient with acute cardiac tamponade will show signs of decreased cardiac output, such as altered mental status, cool, clammy skin, tachycardia, and a falling arterial blood pressure. Venous hypertension also occurs, as evidenced by marked neck-vein distention (unless the patient is hypovolemic) and rising central venous pressure. Distant, muffled heart sounds may not be detectable in the field. Pulsus paradoxus is a fall in the systolic blood pressure greater than 15 mm Hg during normal inspiration.[14]

INTERVENTIONS
The patient needs a patent airway and supplemental oxygen. Intravenous access and continuous assessment for signs of decreasing cardiac output are necessary.

The initial treatment of a patient with suspected cardiac tamponade is a rapid intravenous fluid bolus.[5,15,25] This measure improves filling pressures and temporarily improves cardiac output until pericardiocentesis can be performed. The emergent treatment of choice is pericardiocentesis (Figure 16-6).[10,25] A needle is placed into the pericardial sac and may withdraw as little as 15 to 20 ml of blood to improve the patient's condition. Pericardial blood will generally not clot because it has been defibrinated by heart motion. Pericardiocentesis is extremely challenging to perform during flight because of the confined environment and air turbulence.

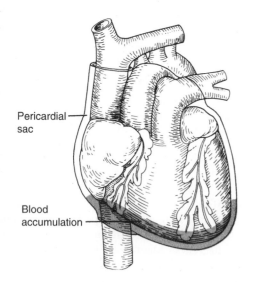

FIGURE 16-5   **Cardiac tamponade.** (From Sheehy SB: *Emergency nursing: principles and practice*, ed 3, St Louis, 1992, Mosby.)

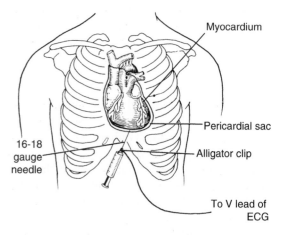

FIGURE 16-6   **Pericardiocentesis.** (From Sheehy SB: *Emergency nursing: principles and practice*, ed 3, St Louis, 1992, Mosby.)

Because the long-term survival rate is less than 10%, aggressive interventions offer the best chance for patient survival. Failure to diagnose and repair aortic injuries within 24 hours of the patient's arrival results in mortality rates of 25% to 40%.[11] The transesophageal echocardiogram has been used as a rapid, accurate, and safe method of aortic transection identification.[20,22] Early recognition of this injury and rapid transport to definitive care is imperative.

EVALUATION

When a trauma patient continues to deteriorate even with aggressive management, the transport team should consider acute pericardial tamponade.

AORTIC RUPTURE
ETIOLOGIC AND PATHOPHYSIOLOGIC FACTORS

Aortic rupture occurs as a result of blunt or penetrating trauma, and death occurs immediately in 80% to 90% of patients, although when the rupture or transection occurs in only the medial and intimal layers, the intact adventitia may prevent exsanguination temporarily.

ASSESSMENT

The patient may not show any external signs of chest trauma. Severe chest and midscapular pain is not uncommon. If conscious, the patient will report dyspnea. Hypertension in the upper extremities is caused by a periaortic hematoma, partial aortic occlusion, or stretching of the cardiac plexus; a harsh systolic murmur can be auscultated along the precordium. If a radiograph of the chest has been done (before interfacility transport), findings that promote a high index of suspicion on the part of the transport team are (1) widening of the superior mediastinum, (2) loss of aortic knob shadow, (3) fracture of the first rib, (4) depression of the left main stem bronchus, (5) deviation of the trachea to the right, (6) pleural capping, and (7) deviation of the gastric tube in the esophagus.[9,25]

INTERVENTIONS

The ABCs of resuscitation are necessary because it is impossible to prevent patient death if complete rupture occurs in flight. An immediate exploratory thoracotomy may be necessary.

MYOCARDIAL RUPTURE
ETIOLOGIC AND PATHOPHYSIOLOGIC FACTORS

Rupture of the heart is the most lethal of blunt thoracic injuries.[18] Death occurs as a result of exsanguination. However, 61 cases of survival of nonpenetrating rupture of the myocardium have been reported; the majority were men who had been involved in motor vehicle accidents.[23]

ASSESSMENT AND INTERVENTIONS

Absent vital signs are key indicators that a fatal event has occurred. Resuscitation efforts are those used for any traumatically injured patient.

POTENTIALLY LIFE-THREATENING INJURIES

MYOCARDIAL CONTUSION
ETIOLOGIC FACTORS

Blunt trauma is the mechanism that produces myocardial contusion. The compression of the heart between the sternum and vertebrae occurs as a result of motor vehicle accidents, falls, or blows to the chest.

PATHOPHYSIOLOGIC FACTORS

Lesions may vary in size from small areas of petechiae to large contusions and necrosis of the myocardium. Bleeding and edema occur at the site of injury.

ASSESSMENT

The patient should be suspected of having a myocardial contusion based on mechanism of injury, for example, blunt trauma to the chest. The patient may be completely asymptomatic or may report chest pain that is characteristically identical to that of angina or acute myocardial infarction. Sinus tachycardia is common, and cardiac arrhythmias may occur. Patients at risk are those who have abnormal initial electrocardiogram findings with ST-T segment changes.[8] Use of cardiac enzymes as a diagnostic tool in patients with suspected myocardial contusions has been found to be of little value.[2]

INTERVENTIONS

Management is similar to that for a patient who has sustained an acute myocardial infarction. Supplemental oxygen, intravenous access, and prophylactic lidocaine are part of the treatment regimen. Recent studies question the efficacy of critical care unit monitoring and lengthy hospitalization for patients with simple myocardial contusions.[6,12]

PULMONARY CONTUSION

ETIOLOGIC FACTORS

Pulmonary contusion occurs as a result of blunt thoracic trauma. It is not uncommon for pulmonary contusion to be associated with a flail chest or other blunt injuries to the chest.

PATHOPHYSIOLOGIC FACTORS

Intraalveolar hemorrhage and edema occur as a result of blunt injury to the lung parenchyma. The alveolar-capillary integrity is lost, and interstitial hemorrhage and edema occur. Systemic hypoxemia is caused by decreased lung compliance and ventilation-perfusion mismatches.[16]

ASSESSMENT

The patient has a history of blunt thoracic trauma and usually demonstrates dyspnea and tachypnea. Tachycardia and anxiety, which may be caused by the stress of injury or hypoxemia, are also not uncommon. Rales and rhonchi are auscultated over the injured area. Lack of improvement in oxygen saturation during transport, despite oxygen therapy, may also indicate a pulmonary contusion. Maximum changes are seen in the chest radiograph from 48 to 72 hours after the injury.[4,25]

INTERVENTIONS

Adequate ventilation with an aggressive pulmonary toilet is necessary. Supplemental oxygen should be administered. Endotracheal intubation is necessary when the P_{O_2} is lower than 60 mm Hg on room air or lower than 80 mm Hg with supplemental oxygen. Intravenous fluids, if not needed for resuscitation of other injuries, should be restricted. Corticosteroid use is controversial but may be used by some trauma surgeons.

DIAPHRAGMATIC RUPTURE

ETIOLOGIC FACTORS

Herniation of abdominal viscera into the chest occurs when there is a traumatic defect in the diaphragm produced by blunt or penetrating trauma to the upper abdomen or lower thorax. If the injury occurred at the time the diaphragm was contracting strongly, a large avulsion tear will result. The vast majority of diaphragmatic ruptures occur on the left side because the liver protects the right hemidiaphragm.[1,4,23]

PATHOPHYSIOLOGIC FACTORS

Herniation of abdominal contents into the thoracic cavity causes compression of the ipsilateral lung and displacement of mediastinal structures. Cardiopulmonary insufficiency results, causing significantly reduced respiratory efficiency. The herniated viscerae are compressed, causing gastric or intestinal obstruction and/or ischemia and gangrene.

ASSESSMENT

The patient may initially be asymptomatic or in severe distress. Abdominal or chest pain radiating to the shoulder may be present; dyspnea and cyanosis are also common signs. A paralytic ileus may accompany the injuries, so detection of bowel sounds may not be possible in the thorax cavity. Breath sounds will be either decreased or absent on the side of the herniation. The abdomen will be markedly scaphoid. There will be a mediastinal shift to the unaffected side.[1,4,5,23,25]

INTERVENTIONS

Hypoxia should be treated, and ventilation must be maintained. The transport team undertakes intravenous access and routine resuscitative measures, and immediate surgery for repair is indicated.

TRACHEOBRONCHIAL DISRUPTION
ETIOLOGIC FACTORS

Tracheobronchial disruption occurs most often from blunt trauma. Penetrating thoracic trauma is a less-common cause.

PATHOPHYSIOLOGIC FACTORS

Air passes through the tear into the pleural space or the mediastinum. In the pleural space it produces a pneumothorax; in the mediastinum it causes mediastinal emphysema. The patient's airway may be maintained initially because the tracheobronchial cartilage holds the lumen open.

ASSESSMENT

Hemoptysis, respiratory distress, and subcutaneous or mediastinal emphysema (or both) are present. A pneumothorax with a persistent air leak or failure of a lung to reexpand after tube thoracostomy should lead the transport team to suspect a tracheobronchial disruption. A tension pneumothorax may be the first visible sign of the problem.

INTERVENTIONS

The transport team performs immediate endotracheal intubation with placement of the tube below the level of injury. Rapid transport for bronchoscopy and chest tube placement should be accomplished as soon as possible.[1,25]

ESOPHAGEAL PERFORATION
ETIOLOGIC FACTORS

The most common cause of esophageal perforation is iatrogenic traumatic instrumentation, although penetrating trauma, ingestion of a foreign body, or blunt trauma also can be causes.[14,24]

PATHOPHYSIOLOGIC FACTORS

Gastric contents and bacteria leaking into the mediastinum can lead not only to mediastinitis but also to fatal, systemic toxicity. Perforation also results in massive fluid loss and can lead to hypovolemic shock.

ASSESSMENT

The location of the perforation will determine the clinical signs and symptoms. Subcutaneous emphysema, dyspnea, dysphagia, fever, hematemesis, and shock are common observations.

INTERVENTIONS

Intravenous access, gastric tube placement, antibiotic administration, and immediate surgery are the interventions of choice for esophageal perforation.

SUMMARY

Transportation of a patient with a traumatic thoracic injury requires anticipatory planning to have all necessary equipment available. The transport team's prompt recognition and treatment of thoracic traumatic injuries may reduce mortality and morbidity, especially ensuring patency of the airway and performing specific measures for blunt or penetrating injuries.

THORACIC TRAUMA CASE STUDY

The transport team was called to the scene of a high-speed single-car rollover motor vehicle crash. The patient was restrained, and because the car suffered extensive damage, he was trapped for more than 45 minutes. The patient was being removed from the vehicle when the transport team arrived by air.

The primary survey completed and reported by the ground emergency medical service personnel revealed that the patient had an open airway, was having slightly labored breathing, and had a weak, palpable pulse. There was no obvious bleeding. His GCS was 7 (E-1 ; V-1; M-5). There were multiple lacerations and abrasions on his face and upper extremities.

The secondary assessment, performed by the flight nurse on arrival at the scene of the accident, showed the following:

Vital signs: BP: 164/110, HR: 96, RR: 36
Pupils: PERL
Airway: Open
No obvious deformities of skull or face

GCS: 7

Chest expansion asymmetric, but breath sounds could be heard over both sides, though they were decreased on the right

Minor abrasions to chest and back area

No other wounds or abnormalities noted

No abdominal wounds or distention noted

No obvious deformity to extremities

The transport team then initiated the following interventions.

The patient was immobilized on a long board with a cervical collar and head blocks.

Emergency medical service personnel initiated two large-bore peripheral intravenous lines in each arm.

Because of the patient's GCS of 7, RSI was used to intubate the patient on the first attempt with a no. 7.5 endotracheal tube. The patient was then hot-loaded for transport to the trauma center.

During flight, it became increasingly difficult for the patient to ventilate. His heart rate dropped to 48. His oxygen saturation decreased to 88%. Because of the limited cabin size (BO105) and the inability to auscultate breath sounds, the flight nurse elected to perform a needle thoracostomy with a no. 14 gauge needle in the second intercostal space on the right side. There was immediate improvement in ventilation, and the patient's heart rate increased to 100.

The patient was hot off-loaded and taken to the trauma bay for resuscitation.

Outcome

The patient was received in the emergency department of the area trauma center by the trauma team and was assessed by the trauma team. A chest tube was immediately inserted in the right chest. A FAST exam revealed fluid and the patient was taken directly to the OR for further evaluation.

REFERENCES

1. American College of Surgeons Committee on Trauma: Thoracic trauma. *Advanced trauma life support student manual,* Chicago, Ill, 1997, American College of Surgeons.

2. Biffl WL et al: Cardiac enzymes are irrelevant in the patient with suspected myocardial contusion, *Am J Surg* 168(6):523, 1994.

3. Blansfield J: Emergency autotransfusion in hypovolemia, *Crit Care Nurs Clin North Am* 2(2):195, 1990.

4. Bledsoe BE, Porter RS, Cherry RA: *Paramedic care: principles and practice: trauma emergencies,* Upper Saddle River, NJ, 2001, Brady/Prentice Hall Health.

5. Campbell JE: *Basic trauma life support,* ed 4, Upper Saddle River, NJ, 2000, Brady/Prentice Hall Health.

6. Christensen MA, Sutton KR: Myocardial contusion: new concepts in diagnosis and management, *Am J Crit Care* 2(1):28, 1993.

7. Cohn SM et al: Exclusion of aortic tear in the unstable trauma patient: the utility of transesophageal echocardiography, *J Trauma* 39(6):1087, 1995.

8. Cooper A: Thoracic injuries, *Semin Pediatr Surg* 4(2):109, 1995.

9. Daleiden A: Clinical manifestations of blunt cardiac injury: a challenge to the critical care nurse, *Crit Care Nurs Q* 17(2):13, 1994.

10. Feczko JD et al: An autopsy case review of 142 nonpenetrating (blunt) injuries of the aorta, *J Trauma* 33(1): 846, 1992.

11. Fildes JJ et al: Limiting cardiac evaluation in patients with suspected myocardial contusion, *Am Surg* 69(9):832, 1995.

12. Herron H, Falcone RE: Prehospital decompression for suspected tension pneumothorax, *Air Med J* 14(2):69, 1995.

13. Klygis LM et al: Esophageal perforations masked by steroids, *Abdom Imaging* 18(1):10, 1993.

14. Krupa D: *Flight nursing core curriculum,* Des Plaines, Ill, 1997, Road Runner Press.

15. Kshettry VR: Chest trauma, assessment, diagnosis, and management, *Clin Chest Med* 15(1):137, 1994.

16. Newberry L. editor: *Sheehy's emergency nursing principles and practice,* ed 4, St Louis, 1998, Mosby.

17. Nichols CG, Larson RE, Schmidt EW, editors: *A practical approach to emergency medicine: autotransfusion,* Boston, 1993, Little, Brown.

18. Pevec WC, Udekwu AO, Peitzman AB: Blunt rupture of myocardium, *Ann Thorac Surg* 48:139, 1989.

19. Rutter KM: Action stat! tension pneumothorax, *Nursing* 25(4):33, 1995.

20. Saletta S et al: Transesophageal echocardiography for the initial evaluation of the widened mediastinum in trauma patients, *J Trauma* 39(1):137, 1995.

21. Schrader KA: Penetrating chest trauma, *Crit Care Nurs Clin North Am* 5(4):687, 1993.

22. Shively BK: Transesophageal echocardiography in the diagnosis of aortic disease, *Semin Ultrasound CT MR* 14(2):106, 1993.

23. Sukul DM, Kats E, Johannes EJ: Sixty-three cases of traumatic injury of the diaphragm, *Injury* 22(4):303, 1991.

24. Tucker JG, Kim HH, Lucas GW: Esophageal perforation caused by coin ingestion, *South Med J* 87(2):269, 1994.

25. Wraa C, editor: *Transport nursing advanced trauma course,* ed 3, Denver, 2001, Air and Surface Transport Nurses Association.

ABDOMINAL TRAUMA

17

COMPETENCIES

1. Perform an organized and focused abdominal assessment.
2. Identify signs of abdominal trauma.
3. Initiate critical interventions and provide appropriate treatment for the patient with an abdominal injury during transport.

Regionalized trauma care has drastically reduced the incidence of death after injury. However, despite improvements in prehospital, resuscitative, surgical, and critical care, unrecognized abdominal injury remains a preventable cause of death after injury.[2] In a retrospective review of 22,577 patients admitted to six trauma centers, significant preventable errors were made in 1032 cases (4%). Of the total errors, 53.4% occurred in the resuscitative phase. Failure to evaluate the abdomen was the single most common error identified in the study.[9] Additional studies acknowledge errors in the resuscitative phase, including inappropriate or delayed diagnosis of intraabdominal injuries, which can lead to preventable trauma deaths.[14]

Exsanguination continues to be a common causes of death from traumatic injury. Because patients with abdominal trauma may have severe hemorrhage, rapid transport can significantly reduce the mortality and morbidity from both blunt and penetrating abdominal injuries. Four common causes of massive bleeding in trauma patients include external injury, massive hemothorax, retroperitoneal injury (e.g., pelvic fracture, renal laceration, or major vessel lesion), and intraperitoneal injury (e.g., liver, spleen, or major vessel laceration).[32] The likelihood of significant intraabdominal injury is high when a patient has hypotension in the field, a major chest injury, or pelvic fracture.[33,37]

Patients with genitourinary injuries alone are not usually in danger of life-threatening hemorrhage. Shock and time elapsed between injury and arrival in the operating room are the major factors affecting survival of abdominally injured patients, and these factors can be ameliorated by intervention of trained transport personnel able to recognize life-threatening injuries, initiate treatment, and rapidly transport the patient to definitive care.

Although genitourinary trauma alone is not immediately life threatening, appropriate transport can significantly affect the recovery time and reduction of complications resulting from these injuries.

Many lower-level facilities are not equipped to diagnose and treat specific genitourinary injuries. Air medical transport may be appropriate when a delay in ground time diminishes the chances of full recovery from renal, bladder, and genital injuries.

ABDOMINAL TRAUMA

ANATOMY OF THE ABDOMEN

The abdomen contains several major organs of the body responsible for digestion, nutrition, and elimination of toxins and waste from the body. Because the spleen filters aged red blood cells and one of the functions of the liver is to eliminate toxic waste from the bloodstream, both organs are vascular in nature. The spleen, liver, and vascular system of the abdomen are the primary sources of exsanguination during abdominal trauma.[32] Injuries to the hollow abdominal organs, such as the small and large intestine, can result in abscess formation, wound infection, and sepsis, especially if trauma to the intestine remains undiagnosed for a period of time. When injuries to the abdomen occur, they may have a large impact on morbidity and mortality.

The abdominal cavity includes all structures and organs between the respiratory diaphragm and the urogenital diaphragm. This space is divided into three compartments: the first, and largest, is the peritoneal cavity; the second is the space within the pelvic structure; and the third is the retroperitoneal space. The peritoneal cavity contains the diaphragm, spleen, liver, stomach, transverse colon, and most of the small intestine and mesentery.

The bony structure of the pelvis contains the rectum, bladder, iliac vessels, and female reproductive organs; the penis and scrotum are located outside the abdominal cavity below the urogenital diaphragm.

The retroperitoneal space is separated from the abdominal cavity by the posterior peritoneum and therefore is not always accessed by peritoneal lavage. Injuries in this area may be difficult to diagnose and are easily overlooked. The organs contained in this space are the aorta, vena cava, distal esophagus, kidneys, ureters, and portions of the duodenum, pancreas, colon, and rectum.

Knowledge of the basic anatomy of the abdomen and position of the organs is crucial because identification of organs possibly injured by blunt or penetrating trauma helps the transport team provide the treatment necessary for those injuries when preparing for or effecting the patient's transport.

CLASSIFICATION OF INJURIES

Abdominal trauma can be blunt or penetrating, depending on the mechanism of injury. Blunt trauma is caused by any type of force being exerted on the abdomen as the result of falls, motor vehicle accidents (MVCs), bicycle and motorcycle accidents, or any force striking the abdomen.[1,6,11] As the body receives an impact, the organs in the abdominal cavity continue moving forward; vessels and tissues tear away from their attachment points.

Patients have fewer fatal injuries with the increased use of seat belts, motorcycle and bicycle helmets, child restraint seats, and air bags and with enforcement of alcohol restraints. However, the majority of blunt abdominal injuries (50% to 75%) are the result of MVCs.[7,11,13] The use of seat belts decreases the possibility of multisystem injuries, but improper placement across the abdomen rather than the pelvis, loose application, or use of only lap belts can result in visceral trauma. The abdominal organs most frequently injured by blunt trauma are the liver, spleen, and kidney, although hollow-organ (intestinal) injury can occur. Abdominal injuries among air bag–protected occupants occur less frequently than head, chest, and lower extremity injuries. However, abdominal injuries may be occult, and deformation of the steering wheel is an indicator of an increased likelihood of internal injury.[3,34]

Trauma is classified as penetrating when an object such as a knife or bullet enters the abdominal cavity, and anything that has penetrated the abdomen and remains in place may be designated as an impaled object. Penetrating injuries of the abdomen are caused by gunshot wounds (GSWs) or stab wounds. The degree of injury of GSW patients depends on the caliber of the gun and its distance from the patient. High-velocity weapons and close-range shotguns cause more destruction to abdominal organs than do low-velocity weapons. However, bullets from low-velocity weapons can deflect off organs and bony prominences and create extensive injuries that are not easily recognized on initial examination. In stab wounds the length of the knife or object, depth of penetration, and angle at which it was inserted determine the amount of injury. The major organs involved in penetrating injuries are the liver, small bowel, colon, stomach, and vascular structures. The large size and anterior position of the liver and bowel in the abdomen make them particularly vulnerable to penetrating trauma.

Objects found impaled in the patient on arrival of the transport team should be left in place and stabilized for transport (Figure 17-1). Removal of the object may cause further injury or increase bleeding. If placing the patient into the transport vehicle is not possible because of the size and position of the object, it may have to be cut off while still in place within the abdominal cavity. The object should be moved as little as possible. In some instances the trauma surgeon must be transported to the scene to assist in the shortening or removal of the object.[39]

PATIENT HISTORY

The history of the injury and the physical examination should be obtained before transport because the information is important to the transport team when they assess and stabilize a patient for transport. The trauma surgeon may use the information when deciding the degree of injury and whether surgery should be performed soon after arrival at the emergency center. When possible, a past medical history, including medications, allergies, illnesses, and events leading up to injury, should be obtained from the patient, family, or referring facility. It is also helpful to know whether the patient has used alcohol or other substances, has a head or neck injury, has psychiatric problems, or has any underlying medical conditions (i.e., cardiovascular disease or coagulapathies).[11,13] Initial vital signs and level of consciousness, intake and output, and treatments done before the arrival of the transport team, as well as any changes or treatments in transport, should be reported to the trauma team at the receiving trauma center.

When a patient with blunt abdominal trauma is transported from a pedestrian accident or MVC, important information to obtain from the prehospital personnel at the site are the time of injury, probable speed of impact, damage to the vehicle (steering wheel, direction of impact on the vehicle), patient's position in the vehicle, and restraint devices used. When time permits, brief inspection of the damage to the vehicle by the transport team may provide more information on possible patient injuries. In patients injured from falls, the height of fall and position of impact will help point to the type of injuries involved. The history of assault victims should include the type of instrument that struck them.[15]

When a patient with a GSW is transported, information on the type and caliber of gun, number and location of wounds, and distance the victim was from the assailant should be determined whenever possible. In stab-wound patients the size and length of the object and number of wounds should be ascertained. Although internal bleeding is difficult to measure in penetrating injuries, the amount of blood lost at the scene should be noted for determination of the fluid replacement needed and indication of the degree of injury.

PHYSICAL EXAMINATION

The physical examination is one of the most important procedures for diagnosis of abdominal injury. It can be effective in determining the blood loss into

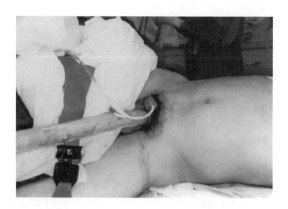

FIGURE 17-1   **Injury resulting from a logging accident.**

the peritoneal cavity or peritoneal irritation. Examination of the abdomen should be as thorough as possible. When a trauma patient who is in hemorrhagic shock is transported from a scene of accident or assault, the only assessment that time may permit is palpation for distention and tenderness. The abdominal assessment should include inspection, auscultation, and palpation before interfacility transport, especially when time and distance are great. Serial abdominal assessments should be done throughout transport because peritoneal irritation and accumulation of blood in the peritoneal cavity may not produce symptoms immediately.

The abdomen should be fully exposed to allow the transport team to inspect for contusions, abrasions, deformity, hematoma formation, open wounds, and penetrating injuries. An ecchymotic discoloration around the umbilicus (Cullen's sign) can indicate intraabdominal or retroperitoneal hemorrhage. When it is possible to examine the patient's back, the team should look for any obvious signs of trauma that would indicate an abdominal or genitourinary injury. Flank bruising may signify retroperitoneal hematoma formation from trauma to the kidneys, major blood vessels, or other organs contained in that space.

Auscultation should be done primarily in a quiet, controlled area because bowel sounds are difficult to hear in the noisy transport environment. Absence of bowel sounds can be an important indicator of an ileus and abdominal injury, and assessment of bowel sounds before an interfacility transfer may alert the transport team to the possibility of abdominal injury. Inspection and palpation of the abdomen are doubly important because hearing bowel sounds in the noisy prehospital environment is difficult, and taking the time to listen for bowel sounds at the scene when rotor noise makes hearing difficult does not alter patient treatment during transport and may delay liftoff. An abdomen that is tender and distended on palpation needs immediate attention; rapid transport with continual observation of vital signs and level of consciousness should be instituted. The major causes of a distended abdomen are gastric dilation and rapid intraabdominal bleeding. Tenderness on palpation with involuntary guarding or rebound tenderness is indicative of peritoneal irritation. Subjective reports of abdominal pain by a trauma patient should always be addressed. Because head-injured patients with a decreased level of consciousness are unable to identify abdominal pain, detection of a distended abdomen on palpation without any obvious signs of trauma may be the only indication of intraabdominal trauma.

The perineum should be visually inspected for any injuries to the genitals, urethra, or rectum. Peroneal hematoma formation can be caused by a retroperitoneal hematoma, pelvic fracture, or direct peritoneal trauma.

DIAGNOSTIC PROCEDURES

There are three diagnostic studies used to evaluate the injured abdomen. These are diagnostic peritoneal lavage (DPL); ultrasound (Focused Abdominal Sonogram for Trauma); and computerized axial tomography (CT).[11]

Diagnostic peritoneal lavage was the standard method used to evaluate abdominal trauma for decades. However, the advent of newer, more accurate and less-invasive technology has made this procedure not as commonly used as it once was. The American College of Surgeons Committee on Trauma recommends that a DPL be performed in an unstable patient if the abdominal exam is suggestive of injury or unreliable.[1,11]

Focused Abdominal Sonogram for Trauma (FAST) is generally used for torso evaluation of patients who suffer multiple traumas.[17] The FAST exam is rapid and noninvasive. There are even machines available that allow evaluation during transport. However, the exam needs to be performed by qualified persons. It also can be distorted by bowel, gas, and subcutaneous air. It does not detect all abdominal injuries.

Computed tomography (CT) of the abdomen for both adults and children offers both high specificity and sensitivity to the detection and location of abdominal injury. CT is effective in demonstrating solid viscous injuries such as spleen or liver lacerations, the presence and quantity of hemoperitoneum, and retroperitoneal injuries such as renal lacerations or hematomas associated with pelvic fractures. The CT has been helpful in decreasing the number of unnecessary laparotomies.[15,24,28]

PATIENT ASSESSMENT, TREATMENT, AND TRANSPORT

In many cases injury is not limited to the abdomen, particularly in patients with blunt-trauma injuries. Once the primary assessment is completed and the patient stabilized, the secondary examination should be done for determination of any other injuries.

In addition to the usual airway and breathing assessment and management, signs and symptoms of cardiovascular system collapse, such as hypotension, delayed capillary refill, and decreased level of consciousness, are important indicators of abdominal injuries. Patients with visceral injuries have the potential for sudden onset of severe hypovolemic shock because of the vascular nature of many organs in the abdominal cavity and the space for occult blood accumulation. Rapid recognition of the possibility of major abdominal injury is of paramount importance. Rapid transport after initial stabilization should be the goal when a patient is in hemorrhagic shock or has impending exsanguination.

Patients in severe shock or near exsanguination exhibit a decreasing level of consciousness as hypoxia increases and pale to mottled skin that is cold, clammy, and possibly profusely diaphoretic (Box 17-1). Mucous membranes may be pasty white, and capillary refill is delayed or absent. When no obvious external bleeding is present, the flight nurse should examine the abdomen. If the abdomen is distended and rigid with no bowel sounds, the transport team member should suspect intraabdominal bleeding. The conscious patient will report severe abdominal pain. If the abdomen is tautly distended, pressure will be exerted on the diaphragm, causing potential shortness of breath and tachypnea. The patient will be tachycardic and hypotensive; a blood pressure reading may not be obtainable even with a weak brachial pulse. If the blood pressure does not respond to fluid administration, exsanguination is a real possibility. The survival of

BOX 17-1	**Symptoms of Shock**

Decreasing consciousness
Pale-to-mottled skin that is cold, clammy, and possibly diaphoretic
Pasty white mucous membranes
Delayed or absent capillary refill
Distended and rigid abdomen with no bowel sounds
Potential shortness of breath and tachypnea
Tachycardia and hypotension
Unobtainable blood pressure reading
Blood pressure that does not respond to fluid administration
Reports of severe abdominal pain

an exsanguinating patient may depend on the amount of time it takes for him or her to be admitted to surgery.

Not all patients with abdominal injuries display all the symptoms described previously. Varying degrees of these symptoms, such as abdominal tenderness without initial distention, decreased but not absent bowel sounds, and tachycardia without hypotension, should alert the flight crew to the possibility of exsanguination.

Initial stabilization at the scene when transport time will be short should consist of airway management, 100% oxygen delivery, and spine immobilization. For the abdominally injured patient, fluid resuscitation should be initiated. This should be done while constantly monitoring the patient during transport. In addition to crystalloids, blood and blood products may need to be administered. The likelihood of significant intraabdominal injury is high when a patient has hypotension in the field, a major chest injury, or pelvic fracture.

Interfacility transfers may incur a longer patient transport time. Patient management should include all the treatment instituted for the short-scene-call transport. In addition, a gastric tube should be inserted for suspected intestinal injury, gastric distention, or aspiration. If massive external or internal hemorrhage is occurring, the referring hospital may have type-specific or O negative blood infusing or ready to send with the patient. If the report before transport indicates hypovolemic shock, the transport team should request that the referring hospital have blood ready for transport on the patient's arrival. For some patients, blood transfusion before arrival at the level I trauma center can be the factor that decreases morbidity and mortality. Hypothermia caused by massive intravenous fluid resuscitation can have a negative influence on patient outcome; therefore warming of intravenous fluids for the administration of many liters of fluid, or at least use of fluids from an emergency department instead of cold fluids in the transport vehicle, can be important. The goals of transport are rapid patient stabilization and transport to the nearest facility capable of treating the abdominally injured patient.

SPECIFIC ABDOMINAL ORGAN INJURIES

DIAPHRAGM

INCIDENCE AND MECHANISM

Blunt injury to the diaphragm, resulting in rupture or partial tear, occurs when a tremendous force is applied to the abdomen. The left diaphragm is injured more often than the right because the liver absorbs the impact of the force on the right side. If a right-sided tear has occurred, liver injury will probably accompany it. Spleen injuries often occur with left-sided diaphragmatic trauma.[8,14,40] Diaphragmatic tears can occur without herniation of bowel into the chest cavity. If an intestinal herniation into the pleural space does occur, intestinal strangulation may develop. A penetrating injury of the diaphragm should be suspected when a knife wound occurs at or below the nipple line anteriorly or at the inferior border of the scapula posteriorly.[8]

ASSESSMENT AND SYMPTOMS

The transport team may not be able to diagnose a diaphragmatic tear that has not resulted in bowel herniation. Further diagnostic procedures may be necessary for him or her to ascertain a diaphragmatic tear. Physical examination of the patient with a diaphragmatic hernia may reveal absent or reduced breath sounds on the affected side. Bowel sounds may be heard in the chest cavity when intestinal contents have herniated into the pleural space.

Respiratory distress may accompany intestinal herniation. If stomach contents are returned when a needle thoracostomy is performed for a believed tension pneumothorax, diaphragmatic hernia should be suspected. When a chest radiograph has been done, it may indicate intestinal herniation by the presence of stomach contents or a curled gastric tube in the chest cavity. Diaphragm injuries missed on diagnostic examination may result in intestinal incarceration or strangulation that occurs weeks to months later. Associated mortality is high.[14]

TREATMENT

Specific treatment for a known or suspected diaphragmatic tear with possible herniation should focus on airway management, oxygenation, and ventilation because of the potentially decreased lung capacity. Intubation and ventilation should be done when respiratory failure occurs. A gastric tube inserted for transport will reduce the possibility of aspiration and gastric dilatation, especially for patients with herniation.

LIVER AND SPLEEN

INCIDENCE AND MECHANISM

The spleen is the most commonly injured organ in blunt abdominal trauma; the liver is second, and they frequently are injured at the same time. In both spleen and liver trauma, early deaths are the result of hemorrhage or other injuries; late deaths result from infection. The mortality rate for liver injuries is 13%, with a higher percentage of deaths occurring from penetrating injury.[15] Penetrating injuries that occur below the nipple level of the thorax or in the upper abdominal cavities may involve the liver or spleen.

The mechanism of injury for liver trauma is direct trauma to the liver itself, causing fractures in the organ, or deceleration forces that may avulse hepatic veins from the inferior vena cava and diaphragm attachments. Tears in the hepatic, arterial, and portal venous vessels from compressive or shearing forces can result in rapid bleeding. The biliary duct system and hepatic vasculature are injured more often in penetrating injuries of the liver than in blunt injuries.

ASSESSMENT AND SYMPTOMS

Both the liver and spleen are vascular in nature. Patients with blunt and penetrating injuries can have symptoms that vary from slight tachycardia with abdominal guarding to profound shock and a distended, taut abdomen when intraabdominal hemorrhage is occurring. A distended abdomen may indicate severe bleeding from either the liver or the spleen. When these patients are assessed, inspection and palpation of the abdomen should be done to locate contusions, abrasions, and pain. Other injuries, such as rib and scapula fractures, are associated with spleen and liver trauma. The amount of force involved in blunt abdominal injuries and the mechanism of injury and location of wounds in penetrating trauma are important indicators of spleen and liver injury.

Subjective symptoms of spleen injury may be localized tenderness in the left upper quadrant. Referred shoulder pain (Kehr's sign) from left hemidiaphragm irritation can also be present, but it is rarely seen. Localized abdominal pain from liver injuries will occur in the right upper quadrant.

TREATMENT

Because exsanguination may be the cause of death immediately after the accident in spleen and liver trauma, specific treatment in these injuries should focus on hemodynamic status. Relay of information to the trauma center when obvious intraabdominal hemorrhage is present can prepare the trauma team for immediate care of the patient.

PANCREAS AND DUODENUM
INCIDENCE AND MECHANISM

Both the pancreas and duodenum lie within the retroperitoneal space; they are in intimate proximity to each other and usually are injured together. Both are well protected and constitute less than 3% to 12% of all abdominal injuries.[14] Mortality and morbidity from pancreatic and duodenal injuries occur more frequently from secondary complications of infection, pseudocyst or fistula formation, gastrointestinal tract malfunction, and chronic pancreatitis. Injury in blunt trauma should be suspected when direct force is applied to the left upper quadrant, as in steering wheel and bicycle handlebar impalement. Injury is caused by compression of these organs against the vertebral column. Injuries to both the pancreas and duodenum occur more frequently from penetrating than from blunt trauma.

ASSESSMENT AND SYMPTOMS

Symptoms of isolated, blunt pancreatic and duodenal injuries may be difficult to observe. If duodenal digestive juices and blood are contained within the retroperitoneal space, the patient may not have many abdominal symptoms. Assessment of the patient will usually show tenderness over the area of the pancreas and the absence of bowel sounds. The patient may be hemodynamically stable, with symptoms associated only with peritonitis (such as abdominal tenderness or guarding), or may have no symptoms at all. These injuries are difficult to diagnose, but careful history taking can assist in their identification.

TREATMENT

The transport treatment for these patients includes a high index of suspicion for injury when the patient has vague abdominal symptoms after trauma. Treatment should include any procedures necessary for patient stabilization and supportive care if the patient's respiratory and cardiovascular status remains stable. If duodenal injury is suspected, gastric tube insertion will reduce the gastric and duodenal juices' infiltration of the peritoneal space. Outlying hospitals may transfer these patients several days after injury when isolated pancreatic and duodenal symptoms occur.

COLON AND SMALL INTESTINE
INCIDENCE AND MECHANISM

Colon and small-intestine damage occurs more frequently in penetrating than in blunt injuries, and in most cases the liver, spleen, or other organs are also injured.[14,16] Colon injuries are caused by penetrating missiles or stabbings 90% of the time. The small intestine is the most commonly injured organ in penetrating injuries; presumably because of the volume it occupies in the abdomen.[15] Blunt injury to the small intestine occurs with crushing of the bowel against the spinal column. Improper use of the seat belt, steering wheel impact, or a blunt object applied to the abdomen can produce this crushing effect. If a victim has a transverse bruise across the lower abdomen from a lap belt, rupture of the small intestine should be considered.[14] Bowel evisceration may occur with penetrating trauma, and bowel contents should be covered with sterile saline solution during transfer.

ASSESSMENT AND SYMPTOMS

The same thorough assessment for abdominal trauma should be done in suspected cases of intestinal injury. The transport team should inspect the location of all entrance and exit sites of patients with GSWs and the entrance wounds of stabbing victims. Examination of the back, buttocks, and perineum is important because wounds to these areas are easily overlooked. Documentation of the locations of wounds should be as accurate as possible. Evisceration of the bowel may be found with penetrating injuries; the color and size of protruding bowel should be noted on the initial examination.

Symptoms of isolated colon injury are associated with peritoneal irritation from blood or feces free in the peritoneum. Pain on palpation with guarding may be present, and symptoms of fever and leukocytosis may increase with time elapsed since injury. Fecal material may be present in the peritoneal lavage fluid when colon disruption has occurred. Abdominal radiographs may reveal free air in the peritoneum or a loss of the psoas shadow.

Symptoms of small-bowel injury include tenderness, patient reluctance to change positions, rebound tenderness, and guarding. In small-intestinal injuries, peritoneal lavage may demonstrate turbid or bile-stained fluid, an elevated white blood cell count, or presence of amylase. Radiographic films may reveal free air in the peritoneum or a small-bowel ileus.

TREATMENT

Because most injuries of the intestine are associated with other more immediate life-threatening injuries, transport management should be prioritized accordingly. While airway and cardiovascular systems are being stabilized, saline dressings should be applied to any eviscerated bowel or dry dressings to any open wounds. The amount of blood loss at the scene should be noted. Most complications of bowel injuries occur later in the patient's course of recovery. The major factors related to morbidity and mortality are sepsis, abscess formation, wound infection, and intraabdominal peritonitis.

GASTRIC AND ESOPHAGEAL TRAUMA
INCIDENCE AND MECHANISM

Gastric and esophageal injuries are uncommon because the esophagus and stomach are well protected within the upper abdominal cavity. The abdominal esophagus is 2 to 4 cm long and lies within the retroperitoneal space, anterior to the aorta. The pliability of the stomach reduces its chances of injury in blunt trauma, although a full stomach is more likely to rupture. The majority of esophageal and gastric injuries are caused by penetrating trauma.

ASSESSMENT AND SYMPTOMS

Symptoms of gastric and esophageal trauma are signs of peritoneal irritation, such as pain and guarding. Gastric tube drainage may show evidence of blood, and that may indicate a gastric rupture in the absence of other obvious sources of bleeding, such as facial trauma, in which the patient may have swallowed blood. Review of the abdominal radiographs at the referring hospital may show free air in the peritoneum, indicating disruption of the intestinal tract, which may involve the esophagus, stomach, or both.

TREATMENT

Diagnosis of gastric and esophageal trauma injuries will most likely be confirmed after arrival at the trauma center. Transport treatment of these patients is similar to that of any other trauma patient with life-threatening injuries. If a gastric rupture is suspected, a nasogastric tube should be carefully inserted for long transports. Time of last food consumption can be useful information to the trauma surgeon, especially in an unconscious patient.

ABDOMINAL VASCULAR INJURIES
INCIDENCE AND MECHANISM
Injuries to the abdominal arterial and venous systems occur more frequently with penetrating trauma than with blunt trauma. A 5-year retrospective study of 530 MVC fatalities revealed that aortic injuries occurred in 18% of victims. The typical victim was a male driver with an elevated blood alcohol level, who was involved in a head-on collision.[39] Compression or deceleration forces applied to the abdomen can result in avulsion of small vessels from the larger vessels from which they branch, and intimal tears within the vessel itself may occur. Intimal tears can result in thrombosis formation, whereas vessel avulsion tears can result in exsanguination. Penetrating injuries of vascular tissue cause lacerations and free bleeding. The major vessels frequently injured are the aorta; inferior vena cava; and the renal, mesenteric, and iliac arteries and veins. Vascular system injury is the primary cause of death in patients who sustain GSWs and stab wounds to the abdomen. Mortality is high, even when patients are not in shock at presentation.[32,38]

ASSESSMENT AND SYMPTOMS
A patient with no obvious active external bleeding source who experiences severe shock shortly after injury probably has arterial injury. Bleeding is profuse, and rapid fluid replacement may not be able to maintain blood pressure and tissue perfusion when intraabdominal arterial lacerations are present. Patients with abdominal vascular injuries may present as or become the exsanguinating patient described earlier, depending on the degree of intraabdominal bleeding and the time elapsed since injury occurred. With arterial injuries the femoral pulse on the affected side may be absent. Major abdominal vein injuries can also produce profound shock, but it may occur up to 30 minutes after the injury instead of immediately. Bleeding from venous injuries may be controlled by direct pressure of the abdominal organs or abdominal pressure itself, limiting the possibility of early exsanguination.

TREATMENT
With abdominal vascular injuries, when exsanguination is imminent, rapid transport to a level I trauma center is critical to patient survival.

Complications after survival of the initial abdominal vascular injury include continued bleeding from vascular reconstruction areas or disseminated intravascular coagulation that develops from massive blood transfusions, liver ischemia, or profound shock. Thrombosis formation can occur and cause tissue ischemia to the kidneys or gastrointestinal tract. When renal or visceral veins are involved, pulmonary embolism can develop.

GENITOURINARY TRAUMA

Genitourinary trauma includes injuries to the kidney, bladder, ureters, urethra, and genitalia and is not usually immediately life threatening, as are the abdominal injuries previously discussed. Because of the position of the urinary and reproductive system within the abdominal cavity, a high index of suspicion for trauma in the genitourinary organs should be maintained when regions of the abdomen and back are injured. The American College of Surgeons Advanced Trauma Life Support Course emphasizes the transport of trauma patients from outlying hospitals without delay for urologic studies. Expeditious treatment of other, more life-threatening injuries at a level I trauma center may be crucial to patient survival.

RENAL AND URETER TRAUMA
INCIDENCE AND MECHANISM
Renal trauma is frequently associated with abdominal injury; the kidney is the third most commonly injured abdominal organ.[9,18] Injuries sustained from blunt mechanisms such as MVCs, falls, contact sports, and assaults account for 70% to 80% of all renal trauma, and 5% of patients may eventually lose renal function.[19] Blunt injuries sustained from sudden acceleration/deceleration result in the stretching of the ureters and renal arteries and veins with the weight of the kidney. Contusions are generally from a direct blow to the

flank. Of all renal and ureter blunt traumas, 85% are minor contusions, and the remaining 15% consist of renal vascular injury, deep cortical lacerations, or shattered kidneys.[18,27]

Penetrating injuries are usually caused by GSWs or stabbings to the back or abdomen, with an 80% incidence of associated injury in other abdominal organs.[6,7,35] Low-velocity bullet injuries are more common than high-velocity bullet injuries (79% versus 8%), and their damage is typically parenchymal laceration. Often a high-velocity GSW injury results in nephrectomy because the kidney explodes from the impact or passage of the bullet.[1,13,35]

Most renal injuries (80% to 85%) are minor and consist of contusions and minor lacerations; 10% are major and extend into the medulla, collecting system, or both, with the possible result of extravasation of urine (Figure 17-2). Vascular injuries occur in 1% to 3% of renal injuries, and retroperitoneal hematoma formation is likely.[4,38]

Ureteral injury, although rare, is generally a result of penetrating trauma such as GSWs or stab wounds. Rapid-deceleration accidents may avulse the ureter from the renal pelvis.[4,23]

ASSESSMENT AND SYMPTOMS

On secondary assessment any contusions, abrasions, or stab penetrations to the back and flank area should alert the flight nurse to the possibility of renal trauma. The patient may complain of flank pain. Kidney damage should always be suspected with gunshot injuries to the abdomen. Hematuria is a marker for both renal and extrarenal abdominal injuries after blunt trauma. All patients with gross hematuria should be evaluated after transfer for both renal and associated abdominal injuries. In addition, patients in shock or with a history of shock and microscopic hematuria after blunt trauma should also be suspected of having abdominal injuries. Studies show that patients with microscopic hematuria but no shock do not demonstrate any major renal injury and are treated successfully without surgical intervention.[21]

TREATMENT

Because renal injuries are not immediately life threatening, the transport team should give supportive care and identify the patient's risk for kidney injury when other life-threatening injuries are absent. If a urinary catheter is in place, the transport team should transport with gravity drainage and monitor urine output. Ureter injury will probably not be diagnosed until full evaluation is completed at the trauma center; therefore no specific intervention exists for air transport. At the receiving hospital, surgery may be indicated for major kidney injuries, ureteral tears, or renal vascular damage, although current literature indicates that the trend in treatment is toward nonsurgical management.[18,35]

BLADDER AND URETHRAL TRAUMA
INCIDENCE AND MECHANISM

Blunt trauma to the bladder is most commonly associated with pelvic fractures (90% of cases of bladder rupture have associated pelvic fractures).

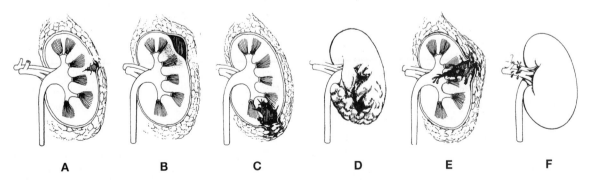

| A | B | C | D | E | F |

FIGURE 17-2 **Renal injuries classified by severity. A** and **B,** Minor injuries. **C, D, E,** and **F,** Major injuries. (Modified from Blaisdell W, Trunkey D, McAninch J: *Trauma management,* vol 2, New York, 1982, Thieme.)

Because the bladder lies within the pelvic girdle, bone fragments from the pelvis can penetrate the bladder. Rupture can also occur when a direct blow to the lower abdomen occurs with a distended bladder. Rupture can cause extravasation of urine into the peritoneal cavity. If diagnosis is not established immediately and the urine is sterile, no symptoms may be noted for several days; if the urine is infected, immediate peritonitis and acute abdominal pain will develop.[23,25]

Urethral injuries are associated with bladder rupture and pelvic fractures and occur more often in men than in women. Shearing forces at the level of the prostate gland usually cause the most severe urethral damage during pelvic fracture; the urethra may be torn near the prostate gland. Straddle injuries caused by bicycle, horse-riding, or gymnastic accidents, as well as direct penetrating trauma, may cause injuries to the lower or more external urethra.

ASSESSMENT AND SYMPTOMS

Identifying patients at risk is the best way for the transport team to determine bladder and urethral injuries in the field. Subjective symptoms in common with both bladder and urethral injuries are lower abdominal pain, groin tenderness, and inability to void. Hematuria will most likely be present with bladder trauma. Shock in these patients is usually associated with other visceral or vascular injuries. Blood at the meatus is the single most important sign of urethral injury.

TREATMENT

Transport treatment of patients with bladder and urethral injuries should emphasize a high index of suspicion for their injuries; life-threatening injuries should take priority. A urinary catheter should not be inserted when blood is found in the urethral meatus. With a urethral tear, further damage can occur if a catheter is improperly inserted, although a prolonged transport time and a distended, painful bladder are indications for careful, controlled insertion of a urinary catheter in these patients. Autonomic hyperreflexia is a serious complication of a prolonged distended bladder that causes

hypertension, bradycardia, and increased intracranial pressure.[25] The transport team should keep these symptoms in mind when transporting a patient with a diagnosed urethral tear and inability to void. When a ruptured bladder is suspected or diagnosed, transport should be accomplished without delay. The diagnosis will be confirmed at the trauma center by retrograde cystography in bladder trauma or retrograde urethrogram in the urethral injury.

GENITAL TRAUMA
INCIDENCE AND MECHANISM

Genital trauma is more common in men than in women. The female reproductive tract is well protected within the pelvic bony structure; consequently, injuries are infrequent with either blunt or penetrating trauma. Bone fragments from a pelvic fracture may pierce the uterus, vagina, or other female organs. Injuries to the exterior female perineum from straddle accidents can result in hematoma formation. Ninety percent of female genital injuries are to the uterus.[39] In men, penetrating trauma to the penis or scrotum is most often caused by a GSW. Urethral disruption may accompany these injuries. Other causes of blunt injury are MVCs, industrial accidents, and assault. Of scrotal injuries, 50% are caused by blunt trauma, and patients usually have contusions, hematomas, avulsions, lacerations, or testicular rupture at presentation.[18]

ASSESSMENT AND SYMPTOMS

Assessment of the patient with genital injuries includes a thorough history and a visual inspection. Respect for dignity should always be maintained. Reports of the event may be embarrassing for the patient, and the flight nurse must be careful to listen without judgment, although discrepancies between history and mechanism of injury should be noted. On physical examination the transport team should visually inspect the perineal area for hematoma formation anywhere on the perineum, scrotum, or penis. If the scrotum is swollen and painful, ruptured testes should be suspected. Rectal injury can also be identified when the perineal area is examined, and the flight nurse should look for any obvious trauma and document any lacerations or avulsions, including the presence and amount of vaginal bleeding. Menstrual history is important for female patients if they are able to provide that information.

TREATMENT

Unless bleeding is profuse, injuries to the genitals are not immediately life threatening. Treatment for transport should consist of saline dressings to avulsions and lacerations, particularly those to the scrotum. Ice packs to both scrotum and penile hematomas help reduce swelling and pain; direct pressure should be applied to the areas of penile injury. In the case of penile or scrotum amputation, the parts should be transported in saline dressings on ice, and the transport team should ensure that the tissue is not in direct contact with the ice, which could cause further tissue damage.

Vaginal bleeding is difficult to control, and pressure dressings should be applied if possible. Exsanguination can occur with major vaginal tears because of the rich blood supply. When severe bleeding and shock are present, rapid transport to the nearest facility capable of treating gynecologic injuries should be the first priority. If objects are impaled in the genitalia, they should be left in place and immobilized.[7] The success rate of repair to genital injuries is high, and even penile reimplantation has been successful with microvascular surgery.[5,29]

SUMMARY

The initial treatment for all patients with suspected abdominal and genitourinary injuries from either blunt or penetrating trauma should include all procedures done for any trauma victim, such as airway control and ventilation, oxygenation, emergency treatment of life-threatening chest injuries, volume replacement and restoration of tissue perfusion, and stabilization of any fractures. The airway should be protected with intubation when needed, and breathing should be supplemented with 100% oxygen, ventilation, or both when the patient's condition warrants it. The patient's circulation should be monitored by assessment of the pulse, blood pressure, capillary refill, and when available, urinary output.

Exsanguination, one of the major causes of death in trauma victims, can take place quickly with an abdominal injury because of the vascular nature of the abdominal organs and the large peritoneal space for blood accumulation. Calculation of the amount of lost blood is difficult in abdominal trauma patients because the abdomen can sequester large volumes of blood before signs of abdominal distention occur. The primary duties of the transport team when transporting patients with abdominal trauma should be recognizing and arresting profound shock and exsanguination by decreasing the blood loss from the intravascular space, replacing circulatory volume, and maintaining tissue perfusion.

Once immediately life-threatening injuries are stabilized, a secondary survey should include assessment for any fractures, major lacerations, and perineal trauma, and initial treatment should be instituted for those injuries present. If bowel evisceration has occurred, a normal saline-soaked dressing should be applied.

Any trauma resulting in hematoma formation to the male or female external genitalia should be treated with ice and pressure dressings. When lacerations are present on the male genitalia, wet saline dressings should be applied, and when bleeding of the penis and scrotum is present, pressure dressings should be applied. Vaginal bleeding should be observed, and a pressure dressing should be applied to the perineum when bleeding is profuse.

Rapid transport reduces the time from injury to definitive treatment. Alerting the trauma center of the patient's condition through radio contact can provide the trauma team with valuable information, which also reduces delay of treatment of specific life-threatening injuries, thereby increasing the patient's chances of survival.

The primary role of the transport team in the management of the patient with abdominal trauma is to identify and manage life-threatening conditions of the airway, cervical spine, respiratory system, and cardiovascular system and to provide rapid transport to the appropriate facility where the patient will receive definitive care.

Patients should receive specialized treatment of their injuries with the least amount of time delay, thereby enhancing their chances for a full recovery.

ABDOMINAL AND GENITOURINARY TRAUMA CASE STUDY

An air medical team was requested to respond to a rural county hospital for a farm tractor rollover, flight time 20 minutes. En route, the faculty physician at the receiving facility relayed the following information to the transport team.

Mr. R is a 75-year-old male who was found by his wife trapped under an overturned tractor for an unknown amount of time. She estimated the time to be approximately 6 hours based on when she had last seen him. Basic EMS responded to the scene, immobilized the patient, and transported him to the closest hospital, which was 10 minutes from the scene of the accident. The referring hospital reports that he has a patent airway, is on 100% oxygen by mask, equal, clear breath sounds, BP 100/70, HR 120R, RR 28. He is complaining of severe abdominal pain.

On arrival at the referring hospital, the transport team performed an assessment and found the following:

AIRWAY

The airway was clear and patent. A nonrebreather mask was in place delivering 100% oxygen. A cervical collar with head blocks was in place.

BREATHING

Respirations were medium depth, equal expansion, and easy, with bilateral clear breath sounds and a respiratory rate of 28. Oxygen saturation of 95% was noted. There was no palpable deformities, crepitus, or subcutaneous air.

CIRCULATION

The patient's radial pulse was weak at a rate of 120, and he had a blood pressure of 80/64. His skin was pale, cool, and dry with a capillary refill of 2 seconds. The cardiac monitor showed sinus tachycardia.

NEUROLOGIC

Mental status remains unchanged with a GCS of 15, PEERL, and he is moving all extremities, although he has limited movement of his left leg. Patient denies any numbness or tingling.

SECONDARY ASSESSMENT

Abdomen

Abdomen was distended, but soft. There was pain with palpation in the upper abdomen both over the right and left quadrants. Patient complained of severe pain with any movement of his pelvis. There was a large bluish area over the left flank area (Grey-Turner's sign). A urinary catheter had drained 25 cc of dark yellow urine, and a gastric tube was draining dark brown liquid. There were no bowel sounds auscultated.

Extremeties

Patient complains of left shoulder pain, but no deformities were palpated on either upper extremity. An open left tib/fib had been immobilized with a splint by the local EMS. Weak peripheral pulses were palpated in both lower extremities.

HISTORY

History of the Event

As previously described.

Past Medical History

Lopressor for treatment of angina.

DIAGNOSTIC INFORMATION

A second line was started, and a fluid bolus of 1 liter of normal saline was begun.

Radiographs

C-spine cleared to C-6.
Chest radiograph is normal.
Pelvic radiograph reveals left pelvic fracture with separation of the sacroiliac joint.
Left leg radiograph: shattered tib/fib.

INTERVENTIONS

While preparing the patient for transport, a second intravenous line is started, and a fluid bolus initiated. The patient is also allowed to see and talk with his family before leaving the emergency department.

TRANSPORT

During transport, Mr. R. lost his radial pulses and became agitated and confused. His skin was clammy. Despite receiving 2 liters of crystalloids, his blood pressure dropped to 64/48. His heart rate continued 120 and above. His abdomen appeared more distended and became firm. Two units of O negative blood were infused, and the trauma center was notified of the patient's deteriorating condition.

On arrival at the trauma center, the patient was hot off-loaded and taken directly to the Shock Resuscitation Unit. The trauma team performed a FAST exam that revealed fluid. The patient was taken to the operating room for immediate repair of his injuries, which included a lacerated spleen and liver, a pelvic fracture, and a left tib/fib fracture.

Recovery in the Surgical Intensive Care Unit (SCICU) was tenuous with disseminated intravascular coagulation (DIC) and two episodes of angina occurring. After 3 weeks he was transferred to the surgical step-down. After an additional uneventful 3 weeks in the hospital, Mr. R. was discharged home.

REFERENCES

1. American College of Surgeons: Abdominal trauma. In *Advanced trauma life support program for physicians,* Chicago, 1997, American College of Surgeons.
2. Augenstein JS et al: Occult abdominal injuries to airbag protected crash victims: a challenge to trauma systems, *J Trauma* 38:502, 1995.
3. Bickell W et al: Immediate versus delayed fluid resuscitation for hypotensive patients with penetrating torso injuries, *N Engl J Med* 331(17):1105, 1994.
4. Blaisdell W, Trunkey D, McAninch J: *Trauma management,* vol 2, Urogenital trauma, New York, 1985, Thieme-Stratton, Thieme Verlag.
5. Bourn M, Bourn S: Genitourinary emergencies: a prehospital perspective, *Emerg Med Clin North Am* 6:379, 1988.
6. Boyd CR, Tolson MA: Mechanisms of abdominal trauma: implications for initial care, *Emerg Care Q* 10:22, 1988.
7. Boyd CR et al: Penetrating abdominal trauma and the basics of ballistics, *J Air Med Transport* 6:6, 1991.
8. Buckman RF et al: Major bowel and diaphragmatic injuries associated with blunt spleen or liver rupture, *J Trauma* 28:1317, 1988.
9. Davis JW et al: An analysis of errors causing morbidity and mortality in a trauma system: a guide for quality improvement, *J Trauma* 32:660, 1992.
10. Emergency Nurses Association: *Standards of emergency nursing practice,* ed 4, St Louis, 2000, Mosby.
11. Emergency Nurses Association: *Trauma nursing core course,* ed 5, Des Plaines, Ill, 2000, Author.
12. Feliciano DV, Marx JA, Sclafani SJA: Abdominal trauma, *Patient Care* 26:44, 1992.
13. Feliciano DV, Rozycki GS: The management of penetrating abdominal trauma, *Adv Surg* 28:1, 1995.
14. Fisher RB, Dearden CH: Improving care of patients with major trauma in the accident and emergency department, *BMJ* 300:1560, 1990.
15. Freshman SP et al: Secondary survey following blunt trauma: a new role for CT scan, *J Trauma* 34:337, 1993.
16. Goins WA, Anderson BB: Abdominal trauma revisited, *J Natl Med Assoc* 83:883, 1991.
17. Gracias VH, Frankel HL, Gupta R et al: Defining the learning curve for the Focused Abdominal Sonogram for Trauma (FAST) examination: implications for credentialing, *Am Surg* 67:364, 2001.
18. Guerriero WG: Etiology, classification, and management of renal trauma, *Surg Clin North Am* 68:1071, 1988.
19. Jacobs LM et al: Prehospital advanced life support: benefits in trauma, *J Trauma* 24:8, 1984.
20. Jacobs L: Timing of fluid resuscitation in trauma, *N Engl J Med* 331(17):1153, 1994.
21. Knudson MM et al: Hematuria, as a predictor of abdominal injury after blunt trauma, *Am J Surg* 164:482, 1992.
22. Leicht MJ et al: Rural interhospital helicopter transport of motor vehicle trauma victims: causes for delays and recommendations, *Ann Emerg Med* 15:450, 1986.
23. Lowe MA et al: Risk factors for urethral injuries in men with traumatic pelvic fractures, *J Urol* 140:506, 1988.

24. Lucciarini P et al: Ultrasonography in the initial evaluation and follow-up of blunt abdominal injury, *Surgery* 114:506, 1993.

25. Macfarlane MT: *Trauma, urology,* Baltimore, 1994, Williams & Wilkins.

26. Maull KI et al: Retroperitoneal injuries: pitfalls in diagnosis and management, *South Med J* 80:1111, 1987.

27. McAninch JW: Injuries to the genitourinary tract. In Tanagho EA, McAninch JW, editors: *Smith's general urology,* Norwalk, Conn, 1992, Appleton & Lange.

28. McKennay M et al: Can ultrasound replace diagnostic peritoneal lavage in the assessment of blunt trauma? *J Trauma* 37:439, 1994.

29. Monstrey SJM et al: Renal trauma and hypertension, *J Trauma* 29:65, 1989.

30. Moylan JA: Impact of helicopters on trauma care and clinical results, *Ann Surg* 28:139, 1988.

31. O'Connell KJ et al: Comparison of low- and high-velocity ballistic trauma to genitourinary organs, *J Trauma* 28:139, 1988.

32. Phillips GR, Kauder DR, Schwab CW: Massive blood loss in trauma patients, *Postgrad Med* 95:61, 1994.

33. Richardson D et al: *Trauma: clinical care and pathophysiology,* St Louis, 1987, Mosby.

34. Rutledge R et al: The cost of not wearing seat belts: a comparison outcome in 3396 patients, *Ann Surg* 217: 122, 1993.

35. Shorr RM et al: Selective management of abdominal stab wounds: importance of the physical examination, *Arch Surg* 16:1141, 1988.

36. Spirnak JP: Pelvic fracture and injury to the lower urinary tract, *Surg Clin North Am* 68:1057, 1988.

37. Wachtel TL: Critical care concepts in the management of abdominal trauma, *Crit Care Nurs Q* 17:34, 1994.

38. Weesner CL et al: Fatal childhood injury patterns in an urban setting, *Ann Emerg Med* 23:231, 1994.

39. Williams JS et al: Aortic injury in vehicular trauma, *Ann Thorac Surg* 57:726, 1994.

40. Worthy SA et al: Diaphragmatic rupture: CT findings in eleven patients, *Radiology* 194:885, 1995.

ORTHOPEDIC TRAUMA

18

1. Perform an assessment of an injured extremity.
2. Appropriately immobilize an injured extremity.
3. Identify and treat potential complications related to musculoskeletal emergencies.

A simple fracture or dislocation can become a devastating injury, resulting in severe, permanent disability. Even a moderate sprain, if inadequately treated, can result in an unnecessarily extended disability and can lead to recurrent injuries.

The hands of a pianist, the elbow of a pitcher, the legs of a dancer are all vital to each of these people. Although musculoskeletal injuries are rarely fatal, they often result in long-term disability that accounts for millions of dollars lost to the economy each year.[12] The first care provided to a patient with a fracture, dislocation, or severe sprain will often determine the ultimate results that occur as a consequence of the injury.[8] The transport team can often prevent permanent disability with a prompt temporary measure, such as immobilization or splinting. This is especially true in patients with multiple traumas when more definitive management must be postponed until life-threatening injuries have been taken care of adequately.

MUSCULOSKELETAL SYSTEM

A basic understanding of the composition and function of the musculoskeletal system is essential to proper management of orthopedic emergencies and ultimately to the welfare of the patient as a whole. The musculoskeletal system is composed of bones, ligaments, muscles, joints, tendons, blood vessels, and nerves. The function of the musculoskeletal system is to allow movement, provide support, and protect internal organs.[7]

Bone is a living structure with its own neurovascular innervation and capacity to heal. Bone is a specialized connective tissue with a calcified collagenous intercellular substance and is either cancellous or compact. The calcium content of bone depends on many factors such as parathyroid hormone and estrogen, dietary intake, and stress. An acid-base balance with a slight decrease in pH can cause bone demineralization.[7]

DEFINITION

An orthopedic injury—a trauma to the axial skeleton—is rarely considered an emergency. However, it does require urgent care. In terms of orthopedic involvement with underlying organs, emergencies can exist. An example is the fracture and/or dislocation of the knee or elbow. Not only are these extremely painful injuries, but they also can cause permanent damage to nerves and vessels distal to the injury if not taken care of immediately. Table 18-1 lists various orthopedic injuries with their possible complications.

CLASSIFICATION OF ORTHOPEDIC INJURIES

When force is applied to a limb, the energy of the impact dissipates to deform supporting structures. If there is an excessive amount of force, more than one structure in the line of force may be damaged.[6] This type of stress to the axial skeleton and its supporting structures can cause various types of injuries, including fractures, dislocations, sprains, tendon injuries, and strains.

FRACTURES

A fracture is defined as any break in the continuity of the bone or cartilage, and it may be either complete or incomplete, depending on the line of fracture through the bone.[2,8,9] Fractures generally are classified as *closed* or *open*. If the skin is unbroken, the fracture is technically closed, regardless of the number of fractures, but if the skin is broken, the fracture is open, even though it may be simple and minor in nature. An open fracture is the more serious because of the risk of infection. Figure 18-1 illustrates nine different types of fractures as defined by their radiographic appearance.

Fractures of the long bone may produce steady, slow bleeding and can result in 750 ml of blood loss from the humerus or tibia and 1500 ml of blood from each femur.[7] These patients must be watched closely for shock, and the long-bone fracture should be immobilized for comfort. Another risk associated with fractures, even uncomplicated ones, is that of fat embolism, which can cause varying degrees of respiratory distress, including respiratory failure. Signs and symptoms of fat embolism are petechial rash, diffuse pulmonary infiltrates, hypoxemia, confusion, fever, tachycardia, and tachypnea. Patients at highest risk of fat embolism are those with long-bone fractures of the lower extremity.[1,4]

DISLOCATIONS

A dislocation is the displacement of the normal articulating ends of two or more bones. A *complete*

TABLE 18-1	**Urgent Complications of Orthopedic Injuries**
Injury	**Possible Complications**
Clavicle fractures	Brachial plexus compression or damage; pneumothorax or hemothorax
Humerus fractures	Injury to brachial artery or radial nerve
Pelvic fractures	Injury to bladder, urethra, rectum
Distal femoral shaft fractures	Femoral or popliteal vessel injury
Proximal tibia fractures	Compression of the anterior tibial compartment; tibial nerve injury
Clavicular head dislocation	Compression of trachea, subclavian, and carotid arteries
Posterior elbow dislocation	Compression of brachial artery
Posterior hip dislocation	Aseptic necrosis of the femoral head and sciatic nerve damage
Knee dislocation	Compression of the popliteal vessel
Ankle dislocation	Compression of the pedal artery

From Perdue P: Abdominal injuries and dangerous fractures, *RN* 44(7):35, 84, 1981.

TYPE OF FRACTURE	DEFINITION
Transverse 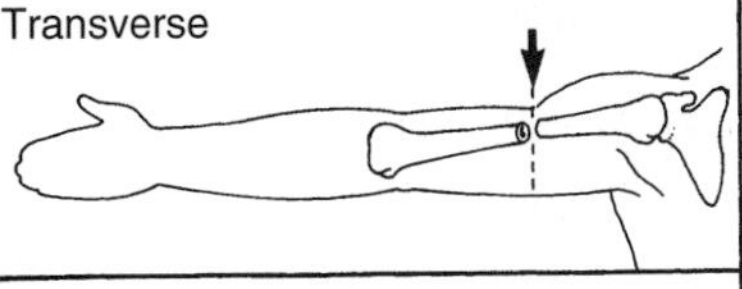	Usually produced by angulating force; once the fragments are aligned and immobilized, stability is ensured
Oblique 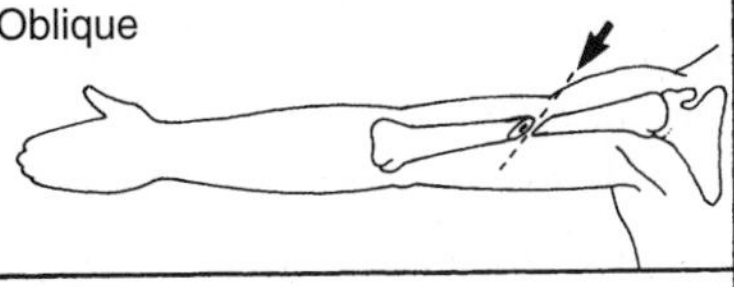	Fragments tend to slip by one another unless traction is maintained
Spiral 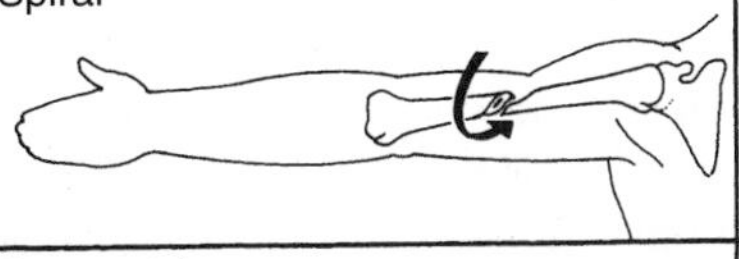	Produced by twisting or rotary force; reduction difficult to maintain
Greenstick 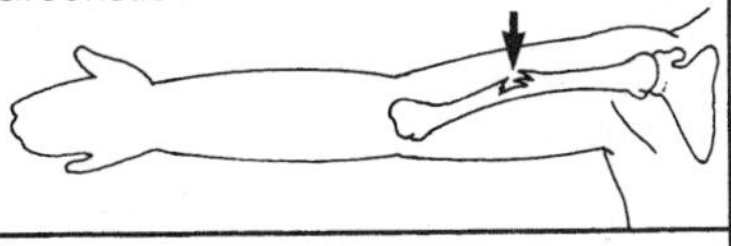	Caused by compression force in long axis of the bone; often seen in children under the age of 10
Compression 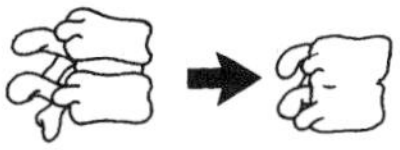	Usually produced by severe violence applied to cancellous bone, such as the spine
Comminuted 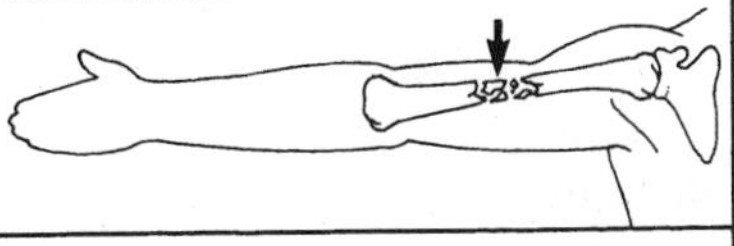	Always more than two fragments
Impacted 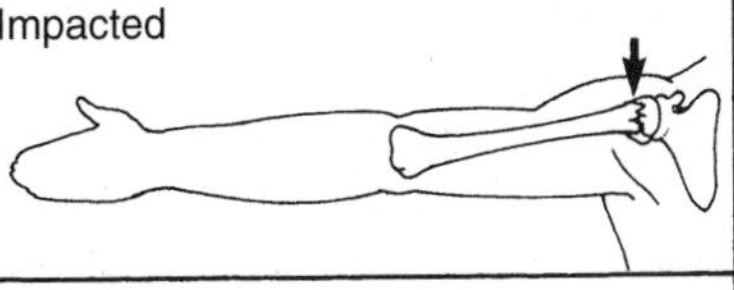	Produced by severe violence, driving bone fragments firmly together
Avulsion 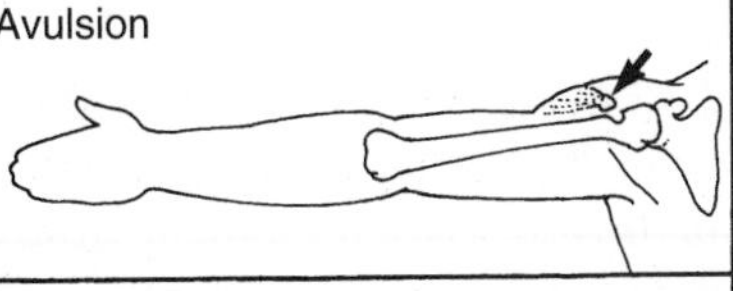	Produced by forcible contraction of a muscle, which pulls off a fragment of bone
Fracture dislocation 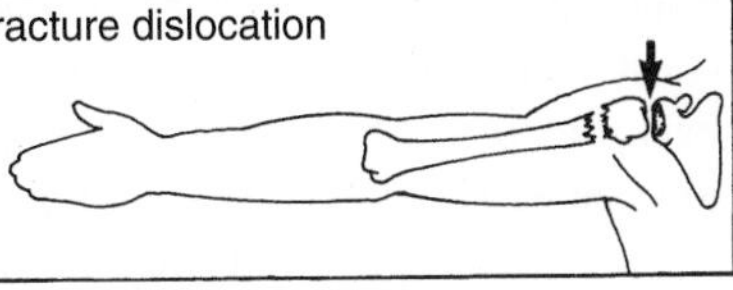	In addition to fracture there is a subluxation or dislocation of the joint

FIGURE 18-1   **Fractures according to their radiographic appearance.**

dislocation causes a tearing of the ligaments. A dislocation may also be described as *compound* when the joint is exposed to the outside air. Joints that are frequently dislocated are shoulders, elbows, fingers, hips, and ankles. Less frequently seen are dislocated wrists or knees. A dislocation is referred to as *subluxated* when the displacement is incomplete.

SPRAINS

A sprain is a partial tearing of a ligament caused by a sudden twisting or stretching of a joint beyond its normal range of motion. Sprains can vary in severity, and the more seriously injured ligaments will resemble a fracture or dislocation because they all present with pain, swelling, discoloration, and impaired movement. No deformity occurs as with dislocation, but a radiograph is required to rule out a fracture. Diagnosing a sprain without radiographic confirmation is dangerous, and treatment should always include proper splinting and referral for definitive care. Two common areas for sprains are the knee and the ankle. A sprained ankle is caused by a sudden twisting inward of the foot.

STRAINS

A strain is an injury to the muscle from overexertion or overextension. This may cause intense pain, some swelling, and decreased movement. Strains are usually seen in backs and arms and are rarely serious.

MECHANISMS OF ORTHOPEDIC INJURIES

There are multiple mechanisms that may cause injury to the musculoskeletal system. These include motor vehicle collisions (one of the most common); falls, particularly to the elderly; sports, such as football and soccer; and routine activities, such as cleaning around the house. Either accelerating or decelerating forces can injure bones, muscles, ligaments, and their surrounding nerves and blood vessels. It is important to remember that when a force is applied to the musculoskeletal system that causes an injury, the surrounding tissue and organs may be injured along with the bones and muscles.[1,7,9,14]

The following describes some of the common mechanisms of injury and their resultant trauma.

HEAD-ON COLLISIONS

In a head-on motor vehicle collision the occupant can follow either a down-and-under pathway or an up-and-over one. In the down-and-under pathway, the occupant slams his or her knees into the dashboard, and that part of the body comes to a fairly rapid stop. The result can be a dislocation of the knee or a fracture along the shaft of the femur. More commonly, however, the pelvis continues its forward motion and the person sustains a posterior fracture or dislocation of the hip. Usually the upper body will also continue forward, with the chest hitting the steering wheel.

In an up-and-over pathway, the body goes up and over the steering wheel, with the head slamming into the windshield. After the head is stopped, the trunk continues forward, causing a hyperflexion, hyperextension, or crushing injury of the cervical spine.

REAR-IMPACT COLLISIONS

In a rear-impact collision, the vehicle is hit from behind, and the energy of the impact is transferred forward. This transfer of energy will also occur with all parts of the body that are in contact with the car. The head, in the absence of a headrest, will snap back, and there will be an energy transfer at vertebra C3 or C4, producing whiplash-type injuries, which are basically sprains and strains of the ligamental supporting structures in that area.

LATERAL-IMPACT COLLISIONS

Lateral-impact collisions generally produce injuries in three areas of the body, all from the side. The first point of impact is the chest. The upper part of the chest will be pushed in as the shoulder is rotated back out of the way. The second point of injury is the pelvis. The greater trochanter receives the initial impact, and the head of the femur will be driven in that direction. The pelvis can also be fractured as it is pushed in, or the head of the femur can be driven through the acetabulum and into the retroperitoneal space. The third point of injury is the head and neck. As with rear-impact collisions, the body is in motion, and the head stays in position. The resulting injury is to the contralateral supporting structures of the neck. Again, these usually are not fractures, but rather they are tears and strains of the ligamental supporting structures.

ROTATIONAL COLLISION

In a rotational collision, the vehicle will rotate around the fixed point of impact. As a result the occupant will sustain a combination of injuries that occur both in a head-on collision and a lateral-impact collision.

ROLLOVER COLLISION

In a rollover collision, it is difficult to predict the type and extent of injuries. Unrestrained occupants will bounce around like pellets in a can, striking various structures in the car.

MOTORCYCLE CRASHES

With motorcycle accidents, injuries sustained are associated with those of head-on collisions and with angular collisions, such as lateral impacts or not-quite-head-on collisions. Also, the rider can receive ejection injuries.

In a head-on collision, when the motorcycle hits, it will tilt up, and the rider will be thrown forward, hitting his or her head, chest, or abdomen on the handlebars. If the rider's feet stay on the pegs, the energy will be absorbed in the midshaft of the femur, probably producing bilateral femur fractures.

In an angular collision, the motorcycle often falls on the rider, crushing the lower leg and often causing open fibular and ankle fractures. In an ejection collision, the rider is thrown free of the motorcycle, and the type and extent of the injuries depend on what part of his or her body collides with what object.

FALLS

Falls are a common mechanism of musculoskeletal injury for both the young and the old. Falls can result in injuries to extremities and more serious injuries, such as pelvic fractures. It is important to consider injuries such as cervical and lumbar spine trauma that may be concurrent with falls.[7,15]

HEALING OF ORTHOPEDIC INJURIES

There are three main stages of repair. In the first stage, a hematoma forms within the first 48 hours. The bone ends and the surrounding soft parts (endosteum, marrow, reticulum, bone chips, periosteum, and extraskeletal tissue that has been lacerated) are bound together by the interlacing mesh of the fibrin formed from the clotted blood that is always present at the site of a fracture.[1,2] The second stage is marked by consolidation or callous formation that restores continuity between fragments. Perivascular connective tissue cells, round cells, and fibroblasts infiltrate the fibrin scaffolding working in a circular motion toward the center to begin the formation of granulation tissue. This mass of cells and tissue then becomes more organized and creates a sleeve of callus, thereby stabilizing the fragments.[1] After about 6 weeks, cartilage is replaced by bone, and at the completion of this stage the fragments are united. Stage 3 occurs with the use and action of normal stresses over a period of months by the provisional callus being removed by remodeling. The dead ends of fragments are reabsorbed, cancellous bone is replaced by compact bone, and the union is complete. This process may take a year or more, but the cast can be removed at the end of stage 2. The rate of union varies from bone to bone and depends on many factors. The healing of fractures is primarily a local phenomenon. A good blood supply to the fragment, adequate proximity of fractured surfaces, and adequate immobilization are the most important prerequisites for healing. However, severe, prolonged negative nitrogen balance, excessive steroids, and a severe lack of vitamin C can impair bone healing. Wound contamination associated with open fractures must also be considered as an impairment to adequate bone repair.[12] Advanced age; diseases such as cancer, osteoporosis, and diabetes; and a disturbance of metabolism should be considered factors affecting the patient's chances of survival, and not factors that might interfere with the healing process.[2]

ASSESSMENT OF AN ORTHOPEDIC INJURY

In patients with multiple trauma, musculoskeletal injuries are rarely life threatening. Thus before assessing possible fractures, the nurse should evaluate associated injuries. The evaluation should begin with attention to airway, breathing, and circulation (the ABCs). Only when the patient has been fully evaluated and is judged stable should an attempt be made to treat an injured limb. The transport team should periodically reassess the patient to make sure that vital functions remain stable.[6] To properly document a musculoskeletal assessment, certain orthopedic terms must be used. Box 18-1 lists common orthopedic terms.

Assessment and monitoring of the trauma patient has four purposes: (1) to monitor the patient's response to the injury, (2) to evaluate the patient's response to treatment, (3) to identify underlying pathologic conditions, and (4) to provide early warnings of complications.[6] To adequately provide this assessment data, a good history is very important. This information can be obtained by talking to the first respondents on the scene or by reading the medical record. As previously discussed, injuries can often be anticipated by knowing the mechanism of injury and the circumstances under which it was sustained.

Open fractures produce greater blood loss and risk of infection than closed fractures, and so demand more immediate attention. However, closed fractures must be carefully monitored, too.[18] The examination for fractures should be organized by body areas, observing first for obvious deformities. If conscious, the patient should be asked to try to move each extremity. If there is a fracture or dislocation, movement or attempted movement is almost always painful or extremely limited with a dislocation. Range of motion, or lack of it, needs to be recorded. Finally, the extremities should be palpated proximally to distally, evaluating for pain, displacement, crepitus, and decreased or absent pulses. The transport team should press down on the iliac

---

BOX 18-1	**Common Orthopedic Terms**

Abduction: movement of a body part away from the body's midline
Adduction: movement of a body part toward the midline
Ankylosis: decreased range of motion caused by stiffening of the joint
Dorsiflexion: movement of the hand or foot upward
Eversion: movement of the ankle outward
Extension: movement of the joint to open it or to maximally increase its angle
External rotation: outward rotation
Flexion: bending of the joint
Hyperextension: extension past neutral
Internal rotation: inward rotation
Inversion: movement of the ankle inward
Kyphosis: round back; increased flexion of the spine
Lordosis: swayback; increased hyperextension of the spine
Plantar flexion: movement of the foot downward
Pronation: movement of the forearm to place the palm downward
Rotation: movement of one bone turning on another
Scoliosis: lateral curvature of the spine
Supination: movement of the forearm to place the palm upward
Torsion: twisting of the bone on its axis
Valgus: deformity causing an outward turning of the foot or toe (e.g., genu valgus or knock-kneed)
Varus: deformity causing an inward turning of the foot or toe (e.g., genu varus or bowlegged)

crests to determine pelvic stability[6] and on the sternum and rib cage to determine stability of the ribs.

The classic signs of musculoskeletal trauma include deformity, localized swelling, pain, pallor, diminished or absent pulses, paresthesia, and paresis or paralysis.[6] If the patient is conscious, the transport team can ask whether the pain is increasing or decreasing and its exact location. Increased swelling, nerve compression, and infiltrated IVs, as well as the actual fracture, can cause an increase in pain. Peripheral pulses (especially those distal to the fracture site) should be checked bilaterally for pressure, strengths, and quality. Paresthesia can be easily checked in the conscious patient by touching or pinching the affected extremity and assessing for altered sensation. Capillary refill needs to be monitored and skin temperature noted.[18] Paralysis at the time of the injury or ensuing paralysis on repeated examination is of great importance in determining definitive care.[1,9]

Also, joints above and below the fracture site or point of injury need to be evaluated. Neurovascular status assessments of the affected extremity should be done frequently, but especially before and after transport.

Children require special consideration in evaluation for musculoskeletal injuries. Because their bones are more flexible than those of adults, greater force is often required to cause a fracture than would be necessary in an adult. Therefore, a child who has sustained even minor rib fractures must be assumed to have sustained serious internal injuries. The transport team should suspect a splenic and/or diaphragmatic injury in a child with low rib fractures. Children are also likely to receive avulsion fractures because of their flexible skeletons.[6]

MANAGEMENT OF ORTHOPEDIC INJURIES

Careless handling of a patient with an injury to the musculoskeletal system may convert a simple problem into a much more serious one. The closed wound may become an open one, a clean wound may become grossly contaminated, or blood vessels and nerves may be seriously injured. There are five

basic principles for managing fractures and/or dislocations: (1) avoid unnecessary handling, (2) immobilize, (3) apply clean dressings to wounds, (4) control hemorrhage with direct pressure, and (5) check for the "5 Ps" distal to the injury—pain, pulselessness, paresthesia, pallor, and paralysis.[7,9]

WOUND MANAGEMENT

Local wound care is initiated by assessing the wound for evidence of severe hemorrhage, debris, and the presence of bone ends protruding through the skin. These findings should be noted on the chart, and a dry, sterile dressing should be applied. So that circulation is not further impaired, there should be no attempt at wound cleansing or pulling the bones back beneath the skin. Severe hemorrhage is generally controllable by direct pressure over the wound or over the arteries just proximal to the wound.[7] Good wound care is as important to the positive outcome of a patient as is good splinting. This technique should not be overlooked. Tetanus status should be noted at some point during patient care.

SPLINTING

Good emergency care rendered to a patient with any type of orthopedic injury will decrease his or her hospital stay, speed recovery, and lessen the chance of serious complications. Because the extent of injury is difficult to assess initially, it is always best to assume a fracture is present and immobilize it until further evaluation can be made by x-ray.

The primary objective of splinting is to prevent motion of fractured bone fragments or dislocated joints and thereby to prevent the following complications.

1. Laceration of the skin by broken bones, which can increase the risk of contamination and infection
2. Damage to local blood vessels causing excessive bleeding into surrounding tissue, ischemia, and even tissue death
3. Restriction of blood flow to an area as a result of pressure of bone ends on blood vessels
4. Damage to nerves by inadvertent excessive traction, contusion, or laceration resulting in

possible permanent loss of sensation and paralysis[15]

5. Damage to muscles with possible subsequent necrosis, scarring, and permanent disability[15]
6. Increased pain associated with movement of bone ends[17]
7. Shock
8. Delayed union or nonunion of fractured bones or dislocated joints

Some basic principles of management for any type of orthopedic injury must be considered in splint application. The first is to splint the patient's fracture immediately. A fracture, dislocation, or sprain should be splinted or traction applied before the patient is moved or transported. Second, pulse, color, pain, and sensation distal to the injury always need to be assessed before and after splinting. Third, if a fracture is open, the transport team should stop the bleeding and dress the wound before applying a splint. No attempts to push the protruding bone back inside should be made. Fourth, with some very important exceptions, a severely angulated fracture should be straightened before splinting to lessen the chance of further damage to vessels and nerves around the fracture site.[17] A fracture or dislocation of the spine, shoulder, elbow, wrist, or knee should not be straightened. The dislocated joint should be splinted above and below the injured site in the position that it is found. For angulated fractures, overlying clothing should be cut or torn away. One should be as gentle as possible because bone ends can break through the skin just from rough handling. The extremity should be gently but firmly grasped by placing one hand just below the fracture site and the other hand farther down the extremity. If possible, someone should apply countertraction by holding the patient in place while a steady downward pull is being exerted. The angle of fracture should not be forcibly changed. A team member should maintain traction until the splint is properly applied. With a traction splint on a lower extremity, manual traction should be continued until the splint has been properly applied. Finally, the splint should be applied firmly but in a way that does not interfere with circulation, and the team should be sure that it is padded sufficiently to prevent pressure points.

The transport team must address certain considerations, including the size of the transport vehicle, the transport vehicle's configuration, and altitude as it relates to the use of splints, when splinting a patient's injuries and preparing the patient for transport.

SOFT SPLINT

A soft splint is one that has no inherent rigidity, such as a pillow or a rolled blanket. Both can provide considerable support when wrapped around an injured part and bandaged.

RIGID SPLINT

A rigid splint has inherent rigidity. It is placed along the side, front, or back of the injured extremity, and when used correctly, it will immobilize the fracture. Examples of rigid splints include backboards, metal splints, hinged splints, cardboard splints, and the pneumatic antishock garment (PSAG). Rigid splints are effective only when they are long enough to allow the entire fractured bone to be immobilized, are padded sufficiently, and are secured firmly to an uninjured part.[18]

When using a rigid splint, the transport team member immobilizes the joints above and below the fracture site. Therefore, a rigid splint must be long enough to extend over joints and immobilize the entire fractured bone. Many items, such as rolled newspapers or pieces of wood, can be used to make a rigid splint. Whatever is used, however, must be long enough, strong enough, and well padded enough to do the job (Box 18-2).

With various other types, depending on the site of the fracture, a rigid splint can be contoured to fit the extremity. For example, wire ladder splints can be bent, cardboard can be cut and taped into the desired form and shape, or a pillow splint can be used with rigid board support.

When using a rigid splint to immobilize a dislocated joint, the transport team member will immobilize the bones above and below the joint. Because one should never try to straighten or reduce a dislocation, many times it is necessary to improvise a

| BOX 18-2 | **General Principles of Splinting** |

Expose and examine the injured extremity. Look for a wound, tenting of the skin, or obvious discoloration that may indicate the presence of or potential for an open fracture.

Support the body part.

Remove jewelry and constrictive items of clothing.

Assess and document sensory and circulatory status before immobilization. If there is no palpable distal pulse, medical control may recommend applying gentle traction along the long axis of the extremity (distal to the injury) until the distal pulse is palpable.

Immobilize the extremity so that the splint includes the joints above and below the fracture or the bones above and below the dislocation. Avoid excessive movement of the body part. (Movement may increase bleeding into the tissue space, increase the risk of fat embolism, or convert a closed fracture to an open fracture.)

NOTE: Immobilization requires a minimum of two rescuers.

When applying splints to the hand or foot, leave the fingers or toes exposed to provide for inspection and evaluation of neurovascular status.

Reevaluate and document sensory and circulatory status after immobilization. If a nerve or pulse deficit develops after splinting, remove the splint and place the extremity in its original position.

From Sanders MJ: *Mosby's paramedic textbook,* St Louis, 1994, Mosby.

splint because of the odd shape of an extremity with a dislocated joint.

TRACTION SPLINT

Traction splints are also rigid splints. However, they are not used to reduce a fracture but rather to align it and immobilize the bone to prevent further damage during movement and transportation.[1,18] The traction splint immobilizes by a steady longitudinal traction pull exerted on the injured extremity. Traction splints should not be used on an injury to an upper extremity because of the danger of further damage or of impeding the circulation. Examples of traction splints are the Thomas half-ring, the Hare traction splint, and the Sager splint.[1] Traction splints immobilize by pulling on the distal portion of the entire extremity below the fracture. When applying a traction splint, the flight nurse watches the patient for signs of pain or relief in his or her face and uses that as a guide for the proper amount of traction.

SPLINTING FRACTURES OF THE UPPER EXTREMITIES

Fractures of the clavicle usually occur at the middle and distal thirds of the bone from a blow to the shoulder. Pain, swelling, and deformity are generally evident. Supporting the arm in a sling and binding it against the chest with a swathe will sufficiently immobilize the fracture. However, injuries that occur in motor vehicle collisions may fracture the bone more medially, pushing it into the thoracic outlet and possibly injuring the long, subclavian artery or vein or the brachioplexus. The pulmonary and neurovascular injuries then become first priority.[7,8]

Fractures of the upper end of the humerus may or may not involve the shoulder joint. There will be pain and tenderness, but severe angulation is less commonly observed. The goals in treating humeral fractures are to maintain shoulder function and achieve fracture union. These goals can best be achieved by treating the problem as a soft tissue injury that happens to involve bone.[8] If there is gross deformity at the fracture site, the arm should be splinted in the position in which it is found with padded boards and pillow splints. In most cases, however, there will be little gross angulation, and the arm may be splinted with a sling and swathe.[18]

Fractures of the midshaft of the humerus endanger the radial nerve. The transport team can check for damage to the radial nerve by observing the patient's ability to spread his or her fingers. If there has been damage, there will be pain on movement and tenderness at the fracture site. If angulation is present, a transport team member should use gentle, constant traction, apply a sling, and with traction still being held, place a padded board along the outer border of the humerus. A swathe is applied around the sling, the padded board, and the injured arm, binding the arm to the chest. A fracture without angulation may be splinted in the same manner.

Fractures of the elbow endanger the radial, ulnar, and median nerves and the brachial artery. The transport team member should check for a pulse, movement, and sensation (Figure 18-2). The fracture should be splinted in the exact position found, using a rigid splint above and below the fracture. If possible, the arm should be bound to the side to offer additional support.

After gentle traction has been applied to any severe angulation of a fracture of the radius or the ulna, a rigid splint should be applied, immobilizing both the elbow and the wrist.

Fractures of the wrist without angulation should be splinted in the same manner as the radius and the ulna. Those fractures with severe angulation, however, should be splinted in the position found.

Severe hand injuries often involve both soft tissue and bone injury. In most cases, the hand should be splinted in the position of function, with the fingers slightly bent and a bulky fluff dressing in the palm of the hand. A rigid splint should also be used to immobilize the wrist.

SPLINTING DISLOCATIONS OF THE UPPER EXTREMITIES

With a shoulder dislocation, the normal rounded appearance of the shoulder is flattened. There are basically two types of shoulder dislocations: anterior and posterior. Most dislocations are anterior. In the anterior dislocation, the patient will hold his or her arm away from the body, and there will be a bony prominence in the front of the shoulder.[6]

A pillow splint, and frequently the help of a second person to hold the arm, can best obtain maximum stability without changing the deformity. With a posterior dislocation, there is little evident deformity, and the arm is held against the chest or abdomen. A sling and swathe are all that is necessary to maintain position. A rare inferior dislocation (the humerus is dislocated downward from the shoulder) may cause the patient to hold his or her arm above the head. The flight nurse splints it in the position found. All of these patients should be transported in a sitting position.

A dislocated elbow may appear as a posterior or anterior dislocation. With a posterior, the more common, the arm is flexed. A long splint with the flexion maintained should be applied. A sling will help to maintain stability. This patient should also be transported in a sitting position. With an anterior

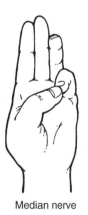

Median nerve

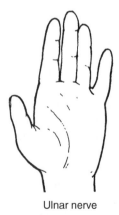

Ulnar nerve

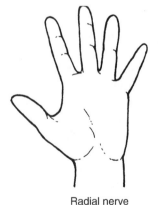

Radial nerve

FIGURE 18-2 **Testing for neurologic function in the upper extremities.**

dislocation, the arm is extended and the joint immovable because of pain. Again, the transport team will splint the injury in the position found.

A dislocated wrist is most often a Colles' fracture, occurring just proximal to the joint. A dislocated wrist will have an obvious deformity, and a well-padded splint should be used. The index finger is the most commonly dislocated finger, with the deformity being obvious and the fingertip slightly cyanotic and cold. A splint is all that is needed to help control pain. Immobilization is all that is needed for both injuries.

SPLINTING FRACTURES OF THE LOWER EXTREMITIES

Fractures of the hip and proximal femur are anatomically divided into two types: fractures of the neck of the femur (transcervical) and fractures through the trochanters (intertrochanteric). Both appear the same clinically, with pain and swelling around the hip, pain on hip motion, and various degrees of shortening and external rotation.[15] The fractured hip is best splinted with pillows in the position found. In assessing a hip injury, there may be associated injuries to the knee, sciatic nerve injury, and ipsilateral femoral shaft fractures.

With fractures of the shaft of the femur, there is a strong contraction of the gluteus medius muscle, which has a tendency to pull the proximal fragment of the femur outward as the adduction causes bowing at the fracture point.[8] These fractures should be splinted immediately with a traction splint and kept in the splint until definitive orthopedic care is rendered. Femoral shaft fractures can cause extensive blood loss that can lead to hypovolemic shock, so an IV also should be initiated in these patients.[7,8]

Fractures of the knee should be splinted as they are found, with no attempt made to correct any angulation. Checking for and reporting changes in pulse, movement, and sensation is especially important with any type of knee injury. Fractures of the patella are recognizable as swelling of the anterior knee with little or no resistance to extension of the joint. A transport team member should splint this kind of fracture with a rigid splint and the patient's knee in extension.

Fractures of the tibia and/or fibula are also best managed with a rigid splint after the application of traction to correct severe angulation. The splint should immobilize both the ankle and knee joints and is best when carried as high as the groin. Great care must be taken with these fractures to prevent penetration of bone ends through the skin.[18]

Severely angulated fractures of the ankle should be straightened by traction applied to the heel and forefoot. A rigid splint should then be applied to immobilize the foot and ankle. If there is any question of a sprain or fracture, the injury should be splinted until a diagnostic radiograph can be made. Another method that can be used to splint some injuries is the application of PASG. A PASG is very effective in the splinting of both long-bone and pelvic fractures and should not be overlooked by the transport team.

SPLINTING DISLOCATIONS OF THE LOWER EXTREMITIES

Differentiating between a dislocated hip and a fractured hip is often impossible, although with a dislocated hip the patient's thigh is sometimes flexed to some extent and turned slightly inward. Treatment for either one is the same. The transport team should splint, using pillows or sheets and blankets, in the position found. Because of the close proximity of the sciatic and femoral nerves, an immediate neurologic assessment of the affected limb is of utmost importance (Figure 18-3).

Dislocations and fractures of the knee are treated the same. Any resistance to attempts to straighten an angulation indicates that it should be splinted in the position found, again paying heed to pulse, movement, and sensation. A rigid splint, preferably a padded board, should be used.

Ankle dislocations rarely occur without associated fractures and should be aligned and splinted exactly the same as ankle fractures. Dislocation of the foot is rare but generally involves more than one joint. It also should be treated the same as fracture of the foot. Toe dislocations are innately stable and need no splinting.[7,9]

Whenever possible after splinting a dislocation or a fracture, the transport team should elevate the

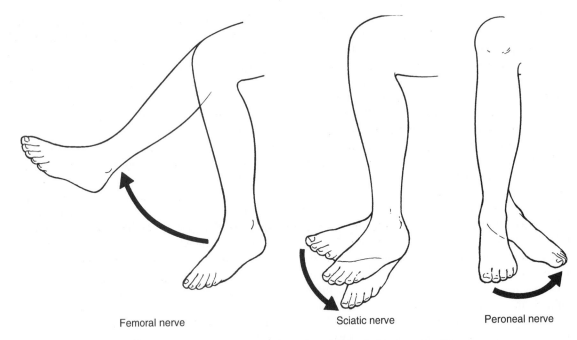

Femoral nerve   Sciatic nerve   Peroneal nerve

FIGURE 18-3   **Testing for neurologic function in the lower extremities.**

affected extremity and apply ice to the injured part. This makes the patient more comfortable and augments the splinting.

PELVIC FRACTURES

A pelvic fracture can be one of the most serious injuries that a patient with multiple injuries can sustain. The major cause of death is hemorrhage from arteries and veins torn by the fracture or dislocation.

The most common form of pelvic fracture results from a severe external force directly on the pelvis or from an indirect force transmitted upward along the shaft of the femur. Minor fractures of the pelvis include breaks of individual bones without a break in the continuity of the pelvic ring. These fractures are relatively stable and rarely require hospitalization. Major pelvic fractures are generally fractured in at least two separate places, and there may be a separation of one or both sacroiliac joints. These fractures are commonly seen in patients with multiple traumas.

Approximately 60% of pelvic fractures should be considered major injuries because of the complications of injury to the structures lying within the pelvis.[5] Besides the danger of damage to the major blood vessels within the pelvic girdle, fractures of the pubic ramus may lacerate the urethra, fractures of the brim of the pelvis may disrupt the ureters, and the bladder itself may rupture.[8] Open fractures of the pelvis occur when there is a direct communication between fracture fragments and a laceration of the skin, vagina, or rectum. This is an uncommon fracture caused by a high-velocity injury, and there is subsequent massive hemorrhage with a 50% mortality rate. Even small amounts of blood on vaginal or rectal examination should indicate the possibility of an open fracture.[5]

Control of bleeding is a top priority.[5,7] Approximately 500 ml of blood loss from each fracture can be expected,[4] so a large-bore intravenous line must also be placed for possible blood transfusion. Patients with pelvic injuries should also be catheterized, unless urethral injury is expected. The indicating symptoms of urethral injury include blood at the meatus, the urge to void but the inability to do so, and in men, a prostate that is positioned high. Many patients with a pelvic injury will have hematuria.

Forces powerful enough to cause pelvic fractures can cause other serious injuries. Associated injuries should be identified from the knees to the chest.

VASCULAR EMERGENCIES

The first crude vascular repair was performed by Hallowell over two centuries ago, and the basic suture techniques as we know them today, including the use of autografts and homografts, were well worked out by the end of the first decade of this century. However, application of these techniques did not occur until the Korean War. Today's relatively optimistic outlook toward peripheral vascular injuries is the result of a variety of innovations including rapid transportation, availability of blood and antibiotics, abandonment of mass tourniquet techniques, a better appreciation of the true nature of certain forms of vessel injury (penetrating, blunt, and fracture-associated injuries), recognition of the importance of fracture stabilization, and many diagnostic and surgical advances.

A major amount of persistent bleeding, either apparent externally or manifested by shock, a hematoma, or a falling hematocrit level demands serious consideration for exploration and hemostasis.

VASCULAR EXAMINATIONS

Vascular abnormalities can be discovered by careful observation, palpation, and auscultation. This examination can be done rapidly and is the basis for immediate treatment.

The patient's general appearance and description of pain is helpful because most arterial obstructions or ruptures are accompanied by severe pain distal to the site. Bilateral arm blood pressures are necessary to rule out an occluded arm.

The transport team should next make a comparison of pulses. This is done by simultaneous or rapid sequential palpation of the temporal, carotid, radial, femoral, popliteal, and pedal or dorsalis pedis pulses.

Auscultation over hematomas with associated arterial or venous injuries may make early diagnosis of an arteriovenous fistula possible. Rounds of turbulence are indicative of communication between an artery and a vein.

Observation of the skin for pallor, cyanosis, sweating, venous collateral engorgement, and edema is important for distinguishing between arterial and venous injuries. Temperature changes on the same extremity or differences in paired extremities may be indicative of impaired circulation. Assessment of capillary refill can also signify circulatory integrity.

Movement and sensation must be observed because traumatic injuries are frequently accompanied by nerve injuries; major arteries and nerves are closely associated anatomically. However, it is vital to note pulses because neurologic deficits will occur as a result of acute obstruction with severe ischemia.

COMPARISON OF ARTERIAL AND VENOUS CONDITIONS

Arterial and venous injuries are pathologically different, and the transport team must be constantly alert during the examination to differentiate between the two. A number of signs and symptoms must be assessed.

An arterial injury will be manifested by continuing copious hemorrhage from an open wound. The hemorrhage may be concealed and appear in the form of a rapid accumulating hematoma. There may be neurologic manifestations, either motor or sensory or spinal cord (produced by acute aortic thrombosis). The patient will report severe pain distal to the site. The temperature of the affected area will be cool, and the color will be pale, blotchy, and/or cyanotic. Blood pressure in the affected extremities will differ, capillary filling will be poor, and pulses will be absent or diminished.[2,9] The transport team must be alert to potential arterial injury with any fracture, especially fracture dislocation.

With venous injury comes potential for major hemorrhage, either from an open or a concealed wound, but bleeding tends to be less severe because of the low pressures involved. There will be edema. Pain will be general and local along the course of the vein. Temperature in the affected area can be either cool or warm, and color may be mottled and show patchy areas of cyanosis. Neurologic manifestations will be paresthesias distal to the site and sweating. Generally, capillary filling will be good, although it can be impaired. Pulses may be diminished because of spasm or impalpable because of edema.[3,10] Pulses are the most important indicator of vascular injury.

PRIMARY CARE OF VASCULAR INJURIES

The most important indication for treatment following vascular injury is external hemorrhaging. This should be controlled initially with direct pressure over the site of injury or the artery proximal to the site (the pressure point). The site should also be immobilized and elevated, if possible. Only after all of this has been done and is ineffective should the use of a tourniquet be considered. The tourniquet should be 3 to 4 inches wide (a blood pressure cuff works well) and should be tightened only enough to stop the bleeding. The prolonged application of a tourniquet gravely jeopardizes the success of reconstructive surgery and may make amputation necessary.

Shock must be combated and volume replaced; therefore large-bore IV lines must be placed. Pulse rate and blood pressure must be closely watched and, if possible, urinary output and hematocrit levels observed.

Finally, expeditious diagnosis and treatment are of paramount importance in any acute vascular injury. The viability of the extremity or organ may depend on the speed with which diagnosis, primary care, and definitive care are undertaken. Although it is recognized that the "golden hour" period is only relative, the results of treatments do correlate well with this concept.

TRAUMATIC AMPUTATIONS

Complete traumatic amputations of extremities occur from time to time from various kinds of trauma, such as motor vehicle collisions, entanglements in farm or industrial machinery, or crushes caused by heavy objects or falls. Excellent emergency care of the patient and the severed extremity will likely result in a successful reimplantation.

A primary assessment must first be made of the patient, and any life-threatening conditions must be addressed. Hemorrhage should be controlled with dry, sterile pressure dressings, and the extremity should be elevated and immobilized. As with any vascular injury, a tourniquet should only be used as a last resort. If bleeding is not a problem, then a transport team member should flush the wound with crystalloid solution depending on the local protocols, apply a dry, sterile dressing and a mild pressure gauze wrap to the extremity, and immobilize and elevate the extremity. The transport team then should flush the amputated part with crystalloid solution, wrap it in a dry, sterile gauze or towel (if unavailable, use a clean sheet), and place it in a plastic bag or container. Then the severed part is put in another container and cooled by another plastic bag containing ice. Dry ice should not be used because it increases necrosis. As with any acute vascular injury, the expediency with which the patient and amputated part reach definitive care directly correlates with the success of reimplantation.

SUMMARY

In most cases, orthopedic and related vascular injuries are not life threatening; however, the long-term outcome for patients who sustain these injuries is greatly influenced by the initial care that they receive. The transport team should approach orthopedic and vascular emergencies with these goals in mind: (1) minimize the complications associated with fractures, both open and closed; (2) decrease complications of immobility caused by these injuries; (3) facilitate the general management of more definitive care; and (4) help to preserve and restore complete function of the affected extremity.[13]

ORTHOPEDIC VASCULAR TRAUMA CASE STUDY

A 25-year-old unrestrained intoxicated male was riding in the front seat of a car that struck the side of a hill. On arrival of the transport team, they found the patient in the back of an ambulance, complaining of severe right leg pain. The patient's ABCs were intact, but his right leg was lying beside his head. When the car had struck the hill, he had his leg crossed over on his knee. The impact of the collision caused dislocation of his right hip and multiple fractures of his leg allowing it to assume this position.

There was no palpable pulse in the extremity. An intravenous line was inserted and conscious sedation was administered using fentanyl and lorazepam. The flight physician then reduced the dislocated hip and splinted the fractures.

The patient was then transported without incident to the trauma center.

REFERENCES

1. Campbell J, editor: *Basic trauma life support for paramedics and other advanced providers,* ed 4, Upper Saddle River, NJ, 2000, Brady/Prentice Hall Health.
2. Committee on Trauma, American College of Surgeons: *Advanced trauma life support course instructor manual,* Chicago, 1997, Author.
3. Fahey VA, Racelis MC: Vascular emergencies. In Kitt S et al, editors: *Emergency nursing,* Philadelphia, 1995, Saunders.
4. Farrell J: The trauma patient with multiple fractures, *RN* 48(6):22, 1985.
5. Harrahill M: Open pelvic fracture: the lethal injury, *J Emerg Nurs* 20(3):243, 1994.
6. Heckman JD: Looking beyond the trees to the forest, *Consultant* 22(2):133, 1982.
7. Jacobs B, Hoyt S, editors: *Trauma nursing core course,* ed 5, Des Plaines, Ill, 2000, Emergency Nurses Association.
8. Jagmin MG: Musculoskeletal emergencies. In Kitt S et al, editors: *Emergency nursing,* Philadelphia, 1995, Saunders.
9. Krupa D, editor: *Flight nursing core curriculum,* Des Plaines, Ill, 1997, Road Runner Press.
10. Lower J: Maxillofacial trauma, *Nurs Clin North Am* 21(4):611, 1986.
11. Mabee JR: Compartment syndrome: a complication of acute extremity trauma, *J Emerg Med* 12(5):651, 1995.
12. Maher AB: Early assessment and management of musculoskeletal injuries, *Nurs Clin North Am* 21(4):717, 1986.
13. McSwain N: To manage multiple injury consider mechanisms, *Emerg Med* 16(4):56, 1984.
14. Pashley J, Wahlstrom NL: Polytrauma: the patient, the family, and the health team, *Nurs Clin North Am* 16(4):721, 1981.
15. Perdue P: Abdominal injuries and dangerous fractures, *RN* 44(7):35, 84, 1981.
16. Proehl J, editor: *Emergency nursing procedures,* ed 2, Philadelphia, 1999, Saunders.
17. Rodts MF: An orthopedic assessment you can do in 15 minutes, *Nurs 83* 13(5):65, 1983.
18. Sanders MJ: *Mosby's paramedic text,* St Louis, 1994, Mosby.

BURN TRAUMA

## 19

COMPETENCIES

1. Calculate percentage of total body surface area burned using both the *rule of nines* and the Lund and Browder charts.
2. Calculate appropriate fluid replacement amounts and rates of administration based on the patient's burn injury and physiologic condition.
3. Prioritize the care of patients who have received thermal, chemical, or electrical burns.
4. Provide appropriate pain management for the patient who has suffered a burn injury.
5. Describe appropriate escharotomy sites.

BURN INJURIES

INCIDENCE AND CAUSATIVE FACTORS

Approximately 1,000,000 individuals sustain burn injuries in the United States each year. Of these, 70,000 require hospitalization, and approximately 4500 will die. The death rate from burns has decreased significantly over the past 20 years.[1,5] The rate of burn injury has also decreased significantly from 10/10,000 to 4.2/10,000 over the past 40 years.[1] The highest risk group for burn injury are people ages 18 to 35 years. However, both young children and older adults are also at risk for burn injuries.

The care of the patient with a major burn requires an organized, educated, and dedicated staff and resources. The transport team will be called to take these patients to burn centers and must be prepared to provide care for them during the transport process.

ETIOLOGY AND EPIDEMIOLOGY

A burn wound is an injury caused by the interaction of an energy form (thermal, chemical, electrical, or radiation) and biologic matter (Figure 19-1).[3] Most burns are thermal: flame burns, scalds, or contacts with hot substances. Frostbite is often included in this category; however, no current statistics are available regarding its incidence.

Chemical injuries occur when the source of energy contacted is capable of causing tissue necrosis. Examples of necrosis-causing chemicals include strong acids, which cause coagulation necrosis from protein precipitation, or alkalis, which cause liquefaction necrosis.

Electrical burns occur when contact is made with a high-voltage current. The current itself is not considered to have any thermal properties while

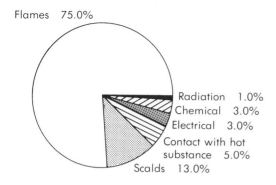

Flames   75.0%

Radiation   1.0%
Chemical   3.0%
Electrical   3.0%
Contact with hot substance   5.0%
Scalds   13.0%

FIGURE 19-1   **Causes of burn injuries.**

traveling through material of low resistance; however, the potential energy of the current is transferred into thermal energy when it meets resistance with biologic tissue and is dispersed throughout that tissue. This action is accomplished primarily by conduction.

Radiation injuries can be caused by both ionizing and nonionizing radiation. Radiation injuries make up a very small percentage of burn injuries.[15,25]

PATHOPHYSIOLOGY OF BURN WOUNDS

The causes of burns may vary, but the local and systemic responses are generally similar. The extent of the injury is influenced by three factors: (1) the intensity of the energy source, (2) the duration of exposure to the energy source, and (3) the conductance of the tissue exposed. The relationship between the duration of exposure to and intensity of the energy source is significant in determining the magnitude of the injury. Increased intensity with increased exposure causes increased amounts of tissue damage. Conductance can be affected by the presence of hair, water content of the tissues, and thickness and pigmentation of the skin.[3,15]

To better understand the pathophysiology of burn wounds, one must know the anatomy and functions of the skin. Skin is composed of two layers, the epidermis and the dermis. The epidermis, the outer layer, consists of the basement layer of cells that migrate upward to become surface keratin. The inner layer, the dermis, consists of collagen and elastic fibers and contains hair follicles, sweat and sebaceous glands, nerve endings, and blood vessels. Beneath the cutaneous layers is a layer of subcutaneous tissue consisting primarily of connective tissue and fat deposits; this layer overlies muscle and bone.[34]

The primary functions of skin include (1) regulation of body temperature through dilation and constriction of the dermal and subcuticular vessels in response to environmental temperature, (2) protection against injury and bacterial invasion, (3) prevention of body fluid loss, and (4) sensory contact with the environment. When a burn injury occurs, it interrupts and compromises these functions.[34]

Responses of the body to thermal injury consist of varying degrees of tissue damage, cellular impairment, and fluid shifts. Locally, there is a brief initial decrease in blood flow to the area, followed by a marked increase in arteriolar vasodilation. A concurrent release of vasoactive substances from the burned tissue causes increased capillary permeability. These combine to produce intravascular fluid loss and wound edema.

Hypoproteinemia resulting from the increase in capillary permeability aggravates edema in the nonburned tissue.[51] Insensible fluid loss from the burn wound increases the basal metabolic rate and, along with fluid shift, leads to hypovolemia.

Many other physiologic responses to burn injuries can compromise patient outcome. With the decrease in circulating plasma comes an increase in hematocrit.[15] This in turn can cause hemoglobinuria when the hemoglobin is filtered through the kidneys and can contribute to renal failure. Increased peripheral vascular resistance leads to a decrease in venous return to the heart, decreased cardiac output, impaired tissue perfusion, and a decrease in renal perfusion, which can also contribute to renal failure.[27]

A decrease in splanchnic blood flow occurs, which increases the occurrence of mucosal hemorrhages in the stomach and duodenum. There may also be increased risk of sepsis from bacterial translocation as a result of diminished mucosal barrier function in the intestine. Patients with burns on more than 20% of their body surface area (BSA) can also experience the problem of adynamic ileus, which can be of special concern for the patient being transported by air at high altitudes.[51]

Decreased immune responses increase the patient's susceptibility to infection. This requires the transport team to take extra precautions to prevent further injury to the burn victim through exposure to contaminated environments. Precautions include covering the burn wound with a dry, clean dressing and, in the case of a large burn wound, placing the patient on one dry, clean sheet and covering him or her with blankets added over the sheets as needed. Wet dressings should not be used because they provide an open pathway for bacteria, cause additional tissue injury, and will leave the patient at risk of becoming hypothermic because of loss of skin integrity from the burn injury.

ASSESSMENT

The assessment of the patient with burn injuries begins with the ABCs of the primary assessment. Burn wounds are often very dramatic in appearance and can lure the transport team's attention away from more immediate life-threatening problems.

The subjective assessment includes obtaining as thorough a history as circumstances permit. The history should include the mechanism and time of the injury and a description of the surrounding environment, such as injuries incurred in an enclosed space, the presence of noxious chemicals, the possibility of smoke inhalation, and any related trauma. The time of the injury is especially important in the calculation of fluid resuscitation. Information regarding tetanus immunization status should also be obtained with the history.[2,15,20,23,51]

The objective assessment of the burn injury itself includes estimating the burn size and depth, associated inhalation injuries, and calculation of fluid resuscitation needs. The size of a burn wound is most frequently estimated by using the *rule of nines* method, which divides the body into multiples of 9% (Figure 19-2). A more accurate assessment can be made of the burn injury, especially for pediatric patients, by using a Lund and Browder chart, which takes into account growth changes (Figure 19-3). For estimating scatter burns, a fairly accurate

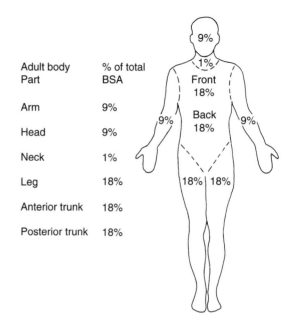

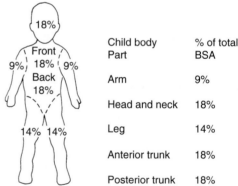

FIGURE 19-2   **The rule of nines.**

approximation can be made using the patient's entire palm size to represent 1% of the total BSA and visualizing that palm over the burned area.[25,46]

Because the depth of a thermal burn wound is determined primarily by the temperature of the burning agent, the duration of exposure, and the conductance of the tissue involved, estimation of injury depth is difficult initially.

Burn wounds typically present in a bull's-eye pattern, with each ring representing a different zone of intensity. A superficial partial-thickness injury or

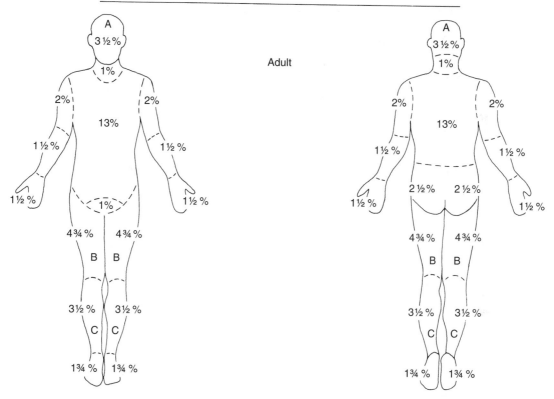

Age	0-1	1-4	5-9	1-14	15
A — ½ of head	9½%	8½%	6½%	5½%	4½%
B — ½ of one thigh	2¾%	3¼%	4%	4¼%	4½%
C — ½ of one thigh	2½%	2½%	2¾%	3%	3¼%

FIGURE 19-3 **Lund and Browder method for calculating percentage of burned body surface area.**

a first-degree burn involves the epidermis and is represented by the outermost ring, the *zone of hyperemia.* This type of injury is usually red in appearance, is painful, and heals in 7 to 10 days.

A deep partial-thickness injury, or second-degree burn, involves both the epidermis and dermis. It is seen as the middle ring and is called the *zone of stasis,* which is potentially viable tissue, despite the heat injury. This wound is characterized by reddened skin that is wet or blistered, is very painful, and generally heals in 14 to 21 days. However, these diagnostic signs can be misleading according to Morgan[20] because it is possible to have a full-thickness burn under a blister.

Full-thickness injuries are the center ring, called the *zone of coagulation.* These injuries encompass third-degree wounds, consisting of both dermal layers and extending into the subcutaneous tissue, and fourth-degree wounds, which extend into muscle and bone. Full-thickness injuries are charred and leathery in appearance or white and waxy, with thrombosed vessels that are easily visible under the surface. They are painless because of destruction of sensory nerves, and there is no epithelial growth for healing. These wounds require grafting.[3,11,34,43,51]

FLUID RESUSCITATION

The goal of initial fluid resuscitation is to restore and maintain adequate tissue perfusion and vital organ function, in addition to preserving heat-injured but viable tissue in the zone of stasis.[11,15] Fluid needs are based on the size of the patient and the extent of the burn. The two most common formulas for estimating fluid needs are the Parkland formula, which is 4 ml/kg/% BSA burned, and the Modified Brooke formula, which is 2 ml/kg/% BSA burned.[3,15,43] These have been combined and presented as the Consensus formula of 2 to 4 ml/kg/% BSA burned.[45] All the formulas call for one half of the total amount to be given over the first 8 hours from the time of the injury and the second half to be given over the following 16 hours.

There is some controversy over the most appropriate fluid to be used in burn resuscitation. There are proponents of various combinations of hypertonic and isotonic solutions, crystalloid, and colloid. Choice of fluid will largely be a matter of local opinion and current research. It is important for the transport team to consult with the physician or burn center that will be accepting the patient to obtain orders for fluids and fluid resuscitation guidelines.

Fluid resuscitation for the pediatric patient should be based on body surface area because the linear relationship between weight and surface area does not apply in children.[20] Taking into account the increased evaporative water loss in the formula for fluid resuscitation for pediatric patients, the Shrine Burn formula calculates 2000 ml × the total BSA + 5000 ml × the total BSA burned for the first 24 hours after the injury. This formula also calls for one half of the total amount to be given over the following 16 hours. This formula is widely used by the Shrine Burn Centers. Emphasis in pediatric fluid resuscitation is shifting to the minimum amount necessary to maintain vital organ function. There is also current research suggesting that children tolerate rapid initial volume infusion, with half the cal-

culated volume given over 4 hours and the remainder given over 20 hours, a formula that differs somewhat from the adult regimen.[12,20,26,41,56]

Monitoring the effectiveness of fluid resuscitation is a very important part of patient management. The parameters most easily available during transport are vital signs, mental status, and urinary output.

VITAL SIGNS

Vital signs are not the most accurate method of monitoring a patient with a large burn because of the pathophysiologic changes that accompany such an injury. Blood pressure may be difficult to ascertain because of increasing generalized edema. An invasive monitoring device may not be accurate because of the peripheral vasoconstriction caused by release of vasoactive mediators such as catecholamines. Pulse may be somewhat more helpful in monitoring the appropriateness of fluid resuscitation. Presence of more than a mild tachycardia or a persistent tachycardia is evidence of hypovolemia. However, even this can be confusing because tachycardia may be the result of pain and the stress response. The transport team should be careful not to overlook young, otherwise healthy adults whose normal resting heart rate may be in the 40 to 60 beats-per-minute range or the elderly patient who may be taking medications, such as beta-blockers, that will interfere with their normal physiologic responses. A heart rate of greater than 70 beats per minute may not indicate the underlying volume deficit for this type of patient.[6]

A decrease in level of consciousness not associated with trauma may also be indicative of hypoxia or hypovolemia. This problem should be alleviated with appropriate adjustments in ventilatory and circulatory support. If the level of consciousness does not improve with increased hydration and oxygenation, other problem sources such as carbon monoxide poisoning or electrolyte imbalance should be suspected and investigated.[11,43]

Urinary output is perhaps the most accurate method of evaluating the effectiveness of fluid replacement. Adults should have an hourly output of 30 to 50 ml.

The urinary output in children should be maintained at 1 to 2 ml/kg/% BSA burned for children under 30 kg. Oliguria is an indication of inadequate fluid volume and should be easily corrected by increasing the rate of fluid administration. When this is ineffective, and fluid volume needs have been accurately assessed and administered, an osmotic diuretic such as mannitol can be given to avoid acute renal failure.[11,46,56]

INHALATION INJURIES

There are three types of identifiable inhalation injuries: (1) asphyxiation from carbon monoxide poisoning; (2) supraglottic injury, which is primarily thermal in nature; and (3) infraglottic injury, which is primarily chemical. Inhalation injuries are the primary cause of death at the scene of a burn injury, and they contribute significantly to the overall morbidity and mortality of burn patients.[21]

Carbon monoxide intoxication occurs when the affinity for carbon monoxide to hemoglobin is markedly greater than that of oxygen; therefore the carbon monoxide binds with the available hemoglobin to form carboxyhemoglobin and causes hypoxia. The signs and symptoms of carbon monoxide poisoning include pink to cherry-red skin, tachycardia, tachypnea, headache, dizziness, and nausea. It is diagnosed by measuring carboxyhemoglobin levels. Levels of 0% to 15% rarely cause symptoms and may be normal, especially for a heavy smoker. Levels of 15% to 40% cause varying amounts of central nervous system disturbances, such as confusion and headache. Levels greater than 40% can cause mental depression and coma.[11,43] Any patient with suspected carbon monoxide injury should be given 100% oxygen.[11,43] The treatment of carbon monoxide poisoning is discussed in both Chapter 22, Pulmonary Emergencies, and Chapter 28, Toxicologic Emergencies.

Supraglottic injury can be suspected when facial burns, singed facial hair, or carbonaceous sputum are present. Other signs and symptoms of upper airway injury include presence of redness or blistering in the posterior pharynx, stridor, wheezing, bronchorrhea, or any other sign of respiratory difficulty. Absence of these indications initially does not exclude the possibility of inhalation injury because upper airway edema may not be present until after the onset of fluid resuscitation.[14,25]

Infraglottic injury is often more difficult to ascertain because the injury is progressive in nature. It is caused by the inhalation of the particulate byproducts of combustion. It is manifested by an increase in both pulmonary vascular resistance and pulmonary capillary permeability, which causes pulmonary edema. The primary symptom is hypoxemia that is resistant to oxygen therapy.[35] Inhalation injuries are unpredictable in onset. Any patient with suspected inhalation injuries should be closely observed for 24 hours for onset of respiratory complications. Some experts advocate fiberoptic bronchoscopy or xenon ventilation-perfusion scanning to identify inhalation injury earlier.[45]

TREATMENT

Transport of a burn victim requires an orderly, prioritized approach. Equipment and supplies should be organized in advance when possible to expedite assessment and stabilization of the burn victim.

Even though supplies and equipment vary among transport programs, depending on protocols and primary service populations, little is required beyond the standard emergency medical supplies to provide quality burn care. Sheets and blankets should be carried even in the summertime to prevent hypothermia during transport.

Management of the burn victim begins with the ABCs of the primary survey, including airway, breathing, and circulation with a brief baseline neurologic examination. While doing assessments and making interventions for life-threatening problems in the primary survey, the transport team should take precautions to maintain cervical spine immobilization if trauma is suspected.[46]

Intubation may need to be accomplished early because it could become impossible later with the onset of edema after the initiation of fluid replacement to manage the burned victim's airway. It is more difficult to assess for dyspnea during transport because of the noise and vibration, so the transport team should learn to rely on other parameters for assessing respiratory status.[25,33]

Securing an endotracheal tube may be difficult because tape, which is most often used, will not adhere to burned skin. Several alternatives are available, such as the use of cotton twill ties or suturing or stapling the tube to the nose or lip.[11,43,51,52]

The transport team must be sure that the burning process has been stopped. This may require copious irrigation of the burn wound, as in the case of chemical burns, or simply removing clothing and jewelry from the patient. It is important to protect the patient from further injury as well as to ensure the safety of the transport team members. The primary survey should then be performed. Humidified oxygen should be used when possible[33] because it helps to keep the airway moist, inhibiting the inspissations of material that could produce atelectatic areas in the lung.

Two IV lines should be initiated peripherally with large-bore catheters. The fluid of choice for initial resuscitation is variable, but crystalloid is the most common.[11,25,28,29,46] Ideally, lines should be placed in nonburned areas but may be placed through the burn if they are the only veins available for cannulation. Intravenous lines should be sutured in place if there is any danger of their being dislodged because venous access may not be available peripherally after the onset of generalized edema. Blood should be obtained for initial lab studies when IV lines are initiated if that has not already been done.[15,43] Vital signs are the next step in readying the patient for transport.

Electrocardiogram monitoring should be instituted on any patient with a large burn, an electrical injury, or preexisting heart disease. Electrode patches may be a problem to place because the adhesive will not stick to burned skin. If alternate sites for placement cannot be found, an option for monitoring is to insert skin staples such as those used for wound closure and attach the monitor leads to them with alligator clips. This provides a stable monitoring system, particularly for the agitated or restless patient who might displace needle electrodes.[11,43] There are burn electrodes available that use needles attached to special cables for monitoring.

A urinary catheter with an urimeter should be placed to accurately monitor urinary output. As with intubation, the catheter should be inserted early, especially for the patient with perineal burns, because edema may make insertion impossible at a later time.[15]

To combat the problem of adynamic[17] ileus, the transport team should insert a gastric tube in all burn victims with significant burns to decompress the stomach. This is especially important for the victim being transported at high altitudes.[15] Initial diagnostic studies should include hematocrit and electrolyte levels, urinalysis, chest x-ray, arterial blood gases with carboxyhemoglobin levels as indicated, and an ECG.[47]

With the exception of escharotomies, open chest wounds, and actively bleeding wounds, wound management in transport consists of simply placing the patient on and covering him or her with clean, dry linen.[25] Wet dressings are contraindicated because of the decreased thermoregulatory capacity of patients sustaining large burns and the possibility of hypothermia. The burn victim should be covered with blankets to avoid hypothermia.[1,2]

Medications should be given intravenously. The generalized edema during this time allows for only sporadic absorption of the medication if given intramuscularly. As fluid shifts reverse, there can be a "dumping" and a potential overdose of any medications that were given intramuscularly.[15] The exception to this is a tetanus booster, which can be given intramuscularly.

For those burn victims who may not be transported until later in their disease process or those who may require long-distance transport to receive care, some debriding and dressings may be required. Mild soap and water may be used to clean simple burns. Blisters should be managed according to the burn center's wound care protocols.

When cleaning burns that are the result of contact with tar or asphalt, mixtures of cool water and mineral oil have been reported to be useful. The removal of these substances stops the burning process and help decrease the patient's pain.[45]

It is essential to have accurate documentation of all treatment provided before and during transport of the burn victim. This information provides the necessary history of the incident and its initial treatment to allow for consistent and quality planning of patient care at the receiving facility.

EVALUATION

Evaluation of the burn victim consists primarily of assessing the effectiveness of problem intervention and the recognition of future potential complications. Not all complications are, however, predictable or correctable.

Circumferential burns to the chest or extremities represent the more easily recognizable complications in burn care. Circumferential burns to the chest wall decrease chest wall compliance, creating respiratory insufficiency and hypoxia, especially in the pediatric population, because chest walls are more pliable. This can be further aggravated by generalized edema. The correction for this problem is an escharotomy, which allows the chest to expand fully for more efficient ventilation (Figure 19-4).

Circumferential burns to the extremities or digits can be equally threatening to the circulatory stability of the affected limb, producing the "five Ps" that represent the signs and symptoms of an arterial injury: pain, pallor, pulselessness, paresthesias, and paralysis. An ultrasonic Doppler device may be helpful in locating pulses in a particularly edematous area.[11,25]

Escharotomies ideally should be performed before transport and should be performed only under the direction of the receiving physician.[46] There are several principles to remember in performing escharotomies. The procedures should be performed in as sterile an environment as possible to avoid seeding bacteria into already compromised tissue. The incisions should be made carefully and deep enough to penetrate the eschar and decompress the area without causing major bleeding in the zone of stasis because the tissue there is often too friable to maintain sutures. When bleeding does occur, the appropriate treatment is direct pressure to the wound. The incisions should extend slightly beyond the constricted area for maximum effect. (See Box 19-1 for possible escharotomy sites.) Major

---

BOX 19-1 | Possible Escharotomy Sites

Chest

Anterior axillary incisions bilaterally joined with a transverse incision along the costal margin (Figure 19-4)

Extremities

Axially on medial and/or lateral aspect. If a single incision is insufficient to relieve the constriction, then an incision on both sides should be performed

Elbow

Medial aspect anterior to the medial epicondyle

Hand

Axially on the dorsum, between the tendons rather than across them

Fingers

Midlateral axial (Figure 19-5)

Ankle

Medial aspect anterior to medial malleolus

Foot

Axially on the dorsum between the tendons rather than across them[34,45]

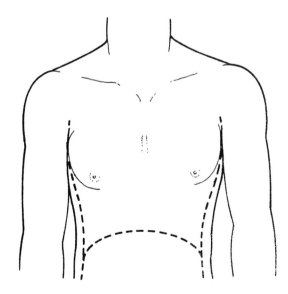

FIGURE 19-4 **Chest escharotomy sites.**

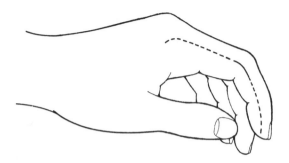

FIGURE 19-5   **Escharotomy site on the finger.**

vessels, nerves, tendons, ligaments, and joints should be avoided because future range of motion can be adversely affected. Results of the escharotomy should be carefully monitored. In most cases relief of the constriction should be immediate.[11,34,46]

Myoglobinuria that occurs from the release of myoglobin after deep muscle damage can precipitate in the renal tubules and cause acute renal failure. This is especially common after electrical burns, and urine should be monitored in such cases for changes, such as to a dark tea color, that would indicate the presence of myoglobin. The treatment for myoglobinuria aims to increase fluid administration rates to maintain a urinary output of at least 100 ml/hr until the pigments clear. If this is not successful, the osmotic diuretic mannitol can be added to the intravenous infusion at the concentration of 12.5 g/L of fluid. Another method of eliminating myoglobin is to alkalinize the urine by administering sodium bicarbonate 1 mEq/kg because myoglobin is more soluble in an alkaline medium.[43,46]

Pulmonary edema can occur from either overzealous fluid resuscitation or smoke inhalation, and the transport team should be careful to monitor respiratory function as fluid administration progresses. This is especially a problem when the transport of the burn victim has been delayed.

Several acid-base and electrolyte imbalances can occur throughout the course of patient management. Acidosis from the increased lactic acid production can occur, and it can be treated with sodium bicarbonate if increased fluid administration is ineffective. Hyperkalemia from potassium

released from the heat-damaged tissues can be reversed in several ways including administration of sodium bicarbonate, glucose and insulin, and/or ion exchange resins. Hyponatremia from fluid replacement does not reflect a true sodium deficiency and seldom requires any type of treatment. Hypoglycemia is a complication that frequently occurs with infants and young children because of their inability to maintain adequate glycogen stores. Blood glucose should be assessed frequently for pediatric patients. Intravenous fluids may be changed to lactated Ringer's with 5% dextrose if hypoglycemia becomes a problem.[46]

IMPACT OF TRANSPORT

For burn victims there are usually two phases of transport. The first is the entry of the burn victim into the EMS system with transport from the scene of the incident to the initial care facility. The second phase is the interfacility transport of the stabilized patient from the initial care facility to a burn center or tertiary care center.[11]

The increasing use of critical care ground and air medical services has had an impact on both phases of burn transport. In early transport, it has made a higher level of medical expertise more rapidly available to a larger service area. This has decreased the amount of time before assessment and resuscitation begins and enables the critically injured patient to reach a definitive care facility quickly. In the second phase of transport, it has markedly decreased the amount of time spent out of a stable environment during transfer to a burn center.[7,33] These changes have had the combined effect of decreasing the morbidity and mortality of burn victims.[11]

The decision to transport to a burn center is made based on the condition of the patient, the size of the burn, and in the case of scene response, the distance to the burn center. Patients who sustain concurrent traumatic injuries should first be evaluated at a trauma center if the traumatic injuries present the greatest immediate risk. If the burn injury is the greater risk to the patient, and initial burn care can be facilitated en route, then transfer to a burn center may be appropriate. The American Burn Association has identified criteria

BOX 19-2	**Burn Unit Referral Criteria**

1. Partial-thickness burns greater than 10% total body surface area (TBSA).
2. Burns that involve the face, hands, feet, genitalia, perineum, or major joints.
3. Third-degree burns in any age group.
4. Electrical burns, including lightening injury.
5. Chemical burns.
6. Inhalation injury.
7. Burn injury in patients with preexisting medical disorders that could complicate management, prolong recovery, or affect mortality.
8. Any patients with burns and concomitant trauma (such as fractures) in which the burn injury poses the greatest risk of morbidity or mortality. In such cases, if trauma poses the greater immediate risk, the patient may be initially be stabilized in a trauma center before being transferred to a burn unit. Physician judgment will be necessary in such situations and should be in concert with the regional medical control plan and triage protocols.
9. Burned children in hospitals without qualified personnel or equipment for the care of children.
10. Burn injury in patients who will require special social, emotional, or long-term rehabilitative intervention.

Modified from American Burn Association: *Burn fact sheet*, 2001, from www.ameriburn.org/pub/factsheet.htm.

for the transfer of burn victims to a burn center (Box 19-2).[1,15,46]

CHEMICAL BURNS

Chemical burns differ from thermal burns in that the burning process continues until the agent is inactivated by reaction with the tissues, is neutralized, or is diluted with water.[11] The degree of damage by a chemical agent depends on the concentration and quantity of the agent, its mechanism of action, and the duration of contact.[3,46]

Treatment of chemical injuries requires removal of all saturated clothing and a copious irrigation of the burn wound. In the otherwise stable patient, wound irrigation takes priority over transportation unless the irrigation can continue en route.[11] The transport team needs to ensure their safety and avoid placing a contaminated patient in a transport vehicle.

Dry chemicals such as lime should be brushed off before irrigation. Water and physiologic saline are the fluids of choice for wound irrigation. The time spent searching for a specific neutralizing agent may be more harmful than simply irrigating with water. The exogenous heat production by neutralization reaction can in itself cause further tissue destruction.[11] In the treatment of chemical burns, the transport team must be aware of the possibility of exposure to the noxious agents and don appropriate protective gear before coming into contact with the patient or the patient's clothing.[46]

RADIATION BURNS

Dealing with radiation burns caused by ionizing radiation is a rare occurrence. Transport following a radiation accident will probably be for more critical injuries than for radiation exposure itself.

Radiation burns are treated like other kinds of burns. Any open wounds should be covered with gauze and fastened with an elastic bandage, never with adhesive.[52] The focus beyond the lifesaving measures is to avoid contaminating the transport team and the transport vehicle. Gross contamination can be avoided if there is time to plan.

SUMMARY

Burn injuries can present a major challenge to transport team members, but an orderly, prioritized approach can greatly simplify their management. A clear understanding of the pathophysiology of burn injuries is essential in providing quality burn care. Not only assessment but also underlying principles of intervention and resuscitation rely on this knowledge base.

The treatment of the burn victim begins with stopping the burning process. This is accomplished by ensuring the safety of the transport team first and then proceeding to provide patient care.

Assessment of the burn victim begins with the primary survey. Life-threatening injuries must be treated first, followed by intervention and control of potentially fatal problems. This activity is followed by appropriate airway control and ventilatory and circulatory support. Special burns such as chemical and electrical injuries have unique consequences that must be observed for early in their management.[43]

ELECTRICAL INJURIES

HISTORY AND INCIDENCE

A Leyden jar was accidentally discharged by Dutch physicians in 1746, causing the first reported man-made electrical shock.[38] The first recorded death by electrical shock occurred in Lyon, France, in 1879, when a stagehand came in contact with a 250-volt current. The first notable electrical injury in the United States occurred in 1881, when an intoxicated citizen touched a DC generator terminal in Buffalo, New York. Because his death appeared painless and quick, that incident led New Yorkers to suggest that electrocution be used as a means of capital punishment in the United States, and in 1890 the first legal electrocution took place in Auburn, New York.[9]

Over 1000 people die each year of electrical accidents. Contact with electricity accounts for approximately 3% of all burns treated in the United States each year. All ages are affected, the most common victims being those who work with electricity professionally. The age group with greatest electrical injury rate is infancy to 4 years of age. These injuries are primarily caused by contact with exposed electrical cords and outlets. The second peak appears from ages 20 to 25. Those injuries occur predominantly in the male population and are caused by work and industrial accidents.[24]

PHYSICS AND PATHOPHYSIOLOGY

Because electrical injury is unique in the field of thermal trauma, a flight nurse needs to appreciate the potential widespread anatomic damage to manage these injuries.[8] Significant factors determining severity of electrical injury are (1) voltage and amperage, (2) resistance of internal body structure and tissue, (3) the type and pathway of current, and (4) duration and intensity of contact.[16,24,55]

OHM'S LAW

The intensity of the electrical current that passes through victims shows a direct correlation to the tissue damage produce. Ohm's Law supports this correlation.[37]

$$\text{Ohm's Law: Resistance (ohms)} = \frac{Voltage}{Amperage}$$

AMPERAGE

Amperage is defined as the number or volume of electrons flowing between two potentials. It cannot be easily measured, although it is actually a better indicator of potential tissue damage than is voltage.[55] This is because the skin's resistance changes as it breaks down and blisters from a burn caused by the electrical injury. This is displayed in Joule's Law:

$$\text{Heat} = \text{Amperage}^2 \times \text{Resistance}$$

VOLTAGE

Voltage is defined as the force with which the electrical movement occurs. High-voltage injuries (> 1000 volts) and low-voltage injuries (< 1000 volts) are both common, and either type can cause death. The higher the voltage, the more significant the injury. Burns, charring, and extensive blistering commonly occur.[32,42] The type of current, alternating (AC) or direct (DC), can also determine the significance of injury. Alternating current produces a tetanic contraction of muscles that "freezes" the victim to the source. This is not seen with direct current, and therefore low-voltage AC exposure, such as to a household current of 110 volts, can be more

TABLE 19-1 **Effects of Amperage by Household Currents (60 Hz AC)**

mAmps	Effect
1-2	Tingling of skin
15-20	Muscle tetany: the "let go" current
50-90	Respiratory arrest (if directed through the medulla)
90-250	Ventricular fibrillation (if the myocardium is transversed)

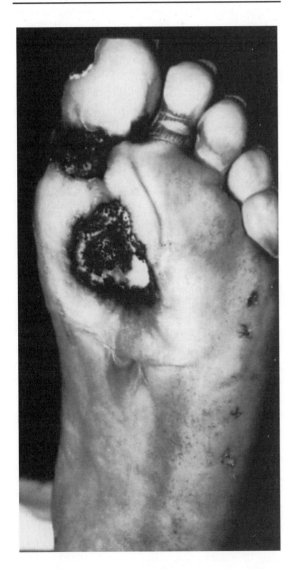

FIGURE 19-6 **Exit wound from direct current.**

dangerous than a low-voltage direct current. The alternating current also has a greater potential to cause ventricular fibrillation from tetanic chest muscle contractions[22] (Table 19-1).

RESISTANCE

Resistance is described as the degree of hindrance to electron flow. Those tissues containing the most electrolyte media, nerves, blood vessels, and muscles transmit current most easily because they have the least resistance. Tissues, tendons, and fat are most resistant and do not allow conduction, causing burning and surrounding deep muscle damage.[49]

CURRENT PATHWAY

The current pathway is very critical because it may determine the severity of injury. Current passing through the head and thorax will involve the respiratory center or heart and is likely to produce instant death.[50]

Current passing from hand to foot may not affect the respiratory center but may damage the heart.[22] From the entry point, the electrical current follows the path of least resistance, causing one or more tracks of damage. The energy collects at the grounding point, causing significant tissue necrosis, and subsequently causing an explosive exit through the skin.[8] The mortality of hand-to-hand current passage is reported to be 60%, hand-to-foot current passage is 20%, and foot-to-foot current passage is 5%.[55] It has been noted that direct current tends to leave a discrete exit wound (Figure 19-6), whereas alternating current tends to be more explosive[18] (Figure 19-7).

DIRECT-CONTACT BURNS

The patient actually becomes part of the circuit in the case of direct-contact burns. These wounds may appear devastating, and they frequently resemble a crush injury rather than a burn (Figure 19-8). The most common point of entry is the hand or skull, and the most common exit site is the feet.[18] The sizes of these entrance and exit wounds are no real indicator of the amount of damage done to internal tissue.

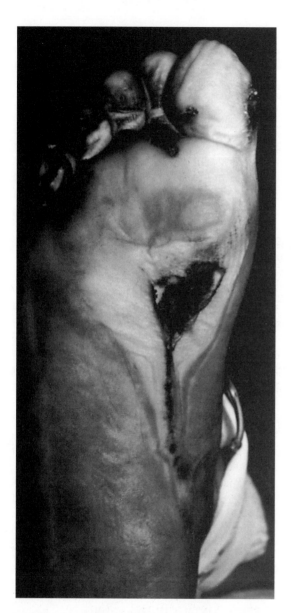

FIGURE 19-7   **Exit wound from alternating current.**

ARC BURNS

Arc burns occur when the current leaves the body on its course to the ground. The arcing current produces extremely high energies, ranging from 3000° C to 20,000° C.[8] Wounds are deeper because the heat intensity is closer to the body. Second- and third-degree thermal burns may be indistinguishable when the heat source is more distant from the body.

FLAME BURNS

Flame burns occur secondary to the ignition of clothing by the current. These wounds could be severe when the victim is unconscious and has a long exposure to the flame. The ignition of clothing usually occurs with high-voltage injuries that are greater than 350 to 1000 volts.[48] Frequently, high-voltage injuries cause combinations of all types of electrical burns, and it may become difficult to determine the proper course of therapy.

CLINICAL MANIFESTATIONS
CUTANEOUS INJURIES

Cutaneous injuries are frequently apparent because the skin is the first point of contact with the electrical current. Dry skin has a greater resistance than wet skin, and thus produces greater generation of heat and subsequently a larger burn.

Flexor crease burns are noted as the hallmark of the true conductive injury.[47] Alternating current produces tetanic contractions of the flexor muscle of the upper extremities, causing the skin layers at the flexed joint to be more closely apposed. As the current path passes through the apposed skin layers, typical arc burns are produced at the wrist, elbow, and antecubital fossa.[48]

Oral commissure burns are commonly seen in children under the age of 2. These burns are typically caused by a child chewing or sucking on a low-tension (110-V) electrical cord. This type of burn is frequently localized but can cause associated injuries to the tongue, palate, and face (Figure 19-9).

CARDIAC INJURIES

As electrical current passes through the body, severe dysrhythmia may occur. Ventricular fibrillation is frequently induced as a 60-cycle alternating current passes through the ventricles. Direct-current injuries predominantly result in asystole by depolarizing the entire myocardium.[31] In addition to those fatal rhythms, other dysrhythmias, such as atrial

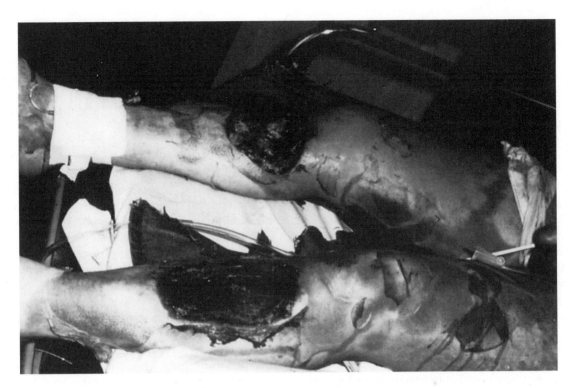

FIGURE 19-8   **Direct-contact burns resembling crush injuries.**

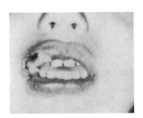 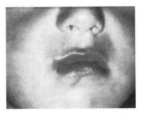

FIGURE 19-9   **Oral commissure burns in a child under age 2.**

fibrillation, sinus bradycardia, ventricular and atrial ectopy, supraventricular tachycardia, bundle branch block, and first- and second-degree block, may occur. Coronary artery spasm, coronary endarteritis, and direct myocardial injury are thought to be the cause of these dysrhythmias.[41,49,50] Damage to the myocardium, including myocardial rupture, is also a result of an electrical injury. These injuries are believed to be caused by the heat generated by the current. Myocardial damage will manifest itself in the same manner as the injury induced by ischemia.[31]

NEUROLOGIC INJURIES

The skull is a common entry point of electrical current, thus the brain stem is often affected and can lead to respiratory arrest and potential cerebral hemorrhage or edema. Nervous system tissue is an excellent conductor of electrical current, and therefore central nervous damage is not uncommon. Effects of electrical injury to the central nervous system are manifested by unconsciousness, seizures, disorientation, or amnesia. Other neurologic complications that have been identified are spinal cord injuries, particularly those associated with electrical current traversing a hand-to-hand or head-to-foot course, and local nerve damage with peripheral neuropathies.[54]

Incomplete spinal cord transection is a common delayed lesion caused by damage to the spinal cord by the heat of the electrical current or by blunt trauma secondary to falls or severe tetanic contractions of the muscles surrounding the cord.[54] Headaches, cerebellar dysfunctions, optic atrophy, ascending paralysis, and transverse myelitis are neurologic sequelae that are delayed.[13]

VASCULAR INJURIES

Extensive necrosis over vessels may precipitate delayed hemorrhage from large blood vessels.[4] Arterial thrombosis, deep vein thrombosis, and abdominal aortic aneurysms may also result. Progressive venous and arterial thrombosis results in muscle damage that is not apparent on first inspection. A major vessel that has been only partially damaged may cause difficulty with hemostasis in open or newly closed wounds.[4,38,41]

GASTROINTESTINAL INJURIES

Intra-abdominal injuries involving major organs may be caused by blunt trauma caused by the electrocution or electrical contact points. Life-threatening injuries involving the abdominal organs must be ruled out during the early interventions. Other injuries to the abdominal cavity commonly identified following electrocution are submucosal hemorrhages in the bowel, liver failure, pancreatitis, nausea and vomiting, paralytic ileus, and various forms and degrees of ulcerative disease.

MUSCULOSKELETAL INJURIES

Long-bone fractures and dislocations and vertebral fractures are caused by the rigorous tetanic muscle contractions that occur. Bilateral scapular fractures have been reported from exposure to a 440-volt, 60-cycle current passing briefly through a person's upper extremities. Bilateral scapula fractures are rare and are usually caused by direct trauma. Because there are multiple muscle attachments that surround the scapula, the severe contractions that occur from the electrical injury lead to stress and subsequent fractures.[10] Amputations have also been the result of severe muscle contractions caused by high-voltage electrical injuries.

OPHTHALMOLOGIC INJURIES

Immediate burns to the eyes, optic atrophy, and the development of cataracts are not uncommon, particularly if the entrance or exit wounds appear on or around the head. Cataracts may develop unilaterally or bilaterally and occur as soon as 4 months or as late as 3 years after the injury.[49]

PREGNANCY

Electrical accidents in pregnant women are rare, and only a few have been reported. Lieberman and Mazor[40] studied six pregnant women who survived electrical injuries. All of the exposures were minimal, and there were no cutaneous burns or loss of consciousness. The current pathways were from hand to foot, and the patients did not seek immediate help. Three of the six fetuses were born prematurely and were stillborn. Another showed hemorrhage to the umbilical cord proximal to the fetus. Otherwise the cord and placenta were normal.

The hand-to-foot pathway of current will invariably pass through the fetus. The amniotic fluid and abundant uteroplacental vascularity have a low resistance to current flow, and the fetus becomes an easy victim of electrical injuries. Regardless of how slight the injury may appear, the mother must be transported to a hospital in which extensive fetal monitoring can be done.

RENAL INJURIES

Acute renal failure is a complication resulting from direct damage to the kidney by the electrical current, by blunt trauma to the kidney, or from myoglobinuria.[21] Myoglobin is released as a result of extensive muscle necrosis, and myoglobinuria is proportionate to the amount of muscle damage incurred. The incidence of renal failure may be reduced significantly with aggressive fluid resuscitation.[50]

MANAGEMENT
PREHOSPITAL

Just with other burn victims, the transport team must be sure that they are safe before beginning patient care. Because of the rotor wash produced by the helicopter, great caution must be used when landing at a scene where live electrical wires may be hanging freely. Communication with ground personnel regarding the type of scene and landing zone is mandatory before approaching.

Removing the victim from the source of current may place rescuers at risk. Wooden poles, rubber gloves, and ropes are not without risk and should be used only by those trained to work with electricity. Extrication is safe only when the power is turned off.[18] It is unfortunate and may even appear cruel not to intervene immediately; however, multiple casualties have occurred when bystanders and rescue workers have attempted to release a victim from electrical current.

Electric lines that have fallen on cars must also be approached with extreme caution. People inside the car are safe as long as they stay inside the car. If victims must be removed immediately because of injury, only trained individuals should attempt to do so. The transport team must not assume that a downed wire is not dangerous because it is not producing sparks and because the surrounding areas are dark. Wires may become jumbled after they are broken; therefore telephone cables, fire alarm wires, cable television lines, street lighting wires, and any other attachment to the pole may be carrying the highest voltage available and must be approached with extreme caution. Electrical lines have a tendency to surge, creating a danger of the line jumping and striking someone. Makeshift equipment (tree limbs, wooden ladders, etc.) should not be used to control downed wires because if the conditions are right, they may actually serve as conductors.[18]

Ground current may be produced with downed wires, and the current increases as one gets closer to the wire. Taking long strides may permit current to pass through the legs; therefore when walking near a live wire, the flight crew should take short shuffling steps to decrease the potential between each foot, thus reducing the risk of injury.[18]

As soon as the scene is secured and the patient is away from the current, the victim's cardiac and respiratory status must be assessed. Arrhythmias must be treated with the same cardiac medications used for any cardiac ischemia, and advanced cardiac life support (ACLS) protocols should be initiated.

The transport team must not allow gross deformities and burns to distract attention from lifesaving interventions. Cervical spine injury is of grave concern because of possible blunt trauma and because of severe tetanic contractions caused by the electrical current. The cervical spine must be immobilized.

Initially, a minimum of two large-bore IVs with normal saline or lactated Ringer's solution should be started. It is difficult to assess the area of surface burns because of the deep injury produced, and multiple liters of fluid may need to be infused. Hemorrhage must be controlled, fractures stabilized, and the patient transported with supplemental oxygen and continuous cardiac monitoring. Patients have been known to recover after long intervals of resuscitation; therefore prolonged resuscitation efforts are recommended.[1,21]

Cervical and thoracic spine immobilization must be maintained. Adequate volume replacement, treatment of acidosis, and management of myoglobinuria must also be initiated. It would be incorrect to use one of the burn formulas as the only means of determining fluid requirements for these patients because of the deep tissue damage seen with the apparently mild cutaneous burns.

It is essential to maintain higher rates of urinary output because hemoglobinuria and myoglobinuria are common with electrical injuries. The fluid resuscitation must be based on actual urine flow. A minimum of 50 to 100 ml/hr of urine must be maintained; however, in the presence of urinary hemochromogen, the fluid volume must be of sufficient quantity to maintain a *minimum* output of 100 ml/hr.[32,37]

Lactic acidosis is common because of the significant muscle damage caused by electrical injury. Sodium bicarbonate must be given until an alkaline urine pH is established. Mannitol, 12.5 g, must also be given in the resuscitative phase to increase urinary output and to minimize acute tubular necrosis.[32,37]

Blood transfusion may be necessary only if there is a significant blood loss caused by secondary trauma or in the event that multiple escharotomies or fasciotomies are performed.[32]

SUMMARY

In summary, the patient with electrical injuries may exhibit a wide spectrum of injuries from minor flesh burns to multiple traumas. The quality of treatment that the victim initially receives may determine his or her ultimate level of rehabilitation. Transportation of these patients to an appropriate hospital and early involvement of a burn care specialist is invaluable.

LIGHTNING INJURIES

There are millions of lightening flashes that strike the ground annually in the United States. An estimated 150 to 300 people are killed by lightning each year in the United States.[5,56] Most lightning injuries occur in the daytime hours of the summer and fall months (Figure 19-10). The outdoors enthusiast, athlete, camper, farmer, or golfer is more prone to lightning injury because of more frequent exposure to the elements. Lightning injuries pose difficult diagnostic problems because they are dissimilar to those caused by high-voltage contact, and therefore the effects and injuries differ.[1,16] A lightning bolt may have a voltage of up to 1 billion volts and induce currents greater than 200,000 amperes. Although the intensity of lightning is much greater than high-voltage electricity, the duration of exposure is much shorter, ranging from 1/100 to 1/1000 of a second. Because of this, skin burns are less severe than those burns seen with

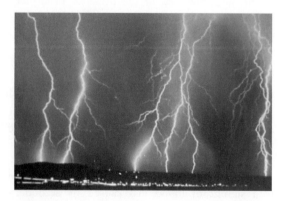

FIGURE 19-10   **Lightning strike demonstrating the power of lightning.**

high-voltage injuries (usually first degree and second degree). Many of the injuries associated with tetanic contractions caused by electrical injuries are not of concern in lightning injuries. Blunt trauma may be caused when the victims are hurled to the ground by the current. A victim may suffer a direct strike from a lightning bolt or may experience a splash injury. The splash injury occurs when lightning strikes an object and the stroke jumps to another object that acts as a better conductor. This is the mechanism that causes multiple lightning strikes in people standing in close proximity to an object or to another individual who has been struck.

TYPES

As stated previously, surface burns are not as severe with lightning injuries because of the short exposure to the current, and third-degree burns are rare. Linear and punctate burns are frequently seen with lightning injuries, and feathering burns are pathognomonic to lightning injuries.[5] With a lightning strike, the electrical current turns moisture on the skin to steam and frequently will blow off or shred clothing or shoes[18] (Figure 19-11).

MINOR

Patients with minor injuries usually are conscious; however, they may have lost consciousness transiently and are frequently confused and amnesic. They rarely exhibit burns or any other signs of injury, and vital signs are usually stable.[5]

MODERATE

Patients with moderate lightning injuries show more obvious altered mentation and may be combative or comatose. They may have fallen or been thrown down forcibly from the current, causing fractures and dislocations.

First- and second-degree burns may be apparent with a moderate lightning strike injury, as may tympanic membrane rupture caused by the explosive force of lightning strike. Difficulty palpating peripheral pulses and a mottled appearance of the patient's lower extremities are caused by arteriospasm and are frequently characteristic with a moderate injury. This usually clears in a few hours.[17]

SEVERE

If lightning current passes through the brain, the direct current or blast effect caused by the strike may damage the brain. The patient will be comatose and may possibly be undergoing a seizure. Closed

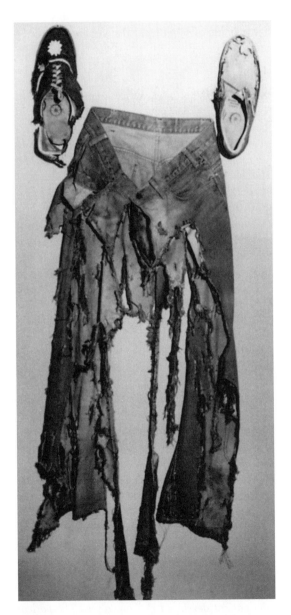

FIGURE 19-11 **Clothing of a patient struck by lightning.**

head injury caused by a fall must also be considered in these cases.[5]

Cardiac arrest with ventricular fibrillation should be anticipated. The most common cause of death in lightning injuries is cardiopulmonary arrest.[5] Lightning may cause paralysis to the medullary respiratory center, first causing respiratory arrest and then cardiac arrest. If immediate ventilation does not occur, a subsequent cardiac arrest will follow, and brain death will occur due to anoxia.[18] Multiple arrhythmias are associated with lightning strikes, including ventricular tachycardia, PVCs, and atrial fibrillation. ST changes associated with ischemia are also common.[36] Many ocular injuries have been reported, including detached retina, hyphema, direct thermal burn, corneal lesion, and cataract. As with electrical injuries, cataracts may appear as late as 2 years after the strike, but they are most commonly present in the first few days after the injury.[6]

Patients must be assessed for other signs of trauma caused by the impact of the strike and for life-threatening injuries.

PREGNANCY

The fetus must be assessed by immediately using fetal heart tones to determine viability. The prognosis of the unborn child is difficult to determine. Half of such pregnancies go on to normal delivery and produce no recognizable abnormality to the child, whereas the other half result in stillbirths.[57]

PREHOSPITAL CARE

Whether the transport team comes by ground or air, scene safety is the first step in the management of a patient struck by lightening. On approaching the scene of a storm, a secured landing site, free from debris and possible downed wires or tree branches, must be immediately established. The patient's cardiopulmonary status must be assessed immediately, and CPR and intubation should be initiated on finding the patient in cardiac arrest. As with any unknown injury, the cervical spine must be immobilized before intubation and transport. The patient's cardiac status must be monitored continuously, and arrhythmias should be treated with standard cardiac therapies (ACLS protocols).

Burns seen with lightning injuries are not as extensive as those seen with high-voltage injuries; therefore massive amounts of fluids are not required unless the patient is in hypovolemic shock. Two IV lines should be established as a "keep open" line and for a medication route. Observation and history taking must be performed with care to treat and transport these victims rapidly.

CASE STUDY 1

03:00   LifeFlight ABC, returning to base after being canceled en route to another scene call, receives a request to respond to the scene of a house fire for a 45-year-old male with a large thermal burn injury. The fire department has just removed the patient and turned him over to the ground EMS, and the municipal police have prepared a landing site for the aircraft.

03:10   Contact was made with the police officer in charge of the LZ, and after checking for hazards, the aircraft lands safely near the scene of the fire. The crew is directed to the ambulance, where the patient is being assessed by EMS.

03:12   Report from EMS: 45-year-old male who fell asleep after assembling his children's toys for Christmas morning. Unfortunately, he was smoking, and the couch caught on fire. The fire quickly spread to the rest of the house. The patient rolled to the floor and tried to crawl out of the house, but collapsed before reaching the door. His wife and children died in the fire. The patient was found to have a large partial- and full-thickness thermal burn injury covering his face, torso, arms, and legs. He was dyspneic, and a 100% nonrebreather oxygen mask has been placed.

PRIMARY ASSESSMENT

Airway/Breathing

The patient has deep partial-thickness burns on his face. His airway is moist, red, with carbonaceous sputum around his mouth. The transport team elected to intubate him because of his altered mental status and inability to protect his airway. No medications were needed to aid intubation.

His ventilations were assisted with 100% oxygen by bag-valve. Twill tape was used to secure the tube.

Circulation

The patient had a rapid carotid pulse. His peripheral pulses were difficult to palpate because of his burn injury. The patient had one antecubital IV initiated.

Disability

After intubation and oxygenation, the patient responded appropriately to commands. The transport team elected to load and go and complete the secondary assessment and additional interventions en route. The patient was covered with a clean sheet and blanket to prevent hypothermia.

03:25   The patient was secured to the transport stretcher and was loaded in the aircraft for a 25-minute transport to the burn center.

03:28   En route, the transport team completed a brief secondary survey. The burn injury was estimated to be 85% TBSA deep partial- and full-thickness burns. No other injuries were noted. The patient weight was estimated at 80 kg. A second IV line was initiated and fluid resuscitation maintained.

Because of his chest burns, the cardiac electrodes would not adhere. A pulse oximeter was used, and the patient maintained saturations of 1005 throughout the flight. Capnography was also used, and $EtCO_2$ levels were maintained between 30 and 34. Vital signs were pulse 112 and regular; and BP 110/60. Morphine sulfate 10 mg was administered for pain.

03:45   Report was called to the burn center.

03:55   The patient was taken directly to the burn unit for assessment and treatment.

Follow-up

The transport crew visited the patient several hours postinjury. The burn injury had been reassessed and determined to be 92% TBSA; within 48 hours, the patient developed rhabdomyolysis. The patient expired 4 days later.

CASE STUDY 2

14:50   The flight team receives a request to respond to an Arctic nursing station for a child with scald injuries from an abusive home situation. The injuries were incurred approximately 1 hour before arrival at the nursing station. The flight nurse relays the request to the pilots so that weather checks can be done while patient information is gathered. The 2-year-old girl is conscious, 12 kg, with 40% total body surface area burned superficial and 10% burned deeper. The flight nurse is also informed that the mother is in police custody and an elderly grandmother is in attendance. The flight nurse advises the nursing station nurse to administer oxygen to the child, cover the wounds with clean, dry dressings, keep her warm, initiate intravenous access, and administer sufficient IV fluids to maintain a urine output of 120 ml/hr.

14:58   The pilots report that the flight can be accepted but that the airstrip is across the lake from the nursing station.

15:20   Airborne! The flight nurse takes advantage of the 2-hour flight to make arrangements for a boat to use for transport across the lake and to obtain updates on the patient's condition.

17:30   Arriving at the airstrip, the flight nurses and equipment are transported across the lake by boat, where they are met by a truck to take them to the nursing station.

17:50   The flight team arrives at the nursing station, where the on-site nurse gives report and introduces them to the patient's grandmother and an aunt, who will accompany the child back to the city.

17:57   Flight nurse assessment: quiet, withdrawn child, tolerating oxygen cannula, IV in place with D$_5$LR infusing at 150 ml/hr. Assessment of injury reveals scald demarcation lines around midchest and thighs indicating a forcible submersion. When questioned, the patient complains of pain. A narcotic analgesic is administered, a Foley catheter with an urimeter is inserted, and the child is transferred onto the aircraft stretcher and covered with a sleeping bag.

18:20   With careful attention to maintaining warmth, the patient and her aunt are transported across the lake to the waiting aircraft. The child is loaded into the aircraft and given a stuffed toy for comfort during the flight.

18:50   Airborne again, the flight nurses monitor the patient's urine output and adjust fluid administration rates to maintain output of 120 ml/hr. A Chemstrip is done to monitor the child's glucose level, and narcotics are administered via IV as needed for complaints of pain. The patient tolerated the flight well and was released to return to her community 2 weeks later, with the aunt named as guardian by social services.

REFERENCES

1. American Burn Association: *Burn fact sheet*, 2001, from www.ameriburn.org/pub/factsheet.htm.
2. American College of Surgeons: *Advanced trauma life support providers' manual*, Chicago, 1997, American College of Surgeons.
3. Archauer B, editor: *Management of the burned patient*, Norwalk, Conn, 1987, Appleton & Lange.
4. Artz CP: Changing concepts of electrical injury, *Am J Surg* 128:600, 1974.
5. Auerbach PS, editor: *Wilderness medicine*, ed 4, St Louis, 2001, Mosby.
6. Bartholome CW, Jacoby WD: Cutaneous manifestations of lightning injury, *Arch Dermatol* 1466, 1975.
7. Baxt WG, Moody P: The impact of a rotorcraft aeromedical emergency care service on trauma mortality, *JAMA* 249:3246, 1983.
8. Baxter CR: Present concepts in the management of major electrical injury, *Surg Clin North Am* 50(6):1401, 1970.
9. Bernstein T: Theories of the cause of death from electricity in the late nineteenth century, *Med Instr* 9:267, 1975.
10. Beswick DR: Bilateral scapular fractures from low voltage electrical injury, *Ann Emerg Med* 11:676, 1982.
11. Boswick JA, editor: *The art and science of burn care*, Rockville, Md, 1987, Aspen.
12. Carvajal HF: Fluid resuscitation of pediatric burn victims: a critical appraisal, *Pediatr Nephrol* 8(3):357, 1994.

13. Christenson JA, Sherman RT: Delayed neurologic injury secondary to high voltage current with recovery, *J Trauma* 20:166, 1980.
14. Clark WR: Smoke inhalation, *Burns* 12:163, 1988.
15. Collini FJ, Kealey GP: Burns: a review and update, *Contemp Surg* 34:160, 1989.
16. Cooper MA: Electrical and lightning injuries, *Emerg Med Clin North Am* 2(3):489, 1984.
17. Cooper MA: Lightning injuries: prognostic signs for death, *Ann Emerg Med* 9:134, 1980.
18. Cooper MA: Lightening injuries, *Emerg Med Clin North Am* 1(3):639-647, 1983.
19. Cooper MA, Sherand M: Enhancing recovery from electrical and lightning injuries, *Emerg Med Rep* 8(8):57, 1983.
20. Deitch EA, Rutan RL: *The challenges of children: the first 48 hours*, Home Study from the American Burn Association from www.aba.org, 2001.
21. Dixon GF: The evaluation and management of electrical injuries, *Crit Care Med* 11(5):384, 1983.
22. Erskine JF: Electrical accidents, *Practitioner* 222:777, 1979.
23. Faldmo L, Kravitz M: Management of acute burns and burn shock resuscitation, *AACN Clin Issues Crit Care Nurs* 4(2):351, 1993.
24. Gant TD: Electrical injuries, with special reference to the upper extremities: a review of 182 cases, *Am J Surg* 134(1):95, 1977.
25. Goldfarb JW: The burn patient, *Air Medical Crew National Standards Curriculum*, Phoenix, 1988, ASH-BEAMS.
26. Herndon DN, Rutan RL, Rutan TC: Management of the pediatric patient with burns, *J Burn Care Rehab* 14(1):3, 1993.
27. Hilton JG, Marullo DS: Effects of thermal trauma of cardiac force of contraction, *Burns* 12:173, 1986.
28. Horton JW, White DJ, Hunt JL: Delayed hypertonic saline dextran administration after burn injury, *J Trauma* 38(2):281, 1995.
29. Housinger TA: A prospective study of myocardial damage in electrical injuries, *J Trauma* 25(2):122, 1985.
30. Huang PP et al: Hypertonic sodium resuscitation is associated with renal failure and death, *Ann Surg* 221(5):543, 1995.
31. Hunt JL: Acute electric burn, *Arch Surg* 115:434, 1980.
32. Hurren JS, Dunn KW: Spontaneous pneumothorax in association with a major burn, *Burns* 20(2):178, 1994.
33. Judkins KC: Aeromedical transfer of burned patients, *Burns* 14:171, 1987.
34. Kemble JVH, Lamb BE: *Practical burns management*, London, 1987, Hodder and Stoughton.
35. Kinsella J: Smoke inhalation, *Burns* 14:150, 1988.
36. Kleiner JP, Welken JH: Cardiac affects of lightning strike, *JAMA* 240:2757, 1978.
37. Kobernick M: Electrical injuries: pathophysiology and emergency management, *Ann Emerg Med*, 11:633, 1982.
38. Kouwenhoven WB: Effects of electricity in the human body, *Electrical Engineering* 68:199, 1949.
39. Kumar P, Jagetia GC: A review of triage and management of burn victims following a nuclear disaster, *Burns* 20(5):397, 1994.
40. Lieberman JR, Mazor JR: Electrical accidents during pregnancy, *Obstet Gynecol* 67(6):861, 1986.
41. Martyn JAJ: *Acute management of the burned patient*, Philadelphia, 1990, Saunders.
42. Masters FW, Robinson DW: Management of electrical burns. In Lynch JB, Lewis F, editors: *Symposium of the treatment of burns*, vol 5, St Louis, 1977, Mosby.
43. Mikhail J: Acute burn care: an update, *J Emerg Nurs* 14:14, 20, 1988.
44. Miller JG et al: Early cardiorespiratory patterns in patients with major burns and pulmonary insufficiency, *Burns* 20(6):542, 1994.
45. Morgan ED, Bledsoe SC, Barker J: Ambulatory management of burns, *Am Family Phy* 62(9): 2015, 2000.
46. Nebraska Burn Institute: *Advanced burn life support provider manual*, Lincoln, Neb, 1987, Author.
47. Puffinbarger NK, Tuggle DW, Smith EI: Rapid isotonic fluid resuscitation in pediatric thermal injury, *J Pediatr Surg* 29(2):339, 1994.
48. Quimby WC: The use of microscopy as a guide to primary excision of high tension electrical burns, *J Trauma* 18:43, 1978.
49. Rosen P, Baker M: *Emergency medicine: concepts of clinical practice*, St Louis, 1992, Mosby.
50. Salem L, Fisher RP: The natural history of electrical injuries, *J Trauma* 17:487, 1977.
51. Shaw A et al: Pathophysiological basis of burn management, *Br J Hosp Med* 52(11):583, 1994.
52. Shaw A et al: The early management of large burns, *Br J Hosp Med* 53(6):247, 1995.
53. Shleien B: *Preparedness and response in radiation accidents*, Rockville, Md, 1983, US Department of Health and Human Services.
54. Taylor PH: The intriguing electrical burns: a review of 321 electrical burn cases, *J Trauma* 2:309, 1962.
55. Thompson MD, Ashway MD: Electrical injuries in children, *Am J Dis Child* 137:231, 1985.

56. Walsh KM, Bennett B, Cooper MA, Holle RL: National athletic trainers' association position statement: lightening safety for athletics and recreation, *Journal of Athletic Training* 35(4):471, 2000.

57. Warden GD: Burn shock resuscitation, *World J Surg* 16(2):16, 1992.

58. Weinstein L: Lightning: a rare cause of intrauterine death with maternal survival, *South Med J* 72:632, 1979.

59. Wilson P: Resolved on burn awareness, *Fire Control Digest* 14:10, 1988.

NEUROLOGIC EMERGENCIES

## 20

COMPETENCIES

1. Perform a focused and comprehensive assessment of the patient with a neurologic emergency.
2. Initiate the critical interventions for the management of the patient with a neurologic emergency during transport.
3. Provide care for the patient with a specific neurologic emergency during transport.

Neurologic emergencies require rapid assessment, stabilization, diagnosis, and transfer to definitive care. The transport team plays an important role in the outcome of these patients; therefore a thorough understanding of the pathophysiology, etiology, and management of these emergencies is crucial.

Neurologic medical emergencies may present either individually or concurrently. Their causes differ, depending on the disorder, but emergency treatment is aimed at controlling the airway, stabilizing and supporting the cardiovascular system, minimizing additional cerebral insult, and protecting the patient from physical harm during expeditious transfer to definitive care.[1]

NEUROLOGIC PATHOPHYSIOLOGY

Alteration in the intracranial pressure (ICP) is the prime concern in the care of patients with neurologic emergencies.[18,23,26,36] Following is a discussion

of how normal ICP is maintained, how it is altered, and how changes in it should be managed.

PRESSURE-VOLUME RELATIONSHIPS

In understanding the diagnosis and management of ICP problems, it is helpful to think of the intracranial contents as having three components: cerebrospinal fluid (CSF), blood volume, and brain. In the average situation, approximately 100 ml of CSF is accompanied by 150 ml of blood and 1250 ml (or grams) of brain. In the normal course of events, brain volume is not altered. However, the average volume of fluid in the CSF and in the blood is rather dynamic, and throughout the day the volumes of these two compartments may vary considerably. These variations occur in response to alterations in ICP.[20,26,33,36]

The way relationships among the volume of CSF, the volume of blood, and the volume of brain maintain a relatively constant ICP is described in the

$$K \sim V_{CSF} + V_{Blood} + V_{Brain}$$

FIGURE 20-1   **Modified Monroe-Kellie hypothesis.**

modified Monroe-Kellie hypothesis, which states that increases and decreases in the volume of one or more compartments will be offset by appropriate reductions or increases in the volume of the other compartment or compartments to maintain a constant ICP (Figure 20-1). Because brain volume changes little (and when it does, it involves mainly interstitial water), most normal variations occur in the volumes of CSF and blood.[20,26,33,36]

Should an intracranial mass or cerebral edema begin to develop, this volume relationship is extremely important early in the insult to compensate for the increase in mass. In the skull, particularly after childhood, when the sutures begin to fuse, the intracranial contents are housed in a nondistensible structure. As a mass or cerebral edema begins to develop, there must be an immediate reduction in the volumes of one or more compartments for ICP not to begin to increase immediately because the contents themselves are largely water and are relatively noncompressible.[35] The viscoelastic properties of the brain are such that if a mass, such as a growing tumor, exerts slowly increasing pressure, the brain may compensate through the slow loss of water or cellular elements through atrophy. However, with acute changes in the size of a mass, such as in an acute epidural hematoma, the brain is relatively noncompressible.

To understand the ability of the intracranial components to compensate for the development of a mass (it is helpful to think of the combined volume of cerebral edema as mass), it is useful to look at the pressure-volume curve[20,26,36,41] (Figure 20-2). It can be seen that at first, as a change in volume of mass occurs, there is no change in ICP. This phenomenon is the result of compliance and is accomplished by reduction in volume of CSF and blood. At some point, however, compliance is lost, and additional changes in volume result in great increases in ICP. In the acute state of cerebral

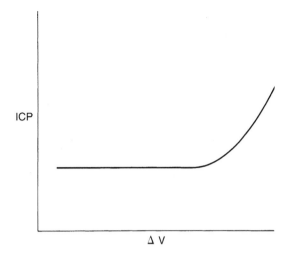

FIGURE 20-2   **Pressure-volume curve.**

edema, or a rapidly developing intracranial hematoma, the total shifts in volume amount to approximately 50 to 75 ml.[20,32,36,42]

CEREBROSPINAL FLUID VOLUME

The volume of CSF is controlled by the rate of production and the rate of absorption of CSF. Production, except in the presence of very high ICP, remains relatively constant in the adult at about 0.35 ml/min. It is a secretory process in which CSF is actively secreted by the choroid plexus in the lateral, third, and fourth ventricles. The fluid leaves the ventricular system and then circulates throughout the subarachnoid space, finally reaching the subarachnoid space overlying the cerebral convexities, where it is absorbed passively by way of the arachnoid granulations located parasagittally along the sagittal sinus. The fluid passes through the structures of the granulation into the cerebral venous system and is carried away with venous blood.[25,32]

Absorption is pressure driven, with the rate of CSF absorption proportional to the ICP. CSF volume is pathologically increased by an interference with absorption.[12,29,38] This increase can be caused by a mass or stricture in the ventricular system that prevents the CSF from exiting into the subarachnoid space. This accumulation of CSF is termed *obstructive* or *noncommunicating hydrocephalus.*[12,36]

Alternatively, after the CSF leaves the ventricular system, its circulation may be disturbed so that the fluid cannot reach the arachnoid granulation, resulting in communicating or nonobstructive hydrocephalus. Because the subarachnoid space is quite large, a focal lesion such as a tumor ordinarily will not produce this type of obstruction. Instead, a widespread disorder such as inflammation of the meninges or increased CSF protein will result in such obstruction.[35]

The management of hydrocephalus, whether acute or chronic, requires the diversion of the CSF around the site of blockage.[3,29,41] In general, this requires a procedure in which the neurosurgeon places a tube in a lateral ventricle by way of a surgically created defect in the skull, through a burr hole made with a small twist-drill trephine. The tube may be left in temporarily if the condition is transient, as in meningitis or if an obstructing tumor is soon to be removed. However, the tube may be made internal, in the form of a ventriculoperitoneal diversion shunt, if the condition is permanent, as in the presence of congenital stenosis of the aqueduct of Sylvius, the small CSF pathway connecting the third ventricle with the fourth ventricle.[3,34,41]

CEREBRAL BLOOD VOLUME

Cerebral blood volume comprises two relatively independent components, the arterial blood volume and the venous blood volume. Arterial blood volume accounts for approximately 25% of the total cerebral blood volume; venous blood volume accounts for the other 75%.[26,27,32]

Arterial cerebral blood flow (and volume) under normal circumstances remains relatively independent of systemic mean arterial blood volume and pressure through a process called *autoregulation.* Autoregulation is influenced by pressure and biochemical parameters.[2,3,22,26] As mean systemic arterial pressure increases, cerebral arterial blood vessels constrict, preventing the increase in blood volume and flow that would normally occur. If the mean systemic arterial blood pressure decreases, the cerebral arteries dilate, increasing cerebral blood flow.

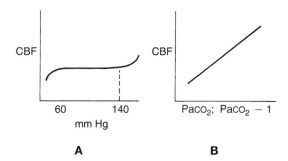

FIGURE 20-3   **A, Autoregulation maintains constant cerebral blood flow. B, Cerebral blood flow increases with increased $Paco_2$.**

Thus between a mean systemic arterial pressure of approximately 60 and 140 mm Hg, cerebral blood flow may be maintained in a constant state (Figure 20-3, *A*).[26,27,36]

Arterial blood volume is also influenced by complex biochemical or metabolic action that can be summarized by the association of $Paco_2$ and blood flow (Figure 20-3, *B*).[30,35,41] Increased $Paco_2$ or decreased Pao_2 results in dilation of the blood vessel, presumably in response to greater cerebral metabolic needs.[26,28,42] As $Paco_2$ decreases, blood volume and flow will be reduced. Thus it can be seen that this component of autoregulation may be influenced by respiratory control, with hyperventilation resulting in decreased cerebral blood flow and hypoventilation resulting in increased cerebral blood flow.[1,2,26] Venous blood volume is passively influenced by the delivery of blood from the arterial side and the ability of the cerebral venous system to drain from the head. This drainage depends on two influences: hydrostatic pressure and central venous pressure. Elevation of the head increases hydrostatic pressure on the venous side, permitting more rapid drainage from the cerebral venous system, mainly through the internal jugular veins bilaterally. Increased central venous pressure, whether caused by increased intrathoracic pressure or by right heart failure, decreases cerebral venous return.[2,26]

Respiratory management can greatly influence the volume of cerebral venous blood. If intrathoracic pressure is increasing because, for example, the patient is straining on an endotracheal tube that is blocked, a decrease in cerebral venous drainage (and thus an increase in cerebral venous blood volume) will occur.[26]

Brain Volume Cerebral Edema

Brain volume, except for a relatively insignificant alteration in interstitial water, does not change under ordinary circumstances. However, with injury, cerebral brain water may accumulate in the form of cerebral edema. This brain water may be found mainly in the cells, where it is called *cytotoxic edema*, or in the interstitial spaces, called *vasogenic edema*.[3,26]

Cytotoxic edema is produced by injury to cells, as occurs in hypoxia and certain metabolic diseases. Under these circumstances, cell membranes are damaged and certain intracellular metabolic processes become deranged. The normal metabolic pumps (e.g., sodium, potassium, calcium) do not function properly, and water, moving along osmotic gradients, accumulates intracellularly.[26,36]

Vasogenic edema is produced mainly by a disruption in the blood-brain barrier, which allows larger molecules than normal to cross from the blood along concentration gradients into the interstitial spaces. This movement of ions and protein alters interstitial osmotic pressure, permitting water to pass into the interstitial spaces of the brain.[26,36]

COMA

All neurologic emergencies discussed in this chapter can lead to coma. The following is a discussion of the precipitating causes, diagnoses, and patient care interventions for the broad categories of coma.

Assessment

The transport team relies on objective data when examining the comatose patient because subjective data can be difficult to obtain. A thorough history including the events preceding coma, medical history, and therapy instituted are important and should be obtained from family and transferring

BOX 20-1	Mnemonic for the Differential Diagnosis of Coma
U	Units of insulin
N	Narcotics
C	Convulsions
O	Oxygen
N	Nonorganic
S	Stroke
C	Cocktail
I	ICP
O	Organism
U	Urea
S	Shock

medical personnel. The transport team's assessment of the comatose patient is crucial in differentiating potential causes of the comatose state and determining the proper treatment protocol.[6,9]

During the assessment, it is useful to use a systematic approach in evaluating the comatose patient and establishing a differential diagnosis.

Differential Diagnosis of the Comatose Patient: UNCONSCIOUS

On the basis of the differential diagnosis, the transport team may institute certain actions in terms of therapy or diagnosis. The components of a reasonable differential diagnosis of the comatose patient may be recalled by remembering the items, the initial letters of which spell the word *unconscious* (Box 20-1).

U = Units of Insulin.   Units of insulin relates to an alteration in the patient's blood sugar. A whole blood glucose should be obtained and glucose administered when indicated. Each transport program should have a glucose level that would trigger the treatment of hypoglycemia.

N = Narcotics.   The word *narcotics* should prompt the transport team to consider any and all drugs, not only narcotics, including street drugs, but also prescription and nonprescription drugs. Naloxone may be useful in the diagnosis of opiate overdose; however, the appropriate management is control of the airway. Appropriate diagnostic studies include blood and urine drug screens.

C = Convulsions.   Seizures of both idiopathic origin and those associated with structural lesions such as stroke, trauma, brain tumor, and arteriovenous malformation should be considered.

O = Oxygen.   Hypoxia and carbon monoxide poisoning should be considered.

N = Nonorganic.   Very rarely, apparent coma will be of psychogenic origin.

S = Stroke.   Ischemic stroke may be the result of thrombi or emboli of cerebrovascular or cardiovascular origin. Assessment of cardiac status in search of arrhythmias and appropriate intervention is important.

C = Cocktail.   The cocktail image should suggest alcohol and its various syndromes to include a postictal state, Wernicke's encephalopathy, and overdose.

I = Intracranial Pressure.   Increase in ICP should be considered.

O = Organism.   Organisms result in infections and manifest bacterial, fungal, and viral causes. They mainly infect the central nervous system or result from systemic sepsis.

U = Urea.   The miscellaneous metabolic causes of coma such as diabetes, liver disease, and kidney failure should be considered. Generally available laboratory examinations that survey blood and urine chemistries are helpful in excluding this category.

S = Shock.   When shock is suspected, the primary concern is hypovolemic shock resulting from trauma or from spontaneous vascular rupture such as dissecting aortic aneurysm. The possibility of trauma should engender the thought of a head injury. Other causes of shock include cardiogenic and sepsis.

PLAN AND IMPLEMENTATION

In developing a plan of care for the comatose patient during transport, the cause of the coma must be considered and care implemented accordingly. A systematic approach should be used in the evaluation and care of the comatose patient, as with any seriously ill or injured patient. Standard precautions should be initiated before contact with any patient.

In the comatose patient, the airway should be secured first, then an IV line should be established. If the cause of the coma is truly unknown, samples for blood work to include blood gases, chemistry studies, drug screens, and toxicology should be drawn while the IV line is being secured.[1,21] Treatment should begin based on the suspected cause of the coma. For example, fluid resuscitation of the patient is hypotensive or dehydrated.

Computed tomography (CT) is the diagnostic procedure of choice for the unconscious patient to rule out a mass lesion, stroke, and hydrocephalus.[24] It may also be useful in the diagnosis of certain forms of encephalitis, particularly that of herpes simplex, which tends to localize in the temporal lobe.[16]

Approximately 60% of patients who are in coma will have some diffuse or systemic problem such as metabolic coma, encephalitis, sepsis, or AIDS. Neurologic symptoms develop in at least 39% of all patients with AIDS; the most common is AIDS encephalopathy.[18] The comatose state indicates a secondary involvement of the brain. The main problem is identification of the underlying systemic or diffuse cause of the patient's illness. Another 25% of patients in coma present as stroke victims; such presentations include not only embolic and ischemic conditions but also subarachnoid hemorrhage and hypertensive hemorrhage into the brain stem. Patients with such disorders require maintenance of the airway and fluids until the definitive diagnosis can be established. The remainder of patients, approximately 15%, has a mass lesion as the underlying cause of coma. Examples of lesions include brain tumors, hematoma, and brain abscesses.[4,6,23,25]

PRACTICAL CONSIDERATIONS IN THE EXAMINATION OF THE COMATOSE PATIENT

In all comatose patients, rapid assessment and diagnosis of the problem are critical to the success of treatment because significant delay will result in major morbidity and mortality.[24,26] Thus it is critical that after examination the unconscious patient be classified in one of the three categories described. This classification requires reevaluation of the patient. Table 15-1 (p. 263) demonstrates a correlation between the anatomic level of the lesion and the physiologic disturbance produced by the lesion, as demonstrated in the neurologic examination.

If repeated examinations demonstrate deterioration of the patient's condition with progressive loss of anatomic and physiologic function, the presence of a dynamic lesion may be assumed; a mass lesion must be immediately excluded.

If reevaluation reveals a stable, unchanging situation, it may be assumed that a static lesion is present, most likely a stroke. For example, pontine hemorrhage is manifested by small, equal-size pupils and abnormal oculocephalic or oculovestibular reflex examination findings, flaccid motor response, and unconsciousness.[5,6,23]

If the repeated examinations reveal a diffusely distributed neurologic picture and, especially, if that picture seems to wax and wane in severity, then a diffuse systemic cause is most likely to blame.[7] For example, a patient with drug intoxication may be lightly stuporous but exhibit pinpoint pupils and near apnea in the absence of significant painful stimulation.

The comatose patient presents a challenge. The patient generally cannot provide a specific history or chief complaint. Therefore a history from family members or bystanders, in addition to clinical data, is necessary for a working diagnosis. All comatose patients require supportive care directed at prevention of complications.[1,6,17] Not infrequently, the comatose patient will require intervention for respiratory support, airway management, cardiovascular

support (to maintain fluid balance and possible dysrhythmia control), and neurologic support (for control of seizures and ICP maintenance).[1,6,17,24]

Serial examinations are vital in the care of a comatose patient. As with all acutely critically ill or injured patients, the neurologically impaired (comatose) patient is not in a static condition. Repeated examination is essential if appropriate and timely interventions are to be instituted.

On the basis of examination findings communicated to the emergency center, CT can be performed on the patient's arrival at the receiving facility. This may require an alteration in the schedule of the CT scan equipment; hence it is important that the patient's needs be prioritized as assessed during the transfer phase.

SEIZURES

Patients with seizures are often transported for definitive care and evaluation. Of primary concern during transport is the safety of the patient and crew, with particular attention to techniques to protect and restrain the patient.

The annual incidence of seizure is estimated to be approximately 0.5% of the population (48 per 100,000) in the United States. Incidence is greater among males, particularly after the age of 20.[3,15,31] This may be due to a higher incidence of head injury with subsequent seizure activity. The highest incidence, however, is among children younger than 5 years (152 per 100,000 population annually). Overall, 650 per 100,000 population are affected by seizure activity in the United States. The prevalence is relatively constant between the ages of 10 and 60 years.[3,15]

PATHOPHYSIOLOGY

The onset of epileptic seizures is associated with several types of generalized and focal brain lesions. The underlying neuropathophysiologic disturbances, however, are poorly understood. Although it is reasonable to believe that an alteration exists in the neuronal pool or in the extracellular environment (both general theories having their advocates), neither laboratory investigations nor clinical experience with specific antiepileptic drugs has yielded a common therapy.[3,19]

It is known, however, that similar-appearing epileptic syndromes may occur, caused by focal lesions such as brain tumors, arteriovenous malformations, stroke, and generalized states such as head trauma and viral or metabolic encephalopathies. Additionally, in some idiopathic epilepsy syndromes, no obvious underlying cause is apparent. With more sophisticated recording techniques, several idiopathic epileptic syndromes are being associated with the presence of focal lesions, such as occult infarcts or sclerosis following birth trauma.[17,19]

Some patients present with status epilepticus syndrome. These patients are to be considered true neurologic emergencies; ischemic changes at the neuronal level, similar to those seen in patients with severe hypoglycemia and cerebral hypoxia, develop.[3,32]

Neuronal ischemic changes were once thought to be caused by decreased respiratory effort. They are theorized to occur in combination with ictal events, including a marked increase in metabolic rate and membrane changes affecting the transport of small ions at the neuronal level.[17,32]

ASSESSMENT

Several classification schemes for epilepsy have been proposed. The one with the most current widespread acceptance is from the International League Against Epilepsy,[3,32] which characterizes the syndromes as (1) partial seizures that begin locally and may or may not spread generally, (2) generalized seizures that begin bilaterally and are symmetrical, (3) a large group of unclassified, poorly understood syndromes, and (4) status epilepticus.

The same assessment criteria should be used regardless of the classification of seizure activity exhibited. The assessment criteria should include a thorough history, physical examination, and neurologic evaluation. The onset, type, and duration of seizure activity should be determined from the history. Additional pertinent information includes allergies, medications, and any recent illness or injury.

In the physical examination the airway is always of primary importance. The examiner must be alert to signs of trauma that may have occurred before or concurrent with the seizure activity. The physical assessment should then include motor, sensory, and psychomotor evaluation. The degree of involvement of these areas will depend on the individual patient presentation. Involvement may range from isolated focal activity to generalized status involvement.[3,6,32]

Regardless of the level of involvement, motor activity is involuntary. It begins with the tonic phase, a continuous tense muscular state. This is followed by a hypertonic phase with hypertension and muscle rigidity. The clonic phase is characterized by rapidly alternating muscle rigidity and relaxation. During the clonic phase sphincter control can be lost, and the patient may be incontinent. Tachycardia, hyperventilation, and salivation result from autonomic discharge during seizure activity. Sensory assessment is subjective because the patient's complaints may include visual, auditory, or proprioceptive phenomena. Psychomotor assessment is the determination of the level of consciousness, which may vary widely depending on the type of seizure activity and the time of evaluation. Other psychomotor observations include amnesia and repetitive behavioral patterns.[11,19,32]

PLAN AND IMPLEMENTATION

A plan of care for the seizure patient requiring transport includes a rapid, thorough assessment; appropriate interventions; and safe transfer to tertiary care.

Implementation of the plan involves management of the airway for prevention of hypoxia, support of the cardiovascular system, control of the seizure activity, and protection of the patient from physical injuries and additional complications associated with the seizure activity. Management of the underlying illness or injury that predisposed the patient to seizures may also be necessary.

Seizure management in the transport setting generally involves the use of a benzodiazepine (lorazepam) and on occasion administration of phenytoin.[8,10] Other medications that have been used to manage seizure activity include phenobarbital, lidocaine, etomidate, propofol, and paraldehyde.

All patients with a generalized presentation of seizures characterized by bilateral tonic-clonic activity, altered level of consciousness, and possibly urinary or fecal incontinence should be treated aggressively. These patients can quickly become relatively hypoxic as a result of the seizure activity. Hypoxia tends to aggravate the seizure disorder and make it more difficult to treat. The hypoxia occurs at two levels: generalized tissue hypoxia and cellular hypoxia. General tissue hypoxia occurs because the intense motor activity of the seizure interferes with adequate respiration. This aspect of the seizure disorder can be managed with the use of neuromuscular blocking agents in association with proper airway management. However, the intense neuronal activity characterized by sustained or rapidly intermittent bursts of neuronal discharge produces additional hypoxia at the cellular level. This hypoxia can result in a more long-term neuronal injury and is the reason for the aggressive use of an antiepileptic drug. The patient with a focal seizure (or partial seizure) characterized, for example, by facial twitching or motor activity limited to one extremity with no alteration of consciousness need not be managed aggressively for short periods of time if attention must be paid to a more serious medical problem. However, it should be recognized that a focal epileptic syndrome could become generalized fairly rapidly, so such a progression should be anticipated.[3,11]

Status epilepticus is the most dangerous syndrome. It is the most refractory to treatment, and the stress of the intense motor activity can cause not only respiratory insufficiency but also, in the elderly, myocardial strain leading to myocardial injury.[8,32] Intense hypertension may also occur during status seizures, resulting in expected complications such as intracerebral hemorrhage.

Practically speaking, the acute management of a generalized seizure syndrome is simple and straightforward. An intravenous line should be placed for administration of the appropriate medication. However, some benzodiazepines are now available in a preparation that can be given rectally if intravenous access is not quickly possible.

Attention to the airway is most important, and intubation should be considered for all patients with generalized seizure activity, especially if a significant alteration in level of consciousness is present. A person in the generalized tonic-clonic seizures, often referred to as grand mal epilepsy, may have such trismus that oral intubation is impossible. Nasal intubation may be attempted.

Generalized epilepsy leading to status epilepticus is most often seen in the acute state in one of two situations: (1) with generalized encephalopathy, including that immediately following trauma, and (2) in patients who are known epileptics, who have reduced drug intake, and whose blood levels have fallen below therapeutic concentrations.[19,32]

Patients with recurrent seizures, whether they are experiencing seizures for the first time or have chronic epilepsy, may be given phenytoin in a relatively rapid loading dose of 18 mg/kg IV (in normal saline solution) at a rate of 50 mg/min. Because this dose can precipitate supraventricular and ventricular arrhythmias, it is wise to observe the patient with a heart monitor. If arrhythmias are noted, administration of the drug should cease. If the cardiac rhythm returns to normal, especially if seizures continue, resumption of the administration of the phenytoin is appropriate at half the previously noted rate of administration.[11,32]

EVALUATION

Obviously, patient outcome depends not only on the intervention but also on precipitating factors and any complications the patient might experience. The optimal goal in caring for the patient with seizures is prompt control of the seizure activity to minimize cerebral insult and prevent complications.

Evaluation data might include arterial blood gas values, chest radiographs, and laboratory results including medication blood levels, and possibly CT or magnetic resonance imaging (MRI) to rule out cerebral pathology on the patient's admission to the receiving facility. In the trauma patient exhibiting seizure activity, radiographs of the skull and cervical spine would also be evaluated.

Patients who present with seizure activity pose special problems. Most obvious is the safety of the uncontrolled seizure patient during transport. The patient, crew, and transport vehicle must be protected from the danger associated with the unpredictable motor responses of the seizure patient. Extra care should be taken in the application of protective patient restraints, and aggressive pharmacologic therapy should be instituted for all seizure patients.

Of particular note are visually induced seizures. The photosensitivity type is most prevalent. These seizures are induced by light flashes[8,11,17]; patients prone to these seizures may experience them in flight as a result of the strobe effect of aircraft lights. Pattern-induced seizures may occur in response to the light-dark pattern caused by a slowly rotating main rotor during start-up and shutdown. (See Case Study in Chapter 6, Transport Physiology.)

CEREBROVASCULAR DISEASE

Cerebrovascular disease frequently results in interference with cerebral blood flow, causing ischemia of brain tissue. The challenge is to recognize when this condition exists and to protect the patient from further decrease in blood flow and poor delivery of oxygen, glucose, and other substrates essential to brain tissue.

Stroke, as it was called in the past, is now termed *brain attack.* This new terminology is purposely used to resemble the term *heart attack* and to underscore the fact that it is a medical emergency.[10,15,19,20]

Atherosclerosis and hypertension lead to approximately half a million strokes annually; approximately 150,000 of those victims survive. According to the American Heart Association, stroke is the leading cause of permanent disability in adults. Approximately 700,000 individuals have a stroke each year in the United States.[10] The need to view stroke as a medical emergency is imperative to improving the outcome of stroke victims. A transport service, particularly air medical transport, is essential for providing rapid transport of the stroke patient to a tertiary care center where screening procedures such as CT, angiography, endovascular techniques, and intra-arterial thrombolytic therapy are available as deemed necessary.[10,12,20]

Regardless of the underlying cause, a cerebrovascular episode requiring transport is frequently abrupt in onset and dynamic in progression. Treatment is directed at life-sustaining intervention, with emphasis on prevention of extension of injury. Prognosis varies depending on the extent of involvement and the affected area of the brain. Recovery may be maximized by the prevention of additional cerebral insult through aggressive airway and cardiovascular support.[10,15,23,24,30]

PATHOPHYSIOLOGY

A knowledge of normal cerebral circulation aids in the understanding of the pathophysiology of cerebrovascular disease. The importance of avoiding hypoxia has been discussed. Because the brain cannot store glucose, this substance must be constantly supplied in the blood flow. Critical reductions in glucose resulting from hypoglycemia or decreased perfusion can cause irreversible cellular damage.

The brain receives its blood from two sets of vessels. Two common carotid arteries in the anterior neck bifurcate, each into an external carotid artery that supplies primarily facial tissue and the internal carotid arteries that provide most of the blood supply to the brain through its major subdivisions, the anterior cerebral and the middle cerebral arteries. In the posterior aspect of the neck on either side lie the vertebral arteries. These combine shortly after they pass through the foramen magnum into the single basilar artery, which mainly supplies the brain stem. The posterior cerebral arteries from the vertebral basilar system communicate through two posterior communicating arteries with the internal carotid arteries. A small anterior artery permits communication between the two anterior cerebral arteries. Thus at the base of the brain a significant collateral circulation called the *circle of Willis* is formed where blood can flow as needed from one internal carotid system to the opposite internal carotid system, or to the vertebral basilar system, or to any combination of connections between the internal carotid systems and the vertebral basilar system.[2,17,26]

In addition, extensive collateral vessels may develop between the external carotid system and the internal carotid system. These collaterals are supplied mainly through facial anastomoses by way of the ophthalmic artery and through anastomoses between scalp vessels and vessels of the dura and arachnoid, called *leptomeningeal vessels.* Beyond this, however, in the depths of the brain, no collaterals assist deficient circulation. Therefore occlusion of smaller vessels from the surface of the brain inward will result in ischemia and infarction.[2]

The main features governing blood flow are summarized only briefly here. In the range of a mean systematic arterial pressure of 60 to 140 mm Hg, cerebral blood flow remains relatively constant through autoregulation (Figure 20-3, *A*). The cerebral blood vessels, especially those of capacitance (in the substance of the brain), constrict or dilate depending on the pressure of blood flow to maintain the constant flow. This system is also governed by metabolic considerations, with increased blood flow occurring with increased Pa_{CO_2} (Figure 20-3, *B*). In the face of increased Pa_{CO_2}, and if cerebral blood flow is impaired, a decrease in Pa_{O_2} will occur and is significant. In a severe hypoxic state, the blood vessels react not mainly on the basis of Pa_{CO_2} but on the basis of Pa_{O_2}, with increased dilation seen as hypoxia worsens.[26,28]

CEREBRAL ISCHEMIA

Cerebral ischemia is the term applied to brain tissue injury resulting from decreased cerebral blood flow.[2] The decrease in blood flow may be caused by systemic problems such as severe hypovolemia and myocardial failure. The primary concern in a cerebral ischemia is decreased regional or local cerebral blood flow resulting from vascular occlusion. The occlusion may be the result of an intraluminal process—that is, the development of a thrombosis or the arrival of an embolus—or it may be the result of extrinsic pressure from a mass in the brain tissue itself.[2,25,26]

The most common cause of vascular occlusion, resulting in the classic appearance of a stroke, is an embolus from some other part of the vascular system. Approximately one third of these emboli (especially in older persons) come from disease in the heart. Previous myocardial infarctions or valvular diseases may result in the development of mural thrombi, which are the source of emboli. In the great vessels a common location for thrombi forma-

tion is the bifurcation of the common carotid into the internal and external carotid. Disease at this location can often be detected by the auscultation of a bruit over the carotid bifurcation at the border of the involved sternocleidomastoid muscle just at the level of the angle of the mandible.[6,28] Auscultation must be performed carefully to prevent the dislodging of thrombi in the underlying vessel.

The next most common cause of cerebral ischemia is spontaneous intracerebral hemorrhage from cerebral aneurysms or arteriovenous malformations; that of accompanying hypertension is the most prevalent. As a result of this hemorrhage, the first vascular response is to contract and constrict to control hemorrhage in the region of the vascular injury. Second, as the hematoma develops in the brain tissue, the mass effect can place significant pressure on the distal arterioles, and capillary blood pressure becomes relatively low. Approximately 85% of hemorrhagic cases involve the cerebral hemispheres, and only a relatively small number occur in the cerebellum and brain stem as a result of involvement of the vertebral basilar system. In the case of hemorrhage in the cerebellum, the fourth ventricle may be acutely obstructed by the hematoma, resulting in sudden increase in ICP caused by impeded CSF flow. This increase will be managed by the neurosurgeon with ventriculostomy drainage.[4,23,25,26]

In the extremely rare instance when such a patient is transferred, the neurosurgeon should be consulted on a case-by-case basis with regard to the care of the ventriculostomy or any other implanted device to monitor ICP before transport.[24,34]

A small subset of hemorrhagic cases involves the rupture of intracranial aneurysms into the subarachnoid space. This subarachnoid hemorrhage, besides causing primary brain injury, may result in cerebral ischemia caused by cerebral vasospasm. There is little to distinguish this condition from other strokes except the complaint of the patient of severe, often focal, headache just before the hemorrhage.[5,910,11,33]

The use of crack cocaine has not only been implicated as a cause of intracranial hemorrhage but has been associated with acute intracranial arterial occlusive disease.[17]

The development of intracerebral thrombi as a cause of cerebral ischemia is relatively uncommon. Such development is most likely when there exists a primary disease of the blood vessels such as occurs with meningitis or with some of the vasculitides that accompany more widespread immunologic conditions, such as rheumatoid arthritis, dermatomyositis, and the polyangiopathies. A small group of patients with primary myopathies may exhibit cerebral symptoms of ischemia. The pathophysiology is not clear, but it may be a combination of cerebrovasospasm and primary thrombosis.[4,25]

The signs and symptoms the patient presents with will depend on the portion of the cerebral circulation involved and the cause. The classic presentation of the embolic state is that of the transient ischemic attack. In this condition, the embolus lodges at the bifurcation of a cerebral blood vessel, temporarily producing decreasing blood flow and symptoms appropriate to the involvement of that part of the brain, such as a contralateral hemiparesis or numbness in the face. After a few minutes or hours, the embolus breaks up, and the material passes more distally, restoring blood flow. Within 24 hours the patient has recovered. If this clearing of the blood flow avenue does not occur, significant injury of the tissue may result, including tissue death; a frank stroke has then occurred. If a small vessel supplying the internal capsule is involved, a dense hemiplegia may develop. Should the embolus lodge in a major branch of the internal carotid artery, such as the anterior cerebral or middle cerebral arteries, the posterior cerebral artery, or the internal carotid itself, major destruction of the hemisphere will occur, and the patient may have an accompanying severe depression of level of consciousness, including coma. If the embolus involves the vertebral basilar system, various combinations of cranial nerve and cerebellar findings may be apparent, but the hallmark of vertebral basilar stroke is sudden coma.[2,25,30]

ASSESSMENT

The transport team can be of help in the initial management of the patient who has had a stroke by performing a directed neurologic assessment once the patient has been stabilized. There are several stroke scales available, including the Cincinnati Prehospital Stroke Scale, the Los Angeles Prehospital Stroke Scale, and the NIH Stroke Scale, that offer a framework for the evaluation of the stroke patient. These scales also assist in patient evaluation when specific therapies such as the administration of fibrinolytics have been begun before transport.[10]

PLAN AND IMPLEMENTATION

As mentioned previously, care of the patient with a cerebrovascular episode is directed toward prevention of additional cerebral insult. Every attempt must be made to maximize cerebral blood flow, to control increased ICP, and to manage associated conditions such as cardiac dysrhythmias and seizures.

If the patient is hypertensive, their blood pressure must be carefully managed. Each transport program should manage hypertension based on a protocol that provides the parameters and medications that should be used to lower the patient's blood pressure. Some medications should not be used in transport unless the patient's blood pressure can accurately be measured. Inappropriate use of antihypertensive medications has been found to be just as detrimental to patient outcome as the stroke itself.[10]

Fibrinolytic therapy has been shown to be beneficial in acute ischemic stroke. Timing is crucial in these patients because evidence suggests that ischemic brain injury occurs when arterial occlusion continues longer than 2 or 3 hours, and an increasing amount of brain is infarcted if occlusion persists beyond this time. Local fibrinolytic therapy should be started in 90 minutes of the time of neurologic deterioration.[10,20] It is important for transport teams to consult experts in the management of stroke before initiating any treatment. Recommendations for treatment are constantly updated, and protocols need to be closely followed.

Once again, airway support is paramount, often requiring intubation and ventilatory support. The use of mechanical ventilation and arterial oxygen-saturation and end-tidal CO_2 ($EtCO_2$) monitoring during transport has proven effective in managing the patient with a neurologic medical emergency. Intravenous access is necessary for fluid maintenance and medication administration. As with all neurologic emergencies, protection of the patient from physical harm is necessary, with particular attention to safety restraints.[22]

Cerebrovascular disease is common in the adult population of the United States. Morbidity and mortality vary, depending on the type and extent of lesion and associated conditions or complications. Patients experiencing cerebrovascular episodes are frequently transferred to tertiary care facilities for further diagnostic studies and intervention. The initiation of life-sustaining care and supportive care throughout the transfer are valuable links in the transfer process. With appropriate and aggressive intervention, the maximal potential for recovery and subsequent rehabilitation can be ensured in the patient who has sustained a cerebrovascular episode.[25]

NEUROLOGIC MEDICAL EMERGENCIES CASE STUDY

The transport team was called to transport a 45-year-old female whose diagnosis was acute ischemic stroke.

HISTORY

The patient had been sitting at her desk when her co-workers observed that she was "slumping" over. The life squad was found, and they performed a Cincinnati Prehospital Stroke Scale. They found:

Left facial droop
No movement of the upper left extremity
Weakness of the left leg
Patient unable to speak
The patient was taken to the local hospital and the Stroke Team activated. A CT showed no evidence of an ischemic stroke, and no risk factors were found for the initiation of fibrinolytics therapy. The transport team was called for rapid transport for further interventions.

ASSESSMENT

On arrival of the transport team, the patient had been started in rt-TPA. Her weight was estimated

to be 65 kg. She had received 6 mg as an IV bolus over 1 minute, and the remaining 54 mg was infusing over 60 minutes. There had been no change in the patient's neurologic assessment. The transport team gave her a NIH Stroke Scale Score of 17.

Her vital signs were stable; she was not hypertensive.

TRANSPORT

During transport, the patient's symptoms began to improve. She was able to move her left arm to command, though it did drift. The patient was also able to say a few words. Her NIH Stroke Scale Score on admission to the receiving facility had improved to 12.

OUTCOME

The patient was taken to the Interventional Radiology Suite. Additional fibrinolytics were given interarterially. Within 24 hours, the patient showed marked improvement, including decreased left-side weakness and improved speech. She was discharged within 4 days to a rehabilitation center.

REFERENCES

1. Albin MS, Babinski M: *Intensive life support of the neurosurgical patient: critical care of neurological and neurosurgical emergencies*, New York, 1980, Raven.
2. Bannister SR: *Brain's clinical neurology*, London, 1985, Oxford University Press.
3. Barker E: *Neuroscience nursing*, St Louis, 1994, Mosby.
4. Barnett HJM et al, editors: *Stroke: pathophysiology, diagnosis and management*, New York, 1986, Churchill Livingstone.
5. Begley D, Newberry L: Neurologic emergencies. In Emergency Nurses Association, editors: *Sheehy's emergency nursing*, ed 4, St Louis, 1998, Mosby.
6. Bickley L, Hoekelman R: *Bate's guide to physical examination and history taking*, Philadelphia, 1999, Lippincott.
7. Biller J et al: Spontaneous subarachnoid hemorrhage in young adults, *Neurosurgery* 21:664, 1987.
8. Bleck T: Seizures in the critically ill. In Ayers S, editor: *Textbook of critical care*, ed 3, Philadelphia, 2000, Saunders.

9. Bubb DI: Neurological problems. In *RN neurological problems: nursing assessment,* series 3, Oradell, NJ, 1984, Medical Economics Books.

10. Carrozzella J, Jauch E: Emergency stroke management: A new era, *Nursing Clin North Am* 37(1), 2002.

11. Clifford DB: The somatosensory system and pain. In Pearlman AL, Collins RC, editors: *Neurological pathophysiology,* ed 3, New York, 1984, Oxford University Press.

12. Daube JR et al: *Medical neurosciences: an approach to anatomy, pathology, and physiology by systems and levels,* ed 2, Boston, 1986, Little, Brown.

13. Doczi T et al: Blood-brain barrier damage during the acute stage of subarachnoid hemorrhage as exemplified by a new animal model, *Neurosurgery* 18:733, 1986.

14. Forster FM, Booker HE: The epilepsies and convulsive disorders. In Baker AB, editor: *Clinical neurology,* vol 3, Philadelphia, 1984, Harper & Row.

15. Garza M: Brain attack, *JEMS* 18(4):60, 1993.

16. Gelb LD: Infections. In Pearlman AL, Collins RC, editors: *Neurological pathophysiology,* ed 3, New York, 1984, Oxford University Press.

17. Gilroy J: *Basic neurology,* ed 2, New York, 1990, Pergamon.

18. Glaser GH: Convulsive disorders (epilepsy). In Merritt H, editor: *A textbook of neurology,* ed 6, Philadelphia, 1979, Lea & Febiger.

19. Greenberg M: Neurologic manifestations of AIDS. In Greenburg M, editor: *Handbook of neurosurgery,* ed 3, Lakeland, Fla, 1994, Greenberg Graphics.

20. Guberman A: *Clinical neurology,* Boston, 1994, Little, Brown.

21. Holleran RS: *Prehospital nursing: a collaborative approach,* St Louis, 1994, Mosby.

22. Krupa D, editor: *Flight nursing core curriculum,* Des Plains, Ill, 1997, Road Runner Press.

23. Lothman EW, Collins RC: Seizures. In Pearlman AL, Collins RC, editors: *Neurological pathophysiology,* ed 3, New York, 1984, Oxford University Press.

24. Lynn-McHale DJ, Carlson KK: *AACN procedure manual for critical care,* Philadelphia, 2001, Saunders.

25. Macabasco AC, Hickman JL: Thrombolytic therapy for brain attack, *J Neurosci Nurs* 27:138, 1995.

26. McCance K, Huether S: *Pathophysiology: the biologic basis of disease in adults and children,* St Louis, 1998, Mosby.

27. McHenry Jr LC: *Cerebral circulation and strokes,* St Louis, 1978, Warren H Green.

28. Merritt H, Houston H: *A textbook of neurology,* ed 6, Philadelphia, 1979, Lea & Febiger.

29. Miller JD, Garabi J, Pichard JD: Induced changes of cerebrospinal fluid volume: effects during continuous monitoring of ventricular fluid pressure, *Arch Neurol* 28:265, 1973.

30. Millikan CH, McDowell F, Easton JD: *Stroke,* Philadelphia, 1987, Lea & Febiger.

31. Overbeeke JJ et al: Higher cortical disorders: an unusual presentation of an arteriovenous malformation, *Neurosurgery* 21:839, 1987.

32. Plum F, Posner JB: *Diagnosis of stupor and coma,* ed 3, Philadelphia, 1983, FA Davis.

33. Powers WJ, Raichle ME: Stroke. In Pearlman AL, Collins RC, editors: *Neurological pathophysiology,* ed 3, New York, 1984, Oxford University Press.

34. Proehl J, editor: *Emergency nursing procedures,* ed 2, Philadelphia, 1999, Saunders.

35. Saper CB: Hypothalamus and brainstem. In Pearlman AL, Collins RC, editors: *Neurological pathophysiology,* ed 3, New York, 1984, Oxford University Press.

36. Schmidley JW: Cerebrospinal fluid, blood-brain barrier, and brain edema. In Pearlman AL, Collins RC, editors: *Neurological pathophysiology,* ed 3, New York, 1984, Oxford University Press.

37. Skinhoj E, Standgoard S: Pathogenesis of hypertensive encephalopathy, *Lancet* 1:461, 1973.

38. Toole JF: Vascular diseases of brain and spinal cord. In Merrit H, editor: *A textbook of neurology,* ed 6, Philadelphia, 1979, Lea & Febiger.

39. Treiman DM, Delgado-Escueta AV: Status epilepticus. In Thompson RA, Green JR, editors: *Critical care of neurological and neurosurgical emergencies,* New York, 1980, Raven Press.

40. Tsemetzis SA: Surgical management of intracerebral hematomas, *Neurosurgery* 16:562, 1985.

41. van Eijndhoven JHM, Avezaat CJ: Cerebrospinal fluid pulse pressure and the pulsatile variation in cerebral blood volume: an experimental study in dogs, *Neurosurgery* 19:507, 1986.

42. Williams FC, Spetzler RF: Hemodynamic management in the neurosurgical intensive care unit. In *Clinical neurosurgery,* 35:101, Baltimore, 1987, Williams & Wilkins.

CARDIOVASCULAR EMERGENCIES

21

COMPETENCIES

1. Perform a detailed cardiovascular assessment before, during, and after transport.
2. Recognize potential for lethal events, and institute appropriate interventions and therapeutic modalities.
3. Identify patients experiencing an acute cardiac event, including acute myocardial infarction, heart failure, cardiogenic shock, primary arrhythmias, and hemodynamic instability.
4. Use invasive monitoring during transport, as indicated, for the purpose of clinical management.
5. Provide treatment for patients with acute cardiac events and hemodynamic abnormalities.
6. Incorporate the use of cardiopulmonary support devices, such as intra-aortic balloon pump (IABP), ventricular assist devices (VAD), and extracorporeal membrane oxygenation (ECMO), as dictated by patient condition as part of patient management.

One of the most challenging aspects for the transport team is caring for critically ill patients who require medical transport because of an acute cardiovascular event. The demand for medical transport of patients who are dependent on invasive devices and new, sophisticated technology continues to increase.[67] This chapter describes advances in clinical care for patients with angina, acute myocardial infarction (AMI), congestive heart failure (CHF), aortic dissection, and other manifestations of cardiovascular disease, with a focus on the assessment and management of these patients relative to the medical transport environment.

Cardiovascular disease is the leading cause of death in the United States, accounting for 1 million deaths annually.[106] Acute coronary syndromes alone are responsible for 95 million emergency department (ED) visits. The diagnostic distribution of 8 million patients seen in emergency departments with "chest pain" as the chief complaint resulted in 5 million hospital admissions, of which 2.5 million were noncardiac, 1 million were caused by AMIs, 1.2 million were found to have unstable angina, and 330,000 died. Of these 8 million people, 3 million were discharged to home from the ED, with 40,000 of them subsequently having a myocardial infarction (MI).[63] Cardiovascular disease, including hypertension, coronary artery disease (CAD), rheumatic heart disease, and stroke, affects over 65 million Americans.

A patient experiencing an acute cardiac event, decompensated CHF, or an aortic dissection in a community-based, limited-resource hospital often requires rapid critical care transfer to a tertiary care facility for further evaluation and emergent intervention. The transport of critically ill cardiovascular patients involves a number of issues, which include but are not limited to the potential effects of altitude and the difficulty associated with initiation of resuscitative interventions in a limited space in an uncontrolled environment.

Early research during the 1980s demonstrated the safety and efficacy of interfacility air medical transport of patients with an evolving MI who had received thrombolytic therapy under the care of a critical care clinician.[47] Current research has established the ability to safely transport patients requiring advanced mechanical circulatory support. Interfacility transfer by air and surface critical care teams of patients dependent on IABPs, VADs, and ECMO can now be accomplished.[67] Previous logistical restrictions, primarily because of the size of these devices and a lack of familiarity by crew members with this new technology, did not permit routine use of these circulatory support devices during transport.

ALTERATIONS OF CARDIOVASCULAR PHYSIOLOGY AT HIGH ALTITUDES

The potential for hypoxia poses one of the greatest risks to a patient with coronary artery disease. Decompensation of patients with acute cardiovascular disease being transported at high altitudes is generally caused by hypoxic hypoxia, which is defined as an oxygen deficiency in the body tissue sufficient to cause impaired function.[9,10] Individual patient tolerances vary, but the patient with cardiovascular compromise may be at risk if cabin pressure is above 6000 feet. For example, at an altitude of 10,000 feet the barometric pressure will decrease from 760 mm Hg at sea level to 523 mm Hg, resulting in a lower partial pressure of oxygen. This reduction in the amount of oxygen in the blood decreases available oxygen to the tissues. As altitude increases, oxygen saturation decreases. If a patient is 98% saturated (Pao_2 103) at sea level, they will be 93% saturated (Pao_2 68.9) at 8000 feet (the level to

which commercial airlines routinely pressurize their cabins).[9,10]

Healthy individuals can easily tolerate the effects of altitude without supplemental oxygen, but the cardiovascularly compromised patient can develop clinical manifestations related to cellular hypoxia with even a change from 0 to 4000 feet. Compensatory mechanisms that occur to maintain adequate oxygen supply to the tissues include increases in respiratory rate, heart rate, and cardiac output. The increased workload on the heart because of these compensatory mechanisms increases myocardial oxygen consumption and necessitates increased blood flow to the heart muscle. In healthy people, cardiac reserve allows the body to compensate and meet the demand for increased blood flow to the tissues by altering heart rate, stroke volume, or both and increases blood flow to the heart muscle by dilating the coronary artery microvasculature. Cardiovascular heart disease and cardiac events limit the compensatory mechanisms available to increase cardiac output in response to increased myocardial oxygen demand. Patients with coronary artery disease may be unable to compensate for the increased workload imposed on the heart by the decreased oxygen tension experienced at high altitude. These patients may develop chest pain, congestive heart failure, pulmonary edema, cardiac arrhythmias, or even cardiac arrest.[9,10]

Patients in cardiogenic shock who are receiving nitroprusside for afterload reduction and susceptible patients on nitroglycerin therapy can develop histotoxic hypoxia because of the potential for cyanide toxicity. Carbon monoxide, cyanide, or alcohol intake can all cause histoxic hypoxia, resulting in the inability of the body to use available oxygen because of poisoning of the cytochrome oxidase enzyme system. Tissue hypoxia occurs because of the formation of *methemoglobin* (which has increased oxygen affinity when compared with normal hemoglobin), and therefore the ability for oxygen to be "unloaded" at the tissue level is decreased. This situation can be made worse in the presence of a low partial pressure of oxygen caused by high altitudes.[9,10,35,47] A patient with adequate available oxygen, who is profoundly anemic, may have such a low hemoglobin concentration that oxygen-carrying capability is reduced to the point that tissue hypoxia develops. This is referred to as hypemic hypoxia, which, again, can be aggravated by the low partial pressure of oxygen that can develop with increases in altitude. This is of special interest to the clinician transporting a patient with a recently placed VAD because of the potential for blood loss during surgical insertion. It is critical that the hemoglobin concentration in these patients be evaluated and optimized prior to departure from the referral institution.[9,10,47]

All patients with cardiovascular disease should receive supplemental oxygen when transported by air. The potential effects of altitude can be minimized if the aircraft is pressurized at or below 4000 feet, along with the delivery of supplemental oxygen. In the fixed-wing population, limiting cabin altitude to a maximum of 6000 feet has been shown to eliminate problems for people with cardiovascular disease. Cabin pressure is not a fixed number and may need to be adjusted to accommodate patient condition. Cabin pressure can be adjusted to as low as sea level; however, a decrease in cabin pressure may come at the expense of traveling at a decreased altitude. Flights at decreased altitude may result in decreased speeds and therefore longer flights with an increased need for refueling during the trip. Decisions regarding altitude limitations must be based on the patient's history, his or her current clinical condition, and pilot expertise and judgment. These decisions may need to be adjusted as a result of continued in-flight patient assessment.[9,10,47,60]

SPECIAL CONSIDERATIONS FOR CARDIOPULMONARY RESUSCITATION IN THE TRANSPORT ENVIRONMENT

Cardiac arrest is of special concern to nurses involved in the transport of critical patients by either air or ground because the performance of cardiopulmonary resuscitation (CPR) in the confined space of an aircraft cabin or ground transport vehicle is often difficult and challenging. The advanced cardiac life support (ACLS) guidelines are the standard of practice for resuscitation of the patient in cardiac arrest and should be used as guidelines in the event of cardiac arrest in the air medical environment. The American Heart Association (AHA) has recently revised its guidelines.[40] Transport team members are expected to have current verification in advanced cardiac life support (ACLS) through the American Heart Association to practice independent patient care in the transport environment.[6,47] Thorough pretransport assessment, planning, and intervention along with prompt correction of dysrhythmias and continuous maintenance of adequate oxygenation may help to prevent the need for in-transport resuscitation. However, the transport team must be prepared in advance for emergencies such as cardiac arrest. Preparation includes ensuring that resuscitation equipment and an adequate oxygen supply are easily accessible. ACLS drugs should be well labeled, not beyond their expiration date, and ready for quick administration. Generally, the number of crew members available to perform basic and advanced life support resuscitation is limited to only two medically trained personnel. To respond effectively and rapidly in the event of an emergency, these team members must establish well-defined roles and responsibilities.

Special consideration should be given to the transport vehicle configuration when anticipating the potential need for CPR during admission. The position and height of the stretcher in relationship to the medical crew's ability to change positions is critical to facilitate proper hand and arm positioning when providing chest compressions. A well-designed configuration will minimize the need for crew members to extend or release their restraint devices when administering therapeutic interventions.[47]

DEFIBRILLATION DURING TRANSPORT

Cardiac arrest as the result of ventricular tachycardia and/or ventricular fibrillation must be treated promptly. The most critical factor in determining the success of a resuscitative effort is the time to restoration of effective spontaneous circulation. Current American Heart Association ACLS standards[40] recommend that defibrillation be immediate in the treatment of confirmed ventricular fibrillation and unstable ventricular tachycardia. The close quarters, metallic composition of transport vehicles, and proximity of vital electronic equipment, particularly in the rotor wing environment, had previously generated concern among transport personnel about initiating defibrillation, especially in the air. Holleran[47] addressed the potential risks of airborne defibrillation and demonstrated that defibrillation with modern equipment in a medically equipped twin-engine helicopter is safe. Despite cramped quarters and sensitive electrical equipment, defibrillation can be carried out without hesitation, whether the aircraft is on the ground or in flight, providing that standard defibrillation precautions are observed. Air medical personnel should follow the ACLS defibrillation standards for selecting energy levels and for placement of self-adhesive monitor/defibrillation pads or handheld paddles. This study[47] demonstrated that self-adhesive monitor/defibrillator pads are superior to standard monitoring leads and handheld electrode paddles in the management of prehospital ventricular defibrillation. Most, if not all, transport cardiac monitors permit "hands-off" defibrillation. When defibrillation pads are appropriately placed and equipment made ready prior to transport, defibrillation can be done more quickly with enhanced effectiveness. These easy-to-perform principles improve safety for both the crew and the patient in the transport environment. It is important to inform the pilot before defibrillation and to maintain clearance from the patient and stretcher when discharging the current. Most defibrillators are monophasic devices. The use of biphasic waveform defibrillators may become more common in the prehospital environment because it allows a lower energy setting, and repeated shocks at these lower energy levels are acceptable by new 2000 ACLS guidelines.

CORONARY ARTERY DISEASE

DEFINITION AND PATHOPHYSIOLOGIC FACTORS

Coronary artery disease remains one of the most common health problems in Western civilization and is directly responsible for half of a million deaths annually.[106] Progressive *atherosclerosis* of the coronary arteries results in a reduction of blood flow to the ventricular myocardium. The innermost layer of the coronary arteries, or endothelium, is responsible for many complex processes in the normal artery, including the secretion of vasodilatory substances and other substances, that mediate of platelet interactions. "Risk factors" for coronary artery disease (i.e., diabetes, hypertension, cigarette smoking, high levels of low-density lipoprotein [LDL], and low levels of high-density lipoprotein [HDL]) contribute to the formation of atherosclerotic plaques by injuring or interfering with the normal function of the vascular endothelium. The "response to injury" theory[87] of the development of atherosclerosis postulates that injury to the endothelium facilitates the subintimal accumulation of lipids. Chronic minimal injury encourages the deposit of lipids in the wall of the coronary artery, resulting in lipid-rich plaques with a fibrous cap.[33] The atherosclerotic *plaque* increases over time and at varying rates, dependent on the degree of vascular injury present. Significant obstruction to flow, as demonstrated by coronary ischemia, occurs when the coronary arteries are narrowed by approximately 70%. At this point, myocardial oxygen blood supply may not be adequate to meet myocardial oxygen demand at times of stress, and ischemia of the myocardium develops.

An area of the ventricular myocardium that becomes ischemic stops contracting normally almost immediately at the onset of ischemia, resulting in decreased left ventricular function.[105] While ischemic, the electrical milieu of the heart is abnormal, and life-threatening ventricular arrhythmias can occur.

PATHOPHYSIOLOGIC FACTORS OF CORONARY ISCHEMIA

Myocardial metabolism is an aerobic process in which the heart extracts about 70% of the available oxygen supplied by the coronary arteries. Increases in myocardial oxygen demand are normally met by increases in blood flow caused by dilation of the numerous microscopic branches of the coronary arteries known as the *microvasculature*.

Angina pectoris or *angina* is a symptom of myocardial ischemia. It is caused by an imbalance between myocardial oxygen supply and demand. The end result is a buildup of metabolites in the ischemic tissue, which activates nerve endings and causes anginal pain.[26]

The myocardial oxygen supply and demand relationship is the basis for understanding both the causes of and the treatment for coronary ischemia. Myocardial oxygen supply is dependent primarily on patent coronary arteries and an adequate hemoglobin concentration to ensure adequate oxygen-carrying capacity. The major determinants of myocardial oxygen demand are heart rate, contractility, and wall stress. The imbalance between myocardial supply and demand can occur for a number of reasons:

1.   Mechanisms that decrease supply:

- A decrease in the caliber of a coronary artery
- Fixed (atherosclerosis)
- Transient (spasm)
- Severe anemia
- Poor perfusion of the coronaries because of profound hypotension

2.   Mechanisms that increase demand:

- Tachycardia
- Hypertension—which increases left ventricular wall stress
- Increased myocardial contractility—caused by increased adrenergic stimuli

Angina can be divided into several categories depending on the onset, severity, duration, and alleviation of symptoms. These categories include classic or stable angina, unstable angina, Prinzmetal's angina or silent angina—more commonly termed *silent ischemia*.

CHRONIC STABLE ANGINA

In the presence of a flow-limiting coronary artery atherosclerotic lesion, myocardial oxygen supply may be inadequate to meet periods of increased myocardial oxygen demand. When a patient with a significant atherosclerotic lesion undertakes an action that increases myocardial demand (such as walking on a treadmill), the patient will begin to demonstrate signs of myocardial ischemia (angina with ST segment depression) when the myocardial oxygen demand begins to outstrip supply. This is the basis of the cardiac "stress test" to diagnose coronary artery disease.

Stable angina is usually precipitated by physical exertion or emotional stress. Chronic stable angina is predictable—patients will develop symptoms at a predictable workload. These symptoms usually last 1 to 5 minutes and are often abated by stopping the exertional activity or by the use of sublingual nitroglycerine (NTG).

UNSTABLE ANGINA

Unstable angina is a clinical *syndrome* and not a specific disease. Unstable angina is routinely classified by using clinical descriptors, such as the presence of chest discomfort at rest.[13] The term *unstable angina* refers to an abrupt change in a patient's anginal symptoms. *Unstable syndromes* include angina with minimal exertion or angina with an exertion level that is much less than usual, new-onset angina, or angina at rest. The abrupt change in symptom pattern can occur as a result of any mechanism that suddenly increases myocardial oxygen demand (tachycardia from pain, fever, hypovolemia, profound hypertension, or thyrotoxicosis) or from a sudden decrease in myocardial oxygen supply (sudden decrease in the caliber of a coronary because of progression of an atherosclerotic plaque or coronary spasm, or anemia from acute bleeding). These symptoms and the ischemic ECG changes that are associated with them are treated by treating the underlying problem.

The most common cause of a sudden decrease in myocardial perfusion is from transient thrombus formation on the surface on a ruptured atherosclerotic plaque. Unstable angina, which is because of an abrupt decrease in the caliber of a coronary artery, falls into the category of "acute coronary syndromes," which will be discussed extensively in a later section of this chapter.

Prinzmetal's angina, or "variant angina," is a form of angina in which spontaneous chest discomfort with ST segment elevation occurs without relationship to exertion. Prinzmetal characterized it in 1959[81] as the result of temporary, increased tone in a coronary artery resulting in a marked reduction in coronary blood flow. Evidence supports focal coronary spasm as the mechanism of transient ST segment elevation and concurrent symptoms. Spasm is usually confined to a single epicardial vessel, but multivessel spasm can occur.[72] Spasm generally occurs in 1 centimeter of an atherosclerotic plaque in a mildly diseased vessel. Patients are generally young and often do not exhibit the classic atherosclerotic "risk factors"—except for cigarette smoking.[97] There is usually a circadian rhythm to anginal attacks, which are often clustered in the early morning hours.[71] During the period of time when the coronary artery is in spasm, these patients are at risk for myocardial necrosis and the life-threatening arrhythmias that are associated with coronary ischemia. The pathophysiology of this disease appears to involve a combination of endothelial dysfunction along with increased reactivity in response to vasoconstrictor substances. Treatment revolves around the use of vasodilator substances, such as NTG and calcium channel blockers, along with risk factor modification.

SILENT ISCHEMIA

Evidence of ischemia in the absence of symptomatic complaints occurs frequently. At least 75% of ischemia occurring in patients with stable angina is "silent," or without clinical manifestations.[76] ST segment changes are often detected on ambulatory monitoring. There are several explanations for the absence of anginal symptoms in patients with silent ischemia, including the observation that patients with this "silent" angina exhibit less sensitivity to pain in general than do patients with reproducible angina.

THE CONTINUUM OF ACUTE CORONARY SYNDROMES

An abrupt change in the caliber of a coronary artery can occur as a result of coronary blood vessel spasm or be due to the abrupt worsening of an atherosclerotic plaque. Atherosclerotic plaques can suddenly become more narrowed as a result of the formation of a hematoma in the wall of the vessel or because of the formation of a thrombus on the surface of a damaged plaque (Figure 21-1).

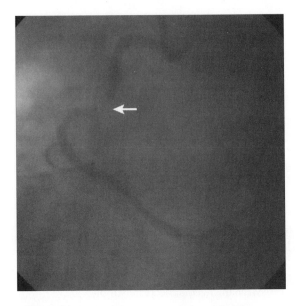

FIGURE 21-1 **Large thrombus in the mid-right coronary artery.** (Courtesy of Cleveland Clinic Foundation Cardiovascular Department, Cleveland, Ohio.)

Atherosclerotic lesions, which are rich in lipids, are susceptible to endothelial damage.[34] Disruption of the protective endothelial lining, known as plaque rupture, leads to a cascade of processes, which are aimed at "healing" this damaged vessel. If these processes become overexuberant, a thrombus can form on the surface of the damaged endothelium, resulting in the total occlusion of the blood vessel (Figure 21-2).

Rupture of vulnerable plaques is responsible for 75% of all acute coronary syndromes, resulting in acute obstruction in blood flow to the myocardium normally served by the occluded coronary artery.[30] Acute coronary syndromes begin with a fissure or disruption of the endothelium overlying an atherosclerotic lesion. The lesions more likely to be involved in acute coronary syndromes are the mild to moderate lesions[72] with thin fibrous tissue caps, and larger lipid concentrations[72] of the underlying coronary vessel wall causes both platelet activation and the stimulation of the clotting cascade to form *thrombin*. Thrombin is a potent stimulant of platelet activation and is responsible for the conversion of

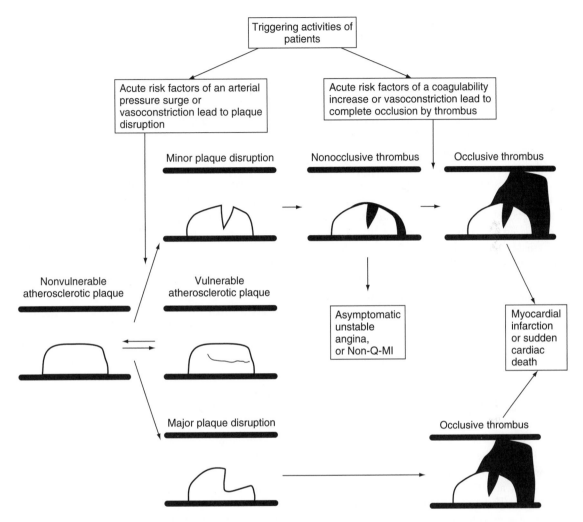

FIGURE 21-2 **Response to injury model.** Illustration of response to injury model of coronary occlusion presenting three triggering mechanisms: (1) physical or mental stress producing hemodynamic changes leading to plaque rupture, (2) activities causing an increase in coagulability, and (3) stimuli leading to vasoconstriction. The scheme depicts the role of coronary thrombosis in unstable angina, MI, and sudden cardiac death has been well described. (The lexicon of a new frontier. Reprinted with permission from the American College of Cardiology, *J Am Coll Cardiol* 23:809, 1994)

fibrinogen in the bloodstream to *fibrin*. Fibrin is responsible for "cross-linking" platelets into a stable thrombus.

Platelets, once activated, bind to exposed areas of the vessel wall. More platelets are drawn to the area, and the activated platelets begin to bind to each other via receptors on their surface, known as *glycoprotein IIb/IIIa receptors*. These platelets eventually form a platelet plug. If large enough,

they can completely occlude the relatively small (3-mm range) coronary arteries and occlude flow in the vessel. Platelet activation also leads to the secretion of vasoconstrictor substances, which limit blood flow in the affected coronary artery. The degree to which a coronary is occluded and whether or not it remains occluded by a platelet plug that is subsequently cross-linked by fibrin determines which part of the continuum of "acute coronary syndromes" an event is classified. For example:

1. Unstable angina caused by an acute change in the caliber of a coronary artery as a result of plaque rupture and thrombus formation. If there is transient occlusion of a coronary by activated platelets at the site of a ruptured plaque with subsequent recanalization of the vessel, the patient may be symptomatic at rest (while the coronary is occluded) and have his/her symptoms resolve spontaneously with recanalization of the vessel. Transient electrocardiogram (ECG) changes may occur while the patient is symptomatic, but the episode is often too short to demonstrate either ECG changes or evidence of myocardial injury (troponin, CPK–MB).

2. An event classified as a "non–Q wave infarction" begins in the same manner, but occlusion of the coronary is either prolonged (with myocardial necrosis) or distal embolization of small platelet clumps occurs, leading to occlusion of smaller, distal coronary branches and therefore myocardial necrosis. Spontaneous recanalization may occur, but there is biochemical evidence of myocardial necrosis (troponin, CPK–MB).

3. In both of these instances a significantly narrowed coronary artery (although recanalized) remains, and therapy is aimed at keeping the activated platelets present on its surface from progressing into a stable thrombus. In the patient whose symptoms resolve with therapy, the question of further management becomes less clear.[11] The data would support the use of either of the following strategies:

4. "Conservative" management—the use of cardiac catheterization with subsequent revascularization only for patients with recurrent symptoms of angina or a positive stress test.

5. "Invasive" management—the performance of a cardiac catheterization with subsequent revascularization in all patients presenting with documented acute coronary syndromes.

6. AMI represents the syndrome of acute plaque rupture, which continues to its ultimate end-

point—an organized thrombus made up of activated platelets cross-linked fibrin, which results in a stable thrombus. These patients present with continued chest pain and associated ST segment elevation because of injury caused by total occlusion of coronary blood flow. At this point, therapy must be aimed at both "deactivation" of platelets and destruction of fibrin.

Chronic Stable Angina: Assessment, Diagnosis, and Treatment. Classic angina is usually described as substernal chest discomfort, "pressure," or "heaviness" that occurs with activity and is resolved with rest. The chest discomfort gradually increases in intensity and often will gradually self-resolve. Occasionally patients may report dyspnea, back, shoulder, arm, or jaw pain without the presence of chest pain. The location of the chest pain is most commonly reported in the middle or lower sternum or the left precordium. Patients may also develop such symptoms as nausea, vomiting, diaphoresis, dyspnea, and fatigue, but in general these symptoms are predictable, and patients "know their limitations." The patients will usually stop exerting themselves or take nitroglycerin (NTG) tablets before their symptoms become severe.

Physical exam in patients with episodes of chronic stable angina is often normal, although many patients will have an S_4 because the ischemic area of the left ventricle is "stiff." In stable angina, the ECG has limited diagnostic value. Transient ST depression may occur *during exertion*. It represents ischemia in the *subendocardium*, the inner surface of the myocardium. This area of the ventricular myocardium, just adjacent to the left ventricular cavity and farthest away from the oxygenated blood supplied from the coronary arteries, is the most susceptible to ischemia. Cardiac arrhythmias, some potentially lethal, may occur with any episode of ischemia caused by alterations in the conductance of electrical activity through the myocardium at times of limited coronary blood flow.

The goal of treatment of chronic stable angina, as with all forms of angina, is to identify the imbalance in the myocardial oxygen supply and demand relationship and subsequently fix that problem. Treatment involves either strategies to increase coronary blood supply, decrease myocardial oxygen demand, or both. This may be accomplished through pharmacologic, percutaneous angioplasty, or surgical interventions.

Medical therapy for chronic stable angina is aimed at decreasing myocardial oxygen demand by controlling heart rate and blood pressure. Chronic therapy includes beta-blockers, ACE inhibitors, transdermal or oral nitrates, and calcium channel blockers. Medical therapy is also aimed at risk factor modification—including smoking cessation and aggressive lipid lowering.

Nitroglycerin can be used in both short-acting and long-acting forms. Sublingual NTG is often used for the initial management of anginal pain and ischemia. It works by relaxing vascular smooth muscle leading to both arterial and venous vasodilation. Venodilation leads to a decrease in preload and therefore a decrease in ventricular wall tension. Arterial vasodilation leads to a decrease in systemic blood pressure. These actions both work to decrease myocardial oxygen consumption or demand. Coronary vasodilation, both epicardial and microvasculature, can help to increase myocardial oxygen supply. Patients using long-acting nitrates should be warned of the "tolerance" effect with this medication and should have at least an 8-hour "drug-free" window to maintain drug efficacy. Patients often use sublingual NTG as prophylaxis before an activity that is known to precipitate an anginal attack.

Beta-blockers work by decreasing myocardial oxygen demand. These agents interrupt sympathetic impulses by competing with the neurotransmitter norepinephrine at the beta-sympathetic nerve endings. Beta-receptor inhibition results in decreased heart rate, myocardial contractility, and slowed impulse transmission through the cardiac conduction system. These effects lead to decreased myocardial oxygen consumption. In addition, beta-blockers decrease MI size and improve survival because of a decreased incidence of myocardial rupture and ventricular fibrillation.[51]

The calcium channel blockers verapamil and diltiazem slow heart rate, decrease blood pressure, and decrease myocardial contractility—each of these contributing to a decrease in myocardial oxygen consumption. Although previously widely used for the management of angina, calcium channel antagonist use has decreased since controversial data was presented in 1995.[82] Beta-blockers should be used as first-line agents unless contraindicated, and calcium channel blocking agents can be added as an alternative or additional therapy if the maximum doses of beta-blockers have been achieved.[40,86]

All patients with coronary artery disease should take 81 mg of aspirin each day,[84] along with following a lifestyle that promotes cardiovascular health. In patients with elevated cholesterol, a "statin" type lipid-lowering agent should be used to achieve an LDL of less than 100 mg/dl.[70]

Percutaneous transluminal angioplasty, with or without intracoronary stenting, can be performed in patients with symptomatic angina and a stress test, which indicates ischemia in the territory of a significantly narrowed coronary artery. In patients with multivessel coronary artery disease, coronary artery bypass surgery may need to be used to revascularize the entire myocardium. Again, aggressive risk factor modification in addition to interventional therapy is indicated.

Patients with chronic stable angina often come into contact with air medical personnel when they are faced with a sudden "stressful" situation—not necessarily a cardiac event. Patients with significant coronary artery disease may be seen in the setting of a trauma, gastrointestinal bleed, or sepsis. The key to the evaluation and treatment of these patients is to ask the question, "What is the underlying problem?" A patient with chest pain and ST segment depression in the setting of a broken pelvis and a hematocrit of 22% is having symptoms caused by an increased myocardial oxygen demand, *not* a sudden change in supply. There has been no change in the caliber of the coronaries, therefore treatment *should not* be aimed at antiplatelet and anticoagulation therapy. The patient is having a "stress test" caused by hypovolemia, anemia, and pain—all leading to increased heart rate and therefore increased myocardial oxygen demand. The goal in treatment is to help get this patient "off the treadmill." The goal is to fix the underlying problem—*not* by giving beta-blockers to cover the problem, but to fix the problem with transfusion, volume replacement, and pain control.

The Acute Coronary Syndromes: Diagnosis, Assessment, and Treatment.

The term *acute coronary syndromes* is applied when referring to patients who present with an abrupt change in their anginal symptoms caused by the sequelae of a *ruptured atherosclerotic plaque*. The continuum of unstable angina, non–Q wave infarction and AMIs are, in truth, varying degrees of the same underlying problem. The problem: a mild to moderate, lipid-laden atherosclerotic plaque suddenly ruptures—exposing the underlying cholesterol "gruel" to the circulating blood and setting in place multiple systems that are responsible for trying to "heal over" the damaged vessel wall. Platelets cover the surface of the injured area, then attach to each other by receptors on their surfaces—called GP IIb/IIIa receptors. The activation of platelets during this process releases regulatory substances, which cause further aggregation of platelets and vasoconstriction. At the same time, the clotting cascade becomes activated, resulting in the formation of *thrombin*, a potent stimulator of platelets. Thrombin is also responsible for the formation of *fibrin* from fibrinogen in the blood. As platelets accumulate in the area, a "platelet plug" forms, which itself can intermittently occlude flow in the coronary. As this mass of platelets becomes organized, fibrin interconnects the platelets into a stable blood clot, or *thrombus*. The continuum of acute coronary syndromes—and the final diagnosis or "label" a patient with an acute coronary syndrome receives—is dependent on the degree to which a platelet plug forms and becomes organized.

Once platelets have aggregated on the surface of a ruptured plaque, the competition between antithrombotic and thrombotic processes in the body becomes intense. The vessel may "reocclude" at any time, or this area may "heal over" without further symptoms, and the ruptured plaque/platelet plug may be incorporated into the atherosclerotic plaque—contributing to the stepwise growth of atherosclerotic coronary artery disease. The goal of treatment in acute coronary syndromes is to augment the anticoagulant properties that the body possesses and interfere with the "clot forming" processes.

Acute coronary syndromes begin primarily as a process mediated by activated platelets; therefore therapeutic strategies are primarily aimed at the inhibition of platelets and interference with platelet–platelet interactions. Efforts aimed at decreasing myocardial oxygen demand, such as beta-blockers, pain control, and NTG, will also help, but do not address the primary problem—activated platelets on the surface of a ruptured plaque.

Aspirin is a potent inhibitor of *thromboxane A2*–stimulated platelet aggregation. There are many other pathways that stimulate platelet aggregation and interactions. Aspirin works at only one part of this process, but its use has clearly been shown to decrease MI and death in patients who present to the hospital with unstable angina.[62] All patients presenting with symptoms consistent with unstable angina and without contraindications should receive at least 160 mg of aspirin.

Ticlopidine and clopidogrel inhibit platelet activation via a different mechanism. These products inhibit *ADP-dependent* platelet activation. This effect does not occur immediately, and there is a risk of neutropenia with their use. These drugs are primarily used in patients with true aspirin allergies and as an adjunct to anticoagulation after intracoronary stent placement.

Heparin is a potent anticoagulant that augments the body's ability to reduce thrombin generation and fibrin formation. Clinical evidence supports the use of heparin in acute coronary syndromes. The dosing and route of administration has become less clear with the addition of glycoprotein IIb/IIIa inhibitors to the armamentarium. The dosage of heparin that is administered along with IIb/IIIa inhibitors continues to change and may also vary by cardiologist. The transport team should follow recommended protocols.

The glycoprotein IIb/IIIa receptors on the surface of platelets are responsible for the attachment of platelets to one another. Inhibitors of this process block the *common final pathway* of platelet aggregation and are therefore potent inhibitors of the formation of thrombus. The agents currently in use, *abciximab, Integrilin*, and *tirofiban*, have different mechanisms of actions, dosing strategies, and half-lives, discussion of which is beyond the scope of this book. These medications, which have become an important part of the treatment of patients with acute coronary syndromes, should be familiar to air medical transport personnel. The new AHA guidelines recommend the use of GP IIb/IIIa inhibitors in addition to aspirin and heparin for patients presenting with a non–ST segment elevation MI and/or refractory ischemia.[40]

In most patients, anticoagulation and antiplatelet therapies cause symptoms and signs of ischemia to abate. For those patients with ongoing signs and symptoms of ischemia not relieved with medical therapy, cardiac catheterization with subsequent *revascularization* should be performed. Dependent on the patient's coronary anatomy, *revascularization* may include angioplasty with or without intracoronary stent placement or coronary artery bypass graft surgery.

An IABP augments coronary flow during diastole. In patients refractory to medical therapy, or those patients who are hemodynamically unstable, intra-aortic balloon counterpulsation may be used in addition to the standard therapies presented. Air medical personnel need to be familiar with the management of an IABP—placed to support a patient with refractory, unstable angina while being transported to a facility with the ability to perform emergency cardiac catheterization with revascularization.

ACUTE MYOCARDIAL INFARCTION: ASSESSMENT, DIAGNOSIS, AND TREATMENT

An AMI occurs because of a coronary artery becoming occluded as a result of a thrombus forming on the surface of a ruptured atherosclerotic plaque. When there is no longer flow in the coronary artery, the entire distribution of that coronary artery is at risk for injury/myocardial cell death. Initially that

wall of the heart becomes "stiff" and then stops moving—resulting in a loss of left ventricular ejection fraction and potentially leading to significant valvular dysfunction and ventricular arrhythmias. The longer the interruption to coronary flow, the more extensive the injury with the subsequent loss of myocardial function.

As with the other acute coronary syndromes, an AMI begins as a platelet problem but evolves into a process that results in the formation of a stable thrombus through the formation and infiltration of the platelet plug by fibrin cross-links. The initial treatment goals are therefore similar to those for other acute coronary syndromes. The adjunctive use of aspirin, heparin, and GP IIb/IIIa inhibitors, in addition to a definitive reperfusion strategy with either fibrinolytic therapy or emergency angioplasty, are the basic concepts of AMI therapy. Fibrinolytic therapy destroys fibrin in the intracoronary thrombus. In doing so, activated platelets are released from the thrombus. These activated platelets can reassemble and reocclude the vessel if adjunctive anticoagulation and antiplatelet strategies are not used. Agents such as beta-blockers, NTG, and morphine sulfate for pain control are important to decrease myocardial oxygen demand; *reperfusion* with restoration of myocardial oxygen supply should be the *primary* goal.

DIAGNOSIS OF ACUTE MYOCARDIAL INFARCTION

Patients who present with an AMI describe chest "heaviness," "discomfort," or "pressure," often associated with shortness of breath, diaphoresis, or nausea. The discomfort may radiate to the neck, jaw, or arms. Ongoing angina associated with an electrocardiogram that demonstrates ST segment elevation in contiguous leads (leads that represent an area of the heart that is supplied by a single coronary) together make the diagnosis of an AMI. ST segment elevation on the surface electrocardiogram represents *injury* with myocardial cell *necrosis* in the area of the occluded coronary artery.

The cardiac blood supply is made up of three principal coronary arteries. These vessels, the first branches off the aorta, originate from the coronary

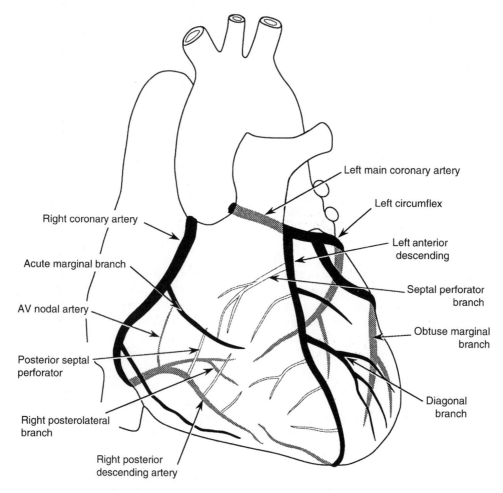

FIGURE 21-3   **Coronary anatomy.** (Courtesy Darell Debowey, Ann Arbor, Mich.)

ostia at the level of the aortic valve cusps. The left main coronary artery divides into the left anterior descending (LAD) and the left circumflex arteries. The LAD supplies the anterior surface of the heart, the anterior two thirds of the septum, and part of the lateral wall (Figure 21-3). The LAD distribution is represented on the surface electrocardiogram in the "V" or chest leads. The circumflex coronary artery supplies branches to the lateral and posterior surfaces of the heart. The circumflex is not well represented on the standard electrocardiogram. Changes caused by ischemia or infarction in the circumflex coronary artery may be seen in the lateral

(V_5, V_6, aVL, and I) leads or in the posterior wall by inference from changes in the V_1 and V_2 leads (Table 21-1).

In 85% of patients the right coronary artery (RCA) is responsible for coronary blood flow to the inferior surface of the heart and to the posterior third of the interventricular septum via one of its branches, the posterior descending coronary artery. These areas of the heart are represented on the electrocardiogram as the "inferior" leads or leads II, III, and aVF. On the way to the inferior surface of the heart, the RCA is also responsible for supplying blood flow to the right ventricle (Figures 21-4 and 21-5).

TABLE 21-1 Location of MI and Associated ST Segment Changes

Location of infarct	Leads with ST segment elevation	Leads with ST segment depression and/or reciprocal changes
Inferior	2, 3, aVF	I, aVL, V_1-V_4
Anterior (extensive)	I, aVL, V_1-V_6	2, 3, aVF, aVR
Anteroseptal	V_1-V_4	
Anterolateral	I, aVL, V_3-V_6	
Lateral	I, aVL, V_5-V_6	2, 3, aVF
High anterolateral	I, aVL	
Posterior	V_6	V_1-V_2

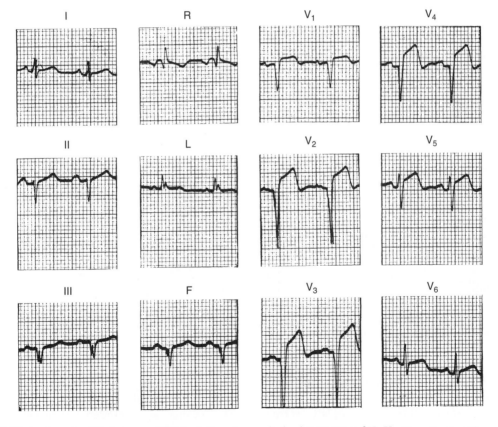

FIGURE 21-4 Anterior MI shown on ECG depicting changes in leads I, II, III and V_1-V_6. (From Conover M: *Understanding electrocardiography*, ed 5, St Louis, 1994, Mosby.)

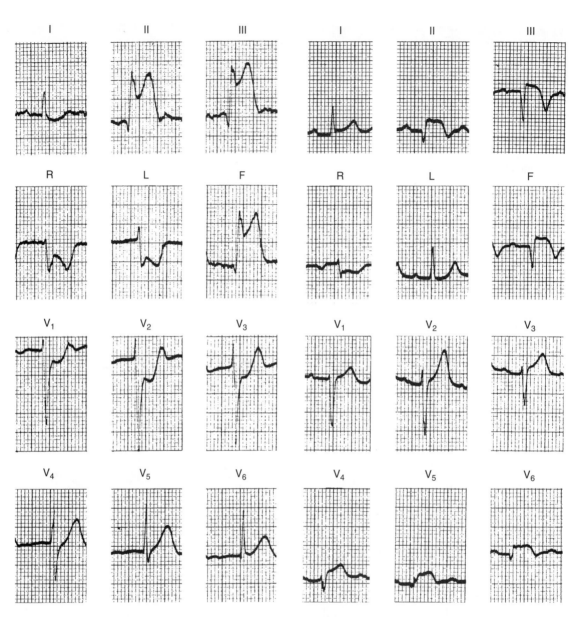

FIGURE 21-5   Inferior MI ECG changes depicting changes in leads I, II, III and V_1-V_6. (From Conover M: *Understanding electrocardiography*, ed 5, St Louis, 1994, Mosby.)

Once the diagnosis of an AMI is clear, it should immediately prompt the decision about which form of reperfusion therapy (angioplasty versus fibrinolytic therapy) will be the best for a particular patient. This decision must be made in a rapid fashion because for each minute the myocardium is devoid of blood flow, more injury will occur. The sooner an occluded coronary artery is reperfused, the less likely the patient is to die from an MI.[37]

Examination of the patient suspected of having an AMI should be focused and include evaluation for contraindications to therapy and a search for complications of the MI. Excessive sympathetic stimulation may result in an elevated blood pressure and an increased heart rate.

The patient should be evaluated for the presence of an S_3, rales, or distended neck veins, which would indicate the presence of congestive heart failure caused by either severe left ventricular failure from the AMI or from "flash" pulmonary edema resulting from the acute onset of severe mitral regurgitation. Mitral regurgitation caused by the abrupt disruption of the mitral valve is often not audible on examination. It occurs as a consequence of occlusion of the blood supply to the lateral surface of the heart. Tachycardia and hypotension in association with the signs of congestive heart failure represent cardiogenic shock. These patients are best treated with emergency angioplasty,[73] ideally after temporary placement of an IABP. It is critical that these patients in cardiogenic shock *DO NOT receive beta-blockers, as their tachycardia is functional because of their severely limited stroke volume from an extensive MI.*

Critical care transport personnel will be involved in the transport of patients with cardiogenic shock to facilities that have the capabilities to perform emergency angioplasty. In patients transported prior to the placement of an IABP, perfusion to the brain and vital organs must be maintained. The use of low-dose dopamine or phenylephrine to maintain blood pressure, albeit at a cost of increased myocardial oxygen demand, should be used. These medications should be used at the lowest dose possible to maintain adequate perfusion of the vital organs (systolic blood pressure [SBP] greater than or equal to 90 mm Hg in the conscious, urinating patient).

Profound bradycardia with complete heart block and hypotension can occur because of occlusion of the blood supply to the inferior surface of the heart. This generally responds to saline infusion and administration of atropine. Rarely will a patient need transcutaneous or transvenous pacing, but the air medical personnel should be well versed in their use should the situation arise.

Hypotension with distended neck veins and clear lungs occurs in patients with right ventricular infarction. This is because of occlusion of the proximal right coronary artery, the blood supply to the right ventricle. Patients with right ventricular infarctions are "volume dependent" because of inadequate *preload* to the left ventricle. Because the right and left ventricles work in circuit, a poorly functional right ventricle is unable to maintain adequate volume back to the left ventricle. The patient develops signs of poor cardiac output despite adequate left ventricular function. The basis of therapy for a right ventricular infarction is large volumes of intravenous fluid.

THERAPY FOR ACUTE MYOCARDIAL INFARCTION

As with the previously described acute coronary syndromes, an AMI begins as a platelet problem, and therefore the same treatment, anticoagulation with antiplatelet therapies, is initiated. Because the patient's thrombus has organized to form fibrin cross-links between platelets, fibrinolytic therapy to help destroy the thrombus or mechanical intervention to disrupt it must also be performed. Remember that even when fibrinolytic therapy or angioplasty is performed, there is still an underlying ruptured plaque, which is prone to reforming thrombus, and adjunctive antiplatelet therapy *must* continue, even after perfusion in the vessel has been restored. Decisions about which form of reperfusion therapy should be performed are based on the pros and cons of each strategy in each individual patient.

Fibrinolytic therapy with tissue plasminogen activator or one of its derivatives has been proven in large, multicenter trials to decrease mortality from AMI.[41] It has also been shown that patients whose blood flow was restored to "normal" (or "TIMI III flow) versus "almost normal" (or "TIMI II)" were more likely to survive.[94] Unfortunately, there is a subgroup of patients who do not respond *at all* to fibrinolytic therapy. In one large study, only 54% of patients receiving tPA achieved TIMI III, or normal flow.[101] Other disadvantage to fibrinolytic therapy include the risk of bleeding complications, especially intracranial hemorrhage and the fact that it

BOX 21-1	**Absolute Contraindications for Thrombolytic Therapy**

History of intracranial neoplasm, arteriovenous malformation, or aneurysm
Active bleeding
Known severe bleeding disorder
History of stroke
Recent noncompressible vascular puncture
Major surgery or trauma in the past 3 months
Systolic blood pressure ≥180 and unresponsive hypertension
Pregnancy and up to 1 month postpartum

cannot be considered in some patients because of contraindications. The major contraindications to fibrinolytic therapy are active bleeding, a history of hemorrhagic stroke, recent trauma or major surgery, prolonged CPR, or uncontrolled hypertension (Box 21-1).

The primary advantage to fibrinolytic therapy is that it can be given intravenously at any medical center or even "in the field" without the need for expensive equipment. Knowing that the time to treatment is proportional to the survival benefit, the goal in any institution for fibrinolytic therapy should be a "door to needle" time of less than 30 minutes. Studies evaluating the use of fibrinolytic therapy "in the field" have collectively shown a 15% reduction in mortality attributed to the 1-hour decrease in time to therapy achieved. At this point, the logistics of staffing, ability for transmission of 12-lead electrocardiograms, and legal concerns have limited the prehospital use of fibrinolytic therapy, but air medical personnel play a crucial part in ensuring that the "door to needle" or the "door to balloon" time is as short as possible.

Current research into medical therapy for MI has focused on the use of newer, longer acting forms of fibrinolytic medications with or without the use of GP IIb/IIIa inhibitors. The combination of lower dose fibrinolytic therapy (with, hopefully, a decreased risk of intracerebral hemorrhage) and the potent antiplatelet effects of the GP IIb/IIIa inhibitors to ensure patency of the vessel appear to be a promising strategy for the future.[18]

Emergency angioplasty or "primary" angioplasty with or without intracoronary stent placement has emerged as an excellent strategy for the treatment of patients with AMI. The advantages of this strategy include the fact that it can be used in patients with contraindications to fibrinolytic therapy, and that it can restore normal (TIMI III) flow in the vessel in 90% of patients at 60 minutes. The primary disadvantages are the logistic difficulty and cost inherent in keeping a cardiac catheterization lab functional for 24 hours a day. Operator training influences patient outcome, and the data achieved in large-scale trials for very experienced operators may not be comparable to operators who are less experienced.[29] Another disadvantage of angioplasty as the primary therapy of AMI is the problem of long-term restenosis that continues to plague this therapy. The use of intracoronary stenting may result in decreased levels of restenosis in the future.

"Rescue angioplasty" is angioplasty performed for a patient who does not reperfuse after fibrinolytic therapy. Critical care transport personnel are crucial in the transport of these patients to institutions with angioplasty facilities in a prompt, safe manner. It is the opinion of the author that any patient transported while "actively infarcting" should be transported with "hands-free" defibrillator patches in place and should not be disconnected from the defibrillator at any time during transport.

Acknowledgment of the presence of an AMI at a referral institution should prompt the receiving institution to activate its cardiac catheterization laboratory staff if reperfusion with thrombolytic therapy has not occurred *or* if the decision for primary angioplasty has been made. This process can be facilitated by air medical personnel. Direct physician-to-physician contact and the timely fax of electrocardiograms can avoid unnecessary delays in reperfusion therapy.

In patients with adequate blood pressure (SBP >110 mm Hg), intravenous morphine sulfate (2-4 mg IV), and IV NTG therapy (goal is to decrease SBP by approximately 10% to 20%) can be used for pain control. Beta-blockers (metoprolol 5 mg IV q 5 minutes for three doses, followed by 50 mg PO, qid in the acute setting) can help decrease myocardial oxygen demand in the patient with no contraindication (i.e., severe congestive heart failure, bradycardia, or diffuse wheezing).

Emergency coronary artery bypass surgery (CABG) is performed in the setting of an AMI for patients with severe left main disease, failed angioplasty, and multivessel coronary artery disease not amenable to percutaneous revascularization. The time required to activate a "pump" team and the time necessary to place patients on bypass limit CABG as an initial strategy to reperfuse an infarcting segment of myocardium.

Only 10% of the hospitals in the United States have cardiac catheterization labs. Critical care transfer of these patients by air or ground is critical. There is data to support transfer to a center equipped with angioplasty facilities for patients with AMIs.[109] These data are often biased by the fact that patients who are transported are "sicker" (i.e., have large, anterior wall MIs) compared to the "average" MI patient. Further research comparing patients treated with fibrinolytic therapy versus patients transferred for emergency angioplasty in a timely fashion need to be assessed.

In the future perhaps the standard of care may be reperfusion at the community hospital with a combination of low-dose fibrinolytics and GP IIb/IIIa inhibitors and then transfer to a center with angioplasty facilities to evaluate the reperfusion status of the vessel. If flow in the vessel is not "normal" or TIMI III, angioplasty would be performed. This strategy, though not adopted at present, would place air medical transport personnel as a critical link in the acute care of the MI patient.

ARRHYTHMIAS

Serious electrical abnormalities of the heart rate and rhythm are classified as arrhythmias. They are described on ECGs as a deviation from the normal sinus rhythm in rate (too fast as in tachycardia or too slow as in bradycardia), regularity (one or more beats occurring earlier or later than expected), or a different pattern of activation of the cardiac muscle.[92] Arrhythmias can originate in any area of the heart. They are usually divided into arrhythmias starting in the atrium, those starting in the atrioventricular (AV) node, and those starting in the ventricle. Identification of the origin of the arrhythmia is based on the following:

1. The relation between the P wave and the QRS complex
2. The width and configuration of the P wave, which indicate how the atria are activated during the arrhythmia
3. The width and configuration of the QRS complex, which indicate how the ventricles are activated during the arrhythmia

Arrhythmias are caused by a variation in the state of discharge of the sinoatrial (SA) node, ectopic impulses that compete with the SA node, or abnormal conduction of impulses from the SA node through the heart. The origin of a normal heartbeat is in the sinus node. The sinus node is located laterally near the junction of the superior vena cava and right atrium. The sinus node is actually a "region"[8] made up of groups of pacemaker cells, which automatically depolarize. The blood flow to this region is variable.

Arrhythmias can be categorized as tachyarrhythmias, which include atrial tachycardia, supraventricular arrhythmias, and ventricular arrhythmias, and bradyarrhythmias, including symptomatic bradycardia and conduction disturbances known as AV (atrioventricular) blocks.

PATHOPHYSIOLOGIC FACTORS

The cells that conduct the electrical current through the heart are known as the *pacemaker* or *automatic* cells. The pacemaker of the heart, the SA node, is located at the junction of the superior vena cava and the right atrium. An electric impulse is initiated at this node, and it travels through the internodal pathways to the AV node. The AV node is located in the right atrium, directly above the tricuspid valve and anterior to the coronary sinus. The electrical impulse travels through the AV node, then moves through a common bundle of His, which divides almost immediately into the right and left bundles. The left bundle divides further to form two direct pathways to the anterior and posterior papillary muscle. The electrical impulse then permeates the many small fibers of the Purkinje network, beginning at the endocardium, and ending in the ventricular myocardium.[57]

Arrhythmias are the result of an irritable focus or foci in the electrical conduction system. There are several contributing mechanisms to the development of arrhythmias. The ischemic process and postnecrotic entities and underlying cardiac disease may enhance myocardial electrical instability. In addition, the development and treatment of myocardial failure result in mechanical dysfunction, metabolic changes, and electrolyte shifts, which contribute to rhythm disturbances. Invasive cardiac instrumentation or pharmacologic therapies also have the potential to provoke serious arrhythmias.

ASSESSMENT, DIAGNOSIS, AND TREATMENT

TACHYARRHYTHMIAS/TACHYCARDIAS

Atrial Tachycardia.   Atrial tachycardias possess a regular rhythm; the impulse formation is in the atrium but outside the sinus node. P waves precede the QRS but are usually obscured because of the rapid heart rate, although AV conduction may be present. The heart rates vary from 140 to 240 beats/min. The incidence of atrial tachycardia seems to increase with age. Current classifications of atrial tachycardia are based on the three mechanisms responsible for the tachycardia.[107]

a. Intra-atrial reentry—the characteristics of the reentrant circuit in atrial tachycardia are still not well understood. Many of these patients have other arrhythmias, specifically

atrial fibrillation, or flutter.[22] Common symptoms expressed are dyspnea, fatigue, and palpitation. Although symptomatic, there is usually no associated homodynamic compromise.[107] Catheter ablation is now the primary therapy for reentrant atrial tachycardia with a suggested success rate of greater than 75%.[22]

b. Ectopic automaticity—these are generated by a single or multiple atrial focus that clusters around the crista terminalis in the right atrium and around the base of the pulmonary veins in the left atrium. This has also been referred to as multiple atrial tachycardia (MAT). This is a descriptive entity that is characterized by an atrial rate of greater than 100 bpm with P wave morphology with varying AV intervals. It is easily confused with atrial fibrillation, and its mechanism is unknown. However, it is seen in patients with acute pulmonary disorders and accompanying hypoxia. Treatment is focused on treatment of the underlying cause. Patients with this mechanism are generally younger in age. Several studies have documented the automatic atrial tachycardia in children.[22,57,92] This tachycardia does not respond to vagal maneuvers and is not be terminated with atrial pacing. Treatment of precipitating causes is advisable. Also, amiodarone has been found to be useful.[79]

c. Triggered activity caused by delayed after depolarization (DADs)—This mechanism is the least common of the types observed. This mechanism appears to be due to DADs from digitalis toxicity. Catecholamines use can also precipitate this mechanism. Verapamil and adenosine have been shown to terminate this type of tachycardia.

Atrial Flutter.   Atrial flutter presents as a series of rapid regular flutter waves, usually described as sawtooth or resembling a picket fence, with a rate from 220 to 350 beats/min. Diagnosis is usually made in leads II, III, and AVF. Conduction through the AV node delays impulses, thus preventing rapid ventricular rates. The QRS complex during atrial flutter is usually the same as during sinus rhythm. Treatment modalities will be addressed in conjunction with fibrillation.

Atrial Fibrillation. Atrial fibrillation represents chaotic atrial activity, with the atrial rate ranging from 300 to 700 beats/min. Impulses are randomly conducted through the AV node to the ventricles, resulting in a typically irregular ventricular response that varies continuously in shape. Atrial fibrillation results in loss of effective atrial contraction, which reduces cardiac output and promotes mural thrombus development.

Treatment for patients with either atrial flutter or fibrillation is based on several clinical factors.

1. Is the patient clinically stable or unstable?
2. Is there impaired cardiac function associated with the flutter/fibrillation?
3. Is Wolff-Parkinson-White syndrome present?
4. Has the flutter or fibrillation been present for more or less than 48 hours?[40]

If the patient is unstable, the patient should be appropriately treated immediately. The objectives of treatment are to control the rate, convert the rhythm, and use anticoagulation when appropriate. There is increased emphasis on assessment of causes of the atrial fibrillation. Some underlying causes include hypoxemia, anemia, hypertension CHF, hypokalemia, and mitral regurgitation. IV verapamil,[78] beta-blockers[93] and diltiazem[91] can be administered to control the heart rate. Adenosine is not an effective agent for common forms of atrial arrhythmias such as atrial flutter or fibrillation.[16] The length of time the patient is in fibrillation or flutter is important because if in such a rhythm for more than 48 hours, there is a risk of systemic embolization on conversion to a sinus rhythm if the patient is not anticoagulated appropriately. If atrial fibrillation patients become unstable, cardioversion at 100 to 200 joules is recommended. If the patient is in atrial flutter, lower joules may be effective at 50 to 100 to convert the patient.

Supraventricular Arrhythmias. Supraventricular arrhythmias originate above the ventricle

and reflect atrial irritability. They can originate from the SA node, the AV node, the penetrating part of the bundle of His, or an accessory pathway.[28] These arrhythmias include premature atrial contractions, atrial tachycardia, atrial flutter, and atrial fibrillation.

Premature Atrial Contractions. Premature atrial contractions are an early atrial depolarization. They are predictors of impending supraventricular arrhythmias and do not require intervention.

Sinus Tachycardia. Sinus tachycardia originates in the sinus node and is characterized by a heart rate greater than 100 beats/min. It is a physiologic response to a demand for a higher cardiac output, and treatment is directed toward correcting the physiologic demand, as opposed to correcting the rapid heart rate. Causes can include infection, anemia, hypotension, and hyperthyroidism. IV or oral beta-blockers may be used when the tachycardia produces symptoms.

Ventricular Arrhythmias. Ventricular ectopic activity is a very common phenomenon in AMI, and ventricular arrhythmias are the major cause of sudden cardiac death in the United States. The most common cause of ventricular arrhythmia is ischemic coronary artery disease. Ventricular arrhythmias arise in the ventricles beyond the bifurcation of the bundle of His.[110]

Death from a ventricular arrhythmia occurs through its interference with the cardiac pumping function. Several conditions occurring during the ventricular arrhythmia contribute to the decrease in cardiac output, which in turn can cause syncope and lead to arrest. The loss of the normal atrioventricular sequence is associated with a significant decrease in cardiac output. The rate of the ventricular arrhythmia also determines hemodynamic instability. A rate below 150 bpm does not usually cause hemodynamic compromise if the duration is short. If the ventricular tachycardia exceeds 200 bpm, significant symptoms are usually present, which can include dyspnea, light-headedness, loss of vision, syncope, and cardiac arrest.[100] Patients demonstrating the presence of ventricular tach-yarrhythmias should be closely monitored because they have an increased risk of progressing to ventricular fibrillation, especially if the there is history of underlying cardiac disease. Refer to the American Heart Association's ACLS guidelines for specific algorithms to treat arrhythmias.

Premature Ventricular Complexes (PVCs) or Ventricular Premature Beats (VPBs).

Premature ventricular complexes or beats represent early ventricular depolarization that occurs before the next sinus beat. A wide, bizarre configuration represents abnormal impulse conduction. PVCs or VPBs are fairly benign and are usually left untreated. They may, however, escalate to ventricular tachycardia or fibrillation, requiring careful observation of patients exhibiting VPBs. Assessment of these patients should include any underlying history of cardiac disease.

Paroxysmal Supraventricular Tachycardia (PSVT).

This is a regular tachycardia exceeding the expected limits of sinus tachycardia at rest (>120 bpm) with or without discernible P waves. It usually has an abrupt onset and termination. It is supraventricular in origin and can be differentiated from atrial or junctional tachycardias by its abrupt onset and termination that the patient describes during assessment.[92] Current recommendations include the use of vagal maneuvers to terminate the PSVT. Adenosine IV is also still recommended, although one should be aware of some of the differing effects of adenosine in patients with asthma being treated with theophylline, in patients prone to bronchospasm caused by reactive airway disease, or in patients with preexisting cardiac disease. If the left ventricular (LV) function is preserved, additional options are amiodarone, calcium channel blockers, or digitalis. Recent evidence suggests, however, that digitalis has a slower onset of action and lower potency relative to other medications recommended. If there is evidence of cardiac compromise (ejection fraction of <40), amiodarone is the drug of choice because of the research evidence provided balancing its effectiveness and side effects. Electric cardioversion should not be used in patients with PSVT that have impaired cardiac function.

Ventricular Tachycardia (VT).

Ventricular tachycardia is three or more premature ventricular beats (PVCs) at an accelerated rate, usually greater than 100 beats/min. The rhythm may be well tolerated or associated with hemodynamic compromise. Current emphasis related to treatment modalities is still placed on whether the patient is deemed stable or nonstable. In assessment of the patient in ventricular tachycardia, instability is determined by symptoms displayed by the patient such as chest pain, hypotension, decreased level of consciousness, shock, shortness of breath, or pulmonary congestion that can be attributed to the rapid heart rate, usually greater than 150 bpm. If the patient is pulseless, immediate defibrillation should be instituted. If the patient is determined to be unstable, immediate synchronized electrical cardioversion is indicated at 100 to 200 joules. If the patient is conscious and stable, assessing what type of VT the patient is experiencing is important for treatment decisions. With monomorphic VT, one needs to know if there is impaired cardiac function. Medications recommended for use are procainamide, sotalol, amiodarone, or lidocaine. When polymorphic VT is diagnosed, the QT baseline interval must be assessed. If the QT baseline interval is prolonged, suggesting torsades de pointe, medications used are magnesium, isoproterenol, phenytoin, or lidocaine with overdrive pacing. This type of VT is seen most often in drug overdose patients. If the polymorphic VT has a normal baseline QT interval, the object is to treat the ischemia and to correct electrolytes. Medications recommended for use are beta-blockers, amiodarone, procainamide, sotalol, or lidocaine.

It is important to remember that the AHA now recommends use of a single medication modality. Research has shown that antiarrhythmics have a significant potential to also be proarrhythmic when used in combination with other antiarrhythmics. Consequently the International Guidelines 2000 recommend only one antiarrhythmic per patient. This should lead to far fewer events in which more than 1 antiarrhythmic causes significant worsening of the patient's condition and a much lower threshold to cardiovert patients nonurgently.[40]

Ventricular Fibrillation (VF). Ventricular fibrillation is chaotic depolarization from multiple areas of the ventricle; no effective contraction occurs resulting in severe hemodynamic compromise. VF is the most common mechanism of cardiac arrest from myocardial ischemia or infarction and leads to sudden death if it is not converted to a more normal rhythm. The best treatment for VF is early defibrillation. Three shocks should be administered, then CPR should be initiated to assist blood flow to the heart and brain. Pharmacologic therapy initiated can include epinephrine 1 mg IV push every 3 to 5 minutes or vasopressin 40 U IV as a one-time single dose. Vasopressin is a natural-substance antidiuretic hormone that becomes a powerful vasoconstrictor when administered at much higher doses than found in the body. It has all the positive effects of epinephrine without the negative effects. Remember, AHA recommendations state that all antiarrhythmics can also behave as proarrhythmics that could generate VF/VT arrest.

Accelerated Idioventricular Rhythm (AIVR). Accelerated idioventricular rhythm is defined as a ventricular rhythm with a rate of 60 to 110 beats/min. Most episodes are of short duration and will terminate abruptly, slow gradually before stopping, or be overdriven by the basic cardiac rhythm. This rhythm is usually not treated but must be observed closely because of its propensity to degenerate into ventricular tachycardia or fibrillation.

BRADYARRHYTHMIAS

Bradycardia. Absolute bradycardia is defined as a heart rate less than 60 beats/min. It is a result of slowing of impulse formation by the sinus node and is most often associated with an inferior or posterior wall MI. It may also result from ischemic effects on the sinus node. The current treatment of choice for symptomatic bradycardia is transcutaneous pacing. This can be accomplished by the application of an external pacemaker (which is preferable in the patient being considered for or receiving thrombolytic therapy). However, transcutaneous pacing is not as readily available as atropine (0.5 to 1.0 mg IV every 3 to 5 minutes to a total dose of 0.03 mg/kg for mildly symptomatic patients). For severe bradycardia a maximum of 0.04 mg/kg is advisable.[40] Atropine enhances sinus node automaticity and AV conduction. Symptomatic bradycardic patients are those exhibiting signs of CHF, hypotension, or refractory ventricular ectopic activity. Dopamine at 2 to 5 µg/kg per minute can be given if there is accompanying hypotension. An epinephrine infusion of 2 to 10 µg/min can be considered if pacing and atropine have failed.[40] The use of lidocaine can be lethal to a bradycardic patient when the bradycardia is a ventricular escape rhythm.

External Pacing. An external pacemaker or noninvasive temporary pacemaker (NTP) provides immediate pacing in an emergency without the risk of complications related to an invasive procedure. Pacing is accomplished by using large electrodes that are placed over the precordium and on the posterior left side of the chest beneath the scapula. Standard electrodes provide the ECG tracing and allow demand-mode operation. The NTP will operate asynchronously if the sensing electrodes are not in place.

Temporary Pacing. Temporary pacing is most commonly used for short-term management of symptomatic bradycardias, either as a bridge to permanent pacing or for self-limited bradycardias.[43] Although the cause and reversibility of the bradyarrhythmia may not be known, prompt institution of external pacing may be crucial to maintain hemodynamic stability. During transport an external pacemaker may be used until a transvenous pacemaker can be inserted. External pacing is performed according to ACLS protocols. Ventricular pacing is used in most clinical situations, although atrial or AV sequential pacing may be indicated. The catheters are inserted using aseptic technique, and the position of the electrode is validated by fluoroscopy.

Some of the complications encountered with temporary cardiac pacing that may occur during air medical transport include sensing problems, failure to capture, myocardial penetration, and cardiac tamponade. Undersensing or "failure to sense" may be caused by malposition of the catheter, poor intracardiac signal quality, or generator malfunction. Undersensing is managed by turning the sensitivity setting of the pulse generator to full-demand position.[38] Oversensing, which results in pauses in paced rhythm, can result from sensing of atrial electrical activity if the pacing lead is positioned near the tricuspid valve, from sensing of T waves, or from sensing voltage transients that are the result of lead wire fracture, environmental influences, or signals from the generator. The problem of oversensing can be resolved by turning the sensitivity setting toward the asynchronous position until the unwanted signals are no longer sensed.[38]

Failure to capture can be related to malposition of the lead or to an increase in the myocardial stimulation threshold. To resolve this, the current output should be increased until consistent capture occurs. If the underlying problem is electrolyte imbalance, that should be corrected. The position of the lead should be checked and repositioned if necessary.

Myocardial penetration or perforation into the pericardial space is usually accompanied by a pericardial friction rub and often by a squeaking systolic sound or murmur. If the pacing has migrated, it should be repositioned. If cardiac tamponade occurs in association with perforation, immediate pericardiocentesis should be performed.

First-Degree AV Block.   First-degree AV block is characterized by prolongation of the PR interval beyond 0.20 seconds in adults and more than 0.18 seconds in children. A QRS complex with a constant, prolonged interval follows each P wave. The usual range for the prolonged PR interval is 0.21 to 0.40, but the interval may extend to as long as 0.80. In this form of AV block, each atrial impulse is conducted to the ventricles. First-degree AV block has been associated with congenital structural heart disease such as endocardial cushion defects. It is rarely treated, but the cause should be determined and corrected.

Second-Degree AV Block.   Mobitz type I (Wenckebach AV block) is characterized by the progressive lengthening of the PR intervals until a single P wave is not followed by a QRS. The RR intervals become progressively shorter until the P wave is blocked, and there is a shortening of the PR interval postblock compared to the PR interval just preceding the blocked cycle. This type of arrhythmia has little clinical significance and is not treated.

Mobitz type II is recognized when the P waves are periodically blocked from conduction to the ventricles without a progressive prolongation of the PR interval or a progressive shortening of the RR interval. In this type of block, the PR interval of all conducted beats is constant, and the P-P intervals remain constant. Mobitz II is usually associated with bundle branch block or bifascicular block. Because Mobitz type II is usually a precursor of complete AV block and is generally irreversible, a permanent pacemaker is usually required. Atropine is not indicated in type II blocks and third-degree blocks with widened QRS complexes.[40]

Third-Degree AV Block or Complete Heart Block.   This potentially lethal conduction abnormality is characterized by separate and independent atrial and ventricular activity. Either sinus or ectopic atrial pacemakers control the atria, and a pacemaker that is distal to the AV block controls the ventricles. The ECG shows completely dissociated P waves and QRS complexes. The heart rate can go as low as 20 to 40 beats/min with this type of block. Treatment almost always involves the use of an transcutaneous or external pacemaker or transvenous pacemaker, if available. Pharmacologic therapy with single agents includes atropine at 0.5 to 1.0 mg or dopamine at 5 to 20 µg/kg per minute. If atropine and pacing fail, epinephrine at 2 to 10 µg/min can be administered.

CARDIOGENIC SHOCK

Cardiogenic shock is defined as a decrease in cardiac output resulting in a critical reduction in tissue perfusion, as evidenced by tissue hypoxia in the presence of adequate intravascular volume.[46,90]

Cardiogenic shock is one of the most severe complications of AMI and is usually the result of extensive ischemic damage to more than 40% of the LV myocardium. Seven percent to 10% of patients with AMI will develop cardiogenic shock with a mortality rate in medically treated patients between 50% and 70%. Although left ventricular failure is the most common cause of cardiogenic shock (78.5%), other common causes are due to mechanical complications, including severe mitral regurgitation (6.9%), ventricular septal rupture (3.9%), isolated right ventricular shock (2.8%), and cardiac tamponade (1.4%). Myocarditis, end-stage cardiomyopathy, myocardial contusion, and septic shock with severe myocardial depression can also deteriorate into cardiogenic shock.[40,42,46,48,90] During the past two decades, the primary goal of therapy for the AMI patient has been to manage or prevent pump failure. Because the amount of ventricular failure is directly related to the extent of infarction, therapies aimed at limiting MI size and early revascularization are imperative in reducing the incidence and extent of pump failure. Prevention of the development of cardiogenic shock by early identification of the preshock state is the primary objective. Treatment should include relief or control of ischemia, prevention of arrhythmias, inotropic hemodynamic support, and administration of glucose-insulin-potassium infusions to support viable myocardial function. Thrombolysis and primary angioplasty have shown to significantly reduce the incidence of cardiogenic shock.[21,90,108] Early intervention reduces the incidence of cardiogenic shock. Initiation of therapy for AMI following the AHA guidelines as soon as possible on presentation becomes very important in the cycle of prevention of pump failure. However, the most extreme form of pump failure after an AMI remains cardiogenic shock.

PATHOPHYSIOLOGIC FACTORS

Inadequate cardiac pumping present in cardiogenic shock results in a decreased cardiac output, hypotension, and inadequate tissue perfusion. Both systolic and diastolic myocardial dysfunction are characteristics of cardiogenic shock. Decreased compliance from ischemia will result in hemodynamic changes that include a decrease in stroke volume (SV), resulting in elevations in left ventricular end-diastolic pressure, left atrial pressure, and pulmonary capillary wedge pressure (PCWP). The concomitant hypotension causes a decrease in coronary artery perfusion, further contributing to myocardial depression. Elevation of left ventricular pressures can result in pulmonary edema and hypoxemia. Clinical cardiogenic shock constitutes the combination of hypotension and pulmonary edema. These changes eventually lead to complete circulatory failure.[46]

ASSESSMENT AND DIAGNOSIS

Patients in cardiogenic shock appear acutely ill and present in acute distress. Physical examination often reveals profound hypotension, signs of peripheral hypoperfusion, hypoxemia, acidosis, rales, and oliguria. They often have an ashen or cyanotic appearance, and their skin is cool and clammy with mottled extremities. Most patients have a depressed sensorium as a result of hypoxemia. Pulses may be irregular if arrhythmias are present and peripheral pulses are faint and rapid. Jugular venous distention is usually present.

Hemodynamically, patients in cardiogenic shock manifest marked hypotension with SBP ≤80 to 85 mm Hg, low cardiac index ≤2.2 L/min/m², decreased urinary output (UO), elevated heart rates, and a pulmonary artery wedge pressure (PAWP) greater than 18 to 20 mm Hg. They also exhibit pulmonary congestion and arterial hypoxemia. Arrhythmias may occur as a result of hypoxemia, with a chest x-ray revealing pulmonary vascular congestion. However, the SHOCK Trial Registry did indicate that 28% of the patients presented only with hypoperfusion and no congestion, whereas 64% of patients presented with the classic symptoms of congestion and hypoperfusion. Mortality rate for both groups were near the same (70% and 60%, respectively).[3]

MANAGEMENT

Specific issues to be addressed include correction of hypoxemia, correction of electrolyte levels and acid/base balance, maximization of volume status, treatment of sustained arrhythmias, inotropic/vasopressor support, early revascularization, and consideration of IABP/VAD support. Oxygenation and airway support are imperative, and correction of hypoxemia may include intubation and mechanical ventilation. Most patients will require intubation with positive-end expiratory pressure (PEEP) if pulmonary congestion is severe. Electrolyte imbalances, such as hypokalemia and hypomagnesemia, create vulnerability to ventricular arrhythmias, whereas acidosis decreases contractility. Maximization of volume status requires fluid resuscitation unless pulmonary edema is present. PAWP should be maintained at 18 to 20 mm Hg. Intake and output should be monitored carefully. Thirty percent of patients with inferior infarction will develop right ventricular infarction. The maintenance of right ventricular preload, with the administration of fluids, is the initial therapy for support of right ventricular infarction. Careful assessment of PCWP and cardiac output is essential. Antiarrhythmic drugs, cardioversion, and pacing should be used promptly as required to correct any arrhythmias or heart blocks that would affect cardiac output. Inotropic agents and vasopressors should be initiated for cardiovascular support in the presence of inadequate tissue perfusion with adequate intravascular volume. Nitrates, beta-blockers, and ACE inhibitors, normally used to improve outcomes after AMI, can worsen hypotension and should be avoided in true cardiac shock. Although thrombolytic therapy has shown to reduce mortality rates in patients with AMI, no significant improvement in outcomes has been demonstrated with established cardiogenic shock. However, even the possibility of saving a small number of lives advocates its use as a potential benefit in a certain high-risk group where both hypotension and tachycardia are present.[90] Aggressive use of vasopressors or IABP has been recommended to enhance the effect of thrombolysis.[90] Revascularization with percutaneous coronary angioplasty (PTCA) or coronary bypass surgery in 24 hours has been shown to significantly decrease mortality rates in the GUSTO–1 trials.[46] Other studies have shown that the placement of coronary stents provides better angiographic results and improves outcomes. Although

CABG surgery demonstrates favorable outcomes as well, the highly beneficial results of PTCA and the higher rates of surgical mortality and morbidity with CABG makes the use of PTCA preferrable.[46] Mechanical circulatory support, IABP, and VADs may be required to stabilize patients until they undergo coronary angioplasty and can be used as a bridge to surgical revascularization or heart transplantation. Early revascularization does significantly improve the outcome of patients in shock resulting from MI. Patients in cardiogenic shock require frequent assessment of hemodynamic parameters including blood pressure (BP), heart rate, and pulmonary artery pressures (if a Swan-Ganz line is present). These patients should be kept in a supine position to improve cerebral blood flow and blood flow to the heart. They should be frequently assessed for peripheral perfusion, presence of edema, color and warmth of skin, blood gases, hemoglobin, and hematocrit to assess oxygen-carrying capacity and function.

PHARMACOLOGIC THERAPY

Pharmacologic management includes the use of inotropic and vasopressor agents such as dopamine and dobutamine to improve cardiac output by increasing contractility. Dobutamine is the initial drug of choice when systolic pressure is greater than 80 mm Hg and is effective without a striking change in heart rate or systemic vascular resistance. Dobutamine can aggravate hypotension and precipitate tachyarrhythmias in some patients. Dopamine has both inotropic and vasopressor effects and is used when the systolic pressures are less than 80 mm Hg. Dopamine can result in tachycardia and an increase in peripheral vascular resistance, exacerbating myocardial ischemia. Dopamine and dobutamine when used in combination may be more effective than when used alone in some patients. When dopamine and dobutamine are ineffective, norepinephrine, a catecholamine with potent alpha- and beta-adrenergic effects, can be administered to improve coronary perfusion and to improve blood pressure. Norepinephrine should be carefully titrated because the combined increase in preload and afterload can threaten myocardial oxygen supply

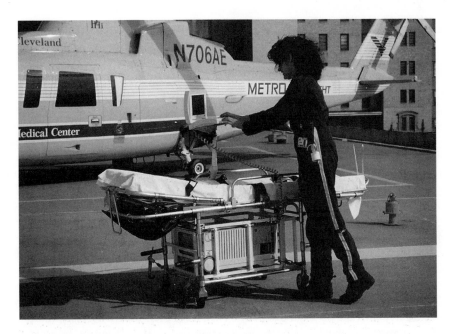

FIGURE 21-6   **Balloon pump from Cleveland Metro Life Flight.** (Courtesy of Metro Life Flight, Cleveland, Ohio.)

and demand, increasing the risk of ischemia and arrhythmia. It can also be used in conjunction with dopamine and dobutamine to allow for lower dosing. Vasodilators should be used with extreme caution because they can cause further hypotension and decrease in coronary blood flow. Vasodilators are used to increase forward flow by reducing afterload; these drugs include nitroprusside and NTG. Sodium nitroprusside reduces afterload by decreasing filling pressures and can also increase stroke volume. NTG reduces PCWP and left ventricular filling pressure and redistributes coronary blood flow to the ischemic area. Diuretic therapy is limited to treating pulmonary congestion and decreasing intravascular volume, thereby improving oxygenation.[32,46]

INTRAAORTIC BALLOON COUNTERPULSATION (IABC)

When pharmacologic support and adjunctive therapies fail to improve low cardiac output and poor perfusion associated with cardiogenic shock, alternative devices are often used, such as the IABP and VADs. IABPs have been used to treat cardiogenic

shock for decades. Results of the recent SHOCK Trial concluded with recommendations that emergency revascularization in conjunction with intraaortic balloon counterpulsation should be used in patients with AMI complicated by cardiogenic shock. Aggressive use of IABP has also been recommended to enhance the effect of thrombolysis. Stabilization with IABP and thrombolysis, followed by transfer to a tertiary care facility, is the treatment option for those facilities without direct angioplasty capability.[46] Air transport of the IABP patient has been done successfully for the past 15 years (Figure 21-6). Current IABP devices such as the Datascope 97 and 98 have been specifically developed for transport. The machine can sense changes in balloon volume caused by the effect of altitude, reduced barometric pressure, and gas expansion and will automatically adjust to these changes. These new balloon pump consoles are Federal Aviation Administration (FAA) approved. They are designed to withstand vibration and shock effects and are shielded from electromagnetic and radio frequency interference (EMI, RFI). This has eliminated previous concerns over IABP transports and the need to purge the pump to avoid over expansion of the balloon.

The counterpulsation action of the IABP decreases the afterload stress of the left ventricle, augments diastolic perfusion pressure, and improves coronary blood flow without increasing oxygen demand. By increasing coronary perfusion it can potentially reduce the risk of ventricular irritability and ventricular arrhythmias.[3,27,31,46] Balloon-pump counterpulsation can augment the cardiac output by as much as 10% to 20%.[85] It accomplishes this by raising the intra-aortic pressure during diastole (diastolic augmentation) and lowering intra-aortic pressure during systole. The insertion procedure involves placing a distensible, nonthrombogenic balloon into the femoral artery percutaneously and advancing it until the balloon lies in the thoracic aorta with the tip 2 cm distal to the aortic arch, just distal to the left subclavian artery and above the renal artery.[83] The balloon is then inflated and deflated in synchrony with the cardiac cycle. During diastole, when the balloon is inflated, blood is displaced both proximally and distally. Proximal displacement enhances coronary artery perfusion and cerebral perfusion; distal displacement improves systemic perfusion. The primary effect of the IABP is to increase myocardial oxygen supply and decrease myocardial oxygen demand while increasing cardiac output and systemic perfusion, resulting in the reduction of left ventricular workload.[54]

Limb ischemia is consistently the most common problem associated with IABP placement and can account for 87% of all complications. Early recognition and aggressive treatment can result in salvage of most of these limbs. Initial treatment will include removal of the balloon pump. Thromboembolectomy or emergency revascularization may by required. Other complications associated with the use of the IABP include emboli, thrombosis, femoral stenosis, thrombocytopenia, infection, visceral and spinal cord ischemia, rupture of the aorta or false aneurysm formation, rupture of the balloon, impaired circulation, bleeding, and inability to wean.[27] Because the IABP is dependent on partial intrinsic ventricular function,

patients who have extremely limited or no intrinsic ventricular function may require more aggressive therapy with a VAD.

VENTRICULAR ASSIST DEVICES

For that 3% to 7% of patients who present with AMI that develops to cardiogenic shock, the prognosis is very poor. Several circulatory assist devices are now available. Indications for these devices include post-cardiotomy ventricular failure, myocarditis, cardiomyopathy idiopathic hypertrophic subaortic stenosis, cardiac transplant rejection, or as a bridge to transplant. The use of a VAD in general is indicated when maximal conventional therapy has failed and profound cardiogenic shock develops.[75] Approximately 60,000 people develop class IV failure or end-stage heart failure annually. Class IV failure is demonstrated when the cardiac myocytes lose all or most of their function. Heart transplant is currently considered the definitive treatment for end-stage heart failure. The number of patients waiting for transplants far exceeds the number of suitable organs available (approximately 2500 hearts are available for transplant each year with approximately 60,000 patients in need), necessitating prevention of end-organ deterioration with the use of mechanical cardiac assist devices.[98] The general principle behind the use of VADs is based on the "stunned myocardium" theory. Severe myocardial ischemia may produce stunned myocardium that is reversible. The myocardium that has minimal or no intrinsic function may be able to regain function if allowed to recover. A VAD allows the myocardium to rest by diverting blood from the natural ventricle to an artificial pump that maintains the circulation.[65] The VAD is a mechanical pumping device that provides support to either the right, left, or both ventricles, with the ultimate goal of improving end-organ blood flow and restoring near normal hemodynamics.[85] Several types of assist devices are available, including VADs that are surgically implanted and those that are inserted percutaneously.

VADs that can be inserted percutaneously have several advantages. They can be inserted quickly and do not require surgical opening of the chest and can even be done at the bedside. This would apply to patients in cardiac arrest to achieve immediate resuscitation that would then be followed by VAD implantation. It provides both cardiac and pulmonary support and allows time to evaluate potential transplant candidates. Insertion involves a simple cutdown procedure of the femoral artery through which a cannula is inserted. Bypass can then be initiated without mobilization of the surgical team.[74]

Extracorporeal membrane oxygenation (ECMO) has been around for some time and is often used to provide emergency circulatory support for patients in cardiogenic shock or respiratory failure.[74] It uses a membrane oxygenator system connected to a heat exchanger and a roller pump system. Venovenous or venoarterial cannulation is used for blood outflow and inflow. Adult ECMO is only indicated in a select group of patients with severe respiratory or cardiac compromise that has not improved with conventional therapy. It is most commonly used with respiratory failure caused by adult respiratory distress syndrome (ARDS), pneumonia, severe asthma, cardiac failure, or trauma. These patients have generally exhausted vigorous respiratory care and are acutely ill with a mortality risk as high as 90%. ECMO is also used for a certain set of patients who are considered high-risk candidates for VAD placement but may benefit from support prior to VAD implantation. This allows for a more adequate evaluation to determine transplant as an option and should improve VAD and posttransplant outcomes and optimize patient survival.[74] There are two major concerns with the use of ECMO. One is that inadequate ventricular decompression may occur and result in pulmonary hypertension, edema, and hemorrhage. A second concern is the limited time that support can be provided on ECMO. Long-term support is associated with poor outcomes. However the use of VADs for long-term bridging to transplant has mostly negated this second concern.

There are several different types of surgically implanted VADs. These include (1) roller pumps that propel blood forward by compressing the blood at a manually set point, creating a nonpulsatile flow; (2) centrifugal devices that circulate high volumes of blood under relatively low pressure; and (3)

pneumatic devices that provide pulsatile flow by using jets of compressed air to drive or eject blood.

A commonly used centrifugal pump is the Biomedicus pump. Because this is a nonpulsatile flow system, patients must be anticoagulated carefully. This is used for very short-term support. Pulsatile VADs such as the BVS systems have shown a survival rate of 43% compared to only a 6% survival rate with centrifugal pumps.[44,53]

The first clinical application of the biventricular support (BVS) system was performed in 1991. Since then the device—BVS 5000 and 5000i—has been approved by the Food and Drug Administration (FDA) for insertion under any cardiac condition where there is a possible chance of myocardial recovery.[89] These conditions include postcardiotomy shock, right ventricular failure after initiation of left ventricular assist device (LVAD) support, failed heart transplant, and any cause of ventricular failure that is reversible.[25] Selection criteria for initiation of BVS support as presented by the Physician Advisory Council includes: technically successful operation, body surface area (BSA) >1.3 m^2, PCWP/LAP >18, CVP >18, C.I. <2.0, SVO$_2$ $<55\%$ (with a corrected hematocrit of 30%), and age <75 years. This criteria must be present despite inotropic and IABP support. Best outcomes have been reported (1) when BVS is initiated after 30 to 45 minutes of treatment with pharmacologic and IABP (optional) support, and the patient remains hemodynamically marginal, (2) when time between first attempt to wean from cardiopulmonary bypass (CPB) is <6 hours, (3) when implant occurs as part of the initial operation, (4) when the amount of support—univentricular versus biventricular—is assessed and initiated appropriately, and (5) when bleeding is controlled in the operating room. Early insertion has demonstrated survival rates between 40% to 50%.[1,53] The BVS 5000 and 5000i are most often used for short-term mechanical support in situations where myocardial recovery is expected (bridge to recovery), or it can be used as bridge to transplant. Although the BVS system is for use with short-term support, patients have been supported for as long as 90 days.[53,89] This device is a pneumatically driven, external pulsatile pump. It requires a sternotomy to achieve vascular access via transthoracic atrial and arterial cannulation. Left atrial cannulation (inflow site) is inserted into the atrium at either the interatrial groove (most frequently used site), the atrial dome, or the left atrial appendage, or it can be inserted in the left ventricular apex when it is undesirable to cannulate the left atrium. The right atrial inflow cannulation site most commonly used is the right atrial midfree wall, but the right atrial appendage is also used. Arterial site (outflow) for right cannulation is the main pulmonary artery, and for left cannulation, it is the ascending aorta. The chest may be left open to allow easier access for control of hemostasis, or it may be closed to promote hemostasis and to decrease the risk of infection.[1,2,53,89] The atrium of the pump fills by gravity, and diastole ensues when pressure from the full atrial bladder opens the AV valve, filling the ventricular bladder. Air is displaced through the driveline to the console as the ventricular bladder is filling. Once the ventricular bladder is full with 80 ml of blood, compressed air is sent back to the pumping chamber, collapsing the ventricular bladder and closing the AV valve. The outflow valve will open, and the ventricular bladder will eject its volume.[2,42,4] The BVS 5000 can provide flows to approximately 5.0 L/min, and the BVS 5000i can provide flows to approximately 6.0 L/min. The console automatically adjusts systole and diastole, beat rate, and flow of each blood pump according to the patient's preload and afterload. This self-adjustment will maintain a stroke volume of 80 ml.[2,64] Biventricular support should be considered when there is a history of RCA disease or right ventricular (RV)/septal infarct, surgery including the right heart, or impaired RV function is observed after initiation of LVAD support. Biventricular support will more completely rest the heart, and it reduces the need for inotropic support. Bleeding is a major complication of VADs and is the major contributor to death postoperatively. Other complications associated with all of the VADs are thromboembolism, hemolysis, mechanical failure, and infection.[2,53,61]

When long-term cardiac support is required as a bridge to transplant, determined by the ability to wean from temporary VAD support and potential for recovery, several implantable left VADs can be used. Novacor and HeartMate are the two primary systems manufactured, and both basically have the same components. These electrical devices with a battery power source allow increased mobility by the patient. It allows them to ambulate, exercise, and frequently to leave the hospital to assume limited activities of daily living. These portable LVADs consist of blood pumps that are implanted in a pocket fashion in the left upper quadrant of the peritoneal cavity. Inflow graft is anastomosed to the left ventricle and outflow graft to the ascending aorta. The blood pump fills passively and in the automatic mode and actively forces blood into the aorta when it is approximately 90% full. Patients who undergo implantable LVAD placement must meet certain criteria as set by FDA guidelines. This criteria includes that the patient (1) must be a transplant candidate; (2) must demonstrate reversible end-stage organ disease; (3) must have body surface area large enough to contain device; (4) meets New York Heart Association Class IV heart failure criteria; (5) has hemodynamic deterioration criteria: cardiac index <2.0 and either mean arterial pressure (MAP) ≤65 or PCWP/PAD (pulmonary artery diastolic) ≥18 or life-threatening arrhythmias nonresponsive to medical treatment; or the patient needs support of two positive inotropes or has an IABP placed; and (6) demonstrates the ability to manage the device or has a support person at all times. New findings indicate mechanical support may assist with cardiac remodeling and actually lead to recovery of the heart in some cases over variable lengths of time. Bleeding and hemorrhage are the major complications associated with LVAD placement.[17,44,64]

Transport of Patients With an IABP or VAD.
Management of the patient in severe cardiogenic shock is challenging and complex. The challenge is further intensified when the patient requires transport to definitive care. The cost and complexity of specialized equipment, the space required for additional staff and equipment, and the need for highly trained personnel all suggest that the air medical transport of patients requiring IABP or LVAD intervention be undertaken only by teams proficient in

the use of these therapies in the air medical environment. The transport vehicle, rotor wing, fixed wing, or ground, must be capable of meeting the requirements for these specialty transports.

The balloon pump has been used for patient transport now for two decades but has limited capabilities in supporting patients in severe cardiogenic shock. During this time, there have been major advances in developing mechanical assist devices that are able to effectively support circulation short term and long term as a bridge to recovery or bridge to transplant. This allows patients to be transferred from smaller cardiovascular surgery facilities and nontransplant centers. Patients have been transported on centrifugal pumps, ECMO, and the ABIOMed BVS systems. These systems are very simple to operate, require minimal operator intervention, and do not require a perfusionist for management of the device. Although the BVS 5000 and 5000i have not been specifically tested for use in

transport, successful air transport has been accomplished. For VAD transports, the vehicle must be able to accommodate the size and weight of the equipment and must be able to accommodate the power requirements of the console (minimum average power consumption of 280 watts) and other medical equipment needed. There must be means to adequately secure the console during transport. The BVS consoles only have 1 hour of battery life, and it will be necessary to use the transport vehicle's electrical system. Time management is imperative during transfer from referring/receiving intensive care units (ICUs) and transport vehicles. Because the BVS system requires that the top of the blood pump chambers be maintained at 4 to 14 inches below the patient's atrium, the helicopter must have enough clearance to maintain the stretcher in an elevated position (Figure 21-7). The blood pump chambers are 22 inches long, and with the 4- to 14-inch height requirement, the patient needs to be elevated at least

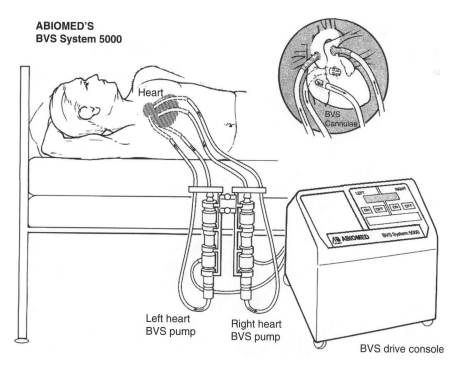

FIGURE 21-7 Schematic drawing of the BVS System 5000 depicting cannula placement and correct height of blood pump chambers from heart. (Courtesy of ABIOMED, Inc., Danvers, MA.)

34 inches from the floor. The helicopter should also allow full access to the patient and have enough room to fully visualize the chest tubes and blood pumps, allow access to the manual foot pump for emergency use, allow enough room to prevent kinking of the driveline, and accommodate the weight of the console and three medical crew members for transport. Organizing a smooth transition from the critical care area to the transport environment requires a team effort to ensure that the hemodynamic stability of the patient is not interrupted. This can be accomplished by organizing the transport team and efficiently using space aboard the aircraft to accommodate equipment and allow the crew to adequately visualize the patient, monitors, and vasoactive medications (Figure 21-8).[67,52,56,89]

Fixed-wing considerations include the size of the aircraft and that it must be medically configured with a pressurized cabin. The BVS 5000 and 5000i console will not fit into the Lear 25, a commonly used aircraft for medical transport, because it will block the egress area. The Lear 35 or King Air will probably be able to accommodate the console, although it may also partially block the egress area in the Lear 35. Loading can be difficult, specifically in the King Air, because of height from ground to door.

In 2001, the BVS 5000t, designed specifically for the transport environment, was approved by the FDA for ground and air patient transport. It provides perfusion equivalent to the BVS 5000i. Because the console is smaller and lighter, it requires less space and can adapt more easily to transport vehicle constraints. The pumps still need to be held 4 to 14 inches below the level of the atrium to accommodate gravity flow. Because it is also vacuum driven, the pumps can be positioned horizontally instead of vertically. This permits less need for cabin height for transport than was previously required with the other BVS 5000 systems, allowing transfer in a wider variety of aircraft. The 5000t transport system does not have flow rates displayed.

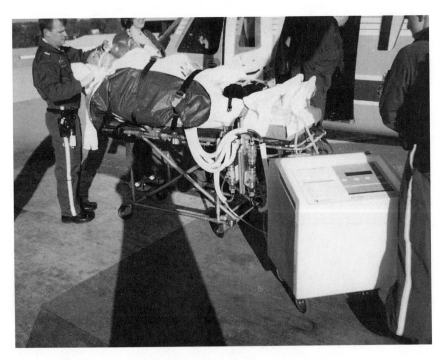

FIGURE 21-8 **Patient on BiVAD getting ready to be loaded into the helicopter.** (Courtesy of Metro Life Flight, Cleveland, Ohio.)

This requires training to focus on clinical presentation and bladder filling and emptying assessments. The first air medical transport with this device, since obtaining FDA approval, was completed by Cleveland Metro Life Flight in November 2000. There were no mechanical- or device-related complications associated with this transfer.[60]

For all VAD transports, thermoregulation requires serious consideration because the patient will have 600 ml of extracorporeal blood going through the tubing and circuit at any time. Transfer to and from the transport vehicles will require insulation around the tubing to assist with maintaining a normothermic state. The aircraft cabin will need to be maintained at temperatures to ensure a warm environment. Blood products and backup equipment for emergency contingencies for any device used should be available during transport.[56,67]

The critical care transport team should have a diverse background in critical care and be well educated on the operation of the VAD and IABP pumps. It is highly recommended that three medical crew members accompany these specialty transports to accommodate the patient and equipment needs and the logistics of movement. The highest possible level of caregivers should be used for transport, with a minimum of two critical care–trained nurses. It is also imperative that adequate oxygen and electrical power are available during all facets of the transport process. To avoid catastrophic inadvertent disconnection of the devices during transport, all equipment must be well secured, and the patient may require sedation.

An additional special consideration is the effect of the hypobaric environment during flight. Fixed-wing aircraft must accelerate to become airborne and will subject the patient to the effects of g-forces. Acceleration during takeoff with the patient positioned head toward the front of the aircraft will result in a decreased preload. When the patient is reversed with head toward the tail, an increase in preload will result. Compensation can be accomplished by loading the patient in the best position to meet cardiovascular needs. Other compensatory actions may be required, such as judicious use of vasoactive drugs and/or adequate intravascular volume prior to takeoff to augment pump capabilities. As discussed, the current IABP models can adjust to balloon volume changes because of the effects of high altitude and acceleration. Pneumatically driven devices such as the BVS 5000 systems show little interference from barometric changes. The effects of high-frequency vibration in fixed-wing aircraft can lead to loose connections in any type of biomedical equipment. Extra caution must be taken to ensure that connections that could work themselves loose are secured.[60,83]

CONGESTIVE HEART FAILURE

DEFINITION AND PATHOPHYSIOLOGIC FACTORS

Heart failure can be difficult to define, but generally it is recognized in the clinical setting. It is a complex clinical syndrome that can be brought on by any form of heart disease, resulting in ventricular failure that prevents adequate blood flow to meet tissue metabolic needs.[42,58] Heart failure has previously been defined as a circulatory disorder secondary to left ventricular dysfunction. Recently, clinicians have recognized the need for a more encompassing definition of heart failure. Specifically, this definition highlights the process of left ventricular (LV) remodeling, the cellular events linked to the remodeling process, such as myocyte hypertrophy, interstitial fibrosis, myocyte dropout, and changes in the genetic expression of specific cardiac cell and subcellular proteins. It is also important to stress that heart failure should not be defined solely on the presence or absence of congestion, but should include a broad spectrum of characteristics such as acute or chronic, right-sided or left-sided failure, systolic or diastolic, and with or without compromised organ perfusion. The hallmark of acute heart failure is demonstrated by a decreased LV function that develops rapidly canceling out the compensatory effect of the sympathetic nervous system. This is can be a result of exacerbation of a chronic condition or as an initial manifestation. When the ventricles cannot adequately deliver their preload, volume will back up in the left ventricle, then the left atrium, and inevitably into the pulmonary circulation. An increase in preload, an increase in afterload, and a decrease in CO_2 are the hemodynamic outcomes of the body's response to myocardial dysfunction. The pathophysiologic processes of heart failure provide the basis for therapy that is directed at decreasing symptoms, promoting clinical stability and decreasing the disease progression.[38,58]

ASSESSMENT AND DIAGNOSIS

A careful history usually reveals the cause of heart failure, such as MI, hypertension, or alcoholism. Left ventricular dysfunction from CAD and advanced ages are the primary risk factors contributing to the development of heart failure. Other risk factors include diabetes, angina, hypertension, history of cigarette smoking, obesity, elevated HDL, abnormally high or low hematocrit, proteinuria, and a history of CAD or previous MI. The patient will experience shortness of breath, which begins initially with exertion and progresses to shortness of breath at rest. In severe heart failure, the patient will develop orthopnea and must sit upright or lean over a table to breathe.

Physical examination reveals elevated central venous pressure, pulsus alternans, or a dicrotic pulse and pulmonary rales that do not clear with coughing and may extend to the lung apices. In right ventricular failure, an S_3 and a holosystolic murmur of tricuspid regurgitation are often heard. Hepatomegaly is felt, and peripheral pitting edema without venous insufficiency is present. In left ventricular failure the apical impulse is usually displaced laterally and downward, and S_1 is diminished. The S_2 is sometimes paradoxically split, and an S_3 gallop is present.[58]

ECG monitoring may show the development of arrhythmias such as arterial fibrillation (AF), complete heart block (CHB), and rapid tachycardias that could exacerbate pump failure. Laboratory data are nonspecific, although arterial hypoxemia and metabolic acidosis are common, and respiratory alkalosis may be present with significant tachypnea. Chest x-ray films reveal cardiomegaly and may show pulmonary vascular congestion and interstitial edema. Because of an increase, invasive monitoring reveals an elevated PAWP, elevated systemic vascular resistance, and low cardiac output.[58]

Flight nurses must remain alert to factors that can aggravate underlying cardiac dysfunction. These factors may be an extension of active ischemia/infarction, uncontrolled hypertension, or heavy alcohol consumption. Viral infections and pneumonias frequently trigger the onset of symptoms and may require weeks of close supervision for recovery, if recovery is even possible. Atrial fibrillation, which can cause or result from worsening failure, warrants the restoration of sinus rhythm to improve cardiac function. Obesity is both a primary cause and an aggravating factor for heart failure. Orthopnea is the most sensitive symptom of elevated filling pressures, and the degree of orthopnea parallels the amount of increased pressure. Jugular venous distention provides the most sensitive symptom of elevated resting filling pressures. Peripheral edema is present in only a few patients with chronic heart failure. Weight gain is another factor, which can indicate an impending episode of failure. Abdominal complaints can result from hepatic congestion.

Once it is determined that the patient is in failure, it must then be determined whether the patient is experiencing hypoperfusion. Physical evidence of hypoperfusion includes low blood pressure, narrow pulse pressure, cool extremities, and occasionally altered mentation, with supporting evidence sometimes provided by decreased sodium levels and worsening renal function and lethargy.[14,39]

MANAGEMENT

Management of acute heart failure focuses on the reduction of preload for relief of pulmonary edema, reduction of afterload with vasodilators to enhance stroke volume, and enhancement of contractile function. Intravenous diuretics and nitrates are used for preload reduction. Afterload reducing agents and angiotensin-converting enzyme inhibitors are used in the chronic, as opposed to the acute, setting. Inotropic agents are rarely used to enhance contractility because of the increase in myocardial oxygen demand, unless shock is present.[14,24] Currently beta-blockers are used to improve LV performance and improvement in survival.[19,39] Continuous ECG monitoring is required (potential ventricular arrhythmias may develop as a result of electrolyte imbalances), and strict intake and output measurements must be maintained and recorded.

CARDIOMYOPATHY

Cardiomyopathy is a general term used to describe disease involving the muscle itself. The cardiomyopathies are unique because they are not the result of ischemic, hypertensive, congenital, valvular, or pericardial diseases.

Cardiomyopathies can be functionally classified into three categories: (1) dilated cardiomyopathy, which is characterized by ventricular dilation, contractile dysfunction, and symptoms of heart failure; (2) hypertrophic cardiomyopathy, which is marked by myocardial hypertrophy, with left and sometimes right ventricular hypertrophy, most commonly involving the interventricular septum; and (3) restrictive cardiomyopathy, characterized by excessively rigid ventricular walls that impede ventricular filling, with the impairment of diastolic filling.[96]

DILATED CARDIOMYOPATHY

Dilated cardiomyopathy, formerly called congestive cardiomyopathy, is characterized by ventricular remodeling producing dilated chambers, contractility dysfunction, and in the majority of cases, heart failure as a result of impairment of systolic pump function. Impaired systolic function can involve left, right, or both ventricles with ejection fraction of <40%. The total mass of the heart is increased, resulting in dilation of the heart. This dilated cardiomyopathy is the end result of myocardial damage produced by a variety of toxic (e.g., cocaine), metabolic, or infectious agents and causes that can be familial, genetic, or idiopathic in origin. Secondary causes that may precipitate dilated cardiomyopathy include alcohol, hypertension, pregnancy, viruses, and hyperthyroidism.[85,96]

PATHOPHYSIOLOGIC FACTORS

Myocardial hypertrophy results in dilation of the heart, and as the disease progresses, the altered hemodynamics of myocardial remodeling are characterized by diminished ejection fraction, decreased stroke volume, and elevated end-systolic volume caused by increased chamber pressure.[85,96] As a compensatory response, cardiac output initially rises but will eventually decline in exercise or stress. Thrombus formation is enhanced because of the retention of blood in the cardiac chambers. The coronary arteries are usually normal. At the end stage of dilated cardiomyopathy, cardiac output declines, and right-sided heart failure occurs, causing biventricular failure and symptoms of CHF.

ASSESSMENT AND DIAGNOSIS

Patients often present with symptoms of low cardiac output or of fluid overload. Congestion is not consistently present, especially in the milder stages. Chest pain is common even in the presence of normal coronaries, and this may be associated with limited coronary vascular reserve or presence of ischemic heart disease. Severe ventricular dysfunction is frequently present with New York Heart Association Class III or IV symptoms. Fatigue and weakness usually accompany these symptoms. Occasionally patients will develop right-sided heart failure, presenting with increased jugular venous distention (JVD), hepatomegaly, splenomegaly, ascites, and peripheral edema. Other clinical features include a persistent S_3 gallop and symptomatic ventricular tachycardia. There may be a reduction in pulse pressure and the presence of systolic murmurs. Patients may also have abdominal pain, a reflection of liver congestion, or gastrointestinal discomfort from mesenteric congestion. Fatigue and weakness will be present because of decreased cardiac output. Arrhythmias and sudden death are not uncommon and may occur at any stage of the disease process.

On physical examination, the patient is breathless at rest or on exertion. The skin may be cool, pale, or cyanotic with peripheral edema. Palpation may reveal ascites, JVD, and pulsatile liver engorgement. An S_3 and an S_4 heart sound is often auscultated as a summation gallop in patients with rapid heart rates.[85,96]

MANAGEMENT

Treatment of dilated cardiomyopathy includes measures to improve the symptoms of heart failure and increase stroke volume. Pharmacologic therapy includes diuretics, digoxin, ACE inhibitors, inotropes, anticoagulants, antiarrhythmias, and beta-blockers. Inotropic agents such as amiodarone, dopamine, and dobutamine are used for their positive inotropic effects to increase contractility and cardiac output. Diuretics decrease blood volume in heart failure patients, and anticoagulation prevents systemic and pulmonary emboli. Beta-blocking agents may be used in patients with tachycardia at rest. Vasodilators can be used to decrease afterload and to improve cardiac output if intravascular volume is normal or high. Nitrates are most commonly used for this purpose. The aggressive use of ACE inhibitors and other therapies has resulted in improved outcomes.[85,96] Unfortunately, all forms of medical treatment are palliative rather than curative in the treatment of dilated cardiomyopathy. VADs may be used as a bridge to transplant to provide systemic support until cardiac transplant is available or other new surgical procedures can be initiated.

HYPERTROPHIC CARDIOMYOPATHY

Hypertrophic cardiomyopathy is characterized by disproportionate left and sometimes right ventricular hypertrophy. This most often involves the septum rather than the left ventricular free wall. Ventricular filling is impaired because of the abnormal stiffness of the ventricular septum. Hypertrophic cardiomyopathy is further characterized by disorganization of cardiac myocytes and myofibrils. The pathology of this disease leads to a gamut of abnormal processes that includes myocardial ischemia, diastolic dysfunction, ventricular and atrial arrhythmias, and congestive heart failure.[85]

PATHOPHYSIOLOGIC FACTORS

Hypertrophic cardiomyopathy (HCM) is usually familial (up to 70%) with an autosomal dominant inheritance. There is evidence that several genetic abnormalities might be associated with this disease. It is characterized by dynamic left ventricular outflow tract obstruction (LVOT) and increased left ventricular systolic performance. Most patients also have diastolic dysfunction as an effect from left ventricular relaxation and distensibility abnormalities.

The high resistance to ventricular filling caused by diastolic dysfunction results in left atrial cavity size enlargement. Patients have demonstrated reduced coronary blood flow that may result in myocardial ischemia, causing chest pain and dyspnea. Hemodynamically, patients with HCM have a high ejection fraction, which can result in increased myocardial oxygen consumption. The stiff ventricle requires high filling pressures, which often produces pulmonary hypertension. Poor outcomes are demonstrated when supraventricular and ventricular tachycardia are present. Sudden death is a common phenomenon, and it occurs in 2% to 4% of adults and in 4% to 6% of children and adolescents per year.[12,50,69,85]

ASSESSMENT AND DIAGNOSIS

Patients with hypertrophic cardiomyopathy are usually young (in their second or third decade of life), active, and athletic, although idiopathic left ventricular hypertrophy is well described in patients over 60. The pattern of disease in this age group differs significantly. Patients with HCM typically are initially seen with a systolic murmur of late onset heard at the left sternal border and apex that radiates to the axilla. The murmur is increased by standing or during the Valsalva maneuver. The arterial pulse is abrupt and has a jerky quality. Patients with significant left ventricular outflow gradients frequently have mitral regurgitation.

The most common symptom is dyspnea; other symptoms include angina as a result of oxygen demand exceeding supply and/or reduced coronary blood flow, syncope from inadequate cardiac output or arrhythmias, palpitations, fatigue, paroxysmal nocturnal dyspnea (PND), heart failure, and vertigo. Most of the symptoms are worsened with exertion. The ECG in hypertrophic cardiomyopathy reflects hypertrophy and atrial abnormality. Approximately 20% of these patients have atrial fibrillation.[69,96] Left ventricular hypertrophy (LVH) has been shown to be present 10 times more often in sudden death events than those without LVH. Autopsy examination on apparently healthy, young athletes succumbing to sudden death has revealed such cardiac diseases as hypertrophic cardiomyopathy. Even in those cases where no apparent cause was found, physiologic LVH is noted to be present.[66]

MANAGEMENT

Management of patients with hypertrophic cardiomyopathy consists of symptom relief and prevention of complications. Pharmacologic interventions that increase or maintain left ventricular end-diastolic volume and reduce ventricular contractility are usually used. Management currently includes beta-blockers and verapamil, dual-chamber pacing, and surgical myectomy. In patients with left ventricular outflow obstruction, beta-blockers to decrease myocardial oxygen consumption, decrease angina, and prevent increase in outflow obstruction with exercise are the first drug of choice. Verapamil can also be used for its negative inotropic effect, and often in high doses it may improve left ventricular relaxation and exercise tolerance in nonobstructive HCM. Dual-chamber pacing using a short program AV delay to maintain constant activation of the right ventricle may improve symptoms in those patients with left ventricular outflow tract gradients. A myectomy to widen the left ventricular outflow tract should be considered in all patients with outflow obstruction >50 mm Hg and symptoms nonresponsive to medical therapy. Percutaneous transluminal septal myocardial ablation (PTSMA) is a novel, nonsurgical approach to ablate hypertrophied septal myocardium by injection of alcohol into the septal branches.[50,69] For long-term management, calcium channel blocking agents are used. The antiarrhythmic agent amiodarone is used for those patients with frequent ventricular ectopy or ventricular tachycardia. Prophylactic antibiotic therapy is indicated both before and after surgical procedures for protection from infective endocarditis.

RESTRICTIVE CARDIOMYOPATHY

Restrictive cardiomyopathy is the least common of the cardiomyopathies. It resembles constrictive pericarditis clinically and is characterized by a normal to slightly enlarged heart, decreased diastolic volumes, and early in the disease process, a normal systolic function.

PATHOPHYSIOLOGIC FACTORS

There is diastolic function impairment resulting from excessively rigid ventricular walls that impede ventricular filling with the consequence of decreased ventricular compliance and filling. The walls of both ventricles are firm, noncompliant, and thickened. There may be mild cardiac enlargement with restrictive cardiomyopathy without significant ventricular dilation. The cause is usually unknown, but many specific pathologic processes may develop into restrictive cardiomyopathy, including myocardial fibrosis, hypertrophy, or infiltration.

ASSESSMENT AND DIAGNOSIS

Patients will present with signs and symptoms of myocardial failure with normal cardiac size. Most patients have chest pain, dyspnea on exertion, and fatigue. Often dyspnea on exertion is the only symptom in patients with early restrictive cardiomyopathy.[69] Because of the heart's inability to increase cardiac output, exercise tolerance is limited. Right-sided clinical presentation is frequently seen in advanced cases: increased jugular venous pressure, ascites, and peripheral edema. Mitral and tricuspid murmurs and S_3 or S_4 heart sounds are usually present. The ECG commonly reveals sinus tachycardia and atrial fibrillation with biventricular hypertrophy and decreased voltage.[85,96]

MANAGEMENT

Medical management of restrictive cardiomyopathy is similar to that for heart failure in that it is symptom limiting. The treatment focuses on fluid restriction, diuretic therapy, anticoagulation, and administration of digitalis if atrial fibrillation is present. Surgical treatment consists of resection of thickened endocardial tissue. Valve replacement surgery is also done when necessary.

VALVULAR DYSFUNCTION

DEFINITION

Valvular dysfunction can result from either congenital or acquired causes that expose the valve to hemodynamic stress and may accelerate the degenerative changes that cause dysfunction. Changes that cause narrowing of the valve orifice are classified as stenosis, which may result in pressure overload. Changes leading to valvular insufficiency because of improper closing of valves are classified as regurgitation and may result in volume overload.[58]

MITRAL STENOSIS
PATHOPHYSIOLOGIC FACTORS

Mitral stenosis most often is a result of rheumatic heart disease usually occurring by the age of 12 years, with the associated murmur heard approximately 20 years later. Although rare, other diseases that result in mitral stenosis include but are not limited to congenital mitral stenosis and infective endocarditis. Mitral stenosis is a narrowing of the mitral orifice associated with abnormal flow patterns resulting from valvulitis and developing into fibrosis and thickening of the mitral valve. The pathologic changes that occur in mitral stenosis are fusion of the commissures, fibrosis and thickening of the leaflets, shortening and fusion of the chordae and papillary muscles or both, and calcification of the leaflets. As the valve area is reduced, the gradient across the valve increases. Critical mitral stenosis occurs when the mitral valve opening is reduced to 1.0 cm^2; the normal mitral valve has an area of 4 to 6 cm^2. The stenosis leads to elevations in left atrial pressure that cause increased pulmonary venous and pulmonary artery wedge pressure.[58]

ASSESSMENT AND DIAGNOSIS

Symptoms develop gradually, with cardiac symptoms usually appearing in the fourth or fifth decade. The principal symptom of severe mitral stenosis is dyspnea with minimal exertion, pulmonary edema and hemoptysis resulting from elevated left atrial, and pulmonary venous and pulmonary capillary pressure. Pulmonary edema develops when the pulmonary capillary pressure is greater 25 mm Hg. Hemoptysis results from ruptured pulmonary venules. AF is a frequently occurring arrhythmia as a result of atrial dilation and hypertrophy, which in return can cause further deterioration of the patient's clinical condition. Systemic embolization and thromboembolism may be a presenting symptom in the presence of atrial fibrillation. Fatigue is a

common symptom, as are palpitations if AF has developed. Systemic venous hypertension with increased JVD develops when severe mitral stenosis leads to pulmonary vascular resistance and right-sided heart failure. Auscultation reveals an increased intensity of the first heart sound described as a snap and a low-pitched diastolic rumbling murmur that is best heard at the apex when the patient is in the left lateral decubitus position.[4]

MANAGEMENT

Medical management of mitral stenosis includes preventing complications such as systemic embolism or bacterial endocarditis and treating AF. Symptomatic patients with dyspnea are treated with diuretics and short- or long-acting nitrate preparations. Those patients with AF should receive prophylactic anticoagulants unless contraindicated. AF is treated with digitalis glycosides. Low-dose beta-blockers can be used to slow ventricular rates if necessary. The development of pulmonary edema secondary to a rapid ventricular response requires urgent intervention with either cardioversion or intravenous procainamide. Prophylactic antibiotics are given prior to dental work, surgery, and other interventions requiring instrumentation procedures to decrease the risk of developing infectious endocarditis. The best treatment for symptomatic mitral stenosis is relief of the valvular obstruction. Surgical management of mitral stenosis includes valvuloplasty or valve replacement, whereas nonsurgical treatment involves balloon valvuloplasty.[4,58]

MITRAL REGURGITATION
PATHOPHYSIOLOGIC FACTORS

Acute mitral regurgitation (MR) is a result of severe mitral incompetence. The mitral valve fails to close completely. This allows blood to flow back into the atrium during ventricular systole. It involves abnormal loading conditions; a sudden volume overload is forced on an ill-equipped left ventricle and left atrium. Preload is elevated; afterload is initially decreased, then eventually increases as left ventricular function deteriorates. Although left ventricular stroke volume increases, a large amount of the flow is forwarded into the left atrium instead of the aorta. This results in an increase in pressure in the noncompliant, nondilated left atrium and ventricle. Acute MR is a potentially fatal occurrence if the disease process includes mitral valve rupture. This valve disruption is caused by rupture of the base of a papillary muscle, usually caused by ischemic necrosis. Rupture of both valve leaflets is incompatible with life; however, if only one leaflet ruptures, resulting in an incompetent valve, prognosis is much better. From acute severe MR, pulmonary edema, left ventricular volume overload, and passive pulmonary hypertension develop. The pulmonary edema and hypertension are a result of left atrial hypertension from acute volume overload in a chamber of normal size and compliance.[4]

ASSESSMENT AND DIAGNOSIS

The symptoms of MR develop very rapidly and are associated with left ventricular failure. Severe dyspnea at rest and angina result from increased left ventricular filling pressures. Tachycardia and tachypnea are common. The MR murmur is of variable intensity; it may be loud if normal left ventricular function is present and soft if left ventricular function is reduced.[4] If both leaflets are involved, the murmur is very loud and widespread.

The ECG may be normal or show evidence of an AMI. The rhythm is usually sinus rhythm; atrial fibrillation is indicative of chronic MR. Invasive monitoring discloses a prominent systolic regurgitant wave in the PAWP tracing.

MANAGEMENT

Surgical intervention (valvuloplasty or replacement) is almost always necessary, and medical management is used to stabilize the patient's condition before surgical treatment. Intravenous nitroprusside therapy is given for vasodilator and afterload reducing affects. It will lower systemic vascular resistance, enhances stroke volume, and is effective in reducing pulmonary vascular congestion. Oral medical therapy includes ACE inhibitors, digoxin, and diuretics. Hypotension is usually treated with dopamine, and hemodynamic support with the IABP or VAD may be necessary.[4]

AORTIC STENOSIS
PATHOPHYSIOLOGIC FACTORS

Aortic stenosis (AS) usually results from a congenital or degenerative origin. The most common cause of adult acquired AS is idiopathic degeneration and calcification of the aortic valve, with symptoms developing in the fifth and sixth decades of life. With rheumatic AS, which occurs in a small minority of patients, symptoms develop in the fourth decade. Congenital AS is diagnosed in childhood in the first decade, although occasionally some of these patients are seen for the first time as adults. The reduction in the valve orifice causes obstruction to the flow of blood from the left ventricle into the aorta during ventricular systole, resulting in eventual ventricular wall thickening. Pressure overload and increased systolic wall stress contribute to the development of left ventricular hypertrophy, which acts as a compensatory mechanism. The progressive pressure overload, increased pressure gradient, and left ventricular hypertrophy can ultimately lead to total left ventricular failure.[20]

ASSESSMENT AND DIAGNOSIS

Both systolic and diastolic myocardial dysfunction may occur in AS, and patients will present with symptoms of heart failure. Angina develops because of myocardial ischemia and abnormalities in oxygen supply and demand. Syncope is suspected of being caused by either an increase in intraventricular pressure during exercise that initiates a vasodepressor response or is caused by supraventricular or ventricular arrhythmias. The presence of a systolic ejection murmur that radiates to the neck is frequently the first suspicion of the presence of AS; the murmur is very loud early in the course of the disease and is associated with a systolic thrill. Later in the disease the murmur is heard loudest at the end of systole and is heard over the aortic area and the apex. Palpation of the carotid arteries will reveal a reduction in amplitude of the carotid upstroke. The palpation of a strong, apical impulse in conjunction with the simultaneous weak and delayed carotid pulse is indicative of severe AS. The ECG may reveal left ventricular hypertrophy and left atrial abnormality, although a patient that is symptomatic can have a fairly normal ECG.[20]

MANAGEMENT

Patients with asymptomatic AS have a nearly normal survival for long latency periods and most often do not require therapy at all other than antibiotic prophylaxis for the prevention of infective endocarditis. Patients with symptomatic AS have an average survival time of 2 to 3 years and will require surgical intervention with aortic valve replacement (AVR).[20,48] For those patients that are not surgical candidates, digitalis and diuretics may be used to treat CHF symptoms, and nitrates may be used with caution to treat angina. Vasodilators and ACE inhibitors, widely used to treat CHF, are contraindicated in patients with AS. Vasodilators will lower peripheral pressure and reduce preload, precipitating dangerous hypotension, without increasing cardiac output. Balloon valvotomy (valvuloplasty) has not shown to reduce mortality in those patients who do not undergo surgery and is used more often for patients that are not candidates for AVR.

AORTIC REGURGITATION

PATHOPHYSIOLOGIC FACTORS

Acute aortic regurgitation (AR) results in a large volume overload at high pressure to the left ventricle, which cannot adapt acutely. The aortic valve fails does not close completely. This allows the blood to flow back into the ventricle during ventricular diastole. Acute AR causes an early impairment in ejection, resulting in low forward stroke output, left atrial hypertension, and pulmonary edema. The most common cause of AR is infective endocarditis and therefore is common in younger patients with a history of intravenous drug use. Other causes include aortic dissection and nonpenetrating chest or upper abdominal trauma.[20,23]

ASSESSMENT AND DIAGNOSIS

The patient with acute AR is acutely ill with tachycardia, peripheral hypoperfusion, and congestive heart failure. Physical examination reveals a widened pulse pressure. S_1 is diminished, and there is no S_4. The diastolic murmur may be of variable intensity. The ECG may be normal or show left ventricular hypertrophy if aortic dissection is present. Infective endocarditis is often mistaken for influenza. A high degree of suspicion should be present when a patient presents with the sudden development of high fever, malaise, and early symptoms of CHF if there is any prior history of an abnormal aortic valve or valve prosthesis.

MANAGEMENT

Medical management for patients with AR is a temporary measure until surgery can be performed. AVR is indicated for both survival and quality of life. Even if the patient is asymptomatic, AVR is indicated to prevent further deterioration into heart failure. Vasodilators may improve symptoms temporarily and assist in preparation for surgery. With endocarditis, broad-spectrum antibiotics should be started initially after blood cultures are drawn. Use of the IABP is contraindicated because it increases AR.[4]

ACUTE PERICARDITIS

Pericarditis refers to inflammation of the pericardium and can have a number of causes. The most common conditions associated with the development of pericarditis include MI, infection, collagen vascular diseases, uremia, malignancy, drug therapy, and trauma.

The pericardium is a closed fibrous sac that envelops the heart. It consists of an inner serous membrane, the visceral pericardium, which closely adheres to the superficial myocardium and coronary vessels. The fibrous outer layer that surrounds the heart is the parietal pericardium. The space between the visceral and parietal layers normally contains between 10 to 20 ml of pericardial fluid that acts as a lubricant between the contracting surfaces. The exact role of the pericardium is not clear. However, it is believed to serve as a lubrication system, ensuring that cardiac motion is unimpaired by surrounding mediastinal structures. Because the pericardium resists stretching, it functions as a protective mechanism to prevent sudden dilation of the heart. The pericardium may also protect the heart from infection.

Pericarditis can be associated with AMI in up to 30% of cases at autopsy. Clinically, it is observed in 7% to 10% of AMIs. It results from an extension of the infarction to the epicardial area and is associated with an inflammatory response localized to the pericardium bordering the infarction. It may also be a delayed response with a more generalized inflammatory response, as with Dressler's syndrome.[45,59]

ASSESSMENT AND DIAGNOSIS

The presentation of pericardial heart disease depends on the pericardium's response to injury and subsequent effect on cardiac function. Diagnosis and recognition of acute pericarditis in the emergent situation are largely dependent on patient history of pleuritic chest pain. Typical chest pain is described as sharp, severe, substernal, and increases with inspiration or in the reclining position. Chest pain caused by acute pericarditis may further be aggravated by coughing or movement and may be relieved when the patient sits up and leans forward. Substernal pain may radiate to the neck, shoulder, and back. The physical examination may reveal a pericardial friction rub, which may be absent when effusion develops. ECG changes may demonstrate atypical T wave abnormalities. ST segment elevation is not common but may be present when pericarditis is more generalized. Diffuse ST segment elevation in conjunction with PR segment depression is the typical ECG presentation. Associated signs and symptoms of pericarditis include (1) fever and leukocytosis, (2) dyspnea related to increased pain with inspiration, (3) dysphagia related to irritation of the esophagus by the posterior pericardium, and (4) sinus tachycardia.

Physical examination reveals a pericardial friction rub that may be heard at various times and in various locations during the patient's course. The friction rub resembles a high-pitched grating or scratching sound. It is best heard with the diaphragm of the stethoscope placed at the lower left sternal border or apex with the patient sitting and leaning forward during held expiration. The presence of a friction rub does not exclude the presence of a large pericardial effusion or tamponade. A normal BP should be present without paradoxical pulse or venous distention. If the flight nurse observes signs of restriction to ventricular filling, he or she should consider the presence of pericardial tamponade or effusion.

Dressler's syndrome appears later and may be related to an autoimmune reaction or may be related to activation of latent viral infections. Pathophysiology involves serosal inflammation and may involve the pleural or peritoneum.[45,59]

Purulent pericarditis is a rare syndrome with fever and hypotension frequently present. It is often mistaken for septic shock. Signs and symptoms associated with this syndrome are chest pain, pericardial friction rub, pulsus, paradoxus, and elevation of jugular venous pressure. Patients only exhibit these classic descriptors 50% of the time, and a high index of suspicion is required to diagnose this disorder.

MANAGEMENT

Evaluation and monitoring of acute pericarditis are important in the emergency setting to establish whether the pericarditis is associated with an underlying problem, such as MI or pericardial effusion, requiring specific therapy. The flight nurse should monitor for complications of pericarditis, such as signs of pericardial effusion that may accumulate rapidly and cause cardiac tamponade.

The chest pain of pericarditis may be managed by analgesics and anti-inflammatory agents, such as aspirin, and nonsteroidal antiinflammatory drugs (NASIDS), such as ibuprofen. Because of the recurrent nature of Dressler's syndrome and the immunologic pathophysiology, steroids may be indicated for this condition.[45,59] The patient should be observed for atrial arrhythmias, such as beats and bursts of atrial tachycardia, which often accompany acute pericarditis.

CARDIAC EFFUSION AND TAMPONADE

Pericardial effusion refers to the development of fluid in the pericardial sac as a response to injury of the parietal pericardium or with all causes of acute pericarditis. Cardiac tamponade occurs when the accumulation of fluid occurs resulting in increased pressure and subsequent compression of the heart, to such an extent that cardiac output is significantly compromised. For emergency practitioners, cardiac tamponade is one of the most dramatic emergencies.

PATHOPHYSIOLOGIC FACTORS

The hemodynamic effects of effusion are related to the speed of accumulation of the fluid. Rapid accumulation of 150 to 200 ml may produce acute cardiac tamponade; in contrast, large pericardial effusions, which develop slowly, can be totally asymptomatic. Under normal conditions, between 15 and 50 ml of fluid may be present in the pericardial space. The development of a larger volume of fluid may result from pericardial inflammation of any cause, heart failure, or traumatic injury to the heart, aortic dissection, or neoplasm. The presence of additional fluid causes the intrapericardial pressure to increase. When intrapericardial pressure is increased, diastolic filling of the ventricles is impeded, resulting in a rise of ventricular pressure and decreased cardiac output. As the increased intrapericardial pressure reaches a critical level, a precipitous decrease in arterial pressure occurs.[59]

ASSESSMENT AND DIAGNOSIS

Mild to moderate pericardial effusion may not produce symptoms. If the fluid accumulates slowly, the fairly noncompliant pericardium stretches to accommodate the increasing volume with little or no rise in intrapericardial pressure until it reaches a size where it can no longer stretch. However, if the fluid accumulates rapidly, a small volume can be life threatening. Clinical symptoms of cardiac tamponade are related to systemic venous congestion, a reduction in cardiac stroke volume, and respiratory effects of impaired ventricular filling. Early tamponade will manifest tachycardia, tachypnea, edema, and elevated venous pressure. The classic signs, described as Beck's triad, include distended neck veins resulting from elevated central venous pressure (CVP), decreased BP, and muffled heart sounds. Pulsus paradoxus (abnormal fall in systolic pressure during inspiration caused by differential filling of the ventricles) may be present. Kussmaul's sign is a true paradoxical venous pressure abnor-

mality associated with tamponade. It is manifested by a rise in venous pressure with inspiration when breathing spontaneously.[5] If early signs of cardiac tamponade are not treated, rapid development of severe hypotension, right atrial and right ventricular collapse with profound circulatory failure, and shock result. Chest x-ray films may demonstrate a widening cardiac silhouette. Echocardiography is the recommended modality for rapid and accurate diagnosis of tamponade.

Cardiac tamponade resulting from trauma is usually the result of penetrating injuries, but blunt injury may also cause the pericardium to fill with blood from either injury to the heart itself or from the surrounding great vessels. Cardiac tamponade should be suspected in any trauma patient that presents in electromechanical dissociation (EMD) or does not respond to volume resuscitation.[5]

PARADOXICAL PULSE

A finding of paradoxical pulse is elicited by measuring BP during quiet respiration. The technique involves pumping the blood pressure cuff above the systolic sounds and slowly deflating the cuff until the first systolic sound is heard. Normally the systolic sound should disappear on inspiration. The flight nurse should continue to deflate the cuff until all systolic sounds can be heard on inspiration and expiration. The paradox is the difference in millimeters of mercury between the pressure where the systolic sound disappears and the pressure at which *all* systolic sounds are heard. A paradox of less than 10 mm Hg is a normal reflection of the inspiratory fall of aortic systolic pressure; however, it is exaggerated in the presence of cardiac tamponade. An inspiratory fall in systolic BP exceeding 10 mm Hg indicates the presence of a paradoxical pulse.[5,47]

MANAGEMENT

Emergent evacuation of the pericardial fluid is definitive therapy in the presence of acute cardiac tamponade. Hemodynamic support during preparation of the patient for pericardiocentesis includes administration of IV fluid—blood, plasma, normal saline, or lactated ringers. Pericardiocentesis is accomplished by needle aspiration of pericardial fluid via the subxiphoid method. Removal of even small amounts of fluid by pericardiocentesis may have extremely beneficial affects and relieve symptoms temporarily. A positive pericardiocentesis caused by trauma will require an open thoracotomy for definitive treatment. Any trauma patient presenting in EMD and not responding to volume resuscitation requires a high index of suspicion for cardiac tamponade.[5]

NONTRAUMATIC AORTIC DISSECTION

One of the most commonly seen life-threatening disorders of the aorta is dissection. Aortic dissection occurs when an intimal tear or separation develops in the aorta, resulting in hematoma formation in its medial layer. Dissections can originate anywhere along the length of the aorta and can be classified according to its location. The most common point of origin, and clinically most urgent, is in the ascending aorta in a few centimeters above the right or left sinus of Valsalva (65%). This can result in aortic valve insufficiency, compromise of a coronary artery, or rupture and cardiac tamponade or exsanguination. Other areas of common dissection include the proximal descending thoracic aorta just beyond the left subclavian artery origin (20%), in the transverse aortic arch (10%), and in the distal thoracic aorta or abdominal aorta (5%). The DeBakey system is the most widely used classification system for acute aortic dissection (Figure 21-9). In type I the dissection originates in the ascending aorta and extends distally; in type II the dissection is limited to the ascending aorta; and in type III the dissection originates near and distally to the left subclavian artery and extends distally. Conditions associated with aortic dissection include systemic hypertension, congenital abnormalities of the aortic valve, advanced age, and heritable disorders of connective tissue such as Marfan's syndrome (a nonatherosclerotic disorder of connective tissue involving massive degeneration of elastic fibers in the aortic media). Complications of aortic dissection include compromise of flow to visceral organs and the extremities and neurologic deficits because of interruption of flow in branch vessels. Acute dissection

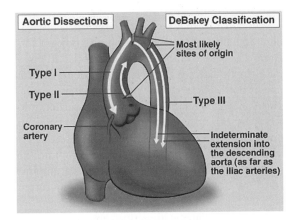

FIGURE 21-9 **Aortic dissections: DeBakey classification.** (Copyright 1995-2002, Challenger Corporation, Artist: Tom Rolain.)

of the ascending aorta that is untreated has a >90% mortality rate. Patients with distal dissection are usually managed medically unless the dissection is complicated by rupture of the aorta or compromise of the blood supply to a vital organ. Surgery, emergent if necessary, is indicated for most patients with proximal dissection.[95,102]

ASSESSMENT AND DIAGNOSIS

The classic symptom of patients with aortic dissection is the sudden onset of pain, described as ripping, searing, and tearing, often originating in the back (interscapular) or substernal area and possibly extending down into the legs. The pain may be migratory and so change in location as the dissection proceeds. Other signs result from obstruction of major vessels originating from the aorta. Depending on the location of the dissection and the compromised vessels involved, the patient may manifest ischemia of various organ systems and signs and symptoms of cardiac disease. MI, cerebral insufficiency, cerebral vascular accident, hemiplegia or paraplegia, renal failure, and intestinal infarction may all be a result of dissection. Because of these diverse presentations and other less-typical symptoms, a delay in diagnosis or misdiagnosis is common.

The patient with acute dissection is in severe distress and will appear to be in shock, with pallor, sweating, peripheral cyanosis, and restlessness.

However, the BP may be normal or elevated, often as high as 200 mm Hg systolic, with a significant difference between both arms. Differential BP and pulses may indicate compromise of blood flow to one or both subclavian arteries. Absence of femoral pulses may indicate extension of the dissection into the aortic bifurcation, compromising circulation to one or both legs. Hypotension in aortic dissection is usually a result of rupture of the dissection into the pericardial space and may lead to cardiac tamponade. Rupture into the pleural space or mediastinum is more common with proximal dissection.[95,102]

Diagnosis of aortic dissection can often be made by physical examination alone. Transport of the acute patient should not be delayed to obtain a chest x-ray. However, if a chest film is available on arrival of the transport team, it may be useful in conjunction with other diagnostic signs. X-ray findings suggestive of an acute aortic dissection are (1) mediastinal widening, (2) extension of the aortic shadow beyond a calcified aortic wall, (3) a localized bulge on the aortic arch, and (4) tracheal deviation, or (5) a left pleural effusion.[95]

MANAGEMENT

Prompt initiation of therapy and transport of patients with acute aortic dissection remains a challenge for flight nurses who are often caring for these patients during the brief interval between the onset of symptoms and the occurrence of life-threatening complications. Interventions are aimed at controlling pain and at halting the progression of the dissecting force by reducing system blood pressure and the rate of change of pressure development. Blood pressure should be aggressively lowered to the lowest level compatible with adequate visceral, renal, and cerebral perfusion. Hypertension is treated with an intravenous beta-adrenergic blocking agent such as propranolol given in conjunction with sodium nitroprusside. It is essential that beta-blockers be given prior to afterload reduction to increase the force of left ventricular ejection, although it may aggravate the dissection. Labetalol can be given in place of a beta-blocker and sodium nitroprusside for short-term therapy for transport. For normotensive patients, beta-blockers can be used alone.

Infusions should be placed on the most accurate delivery pump available for transport, and doses should be titrated to BP response. Expert care and transport to definitive care requires pain relief and continuous ECG and BP monitoring. Pain may be managed with IV narcotic analgesia while the flight nurse constantly observes for signs of respiratory compromise. Type I and type II dissections will require emergent surgical repair with resection and Dacron replacement.[95]

Flight personnel should also be prepared to initiate intubation and assisted ventilation in the event that the patient's condition deteriorates. At least two large-bore IV access sites should be established for transport. Fluids should be kept to a minimum unless severe hypotension or rupture of the aorta occurs in flight. Blood should be available for transfusion during the flight if cardiac output becomes compromised. Inadequate pain or BP control and evidence of progressive dissection indicate an urgent need for surgical intervention. The flight team should not delay transfer to wait for laboratory results, blood products, or x-rays. Coordination of efforts among air medical transport personnel and the referring and receiving hospitals will expedite admission to the surgical department for prompt intervention.

HYPERTENSIVE CRISIS

Hypertension is a common clinical condition affecting approximately 60 million adult Americans. It is considered the most common risk factor for CVD. It is estimated that 50% of the population between the ages of 60 to 74 years have evidence of hypertension. The prevalence of hypertension is expected to increase along with the aging population and increased life expectancy. Recent data from the Framingham Heart Study recognized the importance of elevated systolic blood pressure (SBP) and pulse pressure as significant risk factors for stroke and heart failure. Systolic hypertension and a widening pulse pressure are predominant in the elderly. Major published guidelines for managing hypertension recommend aggressively treating SBP to a target of 140 mm Hg. Epidemiologic data suggests that only 25% of hypertensive patients have adequate blood pressure control and that 50% of the adult population over 65 have SBPs that are too high.[49,55,80,99]

Hypertensive crisis is a potentially life-threatening complication of hypertension. Approximately 600,000 to 800,000 Americans will develop a hypertensive crisis (1% of the 60 million estimated Americans with hypertension). The presence of end-organ damage determines whether the crisis is defined as urgent or emergent. Hypertensive emergency with apparent end-organ damage requires an immediate reduction of blood pressure. The systolic blood pressure will often exceed 200 mm Hg, with a diastolic blood pressure greater than 120 to 130 mm Hg. There are no predetermined criteria for the level of BP necessary to produce a hypertensive emergency. The rate of rise of the blood pressure and the difference between the patient's usual level and that level present during crisis is the more important factor. A hypertensive crisis is a very rapid, progressive rise in BP sufficient to cause potential irreversible damage to vital organs. The major organs at risk are the brain, heart, and kidneys. It may cause aortic dissection, cerebral hemorrhage, renal failure, and left-sided heart failure. Hypertensive crisis may occur in the clinical course of any patient with a persistent BP elevation, or it may occur as the initial presentation of a hypertensive patient. The evidence of organ dysfunction is the basis for diagnosis. When the blood pressure is critically elevated without end-organ damage, it is considered a hypertensive urgency, which can be treated with oral medication over the course of 24 to 48 hours.[7,47,88,99] Patients without prior hypertension may not tolerate BP levels as high as can those patients with chronic hypertension.

ASSESSMENT AND DIAGNOSIS

The underlying pathologic process in accelerated hypertension and subsequent hypertensive crisis begins with arteriolar spasm and later shows fibrinoid necrosis, release of vasoactive substances, continued vasoconstriction, and proliferation of the myointimal. Increased capillary permeability resulting from cerebral arteriole dilation and increased cerebral blood flow or vessel wall damage are the effects of the pathophysiologic changes. The changes in the small arterioles are directly visible in the retina. The pathophysiology underlying specific target organ damage varies. Fluid leakage into the perivascular space from increased blood flow will result in cerebral edema and hypertensive encephalopathy The most devastating complication of hypertension is hypertensive encephalopathy. Hypertensive encephalopathy may be characterized by the presence of progressive central nervous systems signs and symptoms, including severe headache, nausea, vomiting, and visual difficulties. Focal neurologic findings can include blindness, seizures, aphasia, and hemiparesis. If left untreated, symptoms may progress to convulsions, stupor, coma, and death. Hypertensive emergencies are often caused by mismanagement or patient nonadherence. New onset of hypertension with no prior history of elevated blood pressure may be consistent with acute drug reactions.[59,96]

Accelerated hypertension without end-organ damage (hypertensive urgency) is more common than hypertensive emergencies. Alterations in left ventricular performance secondary to increased afterload are the primary mechanism by which an acute rise in pressure affects the cardiovascular system. Left ventricular failure, myocardial ischemia, or both can occur as a result of accelerated hypertension. Retinopathy, congestive heart failure, arrhythmias, or focal neurologic deficits may be present on clinical examination. Palpitations, angina, or congestive failure can present with cardiovascular decompensation. Signs and symptoms of left ventricular failure include chest pain, dyspnea, production of pink frothy sputum, rales, and bronchospasm. Neurologic symptoms may include headache, nausea, seizures, or obtundation.[88,96]

MANAGEMENT

The goal of therapy for patients demonstrating signs of hypertensive encephalopathy or malignant hypertension is to lower the BP in a controlled manner in 30 to 60 minutes to what is "normal" for that patient. It is recommended that blood pressure reduction during the initial treatment should not be more than 25% to avoid the danger of cerebral

TABLE 21-2 **Antihypertensive Therapy in the Management of Hypertensive Emergencies**

Clinical Presentation	Pharmacologic Preference	Avoid or Use Cautiously
Malignant hypertension (no associated disease process)	Diazoxide Nitroprusside Minoxidil	Nifedipine Nicardipine
Intracerebral or subarachnoid hemorrhage	Nitroprusside Labetalol	Diazoxide Methyldopa Reserpine Clonidine
Ischemic heart disease	Nitrates Nitroprusside Labetalol	Diazoxide Hydralazine Minoxidil
Pulmonary edema	Furosemide Morphine, O_2	Beta-blockers Verapamil Diltiazem
Dissecting aortic aneurysm	Nitroprusside + beta-blocker	Diazoxide Hydralazine Minoxidil Diuretics
Renal failure or acute nephritis	Diazoxide Nitroprusside Calcium antagonists	Trimethaphan Beta-blockers
Pregnancy, toxemia	Hydralazine Methyldopa	Trimethaphan Nitrates Thiazides Nifedipine

hypoperfusion. Malignant hypertension may occur with or without associated diseases, such as intracerebral bleed, ischemic heart disease, pulmonary edema, pregnancy induced toxemia, aortic dissection, renal failure, pheochromocytoma, and postoperative hypertension. Therapy should be based on each situation, critical organ involvement, and the desired time frame for lowering the blood pressure. For the flight nurse, the resolution of signs and symptoms should be used as a primary guide in the control of the pressure, in addition to the level of BP, because it may be difficult to obtain frequent accurate BP in flight. Monitoring the patient's cardiac rhythm and BP (by the most accurate means possible), observing the patient's level of consciousness, and assessing for signs of impending pulmonary edema or cardiac failure helps the transport team evaluate whether the antihypertensive agents are

effective. Either nitroprusside or diazoxide may be used when immediate antihypertensive therapy is required. Both of these drugs have a controllable blood pressure reduction action. Other drug therapies should be based on the accompanying disease presenting with the malignant hypertension (Table 21-2). Nifedipine capsules are not recommended for blood pressure reduction because controlled conditions to lower blood pressure cannot be achieved with nifedipine.[88,96]

Sodium nitroprusside acts by direct peripheral vasodilation with balanced effects on arterial and venous blood vessels. The antihypertensive effect of IV sodium nitroprusside is apparent in seconds and is dose dependent. Once the drug is discontinued, the pressure rises rapidly to the previous level in 1 to 10 minutes. Infusion rates must be closely monitored to avoid sudden fluctuations in BP.[35]

TABLE 21-3 Drugs Commonly Used in Hypertensive Emergencies

Drug	Usual Dose	Mechanism and Onset of Action	Duration of Action	Side Effects
Sodium nitroprusside (Nipride)	Prepare 50-100 mg/ 500 ml D$_5$W; administer at rate of 0.05-0.20 mg/min	Arterial and venous vasodilator, immediate onset of action	3-5 min	Severe hypotension, nausea, restlessness, thiocyanate toxicity, methemoglobinemia
Labetalol (Normodyne)	5-50 mg IV every 10 minutes as needed; may be administered as a continuous IV infusion (2 mg/min) thereafter to maximum dose of 300 mg	Alpha- and beta-blocking agent, onset immediate; decrease blood pressure without changing heart rate	2-4 hr	Bradycardia, bronchospasm, profound hypotension
Furosemide (Lasix)	40-80 mg IV over 1-2 min	Diuretic, venous vasodilator, onset 1-5 min	1-12 hr	Electrolyte imbalance

Data from Nissen D, ed: *2001 Mosby's GenRx,* ed 11, St Louis, 2001, Mosby.

Diazoxide exerts its hypotensive effect by reducing arteriolar vascular resistance through direct relaxation of arteriolar smooth muscle. When the drug decreases arterial pressure, baroreceptor reflexes are activated, leading to cardiac stimulation with increased heart rate, stroke volume, and cardiac output, resulting in mechanical stress on the aorta. For this reason diazoxide should not be used for patients with dissection of the aorta and for patients with known CAD. Once the BP is controlled, the BP remains low and returns only gradually over 2 to 12 hours, giving it an advantage over nitroprusside in clinical situations where it is difficult to monitor the patient's condition closely for a long period of time.[35] Other antihypertensive agents useful in the emergent situation are summarized in Table 21-3.

HEMODYNAMIC MONITORING IN CARDIOVASCULAR ASSESSMENT

Accurate hemodynamic assessment is essential during the transport of the patient with cardiovascular compromise. Space limitations, noise levels, and vibration in the air medical environment may preclude the use of sophisticated invasive hemodynamic monitoring equipment during transport in some aircraft. The proficient flight nurse will develop and refine the use of visual and tactile assessment skills to clinically evaluate the patient. These skills should be used in conjunction with hemodynamic monitoring capabilities. Especially valuable are frequent examinations of mental status, skin color and temperature, pulse rate and quality, and UO.

Cardiac Output

The ultimate goal of monitoring and manipulation of hemodynamic parameters is to provide adequate perfusion of the body. This can be accomplished by directing and maintaining adequate cardiac output. Assessing the cardiac output provides a useful measure of the pumping ability of the heart and is one of the major indicators of cardiac output. *Cardiac output* (CO) is defined as the product of the heart rate and stroke volume, which is the amount of blood ejected from the left ventricle with each contraction.

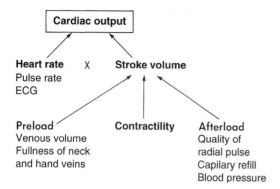

FIGURE 21-10   **Noninvasive assessment of cardiac output.**

Changes in CO result from altering the rate of the heartbeat or the stroke volume. The major factors that influence stroke volume are contractility, preload (venous return or diastolic filling), and afterload (resistance imposed by normal aortic impedance). The normal range for CO is 4 to 8 L per minute. CO is also used to calculate other parameters such as systemic vascular resistance (SVR) and stroke volume (SV) (Figure 21-10).[58]

NONINVASIVE HEMODYNAMIC MONITORING

Noninvasive methods used to assess the hemodynamic status of the patient include the monitoring of the patient's capillary refill, pulse rate and quality, BP, mentation, UO, and skin temperature. Mental status changes are important in determining the patient's overall condition. Significant changes in mentation occur in late shock when flow is compromised to the vital organs. Skin temperature and color, capillary refill, and UO in the absence of renal disease reflect tissue perfusion as it relates to cardiac output and intravascular volume. A combination of noninvasive methods such as capillary refill time, quality of the heart rate, and quality of the pulse or pulse contour should be used in conjunction with percutaneous monitoring and invasive hemodynamic monitoring to assess the adequacy of cardiac output during aeromedical transport of critical patients.

Blood pressure can be obtained noninvasively in the air medical environment by the use of mechanical Doppler augmentation, automated BP devices, or palpation of the radial pulse with a sphygmomanometer and cuff. The cuff pressure measurements are usually adequate for a hemodynamically stable patient; however, direct blood pressure monitoring via an arterial line is more accurate than indirect pressures specifically in the presence of hypertension, hypothermia, and shock. Transducer pressure measures systolic and diastolic from the same heartbeat. Cuff pressure measures systolic from one beat and diastolic from another. Indirect pressures are often difficult to hear in the presence of low CO and peripheral vasoconstriction. Although BP measuring devices can be useful to monitor trends in the patient's hemodynamic status, evaluate the patient's hemodynamic status by multiple methods rather than relying on one specific parameter such as BP.[58]

PERCUTANEOUS DEVICES FOR ASSESSMENT OF OXYGENATION STATUS

The effects of altitude on the cardiovascular system are numerous. Adequate tissue oxygenation remains the highest priority in critically ill patients. The assessment of a patient's oxygenation and hemodynamic status can be augmented by various noninvasive transcutaneous devices that respond to physiologic changes in oxygenation and perfusion. Many monitors are available to monitor pulse oximetry during transport. Pulse oximetry provides continuous noninvasive monitoring of the percentage of oxygen saturation of arterial hemoglobin (SaO_2). A probe or sensor can be placed on a patient's finger or ear lobe and can detect a waveform from pulsatile blood by optical plethysmography. The probe contains red and infrared light emitters on one side and a photodetector on the opposite side. Red and infrared light not absorbed by the blood, bone, and tissue is measured by the photodetector and is converted into a reading indicative of the arterial hemoglobin percentage. An SaO_2 reading of 95% or higher at sea level is considered normal. This percentage will decrease as altitude increases. However, a normal reading does not always mean adequate oxygenation. Some adverse events may not be detected until the event is totally or near irreversible. Several studies have shown pulse oximetry to be accurate and effective in identifying hypoxemia and other undesirable conditions associated with arterial desaturation. Continuous and routine pulse oximetry monitoring should result in fewer episodes of arterial desaturation and more rapid recognition of this event and thus may lower morbidity or mortality. Pulse oximetry is considered to be a standard of care for ground and air medical transport and may be a legal requirement in some states for use with some therapeutic interventions. The most common problem associated with the use of pulse oximetry is failure of signal detection. This can be related to motion, arrhythmia, hypothermia, hypotension/hypoperfusion, and vasoactive drugs. Some errors in detection can be easily resolved by changing or adjusting probe placement. Artifact from motion is more prevalent in the ground transport setting than in the air transport setting.[58,103]

Capnography measures carbon dioxide concentration or partial pressure on those critically ill, intubated patients and reflects the respiratory process. A normal waveform indicates carbon dioxide production, transport, and alveolar ventilation equilibrium. For critical care transport, capnometry can monitor $PaCO_2$, which is usually monitored through ABG analysis. Changes in $EtCO_2$ levels can reflect airway complications and/or equipment problems and may reduce morbidity in the transport environment by early detection of airway and ventilatory difficulty. Monitoring of end-tidal carbon dioxide in critically ill patients, such as those in cardiogenic shock, is recommended in the ICU environment and the prehospital environment when available.[58,103]

INVASIVE HEMODYNAMIC MONITORING

When transporting a patient who has been admitted to a coronary care unit, the goal of transport is to provide a high level of care equal to that in the ICU. Often the patient has invasive intravascular catheters in place. Hemodynamic monitoring in a critically ill patient by means of intravascular catheters placed into a blood vessel and/or a chamber of the heart provides accurate information on initial and continuous cardiovascular status. Parameters will assist with verifying diagnosis and to guide therapy and monitor clinical changes. For example, intra-arterial pressure is more accurate than noninvasive sphygmomanometry in patients who are obese, hypotensive, peripherally vasoconstricted, or severely hypertensive. Hemodynamic monitoring is a valuable aid in assessing patients who require specific interventions such as volume, preload and afterload reducing, or inotropic agents and for patients on IABP. Pulmonary artery (PA) catheters can provide information on both right and left heart pressures. PAWP and PA pressures reflect pressures in the left atrium and left ventricular end-diastolic pressure (LVEDP). These parameters can be used for assessment of left ventricular preload. The CVP is measured independently through a central venous catheter or through the proximal port of a PA catheter. CVP is reduced when preload, or the volume of blood returning to the heart, is reduced. A low CVP may be seen with bleeding, dehydration, drug-induced vasodilation, or overzealous diuresis. An elevated CVP may be seen with fluid overload (overtransfusion, overhydration), right ventricular failure, cardiac tamponade, tricuspid stenosis or insufficiency, or vasoconstrictive states. These parameters can help the flight nurse guide therapy. However, caution should be used not to concentrate on one cardiodynamic variable without a full evaluation of all physiologic information available, such as heart rate, capillary refill, pulse contour, BP, and UO.[58] Before transport, interpretation of intravascular hemodynamic parameters and trends provide the flight nurse with valuable information regarding the cardiovascular status of the patient. To practice safely, flight nurses caring for patients who require invasive hemodynamic monitoring must have knowledge of normal hemodynamic values, understand the significance of changes in these values over time, and demonstrate competency when using hemodynamic equipment. Table 21-4 summarizes the definition, application, and normal values of some of the more commonly seen invasive monitoring devices. Figure 21-11 gives an example of such a device.

TABLE 21-4 **Summary of Frequently Used Hemodynamic Parameters**		
Hemodynamic Pressure	Basic Function	Normal Range
Central venous pressure (CVP)	↓ when blood returning to the heart is reduced as with bleeding, dehydration, vigorous diuresis, or drug-induced vasodilation. ↑ with states of increased blood volume such as overtransfusion or overhydration, right ventricular failure, cardiac tamponade, a vasoconstrictive state, tricuspid stenosis, or insufficiency.	2-6 mm Hg
Pulmonary artery wedge pressure (PAWP)	A reflection of left ventricular filling pressure. Useful as a marker for fluid administration or restriction and used to determine the presence and degree of pulmonary congestion. A normal PAWP in the presence of a normal cardiac output indicates satisfactory ventricular performance.	8-12 mm Hg
Cardiac output (CO)	It is the product of the heart rate and stroke volume and represents the volume of blood pumped by the heart. It reflects the effects of drugs and fluids on the heart.	4-8 L/min (SV × HR)
Stroke volume (SV)	The amount of blood ejected with each heartbeat.	60-135 mL per beat $\dfrac{CO \times 1000}{HR}$
Cardiac index (CI)	Cardiac output calculated to individual body size. CO/CI measurements assess blood flow response to therapeutic intervention. Indications for use include increased pulmonary vascular resistance, right or left ventricular dysfunction, blunt chest trauma, mitral stenosis, mitral regurgitation, cardiogenic shock, volume disturbances, and major cardiothoracic surgical procedures.	2.5-4.2 L/min^2 CI = CO/BSA
Systemic vascular resistance (SVR)	Resistance to left ventricular ejection. Clinically, as SVR rises, cardiac output falls.	800-1200 dynes/sec/cm^5
Pulmonary artery pressure (PAP)	Pulmonary artery systolic pressure represents right ventricular contraction. PA diastolic pressure reflects resistance to flow by small arterioles and pulmonary capillaries. PA diastolic pressure is approximately the same as PAWP in the absence of pulmonary vascular obstruction. A positive difference of 6 mm Hg or more between PAWP and pulmonary diastolic pressure indicates the presence of obstructive vascular disease in the lungs such as pulmonary fibrosis, pulmonary embolus, or cor pulmonale.	PA systolic = 15-25 mm Hg PA diastolic = 8-15 mm Hg
Left atrial pressure (LAP)	Reflects filling pressure in the left ventricle. It is used to determine how efficiently the left ventricle is ejecting its volume. The higher the LAP, the lower the ejection fraction from the left ventricle.	4-12 mm Hg

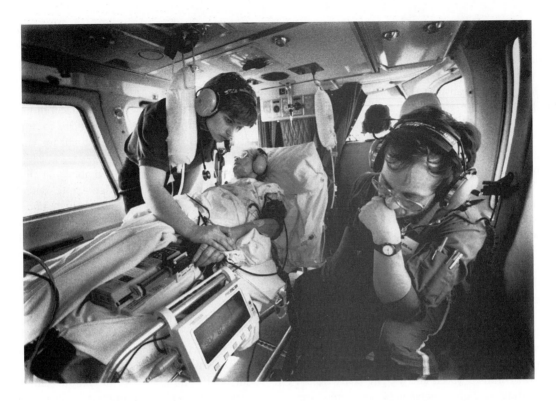

FIGURE 21-11 **The protocol monitor is an example of a multiuse monitor.** This device can monitor the ECG, noninvasive blood pressure, invasive lines such as arterial and pulmonary lines, pulse oximetry, and capnometry. (Photograph by Frank Salle; Courtesy of Metro Life Flight, Cleveland, Ohio.)

Preparation for transport of patients with existing intravascular monitoring lines varies from program to program; however, attention to detail and careful handling of the intravascular line are essential to avoid potential complications. When preparing a patient with intravascular monitoring lines for transport, the flight nurse must label all lines clearly, secure all connections, place sterile caps over all exposed ports, and maintain a heparin flush system during transport. For years, biomedical equipment designed for use in the hospital setting has been used in the transport environment with little research available to substantiate the accuracy of these invasive measures of hemodynamic status during air medical transport. Current biomedical devices developed and marketed for transport systems with features such as compactness, lightness,

durability, and screen lighting conducive to this environment have not all been tested specifically for the air medical industry. The stresses of flight, such as the effect of vibration on biomedical equipment and electromagnetic interference, has not totally been defined.[77,104] This emphasizes the need for the flight nurse to use a combination of invasive and noninvasive assessment methods to evaluate a patient's status throughout the transfer process.

THE NURSING PROCESS AND AIR MEDICAL TRANSPORT OF THE CARDIOVASCULAR PATIENT

The level of care during medical transport should be at the level of the receiving hospital. The goal for critical care transport is to provide equal degrees of monitoring and support as in the hospital ICU. Proper patient preparation, stabilization, and resuscitation will need to be completed to minimize any risk associated with transport. To efficiently organize the care and transport of critically ill patients, the flight nurse's performance must be consistent with the skills and knowledge as performed in an ICU.[15,36] Cognitive knowledge of the nursing process as it relates to the unique air medical environment is imperative. The nursing process helps the flight nurse formulate goals and a plan of action for the complex patients under his or her care. The nursing process-assessment, planning, intervention, and evaluation discussed next are related to air medical transport.

ASSESSMENT

Assessment of the cardiovascular patient begins with the initial information elicited from the referring agency by dispatch personnel. This information can be invaluable when selecting appropriate equipment for the flight (especially when flying in an aircraft with limited space and weight restrictions), anticipating in-flight emergencies, and preparing the receiving agency for the patient. Time en route to the referring agency can be spent developing a preliminary database and plan of care based on initial information obtained from dispatch and the referring agency.

For the cardiovascular patient, assessment and preparation for transport are directed toward recognition, prevention, and correction of hypoxia and maintenance of adequate tissue perfusion and cardiac output. The amount of time spent on assessment of the cardiovascular patient depends on the severity of the illness and the need for rapid intervention. The flight nurse should ascertain as much information as possible in the most efficient way possible to provide safe and efficient transport to a definitive care institution and to ensure continuity of care.[68]

A brief history of the event may be elicited from the patient, family members, or referring agency personnel. A general appraisal of the cardiovascular patient can be made while approaching the bedside and observing, at that time, skin color, diaphoresis, activity or position of comfort, and respiratory distress. The flight nurse should also observe whether IV infusions have been initiated and are running wide open, vasoactive drugs are infusing, and oxygen is being delivered; inspect all invasive catheters; and note what rhythm is on the cardiac monitor. An initial perception of the situation helps to organize and direct management of the patient for efficient and safe transport.[47]

Physical examination is often abbreviated to the situation using skill and judgment to determine what is vital and appropriate to evaluate under the circumstances. Hands-on assessment of the cardiovascular patient includes confirmation of vital signs and hemodynamic readings and the identification of implications for continued emergency care. Initial evaluation of airway, breathing, and circulation is done in accordance with basic cardiac life support guidelines.[40] If the cardiovascular patient is not in immediate need of cardiopulmonary resuscitation, the overall cardiovascular status should be evaluated. Any necessary procedures should be performed at this time, such as intubation, central line insertion, chest thoracostomy tube insertion, or additional therapeutic interventions (initiation or adjustment of medications). Stabilization and management by an appropriate critical care trained medical team takes precedence over speed of transport, unless the illness requires immediate access to the receiving facility (e.g., AAA [abdominal aortic aneurysm] with pending rupture requiring operative intervention).[36,68]

PLANNING AND INTERVENTION

Adequate management and preparation of the patient for air medical transport can greatly reduce the need for resuscitative measures in flight. Planning care for transport of the critical cardiovascular patient includes anticipating complications that may occur as a result of the disease process and preventing the predictable. This requires a strong, critical care knowledge base, orientation, and ongoing competency that encompass the principles and practice of flight nursing and meet the standards of the National Flight Nurses Association (NFNA; now known as the Air and Surface Transport Nurses Association).

EVALUATION

Throughout the transport process, the flight nurse systematically evaluates the patient's progress, analyzes data, and modifies the plan of care based on the patient's response to therapy. In the air medical environment, continual assessment and monitoring of the patient provide data regarding the success or failure of each intervention. The following case study illustrates the nursing process relative to the air medical transport of a patient in cardiogenic shock.

SUMMARY

Technologic advancement is driving the medical industry, which in turn affects air medical transportation programs. The air medical transportation industry must adapt to and be proficient in the ever-changing technology that patients and their families are using in their communities. It is inevitable that one day these patients will need emergent transportation, and it is imperative that the air medical programs be educated and prepared to properly care for them.

CARDIOVASCULAR EMERGENCIES: MANAGEMENT OF THE PATIENT WITH A LVAD

The primary goal of the VE LVAS patient-discharge/outpatient program developed at the Washington Hospital Center is to optimize patients' clinical status to allow them to return to their activities of daily living, as independently as possible, and in their own home environment. Additionally, patients and their significant others serve as the first line of defense should an emergency arise with the LVAD. Patients and their significant others need to be proficient in the daily management of the LVAD and in troubleshooting the device. To achieve this proficiency, an extensive patient education/training program has been developed, with one-on-one teaching of the patient and significant others with the VAD coordinator. The content consists of operational instruction, daily maintenance issues, and alarm troubleshoot-

ing with appropriate activation of the emergency response team. The patient is instructed to carry a travel kit of emergency backup equipment and reference cards at all times. Satisfactory completion of a written examination and return demonstration of specific emergency procedures are required of the patient and companions prior to clearance for hospital discharge.

With the patient independent in the management of the LVAD and prepared for hospital discharge, it is necessary to have the appropriate emergency response program in place for field emergencies. Developing such a plan requires a multidisciplinary approach, which would include at least the cardiac transplant team (i.e., cardiologists, nurse coordinator, nurse practitioner), the transplant surgeon, the VAD coordinator, the emergency transport team (i.e., chief flight nurse, chief paramedic, emergency physician, dispatcher), social services, the hospital's medical board and administrators, and risk management. The team's primary purpose is to develop a plan, discuss individual roles, and develop the necessary policies.

The primary participants in the emergency patient transport are the transplant cardiologist and surgeon, the assist device coordinator, and the flight paramedics and nurses, each with a specific role in the plan. The emergency transport crew, consisting of flight nurses and flight paramedics, is responsible for providing expert critical care, with superb technical knowledge and clinical problem solving during transport. The transport team is available 24 hours per day, 7 days per week, with primary accountability of the patient during the transport.

The development of the emergency transport plan must address the scope of scenarios for transport in the event of an emergency. It is necessary to identify several plans and choose the one(s) that will provide the most accountability for patient care, recognizing that patients are responsible for maintaining their proficiency with LVAD management and for having trained significant others available with them at all times. All plans have several advantages and disadvantages, which must be considered.

EMERGENCY PREPAREDNESS

In dealing with multiple emergency scenarios, each team member's role, including the patient, is to be clearly outlined in the protocols. In preparation for hospital discharge, the patient's power company is requested to mark the patient's home as a high priority for power restoration in power shortage scenarios. Patients are also expected to obtain and wear a medical alert bracelet, which identifies the implanted LVAD and an emergency contact number for trained emergency LVAD staff or transport team. The patient's local EMS jurisdiction and affiliated medical flight programs are identified prior to the patient's discharge to evaluate their involvement in the patient's care. Additionally, the patient is provided with written guidelines on the appropriate actions to take if an alarm indicator light occurs. If the patient is unable to rectify an alarm situation, it becomes the role of the specified emergency transport team to respond to the patient's call and transport the patient safely to a VAD-qualified hospital. In some cases, it may be necessary for a more local emergency room to stabilize a patient until a transport can be safely arranged. The delayed response of the VAD-trained emergency transport team may be due to inclement weather or unavailability of crew who are involved in a concurrent transport.

CREW TRAINING

The flight crew consists of a flight nurse and paramedic certified in management of the LVAD patient. The flight crew members are in-serviced a minimum of every 6 months and are certified in the operational aspects of the VE LVAS and in problem solving. Each crew member receives a copy of the operation manual and the hospital protocols. The VE LVAS training equipment is available on the unit at all times for review, and the VAD clinical specialist is available at all times as a resource for operational issues. It remains, however, the responsibility of each crew member to remain proficient and current with this technology. Each crew member is encouraged to meet the patient prior to discharge. The patient is given a tour of the helicopter and the communication center and meets

each crew member prior to hospital discharge. This helps to alleviate some anxiety for the patient. For the crew members, the opportunity to observe and interface with the device actually connected to a patient, and not a simulator, improves the staff's comfort level in caring for these patients in the field.

MANAGEMENT OF EMERGENCY TRANSPORTS

There are several key factors involved in management of a scene response and interfacility transports. The proper equipment necessary for a response to a patient on an LVAD, whether the problem is the LVAD or the patient, must be available to the crew. This is independent of whether the patient is in the field or at another emergency room. There may also be a significant change in the thought process involved in the response. Typically, the crew is focused on a standard "scoop and run" transport. In the scenario of the LVAD patient, it is crucial to spend the necessary time to ensure proper functioning of the LVAD prior to transporting the patient.

A transport bag is assembled and ready for an emergency call, along with the power base unit. The power base unit is primarily intended for electrical support of the LVAD when batteries are not an option. In the case of an emergency call, it can provide critical information regarding the hemodynamic performance and alarm status of the LVAD, provided that an electrical power source is available. Additional considerations would include alterations in the type of emergency support equipment that is available (e.g., heparin for anticoagulation during persistent, critical low LVAD flows) and the type of defibrillator patches. Medical Control also plays a critical role in these transports because coordination of communication between the transport crew and the LVAD clinical team is essential.

As the crew prepares to transport the patient, additional considerations include transportation of the patient's significant others and positioning of the crew and the patient in the helicopter. Proper positioning serves to optimize access to the patient and the LVAD for emergency interventions and monitoring.

EMERGENCY PROCEDURES

1. Follow advanced cardiac life support (ACLS) guidelines for all lethal arrhythmias except for compressions. This may damage the device and its connections.

2. Patients can be defibrillated, but safety measures must be followed to protect the electronics of the LVAD.

3. All hemodynamically unstable arrhythmias, including atrial arrhythmias, should be aggressively treated, especially if they affect right ventricular performance or preload.

4. External pacing is not recommended because the high voltage may interfere with pump function.

5. Hand pumping, a technique to manually pump the LVAD following mechanical failure, may be affected by high altitudes during air transport. A bulb syringe is used to hand pump air to the diaphragm, allowing for pump ejection and filling. The lower density of air at the high altitudes during air transport may have some effect on refilling of the bulb apparatus, necessitating more frequent refilling of the bulb apparatus.

6. Weight-based heparin is recommended for persistent low stroke volume states to minimize the potential for thrombosis caused by blood stasis.

REFERENCES

1. Abiomed 5000: The new standard of care for ventricular failure, *Abiomed, Inc training manual*, 1997.
2. Abiomed BVS 5000t: *Operator's manual*, Abiomed, Inc 2000.
3. *Acute ischemic syndromes: an interventional perspective*, The International Society for Computerized Electrocardiology 25th Annual Conference, April 29-May 4, 2000, Yosemite Fish Camp, Calif.
4. Alpert J, Sabik J, Cosgrove D: Mitral valve disease. In Topol E et al: *Textbook of cardiovascular medicine*, Philadelphia, 1998, Lippincott-Raven.
5. American College of Surgeons: *Advanced trauma life support for doctors*, ed 6, Chicago, 1997, Author.
6. Bader G, Terhorst M, Heilman P, DePalma J: Characteristics of flight nursing practice, *Air Med J* 14(4):214, 1995.
7. Bales A: Hypertensive crisis: How to tell if it's an emergency or an urgency, *Post Graduate Medicine* 105(5):119, 1999.
8. Benditt D, Sakaguchi S, Goldstein M: Sinus node dysfunction, pathophysiology, clinical features, evaluation and treatment. In Zipes D, Jailife J, editors: *Cardiac electrophysiology: from call to bedside*, New York, 1995, Saunders.
9. Blumen I: Altitude and flight physiology: a reference for air medical physicians, *Air Med Phys Assoc* V, 1994.
10. Blumen I, Rinnert K: Altitude physiology and the stress of flight, *Air Med J* 14(2):87, 1995.
11. Boden W, O'Rourke R, Crawford M, Blaustein A: Outcomes in patients with acute non-Q wave myocardial infarction randomly assigned to an invasive as compared with a conservative management strategy, *New Eng J Med* 338:1785, 1998.
12. Bonaduce D et al: Heart rate variability in patients with hypertrophic cardiomyopathy: association with clinical and echocardiographic features, *Amer Heart J* 134(2):165, 1997.
13. Braunwald E: Unstable angina: a classification, *Circulation* 80:410, 1989.
14. Braunwald E, Bristow M: Congestive heart failure: fifty years of progress, *Circulation* 102:14IV, 2000.
15. Braxton C, Reilly P, Schwab C: The traveling intensive care unit patient, *Surg Clin North Amer* 80(3):949, 2000.
16. Brodsky M et al: Life-threatening alterations in heart rate after the use of adenosine in atrial flutter, *Amer Health J* 130:564, 1993.
17. Camp D: The left ventricular assist device: a bridge to heart transplant, *Crit Care Nur Clin North Amer* 12(1):61, 2000.
18. Cannon C: Overcoming thrombolytic resistance: rationale and initial experience combining thrombolytic therapy and glycoprotein IIb/IIIa receptor inhibition for acute myocardial infarction, *JACC* 34:1395, 1999.
19. Capomolla S et al: Beta blockade therapy in chronic heart failure: diastolic function and mitral regurgitation improvement by carvedilol, *Amer Heart J* 193(4):596, 2000.
20. Carabello B, Stewart W, Crawford F: Aortic valve disease. In Topol E et al: *Textbook of cardiovascular medicine*, Philadelphia, 1998, Lippincott-Raven.
21. Cheitlin M, Macgregor J: Acquired tricuspid and pulmonary valve disease. In Topol E et al: *Textbook of cardiovascular medicine*, Philadelphia, 1998, Lippincott-Raven.

22. Chen S, Chaing C, Yang C: Sustained atrial tachycardia in adult patients: electrophysiological characteristics, pharmacological response, possible mechanisms and effects of radiofrequency ablation, *Circulation* 90:1262, 1994.

23. Cheney M: Medicolegal issues. In Topol E et al: *Textbook of cardiovascular medicine*, Philadelphia, 1998, Lippincott-Raven.

24. Congestive heart failure. In *Clinical resources by topic: cardiovascular disorders*, CCHS Digital Library, Univeristy of Alabama Health Services, accessed 2000.

25. Couper G, Dekkers R, Adams D: The logistics and cost-effectiveness of circulatory support: advantages of the ABIOMED BVS 5000, *Ann Thorac Surg* 68:646, 1999.

26. Crea F, Pupita G, Galassi A: The role of adenosine in the pathogenesis of anginal pain, *Circulation* 81(01):164, 1990.

27. Davidson J, Baumgartner F, Omari B, Milliken J: Intra-aortic balloon pump: indications and complication, *Journal of the National Medical Association* 90(3):137, 1998.

28. Eagan J: Life threatening dysrhythmias, *AACN clinical reference for critical care nursing*, St Louis, 1998, Mosby.

29. Every N, Parson L, Hlatky M: For the myocardial infarction triage and intervention investigators: a comparison of thrombolytic therapy with primary angioplasty for acute myocardial infarction, *New Engl J Med* 335:1253, 1996.

30. Falk E: Stable versus unstable atherosclerosis: clinical aspects, *Amer Heart J* 138(5):421, 1999.

31. Fotopoulos G, Mason M, Jepson N, Patel D, Mitchell P, Paul V: Stabilization of medically refractory ventricular arrhythmia by intra-aortic balloon counterpulsation, *Heart* 82:96, 1999.

32. Francis G: Pathophysiology of the heart failure clinical syndrome. In Topol E et al: *Textbook of cardiovascular medicine*, Philadelphia, 1998, Lippincott-Raven.

33. Fuster V, Badimon L, Badimon J: The pathogenesis of coronary artery disease and the acute coronary syndromes, *New Engl J Med* 326:242, 310, 1992.

34. Fuster V, Gotto A: Risk reduction, *Circulation* 102:94IV, 2000.

35. Gahart B: *Intravenous medications*, ed 15, St Louis, 1999, Mosby.

36. Gebremichael M et al: Interhospital transport of the extremely ill patient: the mobile intensive care unit, *Crit Care Med* 28(1):79, 2000.

37. GISSI: Effectiveness of thrombolytic treatment in acute myocardial infarction, *Lancet* 1:397, 1986.

38. Goldschlager N: Dysrhythmias. In Luce J, Pierson D, editors: *Critical care medicine*, Philadelphia, 1988, Saunders.

39. Grady K et al: Team management of patients with heart failure: a statement for healthcare professionals from the cardiovascular nursing council of the American Heart Association, *Circulation* 102:2443, 2000.

40. Guidelines 2000 for cardiopulmonary resuscitation and emerging cardiovascular care, *Circulation* 102(8):160, 2000.

41. GUSTO Investigators: An international randomized trial comparing four thrombolytic strategies for acute myocardial infarction, *New Engl J Med* 329:673, 1993.

42. Hass G, Young J: Acute heart failure management. In Topol E et al: *The textbook of cardiovascular medicine*, Philadelphia, 1998, Lippincott-Raven.

43. Hayes D: Pacemakers. In Topol E et al: *Textbook of cardiovascular medicine*, Philadelphia, 1998, Lippincott-Raven.

44. Helman D et al: Left ventricular assist device bridge-to-transplant: network improves survival after failed cardiotomy, *Ann Thorac Surg* 68:1187, 1999.

45. Hochman J, Gersh J: Acute myocardial infarction. In Topol E et al: *Textbook of cardiovascular medicine*, Philadelphia, 1998, Lippincott-Raven.

46. Hollenberg S, Kavinsky C, Parrillo J: Cardiogenic shock, *Ann Inter Med* 131:47, 1999.

47. Holleran R: *Flight nursing: principles and practice*, ed 2, St Louis, 1996, Mosby.

48. Cardiogenic shock clinical resources. In *Clinical resources by topic: emergency medicine*, CCHS Digital Library, University of Alabama Health Services, accessed 2000.

49. Hypertension clinical resources. In *Clinical resources by topic: cardiovascular disorders*, CCHS Digital Library, University of Alabama Health Services, accessed 2000.

50. Ince C: Percutaneous transluminal septal myocardial ablation in hypertrophic obstructive cardiomyopathy: acute results and 3-month follow-up in 25 patients, *Cardiology* 02(02), 1998.

51. ISIS–1 Collaborative Group: Mechanisms for the early mortality reduction produced by beta-blockade started early in acute myocardial infarction, *Lancet* 1:921, 1988.

52. Jett G: Left ventricular apical cannulation for circulatory support, *J Cardiac Surg* 13:51, 1998.

53. Jett G: Postcardiotomy support with ventricular assist devices: selection of recipients, *Semin Thorac and Cardiovasc Surg* 6(3):136, 1994.

54. Kahn J: Intra-aortic balloon pumping: theory and clinical applications, Cleveland, Ohio, 1994, Cleveland Metro Hospital.

55. Kannel W: *Risk stratification of hypertension for preventing target-organ damage*, www.medscape.com, 2000.

56. Kelley C, Furlong B, McKee A, Boyce S, McNicholas K: Rotor-wing transport of patients with biventricular assist device: challenging the transport frontiers, *Air Med J* 18(3):121, 1999.

57. Kenney M, Packa D, Dunbar S: *AACN's clinical reference for critical care nursing*, ed 2, New York, 1988, McGraw-Hill.

58. Kinney M, Dunbar S, Brooks-Brunn J, Molter N, Vitello-Cicciu J: *AACN clinical reference for critical care nursing*, ed 4, St Louis, 1998, Mosby.

59. Klein A, Scalia G: Diseases of the pericardium, restrictive cardiomyopathy and diastolic dysfunction. In Topol E et al: *Textbook of cardiovascular medicine*, Philadelphia, 1998 Lippincott-Raven.

60. Kovach B, Polk J: Transport Considerations: Getting from point A to point B on a ventricular support system. Kovach B, Polk J, editors: 2000. Unpublished.

61. Krause T: Abiomed BVS 5000 system: repair of venous cannulation site for excessive bleeding, *Ann Thorac Surg* 66:1817, 1998.

62. Lewis H, Davis J, Archibald D: Protective effects of aspirin against acute myocardial infarction and death in men with unstable angina: results of a Veteran's Administration cooperative study, *New Engl J Med* 309:396, 1983.

63. *Managing cardiac emergencies: year 2000*, Worcester, Mass, 2000, University of Massachusetts Medical School.

64. Marelli D et al: Temporary mechanical support with the BVS 5000 assist device during treatment of acute myocarditis, *J Cardiac Surg* 12:55, 1997.

65. Marelli D et al: Mechanical assist strategy using the BVS 5000i for patients with heart failure, *Ann Thorac Surg* 70:59, 2000.

66. Mayet J et al: QT dispersion in athletic left ventricular hypertrophy, *Amer Heart J* 137(4):678, 1999.

67. McBride L, Lowdermilk G, Fiore A, Moroney D, Brannan J, Swartz M: Transfer of patients receiving advanced mechanical circulatory support, *J Thorac and Cardiovasc Surg* 119:1015, 2000.

68. McCloskey K, Orr R: *Pediatric transport medicine*, St Louis, 1995, Mosby.

69. McKenna W, Elliott P: Hypertrophic cardiomyopathy. In Topol E et al: *The textbook of cardiovascular medicine*, Philadelphia, 1998, Lippincott-Raven.

70. National Cholesterol Education Program: *Detection, evaluation, and treatment of high blood cholesterol in adults* (NHLBI), Bethesda, Md, 1993, National Institute of Health.

71. Ogawa H et al: Circadian variation of plasma fibrinopeptide: a level in patients with variant angina, *Circulation* 80:1617, 1989.

72. Okumura K, Yasue H, Matsuyama K; Diffuse disorder of coronary artery vasomotility in patients with coronary spastic angina: hyperreactivity to the constrictor effects of acetylcholine and the dilator effects of nitroglycerin, *JACC* 27:45, 1996.

73. O'Neil W: Angioplasty for cardiogenic shock: are randomized trials necessary? *JACC* 19, 1992.

74. Pagani F et al: Extracorporeal life support to left ventricular assist device bridge to heart transplant: a strategy to optimize survival and resource utilization, *Circulation* 100:206II, 1999.

75. Park S, Nguyen D, Bank A, Ormaza S, Bolman R: Left ventricular assist device bridge therapy for acute myocardial infraction, *Ann Thorac Surg* 69:1146, 2000.

76. Parker J, Chiong M, West R, Case R: Sequential alterations in myocardial lactate metabolism, ST segments, and left ventricular function during angina induced by atrial pacing, *Circulation* 40:113, 1969.

77. Passini L, Eljaiek L: Verifying the reliability of biomedical equipment, *Air Med* 4(3):34, 1998.

78. Phillips B, Gandhi A, Sanoski C, Just V, Bauman J: Comparison of intravenous diltiazem and verapamil for the acute treatment of atrial fibrillation and atrial flutter, *Pharmacotherapy* 17:1238, 1997.

79. Poty H, Saoudi N, Haissaguerre M: Radiofrequency catheter ablation of atrial tachycardias, *Amer Heart J* 131:481, 1996.

80. *Pressure points: Critical issues behind the new emphasis on systolic blood pressure*, www.medscape.com, 2000.

81. Prinzmetal M, Kennamer R, Merliss R, Wada T, Bor N: Angina pectoris: a variant form of angina pectoris, *Amer J Med* 27:375, 1959.

82. Psaty M, Heckbert S, Koepsell M: The risk of myocardial infarction associated with antihypertensive drug therapies, *JAMA* 274(8):620, 1995.

83. Quaal SJ: Maintaining competence and competency in the care of the intra-aortic balloon pump patient, *Crit Care Nurse Clin North Am* 8:471-476, 1996.

84. Ridker P, Mason J, Gaziano M: Low-dose aspirin therapy for chronic stable angina: a randomized, placebo-controlled clinical trial, *Ann Inter Med* 114(10):835, 1991.

85. Rodkey S, Ratliff N, Young J: Cardiomyopathy and myocardial failure. In Topol E et al: *Textbook of cardiovascular medicine*, Philadelphia, 1998, Lippincott-Raven.

86. Roettig M, Tanabe P: Emergency management of acute coronary syndromes, *J Emerg Nurs* 26:S1, 2000.

87. Ross R: The pathogenesis of atherosclerosis: a perspective for the 1990s, *Nature* 362:801, 1993.

88. Rudd P, Hagar R: Hypertension: mechanisms, diagnosis, and therapy, In Topol E et al: *Textbook of cardiovascular medicine*, Philadelphia, 1998, Lippincott-Raven.

89. Samuels L, Thomas M, Morris J, Wechsler A: Alternative sites for ABIOMED BVS 5000 left ventricular assist device implantation, *J Congestive Heart Failure and Circulatory Support* 1(2):85, 1999.

90. Santoro G, Buonamici P: Reperfusion therapy in cardiogenic shock complicating acute myocardial infarction, *Amer Heart J* 138:S126, 1999.

91. Schneck D, Rivera A, Tricarico V: Emergency management of atrial fibrillation and flutter: intravenous diltiazem versus intravenous digoxin, *Ann Emerg Med* 29:135, 1997.

92. Sgarbossa E, Wagner G: The electrocardiographic diagnosis of arrhythmias. In Topol E et al: *Textbook of cardiovascular medicine*, Philadelphia, 1998, Lippincott-Raven.

93. Shettigar U, Toole J, Appunn D: Combined use of esmolol and digoxin in the acute treatment of atrial fibrillation in flutter, *Amer Heart J* 126:368, 1993.

94. Simes R, Topol E, Holmes D: The links between the angiographic substudy and mortality outcomes in a large randomized trial of myocardial reperfusion: the importance of early and complete infarct artery patency, *Circulation* 91:1923, 1991.

95. Spittell P: Diseases of the aorta. In Topol E et al: *Textbook of cardiovascular medicine*, Philadelphia, 1998, Lippincott-Raven.

96. Steadman E: Cardiovascular transport. In: Krupa D, editor: *Flight nursing core curriculum*, Park Ridge, Ill, 1997, National Flight Nurses Association.

97. Sugiishi M, Takatsu K: Cigarette smoking is a major risk factor for coronary spasm, *Circulation* 87:76, 1993.

98. *Surgical alternatives to transplantation in the patient with heart failure*, www.medscape.com, 2001.

99. *Systolic pressure or pulse pressure as predictors of cardiovascular risk*, www.medscape.com, 2000.

100. Tchou P: Ventricular tachycardia. In Topol E et al: *Textbook of cardiovascular medicine*, Philadelphia, 1998, Lippincott-Raven.

101. The Gusto Angiographic Investigators: The effects of tissue plasminogen activator, streptokinase or both on coronary artery patency, ventricular function and survival after acute myocardial infarction, *New Engl J Med* 329:1615, 1993.

102. Theroux P, Willerson J, Armstrong P: Progress in the treatment of acute coronary syndromes: a 50-year perspective, *Circulation* 102:2IV, 2000.

103. Thomas S, Stone K, Harrison T, Wedel S: Airway management in the air medical setting, *Air Med J* 14(03):129, 1995.

104. Topley D: State of the science: whole body vibration, *Air Med* 5(1):32, 1999.

105. Upton M et al: Detecting abnormalities in left ventricular function during exercise before angina and ST segment depression, *Circulation* 62(2):341, 1980.

106. *Vital Statistics of the United States*, Washington, DC, 1993, Public Health Service, National Center for Health Statistics.

107. Waldo L, Biblo L: AV nodal independent supraventricular tachycardias. In Topol E et al: *Textbook of cardiovascular medicine*, Philadelphia, 1998, Lippincott-Raven.

108. Williams S, Wright L, Tan L: Management of cardiogenic shock complicating acute myocardial infarction towards evidence based practice, *Heart* 83:621, 2000.

109. Zijlstra F, Van't Hof A, Liem A, Hoorntje J, Suryapranata H, deBoer M: Transferring patients for primary angioplasty: a retrospective analysis of 104 selected high risk patients with acute myocardial infarction, *Heart* 78(4):333, 1997.

110. Zipes D: Specific arrhythmias: diagnosis and treatment. In Braunwald E, editor: *Heart disease: a textbook of cardiovascular medicine*, ed 4, Philadelphia, 1992, Saunders.

PULMONARY EMERGENCIES

22

The transport of patients with medical disorders of the pulmonary system can be a significant transport concern. Oxygenation in many patients with pulmonary system disease is already compromised, and altitude or disconnection from set ventilators may have deleterious effects on patients with pulmonary conditions.[1] For the healthy person, alveolar oxygen tension (PaO_2) decreases to 65 mm Hg at 8000 feet with a decrease in arterial oxygen tension (PaO_2) to approximately 60 mm Hg.[2] Patients who have significant pulmonary disease may show signs of hypoxemia at altitudes well below 8000 feet. Severe tissue hypoxia can occur with minimal obvious clinical signs. Thorough physical assessment and the use of pulse oximetry and capnography may help the transport team identify and intervene in impaired oxygenation situations.

Richards studied the effects of commercial air travel on people with cardiovascular disease and respiratory disease.[24] Of 71 passengers with chronic bronchitis and emphysema, 40.9% experienced dyspnea during flight. There were also 3 cases of heart failure after the flight, and 4 people experienced cyanotic episodes during flight. Of 42 patients with asthma, 11 experienced dyspnea in flight. A total of 23 people with postacute pulmonary infections were evaluated; 7 had adverse in-flight effects. None of the passengers was acutely ill, yet most experienced adverse effects from the flights.[3] Patients with acute illness or injury are commonly transported, and the impact of pulmonary disease should be expected.

ANATOMY AND PHYSIOLOGY OVERVIEW

ANATOMY

AIRWAY

The upper airway consists of the nose, mouth, and pharynx. The pharynx extends from the nose to the larynx. The upper airway serves as a conducting system that warms, filters, and humidifies inspired air before it reaches the lungs. The pharynx branches into the larynx and the esophagus. The larynx contains the vocal apparatus, which includes the vocal cords, cartilage, and musculature. External landmarks of this area are the thyroid and cricoid cartilage, which can be palpated in the neck. The cricoid area is often the site for emergency surgical airway access. The epiglottis is a leaf-shaped, flexible cartilage that covers the larynx during swallowing. Its primary function is to prevent food and liquids from entering the trachea and lungs. The lower airway consists of the trachea, the right and left mainstem bronchi, bronchioles, terminal bronchioles, respiratory bronchioles, alveolar ducts, and alveolar sacs.[4]

The trachea originates at the distal margin of the cricoid cartilage at the level of the sixth cervical vertebra. It continues distally to the bifurcation, the carina, which is at the level of the fifth thoracic vertebra. In adults, the length of the trachea is approximately 11 cm with an internal diameter of 12 mm. The trachea accounts for approximately 20% of anatomic dead space (approximately 30 ml).[4]

The mucosal surface of the trachea is made up of columnar epithelium and mucus-secreting cells. The carina branches into the left and right mainstem bronchi. The right mainstem bronchus is straighter and more in line with the trachea than the left mainstem. This may result in the endotracheal tube passing into the right mainstem rather than the left during intubation or suctioning.

The right and left mainstem bronchi branch into bronchioles. The bronchioles have some cartilage, but consist of it less and less as the bronchioles progress distally. Further division gives rise to respiratory bronchioles that are the transitional zones between the bronchioles and the alveolar ducts. This is the transition between conducting airway and gas exchange areas. Alveolar sacs arise from the alveolar duct.[4]

The alveolar sac and pulmonary capillary are in close contact to facilitate gas exchange. The thin alveolar walls are made up of two types of epithelial cells, type I and type II. Type I cells are most abundant and are thin, flat squamous cells across which gas exchange occurs. Type II cells secrete surfactant, a lipoprotein that coats the alveoli. Surfactant facilitates gas exchange by lowering surface tension of the fluids lining the internal surface of the alveoli. This prevents alveolar collapse during expiration.[4]

THORACIC CAGE

The boundaries of the thoracic cavity are the sternum, ribs, and costal cartilage anteriorly and the ribs and thoracic vertebrae posteriorly. The clavicles and diaphragm establish the superior and inferior boundaries. There are two layers of pleura lining the thorax. The visceral pleura cover the outer surface of each lung. The parietal pleura lines the inner surface of the thoracic cavity. Between the two layers of pleural tissue is the pleural space, a potential space containing a small amount of serous fluid. The fluid lubricates the two surfaces to facilitate ease of movement. It also creates a cohesive force that assists in maintaining the negative pressure that allows the lungs to remain inflated. Many organs are found within the thorax, including the heart, great vessels, trachea, esophagus, thymus gland, lymphatics, and nerves.

MUSCLES OF VENTILATION

Ventilation has two phases: inspiration and expiration. Inspiration is an active process. Contraction of the diaphragm and the external intercostal muscles

increases the anterior posterior diameter of the thorax by raising the ribs and lowering the diaphragm.
As chest cavity size increases, a negative pressure
gradient is created, and air is inspired. The muscles
then relax and cause passive expiration.

The accessory muscles used in respiratory distress include the scalene and sternocleidomastoid
muscles, which assist with inhalation. The abdominal wall muscles and the internal intercostal muscles are used during active exhalation.

VOLUMES AND CAPACITIES

To assess the events of pulmonary ventilation the
air in the lungs has been divided into four
different volumes and four different capacities.[4]
Volumes are distinct measurements (Table 22-1).
Total lung capacity (TLC) is the sum of the
volumes. Capacities are combination of volumes
(Table 22-2). Pulmonary volumes and capacities
(Figure 22-1) are approximately 20% to 25%
less in women than in men.[4]

PHYSIOLOGY

Effective ventilation depends on an intact thoracic
cage, patent airway, integrity of the alveolar-capillary membrane, normal compliance, normal airway
resistance, and adequate nutrition.

ALVEOLAR-CAPILLARY MEMBRANE

Gas exchange occurs in the alveolar-capillary membrane. Several structures are involved in this
exchange (Box 22-1). Any change in these components alters gas movement across the respiratory capillary membrane.

TABLE 22-1 Lung Volumes

Lung Volumes	Amount	Definition
Tidal volume	500 ml	Volume of air inspired or expired with a normal breath
Inspiratory reserve volume	3000 ml	Extra air that can be inspired in excess of normal tidal volume
Expiratory reserve volume	1100 ml	Amount of air that can be expired by forceful expiration after normal tidal volume
Residual volume	1200 ml in a 70-kg patient	Volume of air remaining at end of maximum expiration

TABLE 22-2 Capacities

Capacities	Amount	Definition
Inspiratory capacity	3500 ml (~50 ml/kg)	Tidal volume plus inspiratory reserve volume—the amount of air that can be breathed beginning at the normal expiratory level and distending lungs to maximum capacity
Functional residual capacity	2300 ml	Expiratory reserve volume plus residual volume—the amount of air remaining in the lungs at the end of normal exhalation
Vital capacity	4600 ml	Inspiratory reserve volume plus tidal volume—the maximum amount of air that can be expelled from the lungs after filling to the maximum and expiring maximally
Total lung capacity	5800 ml	Maximum volume lung expansion with greatest inspiratory effort

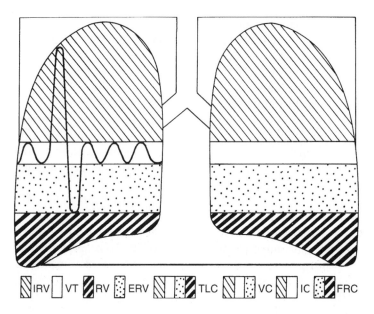

FIGURE 22-1   **Normal lung volumes and capacities.** *IRV,* Inspiratory reserve volume; V_T, tidal volume; *RV,* residual volume; *ERV,* expiratory reserve volume; *TLC,* total lung capacity; *VC,* vital capacity; *IC,* inspiratory capacity; *FRC,* functional residual capacity. (From Des Jardins T, Burton CG: *Clinical manifestations and assessment of respiratory disease,* ed 4, St Louis, 2002, Mosby.)

BOX 22-1	Structures Involved in Gas Exchange

Surfactant
Alveolar membrane
Interstitial space
Capillary membrane
Plasma
Red blood cells

The concepts integral to understanding gas exchange include diffusion, ventilation (V), perfusion (Q), ventilation-perfusion (V/Q) ratio, dead space, and shunts. Diffusion is the movement of gas from an area of higher pressure to an area of lower pressure, simply stated, from a greater concentration to a lesser concentration. Oxygen and carbon dioxide (CO_2) diffuse across the respiratory membrane.

VENTILATION-PERFUSION

Alveolar ventilation is the total volume of new air entering the alveoli each minute. In the normal adult male, alveolar ventilation is approximately 4 L/min.[4]

Perfusion is the amount of blood flow to the respiratory capillaries. Normally the amount of blood perfusing the alveoli is 5 L/min (i.e., cardiac output). In a perfect physiologic state, the ventilation of every alveolus is matched by an equivalent of perfusion, resulting in an equal V/Q ratio.

Various physiologic conditions alter the ventilation and perfusion relationship. When ventilation is less than perfusion, as occurs in atelectasis, more unoxygenated blood enters the systemic circulation. Conditions that result in blood entering the system circulation without passing through a ventilated area of the lung are defined as shunt units.[6] Anatomic shunting is the effect of blood that has not been oxygenated by the lungs traveling from the right to the left side of the heart, as with bronchial circulation.[7] Anatomic shunting normally occurs to less than 5% of cardiac output. Inspiration of 100% oxygen does not correct the shunt unit because all blood does not come in contact with functional alveoli. Shunting is the single cause of hypoxemia that cannot be rectified by delivery of 100% oxygen.[7]

When ventilation is greater than perfusion, a ventilation-perfusion mismatch occurs. A disease state illustrating this situation is a pulmonary embolus. This physiologic occurrence is defined as a dead space unit.[7] Dead space is the inspired volume of air that does not come in contact with pulmonary capillary blood. Anatomic dead space is made up of the conducting airways and is normally 2 ml/kg of ideal body weight.[4]

In the setting of poorly ventilated arterioles, constriction occurs, thereby diverting the blood to better-ventilated areas. Similarly, poorly perfused alveoli collapse, resulting in the diversion of airflow to more effectively perfused areas. This is termed a silent unit and helps to compensate for imbalanced V/Q ratios (Figure 22-2).

TRANSPORTATION OF GASES
Oxygen is transported in the blood as either bound to hemoglobin (97%) or dissolved in the plasma. The oxygen pressure (PO_2) reported on arterial blood gas analysis is a measure of dissolved oxygen only.

OXYGEN-HEMOGLOBIN DISSOCIATION CURVE
The oxygen-hemoglobin dissociation curve illustrates the relationship between hemoglobin saturation and PaO_2. This curve depicts the ability of hemoglobin to bind and release oxygen into the tissues. The relationship between oxygen content and the pressure of oxygen in the blood is not linear (Figure 22-3).

Various physiologic states change the relationship between hemoglobin saturation and PaO_2 (i.e., the oxygen-hemoglobin dissociation curve shifts in position).[8]

A shift to the left indicates an increase in the affinity of oxygen and hemoglobin. Physiologically oxygen does not dissociate from the hemoglobin until tissue oxygen levels are very low because there must be a gradient. Situations that result in a left shift include alkalosis, hypocapnia, hypothermia, and decreased levels of 2,3-diphosphoglycerate (2,3-DPG). 2,3-DPG is an intermediate metabolite of

glucose that assists in the dissociation of oxygen from hemoglobin at the tissue level. Levels of 2,3-DPG may be lower in patients who have received massive transfusions. This is related in part to the fact that stored blood is depleted of 2,3-DPG.[8]

The oxygen-hemoglobin curve shifts to the right in conditions that cause oxygen to dissociate more rapidly. In such cases, hemoglobin has a lessened affinity for oxygen, resulting in increased oxygen delivery at a cellular level. Physiologic conditions that result in a right shift include acidosis, hypercapnia, and hyperthermia (Figure 22-3).

The understanding of this relationship is significant to the flight nurse to allow for the optimum intervention for patients. The amount of oxygen transported per minute is a product of oxygen content and cardiac output. This represents the quality of oxygen transported to the tissues per minute and is contingent on the interaction of the respiratory system, the circulatory system, and the erythropoietic system.[8] These relationships are defined in the formulas in Box 22-2.

OXYGEN CONSUMPTION
The arterial-mixed venous difference in oxygen content is the difference between the arterial oxygen content and the mixed venous oxygen content. This difference indicates the actual sum of oxygen removed from the blood during circulation through the tissue. Normal oxygen transport is 1000 to 1200 ml/min. In normal physiologic conditions, the tissues use 250 to 300 ml. Therefore normal oxygen consumption is 250 to 300 ml. Mixed venous oxygen content values are determined from blood samples from pulmonary artery catheters.[10]

CARBON DIOXIDE
Carbon dioxide is transported in the blood by three mechanisms. CO_2 is dissolved in the plasma. This represents 10% of the CO_2 transported in the blood. Carbon dioxide also is moved by a chemical association with hemoglobin, carbaminohemoglobin. This mechanism affects 30% of the CO_2 transported. It is a rapid system and can bind more CO_2 than oxyhemoglobin. The final and most significant mechanism is a conversion reaction as bicarbonate.

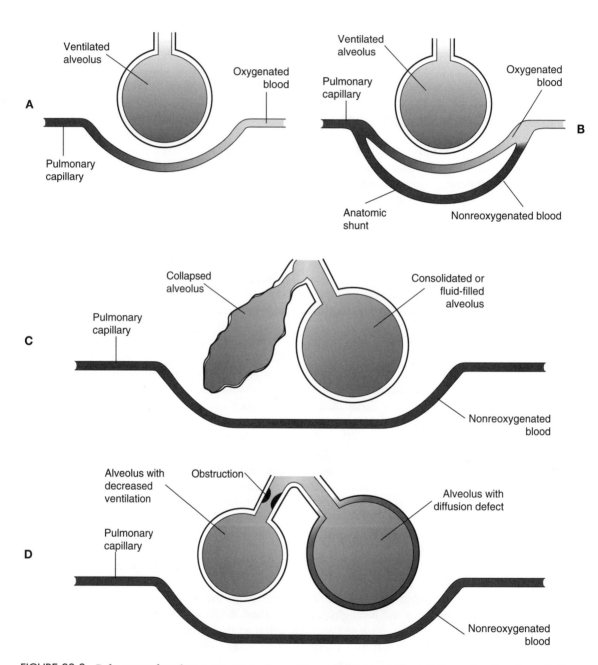

FIGURE 22-2 **Pulmonary shunting.** **A,** Normal alveolar-capillary unit. **B,** Anatomic shunt. **C,** Types of capillary shunts. **D,** Types of shuntlike effects. (Modified from Des Jardins T: *Cardiopulmonary anatomy and physiology: essentials for respiratory care,* ed 2, Albany, NY, 1993, Delmar.)

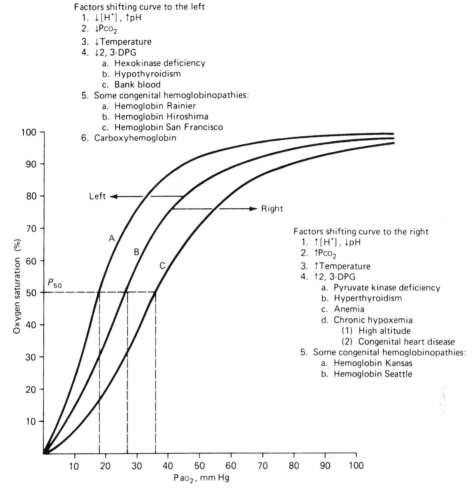

Factors shifting curve to the left
1. $\downarrow[H^+]$, $\uparrow$pH
2. $\downarrow$Pco$_2$
3. $\downarrow$Temperature
4. $\downarrow$2, 3-DPG
   a. Hexokinase deficiency
   b. Hypothyroidism
   c. Bank blood
5. Some congenital hemoglobinopathies:
   a. Hemoglobin Rainier
   b. Hemoglobin Hiroshima
   c. Hemoglobin San Francisco
6. Carboxyhemoglobin

Factors shifting curve to the right
1. $\uparrow[H^+]$, $\downarrow$pH
2. $\uparrow$Pco$_2$
3. $\uparrow$Temperature
4. $\uparrow$2, 3-DPG
   a. Pyruvate kinase deficiency
   b. Hyperthyroidism
   c. Anemia
   d. Chronic hypoxemia
      (1) High altitude
      (2) Congenital heart disease
5. Some congenital hemoglobinopathies:
   a. Hemoglobin Kansas
   b. Hemoglobin Seattle

FIGURE 22-3 Curve B is the standard oxyhemoglobin dissociation curve. Curve A shows the curve shifted to the left because of hemoglobin's increased affinity for oxygen. Curve C shows the curve shifted to the right because of hemoglobin's decreased affinity for oxygen. Factors responsible for shifting the curve are listed adjacent to curves A and C. (From Kinney MR et al: *AACN's clinical reference for critical care nursing,* St Louis, 1988, Mosby.)

BOX 22-2 | Oxygen Content Components

Oxygen content = (Oxygen capacity × oxygen saturation) + (0.0031 × Pa$_{O_2}$)

Oxygen capacity = Maximum amount O$_2$ blood can carry	Stated as milliliters of O$_2$ per 100 ml of blood (vol%)	Multiply hemoglobin by 1.34
Oxygen saturation = % of hemoglobin saturated with oxygen	Stated as percent	Sp$_{O_2}$ or Sv$_{O_2}$

Systemic oxygen transport (ml/min) = Arterial oxygen content (ml/100 ml) × cardiac output × 10 (conversion factor)
= 1000 to 1200 ml/min

TABLE 22-3 Low-Flow Oxygen Systems		
Apparatus	Oxygen Flow Rate (L/min)	Fio_2 (%)
Nasal cannula	1-6	24-45
Simple face mask	4-6	35-45

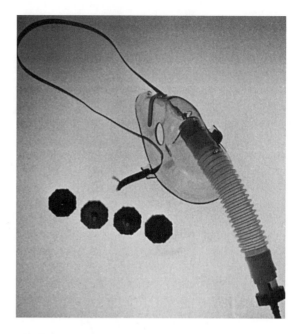

FIGURE 22-4   **Venturi mask and oxygen regulators.**
(Courtesy Richard Lazar, Stanford, Calif.)

This represents 70% of the CO_2 in the body. The bicarbonate reaction is slow in the plasma and rapid in the red blood cells.[10]

RESPIRATORY SYSTEM SUPPORT

OXYGEN THERAPY

Many critically ill and injured patients require oxygen therapy to augment the delivery of adequate tissue oxygenation. The most frequently used initial therapy for hypoxia is oxygen therapy.

Oxygen delivery systems are classified in two categories: high-flow systems and low-flow systems. Low-flow systems include a nasal cannula and simple oxygen face masks. These low-flow systems allow the patient to draw a supplemental amount of oxygen from the apparatus, and the majority of the inspired tidal volume comes from the room air within or around the apparatus. Therefore the amount of oxygen that is inspired varies depending on the patient. The flow of oxygen from a cannula or simple mask is constant. The concentration of inspired oxygen is variable and depends on the patient's minute ventilation[10] (Table 22-3). For example, a cardiac patient with a high minute ventilation inspires less oxygen than a patient with a lower minute ventilation because the patient with high minute ventilation uses a greater amount of room air per minute.[12]

High-flow oxygen systems include Venturi masks and nonrebreather masks. These devices result in the patient inspiring the total present fraction of inspired oxygen (Fio_2). Venturi masks operate by drawing oxygen through a narrow conduit that increases gas velocity and results in more room air being pulled into the mask. This high flow makes the concentration of inspired oxygen less dependent on the patient's ventilatory pattern. Venturi masks can render precise low concentrations of oxygen between 24% and 50%[11] (Figure 22-4).

Nonrebreather masks have a reservoir bag that fills with 100% oxygen. These masks also use a one-way valve that allows inspiration from the reservoir and precludes inspiration of room air. The rebreather ensures that patients inhale basically 100% oxygen, regardless of inspiratory effort[12] (Figure 22-5).

VENTILATORY SUPPORT

Many patients cared for by the transport team require some type of ventilatory support. Patients usually have endotracheal tubes in place and require assistance with a manually powered, self-inflating positive-pressure resuscitator bag system. These bag-valve-mask systems afford the ability to deliver high Fio_2s and effective ventilation when used by experienced practitioners. The percentage of oxygen delivered by simple bags is limited to 40% to 60% because the bag inflation surpasses the oxygen flow rate, resulting in the entrainment of room air.

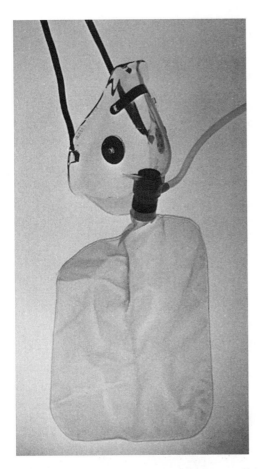

FIGURE 22-5 **Oxygen reservoir mask.** (Courtesy Richard Lazar, Stanford, Calif.)

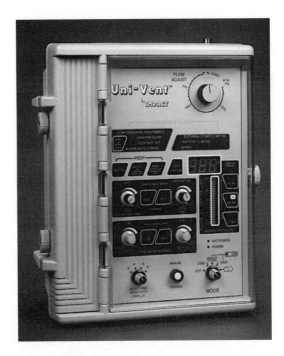

FIGURE 22-6 Example of a transport ventilator. (Courtesy of Impact Instruments, Inc.)

Resuscitator bags with reservoirs are capable of delivering FiO_2s ≥90%, provided that the oxygen flow rate exceeds minute ventilation.[13,16]

The effectiveness of ventilation with a manually powered, self-inflating resuscitator bag depends on the proficiency of the clinician. The transport team must constantly evaluate the compliance, resistance, chest rise, and other monitored parameters to appropriate tidal volume delivery. Spontaneous tidal volumes are approximately 500 ml; however, positive-pressure ventilation affects the distribution of gases in the bronchial tree. Therefore larger tidal volumes are necessary to maintain adequate alveolar ventilation. Typically 10 to 15 ml/kg is used, adjusted according to peak inspiratory pressure,[4] with anatomic dead space of the conducting airways equaling 2 ml/kg of ideal body weight. For a 70-kg patient, these values calculate to 640 ml required to deliver one normal tidal volume. Most manually powered, self-inflating resuscitator bags inflate to 1000 ml; therefore 64% of the bag must be compressed to deliver an effective tidal volume.

Numerous mechanical ventilators are available for transport (Figure 22-6). The primary focus of the transport team must be clinical understanding of mechanical ventilation and operational knowledge of the particular ventilator used.

RESPIRATORY MONITORING METHODS

Measurement of respiratory function during transport assists the team in assessing acute changes in pulmonary function. Chapter 12 contains an in-depth discussion of current methods that can be used to monitor a patient's pulmonary status during transport.[22]

ACUTE RESPIRATORY FAILURE

Acute respiratory failure can occur when chronic pulmonary disease or other factors affect the patient's ability to maintain adequate ventilation. Acute respiratory failure is defined as Po_2 of less than 60 mm Hg and carbon dioxide pressure (Pco_2) greater than 45 to 50 mm Hg.[20] The transport team's initial concern is for adequate oxygenation and ventilation for the patient, followed by management of the underlying process that led to acute respiratory failure.

RESPIRATORY DISTRESS SYNDROME

ETIOLOGY

Respiratory distress syndrome (RDS) is a lung injury that has many causes (Figure 22-7). It may be a complication of other diseases or injuries. It is most commonly seen in patients with direct or indirect acute lung injury (ALS). Direct injuries may include gastric aspiration or inhalation injuries. Indirect injuries result in hypoperfusion of the lung. This may be the result of severe hemorrhage, major burns, sepsis, multiple transfusions, multiple trauma, head injury associated with a change in mental status, pulmonary contusion, multiple fractures, and acute pancreatitis. RDS most commonly

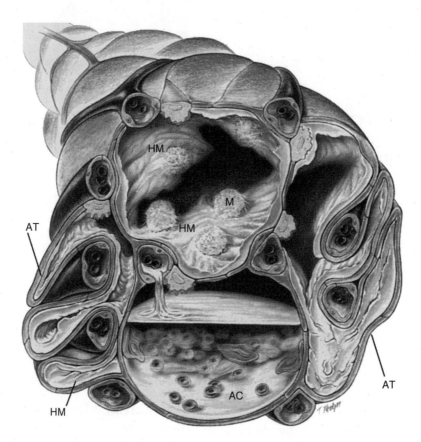

FIGURE 22-7   **Cross-sectional view of alveoli in adult respiratory distress syndrome.** *HM,* Hyaline membrane; *AT,* atelectasis; *AC,* alveolar consolidation; *M,* macrophage. (From Des Jardins T, Burton GG: *Clinical manifestations and assessment of respiratory disease,* ed 4, St Louis, 2002, Mosby.)

occurs in male subjects, and the mortality rate can be as high as 50%.[5]

PATHOPHYSIOLOGIC FACTORS

RDS results from a severe alteration in pulmonary vascular permeability, which leads to a change in lung structure and function. The outstanding characteristic is hypoxemia refractory to oxygen therapy. Fluids and proteins leak through the altered pulmonary capillary membrane, causing pulmonary edema and a decrease in lung compliance without concomitant congestive heart failure. Because RDS is a complication of other illnesses or injuries, the transport team must also consider the pathophysiology of the underlying problem.

ASSESSMENT

Assessment of the patient with RDS includes the history of the present illness to determine the predisposing factors leading up to the diagnosis. Patients with RDS report sudden onset of dyspnea, cyanosis occurs, and intubation with mechanical ventilation often becomes necessary. The patient appears in obvious acute distress. If the transport team is using mechanical ventilatory support for the underlying illness or injury, pulmonary compliance may decrease.[10]

Chest radiographs reveal widespread pulmonary infiltrates. Hypoxemia is present and may be severe. As the process worsens, accumulation of fluid in the alveoli significantly reduces pulmonary compliance. The patient's condition may progress to hypercapnia respiratory failure as the ability to maintain an effective minute ventilation is lost.[11]

INTERVENTION

Management of the patient with RDS is a challenge. Positive end-expiratory pressure (PEEP) is added to mechanical ventilation in an attempt to improve arterial oxygenation. In addition, PEEP increases functional residual capacity (FRC). PEEP is measured in centimeters of water, and the lowest measurement possible should be used to restore FRC. As lung compliance decreases, higher levels of PEEP may be required to maintain oxygenation levels.[5,18,27]

Supplemental oxygen is required because hypoxemia is very significant. Use of 100% supplemental oxygen may be necessary during transport. The oxygen delivery system used depends on the patient's condition.

The use of the pulse oximeter can help the transport team to monitor the patient's oxygen status. Changes in oxygen saturation (SpO_2) will occur with RDS, and subsequent changes may provide useful information for guiding other interventions. Ventilatory support with either a mechanical ventilator or resuscitation bag is required for patients with endotracheal tubes in place. If a resuscitation bag is used, decreased lung compliance, decreased FRC, and impaired gas exchange may make adequate oxygenation difficult.

Capnography may also be used to monitor gas exchange and pulmonary ventilation. Figure 22-8 illustrates a normal capnogram. Both pulse oximetry and capnography assist in patient evaluation and management during transport.[17,18]

Fluids should be restricted unless shock is present. The impaired pulmonary capillary membrane allows fluids to leak into the alveoli. In the presence of shock, fluids must not be withheld. The main pulmonary system goal of air medical transport is to maintain adequate ventilation and oxygenation.

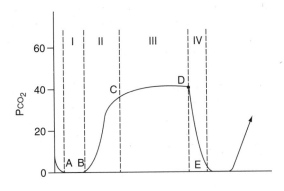

FIGURE 22-8   **Normal capnogram.**

CHRONIC OBSTRUCTIVE PULMONARY DISEASE

Chronic obstructive pulmonary disease (COPD) can be considered a continuum with asthma on one end, chronic bronchitis in the middle, and emphysema on the opposite end.[20] It is not unusual for emphysema and chronic bronchitis to coexist in varying degrees. Although each entity is discussed separately, it is important to remember that different degrees of each can be present in the same patient.

One should not discount the effect of altitude on the patient with COPD because their ability to increase ventilation and cardiac output in response to stress is limited.[31]

ASTHMA

ETIOLOGY

Asthma is an obstructive pulmonary disorder that results from airway inflammation and airway smooth muscle contraction. Asthma may be either intrinsic or extrinsic. Intrinsic asthma is more difficult to treat and usually occurs in patients older than 35 years of age. It is nonatopic in nature and has an unpredictable pattern of occurrence. Skin test results are negative, and the IgE level is normal. Extrinsic asthma is usually of an allergic nature and occurs early in life. Serum IgE is elevated, skin test results are usually positive, and it has a typical seasonal occurrence. Extrinsic asthma is more responsive to therapy than is intrinsic asthma.[11]

PATHOPHYSIOLOGIC FACTORS

Inhalation of pulmonary irritants and pulmonary infections stimulate bronchoconstriction, hypersecretion of mucosal cells, and edema of the airway mucosa (Figure 22-9). The airflow path is narrowed, reversibly, and results in an increased airflow resistance; there is a resultant increased work of breathing leading to increased oxygen consumption and increased oxygen delivery requirements. Alveolar hypoventilation occurs, which leads to hypoxemia and eventually retention of CO_2. The hypoxemia stimulates hyperven-

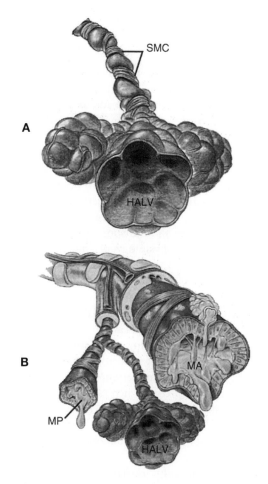

FIGURE 22-9   **Obstructive lung disorders. A,** Bronchial smooth muscle constriction (SMC) accompanied by air trapping. **B,** Tracheobronchial inflammation accompanied by mucous accumulation (MA), partial airway obstruction, and air trapping. MP, Mucus plug. (From Des Jardins T, Burton GG: *Clinical manifestations and assessment of respiratory disease,* ed 3, St Louis, 1995, Mosby.)

tilation with a resultant decrease in the P_{CO_2}. The obstruction of the lower airways by mucous plugs can lead to further alveolar hypoventilation.[9,14,16]

ASSESSMENT

The transport team should elicit a careful history to identify precipitating factors. For example, a viral illness may precede the acute exacerbation of asthma. The patient may report having a cough and dyspnea. A patient with a long history of asthma can usually rank the relative severity of the illness. A thorough medication history with regard to timing and dosage is very helpful. For example, a patient who has been taking steroids will probably require additional steroids during an acute attack.[3]

The physical examination reveals different degrees of respiratory distress based on the severity of the current episode. Tachypnea, wheezing, and a prolonged expiratory phase are not uncommon. If no wheezing is heard and the patient has difficulty talking, the transport team should consider the situation as emergent. Absence of wheezing may indicate that the patient is not able to ventilate sufficiently to produce breath sounds. Inspiratory retractions may be seen, as well as use of accessory muscles. The blood pressure is variable, and pulsus paradoxus may be present. Cyanosis and lethargy are late signs, and the presence of cyanosis or lethargy requires immediate attention.[3]

Diagnostic studies help determine the severity of the asthma. Resistance to airflow is measured by spirometry or a peak flow meter. Spirometric measurement of forced expiratory volume in 1 second (FEV_1) is done before and after treatment to ascertain treatment success. Peak expiratory flow rate (PEFR) can be accomplished with a handheld meter and has been used to determine whether arterial blood gas (ABG) measurement was necessary.[26,28]

In addition to measuring resistance to airflow, a chest radiograph may be done if other parameters are abnormal. Arterial blood gas measurement may be helpful in severe asthmatics. Table 22-4 illustrates the stages of asthma with corresponding ABG results.

INTERVENTION
Ensuring an adequate airway and providing humidified supplemental oxygen are initial interventions. Pharmacologic therapy includes adrenergic agents, anticholinergics, and corticosteroids, which are discussed later in this chapter. Intubation and mechanical ventilation are used only in severe cases. The indications for intubation and mechanical ventilation are listed in Box 22-3. Mortality increases for asthma patients who require intubation.[9]

EVALUATION
The transport team should evaluate the patient's condition at regular intervals to ensure success of therapy. A decrease in dyspnea or in the degree of tachycardia and absence of accessory muscle use are parameters to evaluate success of treatment. Obvious improvement in FEV_1 and PEFR measurements should occur. The patient should also be able to verbalize a subjective improvement in respiratory effort.

CHRONIC BRONCHITIS
ETIOLOGY
Chronic bronchitis is a chronic obstructive pulmonary disease that occurs most often as a result of

Stage	pH	Po_2	Pco_2	Interpretation
I	↑	Normal	↓	Hyperventilation: ED treatment
II	↑	↓	↓	Hyperventilation; ED treatment consists of correcting hypoxemia
III	Normal	↓	Normal	Obstruction prevents hyperventilation; patient may require hospitalization
IV	↓	↓↓	↑	Severe; ICU admission; may require mechanical support of respirations
V	↓	↓↓↓	↑↑	"Crossed" gases: $Pco_2 > Pco_2$; hospitalization and mechanical support of respirations after intubation required

TABLE 22-4 **Stages of Asthma**

From Hammond BB, Lee G: *Quick reference to emergency nursing*, Philadelphia, 1984, Lippincott.
ED, Emergency department; *ICU*, Intensive care unit.

BOX 22-3 | Seven Indications for Intubation and Mechanical Ventilation in the Patient With Asthma

1. Decreased level of consciousness
2. Progressive exhaustion
3. Absent breath sounds or severe wheezing despite therapy
4. pH 7.2
5. P_{CO_2} >55 mm Hg
6. P_{O_2} <60 mm Hg despite high-flow oxygen
7. Vital capacity decreases to level of tidal volume

---

cigarette smoking. Exposure to pollutants in the environment is also a contributor.

PATHOPHYSIOLOGIC FACTORS

The bronchi are the site of illness in the patient with chronic bronchitis. The mucus-secreting cells of the bronchial walls hypersecrete copious amounts of sputum, which prevents airflow into the alveoli. The alveolar gas exchange is normal, but the alveoli are underventilated because of the obstruction of airflow. Hypoventilation results in hypercapnia and hypoxemia. Figure 22-10 illustrates the pathophysiology of chronic bronchitis as well as emphysema.[20]

EMPHYSEMA
ETIOLOGY

Emphysema is a COPD that is defined anatomically as an irreversible increase in the size of air spaces distal to the terminal bronchioles. Most patients with emphysema are either current or past cigarette smokers. COPD develops in approximately 15% of smokers. Diantitrypsin may also play a role in the development of emphysema.[23]

PATHOPHYSIOLOGIC FACTORS

Pathologic changes begin to occur years before the onset of obvious symptoms. The alveoli are destroyed, supporting structures fail to keep the alveoli open, and the air spaces beyond the terminal nonrespiratory bronchioles are increased in size. There is an increase in the ratio of air to lung tissue in the alveoli. The alveolar capillary interface area is decreased, resulting in a decrease in gas

exchange. Air is trapped in the lungs, which increases residual volume. The expiratory phase increases as the increased resistance to airflow continues. The patient's vital capacity is close to normal until the disease has progressed to a severe stage. Retention of CO_2 is also a late finding. Figure 22-10 illustrates the pathophysiology of emphysema.

ASSESSMENT OF CHRONIC BRONCHITIS AND EMPHYSEMA

The assessment of the patient with chronic bronchitis and emphysema is very similar because the two entities often coexist in varying degrees. The history is important in determining the primary etiology of the disease. Exacerbations of stable states may occur with minor pulmonary infections, stress, changes in weather, or continued exposure to environmental pollutants (including smoking). The patient's subjective assessment of his or her condition is important to determine the usual status of the disease. The patient may report increased dyspnea, increased or a change in sputum production, or an increase in the malaise that may accompany the disease.

Physical examination of the patient may reveal rhonchi and/or expiratory wheezes. Rales may be present if the patient has an acute infection. The thorax is hyperresonant to percussion, and the anterior posterior diameter of the chest is increased. Observing the patient's respiratory pattern reveals pursed lips and flaring nostrils. During acute exacerbations, every possible accessory muscle may be used because of the work of

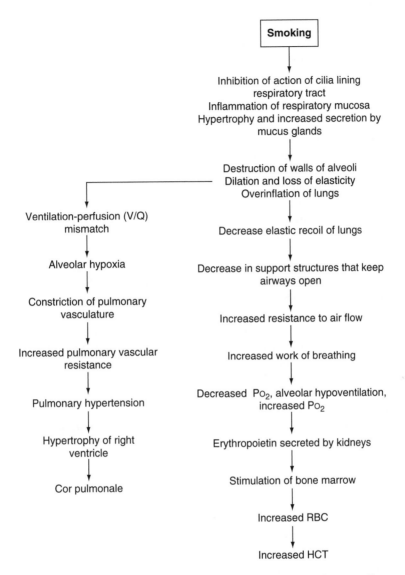

FIGURE 22-10   **Basic pathophysiology of chronic obstructive pulmonary disease.**

breathing. Patients with chronic bronchitis are frequently referred to as "blue bloaters" because they appear edematous and cyanotic. Conversely, emphysema patients are "pink puffers" because they are markedly dyspneic with a pink skin color. Tachycardia and the presence of dysrhythmias are also not uncommon. In the advanced stages of the disease, hemoptysis, fatigue, and weight loss may occur. Breath or heart sounds, or both, may be muffled because of the increased diameter of the patient's thoracic cavity. The patient frequently wants to sit and lean forward to better use accessory muscles.

The patient's mental status is an important component of the transport team's objective assessment of the patient. Retention of CO_2 occurs in the later stages of the disease process. Once the CO_2 level in the arterial circulation increases beyond the baseline level, one of the first signs is behavioral and emotional changes. The mental status changes may vary from confusion, irritability, and decrease in intellectual performance to obtundation.

Diagnostic studies include ABG measurement, chest radiograph, and electrocardiogram (ECG). The ABG results vary depending on the severity of the disease. It is normal for the patient with COPD to have a chronic respiratory acidosis compensated by metabolic alkalosis.[14] Chest radiograph reveals hyperinflation of the lungs, narrow and elongated heart shadow, increased anterior posterior diameter, and flattened hemidiaphragms in a lateral view.[23] The ECG findings are most often normal. However, some alterations that may exist include findings that may show low voltage (again, because of the barrel chest), large peaked P waves in the inferior leads, and right-axis deviation as a result of elongation of the heart, respiratory volume strain, and signs of cor pulmonale. It is not uncommon for atrial and ventricular arrhythmias to be noted on the ECG. Pulmonary studies are vital capacity and FEV_1. If either finding is less than 50% of normal for the patient, respiratory failure is present.

INTERVENTION

Supplemental oxygen is given to attempt correction of the hypoxemia to the patient's baseline level. In the normal person, CO_2 levels in the blood stimulate respirations. In the patient with COPD, the retention of CO_2 has rendered this reflex ineffective, and the drive for respiration becomes hypoxemia. Thus administration of supplemental oxygen should be at low flow rates (≤ 2 L/min) unless the patient is being assisted with respirations by means of a mechanical ventilator or resuscitation bag. Use of humidified oxygen is best to thin secretions.

The patient may require assistance with removal of tracheobronchial secretions. It may be necessary to administer IV fluids for rehydration. IV fluids should be administered cautiously because there is usually some degree of right heart failure. Cardiac monitoring is necessary to detect dysrhythmias. Often treatment with pharmacologic agents may cause dysrhythmia. Life-threatening dysrhythmias should be treated according to standard advanced cardiac life support (ACLS) protocols. Drug therapy is outlined in Table 22-5.[20]

EVALUATION

Evaluation of the patient with COPD includes assessment of the patient's mental status for changes in baseline. Any alterations should be aggressively investigated. ABG results must be matched with the patient's clinical condition. Febrile illnesses are generally treated with antibiotics, and hospitalization may be necessary. If intubation and mechanical ventilation are necessary for respiratory failure in the patient with COPD, aggressive pulmonary toilet measures should be undertaken and evaluated for results.

SPONTANEOUS PNEUMOTHORAX

ETIOLOGY

A pneumothorax is defined as the accumulation of air or gas in the pleural space (Figure 22-11). Spontaneous pneumothorax most frequently occurs in young adult men, but it is not uncommon in older patients who have an underlying obstructive pulmonary disease.[15]

PATHOPHYSIOLOGIC FACTORS

Primary spontaneous pneumothorax most commonly occurs from the rupture of subpleural emphysematous blebs. The blebs are most often located in the apices of the lung.[15] The pathophysiology is similar to that of pneumothorax caused by thoracic trauma. The lung collapses in varying degrees, and hypoxemia may occur. If the pneumothorax is significant, a tension pneumothorax may occur when the air is trapped in the pleural space under pressure.

TABLE 22-5 Drugs Used in Chronic Obstructive Pulmonary Disease

Beta Agonists
Bronchodilation, improve mucociliary clearance

Agent	Dose	Side Effects
Epinephrine 1:1000	0.3 ml SC	Tremor, palpitations, headache, excitement, nausea
Terbutaline sulfate	0.25 mg SC	
Metaproterenol sulfate 5%	0.3 ml/inhaled, nebulizer	
Albuterol	0.5 ml/inhaled, nebulizer	
Isoetharine	0.5 ml/inhaled, nebulizer	

Methylxanthines
Bronchodilation, improve mucociliary clearance, improve diaphragmatic contractility, enhance myocardial contractility, decrease pulmonary vascular resistance and pulmonary artery pressure

Agent	Dose	Side Effects
Aminophylline	5.6 mg/kg IV, loading dose	Nausea, vomiting, tachycardia, arrhythmias, seizures, palpitations
	2.3 mg/kg IV, loading dose (on theophylline prep.)	
	0.2-0.9 mg/kg infusion	

Corticosteroids
Controversial in emphysema, chronic bronchitis; used in asthma; used in acute respiratory failure if pneumonia and sepsis ruled out

Agent	Dose	Side Effects
Hydrocortisone	4-8 mg/kg, q6h	Cataracts, hypertension, diabetes, immunosuppression
Methylprednisolone	60-125 mg IV load	Adrenal insufficiency
	40-60 mg q6h	

Anticholinergics
Decrease in bronchomotor tone, smooth muscle relaxation

Agent	Dose	Side Effects
Atropine	1.2-3.2 mg, nebulizer	Dry mouth, dizziness, blurred vision, urinary retention
Ipratropium bromide	40-80 µg q6h inhaler	Dry mouth

ASSESSMENT

Patients frequently have chest pain and dyspnea. The amount of pain may vary depending on the degree of lung collapse. In the patient with underlying COPD, the patient's condition deteriorates in spite of aggressive therapy. The breath sounds are decreased or absent on the affected side. In the patient with COPD, it may be difficult to determine any change in breath sounds because of the increased anterior posterior diameter. If the hypoxemia becomes severe, changes in mental status can occur.

INTERVENTION

In patients who are asymptomatic with a small collapse of the lung, usually admission to the hospital for observation is all that is necessary. Symptomatic patients are usually treated with a tube thoracostomy.

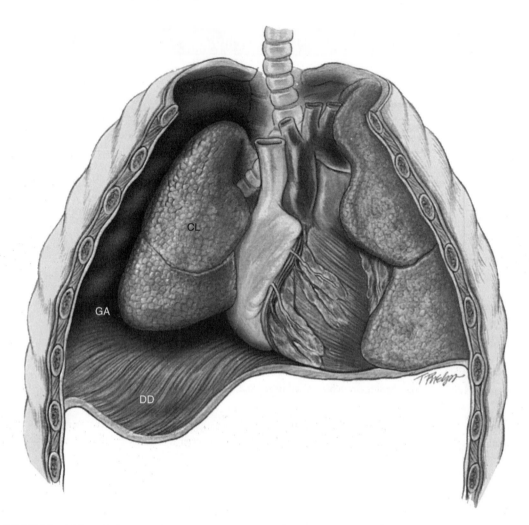

FIGURE 22-11   **Right-sided pneumothorax.** *GA,* Gas accumulation; *DD,* depressed diaphragm; *CL,* collapsed lung. (From Des Jardins T, Burton GG: *Clinical manifestations and assessment of respiratory disease,* ed 4, St Louis, 2002, Mosby.)

A chest tube is placed in the fourth intercostal space, with the anterior axillary line on the affected side.

The implications for transport, particularly air transport, are significant. Gases expand at high altitudes. The transport team should not transport a patient with a pneumothorax, even in a helicopter at low altitudes, without considering whether a chest tube should be inserted. If a chest tube is not inserted before transport, the equipment should be readily available to perform a needle thoracostomy in flight should a tension pneumothorax occur.[1] In transport-

ing a patient with COPD, baseline parameters should be closely assessed before transport. If the patient's condition deteriorates during transport, in spite of aggressive management, the possibility of a pneumothorax should be investigated.

EVALUATION

The evaluation of a patient with a pneumothorax during transport includes reevaluation of mental status, observation of rise and fall of the thorax with respiratory movement, observation for changes in SpO_2, and ensuring patency of the chest tube (if present). Reports of chest pain and dyspnea should also be addressed and reevaluated. Sudden deterioration should lead to an evaluation of signs of tension pneumothorax (tracheal deviation, jugular venous distention, absent breath sounds, or chest movement on the affected side). Any interventions taken during transport should be constantly reassessed.

PULMONARY EMBOLISM

ETIOLOGY

Obstruction of pulmonary flow by emboli can result in alterations in lung tissue function, pulmonary circulation, and heart function. Pulmonary emboli

contribute to the deaths of 50,000 to 100,000 patients annually and account for 5% to 10% of all the deaths in U.S. hospitals.[2] The risk factors include heart disease, cancer, immobility, estrogen therapy, disorders in clotting and fibrinolysis, multiple trauma, obesity, and childbirth.

PATHOPHYSIOLOGIC FACTORS

Once the clot is produced, the lysing system is unable to compensate. The clot travels through the venous system to the right heart and on to the pulmonary vasculature. The obstruction of blood flow in the pulmonary vasculature may be small, massive, or complete. The results vary, depending on the location and size of the clot. Figure 22-12 illustrates

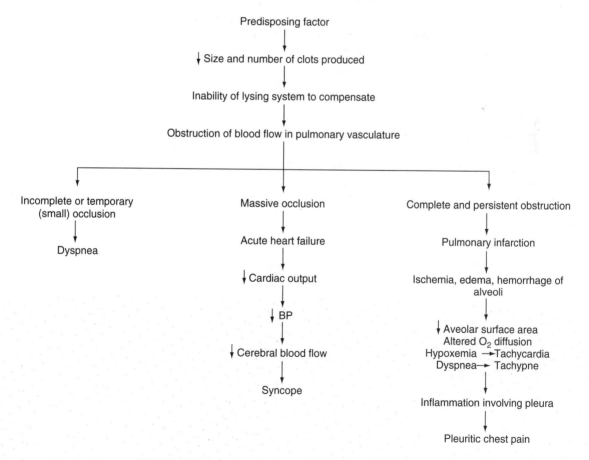

FIGURE 22-12   **Basic pathophysiology of pulmonary embolism.**

the different types of emboli and the resulting symptoms and effects.

ASSESSMENT

Patients with pulmonary embolism report nonspecific and variable symptoms. Lower chest pain, dyspnea, cough, hemoptysis, anxiety, syncope, and diaphoresis are potential symptoms. The transport team should suspect pulmonary embolism in any patient when signs and symptoms of cardiorespiratory problems are not otherwise explained. A thorough history is necessary to determine risk factors.

Physical examination may reveal fever, pleural friction rub, tachypnea, tachycardia, and anxiety. Although the patient exhibits signs of hyperventilation, ABG values reveal hypoxemia. The usual diagnostic tests are generally inconclusive in the patient with pulmonary embolism. The ventilation-perfusion scan (V/Q scan) is the test most often used to diagnose pulmonary embolism. To perform the scan, a small amount of radionuclide-labeled albumin is injected intravenously. After the injection, the labeled albumin particles attach to the pulmonary capillary bed. A pulmonary embolism reveals an area without radionuclide pickup, a perfusion deficit. The ventilation component of the scan assesses ventilatory function with the use of radioactive xenon. The perfusion and ventilation scans are compared, and a perfusion deficit without a correlation on the ventilation scan in the same area is supportive of a pulmonary embolism. If there is low probability and a high index of clinical suspicion, or a high probability scan result, pulmonary angiography is done.

INTERVENTION

Supplemental oxygen should be administered during the diagnostic phase. Cardiac monitoring should be continuous because these patients are at risk of cardiac dysrhythmias. Anticoagulation therapy is started once the diagnosis has been determined; the standard anticoagulant used in treatment is heparin. Some studies of pulmonary emboli reveal thrombolytic therapy is associated with more rapid clot lysis when compared with heparin. As shown in one study, a trend toward a decreased death rate appeared when pulmonary embolism was treated with urokinase followed by heparin compared with patients given heparin alone. However, many practitioners consider the benefits of thrombolytic therapy compared with heparin alone as yet unproved, therefore many patients are treated by anticoagulation therapy alone (current oxygen saturation [SpO_2]). Some physicians use thrombolytic therapy in patients with hypotension and low cardiac output in spite of treatments such as streptokinase, urokinase, and recombinant tissue plasminogen activator that have been used to treat pulmonary embolism. In patients whose conditions cannot be managed with heparin, thrombolytics, or a combination of these two therapies because of the massive size of pulmonary embolism or contraindications to medications, surgical intervention may be required.[30] Intervention may include embolectomy or placement of an inferior vena caval umbrella filter.

EVALUATION

Evaluation of the patient transported with pulmonary embolism includes a thorough history of illness and any treatment started. Samples for baseline coagulation studies should be obtained before the initiation of anticoagulant or thrombolytic therapy. The transport team should assess the patient's cardiopulmonary status constantly during the transport to allow immediate intervention should deterioration occur.

PNEUMONIAS

ETIOLOGY

Pneumonia is an inflammation of the lung parenchyma, caused by either bacterium or viruses (Figure 22-13). Table 22-6 lists the different types of pneumonia with their causative organisms.

PATHOPHYSIOLOGIC FACTORS

Lobar pneumonia is an inflammatory process in which the affected alveoli are diffusely involved. Bacteria, neutrophils, and protein pass from one alveolus to another, producing compact infiltrates. The dense alveolar consolidations prohibit volume loss and produce air bron-

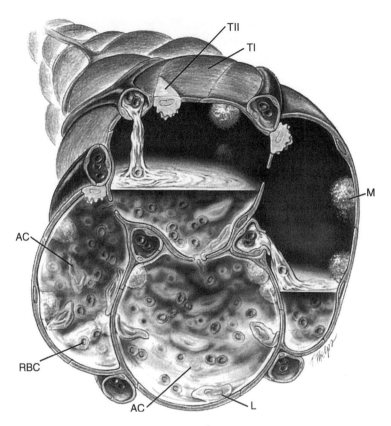

FIGURE 22-13   **Cross-sectional view of alveolar consolidation in pneumonia.** *TI,* Type I cell; *TII,* type II cell; *M,* macrophage; *AC,* alveolar consolidation; *L,* leukocyte; *RBC,* red blood cell. (From Des Jardins T, Burton GG: *Clinical manifestations and assessment of respiratory disease,* ed 4, St Louis, 2002, Mosby.)

chograms on chest radiography. *Streptococcus pneumoniae* and *Klebsiella pneumoniae* are the most common organisms that produce lobar pneumonia.

Bronchopneumonias occur with areas of normal lung parenchyma interspersed with affected lung parenchyma. It is multilobar and bilateral, with areas of atelectasis. *Staphylococcus aureus* is the most common organism. Interstitial pneumonia is the result of an inflammatory process that affects the support structures of the lung.

ASSESSMENT

The history of the patient with suspected pneumonia includes fever and purulent sputum production. The specific signs and symptoms for different types of pneumonia are listed in Table 22-6. In addition to a careful history, a physical examination should include not only a thorough pulmonary assessment but also an assessment of the patient's overall health.

INTERVENTION

The type-specific interventions are summarized in Table 22-6.

EVALUATION

Pulmonary status should be constantly reevaluated during transport of the patient with pneumonia. Mental status, SpO$_2$ readings, cardiac monitoring, and adequate V/Q parameters should be constantly assessed.

TABLE 22-6   Pneumonias

Streptococcus Pneumonia (Pneumococcal)

Organism

Streptococcus pneumoniae: Gram-positive, lancet-shaped *Diplococcus;* aerobe.

Risk Factors

Young, elderly, immunosuppressed, alcoholic, COPD, cardiovascular disease, diabetes mellitus, hyposplenia; highest risk occurring in winter months

Pathophysiology

Bacteria is normal inhabitant of upper respiratory tract; aspiration, inhalation, or hematogenous seeding are routes of entry; damage occurs from overwhelming growth, which impairs gas exchange

Clinical Manifestations

Malaise, sore throat, rhinorrhea, chills, fever, rust-colored sputum, pleuritic chest pain, nausea, vomiting, abdominal pain, tachycardia, tachypnea, dyspnea, decreased breath sounds, dullness, rales, pleural friction rub; in elderly patients change in mental status or congestive heart failure possible presentation

Diagnostic Findings

Leukocytes up to 40,000 ml with left shift
Leukopenia
Liver function tests abnormal
CXR: Homogenous lobar or sublobular infiltrates

Treatment

Antibiotics
Fluids
Oxygen

Staphylococcus Aureus

Organism

Staphylococcus aureus pneumonia: Gram-positive nonmotile spherical organism

Risk Factors

IV drug abuse, immunocompromised patients, and complication of influenza epidemic

Pathophysiology

Aspiration from upper respiratory tract leads to infections; growth occurs rapidly in the debilitated host; hematogenous seeding occurs in the dialysis patient or with IV drug use

Clinical Manifestations

Abrupt onset of fever, chills, cough, dyspnea, pleuritic chest pain; purulent sputum ranging from yellow to pink; frank hemoptysis common; toxic appearance; tachypnea, tachycardia, rales, rhonchi

Diagnostic Findings

WBC >150,000/ml
Positive blood cultures in 20% of cases
CXR: Bilateral lower lobe bronchopneumonia, early abscess formation or pleural effusion possible

Treatment

Antibiotics

TABLE 22-6 Pneumonias—cont'd

Fluids
Oxygen

Klebsiella Pneumoniae

Organism
Klebsiella pneumoniae: Gram-negative, nonmotile, encapsulated rods

Risk Factors
Men, over 50 years of age, alcoholic, heart disease, diabetes mellitus, COPD, aspiration

Pathophysiology
Results in necrosis of alveolar walls, multiple abscesses, loss of lung volume, friable blood vessels

Clinical Manifestations
Fever, rigors, dyspnea, productive cough, hemoptysis, copious purulent sputum that is green or blood streaked

Diagnostic Findings
Leukopenia or leukocytosis
CXR: Lobar consolidation, typically of right upper lobe; rapid appearance of lung abscesses; pleural effusion common; bronchopneumonia in lower lobes

Treatment
Antibiotics
Fluids
Oxygen

Pseudomonas Aeruginosa

Organism
Pseudomonas aeruginosa: Gram-negative motile rod, not encapsulated

Risk Factor
Second most common nosocomial, decreased host defenses or antimicrobial therapy, alcoholism, diabetes mellitus

Pathophysiology
Aspiration, necrosis of alveolar walls, multiple abscesses, loss of lung volume, friable blood vessels

Clinical Manifestations
Same as those for *Klebsiella* infection

Diagnostic Findings
Leukocytosis with left shift
Arterial hypoxemia
Hypocapnia
Positive blood cultures in 33%-50% of cases
CXR: Patchy infiltrates in lower lobes; cavitation, empyema

Treatment
Antibiotics

Continued

TABLE 22-6   **Pneumonias—cont'd**

Fluids
Oxygen

Haemophilus Influenzae

Organism

Haemophilus influenzae: Gram-negative, pleomorphic motile rod; encapsulated and nonencapsulated strains

Risk Factors

50 years of age; >50% have alcoholism, COPD; URI 2-6 wk previously
Encapsulated strain: Alcoholism, diabetes mellitus, COPD, impaired immune system
Nonencapsulated strain: Exacerbation of bronchitis, nonbacteremic pneumonia

Pathophysiology

Bacterial infection that produces inflammation

Clinical Manifestations

Minimal elevations in TPR, dyspnea, rales, rhonchi, pleuritic chest pain, nausea, vomiting

Diagnostic Findings

Leukocytosis
CXR: Bronchopneumonia, lower lobe and multilobular pleural effusions

Treatment

Antibiotics
Fluids
Oxygen

NEAR DROWNING

Each year approximately 4000 people drown in the United States.[6,21] The majority of these victims are pediatric patients and under the age of five. Drowning is the second-leading cause of injury-related death for children ages 1 through 14. However, any age-group can be at risk for drowning or near drowning.

ETIOLOGY

Risk factors for the occurrence of a near drowning include inability to swim, seizures, head injury, hyperventilation, myocardial infraction, and stroke. Alcohol and substance abuse also are great risk factors. Alcohol use has been involved in one quarter of drownings.[6,21] Unfortunately, near drowning may also be an indication of child maltreatment or abuse.

PATHOPHYSIOLOGIC FACTORS

The person who is submersed in a substance, most often water, will panic and hold their breath. They may also hyperventilate, which can lead to aspiration and swallowing of water. Swallowed water may cause vomiting and further aspiration of fluid into the lungs, resulting in direct pulmonary injury and hypoxia.

The primary effect of drowning is generally pulmonary injury followed by hypoxia and cerebral edema. Whether the water aspirated into the lungs is fresh or seawater, the end result is surfactant destruction, alveolitis, and destruction of pulmonary capillary membranes. This results in impaired gas exchange and hypoxia.[21]

BOX 22-4	**Drowning Prevention**

When children are around water (swimming, bathing), they must be watched by an adult at all times.
Never swim alone.
Never drink alcohol or use drugs when swimming or boating.
People with backyard pools, ponds, or who live near bodies of water should learn CPR.
Never use air-filled swimming devices (water wings) in place of life jackets or approved life preservers.
Know the local weather conditions to prevent being caught out on the water in a storm.
Follow beach warnings about dangerous tides, rip currents, or presence of danger in the water.

Modified from Carden DL, Smith JK: *Emerg Med Clin North Am* 7:255, 1989.

ASSESSMENT

The assessment of the near-drowning victim begins with evaluation and management of the patient's airway, breathing, and circulation. The evaluation should include consideration of whether the patient may have sustained a cervical spine injury from falling or jumping into the water.

INTERVENTIONS

The management of a near-drowning victim includes removal of the victim from the water, basic and advanced life support with cervical spine immobilization, and rapid transport. Wet clothing should be removed and dry warm blankets applied to prevent hypothermia.

The primary intervention for near drowning is prevention. Box 22-4[6] contains a summary of interventions to prevent drowning. Teaching and assisting in implementing these prevention strategies should be an important role for transport team members.[6,16,21]

SUMMARY

The transport of the patient with a pulmonary medical emergency requires knowledge of the common disease pathophysiologic changes. The effect of even low altitude on oxygenation in the patient with a chronic pulmonary problem cannot be overemphasized. The transport team must combine the knowledge and skills to affect a safe, expeditious transport of a pulmonary patient to the appropriate facility.

PULMONARY SYSTEM CASE STUDY

HISTORY

The transport team was called to the scene of a near drowning. A 15-year-old male was playing ice hockey with his friends on a farm pond. He suddenly fell through weak ice. He was pulled out by his friends, and CPR was begun.

On arrival of the transport team, the patient was found with a palpable pulse and a GCS of 5 (E–1); (V–1); (M–5), pupils 4 mm and both reacting equally. The patient's airway was secured with endotracheal intubation and RSI after an intravenous access was obtained. His wet clothing was removed, and he was wrapped in a warm blanket. A cervical collar was applied, and the patient was placed in a backboard and prepared for transport to the trauma center.

During transport, lorazepam and fentanyl were administered for agitation. His vital signs were BP 110/50, PR 130R, and assisted ventilations at 16. A pulse oximetry reading could not be obtained because of his cold extremities. His CO_2 was measured at 30 on the end-tidal monitor.

OUTCOME

The patient was admitted to the critical care unit where his LOC continued to improve. However, he developed pneumonia and sepsis, which was felt to be the result of aspiration of the water in the farm pond. Pseudomonas was cultured from his sputum. He required a tracheostomy for ventilatory support. However, after several weeks was able to have his tracheostomy tube removed and eventually made a full recovery.

DISCUSSION

One important point this case makes is the success of basic life support (BLS) at the scene by this patient's friends. Mouth-to-mouth ventilation was started immediately once his friends pulled him out of the water, resulting in a limited amount of time that the patient was without ventilation. Some experts also believe that the water temperature may also increase the chances of survivability.

REFERENCES

1. American College of Surgeons: *Advanced trauma life support-skills procedure, chest trauma management, needle thoracentesis* (student manual), Chicago, 1997, American College of Surgeons.
2. Anderson FA, Wheeler HB: Venous thromboembolism risk factors and prophylaxis, *Clin Chest Med* 16(2):235, 1995.
3. Bickley LS: *Bate's guide to physical examination*, ed 7, Philadelphia, 1999, Lippincott.
4. Bongard FS: Shock and resuscitation. In Bongard FS, Sue DY et al, editors: *Current critical care diagnosis and treatment*, Norwalk, Conn, 1994, Appleton & Lange.
5. Chapman MJ: Adult respiratory distress syndrome—an update, *Anesth Inten Care* 22(3):255, 1994.
6. Centers for Disease and Injury Prevention: *Drowning prevention*, Fact sheet, October 2000.
7. Cottrell JJ: Altitude exposures during aircraft flight, *Chest* 92:81, 1988.
8. Des Jardins T, Burton GG: *Clinical manifestations and assessment of respiratory disease*, ed 3, St Louis, 1995, Mosby.
9. Emergency Nurses Association: *Sheehy's emergency nursing: principles and practice*, ed 4, St Louis, 1998, Mosby.
10. Greene KE, Peters JI: Pathophysiology of acute respiratory failure, *Clin Chest Med* 15(1):1, 1994.
11. Grippi MA: Clinical presentations: pulmonary circulation and pulmonary edema. In Grippi MA, editor: *Lippincott's pathophysiology series pulmonary pathophysiology*, Philadelphia, 1992, Lippincott.
12. Guyton AC: *Textbook of medical physiology, pulmonary ventilation*, Philadelphia, 1991, Lippincott.
13. Jantz MA, Pierson DJ: Pneumothorax and barotrauma, *Clin Chest Med* 15(1):75, 1994.
14. Jordan K, editor: *Emergency nursing core curriculum*, ed 5, Philadelphia, 2000, Saunders.
15. Kirby TJ, Ginsberg RJ: Management of the pneumothorax and barotrauma, *Clin Chest Med* 13(1):97, 1992.
16. Krupa D: *Flight nursing core curriculum*, Des Plaines, Ill, 1997, Road Runner Press.
17. Lake CL, Hines RL, Blitt CD: *Clinical monitoring: practical applications for anesthesia and critical care*, Philadelphia, 2001, Saunders.
18. Lynn-McHale DJ, Carlson K: *AACN procedure manual for critical care*, ed 4, Philadelphia, 2001, Saunders.
19. Mills FJ, Harding RM: Fitness to travel by air: physiological considerations, *Br Med J* 286:1269, 1983.
20. Neagley SR: The pulmonary system. In Alspach JG, editor: *Core curriculum for critical care nursing*, Philadelphia, 1991, Saunders.
21. Newman AB: Submersion incidents. In Auerbach P, editor, *Wilderness medicine*, ed 4, St Louis, 2001, Mosby.
22. Oranato JP et al: Multicenter study of a portable handsize colormetric end-tidal carbon detection device, *Ann Emerg Med* 21(5):518, 1992.
23. Panettieri RA: Chronic obstructive pulmonary disease. In Grippi MA, editor, *Lippincott's pathophysiology series pulmonary pathophysiology*, Philadelphia, 1992, Lippincott.
24. Richards PR: The effects of air travel on passengers with cardiovascular and respiratory disease, *Practitioner* 210:232, 1973.
25. Santa Clara Valley California Poison Control: *Patient management guidelines*, 1995, The Poison Control.
26. Scanlan CL, Spearman CB, Sheldon RL: *Egan's fundamentals of respiratory care*, St Louis, 1990, Mosby.
27. Schwartz AJ, Campbell FW: Cardiopulmonary resuscitation. In Barash PG, Cullen BF, Stoeling RK, editors: *Clinical anesthesia*, ed 2, Philadelphia, 1992, Lippincott.
28. Shapiro BA, Harrison RA, Walton JR: *Clinical application of blood gases*, St Louis, 1982, Mosby.
29. Sue DY: Pulmonary disease. In Bongard FS, Sue DY et al, editors: *Current critical care diagnosis and treatment*, Norwalk, Conn, 1994, Appleton & Lange.
30. Sue DY: Respiratory failure. In Bongard FS, Sue DY et al, editors: *Current critical care diagnosis and treatment*, Norwalk, Conn, 1994, Appleton & Lange.
31. Urden LD, Davie JK, Thelan LA: *Essentials of critical care nursing*, St Louis, 1992, Mosby.

ABDOMINAL EMERGENCIES

1. Perform a comprehensive assessment of the patient with an abdominal emergency.
2. Initiate the critical interventions for the management of the patient with an abdominal emergency during transport.
3. Provide care for the patient with a specific abdominal emergency during transport.

Disorders encountered by transport teams may include esophageal obstruction and varices with rupture; stomach disorders, such as gastric or duodenal hemorrhage, ulceration, perforation, or pyloric obstruction; gallbladder and biliary tract disorders; liver disease; pancreatic disorders; and intestinal obstruction or rupture, ruptured diverticula, and acute appendicitis.

Transport by air may cause specific problems for the patient with an abdominal emergency.[3] The aerodynamics and biophysics that govern air medical care are especially important in relation to the gastrointestinal (GI) system, which encompasses 26 feet of liquid- and gas-producing viscous. Careful patient history, assessment, and preflight planning are imperative for the patient transported by air.

ESOPHAGUS

The esophagus is a hollow tube of striated and smooth muscle that is approximately 10 inches long in an adult. Lying posteriorly to the trachea and closely aligning the left mainstem bronchus, the esophagus exits the thoracic cavity at the diaphragmatic hiatus, or approximately at the T11 level. The esophagus provides the primary functions of peristaltic movement of food bolus, prevention of reflux by lower esophageal sphincter activity, and venting for gastric pressure changes.

Vascular supply to the esophagus is through branches of the descending thoracic aorta. Venous return from the esophagus is through the superior vena cava, azygos system, and portal vein system.

Neurologic intervention is initiated in the medulla and carried out by the vagus nerve. Because the esophagus lies in the thoracic cavity, under normal atmospheric conditions it maintains a subatmospheric pressure of −5 to −10 mm Hg, whereas the stomach, which is in the abdominal cavity, rests at an atmospheric pressure of +5 to +10 mm Hg. Acute esophageal occurrences are esophageal obstruction, esophageal varices, and esophageal rupture.

ESOPHAGEAL OBSTRUCTION

Three areas in the esophagus are narrow and may be potential sites for obstruction and injury. These include the cricoid cartilage, the arch of aorta, and the point at which the esophagus passes through the diaphragm.[2]

Esophageal obstruction is fairly common. Strictures, webs, tumors, diverticula, foreign bodies, achalasia, and lower esophageal rings can all reduce or eliminate the venting property of the esophagus for the upper GI system. When air medical transport of obstructed patients is undertaken, intermittent exposure to variations in altitude is of great importance. Esophageal obstruction and an expanding gastrum can pose a serious threat if rapid decompression occurs at 35,000 feet. The venting property needs to be established before flight and depends on whether rotor-wing or fixed-wing transport is to be used.

ASSESSMENT

The transport team should correlate careful physical assessment with interpretation of radiologic and laboratory data to anticipate any potential problems that may occur during the transport process.

Subjective Data. The transport team should ascertain the patient's chief complaint and past medical history. Included in these subjective data should be the clinical course the patient has taken since the incident occurred. Past medical history will help the transport team identify any other additional problems that may arise during transport.

Objective Data. The flight nurse performs a physical examination that includes assessment of the following:

- Patient's ability to protect their airway
- Ability to clear secretions by swallowing
- Presence and location of pain

DIAGNOSTIC TESTS

Radiographic studies of the obstruction should accompany the patient. If an esophagoscopy has been performed, a report should be provided to the transport team so they can prepare for any potential problems that may occur during transport.

PLAN AND IMPLEMENTATION

If the patient is being transported by air, the plan of care will depend on the anticipated transport altitude. The transport team should carefully evaluate the patient's ability to maintain the airway. Even with aircraft pressurization, ensuring adequate gastric venting is extremely important if high altitude will be maintained. Preflight medications and antiemetic therapy are often helpful not only for the antiemetic effect but also for the associated drowsiness. A gastric tube should be placed (if not contraindicated) and gastric contents emptied before and during transport. If the gastric tube is hooked to suction, its flow and contents should be closely monitored during transport. Continuous monitoring of respiratory status is also necessary.

INTERVENTION

Caution must be exercised when a patient is placed on suction devices during transport; intermittent disconnection of suction from the gastric tube allows the pressures to regurgitate and prevents extreme suction against the gastric wall.

Esophageal obstructions are a common occurrence, and most likely air medical transport is being requested because the patient has an acute condition.

Children with a potential esophageal obstruction may benefit from allowing a parent or other caregiver to accompany them to decrease their anxiety and prevent crying or other movement that may increase the risk of airway compromise.

ESOPHAGEAL VARICES

The most common cause of varices is hepatic congestion. Torturous, fragile, dilated esophageal veins can bleed from spontaneous rupture caused by increased portal hypertension or physical or chemical trauma. Esophageal varices are usually associated with persons with cirrhosis. Varices occur frequently at the distal esophagus and hemorrhoidal plexus, and hemorrhagic shock from an esophageal bleed can occur rapidly.

ASSESSMENT

Sequential history of the patient with esophageal varices will help the transport team anticipate probable needs during transport.

Subjective Data. The transport team should obtain a history related to the cause of the esophageal varices, which can also provide information about other potential problems that could develop during transport. For example, the patient with severe liver disease will also have bleeding problems.

Objective Data. Careful consideration of the patient's most recent preflight laboratory data (hematocrit and hemoglobin levels, PT/PTT or INR, and electrolyte level) will help the transport team anticipate the patient's needs during transport. If the patient is transported directly from the scene, procurement of a blood bank specimen may be of use on admission.

If transport is between medical facilities, a transport team member should review radiologic findings and ensure that adequate interventions have occurred. If a patient has undergone angiography, the transport team must secure the cannulization site before any patient movement and monitor the site frequently throughout transport.

PLAN AND IMPLEMENTATION

The transport team's primary priority is to ensure adequacy of the airway before transport. The transport team should consider the volume that may be needed in the event an acute hemorrhagic episode during transport. Continuous gastric suction can produce large volumes of secretions, and a system to adequately dispose of secretions during transport needs to be ready, such as having available a supply of sealable bags or containers with tight seals.

As with all patient care, standard precautions should be observed. Adequate suction, IV fluids, blood, and irrigating fluid all need to be secured before transport. An experienced transport member must maintain adequate care of esophageal tubes, such as the Sengstaken-Blakemore, Linton, or Minnesota tubes, if one is in place. Even though these devices are rarely used anymore, traction-dependent or specialized esophageal tubes can pose a problem for transport. Traction maintained with a football helmet can be used during transport (Figure 23-1). A plan of care must be predetermined in the event of airway loss.

Airway loss from these particular types of tubes can be from either physiologic deterioration or tracheal obstruction. Saline solution, rather than air, can be used to inflate these cuffs to prevent further expansion during flight.

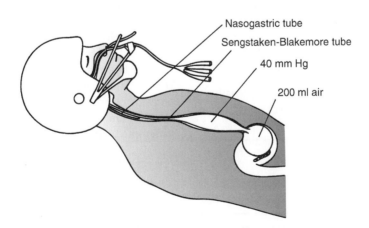

Nasogastric tube

Sengstaken-Blakemore tube

40 mm Hg

200 ml air

FIGURE 23-1   **Traction maintained with football helmet for Sengstaken-Blakemore tube.**

INTERVENTION

If an acute hemorrhagic episode occurs, maintenance of airway and circulating volume is the first priority. Effective pretransport planning to prevent vomiting and ensure adequate venous access and volume resuscitation is crucial.

ESOPHAGEAL RUPTURE

Esophageal rupture commonly results from penetrating trauma but may also result from a blunt insult to the thorax. Rupture from invading lesions, tumors, or caustic exposure also occurs but to a lesser extent. If esophageal rupture has occurred, the venting properties and pathways have been altered. During transport, and with possible altitude changes, the distribution and displacement of gases are no longer circumvented by the appropriate course. Complications of gastric pneumonitis, hemopneumothorax, and alteration in gas exchange may all occur.

ASSESSMENT

The transport team ascertains the history of incidents that led to the current episode. Drugs known to have corrosive effects on the esophagus are doxycycline, tetracycline, acetylsalicylic acid, clindamycin, potassium chloride, quinidine, and ferrous sulfate. Caustic substances can quickly lead to burning or complete erosion of the tissue. Estimation of the degree and size of burns is extremely difficult and can quickly compromise respiratory status. If the rupture is caused by an extravasating tumor, hemorrhage and airway control can become quite difficult.

PLAN AND IMPLEMENTATION PRIORITIES

The transport teams' priorities are as follows:

1. Ascertain adequacy of airway and oxygenation.
2. Maintain adequate venous access and volume support.
3. Place gastric tube with adequate suctioning if it is not contraindicated.

STOMACH

The stomach lies beneath the diaphragm and is secured in the peritoneum by the lesser omentum.

The stomach is subject to alterations in intra-abdominal pressure, unlike the esophagus, which has negative atmospheric pressure. The cardiac sphincter separates the esophagus from the stomach. Vascular supply is from the celiac artery branches, and venous return is through the superior mesenteric, splenic, and portal veins.

The stomach functions as a receptacle of ingested substances and attempts to provide chemical and mechanical breakdown. As the stomach expands, peristaltic action increases. The average time of gastric emptying is 1 to 8 hours. Chyme is then propelled through the pyloric sphincter into the duodenum. Decreased gastric motility and alterations in altitude can lead to complications.

ACUTE GASTRIC OCCURRENCES

Acute gastric occurrences can take the form of gastric duodenal hemorrhage, gastric perforation from both mechanical and chemical means, pyloric obstruction, and gastric and duodenal ulceration.

Bleeding from peptic or duodenal ulceration occurs more frequently than does esophageal variceal bleeding. Several methods may be used to manage the bleeding, including insertion of GI tubes, such as Linton or Minnesota tubes (rarely used anymore for the management of bleeding esophageal varices); pharmacologic management; endoscopy; thermal therapy; and if bleeding is massive and cannot be controlled, surgery.[1,5] Anticipatory planning and thorough preparation can ensure a safe patient transport.

Ulcerative lesions of the stomach or duodenum that lead to bleeding or perforation are in part caused by mucosal membrane erosion. The tissue beneath the mucosa is then subjected to general tissue corrosion. Ulcerations can lead to hemorrhage, perforation, or obstruction and may occur after an attempted repair.

INTERVENTION

In the event of an acute hemorrhagic episode during transport, a transport team member should perform volume resuscitation and gastric saline lavage, and attempts to stop bleeding must be made. Complications may arise if the gastric tube becomes obstructed. Gastric dilation and excessive hydrochloric acid can cause nausea and vomiting, which may mechanically induce hemorrhage. Maintenance of adequate gastric venting is imperative throughout any altitude changes when the patient is transported by air.

Movement can make patients nauseated whether by air or ground. The transport team should provide antiemetics and sedation to decrease the risk of vomiting, which may precipitate bleeding during transport.

GALLBLADDER AND BILIARY TRACT

The primary function of the gallbladder and biliary tract is to receive approximately 2 L of bile a day from the liver. Bile, which is stimulated not only by food ingestion but also by stress and acute illness, flows into the duodenum through the common bile duct. Fluid and electrolyte reabsorption takes place in the gallbladder before the bile enters the duodenum; therefore, with generalized volume deficit, an even more concentrated efficacious bile enters the duodenum.

Bile, which is composed of fatty acids, bile salts, phospholipid, cholesterol, conjugated bilirubin, and water, mixes with the chyme to aid digestion.

The ampulla of Vater and Oddi's sphincter are common sites of disease or injury that dramatically affect the entire tract. The gallbladder and biliary tracts are stimulated sympathetically by the splanchnic nerve and parasympathetically by the vagus. Vascular supply is provided by the hepatic artery and cystic vein.

Gallbladder and biliary disorders that necessitate acute air medical transport are infrequent. However, necrotic gangrenous cholecystitis can progress to septicemia, acute pancreatitis, or gallbladder rupture, hepatic failure, or both, because of obstructional flow of bile production.

PLAN AND IMPLEMENTATION

Transport of patients with gallbladder and biliary tract disorders includes preflight evaluation and determination of adequate drainage of gastric or T tubes or both. Careful observation during transport is imperative for prevention of flow obstruction. As with any major abdominal disease or trauma, effective pulmonary toilet must be maintained, and careful monitoring of oxygen tension and saturation should occur during transport.

LIVER

The incidence of liver disease and its associated illnesses is relatively frequent. Underlying disease processes, trauma, chemical abuse, or drug overdoses—especially acetaminophen—induce liver disease.[4]

An adult liver weighs approximately 3 pounds and is supplied by the hepatic artery and portal vein. The liver contains more than 50,000 lobules of hepatocyte.

Patients with liver disease who are most commonly encountered by air medical transport personnel are those who have cirrhosis, liver failure, or associated biliary atresia, or those who are candidates for liver transplantation.

PLAN AND IMPLEMENTATION

In planning and treating the patient with liver disease, the transport team should apply, as with all patients, standard precautions. It is important to keep in mind when transporting a patient with liver disease what medications may not be effective because of liver dysfunction. For example, benzodiazepines that are used by many transport programs to decrease anxiety related to transport may not be as useful.

PANCREAS

The pancreas, a gland approximately 8 inches long in an adult, is located behind the spleen. The pancreatic body is positioned horizontally across the abdomen. Its vascular supply is through celiac and mesenteric arteries. The pancreas consists of endocrine, alpha, beta, and delta cells. Pancreatic disorders include pancreatitis and hemorrhagic pancreatitis, cancer, and damage caused by trauma. Devastation of this organ leads to difficult care management of fluid and electrolyte balance, hemo-dynamic stability, and pain control.

ASSESSMENT

A sound history is helpful in determination of the cause of the pancreatic disease process. The transport team should also ensure proper airway and venous access before transport. Careful evaluation of electrolyte balance may help the transport team determine additional treatment. A gastric tube must be in place before transport. If the patient has already undergone surgery and drains have been placed, the transport team must ensure proper venting for collection bulbs and surgical dressings. Pain management is an important transport intervention in the care of the patient with pancreatitis.

INTESTINES

The small intestine (duodenum, jejunum, and ileum) is approximately 23 inches long. The primary functions of the intestines are absorption and digestion. The large intestine is composed of the cecum, ascending colon, transverse colon, descending colon, and sigmoid colon. This extensive, enclosed, gas-producing system can pose many difficulties for the flight nurse transporting a patient who has either direct intestinal disease or general acute illness.

The intestinal problems most frequently encountered by transport teams are obstructions, ruptures, ruptured diverticula, acute appendicitis, and mesenteric infarct.[5]

ASSESSMENT

A careful history is necessary to determine whether the intestinal disease is a primary or secondary illness. A physical examination by the flight nurse should check specifically for abdominal distention, hyperactive high-pitched bowel sounds, and rectal blood, and the transport team should assess the patient for signs and symptoms of peritonitis or sepsis. The patient's temperature should be measured before transport.

PLAN AND IMPLEMENTATION

The transport team should evaluate venous access and volume needs before the transport. The patient

in shock may require fluid resuscitation and vasopressors to support his or her blood pressure. During transport, the team must ensure an adequate airway and provide oxygen, consider aircraft altitude or pressurization to reduce gas expansion, and ensure gastric tube patency. Continuous gastric tube suctioning is imperative throughout transport. Patients with stomas will need adequate collection-bag venting.

SUMMARY

Careful planning by the transport team before transport, especially by air, helps provide effective, safe care.

Because patient problems are difficult to predict, the transport team should plan for equipment and treatment modalities that can be applied easily to all patients before transport. Gases that expand with altitude are ever present in the GI system; proper venting mechanisms should be placed before flight, and backup devices should be available on the aircraft. Calculation of flight time, ground time, and unanticipated diversions will help the transport team estimate the amount of volume, battery time, capacities, and therapeutic support needed for the entire transport time.

GASTROINTESTINAL MEDICAL EMERGENCIES CASE STUDY

The helicopter was called to transport an 82-year-old man with an upper GI bleed from a community hospital to a tertiary care center. Refractory massive hemorrhage had occurred during the previous 12 hours, and simple endoscopy by the local community hospital revealed what they believed to be a mass, greater than 13 cm, in the gastric pouch. Because of the size of the mass, clear visualization of the probable hemorrhagic sites was obstructed. This patient had a history of hospital admission 1 week before this occurrence for mild upper GI bleed brought on by food ingestion. A diagnosis of thrombocytopenia and hypertension was made at that time.

TRANSPORT TEAM EXAMINATION

The patient was a mildly obese man, who was pale and diaphoretic, in semi-Fowler's position on an emergency department stretcher. He was actively bleeding from a gastric tube and periodically vomiting large amounts of bright red blood and clots. The patient was visibly anxious and expressed fear of dying.

Cardiovascular: Skin was pale, cool, and diaphoretic, with petechiae over chest, abdomen, and thighs anteriorly.

ECG: Global ischemia with occasional multifocal PVCs was noted. Two large-bore IVs were in upper extremities.

Respiratory: Nasal cannula delivered 4 L/min. Breath sounds revealed faint rales at bilateral bases. The chest radiograph revealed bilateral lower lobe infiltrates and a markedly distended gastrum elevating the left diaphragm. An approximate 13-cm mass with varying densities was seen.

GI-GU: Normoactive bowel sounds were auscultated, and a large mass was palpated in the left upper quadrant. A urinary catheter was in place and draining clear yellow urine. A no. 18 Salem sump was in place and lying posteriorly to the gastric mass draining bright red blood. The emergency department staff was performing saline lavage.

Medications given before the flight crew's arrival were as follows:

Lasix 40 mg IVP
Ativan 2 mg IVP
5 units of packed red blood cells
3200 ml of crystalloid

Laboratory data were as follows: Hct 27, PT 12.9, PTT 22.5; platelets 73,000; ABGs on 4 L/min nasal cannula O_2: pH 7.38, Po_2 68, Pco_2 32; vital signs: BP 110/68; AP 108; respiration 30; temperature 96° F, patient shivering.

Interventions

The transport team prepared the patient for transport and took iced saline solution in a cooler and four additional units of packed red blood cells. The stretcher was prepared with dry, warmed linen and

a space blanket. The oxygen was changed to 100% nonrebreather mask, and the patient was given safety orientation before flight.

The flight time to the tertiary facility was 20 minutes. Vital signs remained stable, and the saline lavage was continued throughout the flight, with noted clearing on landing. Units no. 6 and no. 7 of red packed blood cells were infusing. Patency of the gastric tube during air medical transport was crucial for this patient, and frequent manipulation of the tube was required to prevent occlusion.

Workup of this patient revealed that the gastric mass was a product of small bones, Styrofoam, hair, and paper products. The patient was taken to the operating room for removal of the foreign-body mass. It was noted at that time that the patient had no body hair.

DISCUSSION

Preflight planning for the needs of the patient for both the initial admission time and during the flight to the receiving facility is imperative. This patient continued to receive colloid replacement while being type- and cross-matched at the receiving facility.

The gastric bleeding was caused by mechanical lacerations from small bones. The patient has undergone surgical repair and psychiatric evaluation since admission. In this extremely complicated case, a diagnosis of bezoar was made, and further psychologic evaluations are to follow.

REFERENCES

1. Dinsdale-Novotny V, Andrews L: Gastrointestinal emergencies. In Kitt S et al, editors: *Emergency nursing,* Philadelphia, 1995, Saunders.
2. Finis NM: Abdominal trauma. In Kitt S et al, editors: *Emergency nursing,* Philadelphia, 1995, Saunders.
3. Krupa D, editor: *Flight nursing core curriculum,* Des Plaines, Ill, 1997, Road Runner Press.
4. Reynolds TB: Hepatic failure. In Grevnik A, editor: *Textbook of critical care,* ed 4, Philadelphia, 2001, Saunders.
5. Savides TJ, Jensen DM: Severe gastrointestinal hemorrhage. In Grevnik A, editor: *Textbook of critical care,* ed 4, Philadelphia, 2001, Saunders.

## 24

INFECTIOUS DISEASES

1. Identify risk factors related to infectious disease and transport.
2. Name the agencies involved in governing the management of infectious diseases in the transport environment.
3. Identify the appropriate equipment that should be used to prevent transmission of infection during transport.

Encountering infectious diseases in transport presents a challenge. Infection is frequently not the primary reason why the patient is being transported. Generally, a complication of the infection such as septic shock initiates the need for transport.

The goal of transport is to access multidisciplinary resources not available to the referring hospital. The goals for transport personnel are to provide supportive care to the patient and to prevent the spread of the infectious process. Understanding the infectious process and some of the diseases that transport personnel encounter facilitates accomplishing these two goals.

THE CHAIN OF INFECTION

The causative agent enters a reservoir, which provides an environment that encourages growth. Next, the agent must have a way to exit the reservoir and enter the next host. The means by which the agent

exits one host and enters the next is called a *mode of transmission*. This chain of infection is not only the sequential means that supports a disease but is also the easiest means of "curing" the disease process. Breaking the chain at any one of these intervals prevents the spread of infection (Figure 24-1).

RISKS FOR INFECTION

There are multiple factors that may put people at risk for becoming infected. Some of these include the following[27]:

- Age: young children and older adults are at greater risk for infection and its complications because of their immune systems
- Failure to receive preventative immunizations
- Substance abuse
- Immunocompromised patients either from a disease process such as HIV or from medication

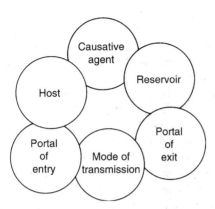

FIGURE 24-1 **The chain of infection.** In the spread of infection, a causative agent passes from a reservoir (such as an infected person) to a susceptible host. The host may then become another reservoir from which the agent can spread.

- Recent out-of-country travel, which allowed the patient to be exposed to infectious diseases common in those countries, for example, hepatitis

MODES OF TRANSMISSION

Healthy skin and tissue are the biggest deterrents to infection. Normal bacteria reside on the skin and in other parts of the body (such as the nasopharynx and the gastrointestinal [GI] tract) as part of the "normal flora." As long as the balance of power is established, the patient does not have a problem with disease. For example, if the skin is healthy but is harboring staphylococci, no disease process has begun. Normal hand washing rids the skin of staphylococci, and the spread of disease is inhibited. If the skin is broken, the balance of power is upset. The microbes now have a mode of entry to a host, and disease processes are encouraged. Frequent hand washing becomes the "cure" for disease and the method to break the chain of infection. Common transmission modes for bacteria are direct contact, droplet infection exposure, organisms colonized on equipment, and percutaneous and mucocutaneous contact.

Nosocomial infections are those contracted in the hospital and are frequently established by direct contact. Sterilization easily prevents transmission of bacteria from equipment, but direct contact and droplet infection as modes of transmission are harder to contain. Staphylococci or other harmful microbes often are colonized in a host that exhibits no infectious process but can pass the disease to the next host. This carrier situation and poor aseptic technique are especially harmful in the hospital setting. There are personnel who are carriers of disease and who come in close contact with patients. Noncompliance with hand washing policies and droplet expulsion by coughing, sneezing, and talking can deliver germs to patients and enhance the spread of disease. An epidemic can be encountered from contact with just one carrier of disease.

Whereas patients in the hospital may be susceptible to nosocomial infections, prehospital and hospital care providers are more susceptible to diseases transmitted by percutaneous and mucocutaneous methods. Hepatitis B virus (HBV), hepatitis C virus (HCV), and human immunodeficiency virus (HIV) are contained in the blood of some of the patients that health-care providers encounter. When the patient harboring the organism sustains trauma, has extensive bleeding, or requires emergent procedures or resuscitation, the transport team becomes susceptible to that microbial transmission. Minor areas of broken skin on a team member's hand can provide a mode of entry and be the reservoir for bacteria.

Any intervention that exposes the transport team to body secretions increases the risk of exposure to an infectious disease. The emergent nature and physical surroundings of the prehospital setting also increase that risk. The lack of light and the limited space of some transport vehicles may increase the risk of exposures. Standard precautions must be used when caring for all patients during transport.

DISEASES AFFECTING TRANSPORT

ACQUIRED IMMUNODEFICIENCY SYNDROME

Acquired immunodeficiency syndrome (AIDS) is caused by infection with the human immunodeficiency virus HIV. HIV attacks and destroys the CD4+ T cells (helper cells). It is characterized by profound immunologic abnormalities, multiple opportunistic infections, and unusual forms of certain malignant neoplasms.[5]

HIV is transmitted percutaneously and mucocutaneously through intravenous (IV) drug use, sexual intercourse with an infected person, from a mother to her unborn or newborn child, and through the major body fluids of blood plasma, semen, vaginal fluid, and possibly saliva. HIV has been isolated in cerebrospinal fluid, tears, breast milk, and saliva, although these have never been proved as sources of disease. The virus has been spread through blood transfusions in the past. New screening techniques were begun in 1985 that decrease the threat of infection through transfusion to only 1 in 50,000 units.[5]

The HIV is classified as a retrovirus, which descriptively carries its genetic material in ribonucleic acid (RNA) rather than deoxyribonucleic acid (DNA). The virus uses the host's reproductive apparatus to reproduce itself. It then kills the host cell and releases more of the virus into the body. The body will produce antibodies to the virus, but these are not protective; they only appear to be an indicator of active infection. Antibody to the virus has been consistently documented in patients with AIDS.

Even though HIV has extensively researched over the past 15 years and medications have been developed that have helped some individuals with AIDS, it continues to challenge the scientific community. Exactly how to prevent and treat HIV remains one of the greatest trials for the twenty-first century. The key to the management of HIV may also be the key that unlocks the human immune system and the prevention of all diseases that afflict mankind.[5]

A report in *Morbidity and Mortality Weekly Report*[6] noted risk factors associated with infection after percutaneous exposure to HIV-infected blood. Three factors were statistically significant: (1) a larger quantity of blood indicated by visible blood on a device, (2) a procedure that involved a needle placed directly in a vein or artery, and (3) a deep injury. The risk was increased when the source patient had terminal illness.

Occult HIV infection poses a risk to health-care providers. The seroprevalence rate of emergency department (ED) patients in the study by Marcus et al[24] was 4.1 to 8.3 per 100 patients. Prehospital care workers in that study did not know the HIV status of the patients they transferred 93.5% of the time. To adequately prevent the spread of infectious diseases, health-care workers should assume that *every* patient is infectious, and standard precautions should be used.

The Centers for Disease Control and Injury Prevention (CDC) has issued guidelines for the management of occupational exposure to HIV.[5] Research has found that people treated in a limited period of time after a significant exposure may decrease the risk of acquiring the virus. The problem in health care is that when a health-care worker suffers a significant exposure, the HIV status of the patient may not immediately be known. These guidelines were proposed as a method of managing a significant exposure until the patient's HIV status could be discovered or assist in the prevention of HIV in the health-care worker if the source of the exposure was never identified.[5,35]

The CDC defined risk of exposure as[5,16,35]:

- Highest risk of exposure: large volume of blood from a deep injury with a large diameter, hollow needle previously in a source patient's vein or artery; blood containing a high titer of HIV
- Increased risk exposure: exposure to larger volume of blood or blood with a higher viral titer of HIV
- No increased risk: exposure neither to larger volume of blood nor blood with a high titer of HIV

Health-care providers with a significant exposure should be treated in 2 hours of exposure. There are recommended medications from the CDC, but these must be given with caution and the health-care provider monitored closely. Each transport service needs to have policies and procedures in place that describe a significant exposure, how it is reported, how it is monitored, and where the team member can receive chemoprophylaxis when it is indicated.[5,16]

HEPATITIS

Viral hepatitis is an infection of the liver caused by multiple viruses. To date, seven distinct hepatitis viruses have been identified that may cause hepatitis. The hepatitis virus may be transmitted in a number of ways, depending on the virus. Hepatitis A, E, and F may be transmitted through oral-fecal contact. Hepatitis B, C, D, and G are bloodborne and may be contracted through sexual contact, perinatal contact, transfusions, and exposure to contaminated body fluids. Hepatitis C is the most common bloodborne infection in the United States. The most accurate means to distinguish the various types of viral hepatitis involves specific serologic testing.[26-28]

HAV is transmitted by the fecal-oral route. This transmission is enhanced by poor personal hygiene and intimate contact. In developed countries, exposure, infection, and subsequent immunity are almost universal in childhood. Childhood infections are frequently subclinical. Adults who contract the disease have symptoms that are more severe. The disease is usually self-limiting.[26-28]

A DNA virus that attacks the liver cells causes HBV. Its incubation period is from 6 weeks to 6 months. Similar to the HIV, HBV is transmitted by percutaneous and mucocutaneous modes: through IV needle use, by sexual intercourse with an infected person, and from a mother to her unborn child through placental transmission or her newborn through breast milk contamination. The major body fluids of blood, plasma, semen, and vaginal fluid are the same primary contaminates as for AIDS. HBV is much more transmissible than HIV and is more environmentally stable. The risk of infection to a health-care provider after percutaneous exposure of an infected source patient is approximately 30% if the exposure is to hepatitis B antigen-positive blood.[26-28]

There are greater than 200 million carriers of hepatitis B surface antigen (HBsAg) in the world. Serum HBsAg is as infrequent as 0.1% to 0.5% in the normal population. HBV is found in 5% to 10% of the volunteer blood donor population. The existence of asymptomatic hepatitis B carriers with normal liver function suggests that the virus is not directly cytopathic. Patients with acute HBV report a percutaneous exposure only 50% of the time.[18] Chronic HBV is present in 5% of the world population. Despite the current focus on HIV risk, hepatitis infection risk is greater in health-care providers because 200 die annually of complications of nosocomially acquired hepatitis B.[33] There has been a decline of HBV in heterosexuals and health-care workers, but the overall incidence has remained constant.[37]

HCV is transmitted primarily through blood transfusions and other percutaneous routes. Other identified risk factors are heterosexual and homosexual contact, household exposure, hemodialysis, IV drug abuse, and occupational exposure. These risk factors parallel that of HBV and HIV. The period that a person can be an asymptomatic carrier without detectable levels of HCV is between 10 weeks and 1.5 years. Infection with HCV has been shown to have substantial morbidity, and 50% or more of these patients have chronic liver disease. One study demonstrated a prevalence of HCV as high as 7.7% in an adult trauma population.[19]

HDV is transmitted by nonpercutaneous means and is endemic in those with HBV. There is a worldwide distribution of the HDV. The epidemiologic pattern is in the Mediterranean countries of Northern Africa, Southern Europe, and the Middle East. In the United States, the HDV is confined to those who are frequently exposed to blood and blood products, drug addicts, and patients with hemophilia.[18]

HEV is the enteric form of non-A, non-B hepatitis. It is rare for a person with HEV to spread the disease to close contacts. HEV occurs after contamination of water supplies and is found primarily in India, Asia, Africa, and Central America. It is not known if HEV is found outside the endemic areas.[18]

The prophylaxis of hepatitis differs with each virus type. The CDC recommends that any person who routinely performs tasks that involve contact with blood, blood-contaminated body fluids, other body fluids, or sharps be vaccinated against hepatitis B.[11] Each transport program needs to ensure that this vaccination is available to the staff.

There must be policies and procedures in place for exposure to the HBV. Table 24-1 contains the latest recommendations from the CDC for postexposure prophylaxis for exposure to hepatitis B virus.[11]

TABLE 24-1. **Recommended Postexposure Prophylaxis for Exposure to Hepatitis B Virus**			
Vaccination and Antibody Response Status of Exposed Workers*	Treatment		
	Source HBsAg[†] Positive	Source HBsAg[†] Negative	Source Unknown or Not Available for Testing
Unvaccinated	HBIG[§] × 1 and initiate HB vaccine series[¶]	Initiate HB vaccine series	Initiate HB vaccine series
Previously vaccinated			
Known responder**	No treatment	No treatment	No treatment
Known nonresponder[††]	HBIG × 1 and initiate revaccination or HBIG × 2[§§]	No treatment	If known high-risk source, treat as if source were HBsAg positive
Antibody response unknown	Test exposed person for anti-HBs[¶¶] 1. If adequate,** no treatment is necessary 2. If inadequate,[††] administer HBIG × 1 and vaccine booster	No treatment	Test exposed person for anti-HBs 1. If adequate,[¶] no treatment is necessary 2. If inadequate,[¶] administer vaccine booster and recheck titer in 1-2 months

From Centers for Disease Control and Prevention: Updated U.S. Public Health Service Buidelines for the Management of occupational Exposures to HBV, HVC, and HIV and Recommendations for Postexposure Prophylaxis, *MMWR* 50(RRH): June 29, 2000.

* Persons who have previously been infected with HBV are immune to reinfection and do not require postexposure prophylaxis.

[†] Hepatitis B surface antigen.

[§] Hepatitis B immune globulin; dose is 0.06 ml/kg intramuscularly.

[¶] Hepatitis B vaccine.

** A responder is a person with adequate levels of serum antibody to HBsAg (i.e., anti-HBs ≥10 mlU/mL).

[††] A nonresponder is a person with inadequate response to vaccination (i.e., serum anti-HBs <10 mlU/mL).

[§§] The option of giving one dose of HBIG and reinitiating the vaccine series is preferred for nonresponders who have not completed a second three-dose vaccine series. For persons who previously completed a second vaccine series but failed to respond, two doses of HBIG are preferred.

[¶¶] Antibody to HBsAg.

TUBERCULOSIS

In the 1980s there was a resurgence of tuberculosis (TB) in the world. The primary cause of this increase is linked to the AIDS epidemic. In 1953 the rate of TB cases was just 5% to 7% a year. In 1985 that rate started to rise, and by 1991 the number of cases had increased to 23% to 25%.[18] It is estimated that between 10 and 15 million people in the United States are infected with TB. In 1993 health-care providers accounted for 3.2% of TB cases.[7]

Fortunately, since the release of guidelines from the CDC in 1994, the rate of TB infection has begun to decrease. However, there has been an increase in the number of multidrug-resistant TB in some areas of the country. Finally, health-care providers who work with patient problems that have a high rate of HIV infection, with a high number of persons from TB endemic countries, and in communities with a high prevalence of TB infection still remain at risk for becoming infected with TB.[11]

The organism that causes TB is *Mycobacterium tuberculosis*. The mode of transmission is by droplet contamination through the respiratory tract. The organism is inhaled and then travels to the alveoli, which provide a good medium for growth of the organism. The risk for infection is proportional to the concentration and the length of the exposure. The *M. tuberculosis* organism is found in the lung about 85% of the time. The organism can also spread through the lymph system to other parts of the body. TB has been found in the peritoneum, meninges, kidneys, and bones.[25]

Once the person is infected with TB, in 2 to 10 weeks cell-mediated immunity responds. The person will have a positive TB skin test result after this immune response is activated. If the immune system prevents further spread of the organism, the patient is said to have tuberculosis infection without the disease. Such patients are not infectious if they do not have the disease. They may be completely asymptomatic, or they may have mild coldlike symptoms. Even if the person is symptomatic, the chest radiograph is often negative. There are no sophisticated methods for diagnosing TB. Smears for acid-fast bacillus (AFB) cultures on patients with TB are estimated to be negative as frequently as 50% of the time.[30]

After exposure to the organism, TB can lie dormant for long periods. It is unclear why the disease later becomes reactivated. Reactivation of the disease is more likely with people who have impaired cell-mediated immunity such as diabetes, renal failure, and HIV. There is a 5% chance of becoming infected in the first 2 years after exposure. The lifetime risk of acquiring active TB once infected is 5% to 10%.

No health-care provider is immune from exposure to TB. After TB outbreaks, Florida and Texas hospital employees had a skin test conversion rate of 20% to 50%.[9] This high rate of conversion indicates that the risk of exposure for health-care workers is significant.

The CDC has issued guidelines to help prevent the spread of TB. First, health-care workers should maintain a high degree of suspicion. Second, the infection should be identified early. Once identified, the infected person should be isolated and treated as early as possible. Most of the guidelines for preventing the spread of TB are directed toward health-care providers who work in hospitals. Placing the person in the proper isolation room with proper airflow ventilation system is recommended. This type of isolation is not possible for infectious patients who require prehospital or interfacility transport.

The close proximity of the health-care providers to the infectious patient in the transport vehicle puts these workers at an increased risk. The CDC[11,35] issued specific guidelines for prehospital personnel and others involved in transport. Because emergency medical services (EMS) and flight personnel work in close quarters, it is recommended that the windows of the vehicle or helicopter be opened whenever possible. If the heating or air conditioner is used, they should be set to nonrecirculating cycles.[35]

OSHA requires the use of certified respirators by health-care providers when respiratory protection is needed. Particulate respirators are designed to filter the air before the health-care provider wearing the respirator inhales it. The use of these respirators poses problems, particularly in an air medical transport where headsets and helmets are worn. Each transport program must carefully evaluate when and how a patient with a diagnosis of tuberculosis should be transported to prevent the potential for exposure.[35]

Different treatment options are available for health-care providers who contract TB. The age of the person and the general health are taken into consideration. It is important to emphasize that once treatment has begun, adherence is important to prevent complications such as the development of drug resistance. Each transport team should also have guidelines for postexposure to tuberculosis, including when the team member may return to work.

Early identification of patients with TB and proper diagnosis prevent the spread of disease. Early drug therapy is essential for a person with TB. Initial steps toward the prevention of MDR-TB include patient education, stressing the importance of completing the drug therapy and appropriate follow-up. Education of health-care workers on the transmission of TB assists them in taking the necessary precautions to avoid contracting or spreading the disease to others.

BACTERIAL MENINGITIS

Bacterial meningitis is a relatively common infection of adults and children. If left untreated, meningitis can be fatal in as few as 6 to 12 hours. The various organisms that cause meningitis, *Streptococcus pneumoniae* and *Neisseria meningitidis*, are the most common in infants of 1 month old up to adults. Group B streptococci and aerobic gram-negative bacilli are common causes of bacterial meningitis in newborns. These organisms are causes of infection in that age-group because individuals may be exposed to them when passing through the birth canal during vaginal deliveries. The incidence of *Haemophilus influenzae* has declined as a causative agent. This is thought to be related to the childhood immunization against *H. influenzae*.[15] Epidemic meningococcal disease since the early 1990s has been caused by serogroup C.[5]

Exercising a high degree of caution when diagnosing or ruling out meningococcal meningitis is necessary. A missed diagnosis can have serious or even fatal repercussions. Classic signs of the disease are new seizure activity, headache, fever, and petechial rash. Absence of the rash does not exclude the diagnosis because the rash may appear in only 50% of the patients. Nuchal rigidity, a positive Kernig's sign (back and leg pain on hip flexion/knee extension), or a positive Brudzinski's sign (back and leg pain on neck flexion) should heighten suspicion of the disease. These last three signs are unreliable in the infant population; therefore a lumbar puncture (LP) may be needed. A differential diagnosis of meningitis should always be considered in a person with an unexplained altered mental status change. This change could be as subtle as a flat affect.[20]

Fulminant meningococcal infection can lead to slight flattening of the gyri cerebri and to polymorphonuclear (PMN) leukocyte accumulation in the meninges and brain. Fibrin may build up in smaller vessels, creating an acute vasculitis resulting in petechial lesions of the meninges.[13] Inflammatory changes in the leptomeninges lead to PMN aggregates and resulting exudate invading the spinal fluid, limiting the entry of solutes, serum proteins, and some antibiotics. Glucose permeability is decreased. Symptoms suggesting this inflammatory process include lethargy and increased intracranial pressure (ICP). The results of fulminant infection can be development of shock, disseminated intravascular coagulopathy, respiratory failure, and electrolyte disturbances. Another nonspecific but important clue in the later stages of the disease is cold extremities caused by peripheral vasoconstriction. This is a compensatory mechanism to support normal central perfusion, and its presence may precede significant hypotension.

The bacterium that causes meningitis is very labile and may be cultured from the blood, spinal fluid, and other normally sterile media. Cultures from the nasopharynx are not helpful because healthy persons have a very high carrier rate. If a referring hospital has already administered antibiotic therapy, cultures should still be obtained from other normally sterile media, such as spinal fluid and blood. The culture results from these areas yield significant conclusive evidence that warrants obtaining them whenever possible. Gram stains help to direct the tertiary care personnel in the course of treatment.

Antibiotics should be administered to a person with suspected bacterial meningitis as soon as possible. Parenteral antibiotics are recommended to be given 30 minutes after presentation. The transport team's medical control will discuss the case with the referring physician. This discussion can be instrumental in initiating the appropriate treatment of performing an LP, obtaining blood cultures, and administering antibiotics before the transport teams arrival. Although obtaining cultures should not delay the transport, antibiotic therapy should be initiated before departure from the referring facility. This is especially important when the disease has progressed to a shock state. It may be possible for the transport nurse, with assistance from the referring physician or nurse, to obtain specimens for blood cultures while the patient is being prepared for the transport.

Many physicians have concerns that the results of cultures can be altered if antibiotic therapy is initiated before obtaining specimens. However, Blazer et al[4] found that cerebral spinal fluid (CSF) cell count and protein remained the same after 2 full days of parenteral antibiotics. This study demonstrated that antibiotics given before the LP do not affect the cell results but may decrease the culture yield. After 2 full days of antibiotic therapy, all of the study cultures were sterile.

If bacterial meningitis is suspected, the transport team must properly protect themselves from transmission, particularly using droplet precautions. This is important because the patient care areas of most transport vehicles are small and have closed quarters. Masks and gloves should always be worn. Other personal protective equipment may be necessary, depending on the cause of the disease in each case.

Antibiotic therapy and supportive care must be instituted without delay. Morbidity and mortality are increased significantly with delays in treatment. Airway management is of great importance for patients with meningitis, especially in the presence of a decreasing level of consciousness. Mannitol may be given for signs of ICP. Fluid and electrolyte management are also important.

The transport team may require postexposure treatment of they have had intensive unprotected contact with infected patients, such as providing mouth-to-mouth resuscitation, endotracheal intubation, or examination of the oropharynx of a patient without mask and gloves. Postexposure treatment should be begun immediately.[5]

OCUPPATIONAL SAFETY AND HEALTH ADMINISTRATION GUIDELINES

The Occupational Safety and Health Administration (OSHA) of the Department of Labor has determined that health-care providers face a significant health risk from the exposure to infectious bloodborne pathogens. OSHA officials believed that this risk could be significantly decreased or even eliminated by establishing work practice controls and guidelines. Therefore the *Occupational Exposure to Bloodborne Pathogens; Final Rule* was developed.[13] The effective date of the standard was March 6, 1992.

In November 2001 OSHA issued a new directive, number CPL 2–2.69.[35] This comprehensive document outlines the enforcement procedures for the occupational exposure to bloodborne pathogens and also includes the revision directed by Public Law 106–430 (Needlestick Safety and Prevention Act). The general focus of this law and its revision is to include new examples of engineering controls, to require that exposure control plans reflect changes in technology that eliminate or reduce exposure to bloodborne pathogens, and to require employers to document annually how they will prevent exposure to bloodborne pathogens by using safer medical devices and how they will monitor exposure to bloodborne pathogens. Employees need to be actively included in the evaluation of process to prevent injuries and exposures.[35]

Work practice laws enacted by OSHA govern most institutions. If OSHA officials find an institution in violation of any portion of the standard, the institution can be fined as little as $7000 up to as much as $70,000 for a single violation.[36] Transport programs may want to determine whether these laws affect their practice. In this chapter, this specific standard is referred to as the OSHA standard.

Every institution that falls under the jurisdiction of OSHA must have a formal infection control plan that covers all areas of the plan. If a transport program is hospital based, the program probably has a well-developed infection control plan that follows the OSHA standard. Flight programs can use the existing plan and modify it to encompass differences in flight nursing practice. Examples of how the OSHA standard is being adapted to patient transport practice appear throughout this chapter.

OSHA defines *bloodborne pathogens* as[35]:

- HBV
- HIV
- Pathogenic microorganisms that can cause:
    - Hepatitis C
    - Malaria
    - Syphilis
    - Babesiosis
    - Brucellosis
    - Leptospirosis
    - Arboviral infections
    - Relapsing fever
    - Creutzfeldt-Jacob disease
    - Adult T-cell leukemia/lymphoma (caused by HTL-I)

- HTLV-I associated myelopathy
- Diseases associated with HTLV-II
- Viral hemorrhagic fever

OSHA defines an occupational *exposure* as reasonably anticipated contact, which includes not only potential but also actual contact with blood or other potentially infectious materials (OPIM). Exposure can occur to nonintact skin such as skin with dermatitis, hangnails, cuts, abrasions, chafing, and acne. "Reasonably anticipated contact" may include: contact with blood, OPIM, and needle sticks. Health-care professionals need to be aware of what constitutes an exposure. Reporting an insignificant exposure such as splashes of blood on clothing is costly, time consuming, and nonproductive. Part of the required yearly training that OSHA mandates is dedicated to the epidemiology and the transmission of the bloodborne pathogens. With increased education, reporting of insignificant exposures should decline. The transport team can be a role model and disseminate information concerning a significant exposure to other medical employees and prehospital care providers. The transport team can assist them in determining the status of an exposure and reporting the significant exposures.[35]

EXPOSURE CONTROL PLAN

OSHA requires that employers have a formal *Exposure Control Plan*. The new record keeping that becomes effective in 2002 states that all employers, whether or not they are covered by the bloodborne pathogens standard, must keep a record of all work-related needle sticks and cuts from sharp objects that are contaminated by blood or OPIM. If the employee later becomes infected, the classification must be changed. Incidents involving splashing or other exposure to blood or OPIM without cut or puncture should also be recorded and changed if the employee becomes infected.[35] It is important to note that the standard allows for a large scope of personnel who may be covered. It essentially states that *"any employee who has occupational exposure to blood or other potentially infectious material will be included within the scope of this standard."*[35]

Figure 24-2 is an example of an exposure documentation form and Figure 24-3 is an example of a form to respond to the prehospital care provider's request for information from a Midwestern teaching hospital. With the information obtained from this form, the hospital can determine whether the exposure is significant enough to warrant further investigation. This facility does not begin testing the source patient's blood unless the exposed healthcare provider completes the exposure documentation form and arranges for testing of his or her own blood. The reporting of insignificant exposures has decreased.

The *Exposure Control Plan* should provide that an employee could obtain confidential medical evaluation and follow-up after reporting an exposure incident. An important part of this plan should include collecting data about how the incident occurred so that plans may be made for prevention of future incidents. Blood should be drawn from the source individual once consent (if it is required) has been obtained. However, if the source is not known, the employer needs to document why. For example, a needle in a laundry bag stuck the employee. The consent of the employee must also be obtained before their blood is drawn.

The employer is not authorized to be informed of the results of the source individual or exposed employee testing. Employees have at least 90 days following baseline blood collection to decide if they wish to have their blood tested for HIV. Employers must provide postexposure prophylaxis for bloodborne pathogens based on the current recommendations from the CDC.[35]

STANDARD PRECAUTIONS (UNIVERSAL PRECAUTIONS)

Use of universal precautions is one approach to infection control. According to OSHA definitions, *universal precautions* means that *all* human blood and certain human body fluids are treated as if known to be infectious for HIV, HBV, and other bloodborne pathogens. The emergent nature of care rendered to patients who are bloody makes use of universal precautions a prudent approach to infection control.

In 2001 the CDC updated their *Guidelines for Isolation Precautions in Hospitals* that separated universal precautions to *standard precautions and transmission-based precautions*.[14] Standard precautions include the major features of universal precautions (blood and body fluids) and body substance isolation (designed to decrease the risk of transmission). Standard precautions include the following:

- Blood
- All body fluids, secretions, and excretions (except sweat), whether they contain visible blood or not
- Nonintact skin
- Mucous membranes

Transmission-based precautions are used for patients diagnosed or suspected to be infected with highly transmissible or epidemiologically important pathogens. They go beyond standard precautions and include the following:

- Airborne precautions
- Droplet precautions
- Contact precautions

An important component of all these precautions includes hand washing. Transport team members do not have access to running water in transport vehicles. An alcohol-based foam soap product can be a replacement to water that can rapidly reduce transient bacteria and the risk of cross infection. The containers for these types of soap are small enough that they can be easily stored in a transport vehicle. These products are antimicrobial and do not require water. After use, hands should be washed with soap and water as soon as possible.

Frequent hand washing can compromise the epidermal barrier and leave the skin susceptible to irritation or allergic contact sensitization. A skin lotion can be used to protect the hands.

PERSONAL PROTECTIVE EQUIPMENT (PPE)

Personal protective equipment (PPE) is meant to prevent blood or other potentially infectious materials (OPIM) from passing to or contacting the employee's work or street clothes, undergarments, skin, eyes, mouth, or mucous membrane. OSHA recommends masks with face shields and eye protection whenever splashes of blood or other potentially infectious materials may be anticipated. These devices should be worn *every time* an intubation or invasive procedure is performed. Even though it is fairly common to see prehospital care providers wearing gloves, these same workers rarely adhere to wearing masks and face shields.

PPE consists of specialized clothing or equipment employees wear to protect themselves against a hazard. The employer is required to supply PPE at no cost to the employee. If employees need special PPE, they are responsible for notifying the employer. The employer is required to purchase the necessary alternative equipment for all employees.

The use of PPE is required when rendering patient care except when the PPE would prevent the proper delivery of health care or public services or would pose an increased hazard to the personal safety of the worker or a co-worker. Headsets and helmets may interfere with face mask and goggles. However, PPE must be used when it is feasible. It is important to not abuse this particular regulation.

PPE must be provided in appropriate sizes and accessible locations. Hypoallergenic gloves, glove liners, powderless gloves, or other similar alternatives must also be available at no cost to the employee who requires them.[35]

Unfortunately, latex allergies are common among health-care providers and patients since the institution and use of universal precautions. An increased demand for gloves may have changed the manufacturing procedure resulting in poor-quality, highly allergenic gloves.[34] The protein in natural rubber is considered to be the responsible antigen.[32] The first documented case of a person with a reaction to latex gloves was in 1979. Approximately 1% of the general population is latex sensitive, and 7% to 10% of health-care workers have a sensitivity. The incidence of sensitivity increases to 12% for operating room personnel. A person with repeated exposure to latex has an increased risk of development of latex allergy. Genetic factors and allergies to certain foods predispose a person to latex allergies.

UNIVERSITY OF CINCINNATI HOSPITAL

REQUEST FOR INFORMATION BY EMERGENCY SERVICES WORKER

<u>PLEASE PRINT</u> - Use Blue or Black Ink - <u>PRESS HARD</u>

REQUEST NO. _____

This form is for use by emergency care workers to request information on the presence of a contagious or infectious disease (if known) of a person, alive or dead, who has been treated, handled, or tranported to University Hospital by an emergency services worker.

Before you can be provided with this information, you must believe that you have suffered significant exposure through contact with the person about whom you are requesting the information. A significant exposure means:

A percutaneous (break in skin or needle stick) or mucous membrane exposure (eyes, nose, mouth) to the blood, semen, vaginal secretions, or spinal (joint, bone, tendon), pleural (lung), peritoneal (abdomen), pericardial (heart), or amniotic fluid of another person.

Deposit top (white) copy in designated Emergency Department QA box. Submit yellow copy to your agency or employer. Retain pink copy.

1. Regarding the exposure, what was

    Name of patient: _____

    Date: _____ Time: _____

    Place: _____

    Manner of exposure:

    _____ Dirty needle stick   _____ Broken skin exposure
    _____ Splash-eye, nose, mouth   _____ Unprotected mouth to mouth
    _____ Other, describe: _____

2. Your name: _____

3. Your address: _____

    City/State/Zip: _____

4. Your telephone number: Home: _____   Work: _____

5. Have you completed more than two (2) injections in Hepatitis B series?   Yes _____   No _____

6. Employer or volunteer agency for whom you were administering health care when exposure occurred:

    Employer or agency: _____

    Address: _____

    City/State/Zip: _____   Phone: _____

7. Name of your chief at above listed place of employment or volunteer agency: _____

This is to attest that the above statements are true and correct to the best of my knowledge and belief.

Your signature: _____   Date: _____

<u>ACKNOWLEDGMENT</u>

Name of person receiving request: _____

Received: Date: _____   Time: _____

White-Emergency Department QA Box   Yellow-Agency/Employer   Pink-Requestor's Copy

FIGURE 24-3 **Examples of forms responding to a prehospital care provider's request for information.**

UNIVERSITY OF CINCINNATI HOSPITAL

REQUEST NO. _____

RESPONSE TO EMERGENCY SERVICES WORKER REQUEST FOR INFORMATION

PLEASE PRINT - Use Blue or Black Ink - PRESS HARD

THIS INFORMATION HAS BEEN DISCLOSED TO YOU FROM CONFIDENTIAL RECORDS PROTECTED FROM DISCLOSURE BY STATE LAW. YOU SHALL MAKE NO FURTHER DISCLOSURE OF THIS INFORMATION WITHOUT THE SPECIFIC, WRITTEN, AND INFORMED RELEASE OF THE INDIVIDUAL TO WHOM IT PERTAINS OR AS OTHERWISE PERMITTED BY STATE LAW. A GENERAL AUTHORIZATION FOR THE RELEASE OF MEDICAL OR OTHER INFORMATION IS NOT SUFFICIENT FOR THE PURPOSE OF THE RELEASE OF HIV TEST RESULTS OR DIAGNOSIS.

Name of ESW: _____

1. Date of oral report: _____

   Person giving report: _____

   Comments: _____
   _____
   _____

2. Date of written report: _____

   Report sent to worker _____ chief _____ chief's name _____

   Person sending report: _____

3. Your request for information has been received. It has been determined that:

   a. _____ There is no known presence of a contagious or infectious disease at this time based upon the following:

   _____ No tests were performed.

   _____ The following tests were performed with negative results:

   _____
   _____
   _____

b. _____ There is the presence of a contagious or infectious disease. Testing on person in question was positive for:

_____

_____

_____

c. _____ The person in question has refused HIV testing.

d. _____ Patient discharged home.

e. _____ Patient discharged to health care facility/coroner's office/funeral home.
Address: _____

THIS RESPONSE PROVIDES ALL INFORMATION AVAILABLE AS OF THE DATE OF THIS WRITTEN RESPONSE.

4. Report included:

_____ Name of disease   _____ Suggested precautions for preventing transmission.
_____ Signs and symptoms of disease   _____ Recommended prophylaxis (if any)
_____ Date of exposure   _____ Suggested follow-up
_____ Incubation period of disease   _____ Appropriate counseling
_____ Mode of transmission

5. It is expected that the worker will consult a physician in cases of true disease exposure. It is understood by provider of report and recipients that decisions related to prophylaxis, treatment, and counseling will be at the discretion of that physician.

White-Requestor's Copy   Yellow-Agency/Employer   Pink-University Hospital Infection Control Committee/Prehospital Training

FIGURE 24-3 *Cont'd*

Reactions to latex range from contact and generalized urticaria to bronchospasm, anaphylaxis, and even death. Most (82%) of the reports are not serious and are classified as a type IV reaction, which presents clinically as contact dermatitis. However, once a person has become sensitized to the allergen, repeated exposures are more severe. The more severe responses are cell mediated by IgE and are classified as type I reactions. Examples of type I reactions are asthma, anaphylaxis, and death.[34]

The treatment for allergies lies in the prevention of exposure. Nonlatex gloves can be worn. As with any allergic response, the person needs to remove the rubber gloves or, with severe reactions, leave the area of exposure. Glove powders easily absorb latex proteins. Powder-free gloves are essential. Depending on the specific person's sensitization and reaction, other employees working with that individual also may have to wear powderless gloves. Cotton liners or barrier creams such as the Proshield help to decrease an allergic reaction. The employer is required to purchase special gloves for an allergic employee's use.

Gowns in the prehospital setting are the least-effective method of protection; they are predictably soiled and soaked with blood or bodily fluids. A better option is to shower and change clothes as soon as possible after care is delivered.

It is the employer's responsibility to provide clean, maintained PPE. Contaminated clothing should not be laundered at home because there is no assurance that the contamination has been properly handled.[35]

Eye protection should be worn as protection against mucocutaneous contact with blood or body fluids through the conjunctiva. It is important to choose glasses that provide peripheral vision. This enhances safety in the transport setting.

PPE should be removed as soon as possible when saturated with blood. It is difficult for the transport team to dispose of contaminated equipment in the helicopter. Bloody PPE can contaminate the transport vehicle. If bloody gloves are worn when entering the transport vehicle, the blood can contaminate the door handles, seat belts, instrument controls, and headsets. A simple alternative is wearing two sets of gloves to the scene. Before entering the transport

vehicle, the outer bloody pair can be removed, and the bottom layer remains in place for protection.

EQUIPMENT

Recapping of needles increases the chance of a percutaneous stick. Experts believe that percutaneous needle sticks are underreported.[23] OSHA mandates that nurses shall *not* recap needles. Recapping needles is likely to be done and is often necessary during transport. Because of the restrictions in space, only a limited amount of drugs can be stored in transport vehicles, and some of the drugs used in the management of the critically ill or injured patients come in multiple does vials or ampules. When needed, the medicine is drawn out of the ampule and into a syringe. If only a small amount of the drug is used, the nurse recaps the needle to keep the remaining drug sterile for future use.

If needles must be recapped, OSHA requires that it be accomplished through the use of a mechanical device or a one-handed technique. With a one-handed technique, the cap is placed on a surface and the syringe is placed inside the cap using one hand.

The Needlestick Safety and Prevention Act of 2000[35] directs that hospitals and others who use needles develop plans to evaluate and implement technology that eliminates or reduces exposure to bloodborne pathogens. A number of needleless products have been developed and are in place in many institutions. There can be problems for transport teams however. One of the greatest problems is that many of the systems are not compatible with others. Also, some do not allow any access with a needle. It is important for the transport team to assess the equipment being used by the referring agency and adapt it as required for safe administration of medications to the patient during transport.

Needles must be placed in needle containers after use. The construction of sharps containers must meet at least four criteria. The NIOSH publication "Selecting and Evaluating and Using Sharps Disposal Containers" contains a description of required criteria. They should be accessible in the transport vehicle and changed and disposed of frequently.[35]

Leakproof sheets or body wraps can be used to contain blood during transport. If a particular part of the patient's body is extremely bloody, that area can be wrapped with a plastic leakproof wrapping. With bloody gunshot wounds and amputations, the area can be surrounded with plastic and towels to absorb some of the blood and prevent it from spreading inside the transport vehicle.

DECONTAMINATION

Contaminated work surfaces must be cleaned as soon as possible after the incident. Transport team members are frequently responsible for decontaminating their own equipment, and they must work quickly after a transport to restock and clean a vehicle to return it to service. It may be necessary for the vehicle to be put on a short delay for the required decontamination. After transport involving extremely bloody patients, all of the equipment may have to be removed from the vehicle to adequately clean its interior surfaces. Fortunately HBV and HIV are known to live for only a short time on environmental surfaces. For decontamination to be successful, surfaces must be cleaned with the appropriate solution for decontamination. Running water from a hose may be necessary for cleanup of a large amount of blood.

Routine cleaning and disinfection of the transport environment is also recommended on a regularly scheduled basis to prevent the transmission of disease. Buckets, mops, and brushes used for decontamination also need to be used on a rotating decontamination schedule. These items need to be clearly marked and used only for decontamination. A record of the cleaning schedules must also be kept.

Transport programs frequently purchase specialized equipment that is exclusive for the needs of the team. Because of budget restraints, sometimes there are no backup pieces of the same equipment; therefore decontamination of the equipment must be done promptly to return it to service. If indicated, the appropriate department in the hospital may be used for assistance in decontaminating equipment. If the equipment is specific to the transport program, the department's name should be clearly labeled on the equipment.

Solutions for disinfection vary in their use according to the equipment on which a particular solution is used. A knowledge of appropriate cleaning solutions and their use is necessary to ensure that adequate decontamination takes place. Bleach solution in 1:10 ml concentration is effective and safe on both soft and hard plastic. The linoleum floors of the ambulance, helicopter, or airplane and the stretcher mattresses can be cleaned with this solution, providing the area is free of dirt and dried blood, although fabric will fade and discolor from use of the bleach solution.[2,35]

Glutaraldehyde 2% also can be used on plastics and vinyl without damage. Acid solutions should not be used around electronic equipment and on stainless steel because corrosion occurs on high-carbon metals with alkalinized solution. Glutaraldehyde should be mixed at the time of use because it is unstable in solution, even though it is very effective.[2] Alcohol is a very effective antiseptic with very short contact on HIV, tubercle bacillus, fungi, and viruses. However, alcohol is flammable and very drying. Alcohol is not recommended for the hands. The surface being cleaned must be free of dirt and blood before the use of alcohol can be effective.[17]

Iodoforms are safe, relatively fast, and effective against many organisms. Cleaning the patient's skin with iodoform and then with alcohol and letting the area dry before an IV skin puncture is often recommended to protect the skin from introduction of bacteria. IV tubings are becoming a source of infection more frequently because more medicines are being introduced into the catheters. Cleaning of the IV ports with alcohol or iodoforms or both definitely helps protect the patient from nosocomial infections.[17]

The pneumatic antishock garment, floor surfaces, and linens can be cleaned with detergent and water before disinfectant application. Cleaning of surfaces with one of the proper chemical disinfectants listed earlier removes the risk from the area.

Laryngoscope blades and handles are reusable and require decontamination after each use. These handles and blades can be properly decontaminated by soaking in an effective antimicrobial solution such as Metricide. This agent is a glutaraldehyde solution used for disinfecting and sterilizing inanimate objects. Surface particles must be cleaned before soaking. The amount of time that the object is soaked determines the effectiveness. HIV is completely inactivated after 10 minutes of soaking. The soaking time must be increased to 20 minutes to provide a 100% effective destruction of the mycobacterium. Because it is difficult to determine which organisms are on the objects, all items should be soaked for at least 20 minutes. Batteries must be removed from handles before soaking. In time, corrosion of various portions of the blade and handle can occur. Because the equipment must soak for 20 minutes, extra laryngoscope blades and handles will be needed for rotation back into the transport vehicle. Rotation of the blades and handles allows the vehicle to be restocked and promptly returned to service. When the blade and handle have been decontaminated, they must be rinsed thoroughly before they are returned to stock.

Disposable laryngoscope blades and handles are available. Disposing of these items after an intubation would definitely decrease the possibility of transmission of infectious organisms. The newer blades and handles are stronger than some of the older models. One disadvantage that may prevent some programs from using disposable laryngoscope blades and handles is their expense.

Transport teams must be aware of other institutions' infection control policies. Contaminated equipment or laundry may need to be disposed of at other institutions. The transport team may have to ask questions at other institutions to follow their specific policies. The development of the OSHA standard has given the industry some consistency and has made following other institutions' policies easier. When the transport team responds to a motor vehicle crash or other incidents where there is a large amount of blood, the site itself has to be decontaminated. Because the transport team is one of the first to leave the scene, the fire department or life squad must assume responsibility to overhaul and decontaminate the area to prevent transmission of infectious diseases to the public.

TRAINING AND EDUCATION

OSHA requires that training be provided at the time of the initial assignment. This training must be at no cost to the employee and be done on the employer's time. The extensive orientation that is required for new transport team members should encompass the infection control procedures that are different or in addition to the hospital's policies. An emphasis should be placed on how infection control practices differ in both the prehospital arena and the closed quarters of the transport vehicle.

All employees must have annual training. If the transport program is hospital based, the hospital-wide infection control program can be used to incorporate all of the teaching requirements of the OSHA standard. There must be a written exposure plan that is accessible to the transport team. This plan must be updated every year or modified to reflect new tasks or procedures that affect occupational exposure. Additional training is required when there are changes or modifications of tasks. The transport team should take an active role in preparing and updating this plan so that it is appropriate for their use.

DISEASE PREVENTION

To break the sequence of events that cause disease and thereby protect the transport team and potential patients from infectious diseases, transport personnel need to apply basic principles to control and reduce the number of infections. Following the OSHA guidelines is essential.

Hand washing is the single most important resource for preventing transmittal of disease; it systematically kills bacteria and is critical in the prevention of disease transmission. Hand washing is required before and after patient care in any category, including IV therapy, catheter insertion, and the administration of medication.

Hepatitis B, measles, flu, and tetanus immunizations for the prehospital and hospital care provider are strongly recommended by the CDC for the prevention of disease, and yearly tuberculin testing also is required.

The HBV vaccination is required for health-care providers in high-risk areas by the OSHA standard. The standard stipulates that the employer is required to notify the employee of the necessity of the vaccination. This vaccination shall be free of charge to the employee. If employees decline the HBV vaccine, they are required to sign a waiver stating their knowledge of the risks and their declination.

Unfortunately, the world we live in today continues to present transport personnel with additional challenges such as the use of infectious diseases as smallpox or anthrax as weapons. Transport personnel need to keep abreast of information that may affect their practice. The Centers for Disease Control and Injury Prevention through its website provides pertinent information about these diseases and others that may be used as terrorist weapons.

As health-care providers, particularly emergency responders, we may find ourselves caring for patients who have been infected, and we need to know how to manage the patient as well as prevent further exposure so that we are able to keep in service.

SUMMARY

Infectious diseases are a challenge for all transport personnel because of the multiple facets of involvement. Health-care providers are inherently exposed to infectious diseases, and flight personnel have an increased risk because of the bloody injuries and the emergent resuscitative measures that their patients require. The close working quarters of transport vehicles add to this risk.

Transport personnel can take up these challenges successfully by collaborative writing of infection control policies between the transport team and the infection control department personnel. Following quality control procedures and enforcing OSHA standards will help to maintain surveillance, control, and prevention of infectious diseases in the transport environment.

Knowledge of the epidemiology and the transmission of infectious diseases decrease the chance of exposure. Since the existence of the OSHA standard, infection control practices have become well defined and universalized. The transport team must make adjustments from hospital to prehospital infection control practices. Use of standard precautions for *all* patient encounters is a prudent way to handle secre-tions and blood. Innovative infection control devices and competent performance of procedures help decrease the risk of exposure in the transport environment. Careful assessment, planning, implementation, and evaluation of treatment are required for the successful outcome of transporting patients with infectious diseases.

INFECTIOUS DISEASES CASE STUDY 1

A request was received to transport a 2-month-old female infant who had been admitted to the emergency department at the referring hospital with a history of poor feeding and lethargy the day of admission. The history was otherwise negative.

On admission, the patient's general appearance was that of a cyanotic, mottled infant. She was lethargic, her pupils were equal and sluggishly reactive, and the anterior fontanelle was soft and slightly depressed. She was tachycardic (pulse 210 beats/min), tachypneic (respirations 96 per minute), and hypotensive (30 mm Hg by palpation), and her rectal temperature was 100° F. Urine output was low the day of admission, and she had none after admission or during transport.

Initial treatment consisted of oxygen by mask at 10 L/min, an IV was started, laboratory results were obtained, including blood cultures, and an LP was performed. The infant was also given a fluid bolus for her hypotension.

The laboratory results were as follows:

CBC	ABG
WBC 3.9	pH 7.15
Hgb 9.7	Pco_2 17.7
Hct 28.2	Po_2 289.1
Poly 19.0	HCO_3^- 6.2
Band 6	BE −20.7
Lymph 75	

ELECTROLYTES	SPINAL FLUID
Na 131*	WBC 14
K+ 5.5*	Mononuclear 9
Cl 100	Polynuclear 5
CO_2 14	RBC 6
Glucose 102	Glucose 58 mg/dl
BUN 22	Protein 36 mg/dl
	*Repeat NA 125; repeat K+ 5.0.

By the time the transport team arrived, the patient's condition had obviously deteriorated. Their examination revealed the infant to be apneic with marked peripheral cyanosis, purpura, and mottling. Her pupils were 4 mm and fixed. She had marked rales and rhonchi bilaterally with a decrease in respiratory effort with a rate of 10 to 20 per minute. Other vital signs showed a regularly irregular heart rate of 105; her blood pressure had increased to 64 mm Hg after the second fluid bolus; and the rectal temperature had dropped to 97.2° F. The only other treatment before transport was intubation and oxygen delivery by bag-valve-mask at a rate of 28 with 100% oxygen.

Because the transport team was not sure of the source of the infant's sepsis, they put on PPE including masks.

During transport the infant had cardiac arrest and pediatric advanced life support protocols were instituted. On arrival at the receiving facility, all efforts to resuscitate the infant failed.

An overwhelming sepsis caused by group A and group B-hemolytic streptococcus *caused her death.*

INFECTIOUS DISEASES CASE STUDY 2

The transport team responded to a small rural hospital to transport a 74-year-old woman with respiratory distress. Her medical history included frequent episodes of pneumonia.

On the helicopter's arrival, the woman was found to be in acute respiratory distress. She was coughing productively thick purulent sputum. She had gasping breaths at a rate of 38 per minute. Her color was pale, and her lips were cyanotic. She was diaphoretic and had a heart rate of 138 beats/min. Po_2 was 47 on 100% nonrebreather mask.

The transport team prepared the patient for intubation. The patient continued to cough productively and required oral tracheal suctioning. The flight team decided to intubate with rapid

induction with succinylcholine. The intubation was uneventful, and the team continued to prepare for the transport.

In flight the patient's color improved and her heart rate decreased. She continued to require endotracheal suctioning for copious amounts of yellow sputum. The remainder of the flight was uneventful, and the patient was admitted directly to the critical care unit.

Follow-up of this patient indicated that her respiratory status had not markedly improved. Sputum culture results revealed M. tuberculosis. Antibiotic therapy was then changed to the appropriate drugs for TB.

Further discussion with the family revealed the patient's history of fatigue, weight loss, anorexia, and a persistent cough. The cough had progressed in severity for the last 2 weeks.

The flight nurse notified the flight physician of the TB diagnosis. Both members of the flight team were exposed to the sputum from the intubation and suctioning. Neither one of the staff used a mask during the intubation, nor did the physician wear gloves because of the emergent nature of the procedure. The team members did not have a high index of suspicion that the woman had an infectious disease such as TB and therefore was not in any of the high-risk categories.

Both flight team members instituted personal follow-up on the exposure with employee health. The flight nurse called the referring hospital to inform them of the infectious disease so they could initiate their own follow-up.

REFERENCES

1. Arankalle VA et al: Non-ABCDE hepatitis: is there another enterically transmitted hepatitis virus? *Hepatol Elsewhere* 256, 2001.
2. Asepsis, *The infection control forum* 2(2):2, 1989.
3. Bradley-Springer L: HIV prevention: what works? *Am J Nurs* 101(6):45, 2001.
4. Blazer S, Berant M, Alon U: Bacterial meningitis: effect of antibiotic treatment on cerebral spinal fluid, *Am J Clin Pathol* 80:386, 1983.

5. Bolyard E, Tablan OC, Pearson ML, Shapiro CN, Deitchman SD, The Hospital Control Practice Advisory Committee: Guideline for infection control in health care personnel, 1998, *AJIC* 26:289, 1998.

6. Case-control study of HIV seroconversion in health-care workers after percutaneous exposure to HIV-infected blood—France, United Kingdom, and United States, *MMWR* 44(50), 1995.

7. Centers for Disease Control and Prevention: Expanded tuberculosis surveillance and tuberculosis morbidity—United States, *MMWR* 43:361, 1994.

8. Centers for Disease Control and Prevention: Guidelines for preventing the transmission of *Mycobacterium tuberculosis* in health-care facilities (recommendation), *MMWR* 43(RR-13):51, 1994.

9. Centers for Disease Control and Prevention: Nosocomial transmission of multidrug-resistant tuberculosis among HIV-infected persons—Florida and New York, 1988-1991, *MMWR* 40:585, 1991.

10. Centers for Disease Control and Prevention: Updated U.S. public health service guidelines for the management of occupational exposures to HBV, HCV, and HIV and recommendations for post exposure prophylaxis, *MMWR* 50(RR-11):1, 2001.

11. Centers for Disease Control and Prevention: Update: evaluation of human T-lymphotropic virus type III/lymphadenopathy-associated virus infection in health care personnel, *MMWR* 31:507, 1985.

12. Dagjartsson A, Ludvigsson P: Bacterial meningitis: diagnosis and initial antibiotic therapy, *Pediatr Clin North Am* 34(1):219, 1987.

13. Department of Labor: 29 CFR part 1910.1030: occupational exposure to bloodborne pathogens (final rule), *Federal Reg*, Dec 6, 1991.

14. Garner JS, Hospital Infection Control Practices Advisory Committee: Guidelines for isolation precautions in hospital, *Am J Infect Control* 24:24, 1996. Updated August 2001.

15. Graham TP, Moran GJ: Meningitis update: pearls, pitfalls, guidelines, and controversies, *Emerg Med Rep* 16(22):213, 1995.

16. Holleran R: CDC guidelines for occupational exposure to HIV, *Air Med J* 17(1):24, 1998.

17. Hoofnagle JH, Lindsay KL: Acute viral hepatitis. In Goldman L, Bennett J, eds: *Cecil textbook of medicine*, Philadelphia, 2000, WB Saunders.

18. *Hospital Infection Control* 16(8):101, 1989.

19. Kaplan AJ et al: The prevalence of hepatitis C in a regional level one trauma center population, *J Trauma* 33(1):126, 1992.

20. Klein NC, Cunha BA: Bacterial meningitis, *Emerg Med* 28, Feb 28, 1994.

21. Lamphear BP et al: Decline of clinical hepatitis B in workers at a general hospital: relation to increasing vaccine-induced immunity, *Clin Infect Dis* 16:10, 1993.

22. Lewandowski C et al: Health care worker exposure to HIV-1 and HTLV I-II in critically ill, resuscitated emergency department patients, *Ann Emerg Med* 21(11):1353, 1992.

23. Mangione C, Gerberding J, Cummings S: Occupational exposure to HIV: frequency and rates of underreporting of percutaneous and mucocutaneous exposures by medical housestaff, *Am J Med* 90:85, 1991.

24. Marcus R et al: Occupational blood contact among prehospital providers, *Ann Emerg Med* 25:776, 1995.

25. Moran GJ: Recognizing and minimizing the risks, *Emerg Med* 37-42, Dec 1994.

26. Perini S: Hepatitis: speaking out about the silent epidemic, *Nursing Management* 32(6):18, 2001.

27. Peabody S: General medical emergencies. In K Jordan, editor: *Emergency nursing core curriculum*, ed 5, Philadelphia, 2000, Saunders.

28. Perry J: The bloodborne pathogens standard 2001: what's changed? *Nursing Management* 32(6):25, 2001.

29. Robert LM, Bell DM: HIV transmission in the health care setting risks to healthcare workers and patients, *Infect Dis Clin North Am* 8(2):319, 1994.

30. Schluger N, Rom W: Current approaches to the diagnosis of active pulmonary tuberculosis, *Am J Respir Crit Care Med* 149:264, 1994.

31. Sepkowitz KA: AIDS, tuberculosis, and the health care worker, *Clin Infect Dis* 20:232, 1995.

32. Simms J: Latex allergy alert, *Can Nurse* 91(2):27, 1995.

33. Sloan EP et al: Human immunodeficiency virus and hepatitis B virus seroprevalence in an urban trauma population, *J Trauma* 38(5):736, 1994.

34. Sussman GL, Beeshold DH: Allergy to latex rubber, *Ann Intern Med* 122(1):43, 1995.

35. U.S. Department of Labor, Occupational Safety and Health Administration: *CPL 2-2.69 enforcement procedures for the occupational exposure to blood-borne pathogens*, Washington, DC, November 2001, Author.

36. West K: The final word, *Emerg Med Serv* 21(1): 54-55, 62, 1992.

37. Wong JB et al: Cost-effectiveness of interferon-alpha 2b treatment for hepatitis B's antigen-positive chronic hepatitis B, *Ann Intern Med* 122(9):664, 1995.

COLD-RELATED EMERGENCIES

25

Hannibal started over the Pyrenean Alps in 218 BC with an army of 46,000, but in 15 days he lost more than 20,000 men to the cold.[7] Statistics have not significantly improved since Hannibal's time. United States' soldiers sustained 90,000 cold-related injuries in World War II, and Germany suffered 100,000. During two winter months in 1942, the Germans performed 15,000 cold-related amputations.[49] During the Korean War, the United States had a 10% cold-related casualty rate.[32,36]

Transport personnel must be aware of the risk of hypothermia regardless of the climate or terrain. A summer-day hiker in the Rocky Mountains, an older person in an unheated home in the Sun Belt, and a sailor stranded off the warm Florida coast are all at equal risk of hypothermia. Studies have shown that cold contributes to 16% of all recreational boating fatalities and 20% of all scuba diving fatalities.[24,43]

HYPOTHERMIA DEFINED

Hypothermia, defined as a core body temperature of less than 35° C, occurs because the body can no longer generate sufficient heat to maintain body functions.[7] Accidental hypothermia, in contrast to iatrogenic hypothermia, is the unintentional decrease in core temperature associated with trauma or exposure to the environment.[1,6,7] Core body temperature can be measured at the rectum, the esophagus, the tympanic membrane, or the bloodstream. Rectal thermometers provide the least reliable measurement of core body temperature. The esophageal and tympanic thermometers are more reliable. Table 25-1 lists thermometric equivalents for Fahrenheit and Celsius temperatures.[12]

CLASSIFICATION

Hypothermia is classified into three categories. *Mild hypothermia* is defined as a core body temperature

TABLE 25-1 **Thermometric Equivalents (Celsius and Fahrenheit)**	
Degrees Celsius	**Degrees Fahrenheit**
15.0	59.0
16.0	60.8
17.0	62.6
18.0	64.4
19.0	66.2
20.0	68.0
21.0	69.8
22.0	71.6
23.0	73.4
24.0	75.2
25.0	77.0
26.0	78.8
27.0	80.6
28.0	82.4
29.0	84.2
30.0	86.0
31.0	87.8
32.0	89.6
33.0	91.4
34.0	93.2
35.0	95.0
36.0	96.8
37.0	98.6
38.0	100.4
39.0	102.2
40.0	104.0

greater than 32° C and less than 35° C and is associated with low morbidity and mortality. *Moderate hypothermia* occurs when the core body temperature is greater than 28° C but less than 32° C. Finally severe hypothermia is defined as a core body temperature of 28° C or less and is associated with a higher morbidity and mortality.[2,17] The classification distinction at 32° C is not arbitrary but is based on profound metabolic and physiologic changes. Heat can still be conserved by vasoconstriction and produced by shivering at core temperatures of 35° C to 32° C. At a core temperature below 32° C, the body no longer tries to conserve or produce heat. At 28° C the body can no longer generate heat by itself and is essentially poikilothermic.[2,17] These changes are summarized in Table 25-2. The lower limit of

survival according to Caroline[3] is 23° C, although she reported one isolated patient who survived a core temperature of 10° C after being in cardiac arrest for 1 hour.[16,30]

Hypothermia can also be classified as acute or chronic, according to length of exposure. Acute hypothermia occurs when body heat is lost over a period of less than 6 hours. Immersion in water colder than 21° C is a common cause of acute hypothermia because water accelerates conductive heat loss. Chronic hypothermia occurs when the patient is exposed to cold for more than 24 hours, and it occurs more frequently on land. Urban hypothermia is a form of chronic hypothermia that is associated with factors such as age, debilitation, drug and alcohol use, predisposing disease, and decreased level of consciousness.[26]

MORTALITY

The mortality rate for severe hypothermia cited in the literature varies from 0% to 50%.[3] Many factors influence the mortality rate, including degree and duration of hypothermia, age, poverty, predisposing disease, and complications. Most victims die of cardiac arrhythmia. The presence of a severe underlying disease is almost always associated with increased mortality. Rankin and Rae[37] noted no correlation between the severity of hypothermia or the rate of rewarming and the clinical outcome but, rather, that mortality was correlated with the presence or absence of severe underlying disease.

The old adage, "the patient is not dead until they are warm and dead" still directs a lot of transport programs. In other words, the patient will probably be transported to definitive care. It is important that transport programs, particularly those that provide service in cold weather or rescue environments, have policies and procedures that control when and how a severely hypothermic patient will be resuscitated and transported.

NORMAL TEMPERATURE REGULATION

Human beings become uncomfortable with even a small deviation in core body temperature from 37.6° C. In *De Re Medicina*, Aurelius Cornelius Celsus

TABLE 25-2 Physiologic Changes Related to Temperature		
Degrees Celsius	Degrees Fahrenheit	Symptoms
38.0	99.6	Normal rectal temperature
37.0	98.6	Normal oral temperature
Mild		
36.0	96.8	Increased basal metabolic rate in an attempt to balance heat loss, tachycardia, increased cardiac output
35.0	95.0	Shivering at the maximum, usually still responsive, but level of consciousness beginning to decrease, regulatory systems beginning to falter
34.0	93.2	Dysarthria, amnesia, blood pressure still normal, oxyhemoglobin curve begins to shift to the left
32.0	91.4	Heart rate decreases to 50-60 beats/min, ataxia, poor coordination, apathy, lethargy
Moderate		
32.0	89.6	Vasoconstriction level of consciousness progressively falls
31.0	87.8	Shivering stops, respirations and blood pressure may be difficult to obtain
30.0	86.0	Mental confusion, delirium, increased muscle rigidity; heart rate and cardiac output begin to decrease, arrhythmias begin to develop (atrial fibrillation)
29.0	84.2	Acidosis, hyperglycemia, metabolic rate decreased by 50%, decreased respirations, bradycardia, decreased stroke volume, decreased cardiac output, pupils dilated
Severe		
28.0	82.4	Hypotension, loss of vasoconstrictive capabilities, ventricular fibrillation if patient handled roughly, increased myocardial irritability
27.0	80.6	Prolonged PR, QRS, and QT intervals; muscle flaccidity; no voluntary movement (appears dead); no pupillary reactions
26.0	78.8	Seldom conscious, areflexic
25.0	77.0	Stuporous, hypoventilation, ventricular fibrillation may appear spontaneously, cerebral blood flow one third of normal, cardiac output 45% of normal
24.0	75.2	Coma, pulmonary edema, respiratory arrest
23.0	73.4	No spontaneous movement, rigor mortis appearance, no corneal reflexes
22.0	71.6	Maximum risk of ventricular fibrillation, 75% decrease in oxygen consumption
21.0	69.8	Apnea
20.0	68.0	Ventricular fibrillation, cardiac standstill/asystole
17.0	62.6	Isoelectric electroencephalogram

described in AD 25 the universal discomfort of cold temperatures as "hurtful to an old or slender man, to a wound, to the precordia, intestines, bladder, ears, hips, shoulders, private parts, teeth, bones, nerves, womb and brain. It also renders the surface of the skin pale, dry, hard and black. From this proceed shudderings and tremors."[5] Normal body temperature is maintained in a narrow range by a delicate balance of heat loss and heat production regulated by a "thermostat" in the preoptic anterior hypothalamus. The hypothalamus is sensitive to temperature changes as small as 0.5° C.[4] Stimuli sent from the hypothalamus to the sympathetic nervous system increase heart rate and dilate muscle blood vessels to increase heat production. In addition, shivering generates heat by increasing muscle activity. At the same time, cutaneous vasoconstriction reduces heat loss by shunting blood from the periphery to the core.[50]

The ability to shiver is affected by hypoglycemia, hypoxia, fatigue, alcohol, and drugs. Shivering is the body's main mechanism of heat production and its strongest defense against hypothermia. However, shivering requires increased blood flow to peripheral muscles and consequently results in a 25% heat loss. Preshivering increases heat production by 50% to 100%. Visible shivering increases heat production by 500%. An average 70-kg person produces about 100 kcal of heat/hr under basal conditions and up to 500 kcal/hr when shivering.[7] This degree of heat production, however, cannot be sustained for long because the patient becomes fatigued once glycogen stores are depleted. Maximum shivering occurs at 35° C and stops below 32° C. Cessation of shivering is a sign that the patient has made the transition from mild to severe hypothermia.

Hypothermia results when the thermoregulation system becomes overwhelmed or damaged centrally at the hypothalamic level or systemically by a decrease in heat production or an increase in heat loss. Thermoregulation is disrupted at the hypothalamic level by head trauma, cerebral neoplasms, cerebrovascular accidents, acute poisoning, acid-base imbalance, Parkinson's disease, and Wernicke's encephalopathy. Acute spinal transection can eliminate vasoconstrictive control by the hypothalamus. Heat production is decreased by malnutrition, hypothyroidism, hypopituitarism, and rheumatoid arthritis. Normally, 90% of the heat produced by the body is lost to the environment by way of conduction, convection, radiation, and evaporation.

METHODS OF HEAT LOSS

Conduction, together with convection, accounts for 15% of heat loss.[16] Conduction occurs when the body comes into direct contact with a heat conductor. Examples of good conductors are water, snow, metal, and damp ground. Normally conduction plays a minor role in heat loss but is an important factor when the patient has been immersed in cold water, lying in a snow bank, or wandering without shoes for an extended period. Heat loss in water is approximately 25 times greater than heat loss in air of the same temperature.[7] Immersion in water in temperatures less than 10° C causes hypothermia in only a few minutes,[7] in contrast to more than an hour in air.

Heat loss by convection occurs when either air or water moves over the patient or the patient moves through air or water. Heat loss is accelerated by increasing air movement (forced convection). The wind, the rotating blades of the helicopter, and the movement required to transport the patient to the transport vehicle all contribute to forced convective heat loss. Figure 25-1 lists temperature differences related to wind chill factors.

Body heat lost by radiation is 45%.[7] Radiant heat transfer occurs when a difference exists between body temperature and ambient temperature. The body absorbs heat when the ambient temperature is higher and emits heat when the ambient temperature is lower. Radiant heat loss, as convection, is directly related to dermal blood flow and percentage of skin surface exposed. Radiant heat loss is accelerated at night or when the sky is overcast.

Evaporation occurs when water on the body surface is converted from a liquid state to a gaseous state.[7] The body is cooled as the vapor moves off the body into the air. The evaporative process accounts for about 25% of heat loss[7] and occurs normally through the skin, lungs, and upper airway. Burns and various skin lesions expose more open, moist surface area and thereby increase evaporative losses. In addition, evaporation increases when the patient is wearing damp clothing or is covered with blood.

Heat loss is inversely proportional to body size and body fat. Fat insulates because it has less blood flow and consequently has less ability to vasodilate and lose heat. Consequently, large people conserve heat better than small people, obese people better than thin people, and adults better than children.

Wind in m.p.h.	Local Temperature in Degrees Fahrenheit										
	32	23	14	5	−4	−13	−22	−31	−40	−49	−58
	Equivalent Temperature (Wind Plus Local Temperature)										
Calm	32	23	14	5	−4	−13	−22	−31	−40	−49	−58
5	29	20	10	1	−9	−18	−28	−37	−47	−56	−65
10	18	7	−4	−15	−26	−37	−48	−59	−70	−81	−92
15	13	−1	−13	−25	−37	−49	−61	−73	−88	−97	−109
20	7	−6	−19	−32	−44	−57	−70	−83	−98	−109	−121
25	3	−10	−24	−37	−50	−64	−77	−90	−104	−117	−130
30	1	−13	−27	−41	−54	−68	−82	−97	−109	−123	−137
35	−1	−15	−29	−43	−57	−71	−85	−99	−113	−127	−142
40	−3	−17	−31	−45	−59	−74	−87	−102	−116	−131	−145
45	−3	−18	−32	−46	−61	−75	−89	−104	−118	−132	−147
50	−4	−18	−33	−47	−62	−76	−91	−105	−120	−134	−148

little danger for those properly clothed ⟶   considerable danger ⟶   extreme danger ⟶

FIGURE 25-1 **Chill factor: temperature plus wind.** (From Vaughn PB: *Milit Med* 5:307, 1980.)

It is important for the transport team to carefully consider risk factors that may place the patient at risk for developing hypothermia. These include[1,2]:

Age: the pediatric patient has less fat, and shivering provides limited heat production. Elderly people may also suffer from similar inabilities to generate heat as children.

Medications such as antidepressants, phenothiazines, narcotics, neuromuscular blocking agents, and NSAIDS are only a few examples of the pharmacologic agents that may interfere with the patient's ability to maintain their body heat.

Preexisting medical problems such as Parkinson's disease, head injury, malnutrition, hypoglycemia and shock place the patient at risk of hypothermia.

Prolonged exposure and weather conditions such as high humidity, brisk winds, and rain or snow may increase patient heat loss.

PHYSIOLOGIC RESPONSE TO HYPOTHERMIA

METABOLIC DERANGEMENTS

Complications of hypothermia result mainly from the sequelae of metabolic derangements. Initially metabolism increases to generate heat. Optimal metabolism begins to decrease at 35° C. Symptoms of mild hypothermia consequently include shivering, hypoglycemia, and increased respiratory rate, heart rate, and cardiac output. A dramatic decrease in metabolic rate occurs between 30° C and 33° C as the patient makes the transition from moderate to severe hypothermia. Every 10° C decrease in temperature decreases metabolism by half.[7] At 28° C all thermoregulation ceases. The metabolic functions of the liver also begin to falter at temperatures below 33° C. The liver no longer efficiently metabolizes fats, proteins, and carbohydrates or drugs, alcohol, and lactic acid. Symptoms of severe hypothermia include absence of shivering, hyperglycemia, and decreased respiratory rate, heart rate, and cardiac output. Bowel sounds are decreased, if not absent, as a result of decreased gastric motility and gastric dilation.[19]

Hypoglycemia is associated with chronic mild hypothermia, whereas hyperglycemia is associated with acute severe hypothermia. Long-term shivering depletes glucose and glucose stored in the form of glycogen. Shivering can stop at temperatures greater than 33° C if glucose or glycogen stores are depleted or if insulin is no longer available. Shivering begins again when the core body temperature increases to 32° C if depleted glucose is replaced. Hyperglycemia occurs at temperatures below 30° C because insulin no longer promotes glucose transport into cells once metabolism significantly decreases.[7,17] Hyperglycemia will not occur if glucose and glycogen stores have been previously depleted but not replaced.

OXYGENATION AND ACID-BASE DISORDERS

Respiratory rate initially increases after sudden exposure to cold but then decreases as body temperature and metabolism decrease.[7,17] At temperatures above 32° C, ventilation is usually adequate. At 30° C, respirations are shallow and difficult to observe. Apnea and respiratory arrest commonly occur at temperatures between 21° C and 24° C. Although carbon dioxide production also decreases to about half the basal level with each 8° C drop in temperature,[17] the decreased respiratory rate is inadequate to effectively excrete CO_2 at a temperature below 33° C. Consequently, a respiratory acidosis develops in the hypothermia victim.

Cellular respiration is impaired by the decrease in metabolism, drop in cardiac output, and left shift on the oxyhemoglobin dissociation curve.

Hypothermia decreases cardiac output by decreasing heart rate and circulating blood volume, as well as by increasing blood viscosity and peripheral vascular resistance. Blood shifting to the core results in a perceived "overhydration," and the body responds by removing the "extra" volume through diuresis. Prolonged hypothermia also causes plasma to leak from the capillaries, thereby increasing blood viscosity by 2% for every 1° C decline.[7,17,45]

Hypothermia begins to shift the oxyhemoglobin dissociation curve to the left at 34° C. Oxygen then binds tenaciously with hemoglobin, resulting in reduced tissue oxygen delivery. In addition, Biddle has noted that oxygen consumption was half of normal at 27° C and at 17° C had fallen to one quarter the normal value.[7,17] Anaerobic metabolism and lactic acid production increases from the combination of decreased cardiac output, oxygen delivery, and oxygen consumption. The increase in lactic acid leads to cardiac arrhythmia and death.

The cardiovascular system is more sensitive to the effects of acid-base disturbances than any other body system. Acidosis is commonly associated with asystole, and alkalosis is associated with ventricular fibrillation.[6,18,19] Hypoventilation and lactic acid production lead to respiratory and metabolic acidosis. Acidosis usually corrects itself once the patient is rewarmed. Hyperkalemia is associated with metabolic acidosis, as well as with muscle damage and kidney failure, which may all be present in the rewarmed hypothermic patient. Iatrogenic respiratory and metabolic alkalosis is difficult to treat and should be avoided.

CENTRAL NERVOUS SYSTEM

The central nervous system (CNS) displays some of the most impressive sequelae in the hypothermic patient. Complete recovery is possible even after prolonged cardiac arrest. Hypothermia protects CNS integrity and allows the brain to withstand long periods of anoxia.[18] Cerebral blood flow decreases 6% to 7% for every 1° C decline until 25° C is reached.[3,6,14] Cerebral oxygen requirements decrease to 50% of normal at 28° C, to 25% of normal at 22° C,[10,37] and to 12.5% of normal at 16° C.[48] Caroline[3] noted that the brain can survive without perfusion for about 10 minutes at 30° C, whereas it can survive for up to 25 to 30 minutes at 20° C.[9] Remarkably, Steinman noted that at 16° C the brain can survive without oxygen for up to 32 to 48 minutes.[44]

Mildly hypothermic patients are clumsy, apathetic, withdrawn, and irritable. Reflexes are hyperactive at temperatures above 32° C. Level of consciousness begins to decrease markedly at 32° C, and the patient becomes lethargic or disoriented and begins to hallucinate. Hypothermia victims will even remove jackets, gloves, shoes, and other protective clothing; "paradoxical undressing" is often one of the first signs that the patient is becoming severely hypothermic. The cough reflex is absent at decreased temperatures, and aspiration of stomach contents can occur. Coma develops between 28° C and 30° C. At temperatures below 30° C, the pupils dilate and become nonreactive. In addition, corneal and deep-tendon reflexes may be absent. The hypothermic patient must be carefully examined to rule out rigor mortis or death. At temperatures below 20° C, the electroencephalogram, if it were available, would be flat.[22,33]

CARDIAC ARRHYTHMIA

The effects of hypothermia on heart rhythm were noted as early as 1912 to produce bradycardia progressing to asystole.[7,17] In 1923 subjects reportedly showed T-wave changes on their ECGs after drinking 600 ml of ice water.[46] It is believed that up to 90% of all hypothermic patients have some electrocardiographic abnormality.[31,47]

The heart initially responds to mild hypothermia with an increase in heart rate as a result of sympathetic stimulation; this response is short lived. Heart rate then decreases to 50 to 60 beats/min at 33° C and at lower temperatures decreases to 20 beats/min.[7,17] Atrial fibrillation with a slow ventricular rate is common at temperatures below 29° C. Okada[29] recently noted that atrial fibrillation was unusual in mild hypothermia (temperature greater than 32° C) and that it was often observed in moderate (32° C to 26° C) and moderately deep (less than 26° C) hypothermia. About half of the cases studied in moderately deep hypothermia remained in sinus, atrial, or junctional rhythm. Okada also noted that

atrial fibrillation usually converted to sinus rhythm spontaneously after return to normothermia.[29]

Changes in the conduction system begin at 27° C and may be observed as a widened QRS interval and prolonged PR and QT intervals. The Osborne, or J, wave is seen clearly at 25° C. The J wave is described as an extra deflection at the junction of the QRS and ST segments (Figure 25-2). The origin of the J wave is unknown. According to Okada, Nishimura, and Yoshiro, the prolongation of the Q-T interval and the presence of J waves are directly related to the severity of the hypothermia.[32] Large J waves are seen at temperatures of less than 30° C, whereas small J waves are seen at higher temperatures.

Several theories have been offered for the presence of J waves in hypothermia. The J wave may represent hypothermia-induced ion fluxes that cause delayed depolarization or early repolarization of the left ventricle. The J wave may also be a hypothalamic or neurogenic factor. It is important to note that J waves may also be seen in patients with central nervous system lesions or cardiac ischemia or who are septic, or even in young healthy people.[17]

Ventricular irritability, occurring at temperatures less than 30° C, is commonly associated with alkalosis and is the most lethal cardiovascular response to hypothermia. At 28° C rough handling, careless intubation, or cardiac compressions can irritate the heart. Ventricular fibrillation can occur spontaneously at 25° C. Unfortunately, arrhythmia at temperatures below 30° C becomes increasingly refractory to drugs and defibrillation.

Asystole occurs at 20° C but has a surprisingly good prognosis if the patient is rewarmed quickly. Asystole is associated with acidosis and appears to be the primary arrhythmia in accidental hypothermia. Rankin and Rae[37] found that asystole was the terminal rhythm in all 22 patients they studied.

FROSTNIP AND FROSTBITE

Frostnip, a superficial form of frostbite usually found on the face, nose, and ears, is manifested by numbness and pallor of the exposed skin. Management consists of warming the area with a warm hand or wrapping or covering the area for protection.

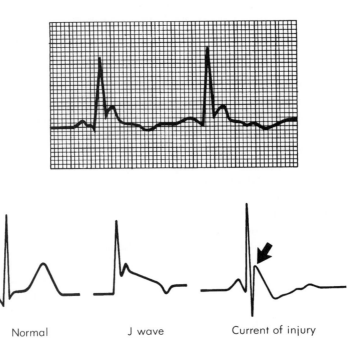

Normal   J wave   Current of injury

FIGURE 25-2   **An ECG tracing showing the characteristic J, or Osborne, wave of hypothermia.**

Frostbite results from the cooling of body tissue to the point of ice crystal formation[27] and most often involves the distal extremities. Destruction of the skin produces a more severe injury than frostnip. Although frostbite is commonly associated with below-freezing temperatures, it can be produced at above-freezing temperatures by wind, altitude, humidity, and prolonged exposure and exacerbated by impaired vascular integrity and decreased cardiac output.[34,51]

The injury caused by frostbite has been divided into four phases. These are the prefreeze phase, the freeze-thaw phase, the vascular stasis phase, and the late ischemic phases. This pathophysiology results in both intracellular and extracellular formation, cell dehydration and shrinkage, abnormal intracellular electrolyte imbalances, thermal shock, and denaturation of the lipid-protein complexes.[25]

Blood cells "sludge" in the vessels, and eventually circulation to the tissue ceases.[25] Frostbite is classified as first, second, or third degree. First-degree injury, superficial freezing without blistering or peeling, is characterized by hyperemia and edema. The tissue becomes mottled, cyanotic, and painful after rewarming. Second-degree frostbite produces blistering or peeling of the skin and is characterized by hyperemia and vesicle/bleb formation. When rewarmed, the skin is deep red, hot, and dry to touch. Third-degree frostbite is characterized by death of the dermis and even deeper tissue such as muscle and bone.[48]

Cauchy, Chetaille, Marchand, and Marsigny recently proposed a new classification for grading the severity of frostbite injuries.[4] It is based on:

- Extent of initial lesion at day 0 after rapid rewarming
- Bone scanning at day 2
- Blisters at day 2
- Prognosis at day 2

This classification system describes the management and potential outcome of the frostbite injury based on the preceding descriptions. The author suggests that the use of this system will[4]:

1. Provide earlier prediction of the final outcome of the frostbite
2. Identify at day 2 the approximate level of amputation
3. Precisely classify the frozen lesions and describe the management of the injury even without any specific knowledge of the topic on the part of the treating health-care provider.

Frostbite management has three stages.[3] The first stage is the most crucial and includes protection of the affected area from trauma or partial thawing. The second stage, rapid rewarming in a whirlpool bath, must occur in a controlled setting with constant observation. The third stage involves provisions for long-term care and follow-up.[25,46]

Prehospital care focuses on protecting the affected area from trauma and partial thawing. Superficial skin injury can be treated by removing any wet clothing and placing warm dry clothing on the injured area. The affected area should be kept frozen if there is any possibility that it will be refrozen. It must never be massaged. The patient should not be allowed to walk if the legs are involved unless it is a matter of survival.

Patients should be given aspirin and fluids and pain management provided.[4] The affected part needs to be carefully immobilized and protected from additional injury. Patients should be transported to a center familiar with the care of frostbite.

EPIDEMIOLOGY

Any individual will become hypothermic given the proper circumstances, but specific groups are particularly vulnerable: infants, older individuals, alcoholic subjects, trauma victims, outdoor people, and those with CNS dysfunction.[8,10,11,13,18] The transport team must always consider hypothermia when assessing patients in these high-risk groups.

INFANTS

Infants and neonates are particularly vulnerable to hypothermia. Mortality rates for neonatal cold injury range from 26% to 45%.[17] Hypothermia must be considered a threat in all out-of-hospital deliveries. The high mortality rate of infants is attributed to several causes:

1. The infant has less tissue insulation than the adult.
2. The large head in proportion to body size allows for greater heat loss.
3. Shivering occurs only at extreme degrees of hypothermia and may go undetected.
4. Limited energy stores are quickly exhausted.
5. Poor motor development may prevent infants from curling into a fetal position for protection.

In addition, the signs and symptoms of hypothermia in the infant are different from the adult and include lethargy, decreased appetite, facial and limb edema, and erythemic rather than blanching skin.

OLDER SUBJECTS

Accidental hypothermia is common and often fatal in older subjects. Urban hypothermia is commonly seen in older subjects who do not have enough money for heat or warm clothing. People 75 years and older are estimated to have a five times greater chance of death from hypothermia than those younger than 75.[17,36] The reasons for the increased susceptibility of the elderly are many.

1. Older subjects normally have a lower basal metabolic rate and body temperature.
2. Older subjects have a decreased ability to adapt to temperature changes by vasoconstriction and shivering.
3. Older subjects have a diminished perception of heat and cold.
4. Older subjects are predisposed to other diseases such as diabetes or pneumonia that make them more susceptible to hypothermia.
5. Older subjects are more susceptible to chronic dehydration.

All confused and lethargic older patients should be assessed for hypothermia in addition to other problems, such as cerebrovascular accident or hypoglycemia.

ALCOHOL AND OTHER TOXIC STATES

Alcohol ingestion has been found to cause serious problems with thermoregulation. Many people consume alcohol with the mistaken belief that it will "warm" them. Many homeless people who become hypothermic are also intoxicated. Alcohol causes vasodilatation, which contributes to additional heat loss. Alcohol ingestion also causes the patient to feel warm, perhaps by altering perception. Hypoglycemia is caused by alcohol ingestion and decreases the patient's ability to shiver and conserve heat. The effects of alcohol on thermoregulation are moderated by the temperature, the amount of alcohol ingested, the patient's nutritional status and body composition, and the patient's ability to tolerate the amount of alcohol ingested.[25]

It is important that alcohol intoxication be recognized as a dangerous cofactor for the hypothermic patient. It is not uncommon for trauma patients to be intoxicated.[11,18]

Other medications also cause hypothermia by impairing centrally mediated vasoconstriction. Barbiturates induce hypothermia in greater than therapeutic doses, whereas phenothiazines induce hypothermia even at therapeutic doses. Other drugs that can contribute to hypothermia include general anesthetics and tricyclic antidepressants. The toxic effects of any drug may not be significant while the person is hypothermic but will become evident when liver, kidney, and metabolic function increase with rewarming. Interestingly, a combination of alcohol, barbiturates, and hypothermia prolongs brain survival even further than hypothermia alone.[53]

TRAUMA PATIENTS

Trauma victims are especially susceptible to hypothermia. Long delays in response time, extrications, stabilization at the scene, and transportation to the hospital contribute to the development of hypothermia. In addition, cold oxygen and IV fluids, removal of clothing, and continuous evaluations by numerous medical personnel add to the problem. The ability of trauma patients to thermoregulate may be disrupted by hypovolemia or head injuries. Burn patients are at high risk because skin integrity has been interrupted. All trauma victims should have temperature closely monitored.[13,14,18,23]

OUTDOOR PEOPLE

Boaters, campers, sailors, hikers, anglers, mountaineers, and other outdoor people are at risk for hypothermia. Generally such people are healthy but become victims of the environment, physical exhaustion, or their own carelessness. Outdoor hypothermia is categorized in two groups: immersion and no immersion. Examples of nonimmersion hypothermia include exposure to wind, rain, snow, and freezing temperatures. Immersion hypothermia occurs more rapidly than nonimmersion hypothermia; heat loss is 35% higher if the patient swims or treads water rather than stays still.[9] A person with immersion hypothermia may drown sooner because the level of consciousness decreases at 30° C.

CENTRAL NERVOUS SYSTEM DYSFUNCTION

Not only does CNS dysfunction increase susceptibility to hypothermia, but hypothermia also mimics the symptoms of CNS dysfunction. Cerebrovascular accidents are the most common CNS dysfunction to cause hypothermia. It is important for the flight nurse to determine if the suspected cerebrovascular accident patient is hypothermic. Schizophrenia and senile dementia are occasionally accompanied by hypothermia. It is unclear whether hypothermia in these states is a consequence of hypothalamic dysfunction[17] or of psychosocial factors such as homelessness and inattention to potential environmental danger.

REWARMING TECHNIQUES

Both Edwards[17] and Bangs and McCauley[25] note that careful review of the literature reveals no evidence supporting one rewarming technique over another. The consensus is that the patient should be rewarmed as quickly as possible because the myocardium is refractory to therapy below 30° C. There are three techniques for rewarming: passive external, active external, and active internal. Only passive external, active external, and limited forms of active internal rewarming can be initiated in the air medical setting. Consequently, rapid transportation to a facility that can provide more extensive rewarming techniques is imperative. Flight personnel must be aware of the existence of these facilities in their service areas.

PASSIVE EXTERNAL REWARMING

Passive external rewarming is simple, inexpensive, and easily instituted. It is used only in mild hypothermia and when the patient can generate heat by shivering and vasoconstriction. The patient is placed in a warm environment, covered with blankets, and allowed to rewarm naturally. Passive external rewarming is available in any transport vehicle with the use of a blanket and a heater. Long-term alcoholic patients have a lower mortality rate when passive external rewarming is used. Passive external rewarming increases core body temperature by 1° C per hour.

ACTIVE EXTERNAL REWARMING

Active external rewarming involves placing heat on the external surface of the body. Heated baths, thermal blankets, and packs to the groin, neck, and axilla and forced air devices such as the Bair Hugger are examples of active rewarming.

Afterdrop is a dangerous phenomenon that can occur in the initial stages of passive and active external rewarming. Afterdrop is defined as a decline of 1° C to 2° C in the core body temperature when cool blood from the extremities moves to the core.[53] Any action that moves blood rapidly from the extremities to the heart, including moving the patient or injudiciously applying heat to the periphery, can cause afterdrop and precipitate ventricular fibrillation. Savard et al[39] suggested another possible explanation for the afterdrop phenomenon: the myocardial irritability of afterdrop is caused by a blood chemical shift and not necessarily from a blood temperature shift.

ACTIVE INTERNAL REWARMING

Active internal rewarming delivers heat directly to the body core, thereby avoiding the dangers of after-drop. The heart, lungs, and brain are warmed first and in turn rewarm of the rest of the body. Heated oxygen, IV fluids, hemodialysis and peritoneal dialysis, gastric lavage, mediastinal lavage (after thoracotomy), and cardiopulmonary bypass are all examples of active internal rewarming. The least-invasive method of active internal rewarming is used when the patient has severe hypothermia but is cardiovascularly stable. On the other hand, the most rapid active internal rewarming methods, such as cardiopulmonary bypass, are recommended if the patient has severe hypothermia and is unstable with cardiovascular collapse unresponsive to drugs and defibrillation.

MANAGEMENT DURING TRANSPORT

Management of hypothermia has been controversial since Napoleon's chief surgeon, Baron Larrey, noted that hypothermic soldiers closest to the fire were the ones who died.[7,17] Hypothermia experiments in human subjects can be safely performed only to 35° C, and those in animals are not equivalent because the physiologic response of animals to hypothermia is different from that of human beings. Consequently, current medical management of the hypothermic patient is based mainly on anecdotal reports in the literature.

All hypothermic patients must be transported, regardless of cardiopulmonary status. Using the old adage, "A patient is not dead until warm and dead,"[14,42] "warm" is defined as 32° C. Severe hypothermia takes priority over any other problem except obstructed airway or major trauma with rapid exsanguination.

Management of the mildly hypothermic patient is relatively uncomplicated; covering the patient with blankets and allowing the patient to warm naturally will prevent further heat loss. Management of the severely hypothermic patient is more complicated and will test the expertise and knowledge of transport personnel.

GENTLE HANDLING

The patient must be handled gently during transport, and stimulation should be minimized. Any movement, including lifting, has been shown to precipitate ventricular fibrillation. Rubbing or massaging the patient is contraindicated. Medical personnel should always cut clothing rather than pull it off. A mildly hypothermic patient must be kept quiet and not allowed to walk or stand. Vehicle vibration can also, theoretically, add to stimulation, but its effects have not been investigated.

PREVENTING FURTHER HEAT LOSS

Prevention of further heat loss is paramount in the management of the hypothermic patient. Limited exposure during assessment will prevent heat loss during examination. The patient's wet clothing should be removed immediately to prevent conductive heat loss. The patient should be removed or protected from any wind source—including helicopter turbulence, which can produce wind up to 100 mph. Insulated and windproofed blankets should be placed under and over the patient, leaving the face exposed, while the patient's head is protected with a wool hat. An electric blanket is contraindicated because this form of active external rewarming can precipitate afterdrop. The cold railings of the stretcher conduct heat and should not be allowed to touch the patient during transport. Warm oral fluids should be considered for the conscious patient only after assessment for an active gag reflex. Aspiration can be a problem, especially if the size of the transport vehicle does not permit the patient to sit upright or at least at a 45-degree angle. Beverages containing alcohol are contraindicated.

ACTIVE INTERNAL REWARMING

The respiratory tract is a major area of heat exchange and evaporative loss. Administration of warm humidified oxygen effectively rewarms the heart, lungs, and brain by way of the bronchial circulation. In addition, the cilia will become more active while being rewarmed and humidified and can assist in decreasing and mobilizing secretions. Warm, humidified oxygen is easy to administer, safe, effective, noninvasive, and readily available in the air medical setting. Mask or bag-valve apparatus at 42° C to 46° C should administer 100% warm humidified oxygen. The rate of rewarming varies

from 0.5° C to 2.0° C/hr[21] to 3.5° C in 20 minutes.[24] A high flow rate is essential for this method to be effective. Core temperature increases an additional 0.3° C/hr by increasing ventilatory rate by 10 liters per minute.[28] McCauley,[25] Danzl,[7] and Slovis and Bachvarov[41] have described various commercial products available.

Rehydration of the hypothermic patient with warm IV fluids increases blood flow to the heart and decreases blood viscosity, vasoconstriction, potential of afterdrop, and the likelihood of cardiac arrhythmias.[7] Hypothermic patients appear to have a better chance of survival when a bolus of warm IV normal saline solution is given before the patient is moved or externally rewarmed.[7] The transport team should establish an IV line in the largest vein available. If needed, a small amount of heat may be applied to the area to facilitate venous access. The fluid of choice is 5% dextrose in normal saline solution (D_5NS) because lactated Ringer's solution is not fully metabolized by the liver in severe hypothermia.[7] D_5NS can be made by adding 2 amps of D50 to 900 ml of normal saline solution. An adult patient may be infused with at least 200 ml/hr and the pediatric patient with at least 4 ml/kg/hr, with adjustment if the patient requires additional fluid resuscitation. Pulmonary edema, jugular vein distention, and other problems associated with fluid overload are monitored. IV fluids are administered at a temperature of 40° C. Fluids can be warmed en route by wrapping them in a shirt, jacket, towel, or an electric blanket or other commercial warming devices. Some transport vehicles now come with environmental drawers that keep fluids warm during transport.

MONITORING VITAL SIGNS

The patient's rectal temperature, heart rate, and respirations should be monitored carefully and on a regular basis. A special thermometer capable of registering to 20° C is required for the hypothermic patient. An esophageal or tympanic thermometer is preferable, but they are impractical in the transport setting. Danzl[7] noted that rectal temperature lags behind actual core temperature and is influenced by leg temperature and placement of the rectal probe.

Volunteers were placed in freezing-cold water for 15 minutes and noted all the classic signs of hypothermia; however, he discovered the body was able to compensate, and core body temperature remained unchanged for at least 15 to 20 minutes.[2,25]

Inaccurate assessment of the patient's respirations can lead to improper management and can precipitate life-threatening arrhythmias. The patient must be observed carefully for at least 1 full minute for the presence of respirations to be determined. A spontaneous respiratory rate of 4 to 6 breaths/min is adequate in hypothermia. An effective cardiac rhythm may be assumed if the patient is breathing spontaneously. Cardiac monitoring may be difficult because of muscle tremors. In fact, baseline oscillations on the ECG may be the only sign that the patient is shivering. Blood pressure may not be obtainable or may be inaccurate because of vasoconstriction. An ultrasound stethoscope may be of use in assessing the presence of a pulse or heartbeat.

AIRWAY

The airway is opened without the use of adjuncts when possible, and intubation is performed only if airway reflexes are absent. Blind nasal intubation may be necessary if trismus is present.[7] The risk of cardiac arrhythmia may be decreased during intubation with preoxygenation and careful technique. Hyperventilation must be avoided because respiratory alkalosis can precipitate ventricular fibrillation. Fewer than 10 breaths/min will successfully oxygenate the hypothermic patient without causing respiratory alkalosis.[7]

CARDIAC RESUSCITATION

Cardiac resuscitation in the hypothermia patient is a controversial topic. The main concern is that chest compressions could be initiated on a patient with a slow but viable rhythm. External cardiac massage on a hypothermic bradycardic heart can precipitate ventricular fibrillation. Established ventricular fibrillation or asystole on the heart monitor is the only indication for prehospital cardiopulmonary resuscitation (CPR) of the severely hypothermic patient.[1,5] Maximal amplification should be used on the cardiac monitor to detect QRS complexes.

Some investigators believe that chest compressions should be withheld in any patient with a core temperature of less than 28° C.[14] Others believe that chest compressions should be reduced to half the recommended rate because metabolic demands are decreased in the hypothermic brain.[3,8] Strong evidence supporting these deviations from advanced cardiac life support (ACLS) guidelines for CPR is lacking. Although hypothermia does protect the brain from anoxic damage, this "safe period" has not been established, and brain damage will occur after cardiac arrest unless CPR is started.[44] Therefore cardiac compressions should be started according to ACLS guidelines once ventricular fibrillation or asystole is established. If spontaneous respirations are present at any rate, a viable rhythm may be assumed, and CPR may be deferred. Danzl and Pozos[7] proposed that CPR be initiated in all cases except the following: (1) a do-not-resuscitate order is confirmed, (2) obviously lethal injuries are noted, (3) chest-wall compression is impossible, (4) rescuers are jeopardized during evacuation, or (5) signs of life are present. Again, a careful assessment of respirations and pulse for at least 1 full minute is imperative to avoid unnecessary and dangerous CPR.

Defibrillation is usually not effective until core temperature is greater than 28° C. However, it is recommended that defibrillation at 200 W seconds be attempted twice and 360 W seconds once and then defibrillation stopped until the patient is warmer.

PHARMACOLOGIC THERAPY

Little clinical evidence to confirm or rule out the effectiveness or complications of pharmacologic therapy has been noted.[6] Medications should be used with extreme caution. Decreased circulation pools medications in the extremities; a toxic reaction can occur when the patient is rewarmed and medication flows to the core. In light of this possibility, several authors have suggested withholding all medications from the hypothermic patient.[3,7] Overzealous correction can precipitate ventricular fibrillation.

Pharmacologic manipulation of pulse, blood pressure, and respiratory rate should be avoided.[7] Medications should not be given orally or intramuscularly because of decreased absorption rates. Other medications should be deferred until the core temperature is 30° C.

SPECIAL CONSIDERATIONS

Transport personnel in the management of cold-related emergencies should consider the following principles:

1. Treat major trauma as the first priority and hypothermia as the second.
2. Remove all wet clothing and get the patient in dry blankets as quickly as possible.
3. Notify the receiving facility while en route to the scene, clinic, or hospital to give the receiving facility time to activate appropriate resources.
4. Insert a urinary catheter and gastric tube for long transports.
5. Avoid vasopressors. Consider them only if rewarming shock is unresponsive to fluids.
6. Continue CPR until the patient is rewarmed to 32° C.

DOCUMENTATION

The history of the incident should be documented, including the time and type of exposure, whether the patient was in cardiopulmonary arrest on arrival of the first responder, what management was initiated before the arrival of transport personnel, and the heart rhythm, drug therapy, and rewarming techniques. Past medical history is important if it is readily available.

Written assessment of the hypothermic patient consists of an initial head-to-toe evaluation including all pertinent findings. The vital signs should be monitored and charted on a regular basis, preferably every 10 to 15 minutes, and should include rectal temperature and heart rhythm with strip readout. The patient and the rewarming techniques should be assessed continuously during transport.

SUMMARY

Almost any treatment mode will suffice in managing the mildly hypothermic patient. Dry, warm blankets or transport blankets should be available in all transport vehicles.

Expertise of transport personnel will be tested when presented with a severely hypothermic patient. Management requires gentle handling, accurate assessment of cardiopulmonary status, passive external rewarming to prevent further heat loss, and active internal rewarming with heated humidified oxygen and IV fluids.

COLD-RELATED EMERGENCIES CASE STUDY

A 7-year-old male passenger in an automobile was thrown from the car, landing in a river. Paramedics were at the scene when the patient was extricated 1 hour later, and primary assessment revealed no breathing and no carotid or femoral pulse. The patient was gently moved to the ambulance, where CPR and ACLS procedures were initiated immediately. The patient was orally intubated using careful technique, and ventilations were assisted with a bag-valve mask. Two IV lines were started: one in the right jugular vein and one in the right antecubital space. Epinephrine was administered intravenously. Warm packs were placed in the groin and armpits to initiate active external rewarming. A gastric tube was placed and a small amount of pale yellow liquid evacuated. Personnel at the scene ordered air medical transport of the patient immediately.

On the arrival of the flight team, reassessment revealed a young male patient (30 kg) lying supine on a backboard in the back of the ambulance; CPR was in progress, the skin was pale and cold to touch, and no capillary refill noted. The patient was orally intubated, and breath sounds were clear. There was good compliance with ventilation. Cardiac monitor displayed pulseless electrical activity rhythm with a rate of 60 to 70 beats/min with no associated femoral or carotid pulses. Rectal temperature was 24° C.

Physical examination revealed the following findings.

Neurologic: Pupils were fixed and dilated at 8 cm. There was no spontaneous movement of extremities, the child was areflexic, and GCS was 3.

Head: Skull and facial bones were grossly intact. The patient had no visible sign of trauma, the nose and ears were clear, and the cervical spine had no palpable deformities. A small amount of pink frothy sputum from the endotracheal tube was seen, and the IV line to the right jugular vein was patent and secure.

Chest: Breath sounds were equal, with scattered rales. The chest wall was intact with no visible trauma.

Abdomen: The abdomen was distended and tense. Nasogastric tube placement was confirmed and secured.

Extremities: The long bones were grossly intact, IV to right antecubital patent and secure.

The patient was gently loaded into the helicopter during continuing CPR and assisted ventilations. The pilot radioed to alert the emergency department of the patient's condition and requested the hypothermia team to remain on standby. In flight the patient was managed in the following manner:

1. Continuous reassessment of condition
2. Continued CPR and assisted ventilations
3. Warm, humidified oxygen administered by bag-valve mask
4. Warm IV fluid provided at a keep-vein-open rate
5. Blankets added to prevent further heat loss
6. Gastric tube to suction
7. Cervical spine immobilization
8. One additional dose of intravenous epinephrine

During the flight the patient remained clinically unchanged. Agonal respirations were noted toward the end of the flight. Rectal temperature rose to 28° C.

On arrival at the emergency department, the patient had a blood pressure of 98/60 mm Hg, with agonal respirations. Rectal temperature was 30° C. An increase in pink frothy sputum from the endotracheal tube was noted, and 3 cm of positive end expiratory pressure (PEEP) was added to the ventilator. A dopamine drip was started by pump

at 16.6 µg/kg/min to maintain a systolic blood pressure between 90 and 100 mm Hg. All fluids were placed on IV warmers. The heart monitor displayed sinus tachycardia with palpable femoral and brachial pulses. Peritoneal lavage was started with warmed normal saline solution as a check for abdominal bleeding and to initiate active internal rewarming.

Initially, arterial blood gas (ABG) values (adjusted for rectal temperature) were pH 7.13, P_{CO_2} 32, P_{O_2} 50, actual HCO_3 11, base deficit 20, O_2 calculated 91, O_2 actual 89, K 2.9. Sodium 10 mEq was given along with potassium chloride 10 mEq IV. Peritoneal lavage was negative for blood. Chest radiography revealed right pneumothorax, which was treated with a chest tube. Computed tomography of the head and neck was negative. The patient was transported to the intensive care unit in fairly stable condition.

In the intensive care unit the patient was maintained on the ventilator with warm humidified oxygen. The dopamine drip was continued to maintain a stable blood pressure between 90 and 100 mm Hg systolic. The patient was placed between hypothermia blankets. The pupils remained fixed and dilated at 8 cm; no corneal reflex was present. There was slight spontaneous flailing of all extremities. ABGs were stabilized throughout the evening with small doses of sodium bicarbonate. The patient's blood pressure was stabilized with 18 µg/kg/min dopamine. Rectal temperature increased slowly, finally stabilizing at 37° C. Four hours after admission to the intensive care unit, the patient suddenly deoxygenated, with the heart monitor displaying bradycardia. The patient's rhythm quickly deteriorated to ventricular fibrillation, and a cardiac arrest situation was called. Unfortunately, efforts failed, and the patient was pronounced dead after 1 hour of aggressive resuscitation.

REFERENCES

1. Bledsoe BE, Porter RS, Cherry RA: *Paramedic care: principles and practice: medical emergencies*, Upper Saddle River, NJ, 2001, Brady Prentice Hall.

2. Butler FK, Zafren K: Tactical management of wilderness casualties in special operations, *Wilder and Environ Med* 9:64, 1998.

3. Caroline NL: *Emergency care in the streets*, ed 2, Boston, 1983, Little, Brown.

4. Cauchy E, Chetaille E, Marchand V, Marsigny B: Retrospective study of 70 cases of severe frostbite lesions: a proposed new classification scheme, *Wilder and Environ Med* 12:248, 2001.

5. Collins KJ: *Hypothermia: the facts*, New York, 1983, Oxford University Press.

6. Danzl D: Accidental hypothermia. In Auerbach P, editor: *Wilderness medicine*, ed 4, St Louis, 2001, Mosby.

7. Danzl DF, Pozos RS: Multicenter hypothermia survey, *Ann Emerg Med* 16(9):1042, 1987.

8. Davies DM, Miller EJ, Miller IA: Accidental hypothermia treated by extracorporeal blood-warming, *Lancet* 1036, May 13, 1967.

9. Department of Transportation/United States Coast Guard: *Hypothermia and cold water survival*, Washington, DC, 1980, GPO.

10. Ehrmantraut WR, Ticktin HE, Fazekras JF: Cerebral hemodynamics and metabolism in accidental hypothermia, *Arch Intern Med* 99:57, 1957.

11. Freund B, O'Brien C, Young A: Alcohol ingestion and temperature regulation during cold exposure, *J Wilderness Med* 5:88, 1994.

12. Gordon AS: Cerebral blood flow and temperature during deep hypothermia for cardiovascular surgery, *J Cardiovasc Surg* 3:299, 1962.

13. Gregory J, Flanbaum I, Townsend M: Incidence and timing of hypothermia in trauma patients, *J Trauma* 31:795, 1991.

14. Gregory RT, Patton JF: Treatment after exposure to cold, *Lancet* 1:377, 1972.

15. Hauty M, Esrig B, Long W: Prognostic factors in severe accidental hypothermia: experience from the Mt. Hood tragedy, *J Trauma* 27:1107, 1987.

16. International Commission of Alpine Rescue, Subcommission of Medicine: *Field and base treatment of cold injuries*. Presented at the Fifth International Symposium on Mountain Medicine, Innsbruck, Austria, Nov 13, 1976.

17. Jolly T, Ghezzi K: Accidental hypothermia, *Emerg Med Clin North Am* 10(2):311, 1992.

18. Jurkovich G, Gaser W, Luterman A: Hypothermia in trauma victims: an ominous sign, *J Trauma* 27:1019, 1987.

19. Knowlton FP, Starling EH: The influence of variations in temperatures and blood pressure on the performance of the isolated mammalian heart, *J Physiol* 44:206, 1912.

20. Krupa D: *Flight nursing core curriculum*, Des Plaines, Ill, 1997, Roadrunner Press.

21. Lloyd EL: Accidental hypothermia treated by central rewarming through the airway, *Br J Anaesth* 45:41, 1973.

22. Lloyd EL, Frankland JC: Accidental hypothermia: central rewarming in the field (correspondence), *Br Med J* 4:717, 1974.

23. Luna G, Maier R, Pavlin E: Incidence and effect of hypothermia in seriously injured patients, *J Trauma* 27:1014, 1987.

24. McAniff JJ: *The incidence of hypothermia in scuba-diving fatalities*, First International Hypothermia Conference, Kingston, Jamaica, Jan 23–27, 1980.

25. McCauley RL, Smith DJ, Robson MC, Heggers JP: Frostbite. In Auerbach P, editor: *Wilderness medicine*, ed 4, St Louis, 2001, Mosby.

26. Miller JW, Danzl DF, Thomas DM: Urban accidental hypothermia: 135 cases, *Ann Emerg Med* 9:456, 1980.

27. Mills WJ, Whaley R: Frostbite: experience with rapid rewarming and ultrasonic therapy. Reprinted in *Lessons from History Wilderness and Environmental Medicine* 9:226, 1998.

28. Morrison JB, Conn ML, Hayward JS: Thermal increment provided by inhalation rewarming from hypothermia, *J Appl Physiol* 46:1061, 1979.

29. Okada M: The cardiac rhythm in accidental hypothermia, *J Electrocardiol* 17:123, 1984.

30. Okada M, Nishimura F, Yoshiro H: The J-wave in accidental hypothermia, *J Electrocardiol* 16:23, 1983.

31. O'Keefe KM: Accidental hypothermia: a review of 62 cases, *JACEP* 6:491, 1977.

32. Orr KD, Fainer DC: *Cold injuries in Korea during winter of 1950–1951*, Fort Knox, Ky, 1951, US Army Medical Research Laboratory.

33. Proehl J: Environmental emergencies. In Kitt S et al, editors: *Emergency nursing*, Philadelphia, 1995, Saunders.

34. Purdue GF, Hunt JL: Cold injury: a collective review, *J Burn Care Rehabil* 7(4):331, 1986.

35. Rango N: Exposure-related hypothermia mortality in the United States, 1970–1979, *Am J Public Health* 74:1159, 1984.

36. Rango N: Old and cold: hypothermia in the elderly, *Geriatrics* 35(11):93, 1980.

37. Rankin AC, Rae AP: Cardiac arrhythmias during rewarming of patients with accidental hypothermia, *Br Med J* 289:874, 1984.

38. Reuler JB: Hypothermia: pathophysiology, clinical settings and management, *Ann Intern Med* 89:519, 1978.

39. Savard GK et al: Peripheral blood flow during rewarming from mild hypothermia in humans, *J Appl Physiol* 58:4, 1985.

40. Holleran RS: *Prehospital nursing*, St Louis, 1994, Mosby.

41. Slovis CM, Bachvarov HL: Heated inhalation treatment of hypothermia, *Am J Emerg Med* 2:533, 1984.

42. Smith DS: Accidental hypothermia: giving "dead" victims the benefit of the doubt, *Postgrad Med* 81(3):38, 1987.

43. Smith DS: *The cold water connection*, First International Hypothermia Conference, Kingston, Jamaica, Jan 23–27, 1980.

44. Steinman AM: The hypothermic code: CPR controversy revisited, *JEMS* 8(10):32, 1983.

45. Steinmann S, Shackford S, Davis J: Implications of admission hypothermia in trauma patients, *J Trauma* 30:200, 1990.

46. Tek D, Mackey S: Non-freezing cold injury in a marine infantry battalion, *J Wilderness Med* 4:353, 1993.

47. Tolman KG, Cohen A: Accidental hypothermia, *Can Med Asso J* 103:1357, 1970.

48. United States Coast Guard Station, UCN 0075, New York, Apr 5, 1982.

49. Vaughn PB: Local cold injury-menace to military operations: a review, *Milit Med* 145:305, 1980.

50. Weast RC, editor: *Handbook of chemistry and physics*, ed 55, Cleveland, Ohio, 1974, CRC Press.

51. Wilkerson JA, Bangs CC, Hayward JS: *Hypothermia, frostbite and other cold injuries*, Seattle, 1986, Mountaineers.

52. Wilson FN, Finch R: The effect of drinking iced water upon the form of the T deflection of the electrocardiogram, *Heart* 10:275, 1923.

53. White JD: Hypothermia: the Bellevue experience, *Ann Emerg Med* 11:417, 1982.

HEAT-RELATED EMERGENCIES

26

COMPETENCIES

1. Identify risk factors that contribute to heat-related illnesses.
2. Identify the different types of heat-related illnesses, including heat exhaustion and heatstroke.
3. Initiate the appropriate management of a patient with a heat-related illness in the transport environment.

Deaths attributed to heat-related illnesses have been reported for centuries. The Bible refers to persons who had heatstroke after working in hot fields 2000 years ago. In 24 BC a Roman army was annihilated in the heat of the Arabian desert. The warriors of the Crusades were ultimately beaten in the Holy Land by heat and fever.[13] Incarceration in the infamous "Black Hole of Calcutta" resulted in high numbers of heat-related deaths.[8] During the summers of 1980, 1983, 1988, and 1995 severe heat waves in the United States resulted in multiple deaths from heatstroke.[4,5] Recent data related to heat illness have been obtained from pilgrims in Mecca, Saudi Arabia, in 1984 and 1985,[13,24] and military experience has provided extensive data on heat illness and the effect of heat on human physiology.[17]

Heatstroke is a true medical emergency that requires rapid diagnosis and treatment. The longer the body remains hyperthermic, the greater the damage and consequent increase in morbidity and mortality. The transport team, by quickly recogniz-ing and immediately treating the heat illness, can do much to combat permanent organ damage and the sequelae of hyperthermia.[6,7]

INCIDENCE AND CAUSATIVE FACTORS

The very young and the elderly are at greatest risk of being afflicted with heat-related illness. Moderate forms of heat-related illness can cause discomfort but are of relatively short duration, with rare seque-lae. Heat exhaustion and heatstroke are the two seri-ous, pathologic states of heat illness.

Even in relatively mild weather, heat illness can affect persons with predisposing risk factors; it can also affect persons who are unacclimatized or unconditioned and who are then pushed rapidly beyond their tolerance or physical capability, as can happen in military "boot camp" and with novice joggers. Even well-conditioned athletes are subject to heat illness if they are not properly acclimatized. Heat illness is second only to head injuries as a cause of death of U.S. athletes.[6,7,15,16,20]

The mortality and morbidity statistics for heat illness do not reflect the true impact of this illness on the civilian population. Civilian statistics can be inferred from military experience. Records show that heat exhaustion affects 280 of 100,000 military recruits undergoing basic training in South Carolina.[15,20]

Many times, death from heatstroke goes unrecorded during heat waves. The patient often has an underlying cardiovascular, pulmonary, renal, or neurologic disease. During heat waves, deaths from myocardial infarction, pneumonia, kidney failure, and stroke climb sharply; these are then recorded as the cause of death. Thus the estimate of heat illness is a "dramatic underrepresentation" of the true magnitude of this problem.[12]

Infants have a relatively small surface area with which to dissipate heat. Parents often prevent heat loss by wrapping infants in blankets and in clothing that is too heavy for a hot environment. The thermoregulatory ability of children lags behind other body systems in maturity and functional ability. Therefore children are more predisposed to heat illness, and recognition and diagnosis of heat pathology are often made more difficult.

Heat illness can develop in elderly persons under conditions that would not generally affect younger persons. As a person's age increases, physiologic ability to regulate temperature decreases. Older persons often do not notice temperature changes less than 2.3° C, probably because of sensory afferent deterioration.[1] The elderly population generally has a higher rate of cardiovascular and pulmonary disease, diabetes, and neurologic pathology, and they often use multiple drugs. All of these conditions contribute to the increased likelihood of heat illness in persons in this age-group.

A person who is obese also has a higher risk of experiencing heat illness. Heat loss is inversely proportional to body size and body weight. Adipose tissue has less ability to lose heat compared to nonadipose tissue because of decreased vascularity. Fat serves as an insulator, which is not conducive to heat loss.

Dehydration occurs because of a decrease in body water. As heat illness progresses, the circulatory blood volume decreases. When heat illness is superimposed on preexisting dehydration, the body has a severely limited volume reserve. The more severe the dehydration, the faster the physiologic compensation will be exhausted. Fluid intake is crucial for the prevention of heat illness.

An increased endogenous heat load will limit the body's ability to maintain normothermia in a hot environment. A classic endogenous heat source is fever. Fever is generally caused by pyrogens released from bacteria or viruses or by breakdown of cells caused by the infectious organism.

It is important to note that two different mechanisms are involved in fever and heat illness. With fever, the thermal set point is elevated because of the induction of prostaglandin synthesis in the thermoregulatory center. Certain medications such as salicylates work well to inhibit the reactions that lead to elevation of the thermal set point and thus relieve hyperthermia caused by fever. With heat illness, the thermal set point remains normal. Hyperthermia occurs because of the body's inability to dissipate heat; normal defense mechanisms designed to protect the set point are overwhelmed. The medications used for fever medication do not work well in this setting and should not be used.[6,7,12]

Hyperactive states demand more energy. The increasing energy demand is met by an increase in metabolic activity. Endogenous heat increases as a by-product of the increased metabolic rate. Strenuous physical exercise and seizures are examples of hyperactive states. Drugs can also lead to a hyperactive state and increase endogenous heat production.

Muscular exertion increases endogenous heat because of increased metabolic demand. Skeletal muscle is one of the major sources of heat production in the body. Muscular exertion often occurs outdoors under conditions in which the ambient temperature exceeds body temperature and high humidity is present. Hyperthermia can occur in this setting. "Weekend warriors," novice hard laborers, military inductees in physical training, football players who practice in the heat, and persons who use hot tubs unwisely can all predispose their bodies to heat illness.

Use of many prescription drugs and alcohol can also predispose a person to heat illness. Anticholinergic drugs reduce sweat gland secretions because of the blocking action of anticholinergics on transmission of sympathetic postganglionic nerve impulses to sweat glands. This cessation of sweating removes the body's chief agent of heat dissipation. Use of tricyclic antidepressants, phenothiazines, butyrophenones, thiothixenes, diuretics, and beta-blockers predispose the patient to heat illness.[12,15]

Other drugs associated with hyperthermia are glutethimide, those that induce hypersensitivity or idiosyncratic reactions (antibiotics, anticonvulsants, and hypertensives), and those that induce direct pyrogenic stimulation (bleomycin).[5,12,14,16]

Psychiatric patients often take anticholinergic drugs. Lithium and haloperidol have been reported to cause fatal hyperthermia. Haloperidol may reduce awareness or recognition of thirst.[13] Thioridazine (Mellaril) overdose is documented to cause hyperthermia.[4] The interaction of monamine oxidase inhibitors with amphetamines, tricyclic antidepressants, or phenothiazines is a well-documented cause of hyperthermia. Psychiatric patients may lack the awareness or desire to care for themselves properly in hot environments.

Alcohol use is known to predispose most persons to heat illness.[12] The exact mechanisms of this phenomenon are complex. Alcohol is a vasodilator and may enhance external heat absorption. Use of alcohol interferes with the judgment and mental acuity necessary to care for oneself. Use of cocaine and LSD has also been documented to cause fatal hyperthermia.[7,12]

One of the major organs that must be functional if heat is to be dissipated is the skin. Any pathologic process that disrupts skin integrity interrupts normal physiologic functions, or both conditions will sharply limit heat dissipation. Sunburn and heat rash are relatively minor conditions that can have a drastic impact on physiologic compensation for heat stress. Major burns cause partial to total loss of skin function. Lack of ability to regulate body temperature is a complication of burn injury. Obviously the burn victim may be a candidate for heat illness.[19]

Patients with cystic fibrosis have a striking elevation of sweat electrolytes; the sodium and chloride content of their sweat is two to five times greater than that of healthy control subjects, and this occurs in 98% to 99% of affected children. These children are subject to massive sodium depletion in hot weather. Today, because of improved early diagnostic measures and treatment, many more patients with cystic fibrosis are living into early adulthood.

Lack of acclimatization predisposes a person to heat illness. On entering a warmer climate, exercise and general activity levels must be gradually increased. Persons vacationing in warm climates often overexert. Even well-conditioned athletes can be affected by heat-related illness if their training programs do not allow sufficient acclimatization before vigorous physical activity in hot, humid weather.

Persons can become acclimated to a hot climate in 10 days with daily exposure to moderate work and heat.[7,12] With a less-zealous routine, acclimatization will occur in several weeks. The recognition of the principle of acclimatization has led to a reduction of the incidence of heat illness for those who are exposed to hot or high-risk environments. Acclimatization can occur at any age; however, its effectiveness can be limited by any of the aforementioned predisposing factors.

The most important physiologic adaptations during the acclimatization period include retention of salt and water, expansion of extracellular fluid volumes, and slight hemodilution.[7,12] Through these processes, sweating mechanisms improve. This is characterized by early onset of sweating, an increase in the volume of sweat, and a lowering of electrolyte concentration in the sweat.[7,12]

The increase in the volume of sweat accompanied by a lowering of the threshold for the onset of sweating results in better heat dissipation. An increase in aldosterone production lowers the sodium content of sweat. Combined with a 7% increase in total body water, the increase in aldosterone lowers sodium content of sweat from 100 mEq/L to 70 mEq/L.[1] The chloride concentration in sweat falls from 40 or 45 mEq/L to as low as 15 or 20 mEq/L, and sweat volume rises from 1 to 3 L/hr.[7,12]

After acclimatization, cardiovascular and metabolic proficiency is improved. Vasodilation occurs earlier and in greater magnitude. The heart rate is lower with a higher stroke volume, thus increasing cardiac output. Biochemical efficiency at the cellular level improves to the point that heat production for a given amount of work is less than in an unacclimatized person. Storage and utilization of glycogen are improved, thus delaying the onset of anaerobic metabolism with resultant lactic acidosis.

PATHOPHYSIOLOGIC FACTORS

NORMAL THERMOGENESIS

Human core temperature is closely regulated by a number of mechanisms to maintain a body core temperature of between 36° C and 38° C. Processes that alter temperature homeostasis result in pathologic changes at the cellular level. Rising body temperature, if unregulated, can exceed the "critical thermal maximum" and cause irreversible organ damage; death quickly ensues. It is well documented that the human thermal maximum is 43° C.

Body core temperature is a species-specific, genetically determined set point that is regulated by the hypothalamus. Temperature regulation is quite precise, with response to temperature changes as small as 0.2° C (1.6° F).[8] A "thermostat" in the preoptic anterior portion of the hypothalamus receives information from various body thermoregulators. Peripheral and core temperature sensors in the skin, viscera, and nervous system tissues produce both thermal and endocrine signals. These signals are transmitted to the hypothalamus via neuronal and circulatory pathways. The "thermostat" then responds through a variety of negative feedback mechanisms to activate processes by which heat is lost or gained. These responses are mediated by means of the sympathetic nervous system.

Body heat production occurs because of two separate processes: endogenous metabolic processes and exogenous environmental exposure. Close regulation of body temperature is critical because the human body is dependent on relatively low temperature biochemical reactions at the microcellular level to sustain life.

Every body process produces exothermic heat. Normal basal cellular metabolism generates 50 to 60 kcal/hr and would cause a rise of 1° C/hr if not dissipated by compensatory mechanisms.[8] Digestion of food is the source of body heat. Major heat-producing organs are the liver and skeletal muscle. Increasing bodywork raises body temperature. Maximum sustained exercise produces 600 to 900 kcal/hr, raising body core temperature 5° C/hr without functional compensatory mechanisms.[20]

Exogenous (external) heat comes from the environment. Exposure to direct sunlight raises body core temperature 150 kcal/hr. The amount of humidity present in the air directly affects the body's ability to disperse heat. Humidity limits cooling by evaporation, which is caused by a lack of an evaporation gradient from skin surface to air.

METHODS OF HEAT LOSS

Thermoregulation by the hypothalamus maintains normothermia by balancing heat production and heat loss. When thermoregulation breaks down because of excess heat generation (endogenous), inability to dissipate heat (pathophysiologic), overwhelming environmental conditions (high ambient temperature with high humidity), or a combination of these factors, hyperthermia results. Under normal conditions, 90% of the heat produced by the body is lost to the environment via the skin surface by conduction, radiation, convection, and evaporation.

Environmental temperature obviously has a direct effect on the patient. The higher the temperature, the more external heat is present. When the environmental temperature is equal to or greater than the body's temperature, passive heat loss through the means of conduction and radiation is decreased. Radiant heat loss occurs when the ambient temperature is lower than the body's temperature; conversely, the body readily absorbs radiant heat from the environment.

When air or water moves across the body surface, heat is lost by convection. Increasing the amount of air moving over the skin (forced convection) increases the amount of heat loss. The drier the air, the better the skin surface to air gradient, and the more heat that is lost.

The primary mechanism for heat dissipation is the evaporation of sweat. Through vaporization from the body surface, loss of 1 ml of sweat reduces body heat load by 1.7 kcal.[7,12,19,20,22] Under conditions of high ambient temperature and high ambient humidity, the skin is unable to provide effective cooling as the evaporation gradient is lost. At 75% humidity, evaporation decreases; at 90% to 95% humidity, evaporation ceases.[7,12]

The average person can produce up to 1.5 L of sweat per hour. Through conditioning and acclimatization, sweat production increases. The well-trained athlete can produce up to 3 L/hr.[7,12,15,20]

Insensible heat loss also occurs; heat is lost with passage of urine and feces, and the respiratory tract can dissipate heat by convection and evaporation.

PHYSIOLOGIC COMPENSATION

Physiologic compensation begins in the hypothalamus. The exact chemical nature of thermoregulation is not yet fully understood. As endocrine and thermal sensors arrive from the heated periphery and core, the hypothalamic "thermostat" reduces bio-amine concentrations. Final common pathway effectors probably include prostaglandins, central nervous system amines, and a host of other hypothesized candidates.[7,12]

On reception of effector "messages" from the hypothalamus and peripheral thermoreceptors, the cardiovascular system responds with peripheral vasodilatation. Vasodilatation maximizes the cooling surface and greatly decreases peripheral vascular resistance. In this manner, the cardiovasculature conducts heat to the surface of the body, where it can be released to the environment. When skin vessels dilate, blood flow shunted through the area can exceed 4 L/min.[7,12] With this increased flow, 97% of cooling occurs at the skin surface.[17]

HEAT PATHOPHYSIOLOGY

The initial response to heatstroke begins on a cellular level. There is subcellular disruption, which directly causes cell destruction. Hypothermia also initiates apoptosis or the programmed cellular destruction. The cells that produce the greatest number of apoptotic cells from hypothermia are the thymus, spleen, lymph nodes and the mucosa of the small intestine.[7]

On exposure to heat, the body initiates compensation by decreasing peripheral vascular resistance, thus shunting blood to the periphery. This action causes an increase in stroke volume and cardiac output, thus increasing demand on the heart. The healthy cardiovascular system can sustain this hyperdynamic state for a limited time; however, it will eventually tax the myocardium.

The purpose of this response is to cool the body. Heat is lost from the skin surface by evaporation of sweat. In severe heat stress, the body loses as much as 1.5 L/hr and even 3 L/hr in extreme cases.[7,12] Over time the circulating blood volume is reduced.

The cardiac output continues to drop as a result of the ensuing hypovolemia. Homeostasis becomes compromised. An altered hemodynamic state may develop that mimics high-output failure, such as that seen in sepsis. This results in hyperdynamic failure. In persons who undergo heatstroke, structural damage to the heart is common, although not extensive. Rarely, acute transmural myocardial infarction or widespread myocardial damage may occur.[7,12]

Cardiac dysrhythmia and myocardial damage may occur because of subendocardial hemorrhage, rupture of muscle fibers, necrosis, and infarction. This pathology is second to increased cardiac workload, thereby increasing myocardial oxygen demand. Not enough oxygen is available because of disruption of oxidative phosphorylation and a resulting shock state. Hypotension is usually a sign of severe or premorbid heat illness.[7,12]

The respiratory system initially responds with an increase in respiratory rate and depth to meet increased oxygen demand. This hyperventilation results in an initial heat loss from an increased volume of air moved over and through the respiratory tract. This evaporative loss decreases with increased respiratory fatigue. A high ambient humidity also limits this evaporative loss. An initial respiratory alkalosis develops as a result of the hyperventilation, with concurrent hypocarbia and the traditional muscle tetany. This tetany is the pathophysiologic basis for the ill-defined syndrome of heat tetany.

Ataxia, dysmetria, and dysarthria may be seen early in the onset of heatstroke because the Purkinje cells of the cerebellum are particularly sensitive to the toxic effects of high temperature. Because these changes are seen in other neurologic events, such as stroke, heatstroke may not be recognized initially. Cerebral edema combined with associated diffuse petechial hemorrhages are often found in fatal cases.

When the hyperthermic insult is associated with status epilepticus and profound hypotension, the energy requirements of the brain increase. This in turn contributes to the spiraling core temperature, increasing up to four times the metabolic rate of the brain. The cerebral vessels dilate maximally, and thus the blood flow is dependent on mean arterial pressure. The added effects of dehydration (hypovolemic source) produce a pathophysiologic state conducive to brain death and damage.

Kidney function is altered from the loss of sodium and water in sweat. The kidneys retain sodium, and thus they retain water and excrete potassium. Renal dysfunction occurs because of hypovolemia and hypoperfusion. Urinary output drops, and acute renal tubular necrosis may ensue. If sodium losses are of sufficient severity, signs of hyponatremia may appear. There is a risk that hypokalemia may develop because of the excretion of potassium in the urine.

The liver, which is particularly sensitive to temperature damage, is affected in nearly every case.[7,10,12] Liver function decreases by 20%. This decrease in function theoretically should aid in heat reduction because the liver is one of the major heat-producing organs. Prothrombin times become prolonged.[2] Reduced hepatic perfusion caused by shunting of blood to the periphery leads to hypoglycemia in 20% of patients with exertional heatstroke.[13] Interestingly, the pancreas is the only organ not damaged by the toxic effects of heat stress.[5]

During heat stress, the gastrointestinal tract undergoes direct thermotoxicity and relative hypoperfusion because of the shunt of blood to the periphery. Ischemic intestinal ulceration can also occur, which may lead to frank gastrointestinal bleeding.[5]

Muscle damage is evidenced by rhabdomyolysis. Muscle degeneration and necrosis occur as a direct result of extremely elevated temperature. Elevated creatine phosphokinase (CPK) values are a diagnostic hallmark of heatstroke because of this rhabdomyolytic process. The release of destructive lysosomal enzymes occurs as a result of extensive skeletal muscle damage. The release of lysosomal enzymes into the circulation may cause widespread capillary injury, leading to disseminated intravascular coagulation, acute respiratory distress syndrome, and acute renal tubular necrosis.[13] Muscle enzymes are greatly elevated.

ASSESSMENT PARAMETERS

The most common forms of heat illness, from least to most severe, are heat cramps, heat exhaustion, and heatstroke.

HEAT CRAMPS

Heat cramps of heavily exercised muscle occur during and after exercise in a hot environment and are an extreme inconvenience to the patient. These cramps usually occur in trained athletes and in physically fit, acclimatized persons. These persons sweat profusely and characteristically replace sweat losses with water and inadequate amounts of salt. Hyponatremia ensues, which hinders muscle relaxation mechanisms. Usually the muscles will show the fasciculations of fatigue. A slight or moderate rise in CPK enzymes in serum is often observed. This rhabdomyolysis has not been shown to constitute an important clinical problem.[13] No permanent effects have been demonstrated from heat cramps.

Heat cramps involve exquisitely painful sustained muscular contractions, most commonly involving the muscles of the lower extremity; however, any muscle group in the body can be affected. The patient usually reports heavy exercise in a hot environment, with onset of cramping after rest.

HEAT EXHAUSTION

Heat exhaustion is an ill-defined syndrome that can affect anyone. Hubbard et al[12] define it as "a derangement of body function encountered when the body temperature is elevated, usually in the 39° C to 41° C [102.2° F to 105.8° F] range." The typical victim of heat exhaustion is usually unacclimatized to the environment and has worked in the heat for several days. Both infants and elderly bedridden patients are at higher risk of experiencing heat exhaustion because of their impaired ability to dissipate heat and communicate thirst.

Heat exhaustion, if allowed to proceed, will result in heatstroke. An essential distinction between the two entities is that cerebral function is unimpaired in persons with heat exhaustion, aside from minor irritability and poor judgment. Body temperatures are lower and the symptoms are less severe in persons experiencing heat exhaustion.

This syndrome results from loss of water, loss of salt, or both. Pure forms of single loss of either water or sodium are rare. Water-depletion heat exhaustion, which results from inadequate fluid replacement, is more serious and develops in a few hours. Salt-depletion heat exhaustion develops over the course of several days.

Heat exhaustion is largely a manifestation of the strain placed on the cardiovascular system when it is attempting to maintain normothermia. With sodium and water loss the patient becomes dehydrated, tachycardic, and syncopal, with orthostatic hypotension. The patient's temperature is usually less than 38° C to 39° C (100.4° F to 102.2° F) and is often normal. The patient retains the ability to sweat, which gives rise to cool, clammy skin. Headache and euphoria commonly occur because of dehydration and hypoperfusion. Mental status remains intact, although minor aberrations may be manifested. Flulike symptoms of nausea, vomiting, and diarrhea with muscle cramps may be present. Subjective complaints include intense thirst, vague malaise, myalgias, and dizziness.

Laboratory values show classic signs of dehydration (elevated hematocrit, blood urea nitrogen [BUN], serum protein, and concentrated urine levels) with hyponatremia and hypokalemia. LDH, AST, and ALT may be elevated. However, this may not occur until 24 to 48 hours after the heat injury.[7]

HEATSTROKE

Heatstroke is a life-threatening medical emergency in which the body's physiologic heat-dissipating mechanisms fail and body temperature rises rapidly and uncontrollably. The central core temperature exceeds 42° C. At 42° C and above, cellular oxygen demands surpass the oxygen supply, and oxidative phosphorylation is disrupted, causing cell and organ damage throughout the body. The duration of the hyperthermic episode and the temperature reached may be the single most important factors in patient survival and prognosis.

The resultant damage of such severe hyperthermia has many causes. Central nervous system disruption with altered mental status is a key diagnostic criterion in heatstroke. Early in the course of heatstroke, some persons appear confused and demonstrate irrational behavior, or even frank psychosis; others become comatose or have seizures. The patient may have hot, flushed skin, with or without sweating, vomiting, and diarrhea. Hyperventilation at rates up to 60 is universally seen. Respiratory alkalosis is often present with tetany and hypokalemia. Pulmonary edema is not uncommon.

The cardiovascular system responds by reaching maximum stroke volume. Because of the shunt through the dilated periphery, tachycardia is the only way to increase cardiac output. Heatstroke results in high output failure, with cardiac output of 20 L or more. Central venous pressure readings are elevated despite hypotension caused by decreased ventricular contractility over 40° C. The hyperdynamic state persists even after cooling. The electrocardiogram (ECG) generally shows nonspecific ST-T changes with various atrial and ventricular arrhythmias.[7,12]

Blood studies should include arterial blood gas, complete blood cell count, platelets, prothrombin time/partial thromboplastin time (PT/PTT), electrolytes, BUN, creatinine, glucose, liver function tests (LVT), CPK, and LDH, and a urinalysis. White blood counts of 30,000 to 50,000 are not uncommon. The platelet count and PT/PTT are monitored for onset of hypocoagulability. Hypofibrinogenemia and fibrinolysis may occur and progress to frank disseminated intravascular coagulation (DIC).

The muscle enzymes (CPK, SGOT, SGPT, and LDH) in heatstroke are elevated in the tens of thousands—a diagnostic hallmark of heatstroke. Muscle breakdown occurs from direct thermal injury, clonic muscle activity, or tissue ischemia. In exertional heatstroke, CPK levels up to 1,500,000 IU/L have been reported. CPK levels greater than 20,000 are ominous and are indicative of later DIC, acute kidney failure, and potentially dangerous hyperkalemia.[7,9,12]

Reduced renal blood flow from shock and dehydration leads to ischemic kidneys. Concentration of the urine may lead to accumulation of uric acid and myoglobin, which have the capacity to crystallize in renal tubules. Crystallization may lead to obstructive uropathy and the development of acute tubular necrosis. BUN levels are frequently elevated. Low serum osmolarity, moderate proteinuria, and machine oil appearance of the urine occurs in patients with exertional heatstroke.[7,9,12,20]

The liver is frequently damaged, and frank jaundice is noted. The development of early jaundice, less than 24 hours after onset, has a worse prognosis than delayed jaundice. The engorged vessels of the gastrointestinal tract may become ulcerated and hemorrhage massively.

PATTERNS OF HEATSTROKE PRESENTATION

Heatstroke is manifested in three distinct patterns: classic, exertional, and drug induced. The three essential elements in the diagnosis of heatstroke are exposure to heat stress, internal or external; central nervous system dysfunction; and increased body temperature greater than 40° C.

Classic heatstroke, which tends to occur in the elderly, the ill, and infants, develops over a period of several days. It often occurs during heat waves and affects persons who do not have access to a cooler environment and fluids. Often the patient is discovered in bed and is unresponsive. In these cases the patient has hot, red, or flushed skin; has usually ceased sweating; and is significantly dehydrated.

Initial symptoms of classic heatstroke are similar to those of heat exhaustion: dizziness, headache, and malaise, progressing to frank confusion and coma. Fever, tachycardia, and hypotension are additional presenting signs. These patients also hyperventilate, which gives rise to respiratory alkalosis.

Exertional heatstroke usually occurs in young, fit, but unacclimatized persons who are often male athletes. Many such patients perform in hot and humid weather conditions that prevent adequate dissipation of generated heat. Of these patients, 50% still sweat profusely from the rapid onset; severe dehydration has not yet had time to occur.

Exertional heatstroke has a prodrome of chills, nausea, throbbing pressure in the head, and piloerection on the chest and upper arms. Concentration wanes, a subjective sense of physical deterioration is noticed, and the person feels increasingly hot, with decreased sweat production. Paresthesia is noted in the hands and feet.

Onset of irrational behavior then occurs. The face turns ashen gray, and the skin may feel relatively cool if sweat is still being produced. This is followed by seizures and collapse. Patients who have exertional heatstroke often have severe respiratory acidosis from lactate caused by muscle exertion and volume depletion. They also have significant rhabdomyolysis.[7,12,20]

Drugs that predispose a person to heatstroke have been previously identified. Anticholinergic drugs such as phenothiazines, tricyclic antidepressants, antihistamines, antiparkinsonian agents, antispasmodics, and glutethimide inhibit sweating, thus interfering with heat dissipation. The side effects of some anticholinergic drugs include hyperkinesis and agitation, resulting in an increase in body temperature. Drugs with cardiovascular actions (beta-blockers, diuretics, and antihypertensives) can inhibit or depress cardiovascular performance during increased demand resulting from heat stress. Diuretics, especially if abused, can lead to dehydration. Amphetamines, neuroleptics, and possibly tricyclic antidepressants induce heatstroke because they increase the endogenous heat load.[19,20] Hyperthermia resulting from interaction of monoamine oxidase inhibitors with tricyclic antidepressants and amphetamines has been noted.

Patients with drug-induced heatstroke have classic signs of heatstroke; the main difficulty is identifying the causative agent. Management should *never* be delayed by attempts to elucidate a comprehensive drug history.

INTERVENTION AND TREATMENT

PRIORITIES

The most critical goal and life-saving measure in heat illness is cooling the victim to *rapidly decrease body temperature.* Immediate treatment often leads to prompt recovery. The more rapid the cooling, the lower the risk of mortality. Morbidity and mortality are directly related to the duration and intensity (temperature maximum) of hyperthermia.

While the patient is being cooled as rapidly as possible, maintenance of the "ABCs" of emergency care must not be forgotten. Because the patient may not have the ability to protect his or her airway, the transport team must effectively ventilate the lungs, oxygenate the blood, and maintain an adequate circulatory volume with an intact pump while carrying out continuous astute assessment through the duration of required therapy.

EQUIPMENT

No special equipment is required to effectively treat patients with heat illness. Standard equipment required for the provision of advanced life-support measures must be available.

Methods for cooling a patient range from use of simple ice packs to elaborate cooling tables. At this time, no method has proved to be superior to any other method. Recognition of the illness and prompt initiation of treatment are the most important tools in the management of heat illness.

INTERVENTIONS—MILD TO INVASIVE

Cooling can be accomplished in the prehospital setting first by removing the patient from the hot environment and especially moving him or her away from hot surfaces, such as concrete and pavement, even if no shaded area is nearby. The transport team should remove the patient's clothing and wet down the patient.

Covering the patient with cool fluid and increasing the movement of air over the patient enhance heat loss by increasing the evaporative gradient. The transport team should open the windows of the ambulance or make use of the air circulation of helicopter rotors during transport to further increase

air movement over the patient. In one study of three cases of heatstroke, the patients were sprayed with lukewarm water while they were exposed to the downwash of a helicopter's rotors.[18,11]

Heat cramps constitute a mild form of heat illness. Treatment consists of fluid and electrolyte replacement. Oral replacement should be started by having the patient drink a balanced electrolyte solution. If oral intake is contraindicated, 1000 ml of normal saline solution is administered intravenously over a 1- to 3-hour period. Mild forms of heat exhaustion are treated in a similar manner. If the patient's body temperature is elevated, the transport team should cool the skin with fans and cool compresses.[9,22]

More severe cases of heat exhaustion require rehydration. Laboratory values (renal electrolytes, BUN, and hematocrit) are best used to guide replacement. Fluid is titrated to cardiovascular status. Normal saline solution, half-normal saline solution, and dextrose-half-normal saline solution have all been used; no evidence exists of a clear superiority of any one of these fluids.[9,22] In 12 hours patients generally should feel well, have normal vital signs, and can be discharged without sequelae.

Heat exhaustion must be regarded on a continuum from the mild case, treated by simple cooling measures, to the severe case, which progresses to full-blown heatstroke. The most important treatment for heat illness is recognizing the hyperthermic insult and rapidly initiating cooling.

Controversy surrounds the question of which method is ideal for cooling the patient with heatstroke. Several methods are considered to be of therapeutic benefit. Packing the patient in ice and immersing the body in cold water are historic methods of cooling.[12] Other therapies involve the use of room-temperature water evaporated from the victim's skin surface by circulating air from a fan. The field treatment measure of ice packs placed in areas of maximum heat transfer (neck, axillae, and inguinal area) may also be continued with caution.

Studies have revealed that dropping the skin surface temperature below 22° to 28° C may actually inhibit cooling because of peripheral vasoconstriction with a marked decrease in cutaneous blood flow. At or below these skin temperatures there is a sevenfold reduction in heat transfer from the body to the environment.[17] Counterproductive shivering may also occur at these skin temperatures. Research has demonstrated that if a patient's temperature has not been decreased in 30 minutes, cold-water immersion should be seriously considered.[7,12,21]

Cooling measures are ceased when body core temperature reaches 39° C (102° F). The core temperature will then continue to fall to the normal range. If normal thermoregulatory mechanisms have been damaged by the thermic insult, a hypothermic overshot could result from further active cooling measures.[10]

Refractory hyperthermia will require more aggressive invasive methods. Ice-water gastric lavage has been reported to be effective both in a controlled canine model[17] and in actual victim treatment.[7,12] Gastric lavage has the advantages of rapid cooling and effective use of readily available equipment. Iced peritoneal lavage, hemodialysis, and cardiopulmonary bypass have been used as end attempts in severely refractory cases.[7,12] These increasingly invasive, operative methods obviously require a great commitment of resources and have higher degrees of risk and complication rates.

TRANSPORT CARE

Heatstroke presents a complex patient management picture. If, when the transport team arrives, cooling measures have not been implemented or require augmentation, institution of the previously discussed interventions must be of the highest priority. As in any life-threatening case, a secured airway, institution of oxygenation, ventilation, and stabilization of cardiovascular status are mandated.

Endotracheal intubation is indicated for any patient who has a depressed sensorium because of the risk of emesis, aspiration, and seizure activity. Patients with heatstroke are often hypotensive because of dehydration and the physiologic compensation of extreme vasodilatation. In the vast number of cases, the hypotension will respond to cooling. Large amounts of fluids and inotropic agents are required only when cooling results in no response.

The choice of intravenous fluid is open to debate. In normotensive patients or those in whom hypotension is readily resolved with cooling, Ringer's lactate or normal saline solution is most often recommended.[7,12] Vasoactive medications may need to be initiated for vascular support when fluid resuscitation is not effective. Because of complications of impaired cardiac function, pulmonary edema, congestive heart failure, adult respiratory distress syndrome, and acute kidney failure, fluid replacement is best guided by placement of a pulmonary catheter. Field guidelines for fluid replacement recommend infusion of normal saline solution until a systolic blood pressure of 90 is obtained.[7,12]

In the light of the axiom that "the best defense is a good offense," monitoring the patient for multiple organ failure and prompt intervention on clinical manifestation of such failure are of utmost importance. Placement of a gastric tube accomplishes gastric decompression and monitors for the onset of gastrointestinal bleeding. H_2 blockers and antacids may be administered to prevent gastrointestinal bleeding.

An in-dwelling urinary catheter should be inserted to monitor hourly urinary output and rhabdomyolysis. Because of the possibility of kidney impairment, the transport team must closely monitor and support kidney function.

Liver failure is a frequent complication of heatstroke. When liver failure is combined with kidney failure, the choice of drugs used in treatment becomes difficult. DIC occurs in severe cases; most patients who die from heatstroke have evidence of DIC.[8] Standard treatment measures are instituted.[10]

Electrolyte and acid-base imbalances may be manifested. Patients with low serum glucose levels are treated with glucose administration. Hyper- and hypokalemia are common. Hypokalemia with respiratory alkalosis is transient and requires no treatment; hypokalemia with acidosis requires replacement therapy.[7,12] Hyperkalemia reflects cellular damage and acidosis.[17]

The recurrence of seizure activity during and after cooling is treated with intravenously administered diazepam or lorazepam. Use of prophylactic treatment has been considered because seizures may increase heat production, metabolic acidosis, and hypoxia.

MALIGNANT HYPERTHERMIA

Malignant hyperthermia is chemically induced either by anesthetic agents or by catecholamine release in stress.[7,8,23] This disease is a genetic myopathy transmitted by an autosomal dominant gene. Malignant hyperthermia occurs in anesthetized patients at a ratio of approximately 1:15,000 in children and 1:50,000 in adults.[1,8] It is most common in male patients between ages 15 and 30. Malignant hyperthermia has been reported in all races but with less frequency in blacks; a muscle-mass sex influence increases the incidence in men. It is uncommon in patients over the age of 50 years and under the age of 2 years.[1,8] The triggering agents are anesthetics: potent inhalant agents (often halothane) and skeletal muscle relaxants (succinylcholine chloride and amide local agents).

The primary disorder is a defect in the sarcoplasmic reticulum in skeletal muscle metabolism. The sarcoplasmic reticulum is a reservoir for calcium storage in the muscle cell. Under normal conditions, the sarcoplasmic reticulum releases calcium ions into the myoplasm, causing skeletal muscle contractions. Contraction is sustained as long as a high concentration of calcium ions exists in the myoplasm. Relaxation occurs when a constantly functional calcium pump in the wall of the sarcoplasmic reticulum pumps calcium ions back into the reticulum.

In malignant hyperthermia, either the sarcoplasmic reticulum is unable to reaccumulate calcium, or an accelerated release of calcium occurs. The increase in intracellular calcium results in sustained muscle contractions, and hypermetabolic state ensues. Increased oxygen consumption leads to decreased tissue oxygen saturation, causing metabolic and respiratory acidosis. Increased heat production leads to hyperthermia.

The loss of muscle cell membrane integrity occurs, which complicates the existing problem. The cell ions and molecules follow their concentration gradients. Calcium continues to move into the myoplasm, sustaining and worsening the muscle contractions. Hyperkalemia, myoglobinemia, and elevated CPK levels occur in the serum.

Malignant hyperthermia is characterized by hyperthermia, sustained tetanic muscle rigidity and contractions, hypermetabolism, and muscle cell destruction. Signs and symptoms are dependent on the use or nonuse of succinylcholine chloride.

With the administration of succinylcholine chloride at induction, rigidity of the masseter muscle may make intubation impossible. Additional doses will only worsen the rigidity. Muscle fasciculations normally observed with use of the drug may not occur. Unmovable joints with hard unindentible bellies may be noted.

Tachycardia is the most consistent first sign of malignant hyperthermia with the use of potent inhalation agents. Tachypnea, which results from hyperventilation caused by increasing acidosis, is the second sign. If the patient is not completely paralyzed, he or she may exhibit ventilatory efforts. Instability of systolic blood pressure is another consistent sign. Cardiac dysrhythmia and ensuing profound hypotension may occur. Cyanotic mottling of the skin, dark blood in the surgical field, and fever are late signs and indicate that the patient is already in crisis.

Immediate reversal of anesthesia and termination of surgery are mandated. Dantrolene sodium (Dantrium) is administered to maximize the survival of the patient. Dantrium, a skeletal muscle relaxant that acts by preventing the release of calcium ions from the sarcoplasmic reticulum, is the drug of choice. Dosage is 1 to 3 mg/kg initially to a maximum dose of 10 mg/kg.[7]

Procainamide is the drug of choice for ventricular arrhythmia because it does not affect myoplasmic calcium. Lidocaine and cardiac glycosides are contraindicated because they increase myoplasmic calcium. Hyperthermia is treated with previously described cooling methods. The standard therapy for hyperkalemia is indicated. Late complications can include pulmonary edema, DIC, kidney failure, and recurrence of malignant hyperthermia that was initially responsive to treatment measures.

SUMMARY

Heat illness presents as a continuum from mild to severe. Heat exhaustion, if untreated, may proceed to frank heatstroke, which is a life-threatening medical emergency. Causes of heat illness encompass endogenous, environmental, and drug-related pathologies. Malignant hyperthermia rarely occurs but has deadly consequences.

Prompt recognition of the problem and rapid cooling limit the severe sequelae associated with heat toxicity. Various cooling methods are used to limit the duration of exposure to hyperthermia. Research shows the length of exposure and maximum temperature reached are two critical criteria in the survival and recovery of patients with heatstroke.

Complications of heatstroke affect every organ system and can lead to multiple organ system failure. Liver and kidney failure are common. Neurologic complications are usually rare with prompt cooling to achieve euthermia. Cerebellar effects are the residual pathologies most often seen.

The onset of DIC, coma lasting more than 8 hours, cardiac dysfunction, hypotension, and high lactate and CPK levels are ominous signs and are usually predictive of mortality. Prevention of heat illness with adequate hydration; recognition of environmental, exertional, and physiologic risk factors; and proper acclimatization are important educational tools for the flight nurse and potential patients.

HEAT-RELATED EMERGENCIES CASE STUDY

The helicopter flight crew was dispatched immediately to a rural hospital a distance of 60 miles from their base hospital. The dispatch information stated that a female patient in her middle 60s had collapsed and was unresponsive. The basic life-support unit reported seizure activity with no change in her level of consciousness after tonic-clonic motor activity. Because the facility has no computed tomography (CT) scan or neurosurgical capabilities, the rural physician was requesting that she be transferred. The patient had not yet arrived at the rural hospital.

The past week had been hot, with temperatures hovering between 90° F and 110° F and humidity registering 80% to 85%.

On arrival at the hospital, the patient's husband reported that they had arrived early that morning at an outlying lake for a fishing trip. He stated that their boat trailer became stuck on the ramp; as a result, he and the patient had to walk about 11 miles to get assistance to launch the boat. The patient tired and sat in the truck while the boat was launched.

After 2 hours of fishing, the patient complained of a headache and nausea, which lasted for an hour. Her husband then noted "really strange behavior—she was talking funny and didn't remember she was in the boat." By the time he reached the shore, the patient was unresponsive. She subsequently had a seizure when the ground ambulance arrived. Because of the location of the boat dock, the weight of the patient, and the ground response time, the patient had been unresponsive for an hour before arrival at the rural hospital.

PHYSICAL FINDINGS

Obese female, weight 100 kg, age 64 years, supine on emergency department (ED) cart with red, flushed skin surfaces. No response noted to any stimuli.

Vital signs: BP 106/62; pulse 152/min regular in rate and rhythm, sinus tachycardia; respirations 40/min; temperature 105.5° F rectally.

HEENT: PERRLA, neck supple, mucous membranes dry, tongue leathery in appearance, upper airway patent.

Thorax: Symmetric expansion on inspiration, breath sounds clear and equal bilaterally, heart sounds normal S_1 and S_2, no murmur or rub noted, no trauma noted.

Abdomen: Obese, soft, no apparent guarding or tenderness, bowel sounds present but decreased, no organomegaly.

Extremities: No obvious trauma, no edema.

Neurologic: Glasgow Coma Score 4 (1–2–1), flaccid tone, no focal deficits noted, Babinski negative bilaterally.

Skin: Hot, dry, red in color, no rashes or other abnormalities noted.

Current interventions: Oxygen 8 L by plain face mask; in-dwelling urinary catheter inserted; patient covered with damp bath blanket.

The patient's husband stated she has no medical allergies; she occasionally takes Lasix for "fluid buildup"; her only past medical history is mild heart failure.

LABORATORY AND X-RAY DATA

CBC: WBC 22,100; RBC 4.2; Hgb/Hct 14.6/42; differential normal.

ABG: pH 7.54; Pco_2 26; Po_2 97; Hco_2 26; O_2 sat 94: B.E. + 2; Na 142; K 3.2; Cl 100; CO_2 17; BUN 32; glucose 62; creatinine 1.2; CPK 25,000; LDH 730; amylase 142. Urinalysis: Color dark greenish-brown; specific gravity 1.042; pH 7; ketones 3+; protein 2+.

PT/PTT and platelets: Within normal limits.

Chest radiograph: Within normal limits with heart size upper side of normal.

ECG (12 lead): Sinus tachycardia without ectopy; nonspecific ST-T changes.

FLIGHT NURSE INTERVENTIONS

Before takeoff, the patient was endotracheally intubated because of neurologic depression and to prevent aspiration; she was placed on a T-piece for supplemental oxygenation. Concurrently with cooling measures, a gastric tube was placed for stomach decompression, and ECG monitoring was instituted.

Immediate cooling measures consisted of stripping the patient and covering her with a wet sheet. Ice packs placed in the axilla, neck, and inguinal areas were promptly replaced when they became warm.

Two large-bore lines were started for IV access because fluid replacement was begun and the patient closely monitored.

An in-dwelling urinary catheter was placed by the referral facility. Urinary output (UO) over the last hour was 20 ml. Because of decreased UO and abnormal urine character as a result of muscle rhabdomyolysis, renal diuresis was indicated; mannitol (1 mg/kg) was given to maintain adequate urine flow.

Further initial treatment was based on a review of the laboratory values. Respiratory alkalosis with hypokalemia was present; hypokalemia should clear with cooling. If signs of hypercarbia became evident the patient would require ventilatory intervention. Hypoglycemia was corrected with the administration of dextrose (D50). CPK values over 20,000 alerted the flight nurse to the probability of the development of DIC and ARDS. Amylase was slightly elevated, perhaps indicative of pending liver failure.

IN-FLIGHT ASSESSMENT

Continuous assessment of this patient for further signs of multiple organ failure was mandatory. Reassessment of the efficacy of cooling measures, airway patency, and neurologic status was especially important in the care of this patient. If seizure activity reoccurred, prompt termination with lorazepam would be indicated.

While in flight the patient was kept moist with water and evaporation that was enhanced by directing air vents onto the body and flying with the windows open (permitted by the rotorcraft's design). The wet sheet was removed once the patient was loaded because it was warm and prevented evaporation. Ice packs were replaced as needed. When the patient's temperature reached 39° C (102° F), cooling measures were stopped.

Airway patency was ensured by frequent suctioning of the endotracheal tube and continuous assessment of respiratory status. If respiratory fatigue had become evident, ventilatory assistance would have been required. Oxygenation was assessed by pulse oximetry. Observation for increased pulmonary secretions, indicating pulmonary edema, was done in flight.

ECG monitoring was required; ACLS protocol was followed in the event of arrhythmia occurrence. Gastric output was observed for the presence of blood because GI bleeding is a frequent complication. Urine character and output were monitored to assess renal function.

Close attention and continuous, ongoing assessment of the patient's condition for presenting signs *of possible complications allowed the flight nurse to promptly initiate corrective and supportive care measures.*

REFERENCES

1. Ayers SM, Keenan RL: The hyperthermic syndromes. In Ayers SM et al, editors: *Textbook of critical care*, Philadelphia, 1995, Saunders.

2. Baker PS et al: Hyperthermia, hypertension, hypertonia, and coma in massive thioridazine overdose, *Am J Emerg Med* 4:346, 1988.

3. Bledsoe BE, Porter R, Cherry RA: *Paramedic care: principles and practice, medical emergencies*, Upper Saddle River, NJ, 2001, Brady Prentice Hall Health.

4. Centers for Disease Control and Prevention: Heat-related illnesses and deaths—United States, 1994–1995, *MMWR* 44(25):465, 1995.

5. Drake DK, Nettina SM: Recognition and management of heat-related illness, *Nurse Pract* 19(8):43, 1994.

6. Gaffin SL, Hubbard R: Experimental approaches to therapy and prophylaxis for heat stress and heatstroke, *Wilder and Environ Med* 4: 312, 1996.

7. Gaffin SL, Moran DS: Pathophysiology of heat-related illnesses. In Auerbach P, editor: *Wilderness medicine: management of wilderness and environmental emergencies*, ed 4, St Louis, 2001, Mosby.

8. Greany D, Brown MM: Malignant hyperthermia: a concern for critical care patients, *Focus Crit Care* 15:49, 1988.

9. Harker J, Gibson P: Heat stroke: a review of rapid cooling techniques, *Intensive Crit Care Nurs* 11(4):198, 1995.

10. Hart LH, Dennis SL: Two hypothermias prevalent in the intensive care unit: fever and heatstroke, *Focus Crit Care* 15(49):235, 1988.

11. Holleran RS: *Prehospital nursing: a collaborative approach*, St Louis, 1994, Mosby.

12. Hubbard RW, Gaffin SL, Squire DL: Heat-related illnesses. In Auerbach P, editor: *Wilderness medicine*, St Louis, 1995, Mosby.

13. Karrimi FA et al: Adult respiratory distress syndrome and disseminated intravascular coagulation complicating heat stroke, *Chest* 9(4):571, 1986.

14. Lee-Chiong TL, Stitt JT: Heatstroke and other heat-related illnesses: the maladies of summer, *Postgrad Med* 98(1):26, 1995.

15. Lim MK: Occupational heat stress, *Ann Acad Med (Singapore)* 23(5):719, 1994.

16. Moran DS, Gaffin SL: Clinical management of heat-related illnesses. In Auerbach P: *Wilderness medicine: management of wilderness and environmental emergencies*, ed 4, St Louis, 2001, Mosby.

17. O'Brien DJ: Heat illness, *J Aeromed Healthcare* 2:6, 1985.

18. Pouton TJ, Walker RA: Helicopter cooling of heat stroke victims, *Aviation, Space Environ Med* 58:358, 1987.

19. Proehl J: Environmental emergencies. In Kitt S et al, editors: *Emergency nursing*, Philadelphia, 1995, Saunders.

20. Sidman RD, Gallagher EJ: Exertional heat stroke in a young woman: gender differences in response to thermal stress, *Acad Emerg Med* 2(4):315, 1995.

21. Syverud SA et al: Iced gastric lavage for treatment of heat stroke: efficacy in a canine model, *Ann Emerg Med* 14:424, 1985.

22. Tek D, Olshaker JS: Heat illness, *Emerg Med Clin North Am* 10(2):299, 1992.

23. Tomarken JL, Britt BA: Malignant hyperthermia, *Ann Emerg Med* 16:1253, 1987.

24. Yaqua BA et al: Heat stroke and the Mekkah pilgrimage: clinical characteristics and course of 30 patients, *Q J Med* 59:523, 1986.

DIVING EMERGENCIES

27

This chapter is dedicated to the memory of Dr. Michael Spadafora.

Scuba (from "self-contained underwater breathing apparatus") diving is an increasingly popular pastime. It is estimated that there are now more than five million recreational divers worldwide. Diving activities are no longer restricted to coastal resorts, but can be found in almost any body of water large enough to hold a diver and equipment. Diving is also a part of many occupations including industry, military, scientific research, and search and rescue.[11,14]

Diving can lead to illnesses and injuries, some of them unique to that environment. The Divers Alert Network (www.diversalertnetwork.com) provides a place where injuries and fatalities from diving may be reported. There are generally about 1000 injuries reported each year, but fatalities vary from year to year.[11]

Manifestations of diving injuries may not be noticed by the diver for 24 to 48 hours after a dive and may, in fact, be seriously potentiated by air travel. Thus patients may present with diving-related problems many hours and many thousands of miles from the original dive site.

Transport personnel encounter many types of scuba-related diving injuries such as marine envenomation, near drowning, decompression illness, arterial gas embolism (AGE), middle-ear squeeze, and other forms of barotrauma. Of these diving injuries, decompression illness and AGE are medical emergencies requiring immediate recompression treatment. Air medical transport of the patient to a hyperbaric chamber is often necessary to avoid the significant morbidity and mortality resulting from delays in treatment of these disorders. Transport personnel must therefore be able to diagnose and manage these diving emergencies in a timely manner.

This chapter provides a brief discussion of diving principles and the pathophysiology, clinical manifestations, and management of diving emergencies likely to be encountered by transport crews.

DIVING PRINCIPLES

To gain a thorough understanding of the pathophysiology underlying decompression illness and air embolism, it is necessary to include a brief discussion of a few physical properties inherent to scuba diving.

At sea level, a 1-square-inch column of air extending upward from the earth's surface to the edge of the atmosphere would weigh 14.7 lb. Thus the pressure exerted by this column of air at sea level is 14.7 lb per square inch (psi), or 760 mm Hg, which is defined as 1 atmosphere of pressure (ATM). As altitude increases, the column of air becomes shorter, and the air pressure decreases. For example, at an altitude of 18,000 feet, the atmospheric pressure is half that at sea level: 380 mm Hg, or 0.5 ATM. On the other hand, water is much denser than air, and a similar 1-square-inch column in seawater would only have to be 33 feet (10 m) to exert the same amount of pressure as a 1-square-inch column of air. Because the density of water is uniform throughout, the proportional relationship of pressure and depth remains constant: pressure increases 1 ATM for every 33-foot (10-m) column of seawater (Figure 27-1). For the scuba diver, the combined weights of the air and water columns must be taken into consideration. At a given depth underwater, the total pressure will be the sum of the barometric pressure exerted by the column of air above plus the hydrostatic pressure exerted by the column of water. This is the concept of absolute pressure or atmospheres absolute (ATA). Therefore a scuba diver at a depth of 33 feet will experience an ambient pressure of 2 ATM absolute pressure, or 2 ATA. Similarly, a scuba diver at 66 feet will experience an ambient pressure of 3 ATA.

As the diver descends from the water's surface the effects of increasing ambient pressure on the scuba diver involve an understanding of the behavior of gases under conditions of varying pressure and volume. The following is a brief discussion of the primary gas laws of diving.

BOYLE'S LAW

The first gas law is Boyle's law, which states that at a constant temperature and mass the volume of a gas is inversely proportional to the total pressure. Simply stated, volume decreases as pressure increases; conversely, the volume increases as pressure decreases. Figure 27-1 depicts the increase of gas volume as the pressure and depth decrease.

HENRY'S LAW

The second gas principle is Henry's law, which states that solubility is proportional to the partial pressure of a gas. As the pressure increases or decreases, the gas goes into or comes out of solution accordingly. This is the "soda bottle" phenomenon. When you release the pressure from the bottle by removing the cap, the dissolved gas comes out of solution (Figure 27-2).

DALTON'S LAW

The last gas principle is Dalton's law of partial pressures, which states that the total pressure of a mixture of gases equals the sum of partial pressures exerted by the constituent gases. The partial pressure is the pressure exerted by a single gas in a mixture as if it were the only gas in the mixture. Air comprises approximately 78% nitrogen, 21% oxygen, and 1% other gases. As illustrated in Figure 27-3, by increasing the total pressure of the mixture, the pressure of each constituent gas is increased proportionately. At a depth of 99 feet (30 m), a scuba diver is under an ambient pressure of 4 ATA and is breathing compressed air with partial pressures of nitrogen and oxygen four times their value at the surface.

PATHOPHYSIOLOGIC FACTORS

Nitrogen is a relatively inert gas that is driven into solution as the diver descends according to Henry's law. The saturation of tissues with nitrogen depends on intrinsic properties, including tissue perfusion and solubility coefficients of the various tissues.[22] The quantity of dissolved nitrogen in the tissues increases with the duration and depth of the dive. If ascent of the scuba diver is too fast or the tissues are oversaturated with gas, the nitrogen is separated from solution rather than being safely transported to the lungs for elimination. Tissue desaturation of nitrogen results in the formation of inert gas bubbles in venous blood and tissues on reduction in ambient pressure.[6]

DECOMPRESSION ILLNESS

The lesion resulting from decompression illness has been a subject of debate for many years, although it is generally accepted that tissue ischemia is the final common pathway.[11] Hallenbeck demonstrated venous congestion by gas bubbles in the epidural venous plexus system of the spinal cord, most frequently in the lumbosacral region. The location of the intravascular lesion was consistent

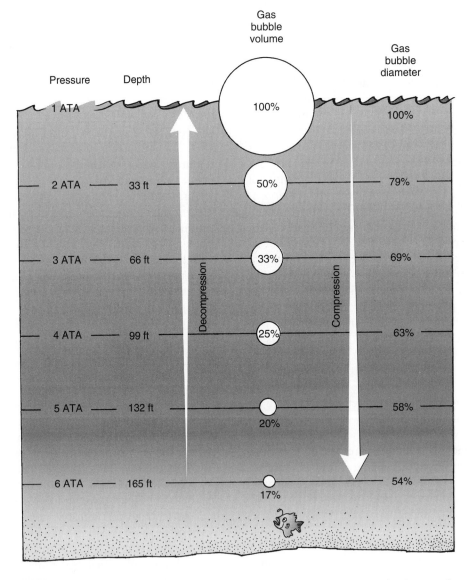

FIGURE 27-1   **Boyle's law.** (From Auerbach PS: *Wilderness medicine: management of wilderness and environmental emergencies,* ed 4, St Louis, 2001, Mosby.)

with the corresponding neurologic symptoms.[9] The formation of bubbles in tissues and venous blood has multiple mechanical and physiologic consequences. Mechanical effects of bubble formation include intravascular or intralymphatic obstruction, cellular distention and rupture, and stretching of ligaments and tendons. These effects result in ischemia or infarction, edema formation, cell death, and pain. The physiologic consequences include activation of the intrinsic clotting pathway, kinins, and the complement system, which all result in platelet aggregation, increased vascular permeability, and microvascular sludging. The end results of all of these events are decreased tissue perfusion and ischemia.[11]

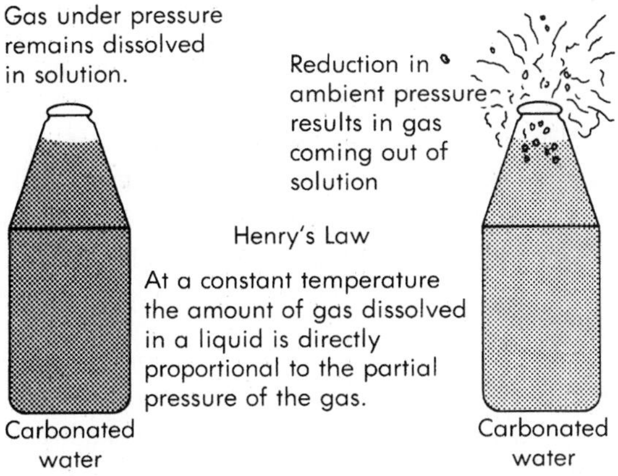

ARTERIAL GAS EMBOLIZATION

By far the most serious manifestation of pressure-related injuries or barotrauma is arterial gas embolization (AGE). AGE is a leading cause of death among scuba divers.[4]

Divers need to exhale continuously when ascending, or several things may occur. Some of the things that may occur include the following:

- Air pushes through the lung tissues and enters the skin in the neck.
- Air pushes through the lung tissues and into the spaces between the lungs and causes a pneumothorax.
- Air is forced from the lungs into blood vessels and carried to vital organs.

In accordance with Boyle's law, gases in the lungs of a scuba diver expand as ambient pressure decreases during ascent. The greatest changes in pressure and volume occur at shallower depths. Pulmonary

Gas under pressure remains dissolved in solution.

Reduction in ambient pressure results in gas coming out of solution

Henry's Law

At a constant temperature the amount of gas dissolved in a liquid is directly proportional to the partial pressure of the gas.

Carbonated water

Carbonated water

FIGURE 27-2 **Henry's law.**

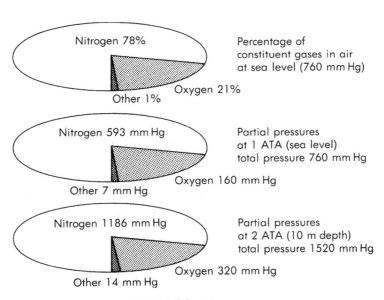

Nitrogen 78%

Oxygen 21%

Other 1%

Percentage of constituent gases in air at sea level (760 mm Hg)

Nitrogen 593 mm Hg

Oxygen 160 mm Hg

Other 7 mm Hg

Partial pressures at 1 ATA (sea level) total pressure 760 mm Hg

Nitrogen 1186 mm Hg

Oxygen 320 mm Hg

Other 14 mm Hg

Partial pressures at 2 ATA (10 m depth) total pressure 1520 mm Hg

FIGURE 27-3 **Dalton's law.**

overpressurization syndrome and alveolar rupture can occur during an ascent from a depth as shallow as 4 feet if compressed air is held in the lungs.[1] Breath holding during an ascent, as with a panicked diver, or air-trapping in a diseased lung results in lung overexpansion and rupture of alveoli. Air bubbles from the ruptured alveoli are free to enter the pulmonary venous return to the left side of the heart for subsequent dissemination through the systemic circulation. Air bubbles can track in the lung parenchyma and tissue planes. The result may be interstitial and mediastinal emphysema or pneumothorax.[1]

Gas bubbles may enter the coronary arteries and produce myocardial ischemia or infarction. However, bubbles most often enter the carotid circulation, producing multiple areas of circulatory occlusion in the brain with resulting ischemia and infarction.

Because multiple cerebrovascular watersheds may be affected, a confusing clinical picture with multiple neurologic deficits may result. The patient may have seizures or become unconscious, which can confuse rescuers as to the seriousness of the patient's problem.

CLINICAL MANIFESTATIONS

Diagnosis of a diving injury is usually made on the basis of the patient's history and clinical presentation.[15] Unfortunately, many of the signs and symptoms of decompression sickness (DCS) and AGE are nonspecific and may mimic other disease processes such as low back pain, arthritis, tendinitis, bronchospasm, stroke, and myocardial infarction. Because of the high morbidity and mortality that can result when treatment of DCS and AGE is delayed, diving accidents and injuries must be treated aggressively. The most common management error of these diving emergencies is failure to treat borderline cases.[16]

DECOMPRESSION SICKNESS

The signs and symptoms of DCS depend on the size and location of the ischemic insult. The most common presentation of decompression sickness may comprise headache, fatigue, limb or joint pain, skin rash and pruritus, and localized swelling. This collection of localized symptomatology is referred to as "pain-only" or type I DCS. The joints commonly affected in type I DCS are the shoulders, elbows, hips, knees, and ankles. Box 27-1 shows a classification scheme based on the systems or tissues involved.[15]

Musculoskeletal decompression sickness, better known as the "bends," is the most common type of decompression sickness. Pain in the shoulders and elbows are a frequent complaint in those affected. The patient may complain of a burning or tearing pain in the effected joint. The joint may also be red and swollen.[11]

The diver may also suffer skin bends or cutaneous decompression sickness. The skin may display a variety of cutaneous manifestations including scarlatiniform or mottled rashes. The patient may also complain of itching or "ants" crawling on their skin.[11]

Type II DCS comprises the more serious manifestations. Symptoms may involve any, or combinations of, the following symptoms: sensory and visual disturbances; dyspnea and nonproductive cough; paresthesia; paresis; fatigue and weakness; headache and nausea; chest, abdominal, or back pain; bowel and bladder dysfunction; shock; and loss of consciousness.

PULMONARY DECOMPRESSION ILLNESS

Otherwise known as the "chokes" or type IV DCS, pulmonary decompression illness is the result of large volumes of emboli occluding end arteries in the pulmonary circulation. If the lesion is large enough, pulmonary artery pressure increases, resulting in symptoms of dyspnea, chest pain, and nonproductive cough.[12] Pulmonary DCS is a rare but life-threatening manifestation of DCS that progress rapidly to shock unless immediate hyperbaric treatment is administered.[6]

ARTERIAL GAS EMBOLISM

Manifestations of AGE usually begin during or in minutes of ascent. As described earlier, AGE is a result of pulmonary overpressurization. Therefore

| BOX 27-1 | **Classification of Decompression Sickness** |

Type I

Local effects only: limb bends (joint or limb pain), skin bends (skin rash or itch), lymphatic obstruction effects

Type II

Cerebral manifestations: fatigue, malaise, visual disturbances, headache, impaired coordination, motor and sensory
  disturbances ranging from minor neurologic impairment to major deficits (e.g., paraplegia, quadriplegia,
  hemiplegia, altered states of consciousness ranging from drowsiness to coma, convulsions, and death)

Type III

Spinal manifestations: any degree of any motor and sensory modality impairment, but commonly weakness and
  numbness of lower limbs and bladder and sphincter impairment

Type IV

Pulmonary chokes: pulmonary dyspnea, pain, cough, altered gas exchange

Type V

Staggers: mild to severe impairment of balance and coordination, often debilitating

Type VI

Dysbaric osteonecrosis: lytic bone lesions resulting from long-term exposure to diving

From Otton J: Medical problems of recreational diving, *Aust Fam Phys* 18(6):674, 1989.

---

symptoms occur at or shortly after the time of the insult. The manifestations of AGE are consistent with strokelike phenomena, and almost any sign of cerebral damage may be observed, ranging from mild dizziness and motor and sensory deficits to severe impairment, coma, and death.[16] In a series of 42 cases analyzed by Kizer,[11] the most common symptom was asymmetric multiplegia or paralysis involving the lower extremities. Other signs of AGE include altered mental status and personality changes, syncope, vertigo, dizziness, cardiac dysrhythmia or cardiac arrest, chest pain, apnea, cough, hemoptysis, and epistaxis.[4,10,17] Transport personnel should always suspect AGE whenever a scuba diver presents with an altered level of consciousness, respiratory distress, or signs of cerebral decompression illness.

MANAGEMENT

Air embolism and decompression illness are medical emergencies and are managed similarly.[10] Recompression in a hyperbaric chamber is the only effective treatment for these diving emergencies. The Divers Alert Network (DAN), located at Duke University in Durham, North Carolina, can be reached by telephone at 919-684-8111 or 919-684-4DAN (collect). DAN can also be reached internationally, and these numbers and additional information is available on the DAN website located at www.diversalertnetwork.org. DAN provides assistance in diagnosis, treatment, and locating the nearest treatment facility. DAN may assist in making ground and air transport arrangements.[3]

The immediate treatment for a patient who is experiencing a diving emergency takes the following sequence:

1. Establish basic life support measures.
2. Place the patient in a supine position. The head-down (Trendelenburg) position and the head-down left lateral decubitus position (Durante position) have been recommended to minimize further passage of air emboli to the brain. The head-down position is no longer recommended for two reasons. First, a

patient placed in a head-down position will sustain an increase in intracranial pressure, which may exacerbate cerebral edema and ischemia. Second, the passage of air emboli throughout the circulatory system is probably more dependent on flow dynamics than on gravity.

3. Administer 100% oxygen at high flow rates (10 to 15 L/min) through a face mask to create a gradient for increased elimination of excess nitrogen.

4. Administer fluid with 5% dextrose in normal saline solution or lactated Ringer's solution to correct underlying fluid deficits and maintain an adequate intravascular.

5. Protect the patient against hypothermia or hyperthermia.

6. Monitor pulmonary, cardiovascular, and neurologic status. Treat developing complications (e.g., pneumothorax, shock, seizures).

7. Avoid rough or excessive handling.

8. Give analgesics as needed.

9. The use of corticosteroids for cerebral edema and endothelial stabilization remains controversial. The recommendation is a combination of dexamethasone and a rapid-acting steroid such as methylprednisolone or hydrocortisone.[11]

10. Transport patient to the nearest hyperbaric treatment facility.

11. Provide the hyperbaric medical personnel with a detailed history of the dive (e.g., depth and duration of dive), timing and onset of symptoms or complications, and treatment rendered. This information will aid the hyperbaric medical personnel in determining proper management such as time and pressure profiles.

12. Always consider the possibility of DCS or AGE in the patient's diving partners as well.

AIR MEDICAL TRANSPORT

Air medical transport of the patient to a hyperbaric chamber is often necessary to avoid significant morbidity and mortality resulting from delays in treatment. However, transportation by air ambulance or even ground ambulance over elevated terrain may exacerbate the patient's condition.[2] Patients should be transported in aircraft with cabins pressurized to 1 ATA, such as the Lear jet, Hercules C-130, Cessna Citation, or many commercial aircraft, but this may require flight at a lower altitude, at considerable fuel expense. If the aircraft cannot be pressurized to 1 ATA (e.g., a helicopter), it should be flown at the lowest and safest altitude possible, preferably below 1000 feet above sea level.[2] In some locations, a portable recompression chamber can be used to transport the patient from the field to the hyperbaric treatment center in a nonpressurized aircraft. The portable unit (with the patient inside) is mated to the larger static hyperbaric chamber while the patient is maintained under pressure.[16]

SUMMARY

The number of scuba-related injuries grows with the increasing number of scuba divers. Of these injuries, DCS and AGE are true medical emergencies that require immediate treatment in the nearest hyperbaric chamber. Delays in the treatment of these diving injuries may result in significant morbidity and mortality. Air medical flight crews may be called on to rapidly assess, manage, and transport patients with these life-threatening injuries. Knowledge of diving principles, pathophysiology, and manifestations of AGE and DCS will aid air medical personnel in developing proper management strategies.

DIVING EMERGENCIES CASE STUDY

An air ambulance was dispatched to the scene where a 19-year-old woman was reported to be unconscious. On arrival the patient was found in a left lateral Trendelenburg position. Bystanders reported that the patient was an inexperienced diver with a history of asthma. She had been scuba diving in a 12-foot swimming pool.

The patient was lethargic and incoherent. Her airway was patent with an intact gag reflex. Her color was pale with no cyanosis. She was dyspneic, with a respiratory rate of 40 breaths/min, heart rate of 120 beats/min, and blood pressure of 150/90 mm Hg. She also had symptoms of a left cerebral infarction including impaired speech; right-sided paresthesia, and decreased motor strength in the right arm. Breath sounds were diminished over the right apex, with occasional expiratory wheezes.

Immediate management included 100% oxygen by mask, IV lactated Ringer's solution at 125 ml/hr, and continuous cardiac, neurologic, and pulmonary monitoring. The patient was placed in a supine position. Cerebral AGE was the most likely diagnosis, but flight personnel observed the patient for a possible closed-head injury as well. The patient was 10 minutes from the nearest recompression chamber, and the decision was made to immediately transport her by helicopter at a low altitude. Initial diagnosis by flight personnel was based solely on history and clinical findings.

On the patient's arrival at the emergency department, assessment remained unchanged. The patient had a blood pressure of 140/86 mm Hg, heart rate of 116 beats/min, and respiratory rate of 42 breaths/min, with an intact airway. Neurologic examination findings were unchanged. Cervical spine radiographs and computed tomography (CT) of the head were negative. The emergency physician confirmed a cerebral AGE. Endotracheal intubation was deferred because the airway was adequate, and the patient was taken immediately to the hyperbaric chamber.

Initial recompression therapy was performed to a depth of 6 ATA. The patient became increasingly coherent, with return of feeling to her right side. Vital signs remained stable during recompression therapy, and a patent airway was maintained. The patient required two additional recompression treatments to a depth of 3 ATA and made a full recovery.

Recreational divers are found in every part of the country. In particular, knowledge of AGE embolism and decompression illness, the two most dangerous diving emergencies, is essential. Before embarking on any flight involving a diving emergency, transport personnel must know the location of the recompression chamber nearest the patient, along with transportation alternatives. This information can be obtained 24 hours a day by calling DAN at (919) 684-8111 or on their website at www.diversalertnetwork.org.

REFERENCES

1. Arthur DC, Margulies RA: A short course in diving medicine, *Ann Emerg Med* 16:689, 1987.
2. Bennett PB et al: Flying after diving: 1987 accidents, *Alert Diver* 5(1):1, 1989.
3. Bennett PB et al: DAN position statement: injury risk in sport diving, *Sources* 1(2):3, 1989.
4. Boettger ML: Scuba diving emergencies: pulmonary overpressure accidents and decompression sickness, *Ann Emerg Med* 12:563, 1983.
5. Bove AA, Davis JC: *Diving medicine*, ed 2, Philadelphia, 1995, Saunders.
6. Davis JC: Decompression sickness in sport scuba diving, *Phys Sportsmed* 16(2):108, 1988.
7. Dick AP, Massey EW: Neurologic presentation of decompression sickness and air embolism in sport divers, *Neurology* 35:667, 1985.
8. Francis TJ, Dutka AJ, Flynn ET: Experimental determination of latency, severity, and outcome in CNS decompression sickness, *Undersea Biomed Res* 15(6):419, 1989.
9. Hallenbeck JM, Bove AA, Elliott DH: Mechanisms underlying spinal cord damage in decompression sickness, *Neurology* 25:308, 1975.
10. Kizer KW: Disorders of the deep, *Emerg Med* 6:18, 1984.
11. Kizer KW: Diving medicine. In Auerbach P, editor: *Wilderness medicine: management of wilderness and environmental emergencies*, ed 4, St Louis, 2001, Mosby.
12. Leveritt SO, Bitter HL, McIver L: *Studies in decompression sickness: circulatory and respiratory changes associated with decompression sickness in anesthetized dogs*, TDR 63–67, Brooks AFB, 1963, TX USAF School of Aerospace Medicine.
13. Mebane GY, Dick AP: *Underwater diving accident manual*, ed 2, Durham, NC, 1982, National Divers Alert Network.
14. Mowatt-Larssen E, Johnson E: The bends-decompression syndromes, *EMedicine Journal*, Accessed December 25, 2001 at www.emedicine.com.
15. Orton J: Medical problems of recreational diving, *Aust Fam Phys* 18:674, 1989.

16. Repogle WH et al: Scuba diving injuries, *Am Fam Pract* 37:135, 1988.

17. Spencer MP: Decompression limits for compressed air determined by ultrasonically detected blood bubbles, *J Appl Physiol* 40:229, 1976.

18. Strauss RH: Diving medicine, *Am Rev Respir Dis* 119:1001, 1979.

19. Ward CA, McCullough D, Fraser WD: Relation between complement activation and susceptibility to decompression sickness, *J Appl Physiol* 62:1160, 1987.

20. Warren JP Jr et al: Neuroimaging of scuba diving injuries to the CNS, *AJR Am J Roentgenol* 151:1003, 1988.

21. Workman RD: *Calculation of decompression schedules for nitrogen-oxygen and helium-oxygen dives,* Washington, DC, 1965, US Navy Experimental Diving Unit, Washington Navy Yard.

TOXICOLOGIC EMERGENCIES

28

COMPETENCIES

1. Identify some of the common sources of poisoning.
2. Describe the care of the poisoned patient during transport.
3. Name three antidotes for specific poisons.

Each year more than 2 million human poison exposures are reported to the American Association of Poison Control Centers (AAPCC). The AAPCC compiles the Toxic Exposure Surveillance System (TESS), the largest database of information about toxic exposures in the United States. More than 90% of these exposures occur in the victim's home. Others occur in locations such as the workplace, health-care facilities, schools, and public areas.[28] Over half of the poisons occur in children less than 6 years of age. The majority of poisons continue to be unintentional. Intentional poisonings are generally related to suicide, misuse, and abuse.[28]

The human environment contains natural and manufactured toxins including plants, animals, chemicals, drugs, and chemotherapeutic agents. Even though there are multiple substances and various sources of toxins and poisons, only a limited number of antidotes are available. Table 28-1 lists most of the available antidotes that may be useful in the management of the poisoned patient.

The most important concept in the care of the patient who has been poisoned is supportive care. In addition to maintenance of the patient's airway, breathing, and circulation, the exposure to the toxin must be quickly stopped to prevent further harm to the patient. It is vital to keep in mind that some toxins can cause injury to caregivers, and appropriate decontamination must be accomplished before transport.

The purpose of this chapter is to discuss the general management of the poisoned patient, identify the pathophysiology of selected drugs, and describe the care of the poisoned patient during transport.

GENERAL CONSIDERATIONS

INTENTIONAL AND UNINTENTIONAL POISONING

Ingestion of or exposure to a toxic substance may be either intentional or unintentional. It is important to determine why the patient has become poisoned because it could make a difference in the care of the

TABLE 28-1   **Antidotes for Selected Poisonings**

Toxin	Antidote
Opiates	Naloxone
Carbon monoxide	Oxygen
Cyanide	Amyl nitrate
	Sodium nitrate
	Sodium thiosulfate
Anticholinesterase	Atropine
Organophosphates	
Carbamates	
Methemoglobinemic	Methylene blue
agents	
Nitrates	
Chlorates	
Nitrobenzene	
Ethylene glycol	Ethanol
Acetaminophen	N-Acetylcysteine
Heavy metals	BAL
	Disodium edetate
	Penicillamine
Iron	Deferoxamine
Anticholinergics	Physostigmine
Diphenhydramine	
Benzotropine	
Anticoagulants	
Coumadin	
Heparin	Vitamin K
Cardiac medications	Protamine
Beta-adrenergic	
blockers	
Calcium-channel	
blockers	Glucagon
Digoxin	Calcium
Tricyclic	
antidepressants	Digoxin Fab antibodies
	Sodium bicarbonate

From Wright RO et al: Poison antidotes: guidelines for rational use in the emergency department, *Emerg Med Rep* 16(21):201, 1995.

patient. A patient who intentionally took a lethal amount of a drug potentially could be a safety risk.

Sources of unintentional exposure include therapeutic error (taking too much of a medication), bites and stings, environmental exposures, and food poisoning. Intentional poison exposures usually result from suicide attempts, abuse, and intentional misuse of medications.

The word *poisoning* denotes a toxic exposure that can be intentional, unintentional, or unknown to the patient. A patient or family member may have misread a label, taken too much of a drug, and accidentally become poisoned. A child may climb up and get into a medicine cabinet, ingest a bottle of aspirin, and be unintentionally poisoned. Criminals do not often use poisonous substances as a method of injuring or killing.[13,15]

An intentional overmedication or ingestion of a toxic substance is considered an *overdose*.[16] Poisoning generally occurs in the pediatric population. Patients who have overdosed or intentionally poisoned themselves are usually 12 years or older, although some cases suggest that children 5 years and older should be evaluated for intentional ingestion.[15]

It is important to make the distinction between accidental and intentional toxic exposure. If the patient is suicidal, the transport team should take additional precautions to ensure a safe environment for the crew and the patient during transport.

GENERAL MANAGEMENT OF THE POISONED PATIENT

The initial management of any poisoned patient includes establishing a patent airway, ventilation, and maintenance of adequate circulation. Further evaluation consists of obtaining a detailed history about the event that led to the poisoning, a thorough physical examination, administration of antidotes as indicated, and transport to an appropriate health-care facility for definitive care. The patient's family should be a part of the initial care because they may be able to offer important information about the incident. The emotional support of the patient, particularly a patient who has attempted suicide, should be included in the planning of care.

INITIAL MANAGEMENT

As with any other critically ill or injured patient, the ABCs (airway-breathing-circulation) take initial precedence. One exception in the case of the poisoned patient is the need to remove the victim from a toxic environment or toxic source before the ABCs can be assessed. If the patient has been sprayed with a toxic substance, or the creature that caused envenomation is still in the immediate vicinity, the environment must be controlled and made safe before patient management so that the health-care providers will not be injured or poisoned.

Many toxins and poisons alter mental status and therefore may compromise the airway. Protecting the airway is particularly important if the toxin is going to be removed by gastric lavage. Mouth-to-mouth resuscitation should always be avoided because of the possibility of contamination of the rescuer with the toxic substance. Endotracheal or nasotracheal intubation is the preferred method of protecting the airway and preventing the possibility of aspiration.

Alterations in the patient's circulatory status may be profound and life threatening. A large-bore IV catheter and appropriate fluid resuscitation initiated. Blood pressure may need to be supported with vasoactive agents.

Depending on the type of poison or toxic exposure, decontamination may need to be carried out before the patient can be transported. Generally, decontamination of the patient can be accomplished by using soap and water. However, there are some toxins that require specific decontaminates. It is important for the transport team to know and follow appropriate procedures to protect both themselves and the patient.[44]

ASSESSMENT
HISTORY
The history of the toxic exposure provides a vital method of identifying the type of substance responsible for the patient's symptoms. Poisoning or an overdose should be suspected in the following types of patients: a psychiatric patient, a trauma victim, a comatose patient with an unknown cause of coma, a young person with a life-threatening arrhythmia of undetermined origin, a patient rescued from a fire, a child with unexplained lethargy, and any person exhibiting suspicious or unusual behavior.[15] The history should include the type of substance or suspected substance that was taken, the exposure

route, the time of the exposure, and size or dosage of the exposure.

The patient may be exposed to a toxin through a number of routes. These include the following:

- Ingestion
- Dermal or skin contact
- Inhalation
- Ocular exposure
- Bite or a sting
- Parenteral
- Aspiration

If a thorough history cannot be obtained, the environment in which the patient was found should be explored for clues to what may have caused the poisoning. The transport team should look for bottles, containers, drug paraphernalia, animals, or items that may provide additional information about a suspected or unknown toxic substance. These items should be transported with the patient. Identification of witnesses to the event can add more information concerning what may have happened to cause the poisoning or toxic exposure.[15]

Past medical history such as allergic reactions, previous surgeries, and past hospitalizations should be noted. When possible, it is important to assess whether the patient has attempted suicide in the past.

In the care of the pediatric or elderly patient, the possibility of abuse or neglect must be kept in mind. A referral may be necessary to outside agencies—perhaps even the police—so that the patient's environment may be evaluated to see if it is appropriate and safe.[16]

SYMPTOMS OF POISONING AND TOXIC EXPOSURES
Certain symptoms without a clear cause may suggest poisoning or overdose. Severe poisoning symptoms include coma, cardiac arrhythmia, metabolic acidosis, seizures, and gastrointestinal (GI) disturbances.[15,44] Many disease states may mimic overdose and should be considered in the differential diagnoses. It is important to keep in mind that head injuries, encephalitis, meningitis, metabolic disturbances, and psychiatric diseases are easily mistaken for poisoning.

PHYSICAL EXAMINATION

The physical examination of a poisoned patient should include assessment of general appearance and pulmonary, cardiovascular, abdominal, and neurologic systems. The information obtained from physical examination will not only help determine the source of the toxic substance but also provide baseline data to follow the effects of the toxic substance and the particular interventions that have been initiated.

Baseline assessment data are particularly important in the determination of any changes in the patient's condition during transport. During transport the toxic effects of the substance should be considered, as well as the success or failure of initial treatments on the patient's condition.

The physical appearance of the patient may give a clue to the type of poison or overdose the patient has taken. The presence of needle tracks, burns, bruises, lacerations, cutaneous bullae, erythema, petechiae, cyanosis, flushed skin, or bite marks may provide information to help diagnose the poison or toxic exposure.[6,16] Breath odors may suggest possible poisoning or help rule it out to another cause. For example, the smell of oil of wintergreen can indicate salicylate poisoning. Table 28-2 lists odors associated with certain poisonings.[15,24,39]

Respiratory rate and pattern are also important assessment parameters. Auscultation of breath sounds is also included in this assessment. Many toxins can cause respiratory arrest and impair the airway, yielding the potential for aspiration.

Assessment of the level of consciousness of the poisoned patient is secondary only to the patient's respiratory assessment and may reveal a spectrum of altered sensorium. Hyperactivity, psychosis, somnolence, or coma may be manifested. Generalized seizures have been reported in many different cases of poisoning or overdose. Level of consciousness, pupillary response, motor and sensory function, and vital signs should also be included in the assessment.

An assessment of the patient's level of consciousness should go beyond orientation to person, place, and time. The patient's interaction with the environment can yield useful information about the patient's level of consciousness. Many drugs and toxic substances cause visual, auditory, or other sensory hallucinations and alter the patient's personality.

Pupil size, shape, and reaction are parts of the neurologic assessment. Constricted or dilated pupils may indicate drug or treatment effects. Motor and sensory functions are usually assessed together and may vary from normal activity to no movement at all. Seizure activity is not an uncommon complication from toxins and should be appropriately documented and treated.

The presence or possibility of an altered mental status occurring during transport requires the use of appropriate safety measures. Restraints and, in some cases, chemical restraint may be warranted to ensure safe transport.

Cardiac monitoring should be performed and blood pressure and pulse quality frequently checked during transport. Hypotension, premature ventricular contractions, prolonged QT intervals, and a widened QRS complex are examples of some of the cardiac arrhythmia that may occur because of cardiac toxicity related to some poisonings.

Certain toxic substances cause GI disturbances such as nausea, vomiting, and severe abdominal pain. Iron, lithium, mercury, phosphorus, arsenic, mushrooms, organophosphates, and fluoride are examples of toxic substances that can cause GI disturbances. Phosphorus poisoning can cause luminescent vomit and flatus.[13] A gastric tube should be inserted before transport to prevent aspiration.

LABORATORY STUDIES

Many substances responsible for adverse reactions, intoxications, and poisoning are difficult to identify.

TABLE 28-2 **Odors Associated With Poisonings**	
Odor	**Possible Poison**
Sweet	Placidyl
	Acetone
	Chloroform
Bitter almond	Cyanide
Pear	Chloral hydrate
Garlic	Arsenic
Wintergreen	Methylsalicylate

Serum levels are not reflective of tissue concentration or receptor interactions. Therefore levels of specific toxins may be incongruous with clinical manifestations.[16]

Laboratory evaluations such as complete blood count, electrolytes, whole blood glucose, liver function tests and coagulation studies are frequently helpful. Many toxins are associated with leukocytosis or electrolyte alterations. An example is the hypokalemia associated with theophylline toxicity. Arterial blood gases are beneficial in determining acidosis or alkalosis. Acidosis can be appreciated in tricyclic poisoning or late methanol or ethylene glycol poisoning, whereas alkalosis occurs in early salicylate intoxication.[15]

The treatment of poisoning with some drugs such as acetaminophen and aspirin necessitates determination of baseline serum levels and a repeat of these levels 3 to 6 hours after ingestion. Levels of some drugs may have to be monitored for several days after ingestion to ensure that they have been eliminated. Any blood, gastric contents, and urine that have been obtained for toxic analysis should accompany the patient for transport.

REMOVAL, ELIMINATION, OR DISRUPTION OF THE TOXIN

Ingestion, parenteral injection, ocular contamination, dermal exposure, inhalation, and envenomation are the major routes of intoxication.[15,28] The method of exposure must be established so that a method of removal or interruption can be chosen. Methods for reversal of the clinical effects of poisons include the use of antidotes, antivenin, supportive therapy, forced diuresis, charcoal, cathartics, whole bowel irrigation, hemoperfusion, and dialysis.[15,24,36] The most common methods of removal are gastric lavage followed by administration of charcoal.

Two types of forced diuresis may be used to enhance the elimination of specific poisons: diuresis with ion trapping and diuresis without ion trapping. In diuresis without ion trapping, the patient is given IV fluid to maintain urine output of 5 ml/min or 300 ml/hr. This method can be dangerous to the patient with any renal or cardiovascular disease.[44]

Ion-trapping diuresis is accomplished by alkalinization and acidification of the poisoned patient's urine. To achieve alkalinization of urine, sodium bicarbonate is added to IV solution, and fluids are administered to yield a urine pH of 7.5. The patient must be monitored closely for complications from fluid and electrolyte imbalances.

If the toxin has been inhaled, the individual should be removed from the source of the exposure. Administration of oxygen may be of use, particularly for the patient who has sustained carbon monoxide (CO) poisoning.

Contact poisons or toxins may enter the body through the skin, eyes, or mucous membranes. Removing the patient from the toxic environment, taking off the patient's clothes, and cleansing the affected area are the most important steps in the initial removal of the poison or toxic substance. It is important to use the correct irrigation fluid or fluids to prevent further injury to the patient. Attention also must be given to the proper disposal of the contaminated fluid and materials to prevent poisoning of the health-care providers and the surrounding environment.

Antivenin administration, hemoperfusion, and dialysis should all be performed under the direction of a trained toxicologist or other health-care professional acquainted with each procedure. Administration of antivenin in the prehospital environment is not recommended because of the potential of severe complications that may not be effectively managed.

SUPPORTIVE AND EMOTIONAL CARE OF THE POISONED PATIENT

As noted earlier, specific antidotes are limited compared with the numbers of the poisons and toxic substances disseminated in the environment. Frequently, supportive care directed at preventing complications from the poison or toxic substance is the most that can be done for the patient.[24] A part of this supportive care may be the transport of the patient to a specific center with additional methods of caring for the patient. Supportive care is based on the previous discussion of initial management, physical examination, and removal, elimination, or interruption of the toxic sequence.

The emotional care of the poisoned patient can be difficult. If the poisoning is intentional, the motive must be quickly discovered so that proper psychiatric and social care can be rendered. All procedures should be explained to the patient and a nonjudgmental attitude imparted when care is provided. If possible, the patient's family should be given some time with the patient before transport.

Protection of the patient from complications and respect for the patient as a human being are important components of the care of the poisoned patient. E.J. Daniels noted how insensitive nursing care can affect the poisoned patient[7]:

> The curtains hadn't been completely closed, and anyone and everyone walking by peered in, adding to my humiliation. I tried staring at everything but Brenda and the gaggy network of tubes in an attempt to keep my mind off the nauseating trauma. Alright. I have to put some medications down you. Try not to gag on it, because you really need it, keep this down. I'd never heard of any medicine that was pitch black! I felt like she had been flushing me out for hours. She hooked up a huge syringe to the end of the tube down inside of me. The thought of the tar going down my throat into my stomach was more repulsive than the gurgling sensation of lavage.

SAFETY ISSUES IN THE TRANSPORT OF THE POISONED PATIENT

Safety is one of the most important issues to be addressed in the care of a poisoned patient during transport. Many intoxicants can cause hallucinations or violent behavior. Physical or chemical restraint to ensure safe transport should be a consideration when preparing the patient for transport.

Both physical and chemical (i.e., medications) restraints provide a means of safely controlling the patient for transport. Decreasing excessive stimulation during transport with ear protectors may also reduce the possibility of dangerous or threatening patient behavior during transport. If neuromuscular blocking agents are used, adequate analgesia and sedation must be provided during transport.

SUMMARY

The care of the poisoned patient who requires transport begins with management of the patient's airway and ventilation and maintenance of the cardiovascular system. Physical examination, including the patient's general appearance; assessment of the neurologic, respiratory, cardiovascular, and gastrointestinal systems; removal, elimination, or interruption of the toxic sequence; and supportive and emotional care are other important components of care of the poisoned patient.

Preparation for the transport of the poisoned patient includes decontamination; sampling of the toxic substance; transfer of laboratory work such as blood, urine, or vomitus; and informing the family of the transport destination.

Box 28-1 summarizes the care for the poisoned patient. It is critical to approach the care of the poi-

---

BOX 28-1   Care of the Poisoned Patient by the Transport Team

1. Provide basic and advanced life support after ensuring that the environment is safe for the transport team.
2. Remove the patient from the toxic environment.
3. When indicated, decontaminate the patient by removing clothing and washing off toxin.
4. Administer appropriate antidote when indicated.
5. Assess respiratory, neurologic, and cardiovascular status frequently.
6. Document or obtain baseline data.
7. Ensure the patient and transport team's safety in transport with the use of chemical or physical restraints. When using chemical restraints, do not forget about analgesia and sedation.
8. Explain to the patient and family what is happening.
9. Transfer appropriate records and specimens.
10. Inform the patient's family of the patient's destination.

soned patient in an organized manner to provide supportive care and prevent complications.

PHARMACOLOGIC PROPERTIES OF DRUGS

Therapeutic dose responses are affected by multiple variables including the rate of absorption, distribution, binding, or localization in tissues and inactivation and excretion. The rate of absorption is defined as the time needed for the chemotherapeutic agent to cross the enterovascular barriers and circulate in the cardiovascular system. Agents dissolved in solution are absorbed more rapidly than those in solid forms. Timed-release, enteric-coated products are engineered to greatly decrease the absorption rate. Medications given in higher concentration are absorbed more rapidly.

Gastric pH may deactivate or precipitate a drug. Areas of increased vascularity, such as the vagina or rectum, tend to absorb agents more rapidly. Topical exposure or inhalation of poisons reaches toxic levels quickly because of the large surface areas exposed to the intoxicants.

The vast majority of drugs are administered orally. Sites of absorption include the oral mucous membranes, stomach, duodenum, and small intestine. Sublingual administration usually promotes quick dissolution and rapid absorption. Absorption in the stomach is a passive process mediated by dissolution and diffusion. The nonionized form of a dissolved medication passes the mucosal barriers and enters the vascular compartment. Most drugs are either weak bases or weak acids. Gastric pH affects both dissolution and diffusion. Weak acids, such as salicylates and barbiturates, are predominantly nonionized in a strongly acidic environment. Therefore they are readily absorbed. Weak bases are in an ionized form in the stomach and are poorly absorbed. The intestinal pH is less acidic than the stomach (pH = 5.3). Weak bases are readily absorbed, but weak acids cross the mucosal barrier less readily. In addition, the gastric mucosa is a lipoid membrane, which absorbs lipid soluble substances, such as alcohol, rapidly. Factors that change gastric emptying time also alter the rate of absorp-

tion of a drug. IV injection is the most immediate and consistent blood concentration for any drug. After injection, a redistribution phase may significantly decrease the blood level of the drug. Absorption of medication given subcutaneously or intramuscularly depends on the site of injection, solubility of the drug, and vascularity of the injection area.

Once the drug is absorbed into the cardiovascular compartment, a redistribution occurs throughout the body. Agents enter or pass through the various body-fluid compartments (plasma, interstitial, transcellular, vitreous, and cellular fluids). Medications are restricted in distribution by their ability to pass through cellular membranes.

Drugs may accumulate in storage depots because of protein binding, fat accumulation, and active transport. Medications are stored in equilibrium and released as plasma concentrations are reduced. Storage depots permit maintenance of plasma levels for long periods, prolonging pharmacologic effects. Anatomic components that act as storage depots include plasma proteins, connective tissues, tissue constituents (such as proteins, phospholipids, or nucleoproteins), adipose tissue, and transcellular fluids.

The mechanism responsible for drug transport across cell membranes may be an active or passive process. Passive transfer is diffusion driven by concentration gradients. Active transport is mediated by a carrier and requires expenditure of energy. The ultimate fate of a drug is metabolism and excretion. Biotransformation involves chemical reactions, classified as either nonsynthetic or synthetic. The nonsynthetic class involves oxidation, reduction, and hydrolysis. The parent drug is changed to a more-active, a less-active, or an inactive metabolite. Hepatocytic enzymes mediate most nonsynthetic reactions. Exceptions include nonenzymatic hydrolysis in the plasma, plasma cholinesterase and pseudocholinesterase, and synaptic metabolism of neurotransmitter analogs.

Synthetic reactions or conjugation occur in the liver or kidney. The process couples parent drug or its metabolites to endogenous substrates (usually carbohydrates, amino acids, or inorganic sulfates).

Conjugated drugs form inactive, highly ionized, water-soluble substances that are excreted in the urine. Conjugation is an active process requiring adenine triphosphate expenditure.

Active parent drugs and metabolites are excreted in the urine as a primary route of disposal. Drugs are also eliminated through excretion of feces. Metabolites are dissolved in bile, secreted into the alimentary tract, and passed through the GI tract. In addition, the unabsorbed parent drug is removed with fecal passage.

This discussion has focused on the incidence of poisoning; general considerations in the care of the poisoned patient; general management of the poisoned patient; signs and symptoms of toxicity; physical examination of the poisoned patient; useful laboratory studies; removal, elimination, or disruption of the poison; supportive and emotional care of the poisoned patient; flight nursing care of the poisoned patient; and the pharmacologic properties of drugs. The next part of this chapter focuses on the toxicity and treatment of toxicity of specific drugs. Information about each of these drugs is presented for quick reference.

TOXICITY AND TREATMENT OF POISONING BY SPECIFIC DRUGS

ACETYLSALICYLIC ACID (ASPIRIN)

Aspirin is one of the oldest nonprescription pharmaceutical agents. Its therapeutic popularity is mainly a result of its antipyretic and analgesic effects. In recent years, the effects of aspirin on platelets have been recognized as a preventive intervention for people who have suffered heart attacks and strokes. Single low doses of aspirin about 80 mg daily are now prescribed.[23]

Aspirin can be taken orally, topically, or rectally. The most common route of toxicity is by ingestion. It is very important to keep in mind that many over-the-counter medications contain aspirin and that multiple sources of poisoning may be involved. Table 28-3 describes a method of assessing the severity of salicylate intoxication.

Salicylate toxicity initially manifests in an increased respiratory rate and hyperventilation. Blood gas analysis usually reflects respiratory alkalosis. Clinical manifestations of mild intoxication include headache, vertigo, tinnitus, mental confusion, sweating, thirst, hyperventilation, nausea, vomiting, and drowsiness. Severe intoxication produces similar symptoms combined with base/electrolyte imbalances. Patients are agitated, restless, and uncommunicative and may have seizures or become comatose. Noncardiac pulmonary edema is observed in severe poisoning, whereas bleeding diatheses are less common.[37]

Treatment of salicylate poisoning involves gastric emptying, administration of oral-activated charcoal, and alkaline diuresis. Charcoal administration without gastric emptying has been found effective in the management of salicylate toxicity.[1,44]

Alkaline diuresis is performed to increase the pH of the patient's urine to improve free salicylate excretion. Supportive care and maintenance of vital

TABLE 28-3 Assessment of the Severity of Salicylate Intoxication Based on the Estimated Dose Ingested	
Ingested Dose (mg/kg)*	Estimated Severity
<150	No toxic reaction expected
150-300	Mild to moderate toxic reaction
300-500	Serious toxic reaction
>500	Potentially lethal toxic reaction

From Haddad L, Shannon M, Winchester J: *Clinical management of poisoning and drug overdose*, Philadelphia, 2000, Saunders.
*Number of tablets ingested times the milligrams of aspirin per tablet divided by patient weight in kilograms equals the acute ingested dose. If a patient has received aspirin therapeutically in the preceding 24 hours, the potential toxicity of the acutely ingested dose will be increased.

functions are mainstays of treatment in this type of poisoning.[24]

The severely poisoned patient may require hemodialysis. Hemodialysis not only enhances the removal of the toxic levels of the salicylate, but it can also correct the fluid, electrolyte, and acid-base imbalances that occur with salicylate toxicity.[15]

ACETAMINOPHEN (TYLENOL)

Acetaminophen, similar to aspirin, has antipyretic and analgesic properties. It is not chemically related to the salicylates. Acetaminophen has become a useful alternative to aspirin because it does not cause the GI and bleeding complications that can occur with aspirin use. Like aspirin, acetaminophen is contained in many over-the-counter drugs and may be administered orally or rectally. The main site of absorption is the small intestine, and the drug is uniformly distributed throughout most body fluids.[22]

Acetaminophen is a drug whose toxicity is increased by the liver, rather than detoxified. The metabolite produced in the liver by metabolism of acetaminophen attaches to the hepatic cell membrane and injures the lipids bilayer if it not neutralized by the antioxidant hepatic glutathione. When hepatic glutathione stores are depleted because of an overdose of acetaminophen, the metabolites are not neutralized and cause injury and death of the hepatic cells.[15]

The classic clinical course of toxic acute acetaminophen poisoning occurs in four stages. The initial stage of toxicity occurs 30 minutes to 24 hours after ingestion and produces anorexia, nausea, vomiting, malaise, pallor, and diaphoresis.

The second stage begins 24 to 48 hours after ingestion. Right upper quadrant pain and tenderness may result from liver enlargement. The levels of liver enzymes, serum bilirubin, and prothrombin time begin to increase 36 hours after ingestion. Oliguria may result from acute tubular necrosis.

The third stage begins 72 to 96 hours after ingestion and is the time of peak liver-function abnormalities. Anorexia, nausea, vomiting, and malaise return and jaundice become apparent. Fatalities from acetaminophen poisoning usually occur during this stage and result from fulminant hepatic necrosis.

The fourth stage, or "resolution period," occurs 4 days to 2 weeks after poisoning. Patients are asymptomatic, and liver function parameters return to baseline values.[38,44]

Ingestions of more than 7.5 g or 150 mg/kg are considered potentially toxic. The serum level of acetaminophen should be measured 4 hours after ingestion in any person who has ingested a potentially toxic dose of acetaminophen. If the acetaminophen level is still toxic at 4 hours after ingestion or the level cannot be assayed before 10 hours have passed since ingestion and the history suggests a toxic ingestion, N-acetylcysteine (NAC) should be administered. NAC is administered orally at an initial dose of 140 mg/kg. A maintenance dose of 70 mg/kg every 4 hours for 17 doses is then given.[38,44] N-Acetylcysteine may be administered intravenously in the critically ill patient. The transport team must consult their policies and procedures to see if they are permitted to do this.

ANTIDEPRESSANTS (TRICYCLICS)

Tricyclic antidepressants (TCAs) are widely prescribed in the United States. Their primary use is in the treatment of endogenous depression in adults; however, recent study has increased their use for school phobia, pain control, obsessive-compulsive behavior, and sleep disorders in children.[20] Overdose statistics demonstrate that cyclic antidepressants are one of the most deadly types of poisoning, with a high degree of morbidity and mortality in significant overdoses. Many tricyclic antidepressants are available throughout the United States.[28]

TCAs are well absorbed in the GI tract. The parent compound and active metabolites are quickly bound to plasma proteins. TCAs exert their effects by inhibiting the amine pump mechanism responsible for the reuptake of norepinephrine and serotonin in adrenergic and serotonergic neurons. Cyclic antidepressants also block cholinergic receptors in the parasympathetic nervous system and exert antihistaminic properties.[5,11,15]

The clinical manifestations of TCA poisoning include mydriasis, tachycardia, dry mucous membranes, urine retention, and decreased peristalsis. Central nervous system (CNS) signs include confusion, agitation, hallucinations, seizures, and coma. Twitching, jerking, and myoclonic movements have also been reported. Generalized tonic clonic seizures are reported in 1% to 20% of TCA poisoning cases. Respiratory depression is common. The enhanced adrenergic stimulation of the myocardium and direct toxic effects of these agents result in many cardiovascular effects. Sinus tachycardia and mild hypertension occur early in poisoning. TCAs exert a quinidinelike cardiac action that depresses conduction velocity. QRS-interval widening, right bundle-branch block, and first-degree heart block are common findings. Acidosis occurs because of cardiac and respiratory depression.[5,11,15]

In TCA poisoning, support of vital functions is essential. Hypotension is initially managed with an IV infusion of saline solution. Pressor agents are used if hypotension is refractory to fluid challenges. α-Adrenergic agents are preferred. Physostigmine is not an antidote to cyclic antidepressant poisoning and should not be used for these patients.

BENZODIAZEPINES

Benzodiazepines became available in the United States in 1963 to control anxiety. These drugs are now used to decrease anxiety and as sedative-hypnotics, muscle-relaxants, and anticonvulsants. Generally, a toxic level of benzodiazepines must be quite high; however, benzodiazepines are often taken in combination with other poisons, such as alcohol, that can cause death.[22]

The syndrome of benzodiazepine toxicity is nonspecific. The clinical picture is usually mild compared with those of other sedative-hypnotic poisonings. Most oral poisonings result in drowsiness and coma.

In contrast, IV diazepam use has been associated with a 1.7% incidence of life-threatening reactions, including hypotension and cardiorespiratory arrest. Diazepam toxicity is markedly increased by the concomitant use of other drugs, particularly alcohol.

The treatment of benzodiazepine poisoning begins with management of the patient's ABCs. Flumazenil can be administered to reverse the sedative, ataxic, anxiolytic, and muscle-relaxant effects of a toxic benzodiazepine ingestion. However, this drug must be administered with caution because many patients who take overdoses take combinations of drugs, some of which may cause seizures at toxic levels, such as TCAs. Flumazenil reverses the anticonvulsant effects of benzodiazepines, which leaves patients with polyoverdoses at risk for lack of seizure management.[44]

DIGITALIS

The term *cardiac glycoside* is used to describe a large group of drugs prescribed to treat heart failure. These drugs have been used throughout history, with early mention of the compound found in ancient writings in the year 1500 BC. Digitalis has become the most familiar of the group. It is derived from the dried leaf of the foxglove plant *Digitalis purpurea*.[15]

Several factors contribute to digitalis poisoning. These include the patient's age, severe heart disease, electrolyte imbalances, and drug therapy such as the use of diuretics.[15]

Clinical manifestations of digitalis toxicity are divided into cardiac and noncardiac. Cardiac manifestations are the result of depression through the sinoatrial and atrioventricular nodes and alteration of impulse formation. Noncardiac signs and symptoms include fatigue, vascular weakness, anorexia, nausea, vomiting, diarrhea, confusion, restlessness, insomnia, drowsiness, hallucinations, frank psychosis, blurred vision, photophobia, and yellow-halo visual effects.[15]

Treatment of digitalis toxicity includes support of vital functions and possible correction of the underlying cause (e.g., correction of an electrolyte imbalance). Advances in immunotherapy have yielded digoxin-specific antibody fragments (Fab), which neutralize digoxin toxicity. Fab fragments are indicated if conventional supportive care to life-threatening dysrhythmias and hyperkalemia fails. Fab fragments bind to digoxin, and the Fab-digoxin complex is excreted in the urine.[42,44]

STREET DRUGS
COCAINE

Cocaine use has reached epidemic proportions in the United States. It has been estimated that more than 30 million Americans have tried cocaine and that about 5 million use it regularly. It was one of the most popular drugs in the 1980s. Thirty percent of men and 20% of women between the ages of 24 and 34 have used cocaine at least once.[17] The cocaine problem varies with geographic location; however, probably few places in the United States have escaped difficulties related to illegal drug use.[32]

Cocaine is a naturally occurring alkaloid, the only source of which is the leaves of the evergreen shrub *Erythroxylon coca*. The leaves contain 0.5% to 2.5% cocaine. The plant is native to Peru, Bolivia, and Colombia but is now a major cultivated cash crop in many Central and South American countries. The crystallized cocaine is extracted from the coca leaf in the hydrochloride salt form. Cocaine hydrochloride is usually transported in a 90% to 95% pure form until it reaches its intended destination, where the drug is diluted and adulterated for street sale. Street cocaine generally varies in potency from 2% to 30% purity. Common adulterants are mannitol, lactose, and local anesthetics such as lidocaine, procaine, and tetracaine. Many times street samples contain no cocaine at all, but are combinations of caffeine, amphetamines, codeine, phencyclidine (PCP), and other local anesthetics.[4,14,32]

There are several routes of cocaine abuse. The easiest and most popular method of misuse is nasal inhalation or "snorting." The blood concentration increases rapidly after snorting for approximately 20 minutes, peaks at 1 hour, and then slowly subsides for several hours. Cocaine may also be injected intravenously. Because blood levels peak after 3 to 5 minutes, this method can be very toxic and lethal. In addition, cocaine is mixed in a mixture that may contain a flammable solvent that is ignited. Smoking cocaine not only may lead to toxicity but also to severe burn injuries.[15]

Crack is the "cooked and dried" version of freebase cocaine. When cocaine is mixed with baking soda and water and then heated in an ordinary pot, the impurities used to cut the drug are removed. The resulting mixture dries into a hard substance that is broken into small chunks or "rocks," which are white or yellowish-white in color. The user then smokes the rocks.[32]

Ingestion of cocaine is not a popular method of abuse. However, oral exposure and poisoning have been observed in the "body-packer" or smuggler. In an effort to hide the illegal substance from authorities, the drug runner ingests a large supply of cocaine that has been packaged in rubber, latex, or similar material. Each individual package may contain 2 to 10 g of pure cocaine; up to 175 bags have been swallowed by one person. If the bag leaks or ruptures, absorption of the cocaine is rapid and often lethal.[6,12,15]

Another popular method of cocaine use is for the male to apply the drug topically to his penis before sexual intercourse. Because cocaine is a local anesthetic, the desired effect of this practice is prolonged erection. Cocaine is absorbed in the female's vagina, and intoxication can occur.[4]

The drug is metabolized by the liver and excreted by the kidney.[13,17] Cocaine stimulates both the peripheral and central adrenergic nervous systems. Cocaine produces euphoria and a mild-to-moderate CNS stimulation manifested by decreased fatigue, excitement, and a general feeling of well-being. The user generally tends to be talkative, physically active, and sociable and may experience a slight tachycardia, mydriasis, slight diaphoresis, and tremor.

Death from cocaine results from cardiovascular and respiratory collapse. Metabolic acidosis, hyperthermia, status epilepticus, or ventricular arrhythmias are seen in the severely poisoned patient. Fatalities may occur from any method of abuse. Unexplained sudden death may occur after IV injection, but most fatal cases follow a progressive downhill course over 30 to 60 minutes. Death can also occur as a result of the effects of agents used to mitigate cocaine effects (especially heroin) or from the untoward effects of adulterants or substituted drugs.[26]

The main objectives in treating acute cocaine poisoning are to support the respiratory system, control hypertension, suppress malignant cardiac arrhythmias, correct metabolic acidosis, reduce hyperthermia, and minimize seizure activity.[4]

HALLUCINOGENS

Two types of drug poisoning that cause hallucinations are PCP and lysergic acid diethylamide (LSD). PCP was initially developed as a general anesthetic in 1958. Because of the postanesthetic reactions that occurred with its use, it has not been used legally since 1965. PCP now is manufactured in "kitchen" laboratories.

The drug may be smoked, snorted, or ingested and is distributed to all tissue compartments, metabolized by the liver, and excreted through the kidneys. Its effects can last up to 48 hours.[16] PCP can produce bizarre and dangerous behavior. In larger doses it can cause psychosis, hostility, and coma. A common neurologic sign of PCP intoxication is nystagmus.[6,44]

Treatment consists of supportive care. Air transportation of patients who have taken PCP demands close observation. Patients may become hostile, belligerent, and destructive. Sedative or neuromuscular blocking agents with airway control may be necessary to safely transport these patients.

LSD is the most potent hallucinogen known. Psychiatrists initially used the drug in the 1950s as an aid in clinical psychotherapy. Abuse became popular during the 1960s, with illicit use reaching epidemic proportions in 1965.[5,36]

LSD can be taken both orally and nasally. The dose required to produce hallucinations is between 0.5 and 1.0 μg/kg, and the intensity of its effect is dose dependent.[13] Absorption of the drug is rapid, and LSD is distributed to all tissues, including the brain. Initial effects occur in 30 to 40 minutes, and peak effects occur in 1 to 2 hours. LSD is metabolized in the liver, and small amounts are excreted unchanged in urine.[15]

Psychologic effects follow ingestion of LSD in 30 to 90 minutes. These effects are generally pleasurable, and the person is usually able to function and is aware that he or she is experiencing a drug-induced illusion. Occasionally a person may have an intense panic reaction ("bad trip"), which includes frightening hallucinations and loss of the knowledge that the symptoms are caused by a transient drug effect. Such a person may become confused, aggressive, suicidal, or violent. Particularly frightening and uncontrollable experiences are linked to the contamination of LSD with other drugs, such as amphetamines.[15]

As with the patient who has taken PCP, extreme caution should be taken during the transport of these patients. Use of ear protectors, sedation, and prophylactic restraints may be necessary before transport.

Designer drugs continue to appear on the street—for example, ecstasy or 3,4-methylenedioxymethamphetamine (MDMA) a substitute amphetamine. Each of these medications causes different signs and symptoms and generally requires supportive care. However, safety must remain the number one concern when transporting these patients for additional care.[23]

ALCOHOL

Alcohol (ethanol) is the most widely used and abused drug in America. It is often involved in poison emergencies because it is frequently used with other drugs.

Ethanol alcohol is rapidly absorbed from the stomach, small intestine, and colon. Food reduces the rate of absorption by 2 to 6 hours. Once ethanol is ingested, equilibration is rapid, and distribution uniformly occurs throughout all bodily tissues and fluids. Passage across the placenta has been documented.[44]

Ethanol metabolism occurs mainly in the liver. Ethanol is oxidized by alcohol. Alcohol is a CNS depressant. Acute intoxication produces psychomotor retardation, reflex slowing, lethargy, sleep, and ultimately, coma and death. Initially, respirations are stimulated as a result of the production of carbon dioxide. However, with increasing concentrations of alcohol, respirations are dangerously depressed. Ethanol enhances cutaneous blood flow, which causes heat loss through vasodilation. Excessive amounts depress the central thermoregulatory mechanism, adding to the hypothermia effects. Ethanol stimulates gastric secretions, which causes an irritation of the gastric mucosa. In addition, ethanol causes diuresis mediated through inhibition of antidiuretic hormone, which decreases renal tubular reabsorption of water.[15,44]

Patients respond differently to alcohol poisoning. Table 28-4 correlates signs and symptoms of alcohol intoxication with blood alcohol levels.[15] The lethal dose of alcohol in children is considered 3 g/kg and in adults 5 to 8 g/kg.

TABLE 28-4	**Signs and Symptoms of Alcohol Intoxication by Blood Alcohol Level**
Blood Alcohol Level	**Signs and Symptoms**
Mild (0.05%-0.15%) 0.5-1.5 mg/ml	Decreased inhibitions
	Slight visual impairments
	Slight muscular incoordination
	Slowing of reaction time
Moderate (0.15%-0.3%) 1.5-3 mg/ml	Definite visual impairment
	Sensory loss
	Muscular incoordination
	Slowing of reaction time
	Slurred speech
Severe (0.3%-0.5%) 3-5 mg/ml	Marked muscular incoordination
	Blurred or double vision
	Approaching stupor
	Sometimes hypoglycemia with hypothermia
	Conjugate deviation of the eyes
	Extensor rigidity of the extremities
	Unilateral or bilateral Babinski sign
	Convulsions and trismus
	Fatalities begin to occur
Coma (>0.5%) >5 mg/ml	Unconsciousness
	Depressed respirations
	Decreased reflexes and complete loss of sensation
	Deaths are frequent

From Dreisbach RH, Robertson WO: *Handbook of poisoning: prevention, diagnosis and treatment*, Norwalk, Conn, 1987, Appleton & Lange.

Care of the alcohol-poisoned patient consists of supportive care. Such patients may become combative, and precautions should be taken for appropriate restraint before transport.

ETHYLENE GLYCOL

Ethylene glycol is an odorless, water-soluble solvent most commonly used in permanent-type antifreezes and coolants. Ingestion usually occurs in the inquisitive toddler or the subject desperate to commit suicide. Ethylene glycol is rapidly absorbed and reaches peak blood levels in 1 to 4 hours after ingestion. Large doses result in an inebriated patient without the odor of alcohol. Ethylene glycol approximates ethanol in CNS toxicity; however, its metabolites produce profound systemic effects.[15,44]

Ethylene glycol is hepatically metabolized. It eventually breaks down into four main by-products that include formic and oxalic acid. Most believe that these by-products are responsible for the pathology seen in ethylene glycol toxicity.[15,44]

Signs and symptoms of ethylene glycol ingestion include nausea, vomiting, ataxia, stupor, coma, convulsions, nystagmus, depressed deep-tendon reflexes, myoclonic jerks, hypothermia, and low-grade fever. A profound anion-gap metabolic acidosis is a hallmark of this poisoning, but it only occurs after metabolism has begun. Severe hypocalcemia resulting from chelation of calcium may produce tetany and cardiac compromise. Other complications of ethylene glycol poisoning include kidney failure and pulmonary edema.[26,44]

Serum/blood levels guide treatment for ethylene glycol ingestion. If history suggests a significant ingestion, an IV ethanol drip should be initiated before the ethylene glycol level is determined. Ethanol blocks the conversion of ethylene glycol to its toxic form. Dialysis is used to remove the ethylene glycol because metabolism is retarded and renal excretion of the parent compound is poor. Thiamine and pyridoxine have also been used to treat ethylene glycol toxicity. Thiamine is administered at 100 μm, and pyroxidine is administered at 50 mg, either intravenously or intramuscularly. There are also case reports of the use of 4-methylpyrazole, a potent inhibitor of alcohol dehydrogenase that prevents the metabolism of methanol and ethylene glycol.[41]

Fomepizole (Antizol)[43] is also an antidote for ethanol toxicity. It prevents the formation of toxic metabolites. The advantages of using fomepizole include the following:

- Intermittent administration
- Decreased mental status changes compared to the use of alcohol
- The patient is less likely to require admission to a critical care unit

The major disadvantage to the use of this therapy is cost. Ethanol therapy is about $100 compared to $5000 for Antizol therapy. However, the decreased need for critical care may balance some of this disadvantage.[43]

CARBON MONOXIDE

Carbon monoxide (CO) is a colorless, odorless, tasteless gas yielded by the incomplete combustion of carbonaceous material. Sources include car exhaust, space heaters, defective fireplace flues, flame-type water heaters, improperly vented gas ranges and furnaces, coal and oil furnaces, poorly ventilated charcoal and gas grills, and fires of all types.[44]

Carbon monoxide poisoning should be suspected in any patient or patients with unexplained symptoms who may have been exposed to machinery running in an enclosed poorly ventilated space, when a furnace is new or run for the first time when the weather changes; exposure to smoke in an enclosed space; or unexplained symptoms in multiple people in the same living space. Animals are more sensitive than humans to CO poisoning and may have been ill long before their human owners.

CO combines with the hemoglobin molecule in the red blood cell. The affinity of hemoglobin for

CO is approximately 200 times that for oxygen. Not only does CO compete with oxygen for hemoglobin, but also the presence of carboxyhemoglobin also greatly impedes the dissociation of oxygen from hemoglobin. This leads to a decreased partial pressure of oxygen in the blood and diminished gradient for oxygen diffusion from the red blood cell to the tissues, resulting in tissue anoxia. Arterial hypoxia results from any of the following reasons: pulmonary venous admixture from an uneven ventilation/perfusion relationship; marked inhibition of the circulatory system; direct effect of CO on the pulmonary tissue, which results in increased capillary permeability and decreased production of surfactant; and a change in the oxyhemoglobin dissociation curve with a shift to the left.[44]

It has been found that that the concentration of CO in the blood relates poorly to the clinical features observed in the person who has been exposed. Figure 28-1 describes the symptomatology of CO poisoning related to CO saturation in the blood.[44]

The treatment of acute CO exposure is oxygen delivery. Carboxyhemoglobin will dissociate and convert to oxyhemoglobin if high concentrations of oxygen are provided. Hyperbaric therapy has also been found to be extremely successful for patients with levels of 40% at the exposure site and emergency unit levels of 25%.[44]

The treatment of the patient in transport with CO poisoning includes management of the patient's airway so that high-flow O_2 can be delivered. It is helpful to perform a neurologic assessment before treatment and once treatment has been begun with high flow oxygen. In addition, the patient must be observed and treated for such hypoxic side effects as seizures.

SNAKEBITES

Responding to the needs of a victim of snakebite may not be one of the most common flights encountered by the flight nurse; however, knowledge of how to care for such patients can decrease complications and save lives. There are many thousands of snakebites reported in the United States each year. Venomous snakes inflict about 7000 to

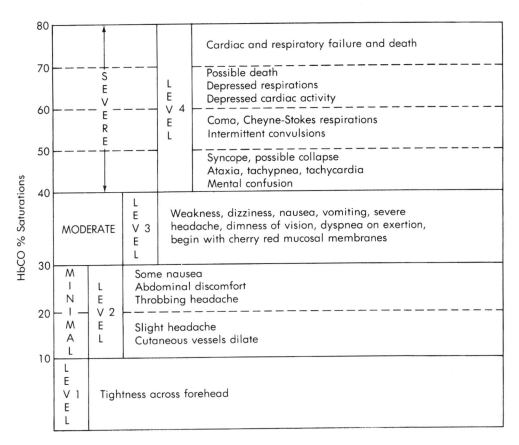

FIGURE 28-1   **Signs and symptoms of various blood levels of HbCO.** (Modified from Elo T: *Carbon monoxide: quick reference to clinical toxicology*, Philadelphia, 1980, Lippincott.)

8000 of them. Unfortunately, people still die from envenomation.[2,8,21,34]

Venom is a special category of poison that must be injected by one organism into another to produce a harmful effect.[14] It is secreted by special epithelial cells in certain organisms and is stored in the lumina or exocrine glands. It comprises multiple substances, some of them toxic. The toxins may affect particular body systems such as the neurologic, hematologic, and cardiovascular systems.[2,27,34]

The effects of venom are dependent on the pharmacologic complexity of the venom and the action that the venom exerts on the tissues. Where the venom is injected also affects the spread of the venom. Bites to the leg are more serious than to

the face because muscle movement will spread the venom throughout the body.[7,40]

The most prevalent venomous snakes in the United States are the pit vipers, which include the true rattlesnakes, the copperheads, and water moccasins. These snakes are found throughout the country with the exception of Maine, Alaska, and Hawaii.[2,34]

The coral snake is another kind of venomous snake found in the United States. The eastern coral snake is found in North and South Carolina, Florida, Louisiana, Mississippi, Alabama, Georgia, and Texas.

In addition to the venomous snakes native to the United States, poisonous snakes have been collected from all over the world. A bite from any one of these snakes may be fraught with complications or may even be instantly fatal.

The following subsections describe the venomous snakes, the initial treatment of snakebites, flight nursing care of snake-bitten patients, and the role of flight transport in the care of these victims.

RECOGNITION OF VENOMOUS BITES

Figure 28-2 compares venomous and nonvenomous snakes. The most prevalent type of venomous snake in the United States is the pit viper. Only trained people should handle live snakes; even a dead snake can envenomate a careless person.[27,34]

Pit vipers, who belong to the Crotalidae family (as shown in Figure 28-2), have a pit midway between the eye and nostril on each side of the head.

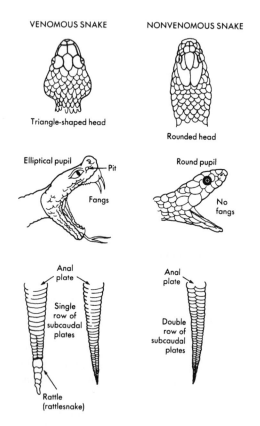

VENOMOUS SNAKE   NONVENOMOUS SNAKE

Triangle-shaped head

Rounded head

Elliptical pupil ──── Pit

Fangs

Round pupil

No fangs

Anal plate

Single row of subcaudal plates

Anal plate

Double row of subcaudal plates

Rattle (rattlesnake)

FIGURE 28-2   **Venomous and nonvenomous snakes.** (From Otten M: Venomous animal injuries. In Rosen P et al, editors: *Emergency medicine,* vol 1, ed 4, St Louis, 1998, Mosby.)

This pit is a heat-sensing organ that helps the snake locate its prey. This particular characteristic, unlike others in Figure 28-2, is a 100% consistent characteristic in the identification of pit vipers.[27,34]

Envenomation by a pit viper usually results in symptoms of localized pain, swelling, and edema in the bitten area. Other symptoms include diaphoresis and chills, paresthesia, nausea, hypotension, faintness, weakness, muscle fasciculations, local ecchymosis, and coagulopathies.[26,34]

The second-largest family of snakes in the world is the Elapidae, which contains some deadly species. These include cobras, mambas, and the eastern coral snakes. One of the distinguishing characteristics of these snakes is their color.

Envenomation by a coral snake may result in a neurotoxic course. Systemic manifestations include drowsiness, euphoria, weakness, nausea, vomiting, fasciculations, dysphagia, salivation, extraocular muscle paresis, hypotension, and cardiopulmonary failure.[26,34]

INITIAL MANAGEMENT OF SNAKEBITES

Just because a snake has bitten a person, it does not always mean that envenomation has occurred. It has been estimated that 20% to 30% of crotalid bites and 50% of elapid bites do not result in penetration; such bites are called "dry bites."[26] There is lengthy and controversial discussion in the literature over the appropriate management of snakebite. As noted by Kunkel,[26] many an emotional discussion has occurred over the appropriate management of a snakebite. In the following discussion of the general management of snakebite patients, it is important to emphasize that experts should be consulted when questions arise about the care of snake-bitten patients. Many of the authors cited in this chapter are available for consultation, as is the local poison control center. It is very important to identify the snake so that appropriate treatment can be initiated. Many patients have received unnecessary treatment for nonvenomous bites.[7,40]

If the snake has not been secured, the patient should be moved to a safe environment. It is important to keep the patient calm and to immobilize the affected part. These two interventions decrease the circulation of venom throughout the patient's system. Specific prehospital care of the snakebite patient is based on the type of envenomation that has occurred. For elapid envenomation the wound should be cleansed, a compressive bandage applied, the extremity immobilized, and the patient transported. The care of viper envenomation should include cleansing of the wound, immobilization of the affected part, no use of compression techniques, and transport of the patient.[7,26,34,40]

The airway, ventilatory, and circulatory status of the patient should be constantly evaluated. Two large-bore IV lines should be started, preferably in an area away from the bite. The patient must be observed closely for progression of symptoms from a localized reaction at the wound site to a systemic reaction.

When possible, blood samples for baseline laboratory work should be drawn before transport. These may include a complete blood count, coagulation studies, electrolytes, blood urea nitrogen, creatinine, and urinalysis. Included in the coagulation studies should be fibrin split products and fibrinogen levels.[2,7,226,34,40]

If the patient exhibits signs of severe envenomation, such as edema that has progressed 30 cm in 1 hour of the bite, shock, kidney failure, pulmonary edema, bleeding, or paralysis, administration of antivenin should be started.[2,7,26,34,40] The size of the patient needs to be considered in relation to the amount of venom that the person may be able to tolerate. A child or small adult may be more severely affected.

Snake antivenin is prepared from the serum of horses hyperimmunized against a specific venom or venoms. Unlike other drugs, the dosage of antivenin should be based on clinical findings rather than on the age and weight of the patient. Skin testing for hypersensitivity with epinephrine at the patient's bedside is recommended before antivenin is administered.[2,34] Administration of steroids and other medications to decrease the risk of anaphylaxis is used by some health-care providers. Again, it cannot be overemphasized that experts are available by a number of communication routes and should be consulted.[7]

When antivenin is given, the package instructions should be followed and resuscitation equipment kept in close range. Patients should be monitored continuously for anaphylactic reactions.

Serum sickness may develop after antivenin administration. The incidence of serum sickness varies from 10% to 80% of all patients given antivenin therapy.[19] The symptoms of serum sickness have occurred up to 3 weeks after antivenin administration. They include fever, rash, nausea, vomiting, and neurologic symptoms. Treatment of serum sickness includes antihistamines and steroids.[2,34]

TRANSPORT CARE OF PATIENTS WITH A SNAKEBITE

The transport team may become involved in the care of the patient with snakebite by directly responding to the scene of the injury or by transporting the patient to more definitive care. Experts in the care of snakebites note that rapid transport of these patients to a hospital or to a person who can manage their injury is imperative in saving lives and preventing complications. Box 28-2 summarizes care to be provided for the patient bitten by a snake.[2,34]

SUMMARY

The transport of the poisoned patient generally involves support of the patient's airway, breathing, and circulation. Few antidotes are available for the poisoned patient, and generally the transport team may have limited resources to determine the cause of the poisoning.

The transport team should always ensure safety before transport begins so they do not become victims of the poison as well. A patient who has deliberately taken poison must be appropriately retrained before transport.

The transport care of the poisoned patient can be interesting (i.e., discovering what poisoned them) as well as challenging (i.e., ensuring that they receive the best care).

| BOX 28-2 | **Transport Care of the Patient Bitten by a Snake** |

1. Provide a safe environment for the transport team and patient.
2. Provide basic and advanced life support.
3. Obtain as much information as possible about the type of snake that has envenomated the patient.
4. Immobilize the affected part.
5. Keep the patient calm.
6. Notify the appropriate receiving facility. Consult an expert when patient management questions arise.
7. Establish a large-bore IV line.
8. Watch for local and systemic effects from the snakebite.
9. Administer analgesia for pain.
10. Bring the dead snake in a secure container for identification, if possible.

TOXICOLOGY CASE STUDY 1

HALLUCINOGENIC TOXICITY

A 16-year-old boy ingested a plant known as monkshood after being told by his friends that he would have a "good trip." The plant that he ingested was a potent alkaloid. He immediately began hallucinating and then went into status epilepticus. The flight team was dispatched to assist in patient care and to transport the patient.

On the arrival of the flight team, the patient's seizures had subsided after administration of 5 mg diazepam. However, the patient was screaming and had be physically restrained. An IV line was started, and the patient was intubated with the use of rapid-sequence induction. Ten milligrams of vecuronium and 2 mg lorazepam were given for safety and sedation.

Blood pressure was 80 mm Hg systolic by palpation, pulse was 130 beats/min and irregular (the monitor showed atrial fibrillation), and respirations were being assisted because of the vecuronium. A fluid bolus of 200 ml of normal saline solution was infused. The patient's blood pressure increased to 100/50 mm Hg. The patient was prepared for transport. Restraints were applied and a headset placed on the patient to decrease outside stimulation.

During transport, the patient sustained cardiac arrest, going into coarse ventricular fibrillation. He was successfully electroconverted with 360 W/sec. Atrial fibrillation continued after resuscitation. A lidocaine bolus was administered and a lidocaine drip initiated per advanced cardiac life support protocol.

The patient experienced no additional problems during transport and was admitted to the medical intensive care unit of the receiving facility. The toxicologist continued supportive care, including correction of the metabolic acidosis and maintenance of sedation. The patient regained consciousness 48 hours later and was discharged home in 5 days of the incident.

TOXICOLOGY CASE STUDY 2

VICTIM OF A SNAKEBITE

The flight team was asked to transport by helicopter a 4-year-old boy who had sustained a snakebite. The child stated he had been playing in a field when a "brown snake with sharp teeth bit him." An adult did not witness this incident.

The child was alert and oriented. His vital signs were stable. The referring physician reported that the child had two puncture wounds at the side of his right foot. Localized swelling was also noted.

The care of this patient included assessment of whether the bite was venomous. Because copperheads are native to the area and fang marks were visible, the flight nurse had to assume that the child had been bitten by a pit viper. The wound had been cleansed and immobilized. The flight nurse placed an IV line and started a cardiac monitor. A tetanus shot was administered because the child had never been immunized.

During flight, the flight nurse monitored the child for signs and symptoms of localized and systemic poisoning, including increasing edema in the bitten extremity, nausea and vomiting, hypotension, and excessive bleeding.

An important role for the flight team in the care of snakebite envenomation is the timely delivery and initiation of antivenin in areas where it is not readily available. However, this child, as in about 50% of snakebites, only sustained a dry bite. He was admitted for observation and discharged later without complications.

REFERENCES

1. Albertson TE et al: Superiority of activated charcoal alone compared with ipecac and activated charcoal in the treatment of acute toxic ingestions, *Ann Emerg Med* 18(1):56, 1989.

2. American Health Consultants. Special report on overdoes patient in the ED, *ED Nursing* 3:77, 2000.

3. Auerbach P, editor: *Wilderness medicine*, ed 4, St Louis, 2001, Mosby.

4. Brabowski J: *Cocaine pharmacology: effects and treatment of abuses*, National Institute on Drug Abuse Research Monograph series, Washington, DC, NIDA Research Monograph 50, 1984.

5. Braden NJ, Jackson JE, Walson PD: Tricyclic antidepressant overdose, *Pediatr Clin North Am* 33:691, 1986.

6. Brent J: Drugs of abuse: an update, *Emerg Med* 7:56, 1995.

7. Callahan M: Challenging paradigms is risky business: reflections on CC Snyder's: a definitive study of snakebite, *Wilder and Environ Med* 12:273, 2001.

8. Curry S et al: The legitimacy of rattlesnake bites in central Arizona, *Ann Emerg Med* 18:658, 1989.

9. Daniels EJ: *Any other song*, Bowie, Md, 1980, Brady.

10. Elo T: Carbon monoxide. In Hanenson IB, editor: *Quick reference to clinical toxicology*, Philadelphia, 1980, Lippincott.

11. Foulke GE: Identifying toxicity risk early after antidepressant overdose, *Am J Emerg Med* 13(2):123, 1995.

12. Gay G: Clinical management of acute and chronic cocaine poisoning, *Ann Emerg Med* 11:562, 1982.

13. Geiderman J: Adverse drug reactions: an emergency department view, *Topics Emerg Med* 9:1, 1986.

14. Goodman L, Gilman A, editors: *The pharmacological basis of therapeutics*, ed 2, New York, 1991, Macmillan.

15. Haddad L, Shannon M, Winchester J, editors: *Clinical management of poisonings and drug overdose*, ed 3, Philadelphia, 1998, Saunders.

16. Haley K, Baker P, Eckles, N, Baker P: *Emergency nursing pediatric course*, Park Ridge, Ill, 1998, Emergency Nurses Association.

17. Hall E. Role of surgical intervention in the management of crotaline snake envenomation, *Ann Emerg Med* 37:175, 2001.

18. Higgins R: Cocaine abuse: what every nurse should know, *J Emerg Nurs* 15:318, 1989.

19. Hoffman RS, Goldfrank LR: The poisoned patient with altered consciousness: controversies in the use of a "coma cocktail," *JAMA* 274(7):562, 1995.

20. Hollander J: The management of cocaine associated myocardial ischemia, *JAMA* 333(19):1267, 1995.

21. Jurkovich G et al: Complications of Crotalidae antivenin therapy, *J Trauma* 28:1032, 1988.

22. Karb V, Queener S, Freeman J: *Handbook of drugs for nursing practice*, ed 2, St Louis, 1996, Mosby.

23. Katzung BG, editor: *Basic and Clinical Pharmacology*, ed 8, New York, 2001, Lange Medical Books/McGraw-Hill.

24. Kitt S et al: *Emergency nursing: a physiologic and clinical perspective*, Philadelphia, 1995, Saunders.

25. Krupa D: *Flight nursing core curriculum*, Park Ridge, Ill, 1997, Road Runner Press.

26. Kulberg A: Substance abuse: clinical identification and management, *Pediatr Clin North Am* 33:325, 1986.

27. Kunkel D et al: Reptile envenomation, *J Toxicol Clin Toxicol* 21:503, 1984.

28. Litovitz T, Klein-Schwartz W, White S, Cobaugh D, Youniss J, Drab A, Benson B: 1999 annual report of the American Association of Poison Control Centers toxic surveillance system, *Am J Emerg Med* 18(5):517, 2000.

29. Matyunas NJ: *Tricyclic antidepressant poisoning*, clinical paper, Lexington, Ky, 1986, Kentucky Regional Poison Center.

30. McDeed C: Toxicological emergencies. In Jordan, K, editor: *Emergency nursing core curriculum*, Philadelphia, 2000, Saunders.

31. Mendenhall CL, Weesner RE: Alcohols and glycols. In Haneson IB, editor: *Quick reference to clinical toxicology*, Philadelphia, 1980, Lippincott.

32. Merigian KS, Roberts JR: *Cocaine*, clinical paper, Cincinnati, 1987, University of Cincinnati Medical Center Department of Emergency Medicine.

33. Merigian KS, Roberts JR: *LSD*, clinical paper, Cincinnati, 1986, University of Cincinnati Medical Center Department of Emergency Medicine.

34. Norris RL, Ling LJ, Wang R: Snake venom poisoning in the United States: assessment and management, *Emerg Med Rep* 16(10):87, 1995.

35. Olson KR et al: Seizures associated with poisoning and drug overdose, *Am J Emerg Med* 11(6):565, 1993.

36. Perrone J, Hoffman RS, Goldfrank LR: Special considerations in gastrointestinal decontamination, *Emerg Med Clin North Am* 12(2):285, 1994.

37. Riggs B: Acetaminophen. In Noji E, Kelen G, editors: *Handbook of toxicologic emergencies*, Chicago, 1989, Mosby.

38. Riggs B: Salicylates. In Nofi E, Kelen G, editors: *Manual of toxicologic emergencies*, Chicago, 1989, Mosby.

39. Sheehy S, Barber J: *Emergency nursing principles and practice*, ed 3, St Louis, 1992, Mosby.

40. Snyder CC, Pickins JE, Knowles RP, Emerson JL, Hines WA: A definitive study of snakebite, *Wilder and Environ Med* 12:276, 2001.

41. Stolpe M et al: Preliminary observations on the effects of hyperbaric oxygen therapy on western diamondback rattlesnake *(Crotalus atrox)* venom poisoning in the rabbit model, *Ann Emerg Med* 18:871, 1989.

42. Sullivan J: Immunotherapy in the poisoned patient: overview of present applications and future trends, *Med Toxicol* 24:47, 1986.

43. Weinman S: A new antidote in review: Fomepizole (Antizol), *J Emerg Nurs* 24:333, 1998.

44. Wright RO et al: Poison antidotes: guidelines for rational use in the emergency department, *Emerg Med Rep* 16(21):201, 1995.

THE PREGNANT PATIENT

COMPETENCIES

1. Perform a focused assessment of the pregnant patient, which includes collecting subjective and objective data related to the patient's pregnancy.
2. Perform a focused assessment of the fetus before and during transport.
3. Initiate appropriate interventions for the patient in preterm labor.

Complications that arise during pregnancy and place the pregnant patient at risk have many causes. Some complications may be related to the pregnancy itself, others are related to preexisting medical conditions that may be aggravated by the pregnancy, and yet others may be related directly to the fetus.

Transport team personnel who provide care for the obstetric patient at risk must be prepared to assess obstetric factors so that stabilizing care can be provided in preparation for transport. The well-being of the fetus and the mother must be considered. Identification of risk factors, early detection of possible complications, and interventions by the team during the transport can ensure a more favorable outcome for both the mother and the fetus. The transport team must be prepared to perform a general obstetric assessment, determine strategies for transport, perform fetal monitoring, and intervene as the situation requires. Complications discovered

can include amniotic fluid embolism, delivery complications, diabetes in pregnancy, hemorrhagic complications, multiple gestation, pregnancy-induced hypertension (PIH) and related disorders, preterm labor (PTL) and related issues, and trauma in pregnancy.[4] The information gained by the general obstetric assessment (Box 29-1) will aid the transport team in setting priorities for care during the transport.[2,4,7,8,13]

DETERMINING TEAM COMPOSITION FOR TRANSPORT OF THE PREGNANT PATIENT

Determining the members of the transport team who will transport the pregnant patient continues to generate controversy. Many pregnant patients are transported by teams composed of personnel who transport a variety of patients.[11] However, there are times when the patient or the fetus's

BOX 29-1	General Obstetric Assessment

1. Age of patient: Age (for teenagers and for women over age 35 years) predisposes the obstetric patient to many complications.
2. Gravida/para: How many times has the patient been pregnant? How many deliveries has she had at or beyond 20 weeks gestation? (Parity is not greater if twins are delivered or less if the fetus is stillborn.)
3. Estimated date of confinement (EDC): The EDC can be estimated from the first day of the last menstrual period (LMP) by using Nägele's rule: Count back 3 months from the LMP and then add 7 days. The due date is accurate within 2 weeks.
4. Ultrasound: Has the patient had an ultrasound? How many? In the event of an uncertain or unknown LMP or irregular menses, an early ultrasound performed between 12 and 30 weeks is reliable for dating the pregnancy in 2 weeks. An ultrasound can confirm the EDC estimated by the LMP. An ultrasound is invaluable if there is any question about placental location, amount of amniotic fluid present, fetal presentation, expected fetal growth, or anomalies.
5. In addition to inquiry into medical history and allergies, obstetric history is of particular significance. The following information may be of some predictive value for the outcome of the current pregnancy:
    a. Did the patient deliver vaginally or by cesarean section? Has she had a vaginal birth after a cesarean section? Observe for the location and extent of any abdominal scars.
    b. Did she or the baby experience any delivery complications?
    c. Did she experience any complications associated with any past pregnancies?
    d. Has she had any preterm deliveries? At what gestation did she deliver, and what was the outcome?
    e. Has she had either spontaneous or elective abortions? Was a dilation and curettage required?
    f. How many living children does she have? What were the birth weight and sex of each child?
    g. Has there been less than 1 year between the last delivery and commencement of the current pregnancy?
    h. What was the length of her last labor?
6. Pertaining to the current pregnancy:
    a. Is the patient having contractions? If so, when did the contractions begin? Has there been a change in the intensity or frequency of contractions? Is there accompanying backache, pelvic, or rectal pressure?
    b. Is any vaginal bleeding or "bloody show" present? Is there active bleeding? Attempt to help the patient quantify the bleeding by the number of towels, pads, or amount of clothing soaked before arrival and observe for evidence of dried blood on the perineum, legs, and soles of the feet. Was the bleeding painless or associated with contractions or abdominal pain? Was the blood bright red or dark? Was mucus combined with the blood (bloody show)? When did the bleeding begin? Was there any previous activity that may have precipitated the bleeding?
    c. Does the patient believe her "bag of waters" has ruptured? Was there a gush or an intermittent trickle? A small leakage of clear fluid may be confused with urinary incontinence. Leakage of amniotic fluid is uncontrollable. What time did it happen? What color was the fluid—meconium-stained, dark (presence of blood in the fluid), or clear? Was an odor present? Is the Chux under the patient wet or pooling with fluid?
    d. Does the patient smoke? If so, how much? Is there any evidence of alcohol or substance abuse? Attempt to ascertain from the patient the frequency and time of last usage.
    e. Has the patient had an adequate weight gain? Does she appear malnourished or obese?
    f. Has the patient had consistent prenatal care, no prenatal care, or limited prenatal care (three or fewer visits)?
    g. Has there been any change in fetal activity in the past several days?
    h. Is the patient currently taking any medications? If so, what is she taking and when was the last dosage?
    i. Is the patient having any current medical problems or problems with this pregnancy?
    j. Have any diagnostic tests been done?
7. Assess initial vital signs, including temperature; the blood pressure (BP), pulse, and respirations should be assessed every 15 minutes or as indicated. The obstetric patient should be positioned in the left lateral recumbent position before the BP is taken. When the patient is in the supine position, the gravid uterus may cause obstruction of the inferior vena cava, diminishing venous return to the heart, and this may lead to supine hypotension. Consequently, uteroplacental blood flow is decreased, placing the fetus at risk for compromise.

| BOX 29-1 | General Obstetric Assessment—cont'd |

8. Fetal heart tones (FHT): If the patient is currently being monitored with electronic fetal monitoring (EFM), evaluate the fetal heart rate (FHR) baseline and variability, observing for accelerations and decelerations. FHR should be assessed by Doppler if EFM is unavailable. FHR auscultations should be assessed every 15 minutes or less if any irregularities are noted. For strip interpretation, refer to the discussion in this chapter on fetal monitoring.

9. Fundal height (FH): FH should be measured in centimeters from the symphysis to the fundus. The fundal height roughly correlates to the gestation of the pregnancy in weeks. In the presence of hydramnios, multiple gestations, a large-for-gestation fetus, or a fetus with intrauterine growth restriction, the fundal height may not correlate with the gestation, signaling the possibility of complications.

10. Lightly palpate the fundus for strength, frequency, and duration of contractions. The fingertips can indent the fundus freely with mild contractions and slightly with moderate contractions; firm tension will be noted with strong contractions. Between contractions, palpate the abdomen for localized or generalized tenderness and observe the patient's coping response to the contractions. Gestures, posture, and facial expressions in response to contractions and verbal description should be noted. If the patient is in labor, observe for indications of advancing labor such as apprehension, restlessness, increasing difficulty coping with the contractions, screaming, nausea and vomiting, bearing-down effort, increase in bloody show, or a bulging perineum.

11. Roughly determine the fetal position by abdominal palpation: With the fingertips and palms, lightly palpate the fundus for the head or buttocks, moving down the sides to identify the fetal spine and small parts, and palpate the lower uterine segment for the presenting part. If the fetal position remains unclear, the fetus may be in a transverse lie. The FHT will be heard most clearly over the fetal spine.

12. Assess cervical status as indicated by the presence of contractions. If the amniotic membranes are intact, cervical status just before departure should be documented. If the membranes are ruptured, a sterile vaginal examination (SVE) should never be attempted unless delivery is deemed imminent. In the presence of hemorrhage, an SVE should never be attempted unless a placenta previa has been ruled out by ultrasound. During transport, an SVE is not indicated unless signs of advancing labor are noted.

13. Observe for the presence of other risk factors that predispose the obstetric patient to complications.

condition may warrant personnel with experience. Some suggested guidelines include the following[15]:

- A patient who is not in labor but requires transport for complications of pregnancy such as mild preeclampsia or stable third-trimester bleeding could probably be transported by a team with maternal and neonatal experience.
- A patient not in labor but with severe preeclampsia should be transported by a maternal transport team.
- A patient in labor may require both a maternal and neonatal transport team.

If the transport team does not routinely transport high-risk obstetrical patients, the Commission on Accreditation of Medical Transport Systems[6] recommends that the team members receive training in neonatal resuscitation. The transport vehicle should allow access to both the mother and the child in the case of a delivery during transport. Each transport program should have a policy and procedure in place that addresses when it is and is not appropriate to transport a pregnant patient and who are the team members that should provide care during transport.

If transport services do include specialty teams as a part of their service, they must be sure that these individuals receive annual training and are equipped and dressed for transport. This training should include[6]:

- Use of restraints systems in the transport vehicle
- Safety and survival skills
- Emergency egress training
- Postaccident/incident training

Contraindications for initiation of maternal transport should be considered before leaving a referring facility. These include the following[15]:

- Inability to stabilize the mother's condition, for example inability to control bleeding
- Acute fetal distress
- Imminent delivery, especially in a vehicle that does not allow access to both the mother and child
- Lack of maternal and neonatal experience by the transport team or no experienced personnel available to accompany the team
- Hazardous weather conditions that may prolong the transport time

GENERAL STRATEGIES FOR TRANSPORT

The primary survey and obstetric physical assessment can be completed in a very short time. Pertinent information obtained from the patient may be gathered as the situation permits during the course of the transport. In a life-threatening situation for the mother, the fetus, or both, lifesaving measures must take precedence. During transport, the team should perform the following assessments and interventions[13]:

1. Place the patient in a left lateral recumbent position or displace the uterus with a wedge if the patient cannot be turned. By displacing the uterus from the inferior vena cava, venous return to the heart is improved.
2. Note the patient's temperature. If possible, assess vital signs every 15 minutes.
3. Note fetal heart tones (FHTs). Initiate continuous electronic fetal monitoring (EFM) if available, or use a Doppler for fetal heart rate (FHR) assessment at least every 15 minutes. Note fetal movement and any contractions.
4. Start an intravenous line with a large-bore 18- or 16-gauge catheter and blood tubing. Use lactated Ringer's solution with an infusion rate of up to 125 ml/hr depending on hydration and renal, cardiac, and pulmonary status.
5. Provide supplemental oxygen with a nonrebreather mask as indicated by FHR pattern or maternal condition.
6. Monitor oxygen status by pulse oximetry, maintaining a level of 98% to 100%.
7. Assess uterine contractions and cervical status.
8. Note and quantify any bleeding or leaking of fluid.

Emotional and psychologic support provided to the obstetric patient at risk and her family is as vital an aspect as the emergency care provided. The team should encourage the patient to express and verbalize her anxiety, fear for the fetus, and concern regarding the complications she is experiencing. The transport team should assess the patient's knowledge of the situation, encourage questions, and use the opportunity for patient education. The vocabulary used should be based on the education and employment background of the patient. Because most patients have never been transported by air or ground ambulance, the team should explain all medications, procedures, and equipment to allay apprehension about the unfamiliar circumstances. The team should also reassure family members about the current condition of the patient and answer any questions they may have regarding the diagnosis, treatment, or destination.

FETAL MONITORING

Fetal monitoring may be accomplished by intermittent Doppler auscultation, which is used most frequently for short transports, and by EFM, used for longer transports (approximately 30 minutes or longer in duration). An external ultrasonographic device records FHTs, and a tocodynamometer detects uterine activity.[14]

Assessment of fetal well-being is best accomplished through the use of EFM. FHTs are recorded simultaneously with uterine activity. Subtle changes in the FHT are often the earliest indication of hypoxia caused by uteroplacental insufficiency or umbilical cord compression. Recognition of normal FHR tracing permits abnormalities to be realized quickly; appropriate intervention should be aimed at correcting or alleviating the source of insult. Baseline FHR (the average FHR) during a 10-minute period should be between 120 and 160.

FETAL HEART RATE ABNORMALITIES
VARIABILITY

Fluctuations in the FHR reflect interplay between the sympathetic and parasympathetic branches of the autonomic nervous system. Normal variability is indicative of an adequately oxygenated autonomic nervous system. Variability is the single most important factor in predicting fetal well-being. Short-term variability is the beat-to-beat irregularity of the FHR and is dominated by the parasympathetic branch; it is described as either present or absent. The parasympathetic branch is more susceptible to hypoxia. Absent short-term variability may be the first indicator of possible fetal hypoxia. The presence of short-term variability has been associated with normal acid-base balance at delivery. Long-term variability is the waviness of the FHR tracing and is dominated by the sympathetic branch; it normally varies from 6 to 25 beats above and below the baseline.[16]

Decreased variability (Figure 29-1), as demonstrated by absent short-term variability or less than five beats during a long-term period, may be precipitated by fetal hypoxia, administration of drugs to the mother, smoking, extreme prematurity, and fetal sleep. The fetus will have frequent sleep periods ranging from 20 to 40 minutes. Increased or marked long-term variability of more than 25 beats may be one of the earliest signs of hypoxia.

When an ultrasound transducer is used, a greater degree of variability may be recorded than is actually present. If there is any question regarding the presence of long-term or short-term variability, use of a fetal scalp electrode is recommended. If the patient has intact membranes, is preterm, or has any other condition that contraindicates internal monitoring at the referring facility, the questionable variability should be presumed to be decreased, with interventions made accordingly. When EFM is used during the transport of an obstetric patient, external monitoring will most frequently be used. The transport should keep in mind that a greater degree of variability may be recorded than is actually present when an ultrasound transducer is used. Because short-term variability cannot be accurately documented, it is not evaluated. Special notice of long-term variability and other reassuring signs must be made. The long-term variability can be assessed as

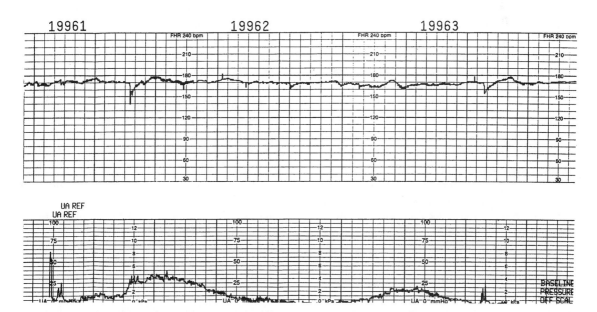

FIGURE 29-1   **Reduced variability and tachycardia.** Note the almost absent beat-to-beat variability and reduced long-term variability as recorded by a fetal scalp electrode; also note the tachycardic baseline.

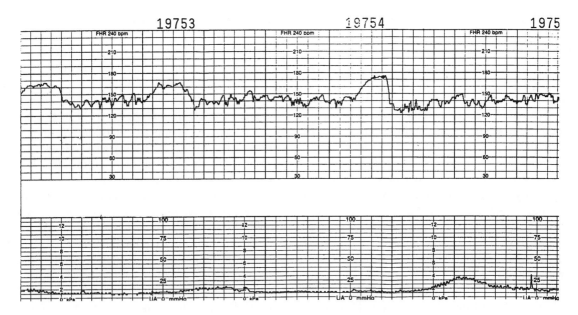

FIGURE 29-2 **Accelerations.** With use of an ultrasound transducer, accelerations of approximately 20 beats above the baseline may be noted. Long-term variability is present, and the FHR baseline range is approximately 135 to 145.

present or absent, and it is reflected in the baseline range.

PERIODIC CHANGES
Periodic changes in the FHR occur in response to stimulation, such as fetal movement and uterine contractions. The FHR may accelerate, decelerate, or not respond.

Acceleration. Accelerations above the baseline are usually associated with fetal movement but may occur during contractions (Figure 29-2). A hypoxic fetus experiencing metabolic acidosis is unable to accelerate its heart rate. The transport team should take note of fetal movements, whether the mother has noticed a decrease, increase, or no change in fetal movement. Decreased fetal movement is indicative of hypoxia.

Variable Deceleration. Variable decelerations can occur at any time during a contraction (Figure 29-3). The shape may also vary and is frequently V-shaped or W-shaped. Cord compression is responsible for these decelerations, which have a

very characteristic appearance; frequently a short acceleration is observed, followed by a rapid deceleration for some seconds, then a rapid rise and a short acceleration before there is a return to the FHR baseline. Cord compression may occur in a variety of circumstances. After the membranes rupture, there is less fluid to cushion the cord. Variables usually occur in response to uterine contractions but also may occur in response to fetal movement in the absence of contractions when membranes are ruptured. If a nuchal cord, short cord, or cord entanglement is present, variables usually result.

These decelerations have commonly been described as mild, moderate, or severe, depending on the drop in FHR. However, it is more conclusive to describe the deceleration. A better indicator of the fetal response is reflected in the FHR baseline, variability, and changes in the variable decelerations. Signs that the fetus is losing its ability to tolerate the stress of repeated cord compression or that the cord compression is becoming more severe include a deeper deceleration that lasts longer, a slow return to baseline, an "overshoot" increase in FHR baseline immediately after the deceleration, loss of shoulders,

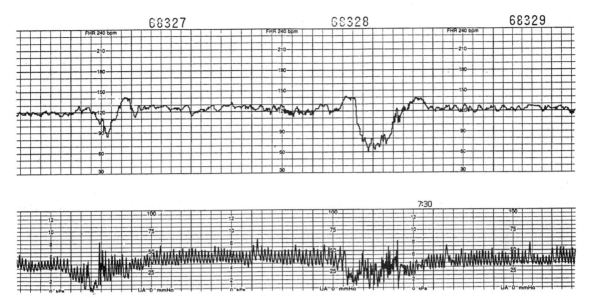

FIGURE 29-3   **Variable decelerations.** Note the variable decelerations in the presence of average variability. The accelerations before and after the deceleration (also called shoulders) are a reflection of adequate variability.

and decreased variability, especially short-term variability. In interpreting the tracing, careful observations of any changes in FHT will reveal more than what has just occurred during the last contraction. The flight nurse should look for answers to these questions: Do the variables occur with every contraction? Were they intermittent for some time? Is the variability decreased? Are the decelerations smoother in appearance? Are shoulders now absent? Does it look as if the FHR attempted to accelerate following the variable and that the baseline is gradually rising? Is the FHR drop during the deceleration lasting longer? Is it a deeper drop?

Late Decelerations.   In reference to the onset of the deceleration in relation to the contraction, a late deceleration is one that begins close to the apex of the contraction, gradually decelerates, and gradually returns to the FHR baseline after the contraction is over (Figure 29-4). Late decelerations always mean uteroplacental insufficiency; there is inadequate oxygen exchange in the placenta during a contraction. When a contraction is stronger, the insufficiency is greater and the deceleration is proportional.

With severe hypoxia, the myocardial depression may be such that the heart is unable to decelerate in response to the stress of the contraction, and very subtle late decelerations will be seen accompanied by a flat FHR baseline.

Uteroplacental insufficiency may result from pregnancy-induced hypertension (PIH), diabetes mellitus (DM), cardiovascular or kidney disease, chorioamnionitis, smoking, and a fetus that is past maturity. Uteroplacental insufficiency may also result from decreased placental perfusion in placental abruption or previa, uterine hypertonus as a result of oxytocin stimulation, and hypotension. As with variable decelerations, evaluation of late decelerations with respect to FHR baseline, variability, and changes noted over time is necessary in evaluating the well-being of the fetus. Signs of fetal decompensation include back-to-back decelerations, loss of variability, lack of spontaneous accelerations, tachycardia, and subtle decelerations.

Early Decelerations.   Early decelerations are innocuous decelerations that begin very close to the beginning of the contraction, appear almost as a

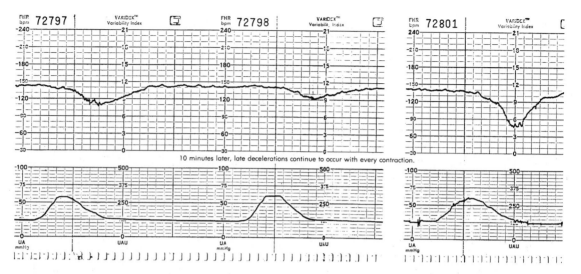

FIGURE 29-4   Late decelerations. Note the onset of deceleration at the apex of the contraction. Also note the minimal variability, slow recovery, and the proportional deceleration observed.

mirror image of the contraction, and end close to the end of the contraction. Head compression with vagus stimulation causes the deceleration. These decelerations frequently occur in active labor when the cervix has dilated 4 to 7 cm. In FHR interpretation, it is essential that late decelerations not be confused with early decelerations. Accurate placement of the tocotransducer over the fundus ensures that contractions are recorded correctly.

Sinusoidal.   A uniform sine wave pattern indicates fetal hypovolemia or anemia and may occur in cases of erythroblastosis fetalis, accidental tap of the umbilical cord during amniocentesis, fetomaternal transfusion, placental abruption, or another type of accident. Variability will be absent or minimal, and accelerations are not seen. When this pattern is recognized, rapid delivery is usually recommended. However, a pseudosinusoidal or undulating pattern (Figure 29-5) may be identified and linked to maternal drug administration.

Bradycardia.   An FHR of less than 120 for a period of 5 to 10 minutes or longer is defined as bradycardia. However, many term fetuses and those past maturity may have a stable baseline between

100 and 120, reflecting a more mature fetal neurologic system. In the absence of hypoxia, adequate variability and accelerations will also be noted.

Bradycardia is a response of increased parasympathetic tone and is reflected by a decrease in fetal cardiac output in the presence of hypoxia. The fetus can tolerate sustained bradycardia for only a short length of time before becoming acidotic. Bradycardia can be a result of severe cord compression and can occur minutes before delivery, when the cord is drawn into the pelvis in the second stage, or with a cord prolapse. Bradycardia can also occur with hypertonic or tetanic contractions and maternal hypotension. When it is a result of chronic hypoxia, bradycardia is usually a late occurrence.

Occasionally, a sterile vaginal examination or application of a fetal electrode will induce a prolonged deceleration, caused by vagal stimulation. The deceleration rarely lasts longer than 90 to 120 seconds. Pushing during the second stage of labor may precipitate end-stage bradycardia, which is characterized by a rapid drop in the FHR baseline. Delivery usually follows in a few minutes. Evaluation of variability will determine how the fetus is tolerating the stress.

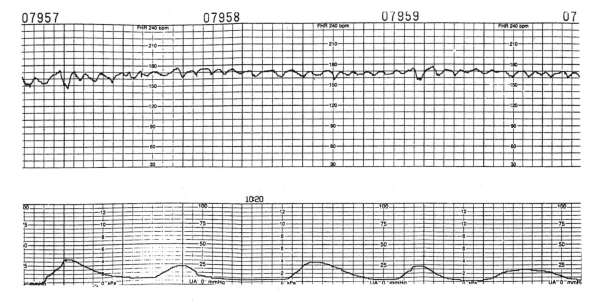

FIGURE 29-5   **Sinusoidal pattern.** Note the jagged, nonuniform pattern observed after intravenous administration of butorphanol (Stadol), 1 mg, which resolved spontaneously after 20 minutes.

Tachycardia.   An FHR of more than 160 for a period of 10 minutes or longer is considered tachycardia. Tachycardia is a response of increased sympathetic tone and is reflected by a compensatory mechanism to increase cardiac output in the presence of transient hypoxia. A decrease in variability is generally associated with tachycardia. Factors that contribute to tachycardia include smoking, maternal fever, use of beta-sympathomimetic agents, fetal anemia, fetal hypovolemia, chorioamnionitis, and maternal hyperthyroidism. Fetal distress is a loose term implying that there are grounds for believing that the fetus is in danger of hypoxia and metabolic acidosis. Late and variable decelerations are sources of stress to the fetus, whereas variability is an indicator of how the fetus is tolerating the stress. Thus, in ruling out fetal distress, the transport team can ask these questions to evaluate the tracing for the following reassuring signs of fetal well-being:

1. Is the baseline FHR in normal range? If so, the fetus is maintaining an adequate cardiac output.

2. Is adequate variability present? If so, the fetus is receiving an adequate oxygen supply.

3. Are any accelerations present? If so, metabolic acidosis can be ruled out.

4. In the presence of tachycardia or bradycardia, is adequate variability present? Are accelerations present? In the presence of late or variable decelerations, assessment of the reassuring signs of fetal well-being can indicate how the fetus is tolerating the stress of the decelerations. If after applying these criteria the team is not confident of the well-being of the fetus, before considering the transport of the obstetric patient, scalp stimulation may be attempted (Figure 29-6). Pressure to the fetal scalp with the fingertips may produce a brisk acceleration of the FHR. Accelerations in response to scalp stimulation have been demonstrated only when a normal acid-base balance is present. Fetal response may also be elicited with acoustic or abdominal stimulation.

Nonreassuring signs of fetal well-being include a significant increase or decrease in the FHR baseline during a period of several hours, a wandering

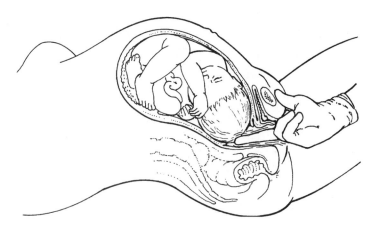

FIGURE 29-6   **Technique for scalp stimulation.**

baseline, a spontaneous decrease in variability or a decrease in variability as labor progresses, bradycardia or tachycardia with reduced variability, subtle late decelerations, or any combination of these signs.

Abnormal FHR tracings will be observed in situations of congenital anomalies. Frequently, variability will be reduced or absent, and tachycardia or bradycardia may be noted. Table 29-1 summarizes comparative signs of acute and chronic distress. Whatever the mechanism of insult to the fetus, the plan of action when presented with possible fetal distress is intrauterine resuscitation.

The "key" formula (LOCK) is as follows:

"L" Place the patient in the left lateral recumbent position.
"O" Provide supplemental oxygen, 100% nonrebreather mask.
"C" Correct or improve contributing factors.
"K" Keep reassessing the FHR and intervene when indicated.

CONTRIBUTING FACTORS TO FETAL DISTRESS

Interventions that must be performed by the transport team when signs and symptoms of fetal distress are present are as follows:

1. Hypotension: Initiate a 500 ml intravenous fluid bolus, depending on the condition of the patient, or correct for supine hypotension with a change to the left lateral position or uterine displacement, if this has not already been done.

2. Hypertonic or tetanic contractions: Discontinue the oxytocin infusion. Oxytocin has a short half-life of approximately 3 minutes, and circulating levels diminish rapidly. Consider the use of terbutaline, 0.25 mg administered subcutaneously or by intravenous push. Check to ensure that the patient's heart rate is less than 120 before administering the medication.

3. Rule out cord prolapse. A sterile vaginal examination will confirm the presence of a cord. Lift the presenting part off the cord to relieve the cord compression and reposition the patient, following recommendations provided in this chapter.

4. Assess for placental abruption or other complications that may affect the FHR.

5. Change the position of the mother. If the left lateral position does not relieve the cord compression as indicated by continued variable decelerations, reposition the mother to the right side, to the hands and knees, or last, to the knee–chest position.

If the patient is located in an outlying area where the transport time is expected to be lengthy, evaluation of the FHT for reassuring signs of fetal well-being will aid in the decision to transport the mother or to

TABLE 29-1 **Comparison of Signs of Chronic and Acute Distress**

Chronic Distress (Occurs Over Time)	Acute Distress (Occurs Suddenly)
Mechanism of insult	
Uteroplacental insufficiency	Umbilical cord compression or uteroplacental insufficiency
Signs of IUGR, decreased fetal movements	Initially, no indication of fetal compromise
Contributing factors	
PIH (preeclampsia)	Cord prolapse
Cardiac or kidney disease	Placental abruption
Severe anemia	Hypotension (vena cava compression, epidural anesthesia, hemorrhage)
DM (class B-R)	Hypertonic contractions
Postdate pregnancy	Placenta previa with hemorrhage
Rh isoimmunization	
Chorioamnionitis	
Smoking	
Fetal response (progression differs depending on circumstances)	
Tachycardia	Variable decelerations
Increased variability	Prolonged decelerations
Decreased variability	Tachycardia
Late decelerations	Increased variability
Bradycardia	Decreased variability
	Late decelerations
	Bradycardia

IUGR, Intrauterine growth restriction.

deliver the fetus at the referring facility to increase the chance of fetal survival. Likewise, if the transport is expected to be short and the time required by the referring facility to prepare for a cesarean section is longer than the estimated transport time, maternal transport is recommended. The intent of the transport is to attain the most expedient delivery of the fetus in a facility most capable of dealing with the fetus at risk.

The transport team may consider use of Doppler auscultations for short transports and EFM for extended transports. Trained and competent individuals must accomplish this monitoring.

COMPLICATIONS OF PREGNANCY AND DELIVERY

In the following discussions regarding complications of pregnancy and delivery, it is assumed that a general obstetric assessment and implementation of general guidelines for transport have already been performed, including assessment of fetal well-being.

AMNIOTIC FLUID EMBOLISM

Amniotic fluid embolism occurs when amniotic fluid gains access to the maternal circulation during labor or delivery or immediately after delivery, resulting in obstruction of the pulmonary vasculature. In addition to amniotic fluid, particulate matter in the fluid such as meconium, lanugo hairs, fetal squamous cells, bile, fat, and mucin may also embolize. In the United States, amniotic fluid embolism causes 10% of maternal deaths. It is a very rare complication and is frequently fatal, with a maternal mortality rate nearing 90%. Amniotic fluid embolism is probably often misdiagnosed, as indicated by the vague clinical picture of surviving patients and missed autopsy findings in fatal cases.

ETIOLOGY AND PATHOPHYSIOLOGIC FACTORS

The route by which amniotic fluid enters the circulatory system of the mother is not clear. The most frequently suggested sites of entry are lacerations in the endocervical veins during cervical dilation and lacerations in the lower uterine segment, the placental site, and uterine veins at sites of uterine trauma. Under the pressure of uterine contractions, amniotic fluid gains access to the circulatory system of the mother and travels quickly to the pulmonary vasculature, where embolization quickly ensues.

Factors that have been associated with amniotic fluid embolism include uterine rupture, cesarean section, and the use of uterine stimulants to induce labor, which produces hypertonic contractions. Other factors that place the obstetric patient at risk are a large fetus, placenta previa, placental abruption, intrauterine fetal death, meconium in the amniotic fluid, multiparity, precipitous delivery, knee-chest position, and maternal age over 30 years.

Disseminated intravascular coagulation (DIC) is a complication that can be expected, although the pathway is unclear. Uterine atony and postpartum hemorrhage are also frequent complications. Acute cor pulmonale, right heart failure, and pulmonary edema follow.

ASSESSMENT

Of the predisposing factors that the patient may have, sudden acute dyspnea is the most characteristic symptom, which is followed by profound cyanosis and sudden shock. Other symptoms may include chest pain, restlessness, anxiety, coughing, vomiting, pulmonary edema with pink, frothy sputum, seizures that are frequently confused with eclamptic seizures, and coma. If the patient has delivered, the transport team should watch for symptoms of postpartum hemorrhage caused by uterine atony.

Because of the extremely rare occurrence of amniotic fluid embolism and the rapidity of onset of symptoms with deterioration, the transport team may be unsure of the clinical picture. If dyspnea appears in a patient who is in a tumultuous labor with ruptured membranes, it is recommended that amniotic fluid embolism be suspected. Tachycardia, hypotension, and tachypnea indicate the severity of the embolic process. Urine output may be decreased (less than 30 ml/hr), indicating inadequate renal perfusion. Blood is shunted away from the uterus to the vital organs, and FHR changes indicative of placental insufficiency will be observed. Severe fetal distress may be present. DIC can be suspected if petechiae, hematuria, bruising, or bleeding from intravenous sites is observed. Coagulation studies confirm DIC. Chest radiograph may show infiltrates.

STRATEGIES FOR TRANSPORT

In the event that an obstetric patient with amniotic fluid embolism is transported, supportive care should be provided. Although the clinical picture may not be clear, treatment focuses on the alleviation of presenting symptoms. The transport team should provide supplemental oxygen with a 100% nonrebreather mask and consider intubation, particularly for a long transport or if the size of the vehicle may impede appropriate care for respiratory arrest. Positive end-expiratory pressure may be required. The transport team can provide circulatory support with additional intravenous fluids and should consider starting a second intravenous line. The transport team may initiate blood replacement in an attempt to correct hypovolemia and blood loss. FHTs should be monitored for signs of severe distress.

If the fetus has been delivered, oxytocin, 20 to 40 units, may be added to 1000 ml intravenous solution for uterine atony. Frequent fundal massage should be performed by supporting the lower uterine segment with one hand while massaging the fundus with the other. Morphine, 2 to 5 mg administered intravenously over a 1- to 2-minute period, may be considered for apprehension and dyspnea. The transport team should expedite the transport in any way possible.[14]

DELIVERY COMPLICATIONS

Delivery complications can be predicted in some situations and may be quite unforeseen in others. A neonatal nurse should always be included on transports when delivery is a possibility. In this case, a nurse with high-risk obstetrics knowledge or skills would be useful.

The information about assessment and suggested transport care that follows makes specific reference to the complication only. It is assumed that general obstetric assessment and the transport team will consider guidelines for transport care as well.

BREECH PRESENTATION

Presentation refers to the portion of the body of the fetus that is in the bony pelvis or is in closest proximity to it and can be felt through the cervix on vaginal examination. With a breech presentation, the buttocks may descend first, with the legs flexed on the fetal abdomen and the feet alongside the buttocks (complete breech); the legs may also be extended upward (frank breech), or one or both feet or knees may be present (footling or incomplete breech). At or near term, the incidence of breech is 3% to 4%. However, before 34 weeks gestation, the incidence is considerably higher.

Etiology and Pathophysiologic Factors.

Breech presentation is more likely to occur in situations in which there are uterine abnormalities, such as a septum extending part or all of the way from the fundus to the cervix (septate uterus), or when the uterus is Y-shaped (bicornuate uterus). It is believed that as the pregnancy progresses, the uterine cavity provides the most room for the fetus's bulkier and more movable parts, with the extremities in the fundus of the uterus and the cephalic presenting. Before 34 weeks gestation, the head of the fetus is disproportionately larger than the body, favoring the breech presentation. For the same reason, the hydrocephalic fetus has a high incidence of breech presentation.[13-16]

Other factors that appear to predispose to the breech presentation are grand multiparity, a previous breech delivery, multiple gestation, hydramnios, oligohydramnios, placenta previa, uterine tumors, congenital anomalies, and implantation of the placenta in either fundal region that is close to the fallopian tube.

Complications associated with breech presentation are inherent because of the position of the fetus. With the buttocks and lower extremities presenting, cord prolapse, cord entanglement around the extremities, and cord compression are more likely to occur. When delivery is managed too forcefully, birth trauma may result. Trauma to the fetal cervical spine and brachial plexus and fractures of the humerus, clavicle, skull, and neck may occur.

The fetus in breech presentation is at higher risk for birth asphyxia (hypoxia, hypercapnia, and metabolic acidosis) compared with the fetus that has a vertex presentation. Head entrapment is a complication that occurs when the buttocks and lower extremities of the premature fetus pass through a cervix that is not completely dilated and is inadequate for the head to be delivered without trauma, asphyxiation, or both for the infant.

Assessment. Although the possibility of breech presentation may be determined either through vaginal examination or ultrasound, this does not have any bearing on the transport of the obstetric patient unless the patient is in active labor or the membranes are ruptured. Labor is frequently slower with a breech presentation, and thus rapid transport should be considered. In the event that vaginal delivery is inevitable, the transport team must be prepared to assist in the delivery. Vaginal delivery is imminent when the buttocks are bulging the perineum and one or both legs are visible.

Strategies for Delivery.   Essentially, the fetus in a breech presentation should not be touched until the umbilicus has spontaneously delivered. At that time the lower end of the scapula will be visible. The team should disengage the legs if one or both have not delivered spontaneously. The cord can be palpated at the umbilicus for the FHR. At this point the arms can usually be delivered by hooking the index finger over each of the baby's shoulders in turn (Figure 29-7). After the shoulders have been delivered, the baby's trunk is rotated so that the back is anterior, and gentle steady downward traction is applied until the hairline is visible. The body can now rest on the palm of one hand and forearm with the index and middle fingers supporting the baby's mouth and chin to maintain

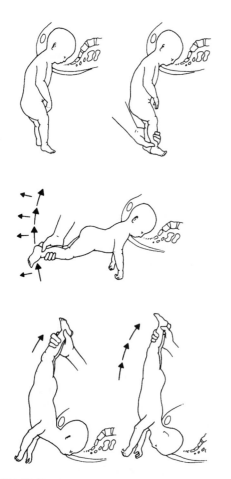

FIGURE 29-7   **Breech extraction.** Upward traction to effect delivery of the posterior shoulder, followed by freeing the posterior arm. (From Hickman M: *Midwifery*, ed 2, Oxford, England, 1985, Blackwell Scientific Publications.)

flexion of the head. With the other hand supporting the back and shoulders, the body can then gently be brought upward while another member of the air medical crew applies suprapubic pressure to facilitate the delivery of the head with a minimum amount of neck traction (Figure 29-8). Care must be taken to achieve slow and controlled delivery of the head, allowing the chin, face, and brow to sweep over the perineum. As soon as the baby's mouth has been delivered, the airway should be cleared with a bulb syringe and then gently and slowly deliver the rest of the head.

Because breech delivery is a rare occurrence for the transport team, there may be a tendency to act in haste when this situation arises. The team should guard against haste because it increases the risk for birth trauma.[13-16]

HEMORRHAGIC DELIVERY COMPLICATIONS

Once excessive bleeding occurs, it is necessary to move quickly to minimize further blood loss. Postpartum hemorrhage, uterine inversion, and uterine rupture are delivery complications that predispose the patient to hypovolemic shock. In addition to proceeding according to the following specific recommendations, the transport team should treat the patient for hypovolemic shock and observe for symptoms of DIC as a complication of hemorrhage.

POSTPARTUM HEMORRHAGE

Blood loss in excess of 500 ml after delivery is defined as postpartum hemorrhage (PPH). The blood loss frequently occurs in the first few hours after delivery but can occur more than 24 hours later. The incidence of PPH occurs in approximately 5% of all deliveries.

Etiology and Pathophysiologic Factors. A blood loss of 500 ml or more frequently results from vaginal delivery and is not necessarily an abnormal event. Estimates of blood loss must be accurate. Some studies have shown that estimated blood loss was approximately half the amount actually lost. Uterine atony is the major cause of postpartum hemorrhage. Normally, bleeding from the placental site is controlled when the interlacing muscle fibers of the uterus contract and retract in conjunction with platelet aggregation and clot formation in the vessels of the decidua. Factors that predispose to uterine atony and prevent compression of the vessels at the implantation site predispose to postpartum hemorrhage. Uterine atony can occur after a prolonged or tumultuous labor or after general anesthetic is used. The uterus that is overdistended as a result of multiple gestation, uterine tumors, hydramnios, or a large fetus is more likely to be

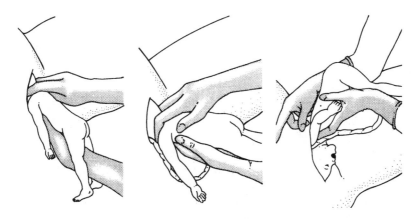

FIGURE 29-8 **Delivery of aftercoming head with use of Mauriceau's maneuver.** Note that as the fetal head is being delivered, flexion of the head is maintained by suprapubic pressure provided by an assistant and simultaneously by pressure on the maxilla by the operator as traction is applied. (From Hickman M: *Midwifery*, ed 2, Oxford, England, 1985, Blackwell Scientific Publications.)

hypotonic after delivery. Multiparity, chorioamnionitis, previous PPH, placenta previa, and use of labor stimulants place the obstetric patient at increased risk for uterine atony and PPH.

As the uterus fills with clots, it is increasingly unable to contract and retract normally, compounding the problem of hemorrhage. In addition, when the placenta and membranes are retained, the same circumstances are created. An abnormally adherent placenta (placenta accreta) or incomplete separation may be the cause.

Another common cause of PPH is lacerations that result from delivery. Undetected lacerations of the cervix, vagina, perineum, or lower uterine segment are all sources for hemorrhage. Hemorrhage as a result of lacerations is usually limited and is rarely severe. However, constant seepage over a few hours can amount to an appreciable loss. Application of forceps may be the reason for the hemorrhage. When a patient has had a previous cesarean section followed by a vaginal delivery, dehiscence of an old uterine scar with hemorrhage may result. Lacerations should be suspected when hemorrhaging occurs in the presence of a firmly contracted uterus. Coagulopathy associated with DIC, placental abruption, and PIH are other causes of PPH. Idiopathic thrombocytopenia or von Willebrand's disease as preexisting coagulopathies predispose to PPH.

Hemorrhage may also result from a combination of sources. Hemorrhage from uterine atony may be coupled with hemorrhage from a cervical laceration.

Assessment. The transport team should determine the source of the hemorrhage. Abdominal palpation may reveal a boggy, enlarged, and soft uterus. Persistent vaginal bleeding from slight to profuse will be noted with uterine atony. The team should also examine the patient for the presence of lacerations in the perineal, cervical, vaginal, and lower uterine segment.

Strategies for Transport. A team member should palpate and vigorously massage the fundus. One hand should cup the fundus, and the other provides support to the lower uterine segment just above the symphysis pubis. Frequently clots will be expressed, and frequent massage alone may be all the stimulation that is required for the uterus to adequately contract and retract. Fundal massage should be performed at least every 5 to 15 minutes, and the location of fundus in relation to the level of the umbilicus, the degree of firmness, and the vaginal flow should be noted.

Rapid infusion of 20 to 40 units of oxytocin in 1000 ml lactated Ringer's solution and/or methylergonovine, 0.2 mg administered intramuscularly or intravenously, is recommended. Methylergonovine should be used cautiously in patients with PIH because of the pressor effects that may result in further elevated blood pressure.

The integrity of the cervix, vagina, perineum, and lower uterine segment should be documented at the referring facility. Inspection of the placenta after delivery will reveal missing fragments, membranes, or both that may be retained. The team should assess blood loss and inspect the perineum; little external bleeding will be observed in the presence of a pelvic hematoma. Blood from lacerations tends to be brighter red.

If atony persists, bimanual uterine compression is recommended. To perform this compression, the uterus is compressed between one hand placed on the abdomen with the other hand clenched as a fist in the vagina; the pressure is maintained for approximately 2 to 5 minutes (Figure 29-9).

UTERINE INVERSION

Complete inversion of the uterus occurs when the entire uterus turns inside out, extends out through the cervix and into the vagina, and is visible. The uterus can partially invert with the fundus turned

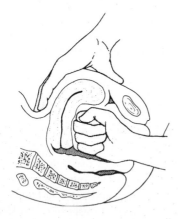

FIGURE 29-9   This technique is very invasive; hence, the transport nurse may avoid use of this procedure. It is a last line of action but is usually effective in controlling PPH as a result of uterine atony. Note the placement of the fist in the anterior fornix. (From Hickman M: *Midwifery,* ed 2, Oxford, England, 1985, Blackwell Scientific Publications.)

inside out. Partial inversion is not as obvious and may initially be more difficult to determine.

ETIOLOGY AND PATHOPHYSIOLOGIC FACTORS
Inversion may occur spontaneously after a contraction or with increased abdominal pressure caused by coughing or sneezing, and it often occurs as the result of overly aggressive management of the third stage of delivery. Predisposing factors include excessive cord traction, fundal pressure, excessive cord traction with a placenta accreta, fundal implantation of the placenta, and uterine atony.

ASSESSMENT
Vaginal bleeding, which may be profuse after delivery and accompanied by sudden and severe lower abdominal pain, may be caused by uterine inversion. Abdominal palpation may reveal a defect in the fundus, or it may not be palpable at all, being nonglobular in shape. Signs of hypovolemic shock may develop quickly.

STRATEGIES FOR TRANSPORT
If uterine inversion is recognized immediately before the uterus has had a chance to contract down and the cervix to constrict, manual replacement can generally be accomplished easily. Without attempting to remove the placenta, pressure should be applied with the fingertips and palm of the hand to push the fundus upward and through the cervical canal (Figure 29-10). This procedure can be extremely painful for the patient. Administering analgesics and explaining the procedure and the necessity for it to the patient while the attempt at manual replacement is being made should be done.[13-16]

If the uterus has contracted, a tocolytic agent such as 10 to 20 mg magnesium sulfate administered intravenously over a 5-minute period will relax the uterus to allow replacement. If the diagnosis is delayed or if the uterus is difficult to replace, anesthesia and surgical management will be required. Rapid transport is recommended.

Removing the placenta before attempting to replace the uterus may increase the hemorrhaging. The placenta will deliver unless there is some degree

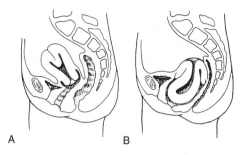

FIGURE 29-10   Uterine inversion. A, First degree; **B,** second degree. Note the abdominal depression where the fundus would normally be and vaginal palpation of the fundus at the cervical opening. Continued pressure with the fingertips will encourage reversion of the fundus. Note the stages of inversion in the inset. (From Hickman M: *Midwifery*, ed 2, Oxford, England, 1985, Blackwell Scientific Publications.)

of placenta accreta, and oxytocin should be administered immediately. The best preventive measure is allowing spontaneous delivery of the placenta.

UTERINE RUPTURE

A spontaneous or traumatic disruption of the uterine wall, known as uterine rupture, can occur. If the laceration is extensive and comes in direct contact with the peritoneal cavity, it is a complete rupture. The rupture most frequently occurs in a weak area of the myometrium, usually at the site of a previous incision.

ETIOLOGY AND PATHOPHYSIOLOGIC FACTORS

Before further discussion of uterine rupture, it is necessary to differentiate between "rupture" and "dehiscence" of a scar. Rupture refers to the separation of an old incision and possibly an extension into previously uninvolved myometrium, with rupture of membranes. Fetal parts may extend through the rupture into the peritoneal cavity. Hemorrhage is usually present from the edges of the separation and may be massive. A dehiscence does not involve the fetal membranes and may not even involve the entire previous scar. Bleeding may be minimal or bloodless. Dehiscence occurs gradually, whereas rupture occurs as a sudden event. A dehiscence may become a rupture with labor or trauma.

Factors that predispose to uterine rupture include previous surgery involving the myometrium, previ-

ous cesarean section with a higher incidence of a "classic" vertical scar being involved, use of labor stimulants, trauma, previous rupture, overdistention of the uterus as a result of multiple gestation or hydramnios, for example, and grand multiparity. Uterine rupture usually occurs during labor but can occur before the onset of labor, with unstimulated labor, with an unscarred uterus, after blunt trauma, after other internal trauma such as perforation with an instrument or difficult forceps delivery, from external pressure such as from an external version of the breech fetus, or from overvigorous fundal pressure during delivery attempts.

In situations in which the patient has had a previous cesarean section, the probability of rupture is much greater when the scar traverses the body of the uterus vertically than when the scar involves the lower uterine section transversely. Dehiscence occurs more frequently without subsequent complications when the scar is low and transverse.

The degree of hemorrhage and extent of possible complications depend on the location and extent of the rupture. If the rupture does not involve the large arteries, the hemorrhage will be less severe. If the rupture is complete, the mortality rate for the fetus is high. Postpartum infection, injury to the bladder, sterility as a result of hysterectomy if the rupture is unable to be adequately repaired, hypovolemic shock, kidney failure, DIC, and death may result.

ASSESSMENT

Signs and symptoms of uterine rupture include severe, sudden, continual abdominal pain and signs of hypovolemic shock. Contractions may cease or may increase in intensity and frequency. Shoulder or chest pain as a result of the collection of blood under the diaphragm, generalized tenderness with rebound, an abdominal mass with fetal parts easily felt, or vaginal bleeding is likely when the rupture occurs in the lower uterine segment. Most bleeding is intra-abdominal, and the abdomen may be distended.

STRATEGIES FOR TRANSPORT

Rapid recognition of the signs and symptoms of uterine rupture will often mean the difference between life and death for the obstetric patient.

Surgical intervention is required, and care is supportive. Oxytocin, 20 to 40 units in a 1000-ml solution administered intravenously, may incite uterine contraction with vessel constriction and reduce the bleeding. Serial abdominal measurements can be made to further assess intraabdominal bleeding. Acute fetal distress with increasingly severe, variable decelerations or absent FHT will be observed.

A history of previous cesarean sections and observation of abdominal scar is of primary importance. Although the scar noted may be low and transverse, documentation is required to determine the location of the scar on the uterus. For the patient in labor who has had a previous cesarean section, the sign of placental abruption may actually be rupture.

PRECIPITATE DELIVERY

Precipitate delivery occurs when the labor is abnormally rapid with strong contractions and rapid cervical dilation and descent of the presenting part. Delivery usually occurs in 2 hours from the start of contractions. The transport team's goal is to prevent an expulsive delivery and minimize trauma to both the mother and the fetus. Possible complications include uterine rupture, amniotic fluid embolism, PPH, and lacerations.

RETAINED PLACENTA

Normally, the placenta separates spontaneously in 5 to 20 minutes after delivery of the fetus. Signs of separation include lengthening of the exposed cord and a gush of blood; the uterus appears to "ball up." Slow, gentle, downward traction is usually all that is required to assist the delivery of the placenta. When no signs of separation occur and hemorrhage is not evident, transport can be accomplished with the placenta retained. When the placenta is partially retained, postpartum hemorrhage will result.

SHOULDER DYSTOCIA

After delivery of the head, the anterior shoulder pushes against the symphysis, creating a situation commonly referred to as *shoulder dystocia*. The condition becomes apparent when the head is pulled down against the perineum and the shoulders do not follow with gentle traction. The incidence of shoulder dystocia increases significantly with birth weight.

ETIOLOGY AND PATHOPHYSIOLOGIC FACTORS

Several predisposing factors have been linked to shoulder dystocia. However, shoulder dystocia can occur quite unexpectedly without obvious associated factors. The complication occurs more frequently with the presence of a large fetus, a macrosomia fetus of a patient with gestational diabetes, a contracted pelvis, maternal obesity, after a prolonged second stage of labor, or after instrumental delivery following a prolonged second stage of labor.

Possible complications of shoulder dystocia include brachial plexus damage and a fractured fetal clavicle. Fetal hypoxia can occur when the cord is drawn into the pelvis and compressed.

ASSESSMENT

In any situation of imminent delivery, unless the fetus is expected to weigh 2500 g or less, shoulder dystocia is a possibility. After the head has been delivered and inspection for a nuchal cord has been performed, the delivery of the anterior shoulder should be accomplished before the nares and mouth are suctioned. Otherwise, precious time may be wasted suctioning before realizing that the shoulder is affected, and because of cord compression, time is of the essence.

Unnecessary haste and overly aggressive force should be avoided because of the increased possibility of birth trauma to the fetus. Excessive lateral flexion of the neck and overly vigorous traction of the head and neck increase the risk of damage to the brachial plexus.

STRATEGIES FOR DELIVERY

Once the team member is aware of the situation, he or she may observe the head retract against the perineum. Fundal pressure aggravates the shoulder impaction and should be avoided. If an episiotomy has not been made, a generous mediolateral episiotomy is recommended. A combination of suprapubic pressure applied by another member of the air medical crew (the shoulder can be palpated suprapubicly) and gentle downward traction of the head should be tried first. The team should not persist if the shoulder does not slip under the symphysis.

The McRoberts maneuver, a simple maneuver that increases the diameter of the pelvis by stretching the pelvic joints, should be tried next. With the patient's legs flexed at the knees, the maternal nurse should help the patient draw her knees up and toward the chest (dorsal knee-chest position) and continue, with gentle downward traction of the head. Once the anterior shoulder clears the symphysis, the posterior shoulder usually delivers without resistance.

Delivery of the posterior shoulder can also be attempted by rotation of the posterior shoulder downward and into the left posterior quadrant. With release of the posterior arm and shoulder, the anterior shoulder will follow. As a last resort, the infant's clavicle may be deliberately broken; however, when this is done the chance of damage to the brachial plexus is increased.

UMBILICAL CORD PROLAPSE

Overt cord prolapse occurs when the cord slips down into the vagina or appears externally after the amniotic membranes have ruptured. When the cord slips down into or near the pelvis, lying adjacent to the presenting part, it is not palpable on vaginal examination (occult prolapse). The cord may also have slipped down to a position in which it is palpable through the cervix, but in intact membranes (forelying prolapse). Varying degrees of prolapse may occur.

ETIOLOGY

Circumstances that cause maladaptation of the presenting part to the lower uterine segment or prevent descent of the presenting part into the pelvis predispose the obstetric patient to cord prolapse. These factors include breech presentation, transverse lie, premature rupture of membrane (PROM), a contracted pelvis, unengaged large fetus multiparity, hydramnios, multiple gestations, a long cord, and preterm labor. Complications include severe fetal distress and fetal death.

ASSESSMENT

Cord prolapse occurs suddenly and requires quick identification of the problem and quick action. Identifying the obstetric patient who is vulnerable to cord prolapse is of primary importance. Clinical signs of prolapse include sudden fetal bradycardia and/or severe recurrent variable decelerations that do not respond to a change in maternal position, administration of oxygen, and hydration. Compression of the cord between the presenting part and the pelvic tissues causes the FHT patterns that are observed.

STRATEGIES FOR TRANSPORT

Actions to take in the event of cord prolapse include elevating the presenting part off the cord with a hand in the vagina to prevent further cord compression and positioning the patient in a Trendelenburg's or knee-chest position to further reduce pressure on the cord. The cord may spontaneously retract, depending on the degree of prolapse, but should never be manually replaced because severe compression may occur. Intervention to elevate the presenting part off the cord must be maintained during the transport.

The transport team should provide supplemental oxygen by nonrebreather mask. A tocolytic agent, such as terbutaline, 0.25 mg administered subcutaneously or by intravenous push, should be given to slow the contractions and reduce the pressure on the cord during contractions. When the cord compression is relieved, the fetus will be able to recover from the hypoxic event in utero as long as the compression does not recur.

If cord prolapse occurs when the patient is en route, the receiving facility should be alerted to prepare for an emergency cesarean section. On occasion the FHR pattern will be normal or show minimal abnormalities, and the only symptom evident is the prolapsed cord; however, the interventions are the same.

DIABETES IN PREGNANCY

Basically, diabates mellitus (DM) is a disease in which the body is unable to produce or sufficiently use insulin to metabolize glucose. The disease is complicated by faulty metabolism of fats and proteins for energy. The course and outcome of a pregnancy complicated by diabetes depend on the severity of the disease process.

ETIOLOGY AND PATHOPHYSIOLOGIC FACTORS

This discussion of diabetes in pregnancy is limited primarily to how diabetes, whether gestational or as a preexisting condition, is affected by the pregnancy and how the pregnancy affects the patient with diabetes. Pregnancy is considered a diabetogenic state in which the patient has an increased need for glucose, and protein and fat are metabolized to aid in the demand for higher glucose levels. During pregnancy, the metabolism of the mother adapts to provide fuel for the growing fetus and for the pregnant woman. Early in pregnancy, during the period of rapid growth of the embryo, the mother's blood glucose level decreases. The obstetric patient who has diabetes may exhibit hypoglycemia.

At approximately 24 weeks of gestation, the diabetogenic effects of pregnancy begin. Increased hormonal activity exerts an anti-insulin effect that results in a decreased responsiveness to insulin and a rise in the level of blood glucose. Increased production of insulin by the pancreas counteracts the anti-insulin effects of the hormones, and normal blood glucose levels are maintained. If, as a result of an acquired or inherited defect in beta cell function, maternal insulin secretion fails to keep pace with the demand, a further increase in blood glucose levels will occur. At this point in the pregnancy, gestational diabetes is frequently recognized and diagnosed. For the woman who is already diabetic, an increase in insulin requirement occurs and remains increased until after delivery.

The obstetric patient with a pregnancy complicated by DM is at an increased risk compared to the remainder of the pregnant population for developing PIH and related disorders, hydramnios, infections such as vaginitis, urinary tract infections, and pyelonephritis. Delivery by cesarean section and preterm delivery also occur with increased frequency because of macrosomia or fetal distress.

The fetus is at increased risk as well when the mother has diabetes. Complications associated with the fetus include congenital anomalies, intrauterine growth restriction (IUGR), macrosomia, delivery trauma, fetal distress, hypoglycemia, hypocalcemia, hyperbilirubinemia, respiratory distress, and intrauterine death. Macrosomia refers to a fetus that is large for gestational age with increased fat deposition and an enlarged spleen and liver. Macrosomia is seen more commonly when the mother has gestational DM or DM without vasculopathy. Congenital anomalies are seen more frequently when pregnant diabetic women are in poor control of their diabetes.[4,13-16]

ASSESSMENT

Assessment of the patient with diabetes includes screening for the presence of risk factors linked to DM. All pregnant women with diabetes need to be assessed so their disease can be classified. Assessment by the flight nurse should include the following:

1. Obstetric history: Assess for the possibility that a previous pregnancy was complicated by undiagnosed diabetes. Has the patient had gestational DM with a previous pregnancy, or is there a family history of DM? Has she delivered an infant weighing more than 4000 g? Has she had unexplained perinatal losses, stillbirths, or traumatic deliveries? Has more than one pregnancy been complicated by PIH? PIH as a multipara? Does she have a history of hydramnios or preterm delivery? Is she older than 35 years?

2. Current pregnancy: Does the patient have signs and symptoms of DM? Is glycosuria present? Are results of a glucose challenge test abnormal? Is the patient obese? Has the patient had recurrent urinary tract infections or vaginitis? Does the patient have chronic hypertension? What are the results of ultrasounds or other diagnostic tests? Is the diabetes controlled by diet or insulin? What is the patient's current insulin regimen?

3. History of preexisting condition: What class is the DM, as determined by the age of onset, duration of the disease, and evidence of vasculopathy? Does the patient have cardiovascular

or kidney disease? Has there been good control of the diabetes during the pregnancy? What is the patient's current insulin regimen?

STRATEGIES FOR TRANSPORT

In addition to following the general guidelines for transport care, careful assessment is required of the obstetric patient with gestational DM or the diabetic obstetric patient because of changing metabolic demands. The transport team should obtain a diabetic history from the patient and assess for complications associated with DM in pregnancy. It is also important to record the time of her last meal and last insulin injection.

If the patient is in labor, simultaneous continuous insulin and glucose infusions will stabilize maternal levels and may reduce neonatal hyperglycemia. The insulin may be adjusted after delivery on the basis of blood sugar levels, and the insulin demand will decrease after delivery. The patient is given nothing by mouth. Blood glucose levels are evaluated every 1 to 2 hours and maintained at a level of 80 to 120 mg/dl with insulin as indicated by the patient's blood sugar.

The transport team should obtain a blood glucose reading just prior to transport. Because labor increases metabolic needs, the team should be aware of the signs and symptoms of hypoglycemia and hyperglycemia and should never administer terbutaline to an insulin-dependent diabetic because of the transient hyperglycemic response seen with terbutaline.

HEMORRHAGIC COMPLICATIONS

PLACENTAL ABRUPTION

Placental abruption can be defined as the premature detachment of a normally implanted placenta from the uterine wall. The separation may occur over a small area with little evidence or can separate totally with devastating results. The incidence of abruption varies widely, depending on the source. Of considerable significance is the incidence of recurrence with subsequent pregnancies.[4]

Etiology. The primary cause of placental abruption is largely unknown. Hypertension, whether chronic or PIH, and previous abruption are two factors that are known to greatly increase the risk of placental abruption. Other factors that place the obstetric patient at risk include abdominal trauma, an unusually short umbilical cord, amniocentesis, multiparity, age over 35 years, uterine anomalies or tumors, sudden uterine decompression when a twin is delivered and the remaining twin is placed at risk or immediately before delivery of single fetus, cigarette smoking, and substance abuse, especially abuse of cocaine.

Pathophysiologic Factors. Hemorrhage occurs from the arterioles that supply the decidua (lining of uterus), causing a retroplacental hematoma. Placental separation takes place at that site and may continue as the hemorrhage continues. As the hemorrhage continues, more vessels are disrupted, leading to increased hemorrhage and further separation. Placental separation can be an avalanche that continues to total separation or suddenly stops for reasons unknown. Sometimes a clot blocks the hemorrhage. The decidua is rich in thromboplastin, and clotting occurs rapidly. When vaginal bleeding is observed, the blood is usually dark because of the rapid clotting. If separation occurs at the margin of the placenta (Figure 29-11) or if the amniotic membranes are dissected from the decidua as a result of the hemorrhage, vaginal bleeding will be observed. No vaginal bleeding will be observed if the hemorrhage is completely concealed behind the placenta.

As the hemorrhage continues and a retroplacental clot forms, enough pressure may be exerted to force blood through the membranes, giving the amniotic fluid a port wine color, or into the myometrium, causing a condition called Couvelaire uterus. The uterine tone is increased, and irritability will be noted. Contractions will frequently be present.

A common complication of placental abruption is DIC. Other complications include postpartum hemorrhage, anemia, postpartum infection, hypovolemic shock, kidney failure, and fetal distress or death. The factors that predispose to placental abruption may occur preterm, predisposing to preterm delivery.

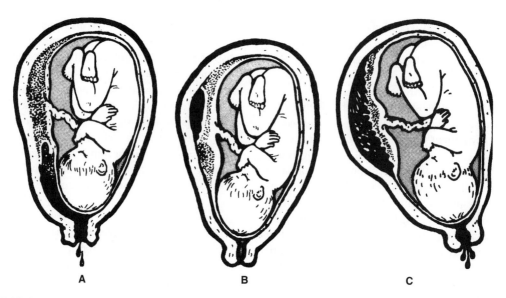

FIGURE 29-11   **Examples of placental abruption. A,** Placental separation occurs at the margin of the placenta; **B** and **C,** separation originates from a central area behind the placenta. (Illustrated by Vincenza Genovese, Phoenix, Arizona. From Gilbert ES, Harmon JS: *High-risk pregnancy and delivery,* St Louis, 1986, Mosby.)

PLACENTA PREVIA

Placenta previa occurs when the placenta becomes implanted in the lower uterine segment and as a result covers or partially covers the internal cervical os. A marginal or low-lying previa extends to or close to but does not cover any part of the internal os. Placenta previa occurs approximately once in every 200 to 400 deliveries. The incidence of placenta previa is higher preterm. As the pregnancy progresses, however, the fundus hypertrophies, the lower uterine segment elongates, and the placenta grows, allowing for placental migration away from the internal os toward the fundus.

Etiology.   Although the exact cause is unknown, there is a higher incidence of placenta previa where uterine scarring is evident. A previous cesarean section or dilatation and curettage, increased parity, multiparity with short intervals, and a previous occurrence of placenta previa can scar the uterus. Other factors that place the obstetric patient at risk for placenta previa include previous chorioamnionitis, multiple gestation for which there is a larger surface area covered by the placenta, fetal erythroblastosis, maternal age over age 35 years, substance abuse, and uterine tumors.

Pathophysiologic Factors.   Normal placental implantation usually occurs in the fundus or body segment of the uterus. It has been suggested that defective perfusion of the decidua may favor implantation of the placenta in the lower uterine segment. Because there is less vascularization in the lower uterine segment, the placenta compensates and tends to grow thinner and larger, thus covering a larger area and thereby increasing perfusion.

Before the onset of labor, the cervix begins to soften, efface, and dilate. These cervical changes disrupt the placental attachment, tearing the vessels, and hemorrhage results. Bright red vaginal bleeding will be observed; it is usually painless and is not initially associated with contractions. The initial episode is usually slight (less than 250 ml of blood is shed) and tends to cease spontaneously as clot formation occurs. Recurrence is unpredictable. Generally, the greater the extent to which the internal os is covered, the sooner the initial episode occurs.

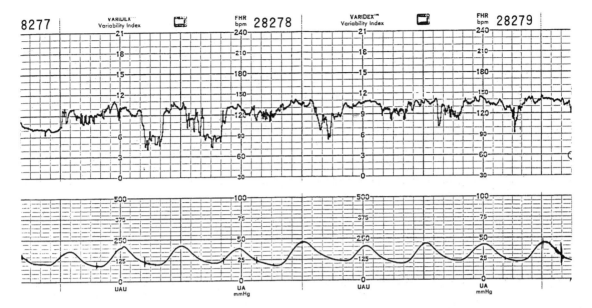

FIGURE 29-12 **Abruption pattern.** Note the increased uterine tone documented with the use of an internal uterine pressure catheter (IUPC). Hypertonic contractions are occurring approximately every minute with virtually no period of relaxation between contractions. Note the distressed fetal response. An emergency cesarean section was performed with Apgar scores of 2 and 7 at 1 and 5 minutes, respectively.

Potential complications of placenta previa include complications similar to those of placental abruption, such as DIC, hypovolemic shock, kidney damage, anemia, postpartum infection, postpartum hemorrhage, and fetal distress or death. Because hemorrhage may occur at any time without warning or precipitating events, the risk is increased with premature delivery. Furthermore, placenta accreta is a rare complication of placenta previa.

ASSESSMENT OF PLACENTAL ABRUPTION AND PLACENTA PREVIA

Generally, the clinical findings of placental abruption vary in degree with the extent of the placental separation and clot formation behind the placenta. Onset of symptoms may be gradual in mild cases to sudden and without warning in severe situations. In cases of vaginal bleeding after 20 weeks of gestation, placenta previa should be considered.

Uterine Assessment (Placental Abruption). Symptoms of placental abruption may range from slight abdominal tenderness and lower back discomfort with a mild abruption to severe unceasing abdominal pain in a severe situation. Sudden severe pain may be indicative of retroplacental hemorrhage into the myometrium. The intensity, frequency, and duration of contractions may vary, from contractions with a slight increase in uterine tone to hypertonic (Figure 29-12) or tetanic contractions (lasting longer than 90 seconds) with a boardlike uterus that fails to relax. With severe abruption, labor tends to progress rapidly. Abdominal palpation for intensity, length, and frequency of contractions and observation of any sustained tone between contractions will aid in the assessment. If it is difficult to determine when a contraction begins or ends and the abdomen is rigid, a severe placental separation should be suspected.

Uterine Assessment (Placenta Previa). Contractions may or may not be present with placenta previa. The onset usually occurs during or after the hemorrhage because of increased uterine irritability.

Assessment of Blood Loss (Placental Abruption). When placental abruption occurs, vaginal bleeding may vary from absent or minimal to profuse. It is essential to realize that the amount of vaginal bleeding is not an indicator of the degree of separation or of total blood loss but of the location of the separation. Assessment of a concealed hemorrhage includes noting any change in fundal height as an indication of continued hemorrhage. The fundus can be marked, providing a quick visual indicator of increasing uterine size. The bleeding usually continues until delivery of the placenta, when the uterus can contract sufficiently to close off the open vessels.

Assessment of Blood Loss (Placenta Previa). Blood loss can be more accurately estimated with placenta previa, for which only external hemorrhage will be observed. Placenta previa is characterized by repetitive and frequently more extensive bleeding episodes.

Ultrasound. An ultrasound can confirm the location of the placenta. If ultrasound is not available, a previa cannot be ruled out. A sterile vaginal examination may stimulate profuse bleeding by dislodging a clot and *should never be done*. With cervical changes that accompany active labor, an increase in bloody show will be noted and may appear excessive, leading the flight nurse to believe that a placenta previa is present. A very gentle examination may be attempted only if delivery appears imminent. An ultrasound can also rule out the presence of an abruption.

Assessment of Vital Signs. Signs of hypovolemic shock may not be present until a blood loss of approximately 30% has occurred. However, before any change in vital signs, shunting away from the placenta occurs, and FHT indicative of placental insufficiency will occur.

Assessment of FHT. Fetal distress as a result of placental separation or placenta previa occurs primarily from placental insufficiency (hypertonic uterus, maternal hemorrhage, or decreased placental perfusion) or fetal hemorrhage as a consequence

of placental separation. The team must observe for late decelerations and bradycardia.

Assessment of Urinary Output. Urinary output of 60 to 100 ml per hour suggests adequate renal perfusion and, indirectly, adequate circulating blood volume. Urinary output of less than 30 ml per hour suggests decreased circulatory volume, in which case insertion of a urinary catheter is recommended.

Assessment of Coagulopathy. The transport team should observe for petechiae, hematuria, bruising, or bleeding from intravenous sites.

Assessment for Impending Shock. Because of the normal physiologic changes of pregnancy, early symptoms of hypovolemia may be masked. Careful assessment of serial vital signs will aid in differentiating expected blood pressure, pulse, and respirations from symptoms of impending shock. Symptoms include tachypnea, decreased blood pressure, increased pulse rate (rapid and thready), oliguria, cyanosis, pallor, and clamminess.[3,18,20]

STRATEGIES FOR TRANSPORT (ABRUPTION AND PREVIA)

The transport team should implement the following strategies for transport of patients with abruption or previa:

1. Implement general guidelines for transport care after the primary survey and obstetric assessment are completed. Assess for contractions, the extent of hemorrhage, and estimated blood loss specific to abruption or previa. Determine fundal height or mark the fundus, reassessing frequently. Recognition of concealed bleeding will be confirmed by noting an increase in the fundal height.
2. Administer tocolytics as recommended. Refer to the discussion in this chapter regarding preterm labor for specifics about labor suppressants.
3. Assess vital signs every 15 minutes or more frequently as needed. Note any subtle

changes that may indicate hypovolemia. Check capillary refill as needed to assess for peripheral perfusion. Initiate EFM, if available, to monitor FHT for changes indicative of impending fetal distress. Provide supplemental oxygen.

4. Observe for signs of DIC. Administration of fluid and blood or blood products may be required for the patient in shock.

5. Expedite transport if the patient's condition deteriorates. If the transport service has a fixed-wing aircraft, consider a rotor-wing transport from the airport to the receiving facility. Notify the medical director and receiving hospital to prepare for a possible emergency cesarean section delivery.

DISSEMINATED INTRAVASCULAR COAGULATION

DIC is a serious and deleterious complication of pregnancy. When accelerated coagulation and activation of the fibrinolytic system occur simultaneously in pregnancy, DIC occurs as a secondary event activated by hemorrhagic complications, such as placental abruption and placenta previa, or by delivery complications, such as a ruptured uterus, uterine inversion, postpartum hemorrhage, traumatic labor and delivery, amniotic fluid embolism, and sepsis. DIC is also a complication of trauma in pregnancy, retained dead fetus syndrome (over 3 weeks since intrauterine death), and hydatidiform mole.

After the delivery of the fetus and after the patient's primary complication has been eliminated or improved, further intervention may not be needed unless the hemorrhage has been severe.[3,18,20]

MULTIPLE GESTATION

A pregnancy with more than one fetus is a multiple gestation. Twins occur in 1 in 80 to 90 births, and triplets occur in 1 in 8000 births. The use of fertility medications and in vitro fertilization has increased the occurrence of multiple gestations.

ETIOLOGY

Embryologically, twins may result from multiple ovulations, in which two distinct ova are fertilized (dizygotic, or fraternal), or from one separate ovum that subsequently divides into two (monozygotic, or identical). Either or both processes can also result in triplets, quadruplets, and so on. The incidence of dizygotic twins is influenced by heredity, maternal age, race, and treatment for infertility, whereas the frequency of monozygotic twins is relatively constant.

In vitro fertilization and fertility medications also contribute to the incidence of multiple fetuses.

Previous delivery of twins or a maternal family history of delivering fraternal twins increases the chance of delivering twins.

PATHOPHYSIOLOGIC FACTORS

Pathophysiology is related to the complications associated with multiple gestations. The large area of the uterine surface covered by the placentas is suspected in several complications. Portions are more likely to implant in the lower uterine segment where there is less vascularity, increasing the chances of IUGR, or at or near the cervical os, increasing the chances of placenta previa. The superabundance of chorionic villi appears to predispose the obstetric patient to PIH, especially if it is her first pregnancy.

Other complications may be caused by uterine overdistention and hemodynamic and endocrinologic changes associated with multiple gestations. The mother is placed at risk for anemia, glucose intolerance, hydramnios, dysfunctional labor associated with uterine overdistention, and dystocia. In addition, multiple gestations predispose to PROM, preterm labor and delivery, placental abruption, cesarean section, uterine atony and resulting postpartum hemorrhage, and malpresentations. The fetuses are at risk for congenital anomalies, cord prolapse or entanglement, vasa previa, twin-twin transfusion, discordant fetal growth, and intrauterine death.

The greatest threat to multiple gestations is premature labor and delivery. The average gestational age for onset of labor is about 36 weeks.[14] Rarer but serious complications include conjoined twins, monoamniotic twins (with a mortality rate of approximately 50% because of knotting and tangling of the cord), and twins locked or compacted, preventing descent or engagement of either twin.

ASSESSMENT

Multiple gestations are usually suspected when a discrepancy develops between the gestational age determined by the obstetric patient's last monthly period and the uterine size determined by regular fundal measurements. When the expected size of approximately 1 cm per week of gestation is exceeded, investigation may be warranted. If twinning is suspected, an ultrasound will confirm or disprove the presence of more than one fetus.

STRATEGIES FOR TRANSPORT

The transport team must be aware that any multiple gestation is a pregnancy at risk and must assess for additional risk factors associated with a multiple gestation.

The primary survey, including general obstetric assessment, is completed initially, followed by the general guidelines for transport care. The fundal height should be noted. EFM should include continuous monitoring, alternating fetuses, unless the transport is of short duration. The FHR of the fetus not currently being monitored can be determined with Doppler auscultation.

The drug of choice in the treatment of preterm labor is $MgSO_4$ because it has been observed that an increased incidence of pulmonary edema is associated with use of beta-sympathomimetic agents in women with multiple gestations.

PIH AND RELATED DISORDERS

PIH refers to a group of hypertensive disorders that have their onset during pregnancy and resolve after pregnancy. Gestational hypertension develops after 20 weeks gestation without evidence of hypertension. Preeclampsia is characterized by hypertension, proteinuria, and edema. PIH may develop before 20 weeks gestation in cases of trophoblastic disease. Eclampsia refers to the development of clonic and tonic seizures in a preeclamptic patient. Persistent hypertension not associated with pregnancy that develops before 20 weeks of gestation is considered to be chronic. Chronic hypertension as a preexisting condition may be complicated during pregnancy by superimposed preeclampsia. HELLP syndrome

(*h*emolysis, *e*levated *l*iver enzymes, and *l*ow *p*latelets) is considered a complication of severe preeclampsia. The incidence of PIH complicates 5% to 10% of pregnancies.[12]

ETIOLOGY

The absolute cause of PIH is unknown. Current theories point to nutritional deficiencies, immunologic deficiencies, genetic predisposition, response to chorionic villi exposure, chronic intravascular coagulation, and other factors. Certain factors are known to predispose the obstetric patient to development of PIH. Primarily, PIH is a disease of the primigravida, the teenaged primigravida, or the primigravida over 35 years of age. The patient with DM, preexisting cardiovascular or kidney disease, hydramnios, family history of PIH, or no prenatal care is also at risk. Other predisposing factors include the pregnancy exposed to a superabundance of chorionic villi, such as with multiple gestation, hydatidiform mole or fetal hydrops, or a poor nutritional status, large fetus, or Rh incompatibility.

PATHOPHYSIOLOGIC FACTORS

To understand the pathophysiology of PIH, it is necessary to have a basic understanding of the magnitude of physiologic changes that normally occur in pregnancy, specifically those pertaining to the pathophysiology of PIH. Briefly, blood volume increases by almost 50%, hemodilution occurs, the pulse rate increases, cardiac output increases, and the glomerular filtration rate increases. Increased vasodilation is seen, peripheral resistance drops, and blood pressure decreases in the second trimester and returns to normal near term. A fluid shift from the intravascular space to the extracellular space in dependent limbs occurs, and the potential for coagulation increases. Resistance to the pressor effects of angiotensin II also occurs.

In patients with PIH, the disease process actually begins many weeks before the onset of any symptoms. A chain reaction of events is initiated as, for unknown reasons, an increased sensitivity to angiotensin II develops. As a result, vasospasm occurs, particularly arteriolar vasospasm, which initiates vasoconstriction, which leads to increased peripheral resistance and eventually to hypertension. Blood perfusion to all body organs is decreased, and the function of the placenta, kidneys, liver, and brain is significantly impaired. Although not forgetting the essential problem of vasospasm, the following pathophysiology is characteristic of PIH.

UTEROPLACENTAL CHANGES

Compromised uterine and placental blood flow can lead to degeneration of the placenta and necrosis. With chronic decreased blood perfusion, IUGR can result. During labor, fetal distress caused by uteroplacental insufficiency (late decelerations) will frequently be seen. As a consequence of decreased uterine blood flow, uterine activity is increased, and uterine irritability and preterm labor may be seen.

RENAL CHANGES

Decreased renal blood flow decreases glomerular filtration rate and decreases urinary output. Cellular changes are observed in the glomerular capillary endothelial cells. The cells swell, producing narrowing of the capillary lumens, and lesions develop, causing the proteinuria (primarily albumin) seen in preeclampsia. Plasma uric acid is typically elevated as a result of the decreased uric acid clearance by the kidneys. In addition, creatinine clearance and blood urea nitrogen aid in the evaluation of kidney function. With decreased kidney function, sodium and water are retained. In conjunction with a decreased circulating albumin and a decrease in colloid osmotic pressure, fluid is shifted from the intravascular space to the extracellular space, giving rise to edema, which may range from slight to severe.

HEMATOLOGIC CHANGES

Because of fluid shifts, hemoconcentration is seen with a rise in hematocrit levels. An increase in the hematocrit level that is noted after an initial assessment may signal a deteriorating condition. The normal hypervolemia of pregnancy is decreased or nearly absent when preeclampsia is present. Also observed is intravascular platelet and fibrin deposition, which occurs in response to vessel wall damage as the disease progresses. In addition, there is some evidence of

hemolysis and coagulopathy in patients with severe preeclampsia that is more frequently associated with HELLP syndrome and the development of DIC as severe complications of preeclampsia.

HEPATIC CHANGES

Reduction in blood flow to the liver impairs liver function. Swelling of the capsule (the fibrous sheath that completely covers the liver) and subcapsular hemorrhage may occur. Necrosis and damage to liver tissue are demonstrated by elevated liver enzymes. In rare cases, subcapsular hemorrhage can be so extensive that the liver capsule can rupture with massive hemorrhage into the peritoneal cavity. Epigastric pain (right upper quadrant pain) is associated with hepatic swelling and subcapsular hemorrhage.

CEREBRAL CHANGES

Although cerebral perfusion is not impaired, vasospasm gives rise to cerebral edema, hemorrhage, and central nervous system irritability, which is evidenced by hyperreflexia, headaches, ankle clonus, nausea and vomiting, and clonic and tonic seizures.

RETINAL CHANGES

Retinal arteriolar spasms, ischemia, and edema as a result of decreased perfusion are the sources of the visual disturbances seen in preeclampsia. Blurring and scotoma (blind or twinkling spots in the vision) and diplopia (double vision) may occur. Retinal detachment is a rare occurrence.

PULMONARY CHANGES

Changes in pulmonary capillary permeability can occur, predisposing to pulmonary edema in severe cases of PIH.

COMPLICATIONS

Complications of PIH, some of which have already been discussed, include eclampsia, placental abruption, pulmonary edema, DIC, HELLP syndrome, hemolytic anemia, thrombocytopenia, preterm delivery and prematurity, and IUGR. Seldom-observed and grave complications include retinal

TABLE 29-2 General Guidelines for Determining the Severity of the Disease Process*			
	Mild	**Severe**	**Impending Eclampsia**
Blood pressure	≥140/90 Diastolic increases ≥15 mm Hg	Diastolic >100 mm Hg	Diastolic >100 mm Hg
Proteinuria (dipstick)	2+/3+	3+/4+	3+/4+
Urinary output	>30 ml/hr	<20-30 ml/hr	<20-30 ml/hr
Edema	+1/+2	+3/+4	+3/+4
Pulmonary edema	Not present	May be present	Present
Headache	Not present	May be present	Present
Visual disturbances	Not present	May be present	Present
Epigastric pain	Not present	May be present	Present
Hyperreflexia and clonus	Not present	May be present	Present

Data from Magee LA: Management of hypertension in pregnancy, *Brit Med J* 318:1332-1336, 1999.
*Some crossover of clinical findings can occur, and not all findings are absolute for each category.

detachment, kidney failure, cerebral hemorrhage, liver rupture, heart failure, intrauterine death, and rarely, maternal death.

As a general rule, the predisposition for the development of complications increases as the disease state deteriorates. Though prompt treatment should stabilize the patient with PIH, complications and progression to eclampsia can occur.[3,12]

ECLAMPSIA

Eclampsia can occur before labor, during labor, or early into the postpartum period. Headache, visual disturbances, epigastric pain, apprehension, anxiety, and hyperreflexia with clonus in a patient with severe preeclampsia are signs of impending eclampsia.

Seizures are characterized by clonic and tonic activity and usually begin around the mouth in the form of facial twitching. The seizure may be so forceful that the patient may fall from the bed. Respirations cease during the seizure but spontaneously resume as the seizure activity quiets. Coma frequently ensues, and the patient remembers little of the events immediately before and after the seizure. The length of the coma varies, with the patient gradually becoming responsive. Frequently, labor spontaneously begins and progresses rapidly. Pulmonary edema may develop. Massive cerebral hemorrhage and death can occur as a result of eclampsia, but the incidence is very rare (Table 29-2).

HELLP SYNDROME

The HELLP syndrome was first identified and described as a serious complication of preeclampsia by Weinstein in 1982. *H* stands for *h*emolysis, which is confirmed by the evidence of red cell fragments and irregularly shaped red cells on peripheral blood smears. It is believed that as red cells pass through the constricted vessels that have sustained wall damage with platelet and fibrin deposition, red cell integrity is altered, and many cells are lysed. As a result, hyperbilirubinemia is frequently seen. *EL* stands for *e*levated *l*iver enzymes. Elevated serum glutamicoxaloacetic transaminase and serum glutamic-pyruvic transaminase are observed. *LP* stands for *l*ow *p*latelet count. Consumptive thrombocytopenia (a platelet count lower than 100,000/mm^3) unaccompanied by any other coagulation factor abnormalities is characteristic of the HELLP syndrome.

ASSESSMENT

The "big three" in assessing PIH includes hypertension, edema, and proteinuria.

HYPERTENSION

Hypertension is a rise in systolic pressure of 30 mm Hg or a rise in diastolic pressure of 15 mm Hg on the basis of previously known pressures or a blood pressure of 140/90 or higher. The diastolic pressure is a more reliable predictor of the disease process.

TABLE 29-3 Assessment of Edema and Hyperreflexia	
Evaluation of Edema	**Score**
Minimal edema of lower extremities	+1
Marked edema of lower extremities	+2
Edema of lower extremities, face, and hands	+3
Generalized massive edema including the abdomen and sacrum	+4
Evaluation of Hyperreflexia	**Grade**
None elicited	0
Sluggish or dull	+1
Active, normal	+2
Brisk	+3
Brisk with transient clonus	+4
Brisk with sustained clonus	+5

Assessment of edema should include description and scoring with regard to location, onset, and duration, any sudden increase in swelling noticed, and any pitting edema.

Assessment of hyperreflexia is usually accomplished by eliciting patellar deep-tendon reflexes. Clonus can be assessed at the same time by swift dorsiflexion of the foot. Clonus indicates neuromuscular irritability, and each beat should be counted.

Data from Seidel HM et al: *Mosby's physical examination handbook,* St Louis, 1999, Mosby.

The blood pressure should be taken with the patient in the left lateral recumbent position. Hypertension associated with PIH is labile and may change in the time it takes to retake the blood pressure.

EDEMA

A sudden excessive weight gain of more than 2 lb in a week or 6 lb in a month is primarily attributable to fluid retention. Nondependent edema of the eyelids, face, and hands is characteristic of PIH. Pitting edema of the lower extremities is common. For evaluation of edema, see Table 29-3.

PROTEINURIA

Proteinuria usually develops after hypertension, and edema is evident when proteinuria is present. The flight nurse should observe the patient for evidence of the following: (1) central nervous system irritability (headache, hyperreflexia evaluated by deep tendon reflexes and ankle clonus [see Table 33-3], nausea, vomiting, apprehension, and anxiety); (2) impaired renal function (oliguria and proteinuria); and (3) hepatic involvement (epigastric pain [unmistakable from uterine contractions], malaise, nausea, vomiting, and jaundice).

The transport team should also assess fetal status by EFM evaluations of FHR baseline, variability, acceleration, and deceleration patterns; observe for fetal activity; observe for evidence of pulmonary involvement (moist rales on auscultation, dyspnea, tachypnea, tachycardia, wheezing or cough, and anxiety), and identify evidence of evolving or impending eclampsia, placental abruption, HELLP syndrome, and DIC.

STRATEGIES FOR TRANSPORT

Protecting the obstetric patient from the effects of vasospasm and hypertension and preventing seizures and other complications are critical. Maintaining or improving uteroplacental blood flow minimizes the risk of insult to the fetus.

The primary survey, including obstetric assessment, is done initially. The transport team should follow general guidelines for transport care and assess for PIH and risk factors and complications associated with PIH. Obtaining a history of the onset of any symptoms provides insight in the consideration of the clinical picture.

The fetus is at increased risk for uteroplacental insufficiency. The maternal transport nurse should observe for late decelerations and reduced variability while monitoring and take note of fetal movement.

The maternal transport nurse should place a urinary catheter to monitor urinary output and proteinuria when symptoms indicate severe preeclampsia. When assessing for proteinuria, the maternal transport nurse should avoid contamination with vaginal discharge (blood, amniotic fluid, and bacteria) to avoid inaccurate results.

Sensory stimulation should be decreased during transport by keeping lights and voices low and sirens turned off, or by turning the cardiac monitor audible signal to low or off. The transport team must be prepared to intervene in the event of an eclamptic seizure. $MgSO_4$, benzodiazepines, and airway supplies should be readily available.[12]

A coagulopathy is suspected if petechiae, hematuria, bruising, or bleeding from intravenous sites is noted. Symptoms of shock may rapidly ensue.

The transport nurse should evaluate pulmonary status for signs of pulmonary edema. If acute pulmonary edema with respiratory distress occurs, morphine (2 to 5 mg administered intravenously over 1 to 2 minutes) and furosemide (20 to 40 mg administered intravenously over 2 to 3 minutes) can be given. The medical plan to control the disease includes a thorough knowledge of the action, dosage, administration, and adverse reactions of the medications that may be used in the management of PIH.

Magnesium Sulfate

$MgSO_4$ acts at the neuromuscular junction to slow transmission of impulses. By displacing calcium, it interferes with the release of acetylcholine, blocking nerve transmission to the muscle and thereby preventing the seizure. Fifty grams of $MgSO_4$ can be added to 500 ml lactated Ringer's solution (or 40 g added to 1000 ml) with a bolus of 4 to 6 g given slowly over 15 to 30 minutes, followed by 2 g per hour, preferably by infusion pump. Therapeutic serum magnesium levels to prevent seizures range from approximately 4 to 8 mEq/L (1.5 to 2.5 mEq/L is normal). When therapeutic levels are achieved, deep tendon reflexes will be depressed but not absent. Loss of deep tendon reflexes indicates a toxic

level. Respiratory arrest and cardiac arrest are seen with highly toxic levels (greater than 15 mEq/L). While a patient is receiving intravenous $MgSO_4$, frequent assessment of deep tendon reflexes is essential. Respirations should also be closely monitored and the infusion stopped if less than 12 per minute are observed. Pulse oximetry should be used during transport.

The antidote for magnesium toxicity is calcium gluconate. Calcium stimulates the release of acetylcholine, stimulating nerve transmission to the muscle. The recommended dosage of calcium gluconate is 1 g of a 10% solution administered intravenously over at least 3 minutes. If administered too rapidly, bradycardia and arrhythmias may occur.

$MgSO_4$ is not an antihypertensive agent. However, a transient drop in blood pressure after initiation of treatment is frequently seen and can be attributed to smooth muscle relaxation. Adverse reactions include flushing, sweating, nausea and vomiting, and drowsiness. A decrease in FHR variability may be observed. Because $MgSO_4$ is primarily excreted in the urine, toxicity may develop rather rapidly in the patient with significantly impaired kidney function. The urinary output should exceed 30 ml per hour while the patient is receiving $MgSO_4$. The infusion should be decreased or stopped if urinary output drops below 30 ml per hour. In cases of kidney or heart disease, $MgSO_4$ should be used cautiously.

Labetalol

Labetalol is a selective beta-blocking agent that decreases systemic vascular resistance without changing cardiac output. The standard dosage, 20 mg administered by intravenous push over 2 minutes, may be repeated every 10 minutes with 40 to 80 mg until the maximum dosage of 300 mg has been given.[12]

Hydralazine

Hydralazine acts by relaxing arterioles and decreasing vasospasm, and as a result, it reduces blood pressure and stimulates cardiac output. Blood perfusion to the brain, kidneys, liver, and uterus is thus improved. To prevent a cerebrovascular accident, hydralazine is recommended when the diastolic pressure is 110 mm Hg or greater. Two milligrams administered intravenously every 5 minutes until the diastolic pressure is in the 90 to 100 mm Hg range is the standard dosage. During administration, the blood pressure should be taken every couple of minutes because the onset of action is 5 to 10 minutes. If the diastolic pressure falls below 90 mm Hg, uterine blood flow may be further reduced, placing the fetus at risk. Adverse reactions include reflex tachycardia, headache, palpitations, dizziness, nausea, and vomiting. Hydralazine is contraindicated in cases of lupus erythematosus and tachycardia.

BENZODIAZEPINES

Benzodiazepines are classified as antianxiety/sedative medications but are known to prevent or arrest seizure activity, although the exact mode of action is not known. They also produce mild sedation and muscular relaxation. They should be administered parentally, but in an extreme emergency when intravenous access is not possible, they may be given rectally. Adverse reactions include transient bradycardia and hypotension.

PRETERM LABOR AND RELATED ISSUES

Regular and rhythmic contractions that produce progressive cervical changes after the 20th week of gestation and before the 37th week are considered to be preterm labor. Preterm delivery occurs in 6% to 9% of all deliveries. Preterm labor does not always result in preterm delivery; however, the rate of preterm delivery has changed little in recent years. With improved prenatal care, elimination or improvement of risk factors, patient education, and earlier diagnosis and treatment of preterm labor, the next decade may realize a decrease in the rate of preterm delivery.

ETIOLOGY

Although many factors predispose the obstetric patient to preterm labor, a few single identifiable causes exist. Infection has been recognized as a primary cause of preterm labor. Although the pathways frequently differ, sources of infection may include urinary tract infection, pyelonephritis, vaginitis (particularly bacterial), chorioamnionitis, and viral infection. Another identifiable cause is PROM (spontaneous rupture before the onset of contractions and before the 37th week). Other factors include previous preterm delivery (the single most frequent contributing factor), uterine anomalies, poor nutritional status, poor perineal hygiene, poor weight gain, no prenatal care, less than 1 year between the last delivery and commencement of the current pregnancy, substance abuse, PIH, cigarette smoking, diabetes, chronic cardiovascular or kidney disease, previous induced or spontaneous abortion, abdominal trauma, a long commute to work, a high stress level at work or home, physical stress, overdistention of the uterus as a result of multiple gestation, hydramnios, uterine tumors, age (teenage or over 40 years), placenta previa or placental abruption, cervical incompetence, women exposed to diethylstilbestrol in utero, a retained intrauterine device, a history of pelvic inflammatory disease, and fetal anomalies, distress, or death.[17]

Only a few or many factors may be implicated in each instance of preterm labor. When multiple factors are present, the obstetric patient is at greater risk.

PATHOPHYSIOLOGIC FACTORS

In any situation in which uterine blood flow is reduced or impaired, an increase in uterine irritability can be noted and may result in the onset of labor. Viral infections with symptoms of fever, nausea, vomiting, or diarrhea may predispose to preterm labor primarily because of dehydration, which reduces uterine blood flow. Other similar conditions in which uteroplacental perfusion is compromised include PIH, diabetes, cardiovascular or kidney disease, overdistention of the uterus, heavy smoking, placental abruption, or placenta previa.

Hormonal influence contributes to increased uterine activity and the onset of labor. Prostaglandin release is associated with PROM, bacterial infections, abdominal trauma, and overdistention of the uterus. In at least half the patients who have PROM, labor begins in 48 hours. Meconium-stained amniotic fluid (indicating possible fetal distress) contains high levels of oxytocin, which can initiate labor.

When a patient has cervical incompetence, the cervix is unable to support and maintain the growing pregnancy to term and often dilates without perceptible contractions. Cervical incompetence is characterized by premature, painless, bloodless cervical dilation in which the membranes bulge and rupture, and delivery rapidly follows. Congenital defects and traumatic injury to the cervix may result in cervical incompetence. Probable causes of cervical injury include trauma during a previous childbirth, cervical dilation after elective or spontaneous abortions, or gynecologic procedures. Other physiologic abnormalities where preterm labor (PTL) is known to occur, especially if it does not allow for uterine growth and expansion during the course of the pregnancy, include exposure to diethylstilbestrol and uterine anomalies.

For many identified risk factors, no single physiologic factor or other pathology can be identified. It appears that numerous issues are involved. Consequently, for many patients, the cause of preterm labor cannot be identified.

The complications associated with preterm labor and delivery predominantly affect the fetus. Birth trauma and the complications associated with the transition to extrauterine life for the premature infant are primary. Neonatal sepsis can result from PROM. The severity of the complications seen depend in a great measure on the gestational age of the neonate.

Maternal complications include adverse reactions to labor-suppressing agents, complications associated with cesarean section (increased incidence with preterm labor), endometritis, septicemia and septic shock related to prolonged PROM and chorioamnionitis, or other complications associated with pre-existing conditions or the current pregnancy.

ASSESSMENT

Preterm labor should be suspected if the patient has a history of contractions 10 minutes apart or less for a period of 1 hour or longer. The transport team should assess for factors associated with preterm labor, remembering that the incidence of preterm labor increases with the number of predisposing factors.

SPONTANEOUS RUPTURE OF MEMBRANES

To assess the status of the amniotic membranes, the transport team should ask the following question: Did contractions begin before or after rupture? If there is any history of possible spontaneous rupture, a sterile speculum examination (SSE) will verify the presence of amniotic fluid leaking from the cervix and collecting in the posterior fornix of the vagina (the area underneath the cervix posteriorly). If an SSE has already been performed, the transport team should note documented results. Three factors, positive pooling, positive Nitrazine, and positive ferning, will definitely confirm spontaneous rupture of the membranes (SROM). Pooling of fluid will be seen in the vaginal vault. If none is seen, the team may encourage the patient to cough; the increased pressure will usually result in the release of amniotic fluid. A sample from a site as close to the posterior fornix as possible will turn Nitrazine paper dark blue (alkaline) in the presence of amniotic fluid. Vaginal secretions are acidic in nature and will not affect the paper. The transport team should use caution because blood, cervical mucus, and povidone-iodine (Betadine) are alkaline in nature and can give a false-positive reading. Finally, a small amount of the fluid can be spread on a slide and allowed to dry completely. A frond crystallization pattern of dried amniotic fluid (with a high concentration of sodium chloride) will be seen under microscopic examination; it looks very similar to a Boston fern in appearance. Because a microscope may not be available in small outlying areas and there may not be time to perform this procedure, the transport team must depend on the presence of pooling and positive results of a test for Nitrazine. If rupture is confirmed, avoid performing a sterile vaginal examination (SVE) unless delivery appears imminent; this will prevent introducing microbes from the vagina into the cervical canal, which can place the patient at an increased risk for infection. If a gross rupture has occurred, if the patient has a history of a large volume loss, or if continual leaking is observed, a sterile speculum examination is not necessary if it does not alter the plan for nursing care. The transport team should keep in mind that with a decreased amount of amniotic fluid, the umbilical cord is at risk for compression and variable decelerations may be seen, with or without contractions.

If a rupture has not occurred, an SVE will confirm if any cervical changes have taken place. The cervix does not have to dilate before changes can be noted. Normally, the cervix is firm, long, and closed. Any softening or effacing, which frequently occurs before dilation, indicates cervical changes.

If this is not the initial episode of preterm labor, the transport team should assess for the history of onset, current medications, other treatment such as home monitoring or bed rest, and patient compliance. Frequently the present episode can be linked to increased activity, failure to take medication altogether, or inconsistency in following the medication regimen.

The transport team should observe the patient for any indications of the presence of infection. Symptoms of a urinary tract infection, pyelonephritis, or both include dysuria, frequency of urination, fever, and flank tenderness, pain, or both. Evidence of poor perineal hygiene may be a factor not only in the development of a urinary tract infection but in vaginal infections and chorioamnionitis as well.

The transport team may assess the patient for possible chorioamnionitis; symptoms include fever, tachycardia, fetal tachycardia, uterine tenderness not associated with contractions, purulent vaginal discharge, and an elevated white blood cell count. If results of laboratory tests done by a referring facility are available, the labs indicated are a complete blood count with differential and cervical cultures for β-hemolytic streptococcus and *Neisseria gonorrhoeae*. However, most are asymptomatic. The most common route for infection is the ascending route from the vagina to the cervix. Evidence indicates that the presence of bacteria in the vagina may locally dissolve the membrane; the bacteria then gain access to the fluid and cause a chorioamnionitis that dissolves the membrane, and SROM results. With no evidence of prior infection, the incidence of infection after SROM greatly increases if the membranes have been ruptured longer than 24 hours.

A history of flulike symptoms and persistent nausea with vomiting, fever, or diarrhea may precipitate PTL, in which case fluid and electrolyte replacement is needed.

The transport team should assess the patient for cervical incompetence. A history of previous pregnancy losses, especially associated with "painless labors," is suspect. Vaginal mucus may be the first sign of cervical dilation. The mucus plug that fills the cervical canal can be dislodged by cervical changes. Other symptoms include lower abdominal discomfort or a sensation of fullness in the vagina. Vague symptoms should not be taken lightly. The transport team should ask whether any interventions have been performed to prevent problems with cervical incompetence.

STRATEGIES FOR TRANSPORT

Primarily supporting the medical plan to suppress labor, maintaining or improving uterine perfusion, and investigating for causes accomplish protection of the obstetric patient and the fetus from the threat of preterm delivery.

The primary survey, including general obstetric assessment, should be done first. The transport team should then follow these general guidelines for transport care:

1. Determine the contraction pattern: Determine the phase of labor and assess whether transport can safely be attempted or whether delivery should be accomplished at the referring facility. In the event of an imminent delivery, call for the neonate team, notify the medical director, and help the referring facility prepare for delivery.

2. Determine the status of the amniotic membranes: If there is questionable history of fluid leakage and contractions have slowed or stopped altogether, absolute determination of rupture is not required before transport if it does not alter the plan for nursing care.

3. Determine cervical status: Determine the number of SSEs done at the referring facility, especially if an SSE was done in the presence of ruptured membranes. Assess the amount

of cervical change accomplished since admission to the referring facility. Remember that once labor is established, the multiparous woman will frequently progress at a faster rate than a primipara and may require rapid transport.

4. Maintain the patient in the left lateral position: Not only does the left lateral position improve uterine perfusion, thus decreasing uterine irritability, but it decreases pressure on the cervix from the presenting part and may protect against further cervical changes. Having the patient stand, sit, or bend can place pressure against the cervix and should be avoided during transport.

5. Assess for infection: Observe for symptoms of urinary tract infection, pyelonephritis, vaginitis, chorioamnionitis, or signs of a viral infection.

6. Assess for cervical incompetence: An incompetent cervix can be suspected if the patient has vague symptoms accompanied by disproportionate cervical changes. Obstetric history in these cases is of particular importance. Placing these patients in the left lateral position in a slight Trendelenburg's position, or with hips slightly elevated, may further reduce any pressure on the cervix.

7. Administer or continue tocolytic agents as prescribed: Suppression of labor is always attempted to "buy time" for the transport. Optimal neonatal outcome can be anticipated when the delivery occurs in a hospital that is prepared for the intensive care of premature infants. If hydration and positioning to the left lateral have not slowed or arrested labor, tocolytic agents can be administered. The medications used most frequently in suppressing labor are $MgSO_4$ or terbutaline.

TRAUMA IN PREGNANCY

Minor accidental injuries are common during pregnancy. The gravid uterus, loosened joints, altered center of gravity, shortness of breath, dizziness, increased fatigue, and edema all contribute to minor accidents.

Serious accidental injuries during pregnancy place not only the obstetric patient but also the fetus at risk. The fetus is well protected in the confines of the uterus because it is surrounded by amniotic fluid, which serves as an excellent shock absorber. It is extremely rare for a fetus to experience physical trauma except as a result of direct penetrating wounds or extensive blunt trauma. The fetus is at greatest risk for fetal distress and intrauterine death as a result of maternal trauma and death. The obstetric patient is more vulnerable to hemorrhage because of the increased vascularity surrounding the gravid uterus. Early signs and symptoms of hypovolemia may be masked by the normal physiologic changes of pregnancy. As a result, blood is shunted away from nonvital organs, including the uterus, threatening the well-being of the fetus. In dealing with a trauma patient who is pregnant, the best interest of the fetus is served by prompt assessment and interventions on behalf of the mother. When the situation is life-threatening, the pregnancy should be ignored.[18,20]

The pregnant trauma patient needs to be appropriately immobilized for transport. Placing a small roll under the right side of the backboard and tipping the backboard 30 degrees displaces the uterus to the left side. Stretcher straps should be placed low over the pelvis.

PERIMORTEM CESAREAN SECTION

There is controversy over whether a perimortem caesarian section is of any value in the transport environment. There have been some anecdotal reports of these types of deliveries, but with limited survival of either the infant or the mother. Indications for this procedure may include the following[18-20]:

- Gestational age of the fetus (24 to 26 weeks)
- Limited amount of time since maternal arrest (some suggest within 5 minutes of maternal arrest)

Experienced personnel should perform the procedure, and they must be prepared to perform neonatal resuscitation.

SUMMARY

The transport of the patient who is pregnant requires experience and skills so that both the mother and fetus may benefit. There is no arguing that if the mother does not receive appropriate care, the baby will suffer, but there are times when the patient or the fetus's condition may warrant personnel with specific abilities not generally obtained by a general transport service.

Each transport service must ensure that they are competent and capable of providing care for both the mother and fetus.

PREGNANT PATIENT CASE STUDY

The transport team was called to the scene of a 23-year-old female involved in a motor vehicle crash. The patient was the restrained driver of a car that was struck on her side by a truck. On arrival of the team, she was still entrapped in the vehicle. The patient was awake, but confused and maintaining her airway. A 100% nonrebreather mask was in place.

She had no peripheral pulses, and her monitor showed a sinus tachycardia at a rate of 144. On removal from the car, the patient was found to have a grossly distended firm abdomen and was wearing maternity pants. The patient confirmed she was pregnant, but was confused and agitated and could not answer how many months.

Because of her signs of decompensated shock, the transport team elected to intubate the patient using RSI before transport and another intravenous line with blood tubing was initiated. A blood pressure could not be palpated. The patient did have a palpable femoral pulse. Blankets were placed under the backboard to place the uterus over to the left.

During transport, one unit of packed red blood cells was started. The patient was hot off-loaded at the receiving trauma center. A pelvic film was obtained and a well-developed fetus was identified along with a severely fractured pelvis.

Because of her instability, the patient was taken immediately to the operating room for a caesarian section and operative management of

her bleeding. A 7-pound female infant was delivered. She did not have any vital signs, and despite aggressive resuscitation, she could not be revived.

The mother suffered a ruptured uterus and a severe pelvic fracture and also, despite aggressive resuscitation, expired in the operating room.

REFERENCES

1. Arnone B: Amniotic fluid embolism: a case report, *J Nurse Midwifery* 34:92, 1989.
2. Benorub GI: *Obstetric and gynecologic emergencies*, Philadelphia, 1993, Lippincott.
3. Brundage SI, Davies JK, Jurkovich G: Trauma to the pregnant patient. In Grenvik A, editor: *Textbook of critical care*, ed 4, Philadelphia, 2000, WB Saunders.
4. Buckley K, Klub N: *High risk pregnancy manual*, Baltimore, 1993, Williams & Wilkins.
5. Clark SL, Cotton DB: *Handbook of critical care obstetrics*, Boston, 1994, Blackwell.
6. Commission on Accreditation of Medical Transport Systems: *Standards*, Andersonville, SC, 2002, Author.
7. Cunningham GF et al: *Williams obstetrics*, ed 19, East Norwalk, Conn, 1993, Appleton-Century-Crofts.
8. Gilbert E, Harmon J: *High-risk pregnancy and delivery: nursing perspectives*, St Louis, 1986, Mosby.
9. Harvey CJ: *Critical care obstetrical nursing*, Gaithersburg, Md, 1991, Aspen.
10. Henderson S, Mallon W: Trauma in pregnancy, *Emerg Med Clin of North Am* 16(1):209, 1998.
11. Krupa D, editor: *Flight nursing core curriculum*, Park Ridge, Ill, 1997, Road Runner Press.
12. Magee LA: Management of hypertension in pregnancy, *Br Med J* 318:1332, 1999.
13. Mandeville LK, Troiano NH: *High risk intrapartum nursing*, Philadelphia, 1992, Lippincott.
14. Mattson S, Smith JE: *Core curriculum for maternal newborn nursing*, Philadelphia, 1993, Saunders.
15. Morton N, Pollack M, Wallace P, editors: *Stabilization and transport of the critically ill*, New York, 1997, Churchill Livingstone.
16. Pritchard JA, MacDonald PC, Gant NF: *Williams obstetrics*, ed 17, East Norwalk, Conn, 1985, Appleton-Century-Crofts.
17. Smith J: The dangers of prenatal cocaine use, *Matern Child Nurs J* 13:174, 1988.

18. Smith LG: The pregnant trauma patient. In McQuillan K, Von Rueden K, Hartsock R, Flynn M, Whalen E, editors: *Trauma nursing: from resuscitation through rehabilitation*, ed 3, Philadelphia, 2002, Saunders.

19. Strong T, Lowe R: Perimortem cesarean section, *A J of Emerg Med* 5:489, 1989.

20. Wraa C, editor: *Transport nursing advanced trauma course*, ed 2, Denver, 2001, Air and Surface Transport Nurses.

1. Perform an initial assessment of the neonatal patient.
2. Perform the necessary interventions to maintain the neonate's airway, breathing, and circulation after delivery.
3. Prepare the neonate for transport using the appropriate equipment for size and need.

The neonate has a unique anatomy, physiology, and pathophysiology. The depth of knowledge required by transport personnel is directly related to the mission of the team as it pertains to the care of neonates. In the case of the infant requiring care in a nonmedical environment, including a home, car, and so on, the needs of the infant are for basic resuscitation and stabilization and expedient transport to the nearest appropriate medical facility. In the case of interfacility transport of newborns, the emphasis should be on providing a level of care during stabilization and transport equivalent to the level of care the infant will obtain at the receiving hospital. This implies that the combined expertise of the referring staff and the transport team can provide that level of assessment and care. The final step in ensuring quality care should include review of all neonatal protocols, procedures, and cases by a designated individual with recognized expertise in that field.

The American Academy of Pediatrics offers some specific criteria for the composition of the neonatal transport team. In addition, they also provide guidelines for what equipment should be used to safely stabilize and transport the neonate. See Box 30-1 for a summary of these recommendations.

FETAL CIRCULATION AND TRANSITION

The scope of this chapter allows only a brief overview of the fetal circulation and transition to extrauterine life. The umbilical vein carries blood with the highest oxygen saturation back to the right atrium via the ductus venosus and the inferior vena cava. A large percentage of this blood is directed across the foramen ovale to the left atrium, left ventricle, and ascending aorta, thus perfusing the coronary arteries and the brain with the most highly oxygenated blood in the fetal circulation. Some of the blood coming from the umbilical vein along with blood returning from the superior vena cava flows through the tricuspid valve to the right ventricle and out through the pulmonary valve. Because

---

BOX 30-1 **Guidelines for Neonatal Transport From the American Academy of Pediatrics**

1. Access to neonatal-pediatric transport services are essential to the health of infants and children.
2. Requirements for neonatal-pediatric interfacility transport should include: patient and team safety, a level and quality of patient care equivalent to the care provided in a critical care unit, quality monitoring, optimal resource allocation, cost effective, and rapid response.
3. Skilled health-care professionals.
4. Adequate volume of patients so that the team remains competent.
5. Maintenance of a database that must include: demographic data, treatment outcomes, and quality improvement data.
6. Communication between the transport system and the communities they serve must be open and expeditious at all times.
7. Encourage transport back to the referring facility when the infant's clinical condition allows it.

Modified from: American Academy of Pediatrics: *Guidelines for air and ground transport of neonatal and pediatric patients,* Elk Grove Village, Ill, 1999, Author.

---

of the high resistance in the peripheral pulmonary vasculature, most of the blood flow from the right ventricle passes from the pulmonary artery through the ductus arteriosus and into the descending aorta, mixing with the remainder of the blood coming from the left side of the heart. In utero, the right and left ventricles both pump at systemic pressures into the aorta (Figure 30-1).[20]

With the expansion of the lungs and improved oxygenation at birth, the pulmonary vascular resistance falls, allowing a rapid increase in pulmonary blood flow and a consequent decrease in flow across the ductus arteriosus. Simultaneously, the umbilical cord is clamped, removing the low-resistance placental circuit and increasing systemic resistance. This increase in afterload, as well as increased return to the left atrium from the pulmonary circuit, closes the flaplike foramen ovale. Neonatal hypoxia, hypoglycemia, hypothermia, sepsis, and acidosis can all interfere with the normal progression of this transition period.[14,31,33] Therefore careful ongoing assessment and early intervention are critical during this time period. Common findings at this time include intermittent grunting, mild retracting, and tachypnea.[41] The infant should be observed closely until all these symptoms have resolved.

DELIVERY ROOM MANAGEMENT

ASSESSMENT

Traditional delivery room assessment includes the assignments of the Apgar score developed in 1953 by Dr. Virginia Apgar (Table 30-1).[1] The Apgar score is a basic rapid evaluation of the infant's immediate adaptation to extrauterine life, which evaluates color, respiratory effort, heart rate, body tone, and responsiveness to stimuli. It is routinely measured at 1 and 5 minutes after birth. If, however, the infant continues to be depressed after 5 minutes of age, it can be useful to continue assigning Apgar for up to 20 minutes after delivery.[26] Early studies correlated low 5-minute Apgar scores with poor neurologic outcome.[12] However, later studies have shown that the Apgar score is not an accurate indicator of neonatal asphyxia as defined by metabolic acidosis.[30,42] In the case of a depressed infant, cord gases should be evaluated whenever possible for the presence of metabolic acidosis. The Apgar score remains, however, an excellent tool for assessing perinatal fetal depression, which may be the result of to a number of etiologies. In addition to perinatal asphyxia, the Apgar score can be affected by maternal medications, prematurity, neuromuscular

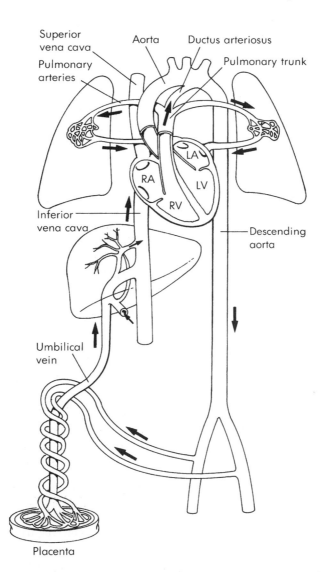

FIGURE 30-1 **The normal fetal circulation and major fetal flow patterns.** (From Heymann MA: Biophysical evaluation of fetal status: fetal cardiovascular physiology. In Creasy RK, Resnik R, editors: *Maternal fetal medicine,* Philadelphia, 1984, Saunders.)

TABLE 30-1 The Apgar Score

		Sign	
Score	0	1	2
*A*ppearance, color	Blue, pale	Centrally pink	Completely pink
*P*ulse, heart rate	None	Less than 100 beats/min	Greater than 100 beats/min
*G*rimace, reflex	No response	Grimace	Cough, gag, cry
*A*ctivity/attitude	Flaccid/limp muscle tone	Some flexion	Well-flexed/active motion
*R*espiratory, effort	None, irritability	Weak/irregular	Good, crying

disorders, previous intrauterine cerebral insults, and central nervous system (CNS) abnormalities, among others. The use of the Apgar score is most helpful in directing the level of intervention required by the infant.

CLEAR THE AIRWAY

Immediately on delivery of the head, the airway should be cleared with either bulb syringe, DeLee, or a 10- to 14-Fr suction catheter using a mechanical suction. Neonatal Resuscitation Program (NRP) recommends that no greater than 100 mm Hg of negative pressure should be used to avoid injury to the neonate.[26] The oropharynx should normally be cleared before suctioning the nose because stimulation of the nares may cause the infant to gasp and aspirate secretions present in the oropharynx. Stimulation of the vagus nerve resulting in severe bradycardia can result from suctioning too vigorously and too deeply. Therefore suctioning after the initial clearing of the airway should be done strictly on an as-needed basis.

It is essential that thorough suctioning of the oropharynx and nasopharynx be completed before the delivery of the thorax and the infant's first breath. The aspiration by the infant of meconium-stained fluid into distal airways contributes significantly to morbidity and mortality. NRP states "Some previous recommendations have suggested that endotracheal suctioning should be determined by whether the meconium has "thick" versus "thin" consistency. While it might be reasonable to speculate that thick meconium might be more hazardous than thin, there are currently no clinical studies that warrant basing suctioning techniques on meconium consistency."[26]

The incidence of meconium aspiration syndrome can be greatly reduced by effective clearing of the airway.[10,46] After delivery with meconium stained amniotic fluid, if the infant has depressed respirations, poor tone, and/or a heart rate less than 100, the trachea should be intubated and suctioned using an endotracheal tube and a meconium aspirator before positive-pressure ventilation is used. If the baby looks good (i.e., breathing well, HR >100,

good muscle tone) and is covered in meconium, just simply suction the mouth/nose. It is not recommended to suction the baby's trachea.[26]

MAINTAIN BODY TEMPERATURE

As soon as possible after delivery, the infant should be dried and a heat source provided. The use of a stocking cap can greatly decrease heat losses. The only circumstance in which drying of the infant should be delayed is in the presence of meconium-stained fluid. In this situation, the baby should not be stimulated until the airway has been cleared, possibly including direct suctioning of the trachea. The cord should also be appropriately clamped and cut.

INITIATE BREATHING

The baby's head should be maintained in the sniffing position and blow-by oxygen may be supplied until the infant is centrally pink. If the infant does not begin spontaneous effective respirations or the heart rate remains below 100 beats/min after clearing of the airway and stimulating the infant, ventilation should be initiated at a rate of 40 to 60 breaths/min. During the resuscitation stage, 100% oxygen should always be used. Adequate ventilation should be evaluated by auscultating breath sounds and observing chest excursion and heart rate. The infant will respond to adequate ventilation with an improvement in color, heart rate, and tone. Ventilating pressures should always be monitored with a manometer. Although pressures up to 30 to 40 cm H_2O may be required in the initial breaths to open the lungs, the lowest pressures possible to maintain good ventilation should be used. Newborn infants are at high risk for pulmonary air leaks during mechanical ventilation. Once the infant has established spontaneous respirations, a heart rate >100 beats/min, and is centrally pink, the flight nurse reevaluates the amount of support required. Support may include blow-by oxygen, face mask or nasal prongs, continuous positive airway pressure (CPAP), continued ventilation, or no additional supplemental oxygen.

If there is no response in heart rate and color after 30 seconds of bag and mask ventilation, then an endotracheal tube if immediately available should be

TABLE 30-2	**Endotracheal Tube Size Selection**		
Weight (kg)	Endotracheal Tube (size)	Depth of Insertion (cm from upper lip)	Suction Cath Size
1	2.5	7	5 Fr
2	3.0	8	6 Fr
3	3.5	9	8 Fr
4	4.0	10	8-10 Fr

placed, otherwise cardiopulmonary resuscitation (CPR) should be initiated while preparations for intubation are being made (Table 30-2). Because there is little room for error in the placement of the endotracheal tube, careful and immediate evaluation for right or left mainstem or esophageal intubation should be done, and adequacy of ventilation should be assessed again. Ventilation should be continued until effective spontaneous respirations have been established.

CHEST COMPRESSIONS

If the heart rate remains below 60 beats/min and does not increase after 30 seconds of ventilation, chest compressions should be initiated. Two methods are recommended for performing chest compressions on the neonate. These are the thumb technique and the two-finger technique.[26]

The thumb technique involves the caregiver encompassing the infant's chest. The caregiver's thumbs are used to depress the infant's sternum. The baby should be placed on a firm surface to deliver effective compressions.

The two-finger technique uses the tips of the caregiver's middle finger and either the index finger or the ring finger of one hand to compress the sternum. The other hand can be used to support the infant's back.

Whether using the thumb or two-finger technique, the infant's chest should be depressed to a depth of approximately one third of the anterior-posterior diameter of the chest. The pressure should then be released so that the heart can refill.[26]

The rate of resuscitation involves 120 "events" per minute. Ninety compressions plus 30 breaths should occur.

The status of the infant should be reassessed after 30 seconds of resuscitation. If the child's heart rate

is above 60, compressions can be stopped. If chest compressions are not effective, epinephrine should be administered.[26]

DRUG SUPPORT

Drugs are rarely needed in the delivery room resuscitation of the newborn if adequate ventilation has been established (Table 30-3). If the heart rate continues below 60 beats/min despite adequate ventilation and compressions for a minimum of 30 seconds, or if there is no heart rate, the transport team should instill 0.1 to 0.3 ml per kg of 1:10,000 solution of epinephrine down the endotracheal tube. To ensure that the epinephrine reaches the lungs, it should be diluted in or flushed with 1 to 2 ml of normal saline. Intraenous (IV) access should be attained as soon as possible and the medication delivered intravenously.

During delivery room resuscitation the umbilical vein is the most accessible parenteral route (Box 30-2). If the heart rate remains below 60 beats/min, a second dose of epinephrine may be given through the endotracheal tube or through the established IV line. Hypovolemia should be suspected when there is a history of bleeding or if the infant demonstrates poor response to resuscitation, pallor, or poor pulse volume despite adequate ventilation. If hypovolemia is thought to be a problem, volume expanders should be given. Once adequate ventilation and tissue perfusion have been established, the transport team may administer sodium bicarbonate 4.2% solution in a dose of 1 to 2 mEq/kg *slowly* over at least 2 to 3 minutes for documented metabolic acidosis. Under transport conditions, documenting blood gas status may be impossible. A decision to administer sodium bicarbonate in the presence of

TABLE 30-3 Neonatal Emergency Drug Dosages

Drug	Indication	Dose	Route*
Naloxone (neonatal Narcan)	Narcotic depression	0.1 mg/kg	IV/UVC/IM/ETT
Epinephrine (1:10,000)	Bradycardia, cardiac arrest	0.1-0.3 ml/kg	ETT/UVC/IV
Sodium bicarbonate, 4.2% (0.5 mEq/ml)	Metabolic acidosis	2 mEq/kg over 2-3 minutes	UVC/IV (always clear line before and after administration)
5% Albumin	Hypotension volume restoration	10 ml/kg over 5-10 minutes	UVC/IV
Lactated Ringer's	Hypotension volume restoration	10 ml/kg over 5-10 minutes	UVC/IV
Dextrose 10%	Hypoglycemia	2-4 ml/kg	UVC/IV

*IV, Intravenous; IM, intramuscular; UVC, umbilical venous catheter.

BOX 30-2 Umbilical Vein Catheterization

The neonatal transport nurses should place the umbilical vein catheter under aseptic technique. The umbilical stump and surrounding skin should first be cleansed using an approved protocol that describes preparation of the area. For example, use alcohol first, then povidone-iodine (Betadine) and let the povidone-iodine dry for at least a minute—povidone-iodine can be wiped off when the procedure is completed. Drapes are then applied to create a sterile filed. A no. 5 Fr catheter is usually adequate and can normally be placed in all sizes of infants; it is prepared by either attaching the catheter directly to a three-way stopcock or trimming the flared end of the catheter and inserting a blunt needle adapter. The blunt needle adapter would then be connected to the three-way stopcock and flushed with solution.

Umbilical tape is tied snugly around the base of the cord to provide control of bleeding during the procedure. The umbilical stump can then be cut approximately 1 cm above the skin line. The neonatal transport nurse can then identify the two thick-walled constricted arteries (4-o'clock and 8-o'clock positions) and the thinner-walled larger vein (12-o'clock position). A pair of curved iris forceps may be helpful in identifying and opening the lumen of the vein.

The neonatal transport nurse then inserts the catheter tip in the lumen and gently advances it. It may be helpful to stabilize the cord by gently holding the cord at the base or applying traction with a clamp on the Wharton's jelly. The umbilical vein normally runs in a cephalad direction. Directing the catheter in that line may assist in ease of entry. The venous catheter should be inserted only as far as necessary to obtain blood return, which is normally 2 to 3 cm. Advancing the catheter further may result in a placement in the liver and consequent hepatic damage from medication injections.

The umbilical catheter can then be secured with a "goalpost" tape bridge. A purse-string suture around the Wharton's jelly and then tied to the catheter will control bleeding, as well as assist in securing the catheter.

Complications of this procedure include infection, hemorrhage, air emboli, and thrombus formation. Therefore the procedure should only be undertaken after appropriate training under supervision and then performed with extreme care.

---

prolonged asphyxia/resuscitation may be made after the earlier steps have been adequately completed. As soon as possible, a blood sample should be evaluated for partial pressure of oxygen (Pao_2), partial pressure of carbon dioxide ($Paco_2$), and pH. If an arterial sample is not available, a venous sample is still valuable, particularly for $Paco_2$ and pH. If the heart rate has not responded to this therapy, epinephrine may be repeated every 3 to 5 minutes and sodium bicarbonate as indicated by blood gas determination. For narcotic depression, naloxone 0.1 mg/kg can be given intravenously, intramuscularly, subcutaneously, or via the endotracheal tube. These infants, however, should respond to ventilation with improved heart rate and color despite their respiratory depression. Naloxone may precipitate severe withdrawal in the infant of a mother with narcotic addiction and should be used with extreme caution by the transport team.[26]

EVALUATION

If the infant has not responded to the measures just discussed, the transport team must reevaluate the clinical assessment and management of the infant. Common reasons for an inadequate response to resuscitation include the following:

1. Mechanical problems
   a. Inadequate oxygen supply
   b. Inadequate ventilatory pressures
2. Tube malposition
   a. Tube in esophagus
   b. Tube in right or left mainstem
   c. Blocked tube
3. Unrecognized clinical problem
   a. Pneumothorax
   b. Diaphragmatic hernia
   c. Hypoplastic lungs

NONINITIATION OR DISCONTINUATION OF RESUSCITATION OF THE NEONATE

The International Guidelines for Neonatal Resuscitation Guidelines for 2000 include recommendations for the noninitiation or discontinuation of resuscitation. These include[35,36]:

- Birthweight less than 500 g
- Confirmed trisomy 13 or 18
- Congenital hydrocephalus
- Gestational age less than 24 weeks
- Severe fetal growth restriction

Each transport team should have policies and procedures that outline how to manage these issues.

STABILIZATION BASICS

The goal of stabilization is an infant who has normal vital signs, normal perfusion, normal blood gases, and normal glucose and electrolyte levels. This goal is not always attainable, but every attempt should be made to achieve it before transport.

THERMOREGULATION

Because of the large surface area compared to body mass and poor thermal insulation, the infant is at high risk for hypothermia. Hypothermia in the neonate can be lethal. It is usually an iatrogenic condition and is almost always preventable. Compared with the adult, the newborn has limited ability to produce heat by shivering. Similarly, the hyperthermic infant has an increased oxygen consumption and a limited ability to dissipate heat through sweating. It is therefore essential to understand the mechanisms of heat production and loss and interventions for maintaining a neutral thermal environment. The neutral thermal environment is that range of environmental temperature at which the baby can maintain a normal body temperature with minimal metabolic activity and oxygen consumption.[7,11,40,43]

The optimal temperature ranges for the newborn are

Skin temperature 36.0° C to 36.5° C
Axillary 36.5° C to 37.0° C
Rectal 36.5° C to 37.0° C

It is essential that skin temperature be continuously monitored in the newborn in addition to intermittent either axillary or rectal temperatures. An infant can have a normal central temperature using axillary or rectal measurements and still be cold stressed with a cool skin temperature. Cold stress increases mortality and morbidity. Side effects of cold stress and hypothermia include increased oxygen consumption, hypoxemia, acidosis, and pulmonary vasoconstriction. In addition, the infant increases his or her glucose consumption, which may result in hypoglycemia. Release of free fatty acids into the blood may contribute to the development of kernicterus at low levels of indirect hyperbilirubinemia.

The neonate maintains his or her body temperature through basal metabolism, muscular activity, and chemical thermogenesis. The infant's primary mechanism of heat production in response to cold stress is chemical thermogenesis using his or her brown fat stores. This process requires increased oxygen consumption.[23] In the presence of decreased brown fat stores (i.e., prematurity) or hypoxia, his or her ability to generate heat production is severely limited.[39]

Heat losses occur through convection, conduction, evaporation, and radiation, as follows:

Radiation: Heat transfer between the body and surrounding objects (e.g., Isolette walls)

Convection: Heat transfer dependent on air flow over the body (e.g., a cold delivery room, emergency department, aircraft, or ground transport vehicle)

Evaporation: Heat transfer to water in the state change from liquid to gas (e.g., a wet infant)

Conduction: Heat transfer between the body and objects in contact (e.g., a scale)

Convection and evaporation are the most important mechanisms of heat loss in newborns. The management of the infant's thermal environment requires a careful balancing of heat losses and heat sources. Interventions for blocking heat loss include keeping the infant dry; swaddling in blankets, foil, or plastic; using heat shields and stocking caps; and preventing drafts. Heat sources may be most effective when used in combination. Available sources include radiant heat, warmed air, and warming pads. During transport the team must anticipate the effects of weather conditions. The newborn can lose significant amounts of heat through radiation to cold Isolette walls. Therefore continuous temperature monitoring during transport is preferable. Lacking this capability, the temperature should be assessed at 15-minute intervals as a minimum standard.

It is important to also ensure that the neonate does not become hyperthermic. Hyperthermia has been associated with perinatal respiratory depression.[35,36]

FLUIDS, CALORIES, AND ELECTROLYTES

Maintaining fluid, electrolyte, and glucose balance in the newborn requires an initial educated guess as to the individual infant's requirements followed by close observation and evaluation. The main components of fluid loss in the newborn are through insensible water loss and urinary output (UO). In the sick newborn, UO should be measured as accurately as possible by means of urine bags, diaper weights, catheterization, and so on. Insensible water loss increases significantly as the level of prematurity increases. Radiant warmers, elevated environmental temperatures, and respiratory distress increase insensible water loss. On the other hand, use of heat shields and warm humidified inspired air on the ventilator can significantly minimize these losses. Fluid balance in newborns on IV therapy should be monitored with daily body weights, UO, specific gravities, and serum electrolytes. The need for electrolyte evaluation before transport must be determined based on the age of the newborn, the length of the transport, and the presence of risk factors for electrolyte imbalance.

The newborn infant normally has a fluid requirement of approximately 60 to 80 ml/kg/day on the first day of life. This requirement increases by approximately 10 ml/kg/day on the first subsequent day of life. (It is important to make sure that one doesn't increase maintenance fluids by 10 ml/kg/day *each* day for each day of life—only the first day or two. Increasing fluid by 10 ml/kg/day each day for a week, would result in 150 ml/kg/day, which is too much fluid.) In the premature infant, particularly <1500 g, special consideration should be given to potential increased fluid needs. The use of the radiant warmer or phototherapy in these infants can increase fluid requirements by as much as 50% for each.[4] As mentioned, use of heat shields or clear plastic covers over the infants may help to control these losses. With appropriate fluid intake, UO should be 1 to 2 ml/kg/hr with specific gravities of approximately 1.008 to 1.012. During the first week of life it should be anticipated that the infant will lose 5 to 15% of birth weight.[4] Subsequent changes in the baby's fluid intake are based on evaluation of these criteria.

The addition of electrolytes to IV fluids is usually not necessary in the first 12 to 24 hours. Serum electrolyte levels should be checked before additions. Potassium should not be added until after the infant has voided. Normal electrolyte supplementation is approximately 3 to 4 mEq/kg/day of sodium and 2 to 3 mEq/kg/day of potassium. Because of the immaturity of the renal system, the premature infant may have comparatively larger sodium losses requiring a corresponding increase in sodium supplementation. In the term infant, normal sodium level is 135 to 145 mEq/L with a normal serum potassium of 3.5 to 6.0 mEq/L. The preterm infant frequently has a serum sodium as low as 130 mEq/L. The flight nurse must precisely calculate the infant's fluid requirement, including any abnormal losses, because either too much or too little fluid can be detrimental to the progress of the infant. High fluid intake in these infants contributes to an increased incidence of patent ductus arteriosus.[4] The extremely low birth weight infant of less than 1000 g may require recalculation of fluid and electrolyte requirements two to three times per day.

GLUCOSE REQUIREMENTS

Newborns are susceptible to hypoglycemia because of immature glucose control mechanisms, decreased glucose substrate stores, or both. The definition of hypoglycemia in the newborn may be variable depending on the reference. In actual practice most clinicians consider a serum glucose of less than 40 mg/dl to represent hypoglycemia.[31,34] The healthy term infant normally reaches the nadir of his or her serum glucose level at approximately 2 hours after birth. It is therefore recommended that glucose screening be conducted in all healthy term infants at 1 to 2 hours of age. However, in the transport setting, the population is generally at higher risk for developing hypoglycemia (Box 30-3). These high-risk infants should have screening glucose levels as soon as possible after delivery and at appropriate intervals thereafter. Most newborns can be maintained on IV fluids of 10% dextrose in water at the fluid levels recommended in the previous section. Glucose levels should be checked every 30 minutes to 1 hour until it has been demonstrated that the amount of glucose provided is adequate to maintain normal serum levels. The infant weighing less than 1000 g should receive 5% dextrose in water because of his or her intolerance of the higher glucose loads, resulting in hyperglycemia.

Hypoglycemia may be treated in several ways depending on the severity of the deficiency. A bolus of 200 to 400 mg/kg (2 to 4 ml/kg) of 10% dextrose in water may be *slowly* given to return the serum glucose to the normal range. It can then be maintained with maintenance IV fluids. If the hypoglycemia is not profound, the transport team may elect to respond by increasing the maintenance fluids to increase glucose delivery without the use of a bolus. A decision as to whether to increase fluid rate or dextrose concentration must be made on the basis of the fluid tolerance of the individual baby. A peripheral vein may be used for glucose concentrations of up to 12.5% dextrose. At concentrations of 12.5% dextrose and higher, a central venous line should be considered. Treatment of extremely resistant hypoglycemia may include the use of corticosteroids, glucagon, epinephrine, and diazoxide. Administration of these drugs, however, is beyond the scope of this chapter.

Hyperglycemia, blood glucose levels greater than 125 mg/dl, is most commonly seen in the infant weighing less than 1000 g or in infants whose hypoglycemia has been overcorrected. Management of

BOX 30-3	**Risk Factors for Hypoglycemia**

Small for gestational age (SGA)
Hypothermia or cold stress
Respiratory distress
Congenital heart disease
Large for gestational age (LGA)
Infant of a diabetic mother
Rh incompatibility
Beckwith-Wiedemann syndrome
Nesidioblastosis
Islet cell adenomas
Sepsis
Asphyxia

hyperglycemia in infants <1000 g can usually be handled with the use of 5% dextrose as a maintenance fluid. Hyperglycemia in the infant who is being treated for hypoglycemia can be avoided by administering the appropriate amount of glucose. In general, hyperglycemia is not a problem that requires further management during transport.

RESPIRATORY MANAGEMENT: GENERAL CONSIDERATIONS

Because most ill neonates requiring transport have some degree of respiratory compromise, it is essential that the transport team perform careful and continuous assessment of their respiratory status. Assessment must include both physical assessment and blood gas and radiographic studies. The presence of retractions, grunting, and flaring indicates a decrease in lung compliance. Both central and peripheral color should be evaluated for the presence of cyanosis. The presence of adequate central oxygenation indicates adequate pulmonary blood flow and gas exchange. The peripheral color may reflect problems with either oxygenation or perfusion. If the infant is centrally oxygenated (pink) but peripherally cyanotic (purple), then he or she should be evaluated to determine the cause of the poor perfusion. This may include poor cardiac output, vasoconstriction, or hypothermia. Auscultation reveals adequacy of air entry and the presence or absence of fluid in the bronchial tree.

The primary component of respiratory management is ensuring correct positioning and clearing of the airway. As a basic principle, sufficient oxygen should be supplied to ensure central oxygenation. Adequacy of central oxygenation should be checked by evaluating mucous membranes of the mouth and the tongue. Oxygen should be considered a drug, with risks and side effects associated with its use. These risks need to be weighed against the complications of hypoxemia in determining what percentage of oxygen to supply. The term or near-term infant is at increased risk for persistent pulmonary hypertension in the presence of hypoxemia/acidosis while having a very low risk for the development of retrolental fibroplasia from hyperoxia. It is prudent to err on the side of hyperoxia in the infant of 35 weeks

and greater gestation. The infant of 34 weeks or less gestational age has a decreased incidence of persistent pulmonary hypertension. However, there is an increased concern of irreversible side effects if these newborns are maintained in a hyperoxic state. It is therefore important to ensure adequate oxygenation in these infants without sustaining long periods of hyperoxia. Current technology including use of transcutaneous monitor and pulse oximetry greatly enhances the ability to supply oxygen for the newborn in an appropriate range.

Oxygen can be supplied by a number of methods. Blow-by or free-flow oxygen near the baby's face can be used on a short-term basis but has severe drawbacks. First, it is impossible to accurately measure the exact percentage of oxygen that the baby is receiving on a continuous basis. Second, the flow of cold oxygen onto the cold-sensitive face may result in increased inappropriate heat-generating maneuvers and vagal stimulation on the part of the baby. Hood oxygen allows for the accurate measurement and stabilization of oxygen supply to the newborn. Its drawback is the lack of accessibility to the newborn's head without disturbing the oxygen concentration. Continuous positive airway pressure can be delivered via alternate modes including nasal prongs, nasopharyngeal tube, and endotracheal tube. An endotracheal tube obviously provides the most effective delivery of CPAP but requires the invasive procedure of intubation. Positive-pressure ventilation requires the placement of an endotracheal tube, with its inherent potential complications, but it can be done safely in the hands of a skilled practitioner. In selecting the mode of oxygen delivery, the flight nurse must weigh both the benefits to be gained and the risks incurred by the selected approach. These are addressed in this chapter under the various disease entities.

Once respiratory support has begun, continuous observation and reevaluation must be accomplished to maintain the correct level of support. Adjustments must be made to accommodate changes in the infant's pulmonary compliance. Diminishing compliance without an appropriate adjustment in oxygen support may result in hypoxia with hypercarbia. Improvement in compliance could result in hyperoxia, hypocarbia, and potentially air leaks with a resultant decrease in cardiac output. Any infant treated with positive pressure is at an automatic increased risk for air leaks including pneumothorax, pneumomediastinum, and pulmonary interstitial emphysema. Uncommonly, pneumoperitoneum and pneumopericardium could also occur. Any sudden deterioration in an infant receiving positive-pressure ventilation should prompt immediate evaluation for a displaced endotracheal tube or pulmonary air leaks. Evaluation should include assessment of breath sounds, shifting of the point of maximal intensity (PMI), transillumination of the chest, and chest radiograph.[38] Mechanical problems with the oxygen delivery system should also be immediately ruled out. It is always important after bag-mask ventilation to ensure that excess air is removed from the stomach because a distended stomach could interfere with adequate ventilation.

BLOOD PRESSURE AND PERFUSION

Hypotension, poor perfusion, or both are also common problems in the neonate. Assessment of this problem should begin with an evaluation of the obstetric history, which would suggest a cause for either hypovolemia or myocardial dysfunction. Historical facts suggestive of hypovolemia as a basis for poor perfusion would include compression of the cord, preferentially obstructing flow to the baby through the umbilical veins while allowing flow from the baby to the placenta through the firm-walled umbilical arteries, and a history of blood loss during the pregnancy, labor, or delivery.

Infants with a history of asphyxia may well have both hypovolemia and myocardial dysfunction. Assessment would include arterial pressures, central venous pressures, extremity versus core temperatures, a capillary refill greater than 3 seconds in the presence of a normal temperature, and evaluation of pulse volume. The presence of a progressive metabolic acidosis in a well-ventilated and oxygenated infant and evidence of cardiomegaly on radiographic films may be indicative of an asphyxial cardiomyopathy.

Treatment is aimed at the return to adequate perfusion of the tissues to prevent continued metabolic acidosis. If the transport team suspects hypovolemia, the treatment would include careful transfusion with 10 ml/kg of an isotonic crystalloid solution such as normal saline or Ringer's lactate solution.[26] Rapid increase in systemic blood pressure carries the risk of sudden rise in pressure in vascular beds. This could cause capillary rupture and hemorrhage and result in intracranial bleeding. If myocardial dysfunction is suspected, the transport team may consider administering inotropic agents. Whichever treatment is instituted, careful monitoring of arterial pressures is essential both to monitor results and to prevent complications.

ASSESSMENT OF THE NEWBORN

Assessment of the newborn includes historical information, clinical examination, and laboratory data. Obstetric information obtained should include the estimated day of confinement (EDC) based on the mother's dates and clinical data, maternal age, gravity, parity, abortions, fetal demises, neonatal deaths, number of living children, length of rupture of membranes, and complications of the pregnancy, labor, or delivery. Neonatal history would include Apgar scores, resuscitation required, initial physical examination, and subsequent course. Laboratory data and radiographic studies must also be reviewed.

GESTATIONAL AGE EXAMINATION

Both Dubowitz[14] and Cappurro[10] have developed assessment tools for gestational aging of the newborn. Cappurro's scale is reproduced here (Figure 30-2). In 1977 Hittner published an assessment of gestational age using the examination of the anterior vascular capsule of the lens.[4] This examination is especially helpful for assessing infants between 27 and 34 weeks gestation. For the infant less than 34 weeks of age, Jacinto Hernandez at The Children's Hospital in Denver, Colorado, has developed a system correlating foot length with gestational age. Using this measurement, the foot is measured from the heel to the tip of the longest toe. A 4.5 cm measurement would equal 25 weeks. For each additional 0.5 cm of length, 2 weeks is added to

A.   VARIABLES

Variable					
Nipple formation	Nipple barely visible; no areola /0	Well-defined nipple; areola <0.75 cm /5	Areola stippled not raised >0.75 cm /10	Areola raised >0.75 cm /15	
Skin texture	Thin, gelatinous /0	Thin and smooth /5	Smooth, medium thickness, superficial peeling /10	Slight thickening, superficial cracking & peeling of hands & feet /15	Thick and parchment like /20
Ear form	Pinna flat & shapeless /0	Incurving of part of edge /8	Partial incurving of whole of upper pinna /16	Well-defined incurving of pinna /24	
Breast size	No breast tissue /6	Diameter <0.5 cm /5	Diameter 0.5-1 cm /10	Diameter >1 cm /15	
Plantar creases	No creases /0	Faint red marks over anterior ½ /5	Definite red marks over anterior ½, indentations over anterior ⅓ /10	Indentations over anterior ½ /15	Deep indentations over more than anterior ½ /20
Scarf sign	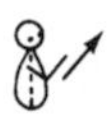 /0	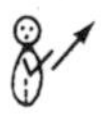 /6	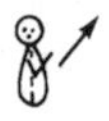 /12	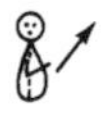 /18	
Head lag	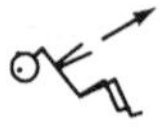 /0	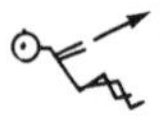 /4	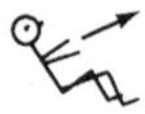 /8	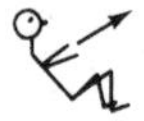 /12	

Left margin labels: A. SOMATIC — B. SOMATIC AND NEUROLOGIC — K= 204 days — K= 200 days

Variables and assigned scores in the modified Dubowitz method for assessment of gestational age. A. Gestational age in days = 204 + total somatic score (for neurologically depressed infants). B. Gestational = 200 + total combined somatic and neurologic score (for healthy infants).

FIGURE 30-2 Cappurro's method for assessing gestational age. (From Cappurro H et al: A simplified method for diagnosis of gestational age in the newborn infant, *J Pediatr* 93:121, 1978.)

the gestational age. These measurements have been well correlated in preterm infants less than or equal to 34 weeks gestation using the Dubowitz examination. However, it is not reliable in the small-for-gestational-age infant. Once the gestational age has been determined according to both historical and clinical data, the weight, length, and head circumference of the infant should be plotted on standardized growth charts.[4,34] The infant with a weight less than the 10th percentile for gestational age is classified as small for gestational age. The infant with a weight greater than 90th percentile for gestational age is classified as large for gestational age. All infants between the 10th and the 90th percentile are classified as appropriate for gestational age.[2,6,26,28,29]

PHYSICAL EXAMINATION

A considerable amount of information can be obtained strictly through observation of the infant. The observation should include:

1. Signs and symptoms of distress
2. Nutritional state
3. Morphology
4. Color
5. Respiratory effort
6. Posture and tone
7. Cry
8. Activity level/behavioral state

Before disturbing the baby by handling, the transport team should evaluate those things for which a quiet infant is required, including the following:

1. Heart: Rate, rhythm, heart sounds, murmurs, extra sounds
2. Chest: Symmetry and adequacy of air entry, rales, rhonchi, wheezes
3. Abdomen: Bowel sounds, organomegaly, masses
4. Femoral pulses: Volume

It is then important to complete the rest of the examination in an organized, systematic approach. For example, the transport team might examine the infant beginning from the head and working downward. The rest of the examination is outlined as follows:

1. Head: Symmetry, shape, caput succedaneum, cephalhematoma
2. Fontanelles/sutures: Fontanelle number, fullness, depression, and size; suture mobility
3. Symmetry of face: Development, shape, movement
4. Eyes: Shape, position, size, pupils, hemorrhages
5. Mouth: Clefts, teeth, movement of tongue
6. Neck: Webbing, length
7. Nose: Symmetry, septum, patency
8. Clavicles: Masses, intactness
9. Chest: Size, symmetry, shape
10. Umbilical cord: Number of vessels
11. Genitals: Development, testes, urethral and vaginal openings
12. Anus: Patency
13. Spine: Masses, symmetry, dimples
14. Extremities: Symmetry, development, movement, pulses
15. Hips: Range of motion
16. Reflexes: Root, suck, Moro's, grasp
17. Tone: Head control when pulled to sit, jitteriness, flexion

In the transport setting the potential value of each part of the examination must be weighed against any stress it may cause to an already compromised infant.

PATHOLOGIC CONDITIONS OF THE NEONATE

One of the major roles of the transport team is to assist in the development of the differential diagnosis and management plan for the newborn requiring transport. In the development of this plan, steps outlined in the section "Assessment of the Newborn" serve as the basics for the differential diagnosis. The history obtained must include the development and timing of symptomatology and the progress of the condition. Integration of historical data with the physical examination and evaluation of laboratory and x-ray data is essential.

RESPIRATORY DISORDERS
DIAPHRAGMATIC HERNIA

Diaphragmatic hernia is caused early in gestation when the pleuroperitoneal cavity fails to close. Abdominal contents migrate into the thoracic cavity, compressing developing lungs and causing pulmonary hypoplasia.

Early detection of this defect is essential to the initiation of appropriate therapy. Classic presentation by these infants includes early onset of respiratory distress with deterioration between the 1- and 5-minute Apgar scores in the delivery room. Clinical signs include dyspnea, unequal breath sounds, a shift in the PMI, and potentially scaphoid abdomen. Although scaphoid abdomen is listed as a classic sign, it is frequently not evident in the delivery room. Because any distention of the bowel further compromises respiratory function, the transport team should insert a large-bore (10 Fr) orogastric tube and initiate suction. Positive-pressure ventilation with a face mask should be avoided. When ventilation is required, immediate endotracheal intubation should be performed.

Diaphragmatic hernia used to be considered a "surgical emergency." Recent studies have supported delaying surgery to allow for a period of physiologic stabilization.[27] The efforts of preoperative stabilization are aimed at optimizing oxygenation, maintaining an adequate systemic blood pressure, and reducing the associated pulmonary hypertension.

These infants are at high risk of severe hypercarbia and pneumothoraces. Therefore ventilatory management is aimed at maximizing ventilation while minimizing barotrauma, if possible. Persistent pulmonary hypertension and shock frequently complicate the management of these infants. In the transport setting, an additional member should be added to the team if it would decrease the stabilization time.

ASPIRATION PNEUMONIAS

Although aspiration of meconium is the most severe form of aspiration pneumonia, the infant may also aspirate amniotic fluid or blood at the time of delivery. The presence of meconium in the amniotic fluid should alert the medical team to the possibility of acute or chronic in utero asphyxia. The airway should be cleared as discussed previously in this chapter. Meconium can be aspirated in utero and therefore may be impossible to prevent in the presence of severe asphyxia. The flight nurse should attempt to clear the meconium from the airway. The presence of meconium in the bronchial tree causes obstruction to airflow and pneumonitis. These infants are usually term or postterm. Common complications in meconium aspiration syndrome include pulmonary air leaks and persistent pulmonary hypertension. Therefore the goals of respiratory management are the maintenance of oxygenation, avoiding acidosis, and minimizing high airway pressures. Antibiotic therapy is frequently started in these infants until sepsis has been ruled out as the reason for the meconium release

predelivery. Common symptoms in these newborns include the appearance of a hyperinflated chest and tachypnea. Radiographic findings can assist significantly by revealing patchy densities bilaterally.

SURFACTANT DEFICIENCY

The most common cause of respiratory distress in the preterm infant is respiratory distress syndrome (RDS), formally known as hyaline membrane disease (HMD). This condition is primarily caused by a deficiency of surfactant. A deficiency of surfactant may also occur in the presence of extreme stress such as severe hypoxia. Surfactant decreases surface tension in the alveolus during expiration, allowing the alveolus to maintain a functional residual capacity. The absence of surfactant results in poor lung compliance and atelectasis. Infants with surfactant deficiency demonstrate progressive increase in symptoms as a result of poor lung compliance. This progression is evidenced by increasing effort at breathing with intercostal retractions, flaring, and grunting. Oxygen requirements continue to increase to maintain an adequate arterial oxygen level. The increased respiratory effort required results in increasing lethargy. Characteristic radiographic findings include reticular granular pattern in the lungs and hypoexpansion. The severity of the illness varies from requiring minimal respiratory support by hood oxygen to maximal support with the ventilator.

The cornerstone of treatment for RDS is supplemental oxygen to maintain a PaO_2 of 60 to 70 mm Hg and an arterial saturation of 92% to 95%.[41] Intubation and ventilation should be undertaken for signs of worsening respiratory distress including partial pressure of oxygen (PaO_2) <60 mm Hg in 70% to 80% fraction of inspired oxygen (FiO_2) or a partial pressure of carbon dioxide ($PaCO_2$) >50 mm Hg. In an effort to avoid intubation, or after surfactant administration and weaning from ventilatory support, continuous positive airway pressure is administered either nasally or by endotracheal tube. Ventilation should be instituted or continued if the infant becomes fatigued, as indicated by worsening arterial blood gases.[26]

Exogenous surfactant was approved for use by the Food and Drug Administration (FDA) in 1990.

Ten years of extensive clinical studies before then showed that exogenous surfactant treatment substantially reduces mortality and the incidence of air leak, although it does not appear to reduce other complications such as bronchopulmonary dysplasia and intraventricular hemorrhage. There are both natural surfactant extracts and synthetic preparations. The primary function of lung surfactant is to lower surface tension at the air-water interface of the alveoli, thereby preventing atelectasis and improving compliance. Administration of exogenous surfactant may result in rapid changes in lung compliance, subsequent overventilation, and air leaks unless close monitoring and adjusting of ventilator settings occur.

Pulmonary interstitial emphysema is common in those infants requiring high levels of ventilatory support. Added complications of the disease include development of chronic lung disease as a result of ventilatory support and a persistent patent ductus arteriosus. These complications may be decreased by using the lowest possible ventilatory settings and avoiding excessive fluid administration during transport.[6,17,19]

PNEUMONIA

Pneumonia is often associated with a history of prolonged rupture of membranes of at least 12 hours before delivery. However, respiratory infection can occur in the fetus even in the presence of intact membranes. Symptoms of amnionitis and fetal infection including maternal fever or elevated white count, purulent or foul-smelling fluid, fetal tachycardia, loss of beat-to-beat variability, or premature labor are also very suggestive. Signs of infection in infants may be present immediately at birth or be delayed for 1 to 2 days. In addition to respiratory symptoms of tachypnea, apnea, grunting, flaring, or retracting, systemic symptoms may also be present. These may include hypotonia, hypotension, poor perfusion, lethargy, and seizures. An elevated or extremely low white blood cell count may or may not be present. Radiographic examination may resemble either RDS with a uniform granularity or aspiration with patchy lung fields. Management includes maintaining adequate oxygenation and ventilation, antibiotic therapy, and cardiovascular support.

PULMONARY AIR LEAKS

Air leaks including pulmonary interstitial emphysema (PIE), pneumothorax, and pneumomediastinum are most commonly related to excessive positive-pressure ventilation used during resuscitation or the use of positive airway pressure treatments.[38] The infant with an air leak may appear nearly asymptomatic, with only muffled heart tones or absent/diminished breath sounds, or the infant's condition may deteriorate rapidly, requiring immediate intervention. Assessment includes evaluation of breath sounds, location of PMI, transillumination of the chest, and x-ray. In the infant requiring immediate resuscitation, there may be no opportunity to delay for x-ray diagnosis, and a diagnostic thoracentesis must be performed. In the milder form with minimal symptoms, no treatment may be necessary, or a one-time needle thoracentesis and hood oxygen may be adequate. In the clinically significant tension pneumothorax, the placement of a chest tube is usually required. In the transport setting, air medical personnel must anticipate increasing symptoms from an untapped pneumothorax if the transport requires moving the child at high altitudes. Before departing the referring hospital, the flight nurse must also evaluate the effectiveness of the use of either a one-way valve or suction on the chest tube.

NEONATAL HEART DISEASE

The diagnosis and management of the infant with congenital heart disease can be a major challenge in the transport setting. Frequently, the referring staff and transport team do not have the benefit of echocardiography and must rely on history, clinical examination, laboratory, and x-ray results. The initial symptoms of serious congenital heart disease in the newborn, in order of frequency, are cyanosis, cyanosis with heart failure, heart failure without cyanosis, cardiogenic shock, and arrhythmias. Because the early signs of congestive heart failure are tachypnea and tachycardia, it is easy to understand the potential difficulty in distinguishing pulmonary from cardiac disease in the cyanotic, tachypneic newborn.

In the transport setting, the critical issues include the differentiation of pulmonary from cardiac disease and the determination of those heart lesions that are dependent on ductal flow. Once the determination has been made that cyanosis in the newborn is caused by a fixed right-to-left shunt, the neonatal transport nurses must still differentiate between shunting caused by persistent pulmonary hypertension and anatomic heart disease. A history containing high-risk factors for persistent pulmonary hypertension and a clinical course demonstrating previous adequate oxygenation in room air is helpful.

It is essential to obtain a detailed history of the onset of symptoms from the referring staff (Table 30-4). The referring nursing staff can frequently provide the most detailed chronologic report. Immediate onset of respiratory symptoms at birth is likely to indicate the presence of pulmonary disease because few babies are born in active heart failure. An obstetric history that would indicate an infant at risk for pulmonary disease is also important to elicit. High-risk factors for pulmonary disease would include prematurity, postmaturity, meconium-stained fluid, prolonged rupture of membranes, maternal diabetes, neonatal asphyxia, or cesarean section.

Clinical examination includes a complete examination of the cardiorespiratory system and a search for evidence of other anomalies. Findings suggestive of cardiac disease include cardiac murmur, hepatomegaly, decreased or unequal pulses, hyperactive pericardium, arrhythmias, and poor perfusion. Tachypnea without other signs of respiratory distress such as grunting and retracting may also be an indication of early heart failure. Clinical signs suggestive of respiratory disease include retractions, grunting, poor air exchange, and unequal air entry.

Laboratory data that may be helpful include a comparison of oxygenation in room air and 100% oxygen. The infant who is hypoxic in room air but demonstrates a partial pressure of oxygen (Po_2), greater than 150 in 100% oxygen is more likely to have pulmonary disease than heart disease with a

TABLE 30-4   The Top Five Diagnoses Presenting at Different Ages

Age on admission: 0-6 days (N = 537)

Diagnosis	%
D-Transposition of great arteries	19
Hypoplastic left ventricle	14
Tetralogy of Fallot	8
Coarctation of aorta	7
Ventricular septal defect	3
Others	49
Total	100

Age on admission: 7-13 days (N = 195)

Diagnosis	%
Coarction of aorta	16
Ventricular septal defect	14
Hypoplastic left ventricle	8
D-Transposition of great arteries	7
Tetralogy of Fallot	7
Others	48
Total	100

Age on admission: 14-28 days (N = 177)

Diagnosis	%
Ventricular septal defect	16
Tetralogy of Fallot	7
Coarctation of aorta	12
D-Transposition of great arteries	7
Patent ductus arteriosus	5
Others	53
Total	100

From Fyler D, Lang P: Neonatal heart disease. In Avery GB, editor: *Neonatology*, Philadelphia, 1987, Lippincott.

fixed right-to-left shunt. Comparison of simultaneous arterial blood gases demonstrating a Pao_2 at least 10 mm higher from a preductal site versus a postductal site indicates right-to-left shunting of desaturated blood at the ductal level.[23]

Those heart defects that may be dependent on ductal patency for pulmonary blood flow would include transposition without ventricular septal defect (VSD), pulmonary or tricuspid atresia, and critical pulmonary stenosis including tetralogy of

Fallot. Coarctation of the aorta and hypoplastic left heart syndrome may also require the use of prostaglandin E$_1$ for stabilization for transport.[16] In these ductal dependent lesions, the prostaglandins are required to maintain adequate systemic blood flow. Prostaglandins are normally used during transport when the patient's condition is deteriorating, as indicated by the presence of metabolic acidosis, or when deterioration is anticipated before completion of the transport. The most common side effect complicating transport with the use of prostaglandin E$_1$ is apnea or hypoventilation. The length of the transport and the difficulty of placing an endotracheal tube during transport must be considered in the decision of whether to place an endotracheal tube before transport when prostaglandins are begun. Other side effects with the use of prostaglandin E$_1$ include fever, vasodilation with flushing, and diarrhea. Uncommonly, the vasodilation may result in systemic hypotension requiring intervention.

Management of the infant with congenital heart disease during transport involves treatment of the symptomatic failing heart. The presence of clinical and laboratory evidence of heart failure dictates the interventions to stabilize the patient's condition during transport. Clinical symptoms would include hepatomegaly, decreased pulses, capillary refill greater than 3 seconds, mottled color, peripheral cyanosis, tachycardia, and cool extremities. Laboratory indications would include cardiomegaly on radiographic findings and metabolic acidosis. The primary intervention available for the failing myocardium is inotropic drug support.

PERSISTENT PULMONARY HYPERTENSION IN THE NEWBORN (PPHN)

PPHN is a syndrome characterized by persistent elevated pulmonary vascular resistance resulting in right-to-left shunt at the ductus arteriosus or the foramen ovale leading to hypoxemia in the presence of a structurally normal heart.[15] This disease process is most commonly seen in near-term infants with severe asphyxia, meconium-aspiration syndrome, congenital diaphragmatic hernia sepsis, or other respiratory distress resulting in hypoxia. It can be very difficult in the transport setting to make the clinical differentiation between cyanotic heart disease and PPHN. Demonstration of right-to-left shunting at the ductus using preductal and postductal simultaneous arterial blood gas levels is helpful in the diagnosis of this problem. Treatment is aimed at maintaining adequate oxygenation until the pulmonary vasculature resistance begins to drop. This normally occurs in the first several days. The more severely affected infants may require extremely high inspiratory pressures and rates to maintain adequate oxygenation. Current treatment therapies include maintaining the infant in an alkalemic state through hyperventilation and the use of blood buffers, sedation or neuromuscular blockade, fluid boluses, and cardiotonic drugs. Alkalemia is believed to enhance the decrease in pulmonary vasculature resistance. Maintenance of the systemic blood pressure (BP) discourages right-to-left shunting. Ongoing studies of the pulmonary vasodilatory effects of inhaled nitric oxide have been promising and are now being used by some transport teams.[26,35,36]

Complications of the ventilatory therapy include pulmonary air leaks and chronic lung disease.

GASTROINTESTINAL DISORDERS

The transport team deals primarily with gastrointestinal disorders related to obstruction, either functional or anatomic, infection, or externalized abdominal contents. Obstructions of the gastrointestinal (GI) tract can occur anywhere from the esophagus through the anus. The management of all of these disorders primarily centers on decompression of the bowel, fluid management, antibiotic therapy, and respiratory support.

ESOPHAGEAL ATRESIA

Findings related to identification of esophageal atresia include inability to pass an oral gastric tube to the stomach, excessive oral secretions, and feeding intolerance. An obstetric history of polyhydramnios should increase suspicion of upper GI obstruction. Of patients with esophageal atresia, 92% have an associated tracheoesophageal fistula. Approximately

85% of fistulas occur between the lower esophageal pouch and the trachea. This fistula allows air to pass from the respiratory tree into the stomach and gastric acids to reflux into the bronchial tree. These infants are at high risk for aspiration either from the oropharynx refluxing from the upper esophageal pouch or aspiration of gastric contents from the lower tracheoesophageal fistula. A transport team who suspects that an infant has esophageal atresia should immediately elevate the head of the bed and place a double-lumen suction tube in the upper esophageal pouch. This tube should be placed to continuous suction. Diagnosis can be confirmed with radiographs taken while having a radiopaque catheter curled in the upper esophageal pouch. The presence of air in the stomach or intestines would confirm the presence of a lower esophageal fistula. Management of these infants during transport should feature the following:

1. Intermittent suction of the upper esophageal pouch
2. Elevation of the head of the bed to prevent gastric reflux
3. Intravenous fluid therapy for fluids and glucose

Positive-pressure ventilation distends the stomach via the fistula and may interfere with ventilation or result in gastric perforation if adequate esophageal/gastric decompression is not maintained.

Approximately 8% of infants with esophageal atresia have no tracheoesophageal fistula. Esophageal atresia with a fistula to the tracheal tree from both the upper and the lower pouch occurs approximately 1% of the time. An H-type fistula that connects an intact esophagus and tracheal tree occurs approximately 4% of the time. These conditions may be more difficult to diagnose, with more subtle initial symptoms of choking or coughing during feedings. They also require more detailed radiographic studies using a contrast-medium dye; this should not be attempted in the transport setting. The infant with esophageal atresia and without air in the abdomen may be considered for transport either prone or even with the head slightly lowered to encourage effective evacuation of the upper esophageal pouch. Careful evaluation of the rest of the GI tract, the cardiovascular system, and the genitourinary system should be completed because of frequent associated anomalies.[18]

INTESTINAL OBSTRUCTIONS

Common initial symptoms for intestinal obstruction include bilious vomiting, abdominal distention, feeding intolerance, large quantities of gastric contents at delivery, absence of an anal opening, and lack of stooling in the first 24 hours. Obstetric history with a high obstruction may reveal polyhydramnios. Although the presence of bilious vomiting may be related to other causes, intestinal obstruction should be presumed until ruled out. Abdominal distention may be present depending on the level of the obstruction. Presence of tenderness, metabolic acidosis, or decreasing platelets may indicate a bowel necrosis or peritonitis and should be treated as an urgent problem.

Diagnosis can usually be made through x-ray evaluation. Contrast studies are rarely, if ever, indicated on transport. X-ray studies should be carefully evaluated for perforation of the bowel. Urgent cases include malrotations with volvulus and those with associated peritonitis, perforation, or suspected bowel necrosis.

Management includes decompression of the bowel with intermittent large-bore gastric suction, IV fluids, antibiotic therapy as indicated, and respiratory support. These infants may have large fluid requirements because of large interstitial fluid losses. Severe abdominal distention may compromise respiratory status. Evaluation of these children should include assessment of their oxygen needs and ventilatory capacity with appropriate measures taken to correct deficits. In severe cases of peritonitis, sepsis and shock may also be present and should be treated appropriately.

NECROTIZING ENTEROCOLITIS

Although the cause of necrotizing enterocolitis (NEC) remains controversial, ischemia of the bowel predisposes the infant to this disease process. Infants at particular risk include those with asphyxia, especially the small, ill, preterm infant.[8] Early recognition of risk factors and symptoms allows for early treatment, minimizing the incidence of necrosis of the bowel. Early symptoms include feeding intolerance with increased gastric aspirates, bile-stained gastric aspirates, abdominal distention, and Hematest-positive stools. Progression of the disease results in increasing abdominal distention to the point of tautness, grossly bloody stools, abdominal wall erythema, and abdominal tenderness. X-ray findings include intestinal distention, thickening of the bowel wall, and the classic sign of air in the bowel wall (pneumatosis intestinalis). The absence of these radiographic findings, however, does not rule out the diagnosis of necrotizing enterocolitis. These infants are at risk for peritonitis, bowel perforation, and disseminated intravascular coagulation.

The infant at risk for NEC as a result of severe birth asphyxia should be maintained on NPO (nil per os) status on IV fluids to allow the bowel to recover. Symptomatic infants should also be placed on NPO status on IV fluids and antibiotics. Any abdominal distention should be treated with intermittent gastric suction to keep the bowel decompressed. The presence of thrombocytopenia may indicate an underlying disseminated intravascular coagulation and may require treatment with platelet infusions.

Omphalocele/Gastroschisis
Although omphalocele and gastroschisis are two separate entities, their treatment during transport is essentially the same. An omphalocele is an arrest of development of the abdominal wall, with the abdominal contents remaining externalized. The defect remains covered by a membrane in utero, although the sac may be broken during delivery. The size of the defect may vary from a small hernia to inclusion of a large percentage of the abdominal contents. Gastroschisis, on the other hand, is a defect in the abdominal wall that has otherwise completed its development. The defect allows for protrusion of abdominal contents. Because the defect is normally very close to the umbilicus, it is frequently mistaken for an omphalocele. This defect, however, is not covered by a membrane. If the defect occurred early in gestation and the intestines have been floating in the amniotic fluid for

some time, they may appear very edematous with adhesions.

Both groups of infants are at risk for infection, large fluid losses, impaired bowel perfusion, and hypothermia. Treatment includes immediate wrapping of the defect with moist saline gauze and plastic wrap or, alternatively, placing the defect in a bowel bag to prevent fluid losses. The infant must obviously remain on NPO status, and gastric suction should be applied to maintain decompression of the bowel. If the abdominal opening is extremely small, the patient may be at a high risk for bowel ischemia as a result of the constriction of blood flow. Caring for the child on his or her side may help to reduce tension on the bowel and improve circulation. Careful monitoring and maintenance of temperature in normal range are essential in the management of these children. This increased need for thermogenesis also places them at risk for hypoglycemia and requires closer observation of blood glucose. They may also require increased fluid intake, particularly in the case of the gastroschisis or omphalocele with ruptured membranes.

Neonatal Infections
The most common neonatal infections requiring treatment on transport include pneumonia, both viral and bacterial, sepsis, and infrequently, meningitis. Pneumonia has been addressed in the subsections featuring respiratory illnesses. The infant with sepsis may have very mild and subtle onset of symptoms or a fulminating course resulting in rapid progression to shock. Symptoms include temperature instability, either hypothermia or hyperthermia, apnea and bradycardia ("A's & B's") lethargy, poor feeding, tachypnea, hypoglycemia, or cyanosis. An infant with any of these symptoms must be evaluated for potential sepsis. If the infant has meningitis, seizures must be added to the list of common presenting signs.

Evaluation of these infants includes a complete blood cell count with differential. A low absolute neutrophil count and elevated ratio of immature to total neutrophils, although not diagnostic, increases the level of suspicion for bacterial sepsis. Samples for blood cultures should be obtained using strict aseptic technique. Although the definitive diagnosis of septicemia requires positive blood culture results, infants with highly suspicious signs should be started on an appropriate antibiotic regimen. In addition to antibiotic therapy, supportive therapy should be provided as needed. Infants with overwhelming sepsis may be in shock, requiring support of blood volume and myocardial function. In the case of meningitis with seizures, examination of the cerebrospinal fluid is indicated but usually can be delayed until after the transport. However, antibiotic therapy and treatment for the seizures should be begun as soon as possible on transport.

Neurologic Disorders

The primary neurologic disorders requiring therapy during transport include cranial enlargement, neural tube defects, and seizures.

Cranial Enlargement

Cranial enlargement may either be benign or caused by a number of pathologic conditions that include hydrocephalus, intracranial hemorrhage, intracranial cysts and tumors, or other encephalopathy. Differentiation of etiology requires careful evaluation of history, skull films, computed tomographic (CT) scan, and transillumination. If the history indicates a difficult delivery and intracranial bleeding is suspected, the infant should be evaluated for anemia. From a transport perspective, management of these disorders is primarily supportive, responding to secondary dysfunctions in the respiratory or cardiovascular systems.

Neural Tube Defects/Encephaloceles

Failure of development of the neural tube early in gestation may result in a number of defects including anencephaly, meningomyelocele, meningocele, and encephalocele. These defects may include nervous tissue. The primary concern during transport is to prevent infection in the case of the open lesion. A moist, sterile dressing should be applied. Otherwise, transport management includes normal supportive therapy. Antibiotics may or may not be ordered.

Seizures

Seizures occur frequently in ill newborns, either as a primary or secondary disorder. Because of the immature nervous system of the newborn, they rarely exhibit the generalized tonic-clonic seizures seen in adults and older children. Seizures in the newborn can be divided into four categories[22]:

1. *Subtle.* This type of seizure is frequently overlooked by caretakers. It may consist of repetitive mouth or tongue movement, bicycling movements, eye deviation, repetitive blinking, staring, or apnea.
2. *Clonic* (multifocal or focal). Clonic seizures are characterized by repetitive jerky movements of the limb(s), which may move from limb-to-limb in a disorganized fashion.
3. *Tonic* (generalized or focal). Tonic seizures may resemble posturing seen in older infants and children and be accompanied by disturbed respiratory patterns and may include tonic extension of limb or limbs or tonic flexion of upper limbs and extension of lower limbs.
4. *Myoclonic.* Myoclonic seizures are characterized by multiple jerking motions of the upper (common) or lower (rare) extremities.

Seizure activity is frequently confused with jitteriness in the newborn. Jitteriness may be distinguished from seizures in the following ways:

1. Jitteriness is sensitive to stimulus, whereas seizures are not.
2. Jitteriness is characterized by tremors rather than the slow and fast phases of seizure activity.
3. Jitteriness can normally be stopped by flexing the limb, as opposed to seizures that will not respond to this maneuver.

To treat neonatal seizures, it is important to attempt to identify the cause (Box 30-4). Careful examination of the obstetric and neonatal history may reveal risk factors for seizure disorders. Physical examination should be performed, along with laboratory studies including glucose, calcium, phosphorus, magnesium, sodium, and potassium. The glucose level should be checked immediately with the bedside test strip. If hypoglycemia is present, it should be corrected

BOX 30-4	**Causes of Neonatal Seizures**

Birth trauma/intracranial hemorrhage
Hypoxic/ischemic encephalopathy
Hypoglycemia
Hypocalcemia
Hypomagnesemia
Hypophosphatemia
Hyponatremia/hypernatremia
Pyridoxine deficiency
Amino acid disturbances
Neonatal injection of caine derivatives
Bacterial meningitis
CNS abnormalities
Drug withdrawal

immediately with an infusion of glucose. If a correctable metabolic cause is not identified, seizures should be treated according to established protocols or after consultation with the appropriate physician. A number of medications including phenobarbital, phenytoin (Dilantin), and Lorazepam (Ativan) may be used. Serious side effects from these drugs may include respiratory or cardiovascular depression.[26]

EQUIPMENT

The transport of the neonate requires a skilled team and proper equipment. Box 30-5 contains a list of neonatal equipment designed for critical care interfacility neonatal transport. The

BOX 30-5	**Neonatal Equipment Inventory**

Respiratory equipment

Laryngoscope handle with blades, sizes Miller 0 and
   Miller 1
Spare laryngoscope bulbs and batteries
Endotracheal tube stylet
Anesthesia resuscitation bag 0.5 L
Anesthesia resuscitation bag 1.0 L
Tubing
Pressure manometer
Infant self-inflating bag
Pediatric self-inflating bag
Masks for resuscitation bags, 1 each, premature, term,
   and infant
Endotracheal tube sizes 2.5, 3.0, 3.5, & 4.0
Benzoin
Tape
Suction catheter and glove sets sizes nos. 5/6 Fr, 8 Fr,
   10 Fr, & 12 Fr
Bulb syringe
Extra-small, small, and large CPAP nasal prongs, 1
   each CPAP hats with ties
Gastric tubes: 10 Fr, 12 Fr
Feeding tubes: 5 Fr and 8 Fr
Thoracentesis
Large-bore catheters
Heimlich valve
Scalpel no. 11
Suture: 3-0 and 4-0 silk
Vaseline gauze

Stopcock
T-connector
Chest tubes 8 Fr and greater

Intravenous therapy equipment

Intravenous fluids
IV pump tubing
Blood tubing
Umbilical artery catheters, sizes 3.5 and 5.0
IV extension tubing
T-connectors
Steri drape
3-tail connector
Syringes, sizes from 1 ml through 60 ml
Peripheral IV catheters: 24 gauge, 22 gauge, and 20
   gauge
Heparin locks
3-way stopcock and stopcock plugs
Intraosseous needles
Medication additive labels
Armboards, sizes premature and infant
Assorted tape
Umbilical tape
Umbilical artery catheterization/thoracotomy set
   including: two sterile drapes, iris forceps, needle
   holders, scissors, curved forceps, tongue tissue
   forceps, sterile 2 × 2s, umbilical tape, scalpel, and
   blade
Blood pressure cuffs: neonate and infant (size 1-5)

Continued

BOX 30-5 Neonatal Equipment Inventory—cont'd

Thermoregulation and monitoring equipment

Stocking hat
Plastic wrap
Portawarmer
Silver swaddler/bubble wrap/plastic wrap
Thermometers
Limb leads
Chest electrodes
Heart monitor lead wires
Capillary tubes
Chemstrips
Lancets
Arterial transducer tubing

Miscellaneous

Blood culture bottles
Scissors and hemostat
Flashlight
2×2s
Limb restraints
Safety pins
Rubber bands
Pacifier
Cotton balls
Christmas tree adapters
Sterile glove packs
Neonatal stethoscope
Trash bag
Sterile plastic bags for gastroschisis, omphalocele and
    dressings for spinal dysraphism
Glass filter needles
Camera with instant film
Parent information books, permits, transport
    documents and maps

Medications

Epinephrine 1:10,000
$NaHCO_3$ 4.2%
Narcan
Dopamine
Dobutamine
Phenobarbital
Phenytoin
Midazolam
Fentanyl
Ketamine
Morphine
Vecuronium
Xylocaine 1%
Heparin 1000/ml
0.9% normal saline dilutent
Sterile water dilutent
Flush solution
Antibiotics
Antivirals
Albumin
$D_{50}W$
Atropine
Amioderone
Calcium gluconate
Calcium chloride
Exogenous surfactant
Methylprednisolone sodium succinate
Furosemide
Amrinone
Isoproterenol
Digoxin
Prostaglandin E_1

equipment selected for a scene-response team could be much abbreviated.[1]

NEONATAL CASE STUDIES

CASE 1

Baby B was a 38-week, 3200 g, appropriate-for-gestational-age female born to a 24-year-old gravida 2, para 1 (now 2), living child 1 (now 2),

A+ married woman. Previous medical history unremarkable. Normal prenatal course during this pregnancy. At 38 weeks by date, an elective repeat cesarean section was performed. Membranes were ruptured at delivery with clear fluid. Apgar scores were 7 at 1 minute and 9 at 5 minutes, requiring suctioning, O_2 blow-by, and stimulation in the delivery room. Baby's early course was reported to be unremarkable in level I. She was breastfeeding in room air. Transport was called at 18 hours of age for sudden deterioration with respiratory rate of 78, pale, cyanotic, poorly perfused infant with diminished pulses. Lower extremity pulses appeared to be weaker than upper extremity pulses. Arterial blood gas in 40% oxygen by hood, PO_2 of 52, PCO_2 of 38, pH 7.28, with a base deficit of 11. Complete blood cell count with differential was in normal limits. Provisional diagnosis was coarctation of the aorta with a closing ductus.

Predeparture differential diagnosis by the transport nurse included the following:

1. Rule out sepsis
2. Respiratory distress/rule out pneumonia vs. PPHN vs. aspiration
3. Rule out congenital heart disease

Transport considerations included the distance of the trip, which was 1600 miles round trip, with an approximate trip time of 8 hours. Prostaglandin E_1 would be taken in the event the child had a ductal-dependent congenital heart defect. The transport team anticipated the need for full support; a neonatal nurse practitioner and a respiratory therapist were dispatched.

On arrival at the referring hospital, the infant was observed to be pale pink in a 78% hood in a crib. Further history from the nursing staff included an early nursery course remarkable for intermittent mild tachypnea with respiratory rates in the 60s and slight duskiness with agitation. The chest x-ray findings at 18 hours of age revealed increased perihilar streaking, fluid in the right fissure, and a normal cardiothoracic ratio. The x-ray film was otherwise unremarkable. Both history and x-ray findings were consistent with mild retained fetal lung fluid and borderline oxygenation.

The infant was placed on a radiant warmer with automatic temperature control. Transcutaneous PO_2 and PCO_2 monitors were placed. Physical examination was remarkable for a lethargic term infant who was pale pink in 78% oxygen by hood. Pulses were decreased in all extremities but equal with upper extremity blood pressures of 58 mm Hg by palpation and lower blood pressure extremities of 50 mm Hg by palpation. Capillary refill was 4 seconds with slight mottling. Heart tones were normal

with no murmur or extra sounds noted. Respiratory rate was 82; breath sounds were equal and clear with shallow air exchange. Peripheral IV was infusing with $D_{10}W$ at 80 ml/kg/day. Blood glucose level was 60. O_2 was increased to 85%, secondary to transcutaneous PO_2 of 50 with an increase to PO_2 of 54 and PCO_2 of 36. After consultation with the attending physician at the receiving hospital, 10 ml/kg of 5% albumin was begun by slow push through the peripheral IV. An umbilical artery catheter was placed and blood culture obtained. Continuous blood pressure monitoring was begun via umbilical catheter. Blood pressure after volume was 64/42 mm Hg, capillary refill 3+ seconds. Simultaneous preductal and postductal pulse oximeters were placed with results of 93% preductal and 85% postductal, indicating a shunting of blood at the ductal level.

Oxygen was increased to 100% by hood with no increase in transcutaneous PO_2. Baby was given 2 mEq/kg of sodium bicarbonate. Blood pressure remained at 60/36 mm Hg. A second 10 ml/kg of 5% albumin was administered with increase in blood pressure to 72/45 mm Hg and decrease in capillary refill time to 3 seconds.

An endotracheal tube was inserted, and hand ventilation was used to test for response to hyperventilation with decrease of $PaCO_2$ to 26. TCM began to increase, rising to transcutaneous PaO_2 of 78, with a transcutaneous $PaCO_2$ of 26. The patient was placed on 24 over 4, a rate of 60, and a 100% attempting to match hand ventilation. Arterial blood gas results revealed a PO_2 of 80, PCO_2 of 25, pH 7.43, and a base deficit of 6. Transport diagnoses included:

Health-care maintenance for a 38-week appropriate-for-gestational-age female. Plan: Fluids of $D_{10}W$ were continued at 80 ml/kg, and blood glucose levels were checked every 1 to 2 hours and remained stable throughout.

Respiratory distress; rule out PPHN. Plan: Blood pressure was monitored continuously throughout transport with a plan to support blood pressure with dopamine and volume as needed to prevent right-to-left shunting. Continued to hyperventilate, maintaining PCO_2 in the mid 20s and PO_2 >60.

Rule out sepsis. Plan: Antibiotics begun before transport.

Care during transport included cardiorespiratory monitor, continuous skin temperature monitoring, continuous blood pressure monitoring, continuous transcutaneous Po_2 and Po_2 monitoring, vital signs with axillary temperature every half hour throughout trip. Oral gastric tube was placed before transport to empty the stomach of any air or contents. The neonatal nurse practitioner and the referring physician spoke with the family, updating the patient's condition, current treatment, potential complications, and risks of transport. Transport consent was signed. The parents were also provided with information regarding intensive care nurseries and the specific information on the receiving nursery, including phone numbers, the attending physician, the policies regarding phone information, and visiting. A Polaroid photograph of the baby was left with the parents. After the baby was put in the transport Isolette, she was taken to the parents' room where the parents were encouraged to see her and touch her before departure. The parents were offered the option of having one parent accompany the baby to the receiving hospital, but this was declined. The baby was in stable condition tolerating the transport well.

CASE 2

Baby H. was a 28-week, 1430 g, appropriate-for-gestational-age male born to a gravida 5, para 3, who had no prenatal care. Previous history includes maternal IV drug abuse but denied use during pregnancy. The mother smokes a half pack of cigarettes per day. Prenatal laboratory data were unavailable.

The mother came to the emergency department in labor, where she was completely dilated with bulging membranes. Terbutaline was given 1 hour before delivery but did not stop labor. Phenobarbital was also given before delivery. The membranes were ruptured 30 minutes before delivery, and an attempt was made at a vaginal delivery, but the baby's presentation had changed to a transverse lie. A cesarean section was performed with the mother receiving epidural anesthesia.

Infant cried spontaneously and appeared to be about 28 weeks of gestational age by examination. Apgar scores were 6 at 1 minute and 8 at 5 minutes. A 2.5 endotracheal tube (ETT) was inserted. Initial ventilator settings were 20/4, rate 50, 100% Fio_2; arterial blood gases were pH 7.18, Pco_2 59, and Po_2 43. Umbilical artery and umbilical vein catheters were placed. Initial chest x-ray films revealed ETT down the left mainstem and air leak around ETT; reintubation with 3.0 ETT. Second chest x-ray film revealed bilateral reticular granular pattern with ETT down the right mainstem; ETT pulled back. The umbilical venous catheter was in the liver and was discontinued. Blood samples for culture and complete blood cell count were sent to the laboratory with these findings: complete blood cell count: white blood cell count 10.1 with 26% neutrophils, 61% leukocytes, 12M 1B, hematocrit 51, hemoglobin 17.1%, platelets 278,000. Initial blood glucose level 80. Antibiotics were given at 3:30 AM.

Attending physician called for transport because of inability to care for a premature infant on a ventilator. Transport team arrived 1 hour and 19 minutes after transport initiated. Predeparture differential diagnosis by transport nurse included:

1. *Premature appropriate-for-gestational-age male infant*
2. *Respiratory distress, probable RDS vs. group B streptococcal pneumonia*
3. *Rule out sepsis*
4. *Rule out maternal drug use*

Transport considerations included ventilatory management and thermoregulation because of the infant's extreme prematurity.

On arrival at the referring hospital, the patient was on a radiant warmer with temperature 37° C axillary, heart rate 163 beats/min, RR with ventilator, blood pressure 46/18 mm/Hg. Ventilator settings were 24/4, rate 60, 60% Fio_2 with arterial blood gases of pH 7.37, Pco_2 34, and Po_2 288. Pulse oximeter reading was 99. The team received report and x-ray films were viewed.

Because the umbilical venous catheter was discontinued, the neonatal nurse practitioner began a *peripheral IV for maintenance fluids. After discussion with the attending physician, it was decided to give exogenous surfactant. In-house time is lengthened because the patient's condition should be monitored in-house for at least a half hour after surfactant is given. Patient's ventilator settings were weaned using physical parameters (i.e., chest excursion, auscultation, and by monitoring transcutaneous readings and pulse oximetry). A second sample was sent for determination of arterial blood gas values 20 minutes after the surfactant. The values were as follows: pH 7.40, Pco_2 29, Po_2 142 on 22/4, rate 50, and 40% Fio_2. Transport diagnosis included:*

1. *Health-care maintenance for a 28-week appropriate-for-gestational-age male. Plan: Fluids of $D_{10}W$ in the PIV and normal saline solution in the umbilical artery catheter continued at 80 ml/kg/day. Blood glucose levels were checked every 1 to 2 hours and remained stable throughout.*
2. *Respiratory distress, presumed HMD. Plan: Continue to wean ventilator as indicated by above physical and monitor observations.*
3. *Rule out sepsis. Plan: Antibiotics were begun during transport.*
4. *Rule out maternal drug use. Plan: A urine toxicology screen would be sent when patient voided.*

Care during transport included all measures mentioned in Case 1. The patient's condition was stable, but he became agitated and began breathing against the ventilator. Fentanyl was given for sedation and the patient did not "fight the vent." On arrival at the hospital, report was given to the attending physician and bedside nurse. Care was transferred to the staff.

REFERENCES

1. American Academy of Pediatrics: *Guidelines for air and ground transport of neonatal and pediatric patients,* Elk Grove Village, Ill, 1999, Author.
2. American Academy of Pediatrics: Emergency drug doses for infants and children and Naloxone use in newborns: clarification, *Pediatrics* 83(5):803, 1989.
3. Apgar V: A proposal for new method of evaluation of the newborn infant, *Anesth/Analg* 32:260, 1953.
4. Babson SG, Behrman RE, Lessel R: Live-born birth weights for gestational age of white middle class infants, *Pediatrics* 45:937, 1970.
5. Bell EF et al: Effect of fluid administration on the development of symptomatic patent ductus arteriosus and congestive heart failure in premature infants, *N Engl J Med* 302:598, 1980.
6. Bell EF, Oh W: Fluid and electrolyte management. In Avery GB, Fletcher MA, MacDonald M, editors: *Neonatology,* ed 4, Philadelphia, 1994, Lippincott.
7. Berg TJ et al: Bronchopulmonary dysplasia and lung rupture in hyaline membrane disease: influence of continuous distending pressure, *Pediatrics* 55:51, 1975.
8. Buetow KC, Klein SW: Effect of maintenance of normal skin temperature on survival of infants of low birthweight, *Pediatrics* 34:163, 1964.
9. Caplan MS, MacKendrick W: Necrotizing enterocolitis: a review of pathogenetic mechanisms and implications for prevention, *Pediatr Pathol* 13:357, 1993.
10. Cappurro H et al: A simplified method for diagnosis of gestational age in the newborn infant, *J Pediatr* 93:120, 1978.
11. Carson BS et al: Combined obstetric and pediatric approach to prevent meconium aspiration syndrome, *Am J Obstet Gynecol* 126:712, 1976.
12. Day RL et al: Body temperature and survival of premature infants, *Pediatrics* 34:171, 1964.
13. Drage JS et al: The Apgar score as an index of infant morbidity: a report from the Collaborative Study of Cerebral Palsy, *Dev Med Child Neurol* 8:141, 1966.
14. Dubowitz LMS, Dubowitz V, Goldberg C: Clinical assessment of gestational age in the newborn infant, *J Pediatr* 77:1, 1970.
15. Flanagan MF, Fyler DC: Cardiac disease. In Avery G, Fletcher MA, MacDonald M, editors: *Neonatology,* ed 4, Philadelphia, 1994, Lippincott.
16. Fox WW, Duara S: Persistent pulmonary hypertension in the neonate: diagnosis and management, *J Pediatr* 98:505, 1983.
17. Freed MD et al: Prostaglandin E1 in infants with ductus arteriosus-dependent congenital heart disease, *Circulation* 64:899, 1981.
18. Greenough A, Dixon AK, Roberton NRC: Pulmonary interstitial emphysema, *Arch Dis Child* 59:1046, 1984.
19. Guzzetta PC et al: Surgery of the neonate. In Avery GB, editor: *Neonatology,* ed 3, Philadelphia, 1987, Lippincott.

20. Hart SM et al: Pulmonary interstitial emphysema in very low birthweight infants, *Arch Dis Child* 58:612, 1983.

21. Heyman MA: Biophysical evaluation of fetal status: fetal cardiovascular physiology. In Creasy RK, Resnik R editors: *Maternal fetal medicine,* Philadelphia, 1984, Saunders.

22. Hill A, Volpe JJ: Neurologic disorders. In Avery G, Fletcher MA, MacDonald M, editors: *Neonatology,* ed 4, Philadelphia, 1994, Lippincott.

23. Hill JR, Rahimtulla KA: Heat balance and the metabolic rate of newborn babies in relation to environmental temperature, and the effect of age and weight on basal metabolic rate, *J Physiol* 180:239, 1965.

24. Jacob J et al: The contribution of PDA in the neonate with severe RDS, *J Pediatr* 96:79, 1980.

25. Jaimovich DG, Vidyasagar D: *Handbook of pediatric and neonatal transport medicine,* St Louis, 1996, Mosby.

26. Kattwinkel J, editor: *Textbook of neonatal resuscitation,* ed 4, Elk Grove Village, Ill, 2000, American Academy of Pediatrics.

27. Kinsella JP, Abman SH: Recent development in the pathophysiology and treatment of persistent pulmonary hypertension of the newborn, *J Pediatr* 126:853, 1995.

28. Koops BL, Morgan LJ, Battaglia FC: Neonatal mortality risk in relation to birth weight and gestational age: update, *J Pediatr* 101:969, 1982.

29. Krupa DT, editor: *Flight nursing core curriculum,* Des Plaines, Ill, 1997, Road Runner Press.

30. Langer J et al: Timing of surgery for congenital diaphragmatic hernia: is emergency operation necessary? *J Pediatr Surg* 23:731, 1988.

31. Lubchenco LO, Hansman C, Boyd E: Intrauterine growth in length and head circumference as estimated from live births at gestational ages from 26 to 42 weeks, *Pediatrics* 37:403, 1966.

32. Lubchenco LO, Searls DT, Brazie JV: Neonatal mortality rate: relationship to birth weight and gestational age, *J Pediatr* 81:814, 1972.

33. Martin M, Paes BA: Birth asphyxia: does the Apgar score have diagnostic value? *Obstet Gynecol* 72:120, 1989.

34. Nelson N: Physiology of transition. In Avery G, Fletcher MA, MacDonald M, editors: *Neonatology,* ed 4, Philadelphia, 1994, Lippincott.

35. Niermeyer S: Evidence-based guidelines for neonatal resuscitation, *NeoReviews* 2:38, 2001.

36. Niermeyer S, Waldemar C, Boyle D, Goldsmith J, Nightengale B, Perlman J, Solimano A, Speer M, Wiswell T: What is on the horizon for neonatal resuscitation? *NeoReviews* 2:51, 2001.

37. Pagliari AS et al: Hypoglycemia in infancy and childhood, *J Pediatr* 82:365, 1973.

38. Phibbs RH: Delivery room management. In Avery G, Fletcher MA, MacDonald M, editors: *Neonatology,* ed 4, Philadelphia, 1994, Lippincott.

39. Philips JB, editor: Neonatal pulmonary hypertension, *Clin Perinatol* 11:515, 1984.

40. Pildes R et al: The incidence of neonatal hypoglycemia-a completed survey, *J Pediatr* 70:76, 1967.

41. Primhak RA: Factors associated with pulmonary air leak in premature infants receiving mechanical ventilation, *J Pediatr* 102:764, 1983.

42. Scopes JW, Ahmed I: Range of critical temperatures in sick and premature newborn babies, *Arch Dis Child* 41:417, 1966.

43. Shaul DB, Horth SB: Temperature regulation in preterm infants: Role of the skin-environment interface, *NeoReviews* 2:282, 2001.

44. Silverman WA, Fertig JW, Berger AP: The influence of the thermal environment upon the survival of newly born premature infants, *Pediatrics* 22:876, 1958.

45. Stoll BJ, Kliegman RM: The fetus and the neonatal infant. In Behrman RE, Kliegman RM, Jenson HB, editors: *Nelson's textbook of pediatrics,* ed 16, Philadelphia, 2000, Saunders.

46. Streeter NS: *High-risk neonatal care,* Rockville, Md, 1986, Aspen.

47. Sykes GS et al: Do Apgar scores indicate asphyxia? *Lancet* 1:494, 1982.

48. Whitfield JM: Neonatal transport. In McCloskey KAL, Orr RA, editors: *Pediatric transport medicine,* St Louis, 1995, Mosby.

49. Whitsett J et al: Acute respiratory disorders. In Avery G, Fletcher MA, MacDonald M, editors: *Neonatology,* ed 4, Philadelphia, 1994, Lippincott.

THE PEDIATRIC PATIENT

COMPETENCIES

1. Identify the differences between the pediatric and adult patient.
2. Perform a primary and secondary assessment of the pediatric patient in preparation for transport.
3. Identify the equipment necessary to perform a competent pediatric transport.

The care and transport of the ill or injured pediatric patient requires an ability to quickly assess and treat acute changes in a child's condition. Consideration of the critical anatomic and physiologic differences in this population is paramount for safe and effective intervention. An understanding of normal growth and development in children is an invaluable tool for the pediatric practitioner.

A DEVELOPMENTAL APPROACH TO PEDIATRIC ASSESSMENT

The assessment of an ill or injured child is for all intents and purposes not dissimilar to the evaluation of adults. The challenge in caring for children is the impact of growth and development on a variety of clinical factors. A child's age can present challenges in their ability to communicate verbally, their response to invasive procedures, and their ability to be separated from a family member, and it may be a risk factor for traumatic injury. To properly treat

children with injuries and, more importantly, be able to teach parents and children to avoid injury, growth and developmental factors must be used as a foundation for clinical care. Table 31-1 summarizes age-specific development and injury patterns.

Although not addressed in Table 31-1, children, regardless of age, are at risk for emergent complications that arise from infectious disease and metabolic/endocrine disorders. These will be discussed briefly later in this chapter. Box 31-1 contains examples of how to approach the pediatric patient using a developmental approach.[5]

PEDIATRIC RESUSCITATION

The resuscitation of the pediatric patient involves knowledge and skills that each transport team member needs to able to provide. Some transport programs use specialty teams to care for the child during transport. However, the majority of pediatric transport still continues to be provided by teams who do not specialize

TABLE 31-1	Age-Specific Development and Injury Patterns	
Age	Development	At-Risk Injuries
Infant 0-4 months	Feeding, holding, bonding/ dependence on caregivers.	Aspiration, SIDS, bathing injuries (burns, near drowning), environmental exposures (heat and cold), abuse/neglect/homicide/sexual assault/ MVCs/ improper vehicle restraint.
Infant 4-8 months	Introduction of solid foods, teething, rolling side to side, sitting up, crawling.	Falls, electrocution from cords/outlets, foreign body aspiration, toxic ingestions, MVCs without proper restraint, burns, near drowning, abuse/neglect/ homicide/sexual assault, lacerations, fractures, head/spine injuries.
Infant 8-12 months	Crawling, walking, increased motor coordination (opening doors, latches, etc.).	Falls, aspiration, foreign body ingestion, toxic ingestion, pedestrian vs. vehicle injuries near drowning, electrocution, MVCs without proper restraint, burns, suffocation, abuse/neglect/homicide lacerations, fractures, head and spine injuries.
Child 15 months- 3 years	Walking well and running, increased climbing skills, increased use of riding toys, use of utensils and cup, advanced motor skills (latches, doorways, match/ lighter use). Emotionally have increased desire for autonomy but have stranger anxiety. Beginning to speak simple sentences.	Falls, strike by vehicle both as pedestrian or bike rider, burns, suffocation, near drowning, toxic ingestions, foreign body aspiration, electrocution, MVCs without proper restraint, abuse/neglect/homicide, lacerations, fractures, head and spine injuries.
Child 4 years- 9 years	Bike riding, swimming skills, entry into school systems, use of tools, firearms, and weapons. Increased exposures to nonfamily members, involvement in team sports. Use of seat belts. Emotionally continue to increase autonomy with heightened body awareness and sensitivity to invasive exams/procedures. Rapidly increasing verbal skills.	Toxic ingestions, foreign body aspiration, electrocution, MVCs without proper restraint, abuse/neglect/ homicide, sexual assault, lacerations, fractures, head and spine injuries.
Child 10 years- 12 years	Rapid physical growth, learning complex social skills, beginning of alcohol/tobacco/drug experimentation, increased sexual experimentation, and involvement in largely physical team sports. Use of motorized vehicles. Emotionally have heightened awareness in gender differences, intense need for privacy, sense of responsibility,	Falls, strikes by vehicle both as pedestrian or vehicle rider, burns, near drowning, toxic ingestions, drug/alcohol overdose, foreign body aspiration, electrocution, MVCs without proper restraint, abuse/neglect/homicide, sexual assault, suicide, complications of pregnancy/contraception, lacerations, fractures, head and spine injuries.

TABLE 31-1	Age-Specific Development and Injury Patterns—cont'd	
Age	Development	At-Risk Injuries
	and need to be involved in decision making. May experience clinical depression.	
Child 12 years- 16 years	Increased incidence of risk-taking behaviors, increased autonomy in decisions of daily living, begin car driving, begin part-time jobs, increased sexual behavior, increased drug/alcohol/tobacco use. Emotionally have increased body image disturbances, increased need for independence/decision making. May suffer from clinical depression.	MVCs, falls, occupational injuries, strikes by vehicle both as pedestrian or bike rider, burns, near drowning, toxic ingestions, drug/alcohol overdose, foreign body aspiration, electrocution, abuse/ neglect/homicide/suicide, sexual assault, complications of pregnancy/contraception, lacerations, fractures, head and spine injuries.

SIDS, Sudden infant death syndrome; *MVC,* motor vechicle.

in pediatrics but have received additional education and training for working with this group of patients.

Pediatric resuscitation begins with the use of the pediatric advanced life support universal algorithm (Figure 31-1). The following is a more detailed description of the components of that algorithm as well as a discussion of the transport of the ill or injured pediatric patient.

PEDIATRIC AIRWAY MANAGEMENT/RESPIRATORY DISTRESS

The most important clinical skill for any clinician involved in pediatric care is the ability to assess respiratory distress and intervene appropriately. Nearly every life-threatening complication in pediatric care is related to inadequate oxygenation and ventilation.

PEDIATRIC AIRWAY ANATOMY

Pediatric airway anatomy differs from adult anatomy in the following ways (see Figure 12-5)[1]:

- Airway diameter in children is smaller when compared to adults.
- The tongue (especially in infants) is proportionately larger.
- The larynx is anteriorly located in infants and children.

- The epiglottis is long and narrow and angled away from the trachea.
- The vocal cords are attached lower anteriorly.
- In children younger than 10 the narrowest portion of the trachea is at the cricoid process.

The clinical implications of these differences are as follows.[1]

- Small amount of edema or obstruction can markedly decrease air exchange.
- Posterior displacement of the tongue may cause airway obstruction.
- Control of the tongue with the laryngoscope may be difficult.
- The angle between the base of the tongue and glottic opening is more acute, making straight blades more efficacious in visualizing the glottis.
- Control of the epiglottis with the laryngoscope blade may be more difficult.
- A blind endotracheal tube placement may become caught at the anterior commissure of the vocal cords.
- Properly sized endotracheal tubes will have an air leak with ventilation.
- Airway adjuncts for respiratory distress are listed in Box 31-2.

BOX 31-1   Developmental Stages and Approach Strategies for Pediatric Patients

Infants
Major fears
Separation and strangers
Approach strategies
Provide consistent caretakers.
Reduce parents' anxiety because it is transmitted to the infant.
Minimize separation from parents.

Toddlers
Major fears
Separation and loss of control
Characteristics of thinking
Primitive
Unable to recognize views of others
Little concept of body integrity
Approach strategies
Keep explanations simple.
Choose words carefully.
Let toddler play with equipment (stethoscope).
Minimize separation from parents.

Preschoolers
Major fears
Bodily injury and mutilation
Loss of control
The unknown and the dark
Being left alone
Characteristics of thinking
Highly literal interpretation of words
Unable to abstract
Primitive ideas about the body (e.g., fear that all blood will "leak out" if a bandage is removed)
Approach strategies
Keep explanations simple and concise.
Choose words carefully.
Emphasize that a procedure will help the child be healthier.
Be honest.

School-Age Children
Major fears
Loss of control
Bodily injury and mutilation

Failure to live up to expectations of others
Death
Characteristics of thinking
Vague or false ideas about physical illness and body structure and function
Able to listen attentively without always comprehending
Reluctant to ask questions about something they think they are expected to know
Increased awareness of significant illness, possible hazards of treatments, lifelong consequences of injury, and the meaning of death
Approach strategies
Ask children to explain what they understand.
Provide as many choices as possible to increase the child's sense of control.
Reassure the child that he or she has done nothing wrong and that necessary procedures are not punishment.
Anticipate and answer questions about long-term consequences (e.g., what the scar will look like, how long activities may be curtailed).

Adolescents
Major fears
Loss of control
Altered body image
Separation from peer group
Characteristics of thinking
Able to think abstractly
Tendency toward hyperresponsiveness to pain (reactions not always in proportion to event)
Little understanding of the structure and workings of the body
Approach strategies
When appropriate, allow adolescents to be a part of decision making about their care.
Give information sensitively.
Express how important their compliance and cooperation are to their treatment.
Be honest about consequences.
Use or teach coping mechanisms such as relaxation, deep breathing, and self-comforting talk.

From Sanders MJ: *Mosby's paramedic textbook*, ed 2, St Louis, 2000, Mosby.

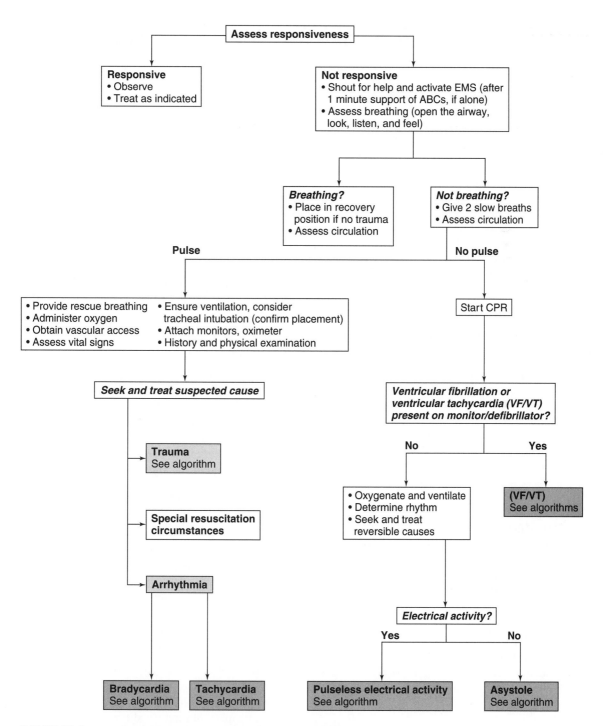

FIGURE 31-1 **Pediatric advanced life support universal algorithm.** (Reproduced with perrmission: *2000 handbook of emergency cardiovascular care,* Dallas, Copyright 2000, American Heart Association.)

BOX 31-2	Airway Adjuncts for Respiratory Distress in the Pediatric Patient

Nasal cannula. Children rarely tolerate flows >4 L/min. Not humidified.

Simple oxygen mask. Can deliver 35%-60% O_2 at 6-10 L/min.

Nonrebreathing mask with reservoir. Can deliver 95%-100% at 10-12 L/min.

Face tent or shield. Can deliver 40% O_2 at 15 L/min. Allows access to face without interrupting oxygen flow.

Oxygen hood. Plastic shell, which encompasses the child's head. Can deliver 80%-90% O_2 at 10-15 L/min. Usually not large enough for children over 1 year old.

Oropharyngeal airway. A plastic flange, which displaces the tongue from the posterior pharynx and provides an oral channel for ventilation and suction. The oral airway should be placed with a tongue depressor and direct visualization in the *unconscious* child in whom other airway maneuvers (jaw thrust/chin lift) have been unsuccessful at opening the airway. The proper size is determined by measuring externally. With the flange at the level of the mouth the tip should reach the angle of the jaw. Airways range from 4-10 cm in length.

Nasopharyngeal airway. A plastic or rubber tube that provides a conduit for air/oxygen from the nares to the posterior pharynx. It also allows for suctioning from the posterior pharynx. These airways are better tolerated in responsive patients. Proper size is again determined externally. The airway is approximated to equal the length from the tip of the nose to the tragus of the ear. A properly sized nasopharyngeal airway should not cause blanching of the external nares. These airways should be lubricated prior to placement.

INITIAL MANAGEMENT OF RESPIRATORY DISTRESS/ARREST IN THE PEDIATRIC PATIENT

- Open the airway. This can be accomplished by a jaw thrust or chin lift maneuver.
- Support breathing. This can be accomplished by using any of the preceding adjuncts dependent on clinical severity of the respiratory distress.

ADVANCED MANAGEMENT OF RESPIRATORY DISTRESS IN THE PEDIATRIC PATIENT

Some patients may present or progress to respiratory distress requiring more aggressive support. These patients can be supported with bag-valve-mask (BVM) ventilation (Box 31-3) with or without endotracheal intubation. A pediatric resuscitation bag is shown in Figure 31-2.

ENDOTRACHEAL INTUBATION

Endotracheal intubation is the most effective and reliable method of airway control for a variety of reasons.[1] These include:

- The airway can be isolated, ensuring adequate ventilation and oxygen delivery.

- The potential for aspiration is decreased.
- Ventilations with chest compressions can be provided more efficiently.
- Inspiratory times and pressures can be controlled.
- Positive end expiratory pressure (PEEP) can be delivered.
- Medications can be administered.
- Pulmonary toilet can be accomplished.

Indications for endotracheal intubation include[1-3]:

- Functional or anatomic airway obstruction
- Loss of airway protective reflexes
- Excessive work of breathing, which may lead to fatigue/respiratory insufficiency
- Need for high inspiratory pressures/PEEP
- Need for mechanical ventilatory support
- Potential for any of the preceding if patient transport is anticipated
- As a route for resuscitative medications

Endotracheal intubation is a skill that requires as much clinical judgment as it does manual skill. Pediatric practitioners must always assess for and anticipate respiratory distress. The ability to determine which patients will require aggressive ventilatory support is an indispensable talent. As

BOX 31-3	**Bag-Valve-Mask Ventilation**

This is a two-handed technique or preferably a two-person technique. With one hand or person securing the mask with an air tight seal, the other provides bag ventilation.

This is best performed with proper positioning. The child should be managed with a head tilt/chin lift maneuver while care is taken not to depress the submental area. Depression of the submental area may cause airway obstruction. Patients with suspected cervical spine injury should be managed with their cervical spine in a neutral position. Infants are often best managed in a neutral sniffing position, whereas toddlers benefit from a roll or towel placed under their head and neck to provide optimal airway patency. It may be necessary to attempt a variety of head and neck positions to find the optimal position for effective ventilation.

All bag-valve-mask ventilation should be provided with 100% oxygen. This is best achieved with the use of self-inflating bag-valve devices with an attached reservoir. Anesthesia ventilation systems may also be used but require greater training and experience to use successfully.

An oropharyngeal or nasopharyngeal airway (depending on the patient's level of consciousness) is helpful in providing more effective oxygenation/ventilation.

Gastric distention is common during bag-valve-mask ventilation. This distention may worsen respiratory embarrassment and lead to emesis. Relief of this distention with a gastric tube is extremely important in the pediatric population.

In the unconscious or extremely sedated patient, application of cricoid pressure (Sellick maneuver) may limit gastric distention and passive regurgitation.

A resuscitation bag should *not* have a pop off valve or one that is easily occluded to properly ventilate patients with poor lung compliance or airway resistance.

A manometer that attaches to the self-inflating bag can be helpful in assessing pressure ventilation during resuscitation.

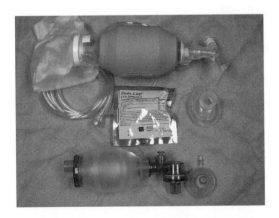

FIGURE 31-2   **Pediatric resuscitation bags.**

discussed earlier, children below the ages of 8 to 10 will have the cricoid process as the narrowest portion of their trachea. Because of this, uncuffed endotracheal tubes are the most appropriate choice in this group. There are a variety of ways to select proper endotracheal tube size. These include:

- Matching the outside diameter of the endotracheal tube to the child's little finger
- Matching the outside diameter of the endotracheal tube to the child's nares
- Use of length based resuscitation tapes (Broselow tapes)
- For children older than 2 years the formula:

$$\text{Endotracheal tube size} = \frac{16 + \text{age in years}}{4}$$

Multiplying the internal diameter of the endotracheal tube by 3 can approximate the proper depth of endotracheal tube placement (i.e., a 3.5-mm ET × 3 would be inserted 10.5 cm).

Preparation for endotracheal intubation is the most overlooked but often the most important part of the procedure. Being properly prepared for problems

Equipment Necessary for Intubation

Oxygen delivery system
Bag-valve resuscitation bag without pop off valve
Resuscitation masks of various pediatric sizes
Oral and nasopharyngeal airways of various pediatric
    sizes
Suction devices including pediatric-sized catheters
Pulse oximeter with pediatric probes
Cardiac monitor
If sedation and paralytics are used rescue meds (i.e.,
    naloxone) should also be available
Pediatric endotracheal tubes (Figure 31-3)/pediatric
    laryngoscope blades
Pediatric stylettes
End-tidal CO_2 detectors (disposable or in line)
Securing tape or device

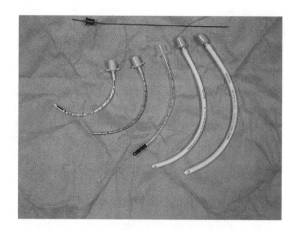

FIGURE 31-3   **Pediatric uncuffed endotracheal tubes.**

that may arise can often prevent life-threatening complications during this procedure. The necessary equipment is listed in Box 31-4.

Immediately after intubation proper tube placement can be verified clinically by a variety of means:

- Observation of symmetrical chest movement
- Auscultation of bilateral breath sounds high in the axillae
- Absence of breath sounds over the stomach
- Positive end-tidal CO_2 readings
- X-ray when clinically possible should verify proper tube placement

Esophageal obturator airways and oxygen-powered breathing devices are both discouraged in the pediatric population because of variability in patient sizes.[1-4]

NEEDLE CRICOTHYROIDOTOMY

A rare occurrence in the pediatric population is the necessity for control of the airway via surgical means.[2] A surgical airway can be placed through the cricothyroid membrane on children over the age of 11 (discussed in Chapter 12), but it is recommended that needle cricothyroidotomy be performed on children under this age (Figure 31-4).

Indications for needle cricothyroidotomy include:

- Complete airway obstruction
- Severe orofacial injuries
- Laryngeal transection
- Inability to secure the airway by less-invasive means

The procedure for needle cricothyroidotomy is shown in Box 31-5.

Complications of needle cricothyroidotomy include:

- Inadequate ventilation leading to hypoxia and death
- Aspiration (blood)
- Esophageal laceration
- Hematoma
- Posterior tracheal wall perforation
- Subcutaneous/mediastinal emphysema
- Thyroid perforation

Needle cricothyroidotomy does not protect the patient's airway from passive aspiration. Also, because of its limited lumen size, it is more effective in oxygenation than in ventilation. Needle cricothyroidotomy is a temporary measure until formal endotracheal tube placement or removal of the obstruction can be achieved.

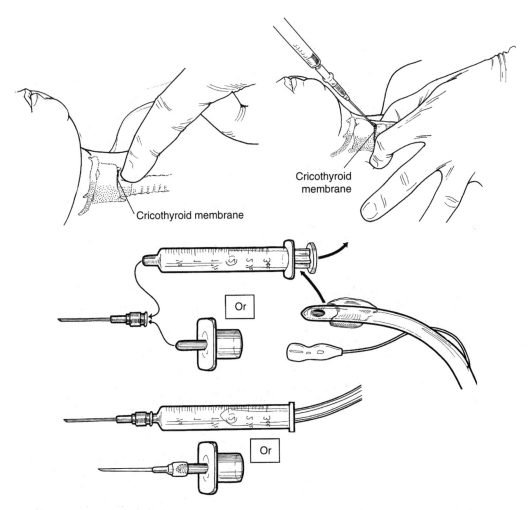

Cricothyroid membrane

Cricothyroid membrane

Or

Or

FIGURE 31-4 **Needle cricothyrotomy.** (From Dieckmann R et al: *Pediatric emergency and critical care procedures,* St Louis, 1997, Mosby.)

SELECTED DIAGNOSES PRESENTING WITH RESPIRATORY DISTRESS IN THE PEDIATRIC POPULATION

The next section of this chapter will deal with specific diagnoses that present with respiratory distress as their primary feature.

ASTHMA

Asthma is the most common chronic illness in the pediatric population. The rate of asthma continues to climb worldwide. A variety of environmental and immunologic factors appear to contribute to this increase.

CLINICAL PRESENTATION

The patient suffering an acute asthmatic attack will have expiratory wheezing as a hallmark finding. In a severe asthma exacerbation air exchange may be so limited that wheezing will not be appreciated. The patient will also have sensitive but nonspecific signs of respiratory distress including retractions, nasal flaring, cyanosis, accessory muscle use, and altered mental status. Peak expiratory flow will also be

BOX 31-5	Needle Cricothyroidotomy

1. Place the patient in a supine position.
2. Assemble a no. 14-gauge, 8.5-cm, over-the-needle catheter to a 10-cc syringe.
3. Surgically prepare the neck using antiseptic swabs.
4. Palpate the cricothyroid membrane between the thyroid and cricoid cartilage.
5. Stabilize the trachea with the thumb and forefinger to prevent lateral movement.
6. Puncture the skin in the midline over the cricothyroid membrane with the no. 14-gauge needle attached to the syringe. A small incision with a no. 11 blade may facilitate passage of the needle.
7. Direct the needle at a 45-degree angle caudally.
8. Carefully insert the needle into the lower half of the cricothyroid membrane, aspirating as the needle is advanced.
9. Aspiration of air signifies entry into the tracheal lumen.
10. Remove the syringe and stylette while gently advancing the catheter downward into position, taking care not to perforate the posterior trachea.
11. Oxygen can then be delivered in a variety of ways. Commercial jet insufflators are available for this purpose. Oxygen can also be supplied by attaching the adapter from a no. 3.0 endotracheal tube to the catheter and ventilating with a resuscitation bag. Finally, oxygen tubing can be cut with a hole toward the end of the tubing, which is then attached to the catheter hub. Once attached to an oxygen source of 50 psi or greater, oxygen can be delivered by occluding the hole with your thumb. Regardless of your oxygen delivery source, inspiration should be provided for 1 second while passive exhalation is provided for 4 seconds.

diminished and should be measured to gauge both acuity and patient's response to therapy. Patient history may reveal past exacerbations requiring the use of home medications. The number and frequency of home treatments is an important indicator of acuity.

TREATMENT

The primary goal of asthma treatment is reversal of hypoxemia as well as control of contributing inflammatory responses. First-line therapy continues to be providing supplemental oxygen and the use of beta-andrenergic and anticholinergic aerosols.[8] The most common are Albuterol or ipratropium bromide delivered via a nebulizer.

The frequency of administration of these medications is a much-debated subject. As with any clinical intervention, patient response should be closely monitored. A key component of asthma therapy is the control of inflammation, which is now felt to contribute to chronic airway changes. Acute inflammation is controlled with steroid therapy, most frequently with methylprednisolone IV or PO.

The use of inhaled steroids and medications that block inflammatory pathways are also being investi-

gated and may be used in the future for acute management.

CROUP

Croup is the common term for a viral infection that affects the larynx but may extend into the trachea and bronchi.

CLINICAL PRESENTATION

Patients generally present with a history of fever and coryza. As the illness progresses inspiratory stridor may be present as well as a characteristic "barking" cough. If the inflammation extends to the bronchi, rhonchi and wheezing may also be present. Care must be taken to rule out epiglottitis and retropharyngeal abscess because the presentations can be similar.

TREATMENT

Treatment for croup is primarily supportive and centers on treating dehydration and the treatment of respiratory distress. In rare severe cases, upper airway edema or obstruction may require endotracheal intubation for ventilation and airway protection.

Medications include Racemic epinephrine aerosols, Dexamethasone, and Prednisolone.

EPIGLOTTITIS

Epiglottitis is a rare but life-threatening bacterial infection of the epiglottis and surrounding structures. Epiglottitis has become increasingly rare with the advent of immunization for *Haemophilus influenzae,* which is the causative agent in 90% of epiglottitis cases.

CLINICAL PRESENTATION

Epiglottitis is second only to croup as a cause for infectious stridor. The course of epiglottitis is differentiated from other presentations because of its abrupt nature. Symptoms often occur rapidly causing parents to seek medical attention in 24 hours of the initial symptoms. Patients present with fever, stridor, labored respirations, and because of supraglottic edema, often present with drooling. The appearance of these children is also helpful in diagnosing epiglottitis. They are often anxious and present in a classic tripod position, sitting forward with their arms supporting them with their jaws thrust forward. This position is assumed by the patient to increase air entry. It is vital that clinicians recognize this presentation because of the life-threatening nature of airway involvement.

TREATMENT

The focus of treatment with epiglottitis is rapid recognition and treatment of airway obstruction. Patients in extremis must have their airway controlled prior to any other intervention. This includes lab work and usually intravenous access. Prior to dealing with these patients, creation of a well-defined epiglottitis algorithm is crucial. A lateral neck x-ray may be helpful in delineating epiglottitis from the much more common causes of stridor and respiratory distress. If endotracheal intubation is indicated, the support from anesthesiologist or ear, nose, and throat (ENT) staffs is invaluable. Use of the operating room with inhalation induction and rapid access to tracheostomy equipment is the optimal method of airway control. In situations without this support, endotracheal intubation should only be undertaken by staff capable of securing the airway, surgically if necessary. It is in the best interest of the patient with epiglottitis to have airway control prior to transport. Current antibiotic recommendations include cefuroxime, cefotaxime, and ceftriaxone.[8]

All patients with epiglottitis require intensive care admission.

FOREIGN BODY ASPIRATION

Aspiration of foreign bodies into the respiratory system can create difficult diagnostic challenges. Aspiration into the upper airway may be immediately life threatening with obvious clinical symptoms, whereas aspiration into the lower respiratory tract may present with varying degrees of severity. Sixty-five percent of lethal aspirations occur before the age of 2, and special consideration for education should be given to parents of these children. Foods most frequently associated with aspiration are hot dogs, candy, nuts, and grapes.

UPPER AIRWAY ASPIRATION

Clinical Presentation.   Patients with upper airway foreign body aspiration generally present in severe respiratory distress. There will be a history of a rapid onset of stridor, tachypnea, and in some cases total airway obstruction.

Treatment.   Complete airway obstruction should be managed initially with basic life support (BLS) measures such as the Heimlich maneuver in older children and chest thrusts in infants. If apneic, attempts at ventilation should also be provided. Failure of BLS measures should be followed by laryngoscopic visualization and attempts at removal. As discussed earlier in this module, unresolved total upper airway obstruction is an indication for needle or surgical cricothyroidotomy depending on the child's age.

LOWER AIRWAY ASPIRATION

The majority of lower airway foreign body aspirations occur in children under 3 years of age. The difficulty in treating these aspirations is the wide range of presentations and the difficulty in imaging nonradio opaque objects. A high index of suspicion must be maintained for at-risk age groups (6 months to 3 years) presenting with respiratory distress.

Clinical Presentation.   As stated earlier presentations can range from essentially asymptomatic to severe respiratory distress. A careful history is often helpful in diagnosing these children. Common presentations include new-onset coughing and wheezing. Less than half of these events are diagnosed on the day of aspiration. If sought, a history of a recent choking or aspiration episode is usually found in 75% of cases.

Treatment.   If an object is found by x-ray or if there is a strong likelihood of aspiration by history, bronchoscopy with removal of the aspirated object is the standard of care for these patients.

BRONCHIOLITIS

Bronchiolitis is a lower respiratory tract infection (primarily viral), which is one of the more common causes of new-onset wheezing in children. Respiratory syncytial virus (RSV) is the causative agent in the majority of cases, but parainfluenzae and *Mycoplasma pneumoniae* have also been isolated.

CLINICAL PRESENTATION

Wheezing is the most common presenting complaint, often with an accompanying 2- to 5-day course of coryza and cough. These patients are often tachypnic, with respiratory rates reaching 80 to 100/min in some cases. Nonspecific signs of respiratory distress such as nasal flaring and intercostal retractions are also present. Most cases occur in the winter months, with the majority of infections in children from ages 2 to 8 months. Apnea in children younger than 3 months is also characteristic of RSV infections.

TREATMENT

Once other causes for wheezing have been ruled out (asthma, foreign body aspiration, pneumonia), care is generally supportive. Supplemental oxygen, antipyretics, and adequate hydration are all helpful for patients in mild distress. Children may benefit from nebulized albuterol aerosols (doses noted earlier) and oral albuterol solution. Oral albuterol solutions are not indicated for patients who do not respond to aerosol therapy. Corticosteroids are not indicated for the treatment of bronchiolitis. There is some evidence the Ribavirin by continuous aerosol may be helpful in ameliorating the clinical course in severely ill, hospitalized children. Ribavirin therapy is difficult to provide in transport. Patients in severe distress who are unresponsive to therapy may require intubation and mechanical ventilation.

PNEUMONIA

Pneumonia, an inflammation of the pulmonary parenchyma, can be caused by a variety of bacterial, fungal, and viral agents. Discussion of all of the causative agents is beyond the scope of this module, so this process will be discussed in general terms.

CLINICAL PRESENTATION

Bacterial pneumonia generally has a rapid onset with accompanying high fevers, chills, and cough. The patient with bacterial pneumonia may also have grunting respirations, decreased breath sounds, and tachypnea, which are all nonspecific signs. Viral pneumonia, in contrast, has a more gradual onset over 2 to 4 days with cough coryza and low-grade fevers. Patients with viral pneumonia may also have rales, grunting respirations, tachypnea, and decreased breath sounds. In truth, bacterial and viral pneumonia are difficult to distinguish based on clinical exam alone. Leukocytosis over 15,000/mm^3 is a more predominant finding in bacterial pneumonia and would weigh against a viral diagnosis. A chest x-ray is often helpful in diagnosing these patients. Bacterial pneumonia will often show a lobar consolidation, whereas viral pneumonia will cause hyperaeration or diffuse interstitial infiltrate without consolidation.

TREATMENT

Treatment for these patients involves supportive measures with appropriate antibiotic therapy for bacterial infections. Dehydration is the most common complication of pneumonia, so adequate intake whether oral or intravenous is essential. Antipyretics will lower fevers as well as increase patient comfort. Drugs most commonly used in children for antipyretics include acetaminophen and ibuprofen.[8]

Sensitivity to these drugs should be determined prior to administration. Currently there is little data on the lower age limits for ibuprofen therapy, so caution should be used in younger children (<6 months). The practice of alternating these medications in patients is also being investigated. Supplemental oxygen for children in distress is also indicated. As with other respiratory illnesses, some children may require intubation and mechanical ventilation, dependent on the severity of pulmonary dysfunction. *Streptococcus pneumoniae* and *H. influenzae* remain the major bacterial causes for pediatric pneumonia. Medication therapy is dependent on the causative microorganism

Children who require hospital admission for pneumonia include[4]:

- Children <1 year old
- Patients with respiratory compromise
- Pleural effusion
- Pneumatocele
- Failure to respond to antibiotic therapy
- Dehydration

CONGENITAL HEART DISEASE AND METABOLIC ACIDOSIS

Two other causes of acute respiratory distress in children that may be encountered by the transport team are congenital heart disease and metabolic acidosis.

CONGENITAL HEART DISEASE

Because of varying rates of closure of the ductus arteriosus, clinical presentations of respiratory distress from congenital heart disease can present anywhere from a few days to 6 weeks after birth. The list of both cyanotic and acyanotic lesions that can cause respiratory distress in the newborns is too lengthy for discussion in this chapter. It remains important to keep cardiac processes on the list of differential diagnoses for children in this age-group.[4]

METABOLIC ACIDOSIS

Tachypnea from metabolic acidosis is a common clinical finding in pediatric patients. Respiratory buffering of acidosis may be the most obvious clinical finding in these situations. Tachypnea without an obvious cardiac or respiratory source should be further investigated to rule out metabolic acidosis.[4]

Causes of metabolic acidosis in children include:

- Diarrheal dehydration (most common cause)
- Diabetic ketoacidosis
- Renal failure (acute or chronic)
- Inborn errors of metabolism
- Poisons (salicylate, ethanol, methanol, ethylene glycol)
- Lactic acidosis (hypoxia, sepsis, shock)
- Hyperalimentation
- Enteric fistulas
- Ureterosigmoidostomy
- Drugs (e.g., mafenide (Sulfamylon), ammonium chloride, amphotericin, acetazolamide)
- Dilution (rapid volume expansion)

Once the cause of metabolic acidosis is identified and treated, respiratory distress should be quickly controlled. Supplemental oxygen including intubation and mechanical ventilation may be necessary during the acute treatment phase of these disorders.

PEDIATRIC TRAUMA

Outside of the immediate perinatal period, trauma and accidents continue to be the leading cause of death in all pediatric age groups. Although this section will focus on specific injuries and treatment, education aimed at the prevention of these avoidable injuries should always be the focus for emergency care providers and transport team members.

PHYSIOLOGIC/PSYCHOLOGIC CONSIDERATIONS

Pediatric patients have several unique physiologic, psychologic, and anatomic characteristics that must be considered when dealing with the acutely injured child.

SIZE/BODY SURFACE AREA

Because of children's smaller size and surface area, energy from traumatic injuries impart more force per unit of body area. The relative lack of body fat, the decreased elasticity of connective tissue, and the close proximity of internal organs to surface tissue all increase the potential for multiple injuries in this population. Increased body surface area also lends itself to increased thermal loss. Hypothermia becomes a major clinical concern for these patients.[1-3]

SKELETAL STRUCTURE

Incomplete calcification of the child's skeleton predisposes them to underlying soft tissue and organ injury without obvious overlying bony deformity. Multiple growth centers in the pediatric skeleton may also have clinical implications in their care. Skeletal fractures in children, especially in the thorax should heighten clinical suspicion of a high-energy injury with resultant trauma to underlying structures.[1-4]

PSYCHOLOGIC

As discussed previously in this chapter, children of different ages will present with very different emotional and developmental needs. Familiarity with these issues will allow the clinician to tailor the clinical approach and anticipate the patient's needs. It is also important to note that injuries and stress may cause regression in psychologic behavior, which in turn can complicate clinical management.

LONG-TERM EFFECTS OF TRAUMATIC INJURY

The effect of traumatic injuries on the growth and development of pediatric patients should never be underestimated. Evidence suggests that over 50% of children with multisystem injuries will have cognitive and personality changes up to a year after injury. Social, affective, and learning disabilities have all been linked to serious injuries in children. Damage to growth plates, amputations, or physical scars can have a lasting impact on not only physical function but emotional well-being as well. Pediatric injuries also create considerable strain to the family. Difficulties with finances, parental relationships, and sibling relationships are common issues when dealing with childhood injuries.[1-3]

Support from family services, social work, and psychologists/psychiatrists is invaluable in these situations.

THE PRIMARY SURVEY

The ABCDE algorithm (airway, breathing, circulation, disability, and exposure) for the initial survey of trauma in adults is also applied to pediatric patients. Again, consideration of their unique physiologic and anatomic differences is critical for proper assessment and care. Just as with the adult patient, the child's cervical spine needs to be appropriately immobilized.

AIRWAY AND CERVICAL SPINE IMMOBILIZATION

As discussed earlier, the establishment and maintenance of an open airway is critical to prevent complications in the pediatric population. Effective oxygenation and ventilation cannot take place until this is achieved.

An open airway is the number one priority in care. In children there is a disproportion in size between the child's head and midface. Placing the child in a "sniffing" position, with the midface placed superiorly and anteriorly, is the optimal alignment for airway protection. With traumatic injuries, care must be taken to maintain a neutral position of the cervical spine while opening the airway. (Immobilization of the cervical spine will be addressed in the disability portion of the primary assessment.) Padding of the backboard under a child's shoulders and posterior thorax will also aid in neutral alignment of the cervical spine (Figure 31-5).

A jaw thrust or chin lift maneuver in the unresponsive patient may be helpful in opening the airway. If the child is profoundly unconscious, an oral airway (as discussed earlier) aids in keeping the tongue out of the hypopharynx. An oral airway should be placed under direct visualization with a tongue blade to prevent oral trauma and subsequent bleeding.

Once the airway is opened and suctioned for debris/secretions, supplemental oxygen should be

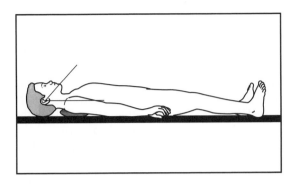

FIGURE 31-5 **Proper positioning of a child on a backboard.** (From Emergency Nurses Association: *Emergency nursing pediatric course: provider manual,* ed 2, Des Plaines, Ill, 1998, Author.)

provided. Patients with inadequate respiratory rates, impaired ventilation, or an inability to protect the airway from secretions/emesis should have their airway protected by endotracheal intubation. Prior to mechanical control of the airway, patients should be oxygenated via face mask or assisted bag-valve-mask ventilations.

Nasal intubations should not be performed on children less than 12 years of age because the acute angle to the glottis makes this an extremely difficult procedure while maintaining neutral cervical spine position. Needle or surgical cricothyroidotomy (dependent on age) may be necessary for airway protection for patients who cannot be successfully intubated.[1]

Many clinicians use as part of the airway management algorithm, rapid sequence intubation (RSI) protocols. Generally speaking, these protocols outline the use of intravenous medications to optimize patient condition for endotracheal intubation. Accurate weights are necessary to provide proper dosages during this procedure. Controversy exists over which specific medications are best for traumatically injured children. Bearing this in mind, most protocols use as the initial medication, atropine sulfate (0.01-0.02 mg/kg with no dose <0.1 mg) to block vagal responses to laryngoscopic instrumentation. Hypoxia is a major cause of bradycardia in the pediatric patient, so bradycardia during any airway procedure should be treated promptly with hyperventilation with supplemental oxygen.

Atropine is then followed by a short-acting sedative and a short-acting neuromuscular blocking agent. There are many medications that fulfill these requirements and can be safely used in children. The medications used in RSI are discussed in Chapter 12.

Under no circumstance should these potent medications be administered by persons unfamiliar with their actions and contraindications. The inability of a clinician to surgically control the airway should also preclude the use of neuromuscular blocking agents.

There is data that suggests lidocaine (1.0-1.5 mg/kg) may blunt increases in intracranial pressure in patients with head injuries requiring endotracheal intubation. Inclusion of lidocaine into the RSI protocol should be considered for patients with documented or suspected increased intracranial pressure.

Rescue airways such as the Combitube and the laryngeal mask airway (LMA) have limitations that may preclude their use in children. Familiarity with the contraindications for use of these devices is necessary before using them for pediatric patients.

BREATHING

After control of the airway and cervical spine has been achieved attention is then turned to oxygenation and ventilation of the patient. All trauma patients will require supplemental oxygen. Assessment of effectiveness of breathing and ventilation can be determined by a variety of factors.

Subtle findings of respiratory distress are often missed in pediatric patients. Respiratory rate is the initial factor assessed. Children have varying normal rates of respiration depending on age. An infant breathes 40 to 60 times per minute, whereas older children have rates of only 20 per minute. Tachypnea is an early but nonspecific sign of respiratory distress. Bradypnea is a late sign of distress and often heralds impending cardiorespiratory arrest. When assessing children, their respiratory rate, when viewed with other physical findings, often provides a much more accurate assessment of ventilation.

Work of breathing increases in children with respiratory distress. Increased work of breathing can present with any of the following clinical findings[3]:

- Nasal flaring
- Retractions (intercostal, subcostal, substernal, clavicular, and suprasternal)
- Head bobbing
- Grunting respirations
- Tripod positioning
- Paradoxical respirations (seesawing respirations with increased dependence on the diaphragm)
- Pallor
- Increased drooling or inability to control secretions
- Decreased gag reflex
- Altered respiratory rate (tachypnea, bradypnea, or apnea)
- Snoring
- Stridor
- Adventitious breath sounds (wheezing, rales, or rhonchi)
- Decreased or absent breath sounds
- Cyanosis (late sign of distress)

As discussed earlier, any of these findings require support with supplemental oxygen and may require, dependent on the severity of distress, assisted ventilation with a bag-valve mask or endotracheal intubation.

Selected Traumatic Injuries That Contribute to Respiratory Distress.

Injuries to the thorax are a common cause of respiratory distress after traumatic injuries. Physiologic differences in children change the patterns of injury. As discussed previously a child's ribs are more cartilaginous, so rib fractures are uncommon, whereas injuries to underlying structures (i.e., pulmonary/cardiac contusions) occur more frequently. The pediatric mediastinum is more mobile and easily shifted, which can contribute to ventilatory and cardiovascular compromise. The thinness of the chest wall makes respiratory assessment more difficult because breath sounds may be referred from one area of the chest to another making it difficult to diagnose atelectasis and pneumothoraces.[3]

Tension Pneumothorax. This occurs when air enters the pleural space on inspiration but cannot escape on expiration. Rapidly rising intrathoracic pressures can lead to rapid ventilatory and cardiovascular collapse. This is a **life-threatening** complication. A tension pneumothorax is characterized by decreased or absent breath sounds on the affected hemothorax, dyspnea, hypotension, neck vein distention, cyanosis, and as a late sign, tracheal deviation. Subcutaneous emphysema may be appreciated with tactile examination of the chest. Intubation and mechanical ventilation may put trauma patients at risk for this complication because intrathoracic pressure will increase with positive-pressure ventilation. Tension pneumothoraces are diagnosed by clinical not radiographic exam.

Treatment for Tension Pneumothorax. Initially treated with needle decompression with a no. 14 to no. 16 Angiocath placed into the intrapleural space at the second intercostal space at the midclavicular line of the affected hemothorax. Tube thoracostomy with a size-/age-appropriate chest tube, at the fifth intercostal space at the anterior mid axillary line of the affected hemothorax is definitive treatment. Chest tubes should have a one-way flutter valve attached or be placed to water seal drainage to prevent reaccumulations of air. Tension pneumothoraces should always be treated prior to transport.

Simple Pneumothorax. Occurs when air enters the pleural space causing a loss of negative pressure between the visceral and parietal pleura. This loss of pressure will lead to partial or total lung collapse. A simple pneumothorax is characterized by decreased breath sounds over the affected hemothorax, dyspnea, hyper-resonance of the affected hemothorax, and chest pain with radiation to the shoulders. Subcutaneous emphysema may be appreciated with tactile examination of the chest.

Treatment for Simple Pneumothorax. Treatment consists of placement of a size-/age-appropriate chest tube to the fifth intercostal space, at the anterior midaxillary line of the affected side. An alternative site for chest tube placement is the second intercostal space at the midclavicular line of the affected hemothorax.

Chest tubes should be attached to one-way flutter valves or water seal drainage to prevent reaccumulation of air. An anterior approach is inappropriate if both air and fluid are suspected in the pleural space. Suspected pneumothoraces not causing severe respiratory or cardiovascular compromise should be confirmed radiographically as other conditions (e.g., diaphragmatic hernia) may present with similar clinical findings. All pneumothoraces greater than 20% or any pneumothorax present in patients requiring positive pressure ventilation should be treated with tube thoracostomy prior to transport.

Open Pneumothorax. Open pneumothorax occurs when an open wound allows free movement of air into and out of the pleural space. Collapse of the lung and impaired ventilation result. An open pneumothorax is characterized by the presence of a penetrating chest wound, dyspnea, chest pain, and hyperresonance and decreased breath sounds over the affected hemothorax. An audible "sucking" sound may be heard during inspiration and expiration.

Treatment for Open Pneumothorax. Treatment of this complication requires the clinician to treat both the lung collapse and the penetrating wound. A sterile occlusive dressing, taped on three sides, should be immediately placed over the wound. It is taped on three sides to allow for venting of the pleural space by lifting the dressing, should reaccumulation of intrapleural air occur. If untreated, reaccumulation of pleural air can lead to tension pneumothorax. After the wound is treated a chest tube should then be inserted as discussed earlier to treat lung collapse and prevent tension pneumothorax during transport. This chest tube should be placed remotely from the penetrating wound to decrease the risk of intrathoracic infection.

Hemothorax. Hemothorax occurs when blood accumulates in the pleural space. When more than 1500 ml of blood accumulates in the pleural space, a hemothorax is deemed massive. A hemothorax is characterized by dyspnea, chest pain, decreased or absent breath sounds over the affected side, and dullness to percussion of the affected hemothorax.

Signs of shock (related to the blood loss) may also be present.

Treatment for Hemothorax. Treatment for this complication also requires a two-pronged clinical approach. The affected hemothorax must be decompressed and drained with an age-/size-appropriate chest tube placed in the fifth intercostal space of the anterior midaxillary line. The chest tube needs then to be placed to water seal drainage with suction. Controversy surrounds how much blood should be drained from the pleural space prior to clamping the thoracostomy tube. Advanced trauma life support (ATLS) guidelines state the tube should be clamped after 1000 ml of blood is removed in adult patients. Pediatric patients have a circulating volume of 80 ml/kg. The 1000 ml in adults represents one fifth of the circulating volume (in an average-sized patient) so a similar 20% loss in children (depending on size) may require thoracostomy tube clamping. It is important to remember that tube clamping is a temporizing measure until open thoracotomy can be performed. Fluid resuscitation for blood loss with crystalloid and possibly transfusion therapy also needs to be initiated in these patients. Fluid resuscitation is discussed in depth in the shock management section of this module.

Flail Chest. Flail chest occurs when rib fractures of more than two ribs at more than two sites causes a segment of the chest to lose continuity with the rest of the thoracic cage. Flail chest injuries are very uncommon in children because of the lack of rib calcification, but they can occur with adolescents. A flail chest is characterized by paradoxical chest wall movement of the affected segment during inspiration and expiration, chest pain, dyspnea, hypoxia, and cyanosis.

Treatment for Flail Chest. Treatment of flail chest injuries centers around support of ventilation, provision of humidified oxygen, and careful fluid administration to prevent overhydration. The underlying pulmonary contusion is the primary concern of this injury. Without the presence of systemic hypotension, great care should be taken to prevent overhydration. These injuries can be very difficult to manage because the affected lung is sensitive to both over- and underresuscitation. Some patients will require intubation for ventilatory support. Analgesia to control the severe pain of this injury is also beneficial in supporting the patient's ventilatory status.

Pulmonary Contusion. Pulmonary contusion occurs when lung parenchyma is traumatically injured causing leakage of blood and fluid into the interstitial spaces. Pulmonary contusions are characterized by dyspnea, tachypnea, bloody sputum, and possibly obvious chest wall injuries. It can be difficult to clinically appreciate pulmonary contusions on exam, and a high index of suspicion should be maintained for patients suffering thoracic injuries or those involved in rapid deceleration injuries. Radiologic changes may not be present until 24 hours postinjury.

Treatment for Pulmonary Contusion. The treatment of this injury involves care fluid resuscitation as noted earlier and support of the patient's ventilatory status. Use of steroids and diuretics for these injuries remains controversial.

Diaphragmatic Rupture. Diaphragmatic rupture occurs when a traumatic injury causes a defect in the diaphragm allowing for herniation of abdominal contents into the thoracic cavity. Some injuries may only cause small diaphragmatic tears that take time (even years) to develop into diaphragmatic herniations. The majority of these injuries occur in the left hemothorax because the liver serves as protection for the right hemidiaphragm. Herniation of abdominal contents causes compression of the ipsilateral lung and possible shift of mediastinal structures. Intestinal or gastric obstruction/ischemia may also occur.

Diaphragmatic ruptures are characterized by dyspnea, dysphagia, chest pain, sharp shoulder pain, auscultation of bowel sounds over the lower thorax, and decreased breath sounds over the affected hemothorax. Radiographic studies may show shift of thoracic structures, the presence of the gastric silhouette above the diaphragm, and if present, the radio opaque gastric tube curled in the lower left chest.

Treatment for Diaphragmatic Rupture. The definitive treatment of diaphragmatic rupture is

surgical repair. Clinical support of ventilation and gastric decompression is necessary prior to surgical intervention/transport.

Tracheobronchial Injuries. Tracheobronchial injuries occur when blunt or penetrating trauma causes a tear in the trachea or bronchus allowing air to enter the pleural space or mediastinum. These injuries are characterized by palpable subcutaneous emphysema (in the neck, face, and thorax), dyspnea, hemoptysis, and absent breath sounds to the affected hemithorax. Hamman's sign, which is a crunching sound auscultated to the anterior chest that is synchronized to the patient's heartbeat, may also be appreciated. A pneumothorax that reaccumulates after chest tube insertion and placement to water seal drainage and suction should heighten a clinician's suspicion for tracheobronchial injuries.

Treatment for Tracheobronchial Injuries. Intubation with placement of the tube distal to the injury site should be accomplished. This can be extremely difficult in the transport setting because the level of injury may be difficult to appreciate and fiber-optic support is rarely available. Patients may require more than one chest tube placed on the affected hemithorax, and they made need them placed both anteriorly and laterally as described earlier. All of these patients must be closely monitored for development of tension pneumothorax during transport. Surgical intervention for repair of these injuries will be required.

Sternal Fractures/Rib Fractures. Both of these injuries are fortunately rare in children but may be present in adolescents. Injuries to these areas with or without fracture should always raise concern for damage to underlying structures (i.e., cardiac and pulmonary contusions, aortic injuries). These injuries are characterized by pain to the injured area, splinting of respirations, dyspnea, ecchymosis, and possibly crepitus.

Treatment for Sternal/Rib Fractures. Treatment for these fractures centers on ventilatory support and providing appropriate analgesia. As discussed, clinical examination for damage to underlying structures should always take place.

CIRCULATION

The third step in trauma assessment is determining the circulatory status of the patient. In traumatic injuries this centers primarily on the estimation and treatment of fluid/blood loss, which accompanies traumatic injuries. Again, physiologic differences in pediatric patients make this assessment more difficult than in adults. Knowledge of the normal parameters of heart rate, blood pressure, and respiratory rates in various age-groups is essential for accurate diagnosis. Physical examination combined with a history of the injury mechanism is extremely helpful in identifying patients requiring circulatory support.

Physical Examination. Clinical signs and symptoms of fluid/blood loss in pediatric patients after traumatic injuries include the following:

- Altered level of consciousness. In preverbal children this may be manifested as an inability to recognize parents/caregivers.
- Decreased response to stimuli or the environment. This is often identified by decreased pain response to procedures such as intravnous (IV) starts or reduction of fractures.
- Restlessness/anxiety.
- Confusion/irritability.
- Dry mucous membranes/absence of tears.
- Tachypnea.
- Tachycardia. In the early stages of shock, tachycardia with a widened pulse pressure may be the only clinical finding in patients with fluid/blood loss.
- Changes in skin color. This includes patients who appear ashen, pale, mottled, or cyanotic.
- Capillary refill greater than 2 to 3 seconds. This can be an extremely sensitive measure of circulatory status in children. Care must be taken when examining the hypothermic patient as hypothermia may increase capillary refill time without fluid/blood loss.
- Changes in the quality of pulse pressures. Peripheral pulses in severe shock will be weak and thready.
- Cool diaphoretic skin.
- Difficulty in obtaining a blood pressure. With vasoconstriction from catecholamines release

and decreased cardiac output, blood pressure readings may be difficult to obtain in pediatric patients. Children can remain normotensive in moderate to severe shock because of sustained catecholamine response. Blood pressures can be the vital sign least reflective of circulatory status in children. Other clinical indicators as listed earlier are often much more sensitive. *Hypotension and bradycardia after traumatic injuries in children are ominous clinical findings and need to be treated aggressively.*

- Decreased or absent breath sounds.
- Decreased urine output. Placement of a urinary catheter early in the care of traumatically injured children is essential for assessment of circulatory status and effectiveness of resuscitation. End organ perfusion (i.e., kidneys) will decrease with fluid/blood loss and will be reflected by oliguria or anuria. Maintenance of 1 to 2 ml/kg/hr of urine output is the goal of circulatory support in the pediatric patient.

Circulatory compromise in children can often be subtle and must be found by a careful physical examination. Waiting for major changes in vital signs or laboratory studies will increase patient morbidity and often make resuscitation more difficult.

Monitoring of the patient is required during assessment and resuscitation of traumatically injured children. Cardiac monitoring and pulse oximetry monitoring can aid in initial assessment and monitoring of ongoing patient status.

A normal pulse oximetry reading does not preclude a patient's need for supplemental oxygen and may not accurately reflect tissue oxygenation.

A laboratory study that may be helpful in assessing the circulatory status of trauma patients includes:

- A complete blood cell count, especially hematocrit levels.
- Serum or finger stick glucose measurement.
- Electrolytes.
- Arterial/venous blood gases. Decreasing pH indicates acidosis developing from oxygen debt and anaerobic metabolism. Elevated $Paco_2$ indicates respiratory acidosis and impaired

ventilation, while a deceased PaO_2 is indicative of hypoxia. Decreased HCO_3^- indicates buffering of acidosis. The blood gas can be a very helpful tool in the initial assessment of ventilation and fluid status in the injured child.

- Lactate level.
- Urinalysis to measure specific gravity.

Diagnostic studies that may be helpful in assessing circulatory status of trauma patients include:

- Chest radiograph to evaluate for hemothorax, aortic injury, and pulmonary contusion
- Head computed tomography (CT) to evaluate intracranial blood loss
- Abdominal/pelvic CT
- Pelvis x-ray to evaluate for pelvic fractures
- Long-bone x-rays, especially of the femurs, which can account for significant blood loss

After determining circulatory status, care is focused on prevention of further fluid loss (i.e., controlling bleeding) and replacement of fluid/blood loss. Fluid resuscitation will be discussed at length in the shock management portion of this chapter.

Selected Traumatic Injuries That Can Lead to Fluid/Blood Loss or Circulatory Compromise.   Any injury that causes bleeding or fluid loss has the potential to cause patient compromise if not treated. The following injuries are of greatest concern for major blood/fluid loss in the pediatric trauma patient.

Head Injuries/Scalp Lacerations.   Epidural bleeding (bleeding between the skull and dural meninges) and subdural bleeding (bleeding between the dura and the brain) can cause lethal amounts of blood loss in pediatric patients. As discussed earlier, pediatric patients have an estimated circulating volume of 80 ml/kg. Combined with the fact that infants have a proportionately larger amount of blood volume in their head, this can lead to hypovolemia with relatively small amounts of intracranial hemorrhage. Infants with fontanelles and open cranial sutures may have increased bleeding and intracranial pressure. The vascularity of the head

and scalp can also lead to hypovolemia from scalp lacerations, and aggressive fluid resuscitation may be required. The support of circulatory status takes precedence over management of increased intracranial pressure by fluid restrictions. (Head injuries will be discussed in depth in the disability section of trauma care.)

Facial/Mandibular Injuries.   As with the scalp, the bony structures of the skull are very vascular and can bleed profusely when injured. Patients with LeForte fractures or open mandibular fractures may require aggressive resuscitation. Clinical findings are often very obvious with frank external bleeding noted. After airway control is achieved some patients may require oral and retropharyngeal packing to control bleeding. Marked facial swelling and ecchymosis may also be present with these injuries.

Treatment of Facial Mandibular Injuries. Treatment is focused on basic support and involves maintenance of a clear and secure airway and bleeding control. Patients will often require fluid resuscitation but may also require transfusion therapy, depending on their response to crystalloid support.

Massive Hemothorax.   This injury was discussed in depth in the preceding section.

Cardiac Injury.   Injuries to the heart can be caused by either blunt, or penetrating traumatic forces, causing a variety of pathologic conditions.

Cardiac Tamponade.   This occurs when blunt or penetrating injury causes bleeding from the heart (cardiac rupture), the pericardial vessels, or the great vessels, to accumulate in the pericardial sac. As little as 15 to 20 ml of blood can interfere with cardiac activity. Fortunately, removal of these same small amounts can drastically improve cardiac function. Clinically, cardiac tamponade is diagnosed by the presence of muffled heart tones, hypotension, and distended neck veins (Beck's triad). It is important to remember that other clinical conditions, such as hypovolemia, or environmental concerns, such as noise, can make this diagnosis difficult.

Cardiac tamponade should be considered in all patients with blunt or penetrating thoracic injuries.

Pulseless electrical activity in the absence of tension pneumothorax and hypovolemia is highly suggestive of cardiac tamponade. Kussmaul's sign (a rise in venous pressure with inspiration) and pulsus paradoxus (a decrease of >10 mm Hg of systolic blood pressure with inspiration) are extremely difficult to assess in the transport setting but are also indicative of cardiac tamponade.

Treatment of Cardiac Tamponade. Treatment of this injury is rapid pericardiocentesis to decompress the pericardium. It is assumed prior to initiation of pericardiocentesis that the patient has not responded to fluid resuscitation to raise venous pressure. A subxiphoid approach with a spinal needle or an over-the-needle catheter attached to a 30-cc syringe with a three-way stopcock is the preferred method of aspiration. The needle is directed to the pericardium at a 45-degree angle while aspirating. Cardiac monitoring to assess for ventricular arrhythmias or irritability is required. Because the pericardium is self-healing, aspiration of a small amount of blood may be all that is necessary as a temporizing measure to definitive surgical care. Controversy surrounds leaving a needle or catheter in place during transport because risks of inadvertent cardiac damage may outweigh the benefits.

Myocardial Contusion. Myocardial contusion occurs when blunt force is delivered to the myocardium, causing injury. With relatively smaller amounts of subcutaneous fat and cartilaginous ribs, children are at great risk for this injury. Patients with this injury often complain of chest pain. Definitive diagnosis can only be made by direct inspection of the myocardium. As this is rarely done, clinicians must assess for complications of myocardial contusion, which include hypotension, conduction abnormalities, or wall motion abnormalities on echocardiography. Common arrhythmias include premature ventricular contractions, unexplained sinus tachycardia, atrial fibrillation, and bundle branch blocks (primarily on the right). Electrocardiographic exams may show ST segment abnormalities and may indicate myocardial infarction.

Treatment of Myocardial Contusion. Treatment of myocardial contusion is supportive.

Patients require at least 24 hours of cardiac monitoring. The risk for sudden arrhythmia decreases greatly after 24 hours. Significant arrhythmias should be treated by ACLS protocols, and cardiology consultation may be indicated.

Traumatic Aortic Disruption. Traumatic aortic disruption occurs when the aorta is damaged from rapid deceleration most common in motor vehicle crashes and falls from great heights. Traumatic aortic disruption is often rapidly fatal, but survival is increased with rapid detection and surgical intervention. Most survivors of this injury have partial lacerations at the level of the ligamentum arteriosum and survive because of contained hematoma at the site. Unexplained persistent hypotension is usually not related to this injury, and other bleeding sources should be sought.

A transected aorta that bleeds freely into the left chest can cause profound hypotension but is quickly fatal (in minutes) without operative intervention. Clinical signs and symptoms of this injury are often absent, and a high index of suspicion must be maintained for patients with mechanisms of injury that involve rapid deceleration. Chest radiograph findings that may be indicative of major vessel injury are listed in Box 31-6.[2]

BOX 31-6	**Chest Radiograph Findings That May Indicate Major Vessel Injury**

A widened mediastinum
Obliteration of the aortic knob
Deviation of the trachea to the right
Obliteration of the space between the pulmonary artery and the aorta
Depression of the left main stem bronchus
Deviation of the esophagus or the gastric tube to the right
Widened paratracheal stripe
Widened paraspinal interfaces
Presence of a pleural or apical cap
Left hemothorax
Fractures of the first or second rib or scapula

False positive and negative radiograph findings are possible, so any patient with the possibility of aortic injury should be further evaluated radiographically. Angiography continues to be the gold standard for diagnosis, but CT of the chest and transesophageal echocardiography may also show aortic injury.

Treatment of Traumatic Aortic Disruption. Treatment of this injury is operative repair either by resection and grafting or primary repair. Hemothoraces should be treated as described earlier, and fluid resuscitation should be provided based on patient need.

Abdominal Injuries.

Blunt trauma is the cause of the majority of abdominal injuries in children. Anatomic differences in children predispose them to injuries. These include a less-developed abdomen resulting in less protection from injury, a more protuberant abdomen placing vital organs closer to impacting forces, and a small thorax with compliant ribs decreasing protection to the liver and spleen.

Abdominal examination can be extremely difficult in the pediatric population because fear from exam or pain from distracting injuries interferes with assessment. Preverbal children are unable to describe or complain of pain. Abdominal findings can be very subtle and are often missed on initial examination. A high index of suspicion should always be maintained with patients suffering multisystem injury.

Spleen and Liver Injuries.   These solid organs are the most commonly injured in pediatric abdominal trauma. Disruption of the vascular supply to these organs can result in massive hemorrhage. Clinical signs may be subtle but may include point and rebound tenderness, radiation of pain to the left shoulder in splenic injuries, ecchymosis or abrasion to the upper quadrants, lower rib fractures, and abdominal distention. Signs of shock may be present with significant injury.

Treatment of Spleen and Liver Injuries. Treatment of these injuries requires fluid resuscitation (discussed in the shock portion of this module) and surgical evaluation. Splenectomy is undesirable in children because of the increased rates of sepsis in children postsplenectomy. Prompt transport to an institution with pediatric surgical capabilities is imperative with these patients.

Stomach Injuries.   Stomach injuries rarely occur as a result of trauma but can occur with lap belt, air bag, and handlebar injuries. A greater concern in the pediatric trauma patient is gastric dilation from hyperventilation or assisted ventilation. Gastric dilation can lead to circulatory and respiratory embarrassment if untreated. All pediatric patients with multisystem injury or requiring assisted ventilation should have their stomachs decompressed with a gastric tube to prevent these complications. Gastric tubes can be used if the patient does not have known or suspected facial or head injuries.

Pancreatic and Duodenal Injuries.   Pancreatic and duodenal injuries occur in children as a result of rapid deceleration, often in conjunction with lap belt use or falls onto handlebars. These injuries are extremely difficult to diagnose clinically and need to be ruled out radiographically in patients at risk. Their clinical examinations can be variable but should be suspected with the previously noted mechanisms or obvious trauma to the abdomen. Treatment of these injuries is supportive and requires surgical evaluation.

Genitourinary Injuries.   Although injuries to the genitourinary system are rarely fatal, they may be accompanied by hemorrhage and shock. The kidneys in pediatric patients are less protected by fat and are more mobile than in adults, increasing their risk for injury. Fortunately, because of its anatomic position in children, the bladder is less likely to be injured by pelvic fractures. The genitourinary system in children can be injured by vehicle restraints in deceleration injuries or by falls with direct blunt trauma.

As with many abdominal injuries, a high index of suspicion must be maintained for patients with mechanisms of injury likely to cause trauma to the genitourinary system. Clinical findings may be subtle, and hematuria is an insensitive predictor of injury. Treatment of these injuries is supportive and requires surgical evaluation.

Pelvic Fractures.

Pelvic fractures are rare in young children but can be common traumatic injuries in late adolescence. Mechanisms of injuries include motor vehicle crashes and falls with direct blunt trauma. Lethal retroperitoneal hemorrhage can accompany these fractures, requiring prompt immobilization and aggressive fluid resuscitation.

Clinical findings include obvious visual asymmetry, instability and pain to palpation, pain with adduction of the legs, and ecchymosis. As noted, these findings may also present with profound hypotension and shock.

Treatment of Pelvic Injuries.   Controversy surrounds the most appropriate method of stabilizing these fractures for transport. MAST trousers (while recognizing their limitations in other areas of resuscitative care) may be the best transport option. Care must be taken that MAST trouser pressure gains and losses with altitude change during air transport are closely monitored.

Stabilization with sheet strapping and external fixators are other splinting options dependent on fracture patterns and orthopedic surgeon availability. Pelvic fractures without hemodynamic instability may only require close observation during transport.

More aggressive immobilization (as discussed previously) should be reserved for patients presenting with clinical signs of fluid loss. Fluid resuscitation with both crystalloids and blood products may be necessary.

Femur Fractures.   Fractures of the femur, much like fractures of the pelvis, can cause significant amounts of blood loss in children. Femur fractures are rarely isolated injuries and are often part of a constellation of multisystem damage. Clinical findings include shortening of the affected leg, obvious deformity of the femur, pain to palpation at the site, and ecchymosis. Wounds in the areas of suspected or obvious fracture should heighten concerns for open fracture at the site.

Treatment of Femur Fractures.   After assessment of neurovascular function, fractured femurs should be aligned and immobilized. Traction splints, air splints, or a variety of commercial splints can be used for immobilization. If air splints are used for transport, it is again important to monitor

for pressure gains and losses during altitude changes. After alignment and immobilization, a neurovascular assessment should be repeated. Fluid resuscitation with crystalloids and blood products may be required. Antibiotic coverage should be considered with the presence of open wounds.

DISABILITY

The fourth step in the primary assessment of injured children is evaluation of injuries that cause patient disability.

Head injuries and spinal cord injuries are the primary sources of disability in the pediatric trauma patient. Head injuries continue to be the leading cause of death in traumatically injured children. Anatomic differences in children that predispose them to head injuries include head size that is disproportionate to body surface area, open fontanelles and cranial sutures that allow for increased intracranial swelling, and poorly developed neck and upper extremity musculature offering less protection to the head and neck.

A rapid neurologic assessment provides immediate information on patient condition and provides a baseline for further evaluations. A neurologic examination is especially important if paralytics or sedatives are utilized in patient care. Factors that are evaluated in a rapid neurologic assessment include level of consciousness, pupillary response, and gross motor function.

Level of Consciousness.   Determining level of consciousness in older verbal children is the same as the assessment in adults. Using the AVPU mnemonic (A = Awake and alert, V = Only responsive to verbal stimuli, P = Only responsive to painful stimuli, and U = completely unresponsive) is a quick and reliable method of primary neurologic assessment.

Evaluation of the preverbal child becomes more challenging. Factors that can be assessed for preverbal children include level of alertness, response to painful stimuli, interaction with caregivers and family members, ability to be consoled, the presence of abnormal eye movements (i.e., disconjugate gaze), and motor responses to tactile stimuli.

A modified Glasgow coma score for infants may be helpful in this assessment. Presence of a high-pitched cry and bulging, tense fontanelles are also indicative of head injuries in infants. Continued emesis after traumatic injury is also suggestive of head trauma.

Pupillary Response. The pupils should be assessed for size, equality, and light response. Unequal pupils and sluggish or no reaction to light may be indicative of intracranial hypertension. Direct trauma to the eye may also cause pupillary dysfunction, so ocular findings should be correlated with the rest of the neurologic evaluation.

Motor Responses. Children with intracranial hypertension may have decreased or abnormal responses to pain. Decorticate and decerebrate posturing may be present. Flaccidity with severe head injury and paralysis from spinal cord injuries may be found on initial examination. Inspection and palpation of the head, neck, and spine should be performed to assess for lacerations, hematoma, cerebral spinal fluid (CSF) or bloody drainage from the ears or nose, depressed skull fractures, or step off in the spinal column.

All inspection and palpation should be performed with manual stabilization of the cervical spine and logrolling with spinal precautions. Although evaluation of the spine and back are not technically part of the primary survey, these assessments are best performed when placing the patient on a backboard, which is necessary for transport stabilization of the cervical spine. Specific head injuries are discussed in an earlier section of this curriculum, so this section will focus on treatment specific to pediatric patients with head injuries.

Airway Control and Ventilation. Children with Glasgow Coma Scores of 8 or less, children with ongoing seizure activity, or those with deteriorating neurologic status should be intubated so that adequate oxygenation is assured. Care must be taken to prevent the development of low CO_2 levels or hypercapnia because both can be detrimental to

resuscitation. The use of capnography during transport can be very helpful in these patients.

Circulation. An overlooked facet of treatment in the head-injured patient is blood pressure support. Hypoxia and hypotension are the leading causes of neurologic deterioration in the head-injured patient. As noted earlier, hypotension can be caused directly from head injury. Blood loss in the head or from other injuries and injuries that impede circulation should be treated appropriately. Preservation of stable mean arterial pressures is important to provide adequate cerebral perfusion and oxygenation.

Diuresis and Seizure Control. Diuresis and the control of posttraumatic seizures are extremely controversial topics in the care of pediatric head injury. Little consensus on the application of these measures without CT results can be found in the literature. If diuresis and seizure control are deemed necessary, the medications listed in Box 31-7 have been safely used in children. These agents should be used with neurosurgeon consultation.

Positioning. Elevation of the backboard to 30 degrees unless precluded by other injuries may aid in decreasing intracranial pressure.

| BOX 31-7 | **Drugs Used for Diuresis and Seizure Control** |

Diuresis
Mannitol 20% solution
Furosemide

Seizure control
Lorazepam
Diazepam: may be given rectally
Phenytoin
Phenobarbital
Caution should be used in the hypotensive patient because these agents can aggravate hypovolemia. Electrolyte imbalances may also result and should be monitored.

Environmental Issues. Control of noise, especially in the transport setting, is very important in controlling acute elevations in intracranial pressures. Unless precluded by patient injury earplugs or muffs can decrease noise stress on patients. Sedation and pain management can decrease intracranial pressure.

Reevaluation. Constant monitoring and reevaluation of the neurologically impaired patient is necessary in transport to assess both for deterioration of patient status and effectiveness of medical interventions.

Spinal Cord Injuries. Spinal cord injuries are rare in children, but their prevalence increases in adolescents. These devastating and often preventable injuries are rarely seen as an isolated injury but often are combined with complex injury patterns. Careful patient assessment becomes critical in identifying injuries because patients may not be able to assist with the exam.

Specific to children, spinal cord injury without radiographic abnormality is not uncommon. Any child with neurologic dysfunction on exam requires neurosurgical evaluation.

As with many injuries, anatomic differences in children may predispose them to specific spinal injuries. These differences include a large head with weak neck muscles resulting in less protection of the cervical spine and horizontal facets combined with ligamentous laxity allowing more movement of the spine.

Clinical findings of any level of motor or sensory impairment should heighten concern for spinal injury. Spinal care specific to pediatric patients will be discussed next.

Spinal Immobilization. The most important intervention in the transport of children with known or suspected spinal cord injury is proper spine immobilization. Prior to application of cervical collars and a backboard, jewelry and necklaces should be removed. This prevents interference with radiologic examinations and possible pressure injuries. Care should also be taken to remove sharp debris such as glass from the patient to prevent further injury.

A firm cervical collar should then be placed while a second person maintains manual stabilization of the cervical spine. An improperly sized collar can interfere with respiration or cause inappropriate extension of the cervical spine. A properly fitted cervical collar will have the child's chin resting in the chin piece; the collar will be below the child's ears and will rest on the clavicles. Infants may be too small for a properly fitted cervical collar. In these circumstances a towel roll may be used to immobilize the cervical spine. A towel roll must prevent flexion and extension as well as align the cervical spine in a neutral position. If a towel roll cannot achieve these goals, manual control may need to be continued.

Once a cervical collar has been applied, the child is then logrolled onto a backboard (see Figure 31-5). There should be one person providing manual control of the collared cervical spine, one person at the child's shoulders and hips, and one person at the child's hips and legs. Opposite the patient, one person should be in place to position the backboard. The person controlling the cervical spine may then lead the command to turn the patient as a unit onto his or her side. As stated previously, this is an opportune time for a caregiver not involved in logrolling the patient to inspect and palpate the patient's back and spine, assessing for injuries or pain.

Children younger than age 8 have disproportionately large heads, so padding beneath the shoulders on the board will be necessary to keep the cervical spine in a neutral position. The backboard can be positioned at a 30- to 45-degree angle and the child then rolled onto it.

Once centered on the board, lateral stabilization of the cervical spine with blanket rolls or blocks and securing of the head with straps or tape should be performed. The final step in spinal immobilization is securing the body to the board with straps (securing the chest, hips, and knees). Straps should be secure enough to allow turning the board from side to side without movement of the patient's body. This turning may be necessary in the nonintubated patient who suffers periods of emesis during transport.

Suction should be readily available for any patient secured to a backboard. A neurologic examination should precede and follow all spinal immobilization procedures.

Removing a Child From a Child Safety Seat While Maintaining Spinal Immobilization. Children that have an unstable airway or that are experiencing respiratory or circulatory compromise should be removed from their safety seat to a backboard to allow for appropriate intervention.[3] The procedure for accomplishing this is as follows.

- Initiate manual control of the cervical spine.
- Remove or cut the shoulder harness, and move the safety bar out of the way.
- Position the child safety seat at the foot of the backboard. Tip the child safety seat back, and lay it down on the backboard.
- One person will then slide his or her hands along each side of the patient's head until they are behind the patient's shoulders. The head and neck are now supported laterally by that person's arms. A second person should then take control of the patient's body.
- On the instruction of the person holding the head, slide the child out of the safety seat to the backboard and immobilize as described previously.
- Instruct parents or caregivers to replace the seat involved in the crash. Some auto insurance companies will reimburse this cost.

Methylprednisolone Therapy. Methylprednisolone therapy is now standard care for patients suffering spinal cord injuries. (See Chapter 15, Neurologic Trauma, for a discussion of methylprednisolone therapy.) Children will also receive this therapy at dosages appropriate to their weight.

EXPOSURE/ENVIRONMENT

The fifth and final portion of the primary exam of traumatically injured children is exposure (to identify obvious injuries) and assessment of environmental issues on patient condition.

Hypothermia. The most pressing environmental concern for pediatric patients is the effects of hypothermia. Hypothermia may be caused both by environmental exposure and by therapeutic interventions such as rapid fluid infusion.

Hypothermic insults can be rapid as with submersion injuries or gradual as a result of exposure to ambient temperature. The clinical signs of hypothermia are subtle, especially in the unresponsive patient, and a high index of suspicion in patients at risk is essential. The effects of hypothermia in children can be devastating, particularly during resuscitation. Diagnosis and treatment of hypothermia from both injury and therapy requires vigilance by clinicians.

The increased body surface area of children combined with their decreased energy stores puts them at greater risk for hypothermia. Hypothermia can be described as mild (35° to 32° C), moderate (32° to 30° C), or severe (temperature <30° C). Clinical signs of hypothermia are listed in Box 31-8.

| BOX 31-8 | **Clinical Signs of Hypothermia** |

Decreased core temperature (below 35° C). Temperatures should be measured rectally or with temperature-sensing indwelling catheters to provide the most accurate clinical information. Some clinicians feel any level of hypothermia in the pediatric trauma patient is detrimental and requires treatment.
Changes in mental status.
Cool, mottled skin.
Shivering in mild to moderate hypothermia. Children have limited energy stores for effective shivering, and the absence of shivering in patients with decreased core temperatures is concerning.
Variable vital signs (dependent on level of hypothermia). Cardiorespiratory arrest is not uncommon in severe hypothermia.
Coagulopathies with moderate to severe hypothermia.

Management of Hypothermia. Management of hypothermia is dependent on the level of hypothermia encountered. Attention to the ABCDE's of the primary survey remains important. Intubation, CPR, and intravenous access may be required for patients in cardiorespiratory arrest. Chest compressions may cause organized cardiac rhythms to convert to ventricular fibrillation. The existence of an organized rhythm may represent sufficient circulation in patients with decreased metabolism, and CPR may not be indicated. In the absence of an organized cardiac rhythm, CPR should be initiated and continued throughout the rewarming process. The exact role and benefit of CPR in the hypothermic arrest remains controversial.

The initial and often most overlooked factor in rewarming is the removal of the patient from cold stresses. Patients should be removed from the cold environment, have wet clothing removed, and be covered with warm blankets. Supplemental oxygen should be provided by mask if spontaneous respirations are present or by bag-valve mask if respiratory support is indicated. Contributing factors to hypothermia such as hypoglycemia, shock, and occult injuries should be considered and treated if present. Mild and moderate hypothermia is treated with passive external rewarming, whereas severe hypothermia requires active core rewarming (Box 31-9).

BOX 31-9 | **Rewarming Measures for Hypothermia**

Passive external rewarming measures
Placement in a warm room environment
Warmed humidified oxygen
Warm blankets and clothing
Warmed intravenous fluid
Active core rewarming measures
Warmed peritoneal lavage
Warmed thoracic/pleural lavage
Hemodialysis/extracorporeal membrane oxygenation
Cardiopulmonary bypass

*Active core rewarming is best performed in a critical care setting.

Cardiac irritability and asystole are not uncommon in severe hypothermia. Cardiac drugs and defibrillation are usually not effective in core temperatures below 28° C. Rewarming to temperatures above 28° C is therefore recommended prior to initiating these interventions. Ventricular fibrillation in the hypothermic patient is best treated with bretylium tosylate because lidocaine is reportedly ineffective in this setting. Dopamine is the only inotrope that retains some degree of action in the hypothermic patient. Attempts at rewarming should not delay transport to a critical care setting.

Heatstroke. Another environmental emergency in children that merits discussion is heatstroke. Heatstroke is a life-threatening complication of environmental thermal stress. Mortality has been reported in ranges from 17% to 70%, depending on the patient's age and the degree of heat stress. Children left in cars for extended periods, athletes, children with cystic fibrosis, and children intoxicated with drugs or alcohol are at increased risk related to impairment of heat dissipation.

Clinical Presentation of Heatstroke. The symptoms of heatstroke include:

- Core temperature >41° C
- Hot dry skin
- Circulatory collapse
- Severe CNS dysfunction/seizures
- Rhabdomyolysis/acute renal failure

Treatment of Heatstroke. Treatment for heatstroke is as follows:

- Remove from heat stress, remove clothing, and immerse in cool or iced water. All patients should be transported in air-conditioned vehicles. Monitor and protect airway during immersion therapy.
- Moisten skin with water and direct fans onto the patient's skin to increase convection and evaporative heat losses.
- Support circulation with crystalloid infusion initially. Inotropic support with dopamine or dobutamine may also be required.

- Although rare, electrolyte/glucose imbalances should be evaluated and treated.
- Myoglobinuria not cleared by fluid resuscitation may require diuresis with mannitol or furosemide.

Patients suffering from heatstroke should be rapidly transported to a critical care setting. Cooling procedures should continue during transport.

Near Drowning.   Near drowning is an environmental emergency that, although not exclusive to the pediatric population, is responsible for a large number of pediatric deaths and morbidity. Drowning is often the second or third leading cause of death in warm and water oriented portions of the country. Males are much more frequently injured than females, and older infants and toddlers represent a disproportionate number of cases. Although swimming pools and natural bodies of water are often recognized as dangerous, other more innocuous situations such as bathtubs, water pails, and rain barrels are overlooked. Teaching to parents and at-risk age-groups as described earlier in this module is imperative because of the frequently poor outcome of these injuries.

After submersion, patients may or may not aspirate fluid. Regardless of aspiration, hypoxemia is the major contributing factor to death and disability in these children. Although many body systems can be affected, the primary sites of insult are the central nervous and pulmonary systems. If fluid is aspirated, pulmonary gas exchange is impaired and quite often, capillary permeability leads to pulmonary edema. The aspirated fluid and resultant pulmonary edema leads to decreased pulmonary compliance, increased airway resistance, elevated pulmonary artery pressures, and decreased pulmonary flow. These factors cause a rapid decrease in the partial pressure of arterial oxygen related to the perfusion of nonventilated alveoli. Metabolic acidosis will then follow the marked tissue hypoxia.

Hypoxemia will rapidly be followed by unconsciousness and anoxia. Irreversible damage to the central nervous system (CNS) will occur in 4 to 6 minutes. The role of the diving reflex in CNS preservation in these injuries is controversial. Although this reflex is much stronger in pediatric patients, many authors now feel that the diving reflex may only be helpful in those patients who become rapidly hypothermic as a result of cold-water submersion. Cardiovascular complications such as dysrhythmias and myocardial depression occur as a result of myocardial ischemia, acidosis, hypothermia, and intravascular volume changes.

Management of the Near-Drowning Patient.
Pediatric survivors of near drowning almost universally have two things in common, limited submersion times and excellent initial resuscitative care.

On removal from the water the airway should be secured and supplemental oxygen (100%) applied. Oxygen can be delivered via mask, BVM, or endotracheal intubation, depending on the patient's respiratory effort. Even patients who are awake and seemingly uninjured should receive supplemental oxygen to minimize the risk of hypoxemia and its related complications. If intubated, PEEP should be provided in an attempt to ameliorate atelectasis.

After oxygen and ventilatory support, reversal of metabolic acidosis should be addressed. This may improve with adequate ventilation but may also require fluid resuscitation, inotropic support, and sodium bicarbonate therapy. Arterial blood gases are invaluable in guiding therapy and assessing the effectiveness of interventions.

Almost all children involved in submersion injuries, regardless of the time of year, will suffer from hypothermia. Rewarming as outlined earlier should be provided for these patients.

After stabilization of the blood pressure, fluid restriction (to one half maintenance) and diuresis with furosemide (0.5 to 1.0 mg/kg/IV) for pulmonary edema may be indicated. Antibiotics are not indicated unless bacterial infection is documented.

Steroids in the initial resuscitation of these patients are also not indicated. Rarely ongoing hemoglobinuria will require forced diuresis in these patients. Hyperglycemia and hypercapnia should be avoided as they contribute to CNS complications.

Predicting the eventual prognosis for these patients is extremely difficult in the acute setting.

Many factors including submersion time, water temperature, speed of resuscitation, and age of the child seem to play a role in recovery. Emotional support of families during this period is a vital component of patient care.

SECONDARY SURVEY

After completion of the primary survey, a complete head-to-toe evaluation should be completed to assess for non–life-threatening injuries. This evaluation requires inspection, palpation, and where appropriate, auscultation and percussion of all body regions. Ideally, this should take place during transport rather than at the scene of injury.

Assessment for lacerations, fractures, abrasions, ecchymosis, ocular and dental injuries, and areas of swelling/edema are included in the secondary survey. Any part of the body not fully assessed during the primary survey should now be evaluated for injury. A full set of vital signs should also be completed.

If time permits, dressing of wounds and immobilization of fractures can now take place. Frequent reassessment of the patient's primary survey and effectiveness of medical interventions should be ongoing during transport. Neurovascular assessments before and after immobilization of fractures is required.

A patient weight either by caregiver history or by use of a length-based resuscitation tape (Broselow tape) should be ascertained. Cardiac monitors and pulse oximeters (if not already in place) should be applied. A radio report to receiving facilities should also be completed at this time.

NONACCIDENTAL TRAUMA/NEGLECT

The ability to detect maltreatment and neglect is, unfortunately, a necessary skill for any person involved in the care of children. Careful consideration of patient findings and caregiver history is crucial in identifying children in need of intervention.

Abuse can be physical, emotional, or sexual. Acts that deprive children of their basic needs (e.g., food, clothing) are more appropriately termed neglect. All states have statutes that require the reporting of suspected maltreatment or neglect. It is important to familiarize yourself with your local statutes and community support options.

Physicians, nurses, police officers, social workers, prehospital personnel, and other adults who interact with children should all be aware of historical and physical findings that are indicators for abuse or neglect. These are listed in Box 31-10. It is important to keep in mind that some of these injuries can occur in the absence of abuse. A careful history of mechanisms and supervision is critical in children with these clinical findings.

SEXUAL ABUSE

Children who suffer sexual abuse may present vague somatic complaints or behavioral changes. Sexual abuse should always be considered in patients with equivocal clinical findings. Other children may present for care after revealing abuse to their caregiver.[3]

Sign and symptoms of sexual abuse include the following:

- There may be an absence of clinical signs.
- Trauma to the genitals or rectum.
- Abnormal discharge from the vagina or penis.
- Bleeding from the rectum or abnormal bleeding from the vagina.
- Foreign bodies to the vagina, urethra, or rectum.
- Vaginal or rectal pain, itching, or discomfort.
- Sexually transmitted diseases beyond the period of the newborn.
- Pregnancy in young adolescents.
- Psychologic issues, which could include low self-esteem, feelings of detachment, helplessness and self-blame, fear of criticism or rejection, or intrusive images.

Care in the transport setting should include treatment of medical issues with psychologic support of the patient.

SHOCK AND SHOCK MANAGEMENT

The clinical presentation of shock in the pediatric patient can be extremely subtle. It is therefore necessary for clinicians to be proficient in both history taking and physical examination to allow for prompt

BOX 31-10   Indicators of Child Abuse or Neglect

Historical indicators of maltreatment:
Caregiver history incongruent with the mechanism of injury and actual injuries
Caregiver history incongruent with child's developmental abilities
Delay in seeking medical treatment
Patterned or unusual marks on the child's body
Injuries of various age or injuries of multiple types
A caregiver who denies knowledge of how an injury occurred
A caregiver whose response to the child's injury is not appropriate
A caregiver who expresses over- or underconcern for the seriousness of the child's injury
A recent change in caregivers
No preexisting medical condition that would describe the child's injury
Inconsistencies or changes in the history provided
Emphasis of unimportant details or unrelated minor problems by the caregiver
Previous treatment for suspicious or unexplained injuries
Caregivers who seek medical attention for the child's injuries in other area hospitals
Bypassing a closer emergency department to seek care at a department further away
Tension/hostility between caregivers or tension/hostility directed at the child or staff
An uncooperative caregiver
Injuries that could have been prevented by closer supervision
Clinical signs and symptoms of maltreatment
Behavioral
Inappropriate reactions to procedures
Frightened of caregiver
Goes easily to strangers; uncharacteristic for child's age
Extreme apprehension with other children's crying
Bruises
- Potentially inflicted bruises include
- Bruises to the face neck, chest, abdomen, back, flank, thighs, or genitalia
- Bruises in various stages of healing
- Bruises suggestive of being struck by an object
- Pinch marks; pairs of crescent shaped bruises
- Fingerprint or thumb patterns
- Bruises suggestive of being kicked
- Bruises to the mouth, gums, or buccal mucosa
Multiple or symmetric bruises or marks
Burns
Characteristics of intentionally inflicted burns include:
- Immersion burn; circumferential and often symmetric "stocking" pattern burns to the feet, "glovelike" pattern burns to hands, doughnut pattern burn to buttocks
- Burns with sharply demarcated edges without splash burns
- Ligature or rope burns to wrists, ankles, torso, or neck
- Cigarette or cigar burns, especially on typically concealed areas
- Contact burns. Dry uniform print may be in configuration of an object used to cause the burn (e.g., grill) Symmetric burns
- Splash patterns in unusual sites (e.g., genitalia) or splash patterns with separated areas
- Burn to the dorsum of the hand
Delays in seeking treatment

BOX 31-10	Indicators of Child Abuse or Neglect—cont'd

Bites and other marks

Characteristics of potentially inflicted marks include:

- Down-turned lesions at the corners of the mouth, caused by being gagged
- Human bites; crescent-shaped bruises with circular lesions; individual tooth marks may be present. A distance greater than 3 cm between the third tooth or canine on each side indicates a bite caused by an adult or child greater than 8 years of age

Head injuries suggestive of abuse

Skull fractures; multiple complex or bilateral skull fractures in an infant

Cerebral edema with retinal hemorrhage (common in shaken baby syndrome)

Subdural hematoma or subarachnoid hemorrhage

Traction alopecia and scalp swelling from hair pulling

Skeletal fractures suggestive of abuse

Multiple fractures in different stages of healing or untreated healing fractures

Unusual fractures; ribs, scapula, sternum, vertebrae, distal clavicle

Metaphyseal injuries that have the appearance of tufts, chips, or "bucket handles" causing arcs of bone

Spiral fractures of long bones

Transverse fractures

Repeated fractures at the same site

Multiple, bilateral, or symmetric fractures

Modified from Emergency Nurses Association: *Emergency nursing pediatric course: provider manual*, ed 2, Des Plaines, Ill, 1998, Author.

and effective intervention. Although there are many etiologies of shock, the underlying pathology is inadequate tissue oxygenation. The goal of all shock management is the support of both oxygen delivery and cardiac output.

ETIOLOGIES OF SHOCK

There are several etiologies of shock:

- Hypovolemic: Caused by a decrease in circulating blood or fluid volumes. Common causes include hemorrhage, vomiting, diarrhea, diabetic ketoacidosis, and burns.
- Cardiogenic: Caused by an inability of the myocardial tissue to provide an adequate cardiac output. Common causes include post-open-heart surgery, cardiomyopathy, drug intoxication, or cardiac arrhythmia.
- Distributive: Caused by vasodilatation and peripheral pooling of blood. Common causes include sepsis, neurologic injuries, brain stem injury, anesthetic agents, and drug intoxication.

- Obstructive: Caused by obstruction in or compression of the great vessels, the aorta, or the heart. Common causes include pericardial tamponade, tension pneumothorax, mediastinal masses, or congenital anomalies.

ASSESSMENT AND DIAGNOSIS

Because of the subtle presentation in the early stages of shock, a careful history is extremely important in patients with suspected shock.[3] Important historical data includes:

- Obvious bleeding or history of blood loss
- Vomiting and diarrhea
- Decreased fluid intake
- Obvious sites of fluid loss such as burn injuries
- Congenital heart disease
- Potential source or risk factors for infection.

Clinical signs and symptoms of shock include[1-3]:

- Altered level of consciousness. This can present in a variety of ways. Any alteration in level of consciousness should be attributed to decreased cerebral perfusion unless proved otherwise. Possible presentations of altered levels of consciousness include an inability to recognize caregivers, decreased levels of responsiveness to the environment, restlessness, anxiety, confusion, and irritability.

- Tachypnea.
- Tachycardia.
- Hypotension. This is an extremely late sign of shock in the pediatric patient because of their aggressive response to catecholamine release. In early shock the patient may be normotensive or have only a widened pulse pressure. Hypotension and bradycardia should always be recognized as ominous signs and aggressively treated.
- Changes in skin color. Similar to level of consciousness, skin changes have variable presentations. Children in shock may present with pale, mottled, ashen, or cyanotic skin. Environmental temperature can also cause skin color changes, so these findings should be taken into context with the remainder of the physical examination.
- Changes in pulse quality. Pulses may become weak, thready, or absent.
- Cool diaphoretic skin.
- Difficulty in obtaining a blood pressure.
- Decreased or absent bowel sounds.
- Decreased or absent urinary output.

Many of the preceding clinical signs and symptoms are not specific to shock and need to be considered in relation to history and patient presentation. Measures of end-organ perfusion such as level of consciousness, urinary output, heart rate, and pulse quality may be the most helpful assessment factors in patients with suspected shock.

Diagnostic aids for children in shock include:

- Cardiac monitor.
- Pulse oximeter. Poor perfusion may impede accurate oximetry readings. A normal oximetry reading does not preclude a patient's need for supplemental oxygen because oximetry is not a true measure of tissue oxygenation.

- Chest radiograph to rule out cardiomegaly, pulmonary infection, or the presence of pneumothorax or hemothorax.
- Laboratory studies to assess complete blood count, glucose, and electrolyte levels.
- Urinary catheter for accurate measurement of urinary output.
- Arterial or capillary blood gases are very helpful in assessing acidosis caused by oxygen debt and anaerobic metabolism. They also assist with determining the ventilatory status of the patient. Serial blood gases can gauge the effectiveness of clinical intervention.
- Cultures of blood, body fluids, sputum, cerebrospinal fluid, wounds, and indwelling devices to determine sources of potential infection.
- Urinalysis to assess for the presence of blood, ketones, bacteria, glucose, and for specific gravity measurements.

TREATMENT OF SHOCK

Regardless of the etiologic basis for shock, the basic tenets of care remain the same—provision of supplemental oxygen, support of ventilation, and support of an adequate cardiac output. The manner in which these goals are achieved is dependent on patient illness or injury. Methods of oxygenation and ventilation and treatment for specific injuries (i.e., tension pneumothorax) have been discussed previously in this module. The direct cause of shock should be treated while patient support is provided. This section will deal with fluid resuscitation and support of cardiac output.

HYPOVOLEMIC SHOCK

The goal in supporting cardiac output in hypovolemic shock is the replacement of lost circulating volume. A child only has 80 ml/kg of circulating volume, so small amounts of fluid or blood loss can cause serious physiologic effects. Before fluid resuscitation can begin, venous access must be obtained. Sites for venous access in children include[2]:

- Percutaneous peripheral attempts (limited to two attempts).
- Intraosseous needle placement.

- Saphenous vein cutdown.
- Percutaneous placement in the femoral vein.
- Percutaneous placement in the subclavian vein.
- Percutaneous placement in the external jugular vein. This site should not be used if a cervical collar is applied.
- Percutaneous placement in the internal jugular vein.

Fluid Resuscitation in Hypovolemic Shock.

After venous access is obtained resuscitation should quickly follow. Resuscitation begins with a 20-ml/kg bolus of warmed Ringer's lactate or normal saline. Because only approximately one third of crystalloid infusions remain in the intravascular space, this bolus may need to be repeated two or three times.

When beginning the third fluid bolus, consideration to giving 10 ml/kg of type specific or O negative packed red blood cells should be entertained. Children requiring aggressive fluid resuscitation as described need consultation with a pediatric surgeon or intensivist, depending on the etiology of the hypovolemia. Transfer to an appropriate center should not be delayed. Fluid resuscitation can be continued during transport.

Children should be closely monitored for improvement in their hemodynamic status while being fluid resuscitated. Signs of hemodynamic improvement include[2]:

- Slowing of the heart rate to 130 beats/min with improvement in other physiologic signs.
- Increased pulse pressure.
- Return of normal skin color.
- Increased warmth of extremities.
- Clearing of sensorium.
- Increased systolic blood pressure (>80 mm Hg).
- Urinary output of 1 to 2 ml/kg/hr. Urinary output varies with age. Urinary output for newborns to 1 year of age is 2 ml/kg/hr, for toddlers 1.5 ml/kg/hr, and for older children 1 ml/kg/hr.

After fluid resuscitation, maintenance fluids must be provided on a kilogram body weight basis.

The formula for calculation of intravenous maintenance fluid is:

First 10 kg of body weight	100 ml/kg/24 hours
Second 10 kg of body weight	50 ml/kg/24 hours
Any weight greater than 20 kg	20 ml/kg/24 hours

Following this formula a 40 kg child would require 1900 ml over 24 hours (1000 ml for the first 10 kg, 500 ml for the second 10 kg, and 400 ml for the remaining 20 kg) or an hourly IV rate of 80 ml/hr.

Prevention of hypothermia as a result of fluid resuscitation is imperative. The use of warmed fluids, warmed room environments, and judicious patient exposure should all be included in the care of these patients.

CARDIOGENIC SHOCK

Support of patients suffering from cardiogenic shock is focused on the improvement of cardiac output. In comparison to hypovolemic shock, these patients more often require intravenous inotropic medications for output support. The need for inotropic support does not preclude the need for fluid resuscitation.

The role of fluid resuscitation may be difficult to ascertain in patients with cardiac dysfunction. An initial 20-ml/kg bolus of Ringer's lactate is generally safe in most patients. Colloids may be more efficient volume expanders in patients with cardiac dysfunction, but the risk of sensitivity reactions and complications of colloid administration should be considered. Obviously if the cardiac output is compromised by cardiac arrhythmia, prompt correction of the arrhythmia following ACLS/PALS protocols is indicated.

Patients at risk (post–open heart, viral cardiomyopathy, drug ingestions) should all have consideration given for inotropic support early in the course of their care. Correction of electrolyte imbalances and acid-base imbalances may also be required in these patients. Laboratory studies are necessary to aid in diagnosis and treatment.

Inotropic agents that may be indicated for the treatment of cardiogenic shock include epinephrine hydrochloride, dopamine hydrochloride, and dobutamine hydrochloride. Other medications that may be indicated in the treatment of patients with cardiogenic shock include lidocaine hydrochloride, sodium bicarbonate, and glucose. Blood gases should be used as guide. Hypoglycemia should be monitored by evaluating whole blood glucose.

Invasive monitoring, which allows for central venous pressure monitoring, arterial pressure measurement, and cardiac pressure monitoring, can be extremely helpful in both diagnosis and treatment of these patients. Measures of patient improvement are identical to those discussed with hypovolemic shock. Maintenance fluids may be decreased depending on underlying cardiac function.

DISTRIBUTIVE SHOCK

Management of patients with distributive shock requires an astute and skilled pediatric clinician. Distributive shock often combines the need for fluid resuscitation as well as inotropic support. The balancing of these interventions can vary dramatically from patient to patient. Sepsis is by far the most common cause of distributive shock, but CNS dysfunction in the poisoned or traumatically injured patient should also be considered.

As in hypovolemia, fluid replacement is always necessary in patients suffering from distributive shock. The underlying cause of the shock should be addressed while fluid and inotropic support are provided. If sepsis is suspected, antibiotic therapy should be anticipated and discussed with both the referring and receiving physician. The range of possible infectious sources in pediatric patients is beyond the scope of this module, but concern for caregiver exposure in transport bears discussion.

Any transport team member exposed to body fluids during transport of a septic patient should be evaluated by a physician to determine if prophylactic treatment is indicated. This is especially true, but not limited to, patients with HIV, tuberculosis, and meningitis.

As in cardiogenic shock, invasive pressure monitoring can be extremely helpful in determining the appropriateness and effectiveness of fluid and/or inotropic agents. The method of fluid administration and the inotropic agents that may be used were outlined previously.

The use of antipyretics (acetaminophen/ibuprofen) in sepsis and methylprednisolone in acute spinal injuries may also be indicated. In addition to the laboratory values discussed previously, evaluation of leukocytosis and white blood cell count differentials are also indicated in the patient with suspected sepsis.

OBSTRUCTIVE SHOCK

The initial goal in management of obstructive shock is the determination of the etiology of the obstruction. Some etiologies will be amenable to emergent intervention (i.e., tension pneumothorax or pericardial tamponade), whereas others will be much more complicated (i.e., coarctation of the aorta in a newborn). As with most shock therapies, patients with obstructive shock will usually be helped with judicious fluid resuscitation and some may require inotropic support.

The role of fluid resuscitation and inotropic support will vary dependent on the etiology of the obstruction and the ability of the clinician to treat the obstruction. The most important factor is prompt diagnosis of the obstruction and emergent intervention. In the trauma patient careful physical examination coupled with a patient and injury history can assist in diagnosis.

The prompt diagnosis of shock and appropriate clinical intervention are valuable skills in any clinician involved in the care of children

PREPARATION FOR TRANSPORT

The preparation for transport of the pediatric patient should include use of the appropriate restraint system for transport as well as include the family. Each state has regulations that describe the type of device that should be used, based on the weight of the child. This can be particularly challenging depending on what illness or injuries the child has. However, it is important for transport team to ensure that the child is appropriately restrained (Figure 31-6) whether they are transported by ground or air.

essential for reducing pediatric morbidity and mortality.

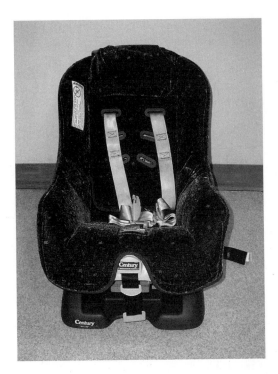

FIGURE 31-6   **Infant and toddler car seat.**

There is probably no greater cause of fear and anxiety in a parent than the illness or injury of their child. Even though as transport personnel we must focus on the needs of the child, the family cannot be ignored. Each program determines whether a family member can accompany the child during transport. Polices and procedures should be in place related to providing information for the family and if they are allowed to accompany the child how can this be accomplished. A further discussion of the role of the family in transport is contained in Chapter 34.

SUMMARY

The care of ill and injured children is a challenging facet of transport care. Decisions based on an understanding of growth and development and physiologic differences in this population are

CASE STUDY

An 8-year-old nonhelmeted bicycle rider was struck on a residential road by a passenger car traveling at approximately 35 miles per hour. Local EMS arrived 8 minutes after the incident, and helicopter transport was requested. The transport crew arrived on the scene 15 minutes after the crash to find an 8-year-old female supine on the roadway and receiving assisted ventilation by EMS. Decerebrate posturing is also noted on initial examination. The patient has, by EMS report, suffered two episodes of emesis, and suctioning of the airway is difficult because of trismus.

The patient's airway is partially obstructed with emesis, and modified jaw lift maneuvers do little to improve her airway patency. The patient is spontaneously breathing at 6 to 8 breaths per minute but is being supported by EMS at a rate of 16 to 18 breaths per minute with a bag-valve mask and 100% oxygen. Cervical immobilization is provided manually by EMS. A strong radial pulse is palpated and at a rate of 140 per minute. The child's skin is moist and cool with a capillary refill of 5 seconds.

Using a Broselow tape, the child's weight is estimated at 24 kg, and preparation for rapid sequence induction and endotracheal intubation is begun. An IV of 1000 cc 0.9 normal saline had been initiated by first responders with an 18-gauge needle in the patient's right antecubital area and is infusing at 100 cc/hr.

An intravenous dose of atropine 0.5 mg is given, followed by lidocaine 36 mg. Etomidate 5 mg is given IVP, and cricoid pressure is applied. Following etomidate administration, succinylcholine 48 mg is also given intravenously, and flaccid paralysis is quickly achieved. After effective neuromuscular block, suction of the oropharynx is performed, and the patient is orally intubated with a 6.0 endotracheal tube, secured at the lip line at 18 cm. Following intubation breath sounds are auscultated bilaterally, and chest expansion is equal. No breath sounds are auscultated over the epigastrium, and end-tidal carbon dioxide is detected with a disposable CO_2 detector.

While a cervical collar and lateral immobilization are placed and this patient secured to a padded backboard, a repeat primary survey reveals an airway protected by an endotracheal tube, a respiratory rate of 16 by bag-valve-mask ventilation with 100% oxygen, and a pulse rate of 150. The skin remains moist and cool with a 5- to 7-second capillary refill. A saline bolus of 500 cc is begun. The patient remains decerebrate with midrange reactive pupils. At this point the child is loaded to the aircraft and evacuated from the scene.

En route to the hospital a second intravenous line is initiated with 1000 cc 0.9 normal saline and an 18-gauge needle in the patient's right forearm. The second IV infuses at 100 cc/hr while the 500-cc bolus continues. A secondary survey of the patient reveals a large hematoma to the left temporoparietal area with bloody drainage from the left ear. No Battle's sign or raccoon eyes are appreciated. No nasal discharge is noted. The face and teeth are stable to palpation. The neck is supple, and the trachea is midline. The clavicles and shoulders are without obvious injury. The chest continues to expand symmetrically, and no crepitus or instability is appreciated. The patient's abdomen is flat with abrasions to the left upper quadrant. The pelvis is stable to palpation, and femoral pulses are weak but palpable. There is no obvious injury to the lower extremities, but decerebrate posturing continues. Examination of the upper extremities reveals a deformity of the left forearm, but all peripheral pulses are palpable.

Following completion of the 500-cc bolus, vital signs are B/P 114/60, pulse 110, and respiratory rate of 16 by bag-valve-mask ventilation. The end-tidal CO_2 detector continues to detect exhaled carbon dioxide. The IV rates are decreased to a total of 75 cc/hr.

Five minutes from arrival at the pediatric trauma center the patient suffers a generalized tonic-clonic seizure that is quickly resolved by administration of 2.4 mg of intravenous lorazepam. A repeat neurologic exam reveals continued decerebrate posturing and a dilated, 8-mm left pupil and a right pupil of 2 mm.

Neither pupil is reactive to light. After report to the receiving facility the patient is hot off loaded from the aircraft and admitted directly to the emergency department for evaluation.

An emergent CT scan reveals a large left epidural hemorrhage requiring emergent operative evacuation. An abdominal CT scan after evacuation of the epidural reveals a small splenic laceration that did not require operative intervention. A radial/ulnar fracture of the left arm required closed reduction and was casted.

The patient was extubated on postoperative day 2 and was transferred from the intensive care unit on postoperative day 4. Ten days after injury this patient was discharged home neurologically intact. Her prognosis for a full recovery is excellent.

REFERENCES

1. American Academy of Pediatric and American Heart Association: *Pediatric advanced life support manual,* Dallas, 1997, American Heart Association.
2. American College of Surgeons, Committee on Trauma: *Pediatric trauma. Advanced trauma life support: student manual,* ed 6, Chicago, 1997, American College of Surgeons.
3. Emergency Nurses Association: *Emergency nursing pediatric course: provider manual,* ed 2, Des Plaines, Ill, 1998, Author.
4. Fleisher GR, Ludwig S: *Pediatric emergency medicine,* ed 4, Philadelphia, 2000, Lippincott, Williams & Wilkins.
5. Hazinski MF, Cummins R, Field J: *2000 handbook of emergency cardiovascular care,* Dallas, 2000, American Heart Association.
6. Needlman RD: Growth and development. In Behrman, RE, Kleigman, RM, Jenson, HB, editors: *Nelson's textbook of pediatrics,* ed 16, Philadelphia, 2000, Saunders.
7. Sanders M: *Mosby's paramedic textbook,* St Louis, 1994, Mosby.
8. Turkoski BB, Lance BR: *Drug information handbook for advanced practice,* Hudson, Ohio, 2001, Lexi-Comp, Inc.

LEGAL ISSUES

32

1. Identify the elements of malpractice.
2. Describe the impact of COBRA/EMTLA on patient transport.
3. Identify the components of professional practice.

Knowledge of legal principles is necessary for members of the transport team. Flight nurses and other members of the transport team practice in a unique setting. There are myriad legal principles and laws with which one must become familiar. Examples include the scope of practice of transport team members, Federal Aviation Administration (FAA) and Federal Communications Commission (FCC) regulations, and state and local regulations that direct ground transport vehicles. The education and training of the transport team must include information on the various laws and regulations pertinent to their practice. Specific laws such as the Consolidated Omnibus Reconciliation Act (COBRA) and EMTALA provide guidelines and regulations that the transport team must be aware of to provide safe and competent patient care.

AN OVERVIEW OF THE LAW

Law comprises all of the rules and regulations by which a society is governed. Statutes are laws made by governmental bodies, and they vary from state to state. Statutes must comply with applicable federal law. The State Nurse Practice Acts are examples of statutory law. Statutes frequently require written rules and regulations for enforcement. Administrative agencies write administrative law, the rules and regulations that enforce the statute. The State Boards of Nursing are administrative agencies that promulgate administrative law.[8] Case law, or judicial law, varies from state to state. Legal issues brought before the courts are interpreted based on the facts of a particular case.

Criminal law permits legal action to be filed by the state for behavior that is offensive or harmful to society. Transport nurses may be charged with a criminal offense if there is violation of either the State Nurse Practice Act or safe nursing practices. Civil law, in contrast to criminal law, permits an action to be filed by an individual for monetary compensation. Tort law is used most commonly in civil cases related to medical and nursing care.

BOX 32-1	Elements of a Malpractice Case

Presence of duty
Breach of duty
Foreseeability
Causation
Injury
Damages

Compensation is requested for the person(s) wrongfully injured by the actions of another.[6,8]

Negligence and malpractice are often incorrectly used as interchangeable terms. *Negligence* is a deviation from accepted standards of performance.[6,8,11,12] *Malpractice* is based on a professional standard of care, as well as the professional statutes of the care giver.[11,12] The same types of acts form the basis for negligence and malpractice.

ELEMENTS OF MALPRACTICE

The elements of malpractice that must be present are presented in order of priority in Box 32-1. First, a *duty* must be present. The duty may be a contract, statute, or when a flight nurse voluntarily assumes care of a patient.[6,8,11,12] A duty is created by the development of a nurse-patient relationship and not merely employment status.[6]

Once it is established that a duty exists, the second element is a *breach of duty.* Breach of duty may occur as a result of malfeasance (act of commission) or nonfeasance (act of omission).[6,8] Administering the wrong medication would be malfeasance, whereas failure to follow a procedure would be nonfeasance.

The third element is *foreseeability;* that is, one could reasonably expect certain events to cause specific results.[4,6]

The fourth element in malpractice is *causation.* There must be a reasonable cause-and-effect relationship between the breach of duty and injury.[4,5,6,11,12] There are two types of causation: (1) in fact and (2) proximate. Proximate cause occurs when the result is directly related to the act. Cause in

fact occurs when the breach of duty owed causes the injury.

The fifth element is *injury.* The patient must be harmed either physically, financially, or emotionally in a discernible way.[4,5,6,11,12]

The sixth element is *damages.* Damages are compensatory in nature and may be of different types. General damages are inherent to the injury itself. Special damages are losses and expenses incurred as a result of stress and emotional pain produced by the injury. Punitive damages are requested when there was alleged malicious intent, or willful or wanton misconduct.[6]

In certain circumstances the doctrine of *res ipsa loquitor,* "let the thing speak for itself," is used. The elements that must be proved are causation, injury, and damages. Commonly, *res ipsa loquitor* is used in situations where the patient was unconscious or in surgery at the time the injury occurred.[4,5,6,11,12]

STATUTE OF LIMITATIONS

Filing a lawsuit is under a statute of time limitations. Generally, if malpractice is alleged after a traumatic injury, the statute of limitations is 2 years, whereas in cases of disease it is at the time discovered.[4,6] The exception is in pediatric cases. The statute of limitations is extended until the minor is emancipated or reaches the age of majority (established by state law).[6]

TYPES OF LIABILITY
INTENTIONAL TORTS OR CRIMINAL ACTS

Assault or battery, or both, may be either criminal or tort (civil). *Assault* is placing an individual without consent in a situation in which he or she fears immediate bodily harm. *Battery* is the touching of a person without his or her consent. Battery can also occur with the touching of anything connected with a person (clothing, purse, jewelry) without consent.[3,4] Damages for battery may be punitive or nominal as well as compensatory.[6]

Other types of intentional torts are, briefly, false imprisonment, the unjustifiable detention of a person without his or her consent, and invasion of privacy, a key concept in issues related to confidentiality. The patient has the right to privacy of medical information. Photographs may not be taken and information may not be released without consent. There are some situations that are newsworthy, and the public's right to know can exceed the patient's right to privacy.[6] Obviously, knowledge of statutes related to consent is vital. Defenses used against intentional torts are consent (discussed later in this chapter), self-defense, defense of others, and necessity.[6]

VICARIOUS LIABILITY

Vicarious liability is defined as one party being responsible for the actions of another. The doctrine of *respondeat superior,* "let the master respond," has been used frequently when nurses are accused of malpractice. As a result of this doctrine, the employer has an obligation to ensure that employees perform duties in a competent, safe manner. Two elements must be demonstrated: (1) the injured party must prove that the employer had control over the employee, and (2) the negligent act occurred in the scope and course of the employment.[6] Vicarious liability can occur for either malfeasance or nonfeasance.

Recently courts have attached judgments directly against institutions for corporate negligence. Hospitals have found themselves accountable as an entity when the duty is owed directly to the patient and not through employees. Types of corporate duties attached directly to the institution are outlined in Box 32-2.[11,12]

PRODUCT LIABILITY

There has been an increase in product liability cases, which are mixtures of tort and contract law. The sale of a product places the manufacturer, processor, or nonmanufacturing seller at risk for a product liability case should injury to a person or person's property occur. Delivery of a service without the sale of the product is generally not substantial enough for a successful product liability suit. However, court decisions have been inconsistent in separating the sale of product from delivery of a service.[6] Collective liability may occur when several manufacturers have participated in a cooperative activity. Alternative liability occurs when two or more manufacturers commit separate acts.

ABANDONMENT

The principles related to abandonment are important to flight nurse practice. Abandonment occurs with unilateral termination of the nurse-patient relationship without consent from the patient.[3] Abandonment can also occur if the care of the patient is transferred to someone less qualified.[7,9] Questions may arise regarding abandonment any time there is a demonstration of disregard for the patient's welfare, unreasonable practices, or both.[3] The various types of air medical transports should be reviewed by each program and evaluated to ensure that potential abandonment issues are addressed. George suggested that the act of dispatching an ambulance was presumptive of voluntary assumption of a duty to a patient.[5] This should be considered when developing communication center protocols.

CONSENT ISSUES

Many medical tort claims are related to consent issues.[4] Informed consent requires more than a patient's signature on a consent form. The suggested treatment must be presented to the patient with a discussion of risks, consequences, and available alternatives.[1-8] If the patient refuses the first treatment option, other treatment options should be

---

BOX 32-2	**Examples of Corporate Duties Owed Directly to Patient**

Duty of reasonable care in maintenance and use of equipment
Availability of equipment and services
Duty of reasonable care in selecting and retaining employees
Adoption and assurance of compliance with rules related to administrative responsibility for patient care
Selection and retention of medical staff

explained. Informed consent requires *understanding* on the part of the patient.

Consent can be written or oral. Nurses are frequently asked to obtain signatures on consent forms. Before having the patient sign, one should determine that he or she understands the purpose of the consent. *Expressed consent* occurs with written or oral acknowledgment. *Implied consent* occurs when a patient is compliant with a request (extending arm for phlebotomy, allowing placement of nasal prongs, and so on). Implied consent is frequently operational in emergency situations. Most consent statutes allow for treatment of life-threatening emergencies if the patient is unable to consent because it is the reasonable thing to do.[4,5] One should be cautious, however, not to exceed the limits of implied consent. If the patient is physically or mentally incapable of consenting, implied consent is operative in the case of a true emergency. Absent a true emergency, consent should be obtained before treatment from a person whose relationship is such that he or she is authorized to consent.[5]

Consent for treatment of minors is reserved for a parent or legal guardian. Implied consent is used for minors with life-threatening, emergency conditions. The parent(s) or legal guardian should be contacted as soon as possible for notification and consent. Most states have laws related to emancipated minors who can consent before the age of majority. In addition, minors may be allowed to consent for treatment of certain conditions such as sexually transmitted diseases, pregnancy, and substance abuse.[4,5]

Refusal to consent or withdrawal of consent is sometimes a murky question. A common issue is the refusal of a blood transfusion because of religious beliefs. If it is the opinion of the treating physician that a blood transfusion is necessary and the patient refuses, an attempt can be made to obtain a court order. However, in the field, the competent patient's wishes must be respected. The court uses a balancing test to weigh one right against the other. The court leans to the right of the patient to make a knowing choice in refusing consent. The exception is in the case of minors. If the court is convinced a child requires lifesaving measures, compelling state's interest in the child usually overrides the parent's interest.

DOCUMENTATION

The purpose of documentation is to document continuity of care, establish a record of patient care so that it can be reviewed for continuity, continue education and research, provide data for reimbursement and cost analysis, and legally protect the caregiver.

The medical record of a patient belongs to the hospital or transport service, although the patient has a right to the information contained therein.[4,6,14] The medical record is the documentation of the patient's course of treatment. It serves as a means of communication between various providers of service. It protects the legal interests of the patient, the hospital, and the health-care practitioner.[6,14] The medical record may also be used for research and continuing education. It is important to be sure to that the patient's privacy is protected in these situations. The contents of the medical record should be factual and based on objective data.[14]

The medical record should be:

- Brief and concise
- Clearly written and legible
- Avoid judgmental terms such as *cooperative* or *drunk*
- Timely

Standard abbreviations may be used. The entries should be readable, concise, and complete.[6] The patient should be described objectively. The patient's appearance, signs and symptoms, interventions, and responses to them should be documented in a timely fashion. If an untoward incident occurs, an incident report should be completed and appropriate personnel notified.

Designated personnel should review charts, and information in those records should not be shared. Patient privacy has become a significant issue over the past years, particularly with the advent of electronic accessible medical records. New rules are being proposed and implemented to protect patient privacy. Transport team members need to be aware of these regulations and their implication to their practice.

COBRA/EMTALA

The Consolidated Omnibus Budget Reconciliation Act was passed in 1986. This contained the Emergency Medical Treatment and Active Labor Act of 1986.[1,9,11,12] In this law is the Emergency Medical and Active Labor Act (EMTALA). This is the antidumping statute. The essential components of the EMTALA include[9]:

1. All patients who present to an emergency department should receive a nondiscriminatory medical screening to determine whether a medical emergency is present.
2. A patient with a medical emergency must be stabilized in the capabilities of the emergency department to which they presented.
3. If the patient must be transferred for further care, there must be a receiving hospital that has accepted the patient if a bed and personal are available to care for the patient.
4. The referring hospitals must send all copies of medical records, diagnostic studies, informed consent documents, and physician transfer certifications.
5. The patient must be transported by qualified personnel, with appropriate equipment, and by the most suitable mode (ground vs. air).

In 1990 the COBRA law underwent further revisions that broadened who is subject to the law. The law now includes all participating physicians and any other physician responsible for the examination, treatment, or the transfer of the participating hospital.[9] Violations of COBRA/EMTALA legislation include financial penalties and potential loss of government funding.

The transport team needs to be aware when a potential violation is occurring, for example, recognizing when a transfer may be based on financial reasons instead of patient need and notify the appropriate authorities when a violation has occurred.[9]

MEDICAL DIRECTION DURING INTERFACILITY PATIENT TRANSFERS

Who is responsible for the patient during transport is an important legal concept that must be understood by transport team members. Transfer of patients from one institution to another has become a fundamental part of patient care today. The chapter on patient preparation for transport identified some of the multiple reasons a patient may require transfer and transport. The section in this chapter describes the federal regulations related to patient transfer and transport as pointed out by EMTALA. According to COBRA/EMTALA, unless otherwise specified, patient care during transport is the responsibility of the transferring physician and hospital. The transferring physician is responsible for[1,13,15,16]:

- Identifying the appropriate receiving facility
- Writing transfer orders
- Identifying the appropriate transport team, equipment, and treatment that will be needed during the transport process

The authority that governs patient care during transport varies from state to state and is based on the type of transport crew that is with the patient. Medical responsibility for the patient should be arranged before the transport process is initiated. For example, our transport team is composed of a nurse and a physician. Because there is physician present, medical direction can come from that person. Other options for medical direction during transport include:

- Transferring physician assumes medical direction.
- Receiving physician assumes medical direction.
- Medical director of the transport service assumes medical direction.
- There may be a shared predefined responsibility with a transfer of medical direction en route because of long distances—for example, on international transports.

Transport teams should have policies, procedures, and protocols in place to address medical direction

---

BOX 32-3 | **Elements of Nurse Practice Acts**

Definition of professional nursing
Requirements for licensure
Exemptions
Licensure across jurisdictions
Disciplinary action and due process requirements
Creation of Board of Nursing
Penalties for practicing without a license

---

during transport. The transport service and their medical director are responsible for providing safe, competent care during the process.

SCOPE OF PRACTICE

Statutes, rules, or a combination of the two defines the scope of practice. Some of the statutes that govern members of the transport team include the scope of practice as stated in State Nurse Practice Acts or Emergency Medical Services statutes. The Nurse Practice Acts establish licensure requirements for nurses. Most states require mandatory licensure before either the title or actions are permitted. Exceptions are generally related to students, new graduates, and transport through a state's jurisdiction.[6] Box 32-3 illustrates the common elements of nurse practice acts as an example of a scope of practice.[6]

Chapter 1 describes the roles of specific members of the transport team. Most of these members are practicing in an expanded role. Before practicing in an expanded role, transport team members should review the pertinent nurse, emergency medical services, medical, and pharmacy practice acts; attorney general's opinions; and recent judicial decisions that govern their practice.[6] The institution's policies and procedures should be investigated and followed to ensure that the scope of practice for the transport team is clearly defined. This is also done with the transport services medical director. The Commission on Accreditation of Medical Transport Systems (CAMTS) outlines in its standards the role of the medical director.

In addition to scope of practice, the standards of care that govern the professional practice of the transport team members must be reviewed. Internal standards are set by the role of the team member, job descriptions, and policies and procedures. External standards are established by state boards of nursing, professional and specialty organizations, and federal guidelines.[6] In cases of purported deviation from the standard of care, the external standards may be submitted as evidence, expert witnesses used, or both. Professional publications may be submitted to assist the jury in understanding the expected standard of care.[4]

The Air And Surface Transport Nurses revised "Practice Standards for Flight Nursing" in 1995. A summary of these standards is presented in Box 32-4. The flight nurse practice standards are an example of external standards. The National Flight Paramedics Association and the Association of Air Medical Physicians are additional examples of external standards that guide the practice of patient transport.[7]

SUMMARY

Knowledge of the law and legal doctrine is necessary component of the transport process. Transport team members must be familiar with both the internal and professional standards that describe their scope of practice and profession. Ignorance of the law harms not only the healthcare provider, but also the patients that they serve.

BOX 32-4	**Standards of Professional Performance**

Standard I. Quality of care

The flight nurse systematically and continuously evaluates the quality, appropriateness, and effectiveness of client care and nursing practice in the air medical transport environment.

Measurement criteria:

1. The flight nurse participates in quality management activities to evaluate care in the transport environment. Such activities may include but are not limited to:
   A. Delineation of scope of care
   B. Development of standards of care
   C. Identification of aspects of care important for quality monitoring
   D. Identification of indicators used to monitor quality and effectiveness of care delivered by flight nurses
   E. Data collection to monitor quality and effectiveness of client care
   F. Data assessment to identify opportunities for improving flight nursing practice and client care
   G. Formulation of recommendations to improve flight nursing practice and client outcomes
   H. Action to improve care and service
   I. Evaluation
   J. Report of findings
2. The flight nurse uses the results of the quality management activities to initiate appropriate changes in client care procedures and flight nursing practice.
3. The flight nurse utilizes the results of the quality management activities to initiate appropriate changes in air medical services.
4. The flight nurse uses the results of the quality management activities to initiate appropriate changes throughout the health care delivery system.
5. The flight nurse identifies safety concerns.
6. The flight nurse ensures that appropriate infection control measures are implemented according to: (a) Centers for Disease Control and Prevention (CDCP) guidelines; (b) Occupational Safety Health Administration (OSHA) standards; (c) individual program and institution procedures.
7. The flight nurse advises appropriate personnel if actual or potential risk exists from exposure to infectious organisms.
8. The flight nurse participates in ongoing infection control educational activities.

Standard II. Performance appraisal

Flight nurse evaluates his/her own nursing practice.

Measurement criteria:

1. The flight nurse engages in performance appraisal on a regular basis, identifying areas of strength as well as areas for professional/practice development.
2. The nurse seeks constructive feedback regarding his/her own practice.
3. The flight nurse takes steps to achieve goals identified during performance appraisal.
4. The flight nurse participates in peer review as appropriate.

Standard III. Education

The flight nurse acquires and maintains knowledge necessary for competent flight nursing practice.

Measurement criteria:

1. The flight nurse successfully completes an initial training/orientation program, which includes didactic and clinical topics pertinent to flight nursing practice and specialty area(s) of practice.
2. The flight nurse participates in ongoing educational activities pertinent to flight nursing practice and specialty area(s).

Continued

BOX 32-4   Standards of Professional Performance—cont'd

3. The flight nurse seeks learning experiences to maintain a knowledge base and clinical skills necessary for flight nursing practice.
4. The flight nurse maintains documentation of educational activities

Excellence criteria:

1. The flight nurse independently seeks advanced learning experiences to expand knowledge base and clinical skills to enhance flight nursing practice.
2. The flight nurse attains advanced educational degrees.

Standard IV. Collegiality

The flight nurse contributes to the knowledge base of peers, colleagues, and health care providers.

Measurement criteria:

1. The flight nurse shares knowledge and skills with colleagues and other health care providers.
2. The flight nurse provides peers with constructive feedback regarding their flight nurse practice.
3. The flight nurse contributes to an environment that is conducive to clinical education of other health care providers.

Excellence criteria:

1. The flight nurse organizes educational presentations for other health care providers to promote optimal health care for the community.

Standard V. Ethics

The flight nurse's decisions and actions on behalf of clients are determined in an ethical manner.

Measurement criteria:

1. Flight nurse practice is guided by the American Nurses Association's Code of Ethics.
2. Flight nursing practice is guided by the Nurse Practice Act as defined by each state.
3. The flight nurse delivers care in a nonjudgmental and nondiscriminatory manner that is sensitive to client diversities.
4. The flight nurse provides information to assist the client or significant other in making an informed decision for transfer.
5. The flight nurse will be a client advocate.
6. The flight nurse maintains client confidentiality at all times.
7. The flight nurse delivers care in a manner that preserves/protects client autonomy, dignity, and rights.
8. The flight nurse uses available resources to help formulate ethical decisions.
9. The flight nurse uses available mechanisms to identify and resolve ethical issues related to client care.

Standard VI. Collaboration

The flight nurse collaborates with the client, significant others, and other health care providers in providing client care.

Measurement criteria:

1. The flight nurse communicates with the client, significant others, and health care professionals regarding client care and nursing's role in the provision of care.
2. The flight nurse consults with health care providers for client care, as needed.
3. The flight nurse makes referrals, including provisions for continuity of care, as needed.

Standard VII. Research

The flight nurse enhances and supports practice through the use of research findings.

| BOX 32-4 | **Standards of Professional Performance—cont'd** |

Measurement criteria:

1. The flight nurse incorporates into practice validated research outcomes.
2. The flight nurse disseminates validated research findings to others.
3. The flight nurse complies with ethical research principles.
4. The flight nurse utilizes the results of validated research to initiate changes in air medical services.

Excellence criteria:

1. The flight nurse initiates and actively participates in formal research through participation in one or more of the following areas: (a) research design; (b) grant application; (c) research analysis; (d) abstract presentation; (e) research contribution to literature.

Standard VIII. Resource utilization

The flight nurse considers factors related to safety, effectiveness, and cost in planning and delivering care.

Measurement criteria:

1. The flight nurse practices safety measures through applied knowledge of:
   A. General aviation safety procedures
   B. FAA rules and regulations pertaining to safety
   C. Emergency aircraft equipment and procedures
   D. Ground operations
   E. Safe use of client care procedures and equipment used in the aircraft environment
   F. Scene hazards
2. The flight nurse evaluates factors related to safety, effectiveness, and cost when two or more practice options would result in the same expected client outcomes.
3. The flight nurse assigns or delegates care based on the needs of the client and the knowledge and skill of the provider.
4. The flight nurse assists the client and significant others to identify and secure appropriate services.

From National Flight Nurses Association: *Standards of flight nursing practice*, St Louis, 1995, Mosby.

REFERENCES

1. Bitterman RA: *Providing emergency acre under federal law: EMTALA,* Dallas, 2000, American College of Emergency Physicians.
2. Cisar NS: Informed consent: an ethical dilemma, *Nurs Forum* 30(303):20, 1995.
3. Commission on Accreditation of Medical Transport Systems (CAMTS): *Standards,* ed 5, Andersonville, SC, 2002, Author.
4. Cushing M: *Nursing jurisprudence,* East Norwalk, Conn, 1988, Appleton & Lange.
5. George JE: *Law and emergency care,* St Louis, 1980, Mosby.
6. Guido GW: *Legal issues in nursing: source book for practice,* East Norwalk, Conn, 1988, Appleton & Lange.
7. Hepp R: *Standards of flight nursing practice,* St Louis, 1995, Mosby.
8. Lazar RA: *EMS law: a guide for EMS professionals,* Rockville, Md, 1989, Aspen.
9. Mitchiner JC, Yeh CS: Emergency medical treatment and active labor act, *Nurs Clin North Am* 37(1): 19-34, 2002.
10. Shelton SL, Swor RA, Domeier RM, Lucas R: *Medical direction of interfacility transports,* Lenexa, Kan, 2000, NAEMSP.

11. Southard P: COBRA legislation: complying with ED provisions, *J Emerg Nurs* 15:23, 1989.

12. Southwick AF: *The law of hospital and health administration,* ed 2, Ann Arbor, Mich, 1988, Health Administration Press.

13. Swor RA, Storer D, Domeier R, Hunt R, Krohmer J, Benson N, Stueland D, Raife J, Schultz C: *Medical direction of interfacility patient transfers.* Dallas, Texas, 1997, American College of Emergency Physicians.

14. Wraa C, editor: *Transport nursing advanced trauma course,* ed 3, Denver, 2001, Air and Surface Transport Nurses Association.

15. Youngberg BJ: Medical-legal considerations involved in the transport of critically ill patients, *Crit Care Clin* 8(3):501, 1992.

16. Youngberg BJ: Legal issues related to transport. In McCloskey K, Orr RA, editors: *Pediatric transport medicine,* St Louis, 1995, Mosby.

ETHICAL ISSUES

33

COMPETENCIES

1. Identify ethical issues related to patient transport.
2. Describe a framework for ethical decision making.
3. Participate in the development and implementation of protocols for "no patient transport."

Many of us went through our professional training with limited exposure to ethical decision making. Then we went through training that persuaded us that we could save everyone. So when we have had to make difficult transport decisions, we have had to do it based on previous experience or using preestablished protocols that may or may have not allowed us to participate in their development.

Today transport team members are faced with many ethical dilemmas. One of the common is when not to transport a patient. Research has documented that the outcomes of patients who sustain cardiac arrest before reaching the hospital are dismal, and patient transport is expensive.[2-7] Currently, transport programs make "no-transport" decisions on the basis of a number of factors.

Other ethical challenges may include being asked to transport patients in unsafe environments, for example when the weather is less than optimal. Some transport teams are forced to make decisions about whether to transport a patient with equipment or problems that they have inadequate experi-ence handling because of competition or fear of revenue loss.

This chapter offers an example of a framework that may be used to make ethical decisions. It also contains information about a common problem encountered in the transport environment—to transport or not to transport. The case study at the end of this chapter provides an outline that may be used to generate discussion about ethical problems that may be encountered by the transport team.

ETHICAL DECISION MAKING IN THE TRANSPORT ENVIRONMENT

Ethical decisions are generally made based on a set of specific values. These include[1,9]:

- Patient autonomy: allowing patients to make decisions about their health care.
- Beneficence versus malfeasance: the benefit of the transport outweighs the potential harm the transport could cause.

633

- Veracity: honesty, telling the truth, open patient care and health-care provider relationships. This should also extend to what the transport program states their purpose is.
- Justice: fairness for the patient and at times the community that the transport program serves.

The American Nurses Association[1] has provided a Code of Ethics for Nurses for decades. The most recent version offers a framework on which a nurse may practice. Concepts expressed include:

- Nurses must practice with compassion and respect for the inherent dignity, worth, and uniqueness of every individual unrestricted by their diversity.
- A nurse's primary commitment is to the patient.
- Nurses must strive to protect the health, safety, and rights of the patient.
- The nurse is responsible and accountable for their nursing practice.
- The nurse owes the same duties to themselves as to their patients to preserve integrity and safety, maintain competence, and continue personal and professional growth.

It is important to examine these values when making decisions about patient care in the transport environment. Unfortunately, there are multiple demands that may influence how one may make a transport decision, including competition, lack of experience, and concern about employment.

The availability of equipment, advanced life support skills, and personnel has contributed to the development of a "technologic imperative."[4,9] In other words, because we have it, we must use it. Patients, families, and communities have come to expect that everything is available for everyone.

Iserson et al[9] have developed a model that can be used to make ethical decisions in the transport environment. This model includes:

- Problem perception: Is there a problem?
- List alternatives: Identify solutions as well as barriers.
- Choose an alternative.
- List the consequences of the actions chosen.

- Consider one's own personal beliefs when making the decision.
- Evaluate the decision.

It is important to note that ethical decision making is a dynamic process. The transport team cannot ignore previous experience as well as the personal beliefs of the team members and those with whom the team is working. These things are never easy, but they cannot be overlooked.

TO TRANSPORT OR NOT TO TRANSPORT

As health-care costs continue to increase, the cost of patient transport and appropriate use of services have become important issues that many transport programs must address. Deciding when to transport patients who have sustained cardiac arrest, whether as a result of trauma or a medical problem, continues to be one of the most difficult dilemmas faced by many transport programs. Research has demonstrated that survival rates of patients who have out-of-hospital cardiac arrests range from 1.9% to 5%. Many survivors sustain severe neurologic injury, and the quality of their life is impaired.[7-15]

Data from a 10-year period of transporting patients who required cardiopulmonary resuscitation during air medical transport indicated that only 1.9% of these patients survived. The injuries sustained by the patients ranged from those resulting from motor vehicle crashes to gunshot wounds to the head. The only intervention provided by the flight team that was not provided by emergency medical services was the administration of blood. The average cost of each flight was $2671.[7]

In a study from the University of Louisville,[8] researchers found that six patients, or 2.4% of patients with traumatic arrest, survived. The air medical costs for these patients averaged $2600. The researchers concluded that patients with cardiac arrest who have obvious severe brain injury and those who have been in arrest for longer than 30 minutes should not be resuscitated.[8]

Whether to transport a patient who may be "dead" in the field remains a difficult decision and has profound ethical implications. Air medical transport illustrates one example of a technologic imperative, or the "unquestioning impulse to use any available technologic intervention."[4] The public also has come to expect both emergency medical services and flight programs to come to the rescue of all who need medical assistance, which attaches additional pressure to the decisions that must be made related to the transport of a patient who is in full arrest.

An ethical practice model suggested by Drought and Liaschenko[4] may serve as a framework for making the decision of whether to transport or pronounce the patient dead and not transport. The practice model is based on the practice account of morality and is composed of the following: (1) the practice knowledge is obtained from dealing with concrete problems, not abstract or hypothetical situations (e.g., the knowledge that patients who sustain blunt cardiac arrest in the field have less than a 1% chance of surviving has been obtained from actual cases); (2) the knowledge that is obtained from practice is shared with other practitioners, such as the fact that multiple studies have demonstrated that the survival rate of patients who have an out-of-hospital arrest is less than 5%[2,3,7-15]; (3) this knowledge has implications for all types of transported patients; and (4) it is dynamic, that is, research is continuous to describe the problem.[4]

The transport team must always be critical when making an ethical decision related to the transport of patients who have sustained cardiac arrest. In other words, "critical" means being thoughtful and reflective of the means, goals, and implications of this practice.[4] The transport team must consider the feelings of those who have been caring for the patient, the wishes of the patient's family, if present, and whether everything has truly been "done" for the patient.

Education, critical examination of the facts, and evaluation of one's personal values related to death and dying should assist the transport team in developing guidelines for when not to transport and with making difficult transport decisions. Case presentations, literature reviews, and the use of clinical guidelines are some methods that may be used to make moral practice decisions. Figure 33-1 presents a protocol that is used to pronounce patients dead in the field. As pointed out by Mattox,[13] "both society and trauma resuscitators [must] accept that the patient who has a fatal injury [should] die with dignity, not being subject to extensive and expensive resurrection techniques."

SUMMARY

Ethical decision making can be very challenging in the transport environment. It must encompass care values, compassion, accountability, and commitment to the people served by the transport service. Transport teams should discuss troubling patient transports. Decision-making protocols should include all members of the transport team, the patients, and the communities that they serve.

As we move into a new century and health-care technology progresses, we must never lose sight of the rights of our patients. In addition, we must never lose sight of our duties to ourselves to provide care in a safe, supportive, professional transport environment.

CASE STUDY

The transport team of a large tertiary care facility has been requested to perform intra-aortic balloon pump (IABP) transports from a small community hospital. The team has already had several complicated referrals from the cardiologist at the referring community hospital, including care that had been initiated by the referring cardiologist that was actually harmful to patients. The cardiologist wishes to insert the IABP, and the team is concerned about the safety and consequences of his request. In addition, a machine would have to be purchased and the transport team trained in its use.

Using the model suggested by Iserson[9] and his colleagues, the transport team discussed this issue.

Problem perception:

Is there a need for this service to implement an IABP transport program?

UNIVERSITY OF CINCINNATI HOSPITAL
UNIVERSITY AIR CARE NURSING

Policy   Page __1__ of ____

Policy: Pronouncing Patients Dead-Scene

File: p-10-a	**Date Originated:** 11/86
Revised: 5/90	**Reviewed:** 4/92, 4/94, 4/95,
Previous Reviews/Revisions: 11/86 - 11/91	4/98, 4/00, 4/02

Precautions:

Responsibility:

Equipment:

Purpose:
To provide guidelines for the pronouncing dead of patients by the University Air Care Flight Physician at the scene of an accident, injury, or illness.

Procedure:
A. Due to the presence of a physician on the University Air Care Team, a patient may be pronounced dead in the field in the following circumstances:
 1. If in the judgment of the University Air Care Physician the patient is clinically dead with no chance of survival.
 2. The requesting agency, rescue personnel, and family members *if and when present* are comfortable with the decision to terminate resuscitative efforts.
 3. There are no medical-legal contraindications to pronouncing the patient dead in the field, such as in homicide or suicide cases.
B. The following are specific situations that if present would generally prohibit pronouncing a patient dead in the field:
 1. Rescue personnel have been working diligently to save the victim's life and feel that the patient should be transported to a higher level of care.
 2. Invasive surgical procedures such as chest tube insertion have been accomplished by the University Air Care Team.
 3. Advanced skills for establishing an adequate airway such as endotracheal intubation and cricothyrotomy may be necessary to determine the likelihood of survival for a patient. These procedures do not preclude pronouncing a patient dead in the field but if accomplished should cause the University Air Care Team to carefully consider all the factors associated with pronouncing a patient dead in the field.
 4. A patient **may not** at any time be pronounced dead in the aircraft or on the helipad.
 5. In the event that a flight nurse is flying without a physician, they **cannot** pronounce a patient dead.
 6. Whenever there is a question as to whether a patient should be pronounced dead in the field, contact should be made with the Emergency Medicine Faculty.

Reviewed by: _____

_____
Senior Administrator, Patient Care Services

FIGURE 33-1   Example of a protocol used in an air medical program when it is necessary to pronounce a patient dead.

List alternatives:

> There are two services that can currently pro-vide IABP transport, but they are not under the direction of the cardiologist at the terti-ary center.

> The cardiologist at the referring hospital has guar-anteed the receiving cardiologist at least 175 patients who may require open heart surgery if IABP transport was available.

> A machine would have to be purchased.

> The transport team would have to be trained.

> Increase the amount of transports that the service may do.

List the ethical values that may be related to the problem:

> Patient autonomy: the patient may not receive all the facts to make a decision or be afforded the opportunity to do so.

> Beneficence v. malfeasance:

> The flight time to the referring facility is less than 20 minutes. Patient delay to transfer is greater than 60 minutes to the receiving facility when the IABP is put in.

> Preparation for transport is greater with the machine in place.

> The referring cardiologist could offer only one study that suggested that this procedure is beneficial in stable patients.

Choose one alternative:

> An individual trained in the use of the equip-ment should be on each transport.

List consequences:

> 30-minute delay in transport waiting for addi-tional team member.

Scan personal values:

> Professional: this type of transport requires training and competencies not readily avail-able at the receiving facility. Most programs that do the transport recommend that the service complete a minimum of 60 transports per year.

Compare consequences with values:

> Potential for patient injury because of lack of experience.

Make the decision:

> A trained person must accompany each IABP transport.

Evaluation:

> Only five transports have been completed. Transport team members feel comfortable with their decision.

REFERENCES

1. American Nurses Association: *Code of ethics for nurses with imperative statements,* Washington DC, 2001, American Nurses Publishing.
2. Cummins RO, Hazinski MF: The most important changes in the ECC and CPR guidelines 2000, *Resuscitation* 23:431, 2000.
3. Dries D: Recent progress in ACLS, *Air Med J* 19:38, 2000.
4. Drought TS, Liaschenko J: Ethical practice in a tech-nological age, *Crit Care Nurs Clin North Am* 7(2):297, 1995.
5. Eisenberg M: Charles Kite's essay on the recovery on the apparently dead: The first scientific study of sud-den death, *Ann Emerg Med* 23:1049, 1994.
6. Eisenberg M, Pantridge J, Cobb L, Geddes J: The rev-olution and evolution of cardiac care, *Arch Internal Med* 12:1, 1996.
7. Falcone RE et al: Air medical transport for the trauma patient requiring cardiopulmonary resuscitation: a 10- year experience, *Air Med J* 14:197, 1995.
8. Fulton R, Voigt W, Hilakos A: Confusion surrounding the treatment of traumatic arrest, *J Coll Surg* 181:209, 1995.
9. Iserson K, Sanders A, Mathieu D: *Ethics in emergency medicine,* Tucson, Ariz, 1995, Galen Press.
10. Jecker N: Ceasing futile resuscitation in the field: eth-ical considerations, *Arch Internal Med* 152(2):3035, 1992.

11. Marco C: Resuscitation research: Future directions and ethical issues, *Academic Emerg Med* 8:839, 2001.

13. Mattox K: "Ideal" post traumatic parameters, *J Trauma* 34(5):734, 1993.

14. Naess AC, Steen E, Steen P: Ethics in treatment decisions during out-of-hospital resuscitation, *Resuscitation* 33:245, 1997.

15. Safar P: On the future of reanimatology, *Academic Emerg Med* 7:75, 2000.

THE FAMILY AND TRANSPORT

34

1. Perform a focused assessment of the needs of families before, during, and after transport.
2. Identify the advantages and disadvantages to allowing the family to accompany the patient during transport.
3. Describe methods to meet the needs of the family.

Patient care during transport is generally focused on meeting the physiologic needs of an acutely ill or injured patient. However, the patient is generally a part of a "family" even though the definition of the term may vary. A family may be described in legal, cultural, religious, or personal terms. The families of today are as diverse as the people who live in them.[5]

Although transport team members are accustomed to the transport environment and process, they should not forget that this is a new and often frightening experience for the family members of a seriously ill or injured person. The transport team must consider care of the family to be an extension of patient care and not an additional task that needs to be accomplished. The support that health-care professionals provide to the patient's family during the initial stages of the patient's crisis can be invaluable. Contact with a transport team or emergency department (ED) employees may be the family's first interaction with health-care personnel in this

emergency. How the family perceives the response of these health-care providers can be the impetus to either healthy or ineffective coping. Ideally, early interventions aimed at decreasing the family's stress should be performed to prevent the breakdown of the family structure.[9,10]

Death of the patient, unfortunately, is an inherent part of the transport process. Some patients die before transport, and the role the family may play in this dying process can make patient care particularly arduous for the transport team. Whether to allow the family to be present during resuscitation attempts is an issue that has been gaining attention from both health-care professionals and the public. Families are now demanding to be a part of the resuscitation so that they can at least say good-bye to their loved ones no matter where the resuscitation is taking place.[23]

This chapter presents the advantages and disadvantages of allowing the family to accompany the patient during transport, the importance of family presence, and how to meet the needs of the family involved in transport.

FAMILY ISSUES RELATING TO TRANSPORT OF THE PATIENT

Family members of critically ill or injured patients are already under stress,[3] and the need to transport the patient on a fixed-wing aircraft, helicopter, or ground vehicle adds to the level of stress they may already be experiencing.[16] Decisions concerning care must be made quickly, and the patient's family members often feel uninformed and unsure, especially if they have limited medical knowledge. Because time is a factor, the family has no opportunity to elicit medical information and request second opinions.

Family members may feel uncomfortable about relaying concerns about the transport to the healthcare providers and transport team. Some such concerns are related to the medical treatment rendered or even the safety of transport (Figure 34-1). Other concerns may include[16,22]:

- Separation from their loved one for the duration or distance of the transport
- Not knowing exactly what happened that necessitated transfer and transport of the patient
- Lack of understanding of the medical diagnosis
- The referring physicians, nurses, and transport team members are unfamiliar to the family and patient

Because most patients who require critical care transport have injuries or illnesses that are sudden and unplanned, family members usually do not have time to prepare for the emergency. If they have never been exposed to this type of crisis, they may not have the coping skills needed to effectively manage the stress entailed.[10]

REFERRING FACILITY

The transport team should make every effort to speak with the patient's family before leaving the referring facility. This interaction may be as simple as an introduction, such as "Hi, my name is Jane Doe and I am the transport nurse who will be

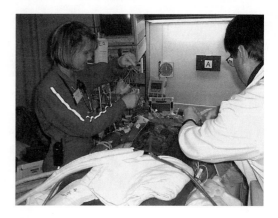

FIGURE 34-1 An example of a critically ill patient on a left ventricular assist device who needs to be transferred to another facility for care. (Courtesy Stanford Life Flight.)

with your family member during the transport." During this interaction the team can assess the family. The team can then alert personnel at the receiving hospital's social or pastoral service department if it appears that the family may need their assistance. The transport team can also take this opportunity to determine the family's plans for traveling to the receiving hospital and get an estimate of their time en route. Family members should be notified of the transport vehicle's intended destination, and they should be told where to report once they arrive at the receiving facility. If necessary, directions to the receiving hospital can be given to the family. Many transport programs provide individual maps for this purpose. It is also helpful when possible to provide the family with a specific individual name or place they may ask for when arriving at the receiving facility.

It is appropriate for the transport team to pause before leaving the institution to allow family members to say goodbye to the patient; this is especially important if the patient's injuries are life threatening, because if this is the case, the family may not have another opportunity to speak to the patient before he or she dies. In this author's experience, the opportunity to say goodbye to the patient

Family Needs of Patients Transported by Helicopter

Family members of patients requiring helicopter transport perceived that they lacked the following:
1. The opportunity to see the patient before he or she was put in the helicopter
2. Information about who would take care of the patient in flight
3. Information about the safety of air transport
4. Directions to the receiving hospital
5. Knowledge about how the patient fared during the flight

From Fultz JH et al: Air medical transport: what the family wants to know, *J Air Med Trans* 431, Nov/Dec 1993.

is greatly appreciated by the family. In most cases, depending on the severity of the patient's injuries, the transport can be delayed for a few minutes without negatively affecting the patient's outcome. These simple interactions between the family and the transport team are invaluable in helping to alleviate the family's stress.

Fultz[13] conducted a study to identify the information needs of family members regarding air medical transport. The information needs rated as very important by family members included what was wrong with the patient, why the patient had to be flown to another facility, and where the patient could be found at the receiving hospital. Box 34-1 lists important needs that most family members perceived as being unmet.[13] The results of this research are important no matter how the patient is transported. Transport programs should use this information as a guide when providing care to the family to better care for the needs of the patient's family.

RECEIVING FACILITY

Information concerning the patient's family members should be communicated to the receiving hospital to facilitate continuity of care. The social services department of the receiving hospital can be alerted to cases in which their services may be especially needed. Personnel at receiving hospitals will want to know whether the family plans to travel to their hospital. Because large distances must sometimes be covered by ground, an estimated time of arrival is useful. Knowing the family's plans can be helpful in case the patient's

condition deteriorates and consent to perform particular procedures is needed. The hospital may need to know the family's wishes for treatment if the patient's condition is life threatening. Organ procurement issues can be considered if the staff knows when and if the family intends to arrive. These issues are particularly important if the patient is a minor.

Family members frequently leave the referring facility as soon as the decision is made to transfer the patient, and they may arrive at the receiving hospital ahead of the patient. In this case the referring nurse can notify the receiving hospital of the family's departure for their facility. If the receiving hospital is aware of the family's intended time of arrival, they can direct the family to the appropriate area in the hospital.

TRANSPORTING FAMILY MEMBERS

Family members frequently ask if they can travel to the receiving facility with the patient. In this era, patients and families are more assertive in making their requests known to the medical community. Research continues to show that patients, families, and health-care providers can benefit from family presence.[1,2,21,22]

The decision to transport a family member is based on multiple factors, some more important than others. The personal feelings of a team member should not interfere with making a decision that is best for the patient and family. The entire transport team should provide input, but safety should always be the overriding principle. In air medical transport, the pilot will have the final

---

BOX 34-2   Examples of Inclusion/Exclusion Criteria for Determining Whether Family Members Should Accompany a Patient During Air Medical Transport

Inclusion of family members during air medical transport may be desirable in the following cases:
The referring facility is far from the receiving facility and the family has no other means of transportation.
The patient is near death and the family wishes to be with the patient during his or her last moments.
The patient is a child and it would be beneficial for a parent to accompany the child.
The family and the patient both strongly want the family to accompany the patient.
Exclusion of family members during air medical transport may be desirable in the following cases:
Inclusion of the family member will interfere with patient care.
The family member's weight exceeds permissible parameters.
The family member is overly anxious and poses a danger to the safety of the transport.
The LZ is walled in on three sides and the pilot must do a vertical takeoff.
A crew member has a concern about a family member.
Marginal weather.
The family member has a fear of flying.
The family member gets motion sickness.
The distance between the two facilities is short.
The patient is unstable and requires extensive care.

---

word. Safety for the entire team is the primary factor on which to base this decision when there is concern about the possibility of the family interfering.

Other factors the team may take into consideration when deciding whether to transport members of the patient's family are the patient's age, the seriousness of the patient's condition, other transportation available to the family, and the length of the transport time. Box 34-2 provides examples of inclusion and exclusion criteria for transporting family members.

Some transport vehicles, particularly air medical, are not capable of carrying an additional passenger because of performance factors or space limitations. Even though the aircraft may have the capability of carrying extra passengers some limitations, including engine power, effects of weather on equipment performance, and the amount of weight the aircraft can safely carry will determine whether an additional passenger can be brought aboard.

Parents often ask if they can accompany their child on the transport. It is important to determine whether the presence of the family member will pose a problem during transport because of an inappropriate level of anxiety. All family members will exhibit some anxiety, and thus it should not rule out the possibility of the person going on the transport. The determination must be made on the basis of whether inclusion of the family members will interrupt the transport team's duties if they sit in the front or interfere with care to the patient if they sit in the back. It cannot be stressed enough that if transporting the family member in any way jeopardizes safety or care, the person should not be transported.

The transport team may want to exclude the family from the transport when the weather is marginal. This can apply to either a ground or air vehicle. Diversions or precautionary landings require extra concentration on the part of the pilot; thus it could interfere with flying if the pilot had to explain what was happening or calm a worried passenger. Ground vehicle drivers need to be able to address their full concentration on roads that may be ice covered or if visibility is impaired by fog.

Once the determination is made that family members can be transported, they will require a safety briefing by the pilot in an air medical vehicle or the driver in a ground vehicle. The family

---

BOX 34-3 | **Reasons for Deciding Not to Transport Family Members**

Liability concerns
Lack of useful load on the aircraft
Exposure of the family to invasive medical procedures
Operator restrictions
Lack of insurance for passengers
Prohibition by the program's operations manual
Concerns about a lack of time to properly brief family members
Concerns about increased stress for the medical team as a result of having a family member on the aircraft

From Edgington BH: Transporting the family and other concerned parties aboard air medical aircraft, *J Air Med Trans* Feb 11-13, 1992.

BOX 34-4 | **Benefits of Transporting a Family Member**

The family member may provide emotional support for the patient.
The family member will be available to sign releases for further treatment and to fill in gaps in the patient's medical history.
The family member may be able to act as a translator.
Organ procurement questions can be resolved more quickly.
The medical team may have the opportunity to explain the patient's prognosis and disposition to the family.

From Edgington BH: Transporting the family and other concerned parties aboard air medical aircraft, *J Air Med Trans* Feb 11-13, 1992.

---

member should be directed to the transport vehicle for the briefing while the patient is being prepared for the transport; this will give the pilot or driver an appropriate amount of time to conduct the safety briefing. The extra passenger can be belted in the seat and be ready for departure. If this is done before the patient reaches the vehicle, the transport will not be delayed.

Edgington[8] conducted a survey of all air medical programs in North America concerning whether family or friends are taken on transports. The results demonstrated that 60% of the programs carry extra passengers. The helicopter programs that carried family members did not advertise that they did so, and they transported them on less than 5% of their flights. Extra passengers were taken more frequently on transports of children. Fixed-wing aircraft programs transported family members on 35% to 95% of their flights. One fixed-wing aircraft program located in the Midwest claimed to carry family members on almost every flight. A program located

in the West indicated that offering to transport family members was important because their transferring sites were so remote that the family refused to consent to the transfer unless they were allowed to accompany the patient.[8]

Forty percent of the programs surveyed did not transport family members. Box 34-3 summarizes the reasons that influenced the decision by these programs not to transport family members. Of the programs surveyed, the ones that carry extra passengers listed the benefits of transporting family members. Box 34-4 lists some of these benefits. Problems with the transfers were rare; only three problems were listed. On one flight a child experienced respiratory arrest and the parent was asked to assist in ventilation. In the other two cases, the passengers experienced airsickness. One program in Oregon has a preflight screening form to determine a prospective rider's suitability for transport. The form included questions about whether the potential passenger had had "recent alcohol or drug consumption, inner ear problems, pregnancy, back or joint trouble, and recent blood donation or dental work."[8]

Many times the transport team must make a split-second decision as to whether the family can be transported with the patient. Experience helps to make this decision process easier. No specific rules exist for including or excluding the family. Each situation must be assessed separately. In many instances, family members will not be allowed to accompany the transport team. The possibility of transporting family members should not automatically be ruled out by the transport team because at times it is appropriate, and it would be good if the team made an effort to include the family.

If family members accompany the transport team, there is always the risk of increased emotional difficulty for the transport team. However, the benefits to the patient and family when emotional support is provided far outweigh the emotional risks to the transport team. One must always look at each situation for what provides the best care for both patient and family.

FAMILY PRESENCE DURING RESUSCITATION

Having family members present while attempts are made to resuscitate a patient is an emotionally charged topic that is gaining the attention of health-care practitioners and the public. Whether families should be allowed to view resuscitation is a topic of controversy among the medical community. Providing emotional support for family members can be difficult. Before health-care providers determine the stance they will take on this issue, they should familiarize themselves with the literature, discuss the issue with others who have participated in a resuscitation attempt with family members present, and ask themselves the following question: "If my child or family member needed to be resuscitated, would I want to be there?" Box 34-5 lists other questions that practitioners should consider when dealing with this issue. A major point to keep in mind is that in most situations, the risks to the health-care provider in emotionally supporting the family do not outweigh the benefits that are provided for the family.

The mission statement or philosophy of most institutions is probably amenable to having family members present during a resuscitation attempt. The practice standards of the Air and Surface Transport Nurses Association state that the flight nurse should possess the skills to effectively communicate with the patient's family.[19] This easily applies to all members of the transport team.

The Emergency Nurses Association (ENA) has issued a position statement in support of the option of family members being present during invasive procedures or resuscitation attempts.[9] The ENA believes that allowing family members to be present during resuscitation attempts facilitates the grieving process. The ENA also believes that families have a right to be together and that this

---

BOX 34-5 | **Questions To Be Considered by Health-Care Providers When Evaluating Whether Family Members Should Be Allowed To Be Present During Resuscitation Attempts**

1. How do you feel about allowing family members to participate in a resuscitation attempt?
2. Have you ever facilitated family participation in a resuscitation attempt?
3. Have you ever experienced a situation in which family members participated in a resuscitation attempt?
4. What, if anything, makes you feel uncomfortable about participation of family members in a resuscitation attempt?
5. What, if anything, would make you feel more comfortable about participation of family members in a resuscitation attempt?

From Emergency Nurses Association: *Presenting the option for family presence*, Park Ridge, Ill, 1995, The Association.

allows the patient and family members to support each other.[6]

The vision of the American Association of Critical Care Nurses (AACN) is that they will work toward a patient-driven health-care system in which critical care nurses make their optimal contribution. The AACN interviewed many nurses who indicated that listening and learning from patients and families is the key to accomplishing this vision. The information obtained from patients and families could then be used to challenge conventional care and ultimately change individual practice. The AACN realizes that activities that alter both the system and individuals are necessary for this vision to come true. The AACN wants nurses to look at the hospital experience "through the patient's eyes," which, they realize, requires enormous effort.[13]

Although nurses have historically professed to be patient and family advocates, very little research supports this statement. When Gorden[14] interviewed Dracup, she cited her previous study on family visitation issues, which found that nurses and families were not in concert with each other. Dracup and Beau examined whether nurses' perceptions of family needs were similar to the actual needs of the families. The results of their survey demonstrated that nurses did not always know what the family wanted. The recommendation was made that nurses continually ask family members what they want, instead of nurses assuming they know what the family wants. Dracup discussed two other issues with Gorden: first, families want to visit patients more frequently in the intensive care unit, yet 80% of hospitals continue to successfully restrict visiting hours; and second, regarding the issue of family members being present during resuscitation attempts, being in the room during a code or when the patient dies is far less upsetting for some persons than sitting alone and frightened in a waiting room or living with the haunting memory that a husband, wife, or child had died alone.[14]

It is important to note that nurses' persistence and vision have now influenced other organizations such as the American Heart Association and the American College of Surgeons. In new guidelines the role of the family is expanded, and their presence is an important consideration to the delivery care.[5]

When family members are encouraged to become involved in the situation, they feel supported, feel useful, and have a sense of some control. When this happens, the health-care provider–family relationship is enhanced. Family members who are frustrated and angry because they do not know what is happening to the patient are actually harder to manage and take more time than those who are kept informed. Health-care providers must keep in mind that family members may not feel comfortable expressing their feelings, especially if they think these feelings are contradictory to the nurse's feelings. Asking family members what is best for them will help the transport team attain the goal of being a family advocate.[6,7,8]

Time and societal influences have changed views about health care and health-care management. Most family members like to be involved in every aspect of the patient's life except when it comes to hospitalization. Health care has marginalized the role of both the patient and family in their care.[23]

At one time, the issue of whether a father should be allowed in the delivery room during the birth of his baby was controversial; many health-care professionals voiced their opposition and resisted this change in policy. Currently, fathers, siblings, and extended family members are often present in birthing rooms. Fathers are even allowed in the operating room when a cesarean section is being performed. This routine practice is not questioned today, and families and health-care providers have adjusted to this change in practice. It would be unheard of today for an obstetric nurse to deny a family member access to a mother giving birth. It appears that it may be just a matter of time before it will be common practice for family members to be present during a resuscitation attempt; it is hoped for the family's benefit that this process of change will begin sooner rather than later.[23]

FAMILY PRESENCE PROGRAM

Foote Hospital in Michigan[6] is a pioneer in the family presence program. The Foote Hospital program was initiated because of two instances in which family members refused to leave the patient during a resuscitation attempt. After these two instances occurred, a survey was sent to the families of patients who had been resuscitated in the Foote Hospital ED. The survey asked if they would have wanted to be present during the resuscitation attempt of their family member if they had been given the opportunity. Seventy-two percent of the respondents indicated that they would have liked to have been present. These results demonstrated to the staff at Foote Hospital that there was a need for a formalized family presence program.[6] Foote Hospital approached the issue by developing a formalized program. Initially a chaplain or social worker provides the family with information about the condition of the patient and determines if the family would like to view the resuscitation attempt. During the time that the chaplain or social worker is with the family, the medical personnel are performing any necessary invasive procedures required by the patient. After the invasive procedures have been completed, the chaplain or social worker accompanies the family into the resuscitation room and stays with them to provide support and information. Because the medical staff has very little responsibility for providing support to the family, they can then keep their attention focused on the resuscitation. If further invasive procedures are needed, family members are asked to step out of the room.[6]

The nurses at Foote Hospital, who were informally surveyed before the program was initiated, had two main concerns: that the family would interrupt patient care and that outward expressions of grief by family members would make it difficult for nurses to perform their job. They also had a fear that they would be observed doing or saying something that would upset the family.[4] Box 34-6 lists reasons that health-care providers give for not wanting family members to be present during resuscitation attempts. Stress for the family is another concern cited by nurses.

The literature confirms that family members have a desire to be present during resuscitation attempts and that this process helps them in their grief work.[6] After Foote Hospital's program was established, a survey revealed that three out of four staff members supported the program. They believed that the program benefited the family even if it was emotionally harder for the staff. Follow-up research with family members who were present during resuscitation attempts demonstrated that the program was successful and that it helped them in their grief process. Many family members commented that they were glad to be able to see that everything possible was done for their loved one. One family member commented that he was glad to be able to say goodbye before the person died.[6]

IMPLICATIONS FOR PATIENT TRANSPORT

All health-care providers have opinions on the issue of whether family members should be present during a resuscitation attempt. Most beliefs on this issue are at opposite ends of the spectrum; few people have middle-of-the-road opinions. Many of those who oppose family presence have admitted that they have never participated in a resuscitation attempt with a family member present. Their feelings are based on what they perceive might happen instead of on reality. Persons who have experience

---

BOX 34-6	**Reasons Given by Health-Care Providers for Excluding Family Members During Resuscitation Attempts**

The family may disrupt or interfere with patient care.

Outward expressions of grief by family members might make it difficult or impossible for staff members to control their own emotions.

The experience may be too traumatic for the family.

From Emergency Nurses Association: *Resolution 93-02: family presence at the bedside during invasive procedures and/or resuscitation,* Park Ridge, Ill, 1993, The Association.

with resuscitation with family members present generally state that they believe it is good for the family and that they only occasionally have problems with the family.

Anecdotes from the Foote Hospital program recount families who have actually been involved in the decision to end a resuscitation attempt. The family was witness to the attempt and was able to say, "Yes, everything was done for my family member. Everyone worked very hard, and it is obvious that the attempts to save the life were futile."[6] This scenario would never happen if family members were left alone in a waiting room and were not informed about what was happening. Difficulty in grasping the reality of the unknown hinders the grieving process.

Some health-care providers are more comfortable with providing emotional care than are others. Some nurses allow family members to visit patients for extended periods of time, whereas others restrict visits to the exact amount of time mandated by the facility or even less. Some doctors take the time to talk to the patient's family members and keep them updated, whereas others avoid contact with the family. If family presence programs are to be successful, everyone's needs must be addressed. Physicians and nurses who find it difficult to provide emotional care will have the most difficult time adjusting to this change. Helping them with the transition will be essential.

Campbell et al[4] found that nurses and physicians differ on how they handle death. Nurses tend to view death more as a natural part of life and associate it with positive terminology, such as rebirth, tranquility, and victory. Physicians, who tend to view death negatively, use words such as unsafe, alone, forgotten, and cold to describe the experience. Gender was not differentiated in this study. An argument could be made that gender instead of the profession of the respondents was the factor that led to different attitudes toward death because the majority of nurses are women and the majority of physicians are men. In addition, male nurses have been influenced in their education mainly by female professors, and female physicians have been influenced mainly by male professors. Historically,

women take a different approach to interpersonal and emotional events than do men. In general, men are much more uncomfortable handling and discussing issues surrounding death than are women. When this is taken into consideration, it appears that in general nurses are best equipped to be patient and family advocates and to assist physicians in determining what is best for the family. Nurses should be the family's voice when communicating with physicians and, if necessary, they should create the atmosphere necessary to have family members present.

Transport team members and emergency personnel, because of the nature of their work, are exposed to situations in which family members may be in close proximity during the resuscitation process. Nurses have a wealth of information on this topic that comes from personal experience, and they should relate these experiences to other health-care providers. Nurses should be on the forefront of supporting family presence; this support can play an important role in changing practice.

If family members are to be allowed in the resuscitation room, the code scenario of hospitals will have to change. The code scenarios of transport teams would be a good example for them to follow. When transport teams resuscitate a patient outside the helicopter or fixed-wing aircraft in the presence of prehospital care providers or referring hospital personnel, the code is conducted in a professional manner. Because flight team members are never on their "own turf" the care they provide is open for scrutiny by all bystanders. Less noise and chaos are generally present during a resuscitation attempt by a flight team than in a hospital simply because fewer people are present. Flight nurses can attest to the fact that a code can be successfully run with fewer people than are used in a hospital. Speaking in normal, calm tones during a code seems to have a calming effect on those present; thus simply decreasing the noise level during a resuscitation attempt will lessen the degree of chaos.

One factor the flight team must consider when giving emotional care to the family outside the hospital is the lack of ancillary support services, such as social services or pastoral care. The flight team must

TABLE 34-1	**Interventions for Initial Family Responses to Crisis**
Family responses	**Interventions**
Anxiety, shock, fright	Give information that is brief, concise, explicit, and concrete.
	Repeat information and frequently reinforce; encourage families to record important facts in writing.
	Ascertain comprehension by asking family members to repeat the information they have been given.
	Encourage or allow ventilation of feelings, even if they are extreme.
	Maintain constant, nonanxious presence in the face of a highly anxious family.
	Inform the family as to the potential range of behaviors and feelings that are in the "norm" for crisis.
	Maximize control in the hospital environment as much as possible.
Denial	Identify the purpose that denial is serving for family (e.g., is it buying them "psychologic time" for future coping and mobilization of resources?).
	Evaluate the appropriateness of the use of denial in terms of time; denial becomes inappropriate when it inhibits the family from taking necessary actions or when it is impinging on the course of treatment.
	Do not actively support denial but neither dash hopes for the future (e.g., "It must be very difficult for you to believe your son is nonresponsive and in a trauma unit").
	If denial is prolonged and dysfunctional, more direct and specific factual representation may be essential.
Anger, hostility, distrust	Allow for ventilation of angry feelings, clarifying the thoughts, fears, and beliefs that are behind the anger; let them know it is "OK" to be angry.
	Do not personalize the family's expression of these strong emotions.
	Institute family control in the hospital environment when possible (e.g., arrange for a set time[s] and set person[s] to give them information about the patient and answer their questions).
	Remain available to families while they vent these emotions.
	Ask families how they can take the energy in their anger and put it to positive use for themselves, for the patients, and for the situation.

adjust to this lack of support services and find other innovative ways to provide care to the family without jeopardizing patient care.

Birth and death are both private life processes that belong to the patients and their families. Health-care providers do not have the right to interfere in either of these processes. People should be able to die with peace and dignity with their families at their sides.

Although not everyone is prepared to view resuscitation attempts, the literature supports the fact that many persons wish families to be present when attempts are made to resuscitate a family member. It is also well documented that being present at resuscitation attempts is helpful for their grief work.

Flight nurses and all transport team members should be patient advocates in the true sense of the word by asking the family what they want and by helping them to achieve their goals.

BEREAVEMENT AFTER SUDDEN DEATH IN THE FIELD

When patients are pronounced dead in the field or are not transported from a referring facility, their families may not be able to benefit from support services available when patients are taken to the receiving facility. Family members often have many questions after the death of a loved one. If family members are at the scene, the transport team should

TABLE 34-1	**Interventions for Initial Family Responses to Crisis—cont'd**
Family responses	**Interventions**
Remorse and guilt	Do not try to "rationalize away" guilt for families.
	Listen, support their expression of feeling and verbalizations (e.g., "I can understand how or why you might feel that way; however . . .").
	Follow the "however" with careful, reality oriented statements or questions (e.g., "None of us can truly control another's behavior"; "Kids make their own choices despite what parents think and want"; "How successful were you when you tried to control _____'s behavior with that before?" "So many things have happened for which there are no absolute answers.")
Grief and depression	Acknowledge the family's grief and depression.
	Encourage family members to be precise about what it is they are grieving and depressed about; give grief and depression a context.
	Allow the family appropriate time for grief.
	Recognize that grieving is an essential step for future adaptation; do not try to rush the grief process.
	Remain sensitive to your own unfinished business and, hence, comfort/discomfort with the family's grieving and depression.
Hope	Clarify with family members what their hopes are, individually, and with one another.
	Clarify with families what their worst fears are in reference to the situation; are the hopes/fears congruent? Realistic? Unrealistic?
	Support realistic hope.
	Offer gentle factual information to reframe unrealistic hope (e.g., "With the information you have or the observations you have made, do you think that is still possible?").
	Assist families in reframing unrealistic hope in some other fashion (e.g., "What do you think others will have learned from _____ if he doesn't make it?" "How do you think _____ would like for you to remember him/her?").

From Kleeman KM: Families in crisis due to multiple trauma, *Crit Care Nurs North Am* 1(1):25, 1989.

make an attempt to interact with them. If at all possible, the family should be encouraged to view the patient's body at the scene.

The initial shock experienced by family members may prevent them from knowing what questions to ask. The team can talk to the family about the facts that led up to the incident and explain the possible injuries that caused the death. Family members often do not remember what was said to them as much as they remember the attitude of the person who was talking to them. Table 34-1 lists interventions that health-care professionals may use in their initial responses to crises.

Common responses of family members to the death of a patient are anger and hostility. These feelings are the result of a lack of control, frustration, and helplessness over the events surrounding the illness and death. Expressed anger often disguises underlying fears and anxieties that need to be addressed. Angry persons often discourage health-care professionals from helping them, thus leaving them feeling lonely and isolated. Rando[20] believes that if the family accepts the death, the grief experience will be more quickly resolved, and the feelings of anger, hostility, and guilt will be diminished.[20]

Transport teams can help the family to understand that the advanced care that their team delivered was the best care possible. The public may not be aware that the transport team is capable of providing the same care that would have been delivered in an ED; they may be under the impression that the best care possible is that which is given in the hospital. They may believe that the role of the transport team is to provide rapid transport and that the gold standard of care is provided in the hospital.

The transport team is responsible for giving care to the victim and emotional care to the family. If at all possible, the transport team should assist the pre-hospital care providers in talking with the family. Because of the nature of transport operations, it is not always possible for the team to stay at the scene and assist the family. If the team cannot stay, the team's assessment of the family may be an impetus for initiating a referral for follow-up. If the base station is associated with a hospital, the social services department may be able to assist with the follow-up. The team may get involved with this follow-up at a later date by calling the family and repeating some of the medical information that the family either did not understand or were not capable of comprehending at the time of the patient's death.

SUMMARY

Emotional care of the family is an important part of patient transport. The transport team may need additional education and increased awareness of their potential impact in this area. Understanding the diversity of patients and their family will aid in providing care. The development of policies and procedures that address the needs of families' related to transport must be a part of every transport program. Family care is an integral part of transport practice and that advocacy role is what makes a difference in what we do.

THE FAMILY AND TRANSPORT CASE STUDY

A 68-year-old man with a history of a leaking abdominal aneurysm was to be transferred to another facility for repair of his aneurysm. On arrival of the transport team, they found a gravely ill man in hypovolemic shock. He was alert but in severe distress. The transport team decided to intu-

bate the patient to assist with oxygenation and beginning administration of packed red blood cells. The patient requested to speak with his daughter before intubation. A few minutes were provided, and the patient was able to ensure that his wife's needs would be met if he should die.

The daughter, who was a nurse at the referring facility, asked to accompany the patient in flight. The pilot approved this, and she was briefed and placed in the front seat of the BK 117. During transport, the patient's condition improved. He arrived at the referring facility with stable vital signs. However, when in transport to the operating room, his blood pressure markedly decreased and he became bradycardiac. His daughter accompanied the flight team to the operating room. She held her father's hand and spoke to him. The patient did well in surgery and both he and his daughter returned to visit the team. Both felt that her presence made a difference in his survival.

REFERENCES

1. Bassler PC: The impact of education on nurses' beliefs regarding family presence in a resuscitation room, *J Nurses Staff Dev* 15:126, 1999.
2. Boie ET, Moore GP, Brommett C et al: Do parents want to be present during invasive procedures performed on their children in the emergency department? A survey of 400 parents, *Ann Emerg Med* 34:70, 1999.
3. Caine RM: Families in crisis: making the critical difference, *Focus Crit Care* 6:184, 1989.
4. Campbell TW, Abernethy V, Waterhouse GJ: Do death attitudes of nurses and physicians differ? *Omega* 14(1):43, 1983.
5. Cummins RO, Hazinski MF: The most important changes in the international ECC and CPR guidelines 2000, *Resuscitation* 46(1-3):431, 2000.
6. Doyle CJ et al: Family participation during resuscitation: an option, *Ann Emerg Med* 16:673, June 1987.
7. Drought TS, Liaschenko J: Ethical practice in a technological age, *Crit Care Nurs Clin North Am* 7(2):297, 1995.

8. Edgington BH: Transporting the family and other concerned parties aboard air medical aircraft, *J Air Med Trans* 11(2):11, 1992.

9. Emergency Nurses Association: *Family presence*, Park Ridge, Ill, 1993, Emergency Nurses Association.

10. Emergency Nurses Association: *Trauma nursing core course*, ed 5, Des Plaines, Ill, 2000, ENA.

11. Falcone RE et al: Air medical transport for the trauma patient requiring cardiopulmonary resuscitation: a 10- year experience, *Air Med J* 14:197, 1995.

12. Fulton R, Voigt W, Hilakos A: Confusion surrounding the treatment of traumatic cardiac arrest, *J Am Coll Surg* 181:209, 1995.

13. Fultz JH et al: Air medical transport: what the family wants to know, *J Air Med Trans* 12(11-12):431, 1993.

14. Gorden S: Inside the patient-driven system, *Crit Care Nurse* (suppl 3-28), June 1994.

15. Jecker N: Ceasing futile resuscitation in the field: ethical considerations, *Arch Int Med* 152(2):3035, 1992.

16. Kleeman KM: Families in crisis due to multiple trauma, *Crit Care Nurs Clin North Am* 1(1):25, 1989.

17. Mattox K: "Ideal" post traumatic parameters, *J Trauma* 34(5):734, 1993.

18. Meyers TA, Eichhorn DJ, Guzzetta CE et al: Family presence during invasive procedures and resuscitation, *Am J Nurse* 100:32, 2000.

19. National Flight Nurses Association: *Flight nursing practice standards*, St Louis, 1995, Mosby.

20. Rando T: *Grief, dying and death: clinical interventions for care givers*, Champaign, Ill, 1984, Research Press Co.

21. Sacchetti A, Carraccio C, Leva E et al: Acceptance of family member presence during pediatric resuscitation in the emergency department: Effect of personal experience, *Pediatr Emerg Care* 16:85, 2000.

22. Von Rueden KT, Hartsock R: Nursing practice through the cycle of trauma. In McQuillan KA, Von Rueden K, Hartsock R, Flynn MB, Whalen E, editors: *Trauma nursing: from resuscitation through rehabilitation*, ed 3, Philadelphia, 2002, Saunders.

23. Williams J: Family presence during resuscitation: to see or not to see, *Nurs Clin North Am* 37(1):211-220, 2002.

MARKETING THE TRANSPORT PROGRAM

35

This chapter presents an overview of the marketing process components and how marketing relates to the transport program.

Marketing is a planned, multistep, strategic process and not a single or isolated event. Each component is one carefully interwoven building block in the overall marketing plan. The main components are the mission statement of the program, market research, market planning, and public relations. Two critical elements of the marketing process are quality of service and customer relations. Marketing plans, just like continuous quality improvement programs, need to be continuously evaluated.

Marketing activities should be designed so that the end results are measurable. This is important for the transport manager in evaluating current and past marketing activities and setting strategy for future market potentials. Marketing is not the distribution of program paraphernalia such as calendars, pens, and buttons. The expenditure of resources for such materials must be carefully planned, budgeted, and evaluated in terms of other marketing activities that are significantly more important. Marketing is not primarily a sales activity. Rather, it is the preparation and delivery of information and support to those on whom the program depends. Through marketing, the program attempts to influence the decision-making and buying practices of the users. The air medical program has no control over these external agencies.

However, through the informational value of the marketing program's public relations function, the nurse manager can influence user selection.[3,4]

The Commission on Accreditation of Medical Transport Systems[1] recommends that each transport program have a professional and community education program and/or printed information with the target audience to be defined by the medical transport service. The information provided by the transport service should be "trustworthy" and may include:

- Hours of operation
- Capabilities of the medical transport personnel
- Types of aircraft/ground interfacility vehicle(s) used and operational protocols specific to type
- Coverage area for the transport service
- Preparation and stabilization of the patient

A marketing plan is a written document that identifies the more promising growth opportunities for the program. It describes the strategies necessary to successfully penetrate, capture, and retain "market share" of the patient referral area. Essentially, it is the foundation on which the transport program's other operating plans are built.

Unfortunately, transport programs have a history of initiating operations with a limited scope of market planning. From inception, marketing may be viewed administratively as a luxury to be addressed later because it requires time and financial support.

Quick program start-ups as a response to competition have often left strategic planning processes on the back burner.

It is not unusual to find the budget line item for marketing, advertising and public relations, and program promotion to be the lowest allocation in the overall transport program. In addition, the sponsor hospital's marketing resources and marketing departments, which are assigned responsibility for promoting the transport service along with an array of other hospital services and programs, often neutralize transport managers. Thus the involvement of the transport manager is limited and often quite latent. At a minimum, the transport program leader must strive to influence the informational environment in which the "marketing department" makes decisions that can affect the program's success.

MISSION OF THE TRANSPORT PROGRAM

A program's mission is generally expressed as a broad statement that defines the roles and purpose of the organization and the environment in which it will operate. The mission reflects the primary reasons for the organization's existence.

Mission and scope may refer to the nature of the program's product and activities in terms of its ability to serve its market area. The mission statement should address the basic questions "What business are we in?" and "What markets should we serve?"

In defining the transport program's mission, the nurse manager should consider the following key questions:

1. What groups will our organization initially serve and need to serve in the future?
2. What are the requirements and characteristics of these groups?
3. Are these groups satisfied with the services they are receiving?
4. Are there any individuals, groups, organizations, or agencies that our program is not servicing but should be?
5. What should the program's posture be toward competition?

6. Is the present mission of our sponsor organization (hospital) patient service mix adequate to meet the needs of the transport program's market?
7. What is our program's responsibility for controlling prehospital care costs and services?

The transport manager must also be able to see the mission of the program through the eyes of the chief executive officers, board of directors, and administrators of the sponsor organization(s). By understanding their expectations for the service and operations, the transport manager can then begin to plan marketing strategies and activities that will support that mission or help to reshape administrative thinking.

For example, administration's priorities and expectations may be to bring 90% of the patients transported back to the sponsoring hospital. The transport manager may need to balance administration's expectations, the institution's clinical resources and expertise, and the projected transport patient market. If in the patient service area there is a high incidence of coronary artery disease, and the institution has very limited specialties in cardiology, the market and the resources may not match to yield the expected transport share for the institution. Integrating the institution's strengths into the program's mission will enhance the success of both. This is especially important today when beds and staff to care for them continue to shrink.

Another common area of confusion in addressing the mission of the transport program is found in the expectations regarding service scene versus interhospital transports. The transport manager might see the mission of the program as being primarily a second responder to scene requests. Thus energies can be focused on this market segment, whereas administration's priorities have been placed exclusively on the interhospital transport market.

The mission statement will give clarity to the transport program with regard to what it does and whom it serves. Through the mission, the program can communicate its identity to its members and the outside community. In essence, the mission statement is the foundation for the behavior of the organization.

The mission statement should drive the goals of the transport program. They are an ideal condition or end result. Goals state the overall long-term intent of the program's management. They define areas of concentration for the organization's financial and human resources.

The goals, or the specific desired results of the program's operating plan, should be driven by what the program sees itself doing in the future, as well as whom it will serve in the future. Clarity of the mission enables the transport manager to set goals that will be supported by the administration.

The goals specified for the accomplishment of the program's mission should include projected results from each of the defined market segments.

MARKET SEGMENTATION: IDENTIFY THE CLIENT BASE

Identifying a market is generally based on demand. Examples of demand include[2,4]:

- Latent: no existing service is currently available that can meet the consumers' needs: the closest transport service is hundreds of miles away.
- Failing: declining interest in the service currently available: the current service has decreased marketing or changed the way they deliver service.
- Irregular: the service is not always available when needed: lack of beds at the receiving facility.
- Full: the current service cannot handle all of the business: current service is always busy and not available when called.
- Unwholesome: discouraging the use of a current service for a particular reason: current program is unsafe or crew configuration dissatisfactory to consumers.

Market segmentation is concerned with finding, identifying, and serving consumer and user groups in the organization's service area. A transport program's service area can be divided into groups of people with similar needs and characteristics to which the program can provide specific services. For example, a program goal may be to provide rapid transport services to a group of people aged 40 to 65 years with a high incidence of coronary artery disease. Thus the market segment, defined in this case by age, is targeted for education regarding heart disease and the role of helicopter transport.

A primary mode for success in marketing is to segment the multiple macromarkets into homogeneous micromarket segments. This subclassification allows implementation by the management of an affordable, focused plan of action. Market segmentation reveals who the customers are and prioritizes the provision of information addressed to their specific needs.

Transport programs have two groups of people they generally serve: patients who receive direct care and program activators who initiate the transport program response. The challenge is to serve the patients clinically and provide the education and training, followed with timely, appropriate, and supportive feedback to the system activators.

Program activators are generally the primary targets of the marketing plan. Because transport programs are generally not accessed directly by patients, an activator network must be created or focused on. The following section discusses the development of an effective network for activators to access the service and patient systems provided by the transport program.

CREATING THE "WEB" OF AN EFFECTIVE MARKETING PLAN

The transport manager must first identify the potential activators of the service. The identification process evaluates the external and internal environments in which the program will operate. The most objective means to gather data to service these environments is through market research.

MARKET RESEARCH

Market research is a systematic analysis of the market to obtain objective data relevant to the goals or objectives of the air medical program. Market research facilitates informed management decision making. Data from market research will help identify and solve marketing problems, but these data are not a substitute for management decision making.[3,4]

With respect to the transport program, market research is focused on people from agencies that would activate a patient transport. Having projected the largest potential group of activators, a survey instrument such as a questionnaire can be developed to obtain information from each specific market segment (physicians, law enforcement agencies, and so on) about the perceived servicing needs of the transport program. From this information, marketing strategies can be formulated.

In addition to the questionnaire, the transport manager can use staff to interact with activators in a community. For example, brief discussions at local hospital medical staff meetings, or in groups as small as a specific physician practice group, may elicit information from the physician activators. Whether the interview method or survey instrument is used, questions should be constructed in such a manner that an objective analysis can be made on the data gathered. Reliability of the instrument must be carefully considered before management decisions on the basis of the information derived are weighted.

In the case of competing programs, market research can objectively identify the perceived strengths and weakness of each of the transport services. It can also identify the parameters by which activators decide that medical transport is most appropriate, which helps the transport manager plan how to sway those not firmly convinced of the efficiency of a specific type of transport; for example, rotor-wing versus ground transport.

INTERNAL ENVIRONMENTAL SUPPORT

Although the external environment is the main user of the transport service, the internal environment—the hospital organization(s) sponsoring the service—must also be addressed. This internal environment allocates the resources that support the transport service, as well as what areas are lacking in resources.

The influence of physicians of the sponsor institution is often overlooked. This component of the internal environment needs as much care, support, and organizational framework to function in as possible. Key physician leaders should be brought on board to help develop marketing strategies for the transport service, as well as be encouraged and reimbursed by the sponsor organizations for their time in developing physician outreach, networking, or physician speaker bureaus. Other institutional resources such as the marketing department or training and development can be used in planning to develop marketing strategies for establishing collaborative relationships with neighboring and system hospitals. The sponsor institutions' resources or strengths in marketing or staff development may well be a supportive asset to the smaller community hospitals' development and/or participation in a health-care network/system.

EXTERNAL MARKET STRATEGIES

External groups are generally hospitals, physicians, and public safety agencies such as ambulance services, fire departments, county sheriff departments, and special rescue teams. A major force supporting or obstructing interhospital transports is the hospital networking and physician-to-physician bridge building that takes place. Experience demonstrates that patients have strong preference for their personal physician and generally prefer to remain in the local community for health-care services. Both of these factors can work as significant obstacles if ignored by the transport program. The role of the transport manager is to develop the appropriate policies that support these natural patient linkages and keep patients in their defined health-care system as is appropriate.

The transport manager must identify and overcome a hospital's resistance to referral. A key resistance may arise from economic issues—specifically, the perceived loss of patient revenue. Intense economic pressure and a patient's strong desire to remain close to home at a time of illness or injury may hamper a transport intervention even when it is most appropriate. Also to be considered is the difficulty for many smaller community and rural hospital employees to have "a patient taken away because we couldn't do the job," and their personal financial effect in realizing the institution's need to keep patients and the revenues that they generate. This may be perceived as an equivalent to the admission of failure.

Given these obstacles, the transport manager can develop several strategies for smaller community and/or rural hospital team participation in the transport service. First is the emphasis on the health-care team. Referring hospital staff must have a participatory role in the patient's road to recovery, rather than that of an inadequate health-care provider. The transport program can implement several different types of strategies to include and enhance rural hospital team participation. Several of the strategies are:

1. *Patient returns home for recovery.* In this program, patients are returned to their local community hospitals for the rehabilitative or final recovery stage of their illness or injury. Strategy must be carefully planned to ensure that the program does not compromise reimbursements by payers. However, such a program encourages the continuum of health care and appropriate use of tertiary health care services and supports the linkage between the patient, the private physician, and the community. It also supports a critical objective of health-care systems and managed care organizations: matching the intensity of the health-care resources with the intensity of the patient's health-care needs. Many neonatal and pediatric transport systems provide return transport to the referring facility for further care once the infant or child is stable enough to go back.

2. *Enhancing the lines of communication.* Each outlying hospital brought on board as a participant in the transport program should be given "preferred status" reception each time they request support. The conveyance of this attitude begins with the initial interaction with the communications center. Responding to the hospital that has the preferred status begins with a service-oriented attitude reflected by the communications staff on the radio and on the telephone with the hospital team. A request for the services of the transport program should be a two-sided, participatory event. Special phone lines can be an asset in conveying the

preferred status to the rural hospital network. The transport manager should streamline the information required to ensure a simple, easy way for the outlying hospitals to access the medical helicopter, airplane, or ground transport vehicle. A "no-questions-asked" approach is afforded if the time is taken proactively to compile the referring institution's information and have it quickly available in the communications center.

3. *Proactive involvement.* Proactively involving the transport program with the health-care team at the outlying hospital can be accomplished through physicians' speaker's bureau, continued education courses or seminars, and visible support of the hospital's marketing efforts. The transport program can gain positive goodwill exposure by assisting the rural hospitals in marketing and promoting *their* services.

4. *Promote training and education about the service.* The transport service needs to provide the referring hospital with education about the appropriate vehicle for transport of patients. For example, not everyone needs to be transported by air. In addition, the transport service needs to provide safety training for the hospital personnel using their service including helipad safety, loading and unloading the aircraft, or ground transport vehicle.

5. *Provide follow-up information about the patient.* Each transport program should have a mechanism to provide follow-up information about patient outcome. This mechanism can also provide a method of continuing education for the referring facility. This information should be provided on a timely basis and given directly to those who cared for the patient at the referring facility.

PATIENTS AND THEIR FAMILIES

Patients being transferred have a unique set of needs. The first is the need for clinical intervention; the second, often overlooked, is for emotional support. Often, patients have not made or even been involved in the decision to be transferred to another institution for care. This factor can be a major obstacle during the transfer of the patient. The transport manager must prepare the staff for dealing with this on a proactive, rather than reactive, basis. The team should take time to meet the needs of the patients and their families before transporting. In the crisis of the moment, this will tend to be a very hurried and rushed encounter. Using the resources at the referring institution, such as other health team members, can facilitate the transport staff's explanations to patients and families if they are informed and encouraged to assist. Taking a few extra minutes to discuss with the family their fears or concerns and to provide written directions to the destination hospital can be most helpful. The transport team should explain the nature of the transport, the length of time of the transport, and most important, the clinical care to be delivered during the transport. It is often helpful to have maps already prepared to direct the family to the destination hospital. The family should know how to reconnect with the transport team after the transport, and the team members should schedule a follow-up visit as soon as they return. This may be more difficult if the destination hospital is not a participating hospital, and the follow-up visit may be limited to telephone contact.

PREHOSPITAL PERSONNEL

The major transport service used by prehospital personnel is air medical transport. Prehospital personnel use of the air medical service is usually less than that of the hospital and physician network. Marketing activities and resources should be proportionately focused on this group.

Prehospital decision-making algorithms should be collaboratively established with each public service and EMS service entity in the patient service area. These should outline a mutual set of expectations for when the helicopter will be called directly to the scene or when interception at the closest hospital is more appropriate.

In meeting with the prehospital personnel, it is highly advantageous to involve local hospital personnel and local physicians, particularly the medical

directors of the prehospital emergency medical services, as well. Thus the hospital staff and physician community will be less likely to perceive the air medical program as a threat, again emphasizing the strategy for team participation with the air medical service as one of the members. The development of objective scoring systems for prehospital use when triaging or decision making for air medical transport is also highly encouraged. Application of guidelines published by national associations representing air medical transport is encouraged. It is important to emphasize the involvement and input of the hospital and local physicians.

Seminars are often efficient marketing tools. Generally they work because they offer the personal contact needed to present the program's expertise and services in a low-key, nonthreatening environment (Figure 35-1). The training and education of prehospital personnel, if considered part of an overall marketing plan, may create unfounded expectations for increased numbers of calls. These expectations may color and consequently defeat the goals of the educational programs. It may also leave prehospital personnel feeling used or propositioned: "They are only doing this so we'll call them."

Training and education can be separate activities of the air medical program yet complement marketing strategies. By identifying the needs of prehospital personnel through surveys or personal communication, the nurse manager may discover a market demand for specific programs to improve the level of prehospital care. Many of these programs should be conducted in conjunction with local training, physicians, or community hospitals. Specifically in the rural communities, hospitals may appreciate and need the additional support of the air medical team and its sponsor hospital resources to provide continuing education opportunities for prehospital and hospital staff. Networking programs such as these have a subtle but positive public relations effect. They can have a dramatic impact on creating the desired team approach and collaboration with the air medical service through recognition of the valued role of each primary caregiver.

CAMTS[1] recommends that each program have a Community Outreach Program. As a part of this,

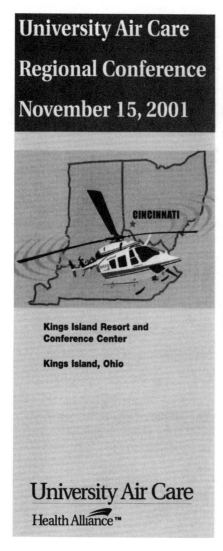

University Air Care Regional Conference November 15, 2001

CINCINNATI

Kings Island Resort and Conference Center

Kings Island, Ohio

University Air Care

Health Alliance™

University Air Care

is pleased to offer

a one-day conference for

emergency medical personnel.

This conference will cover a

variety of topics including:

- air transport

- adult trauma care

- pediatric trauma care

- research

- two skills labs

- a panel discussion

- EMS case presentations

FIGURE 35-1   **An example of a seminar.** (Courtesy of University Air Care, Cincinnati, Ohio.)

the air medical service should support joint continuing education programs and operational programs that may include:

- Hazardous materials recognition and response
- Disaster response/triage
- Advanced trauma care
- Interface of the air medical team with other regional resources

- Crash recovery (extricating personnel from specific types of aircraft and knowledge of the location of certain components in an airframe of specific aircraft make and model)

The team approach must also be emphasized on any scene response. Before the initiation of the request for service, the air medical program personnel and prehospital personnel should have decided who is in charge. Coordination on the scene will directly reflect collaboration that has already taken place.

Many air medical services have follow-up and callback programs for user agencies. These programs should be constructed so that they focus on quality improvement (QI) activities for both organizations. A comprehensive QI program will review the clinical, operational, and aviation components of each mission. The services should each independently evaluate performance against mutually developed standards and share their discoveries about the positive areas and areas for future improvement. The nurse manager should develop the comprehensive, collaborative quality improvement program with a progressive and positive tone. Focusing feedback on predetermined standards, rather than on emotionally charged assumptions, creates clarity for communicating and avoids a negative, policing attitude that might otherwise be conveyed.

Each air medical program also needs a planned and structured safety program that is provided on a regular basis to agencies that use the air transport service. The components of this program should include[1]:

- Identifying, designating, and preparing an appropriate landing zone (LZ)
- Personal safety in and around the helicopter for all ground personnel
- Procedures for daylight operations, conducted by the air medical team, specific to the aircraft
- High and low reconnaissance
- Two-way communication between helicopter and ground personnel to identify approach and departure obstacles and wind direction
- Approach and departure path selection
- Procedures for the pilot to ensure safety during ground operations in a landing zone with or without engines running
- Procedures for the pilot to have ground control during engine start and departure from a landing site

Many of the marketing strategies involve the external environment of the air medical service. In brief, it looks at opportunities for expansion of services, as well as carefully critiquing areas in which services may be threatened. The air medical program depends on external sources over which it has little control. Without control, the focus turns to providing information, influence, and support to achieve the desired outcomes. The external environment is the main user of the air medical service, but the internal environment, the hospital organization sponsoring the service, must also be addressed.

PUBLIC RELATIONS: CREATING THE PROGRAM'S IMAGE

Marketing activities and public relations efforts are often confused. They are not one and the same. The transport manager should consider public relations a part of the overall marketing plan. The public relations activities of the transport program involve those tasks that foster positive regard for the program. It is the building of goodwill and the enhancement of relations with patients and users of the service. It is, in effect, the "image-building" aspect of the overall marketing plan.

Public relations policy should be consistent with and driven by the organization's mission and goals. The policy objectives should ensure two-way communication between the program and the internal and external communities. Image building results of a good public relations program may be difficult to measure. This is the biggest obstacle for the transport manager to overcome in justifying the budget needs for the public relations aspect of the marketing plan.

The benefits of public relations are important not only to sales but also to cooperation and two-way communication with the community. There are two basic elements of the public relations program to be explored. They are community involvement and publicity.

COMMUNITY INVOLVEMENT

Obtaining successful community support uses the same techniques used in networking with hospitals. Enlisting local resources such as government representatives by making them part of the team essentially makes or breaks the service's welcome to their jurisdiction. The transport manager should be knowledgeable about local government activities and recognize opportunities for transport personnel to support these activities.

The goal of the community-involvement aspect of the public relations program is to have the transport team and management contribute to the community's social and economic development. In an effective program, program representatives become active in the community, and community members are invited to participate in the transport program.

The range of community activities for involvement of the team is limited only by management's imagination. Possible areas include[4]:

1. *Medical programs.* The program can cosponsor CPR or wellness training with local emergency medical services (EMS), fire department, and hospital personnel. Opportunities to support primary health-care activities such as immunization clinics in remote areas should also be considered, or injury prevention programs such as Prom Promises should be supported.
2. *Educational assistance.* An effective method for promoting goodwill is to provide scholarships, speakers, equipment, and other assistance to local high schools, colleges, and universities.
3. *Recreation and sports.* Sponsoring sporting events such as golf outings or long-distance runs to raise money for charity can enhance the organization's image in the communities it serves.
4. *Fund-raising drives.* Participation by the organization in fund-raising activities to support local charities is good PR.
5. *Leadership activities.* Transport personnel can become active in the Chamber of Commerce, professional associations, and political advisory groups.
6. *Cultural activities.* The organization can demonstrate goodwill through sponsoring cultural activities such as concerts, plays, or excursions and field trips for the disadvantaged or disabled.
7. *A ride-along program:* Allows members of referring EMS agencies or hospitals the opportunity

to observe a patient transport and tour the transport team's facilities.

PUBLICITY

Through publicity, the program can develop good relations with media audiences by informing them about the organization, its services, and its contributions to the communities. To be effective, publicity must be newsworthy and have special interest for the media's audiences.

Publicity begins with the development of appropriate topics that will enable the organization to translate corporate mission and goals into publicity goals. Such goals may include gaining the competitive edge over other services, influencing the decisions of service users, and improving relations in specific communities.

Through a strategic use of publicity, the organization can maintain a continuous flow of program information to the community. Publicity is a proven technique for achieving specific corporate objectives with a smaller financial investment than other marketing methods. "Free" publicity that is used in conjunction with paid advertising and other marketing methods is especially effective. It is important to remember, however, that the success of a publicity program is reflective of its role in the overall marketing plan.

Working with the press and media has often been outside the responsibilities of the transport manager. However, inadequate or inappropriate press relations will directly reflect the transport program. Thus the transport manager must become involved with the press and media either directly or indirectly through the hospital's normal network. Proactively, it is important that the transport manager form a positive relationship between the media and the program.

METHODS OF PUBLICITY

The transport manager has several options for effectively communicating the objectives and performance of the program through the use of the media. Several methods for obtaining publicity are as follows.

Press Releases.   The press release is the foundation of the publicity program. It is an inexpensive method for the dissemination of program news through the media. Releases contain a brief description of the subject, often accompanied by a diagram.

The media generally welcomes press releases, and releases can be an especially successful means of stimulating positive coverage and increasing the visibility of the program. One can significantly increase the chances of generating coverage of events that are of marginal news value by minimizing the effort needed by reporters. The release should be well written in a style appropriate for the media. The transport manager should meet the media contacts personally and, after sending releases, make follow-up courtesy calls. Releases should be sent as far in advance of the event as possible to facilitate scheduling. Including photographs of the program in action may increase the likelihood of media coverage, especially in smaller newspapers.

Feature Articles.   Generally longer than press releases, feature articles include materials such as a case history of the program (or product news item), an explanation of how the product is properly used, or a description of how the product helped solve a specific problem. Providing photographs is an asset to your article.

The chances of having an article accepted are dramatically increased by developing strong working relationships in the media. A major part of publicity work is in establishing and maintaining rapport with the media representatives.

Press Conferences.   Through effective press conferences, program management has the opportunity to disseminate news about the program and its services. These events can be somewhat complex and intimidating, and therefore require extensive planning and preparation to successfully execute. Transport managers should look to their sponsor hospital or agencies resources for involvement in planning and executing a press conference.

Trade Shows.   The opportunity to disseminate information about the program to a specific audience can be enhanced by participation at trade shows. The types of shows to consider including in the public relations budget should be reflective of the primary users of the program, such as hospital associations, physicians' conferences, EMS conferences, and public safety agency trade shows.

Public Speaking Engagements.   Participation as a public speaker is important to both community involvement and publicity aspects of the public relations program. This public relations tool can keep the transport program's name visible in the community while enabling the program to publicize its objectives. Steps involved in the process of using speakers from the sponsor and/or participating hospital effectively include identifying speaker opportunities accessing the primary program users, constructing presentations to ensure consistency in the message delivered, and developing the list of probable questions that will be asked.

Press Relations Day.   Representatives of the media can be invited for a formal luncheon to encourage open dialogue and conversation. The agenda should include expectations of both the transport program and media in terms of information that is needed for a successful news release and explanation of why some information cannot be made available (i.e., patient confidentiality). The transport manager can create the appropriate environment in which the media learns that the program will provide the information needed in the constraints of patient privacy. The media can provide feedback on how best to supply information, including the framework and content for news releases, as well as how to hold a press conference. Establishing a collaborative relationship between the press and the program will aid in future coverage but should not carry expectation that the program will be shown favoritism by the news media.

EVALUATING RESULTS IN A PUBLIC RELATIONS PROGRAM

The means by which to monitor and evaluate the public relations program are recording activities and measuring success. The record of activities should include the number of press releases mailed versus the number used and by whom; press conferences and speaking engagements, including numbers and lists of participants for future follow-up; and newsletters and brochures produced with documentation of follow-up activities, including solicitation of feedback regarding material content.

Measuring the success of the public relations program is somewhat difficult in that the results are generally seen in changes of attitudes of the program activators. A successful program may result in increased service utilization, but this is not a reliable indicator because it is dependent on an event that is triggered external to the targeted audience. Success may be measured through appropriate use, tracking the numbers of times one service is used versus that of a competitor, and monitoring ground transports that potentially were appropriate to be flown. Other program outputs can be measured on the basis of projections of the response expected through marketing the speaker's bureau versus actual numbers of programs delivered.

THE MARKETING PROCESS

The marketing plan begins with an analysis of the results of market research, public relations activities, strengths identified in the internal and external environment, identification of the market segments, program goals, and ultimately the program mission. Specific objectives are derived from this information that focus program management and staff on the development of a plan that will have specific, measurable outcomes.

Writing a marketing plan is similar to developing a nursing care plan. It involves assessment, identification of objectives, and development of a plan of action, monitoring, and reevaluation. Tools for measuring results must also be established. There is no secret ingredient to a marketing plan outside of commitment to documenting and following it. The marketing plan should be simple, clear, and open to accommodating new strategies. The effectiveness of the plan should be evaluated on a regularly scheduled basis.

Major pitfalls in strategic marketing or planning generally derive from incomplete market information and failure to follow through. Poor communication of the marketing plan also adds to the demise of successful marketing strategies. A collaborative goal-setting and strategic-planning process involving internal and external organizational players is critical to the success of the plan.

Advertising must be carefully integrated and should support the objectives of the marketing plan. For example, the advertising budget should reflect both indirect and direct costs of advertising and marketing. Creative methods to maximize the budget dollar involve use of existing overhead (personnel salaries) to accomplish the marketing plan. Advertising and publicity can be a perfect union for a low-dollar high-impact marketing strategy. Detailed programs should be formulated and evaluated in terms of the following factors:

1. Profitability
2. Market share
3. Continued program use
4. The overall marketing objectives

SUMMARY

Approaching marketing as a process with each of the components developed to support the transport program's mission and goals is important. Integrated into the marketing process are strategies specific to the activities of the transport program. Patient transport involves a great deal of one-on-one contact with EMS agencies and hospitals. Perception of how the transport team works with the referring personnel is a primary component of marketing the transport program. An important theme the transport team can convey is captured in one sentence: "How may we help you?" This is one of the strongest marketing tools that each program has.

Providing transport in a timely, seamless way based on the mission of the transport program is the best way transport programs can serve their patients and those who use their services.

REFERENCES

1. Commission on Accreditation of Medical Transport Systems: *Standards*, Andersonville, SC, 2002, Author.

2. Cowan-Danovaro M, Griffith R: CALSTAR celebrates 15 years of community service, *Air Med* 4(3):18, 1998.

3. Rodenberg JH, Rodenberg H: Part 3: The business plan: Cornerstone of success, *Air Med J* 17(4):174, 1998.

4. Task Force on Interhospital Transport American Academy of Pediatrics: *Guidelines for air and ground transport of neonatal and pediatrics*, Elk Grove Village, Ill, 1999, Author.

36

ACCREDITATION FOR AIR AND GROUND MEDICAL TRANSPORTATION

Accreditation means to give authority or reputation; to trust; to accept as valid or credible. Most medical professionals are familiar with the term accreditation because of the organization that accredits hospitals—Joint Commission on Accreditation of Healthcare Organizations (JCAHO). To understand the history of how accreditation came about for hospitals is interesting and laid the foundation for other accrediting agencies to follow.

HISTORY OF JCAH

In 1915 the American College of Surgeons (ACS), recognizing the need to standardize patient care in hospitals, allocated $500.00 to establish standards to promote quality patient care.[5] Hospitals in 1915—the year ACS recognized the need for standards—were not necessarily places that cured patients but places patients went to when they were about to die. Medical knowledge was minuscule compared to today's world. Penicillin had not yet been discovered and although aseptic technique was used in surgery, there were no effective medications to manage postoperative infections.[7]

By 1917 ACS developed a one-page list of requirements they called *Minimum Standards for Hospitals.*

In 1918 an on-site inspection was developed by ACS to see if hospitals with more than 100 beds could meet compliance with the *Minimum Standards for Hospitals.* More than 700 hospitals throughout the United States were evaluated in the first year, and only 89, or 13%, met the requirements of the *Minimum Standards.* Although these results were dismal, it raised the awareness of the medical community, who were ready to accept the need for standardization and a verification process to improve quality.

By 1951 there were more than 3000 hospitals voluntarily surveyed. With the growth and overwhelming success of voluntary accreditation for hospitals, the ACS organization became overwhelmed and invited other organizations to participate. The Joint Commission on Accreditation of Hospitals (JCAH) was chartered in 1951 with ACS plus the following participating organizations: the American College of Physicians, the American Medical Association, the Canadian Medical Association, and the American Hospital Association.

Later in the 1950s the Canadian Medical Association withdrew to form their own national organization, and JCAH expanded to include health care outside the hospital environment such as home health, mental health, and ambulatory health care. This eventually resulted in a name change to the Joint Commission on Accreditation of Healthcare Organizations (JCAHO), as the organization is known today.

THE "WHITE PAPER" CALLS FOR IMPROVED EMERGENCY MEDICAL SERVICES

So JCAHO was well established before there were even standards for medical transport. In fact, it was not until 1966 when the *White Paper* entitled "Accidental Death and Disability—The Neglected Disease of Modern Society"[2] was published by the National Academy of Science that problems were identified in transport. At that time, helicopter transport for the civilian population was unheard of, and there was no standardization for ground transport vehicles or for the medical attendants who accompanied patients. Untrained personnel in the back of a mortician's vehicle did 50% of ground transports. Fire, police, or volunteer groups did the other 50% of the transports.

The *White Paper* triggered legislation that specifically addressed Emergency Medical Services and even suggested the use of helicopters.[4]

The Maryland State Police Aviation Division developed the earliest known public service helicopter system in 1969. There were a few hospital-based helicopter programs by the mid 1970s, but the growth of these types of services did not really peak until the mid 1980s. At this point in time, hospitals were regionalizing, with specific hospitals recognized as centers of excellence in one or more specialty areas. Trauma center designation often included a helicopter program or access to a helicopter program, which was an added impetus to the growth in the number of helicopter services.

Also, the Vietnam experience proved a sharp decrease in mortality rates because of the rapid response of helicopters in transporting the injured from the field to definitive care. From a civilian perspective, the "Golden Hour" theory by Dr. R. Adams Cowley of the Shock Trauma Unit of Baltimore supposed that a critically injured patient had a precious 60 minutes to obtain definitive surgical treatment following an injury to survive.[8] The "Golden Hour" theory and the Vietnam experience[6] were frequently touted as reasons for a hospital, especially a trauma center, to start a helicopter service.

In 1980 a new organization, the Association of Hospital Based Emergency Air Medical Services (ASHBEAMS—the name was later changed to the Association of Air Medical Services [AAMS]), was formed. This organization started as a way to create a forum for administrators and personnel to get together and network with other hospital-based helicopter programs. There were no standards at this time, so those assigned to start up a hospital-based helicopter program usually had no air transport experience, no pattern to follow, no awareness of the potential hazards, and managers who understood the risks even less. The aviation component—aircraft, pilots, and maintenance—was contracted from an aviation vendor. Pilots were usually Vietnam survivors who were still operating under the oath they practiced in the military—*complete the mission.* Care providers were thrust into the unfamiliar aviation environment without standardized transport training and with the ingrained attitude that the patient, not safety, always comes first. Clearly all were well intentioned, but as more and more accidents began to occur, it was recognized that the profession needed standardization—not unlike the ACS recognizing the need for standards in hospitals in the early 1900s mentioned earlier.

In 1985 there were 16 air medical accidents with 12 fatalities.[3] The FAA was concerned, and the press began to alert the public. At the time ASHBEAMS had minimal guidelines addressing patient care issues, but when the press started to focus on the number of air medical accidents, AHBEAMS started to meet with other national groups, such as the Helicopter Association International (HAI), the National Flight Nurses Association (NFNA), National Flight Paramedics Association (NFPA), and the National EMS Pilots Association (NEMSPA) to develop consensus standards on safety and operational practices.

In 1986 The ASHBEAMS Safety Committee started a peer review safety audit called Priority

One, using the safety guidelines that had been developed through the consensus process of the organizations listed in the previous paragraph. Priority One was beta-tested at Duke University in Durham, North Carolina, and at the Staff for Life Program in Columbia, Missouri. As a result of these visits, the Safety Committee found that patient care standards specific to the transport environment were needed as well as the safety guidelines to make the process complete. Therefore, a feasibility study was performed to determine the need and viability of an accreditation program specifically for air medial transport.

Part of the feasibility study involved dialogue with JCAHO and other accrediting bodies. Many organizational leaders felt that JCAHO should be able to incorporate transport standards into its accreditation process and then be able to layer in the air medical profession. This would negate the expense and effort needed to create another accrediting agency. However, JCAHO was not interested in being responsible for standards addressing the aviation environment, stating this was completely out of their field of expertise. Also, in the late 1980s, helicopter services were starting to be outsourced or privately owned and no longer sponsored or based at hospitals. Typically, fixed-wing medical transport services were privately owned and operated by an aviation company with no connections to hospitals. Both types of services were completely outside the realm of JCAHO.

ACCREDITATION ORGANIZATION FOUNDED FOR AIR MEDICAL TRANSPORT

In 1989, with the feasibility study completed and presented, ASHBEAMS members voted to fund start-up costs for an air medical accreditation agency. Conceptually, this organization would be separate and independent of ASHBEAMS and would be made up of member organizations, so each member organization had equal representation on the Board of Directors.

Seven organizations met on July 13, 1990 in Kansas City, Missouri, to form the Commission on Accreditation of Air Medical Services (CAAMS) as follows: the American College of Emergency Physicians, the Association of Air Medical Services, the National Association of Air Medical Communication Specialists, the National Association of EMS Physicians, the National EMS Pilots Association, the National Flight Nurses Association (now called Air & Surface Transport Nurses Association [ASTNA]), and the National Flight Paramedics Association.

CAAMS was formally incorporated in the state of Pennsylvania as a nonprofit organization. The mission of CAAMS was *and is* to improve the quality of patient care and safety of the transport environment. Along with developing the tools for the new organization's foundation, such as the articles of incorporation, policies, and bylaws, the most important task for the new board was to develop the accreditation standards.

All accrediting organizations have a similar process of site visits, usually every 3 years, to verify compliance with standards. But it is the standards that define the site survey process. Medical transport services that apply for accreditation are awarded or are withheld from accreditation based on compliance with the accreditation standards. Therefore the standards must be attainable, measurable, and consistent with current practice.

ACCREDITATION STANDARDS

To gain acceptance of the accreditation standards, CAAMS used guidelines and standards from many of the organizations mentioned previously—the ASHBEAMS, HAI, NFNA, NEMSPA, and NFPA—to begin the process. In trying to create a document that would address both safety and patient care issues, the CAAMS board studied the National Transportation Safety Board's (NTSB) accident reports to determine if a standardized practice, policy, or procedure could have prevented an accident. The CAAMS board also worked with officials from the Federal Aviation Administration (FAA) who were specifically assigned to be a liaison with the air medical profession.

In some cases the accreditation standards exceeded Federal Aviation Regulations, and in some cases the regulation was copied into a standard to provide needed emphasis on a particular issue. For example, it is a Federal Aviation Regulation that personnel and passengers must be seat belted in for all takeoffs and landings.[1] However, during site visits medical personnel would often tell site surveyors that if they were busy with the patient on liftoff or landing, they did not bother with the seat belts. Indeed, in some of the survivable air medical accidents, several medical attendants received serious back and spinal injuries because they were not secured in their seat belts on liftoff.

Prior to publishing the first edition of Accreditation Standards in 1991, there were numerous drafts mailed to organizations and individuals affiliated with the air medical transport profession. CAAMS also held a public hearing at the air medical transport conference in September 1990 in Nashville, Tennessee, to gather opinions and suggestions for the draft of standards that were distributed.

Accreditation Standards are revised every 3 years to keep abreast of current practice. The following broad topics included in the Accreditation Standards are each supported by specific criteria (Box 36-1).

SITE SURVEYORS

Several accrediting agencies in related health-care fields were willing to share copies of their policies and qualifications for site surveyors when CAAMS was developing its new accrediting agency. One of those organizations, the Commission on Accreditation of Rehabilitation Facilities (CARF), was very generous and allowed the Executive Director of CAAMS to participate in its site surveyor training course. Subsequently, the course developed by the CAAMS Site Surveyor Selection Committee was based on the principles of CARF's program. Originally in 1991 there were 35 applicants for the 12 site surveyor positions. Applicants were chosen based on the requirements and on their level of experience. Applicants were required to have a minimum of 4 years experience and a background in 2 of the four following categories: aviation, communications, medical, and manage-

---

BOX 36-1 | Accreditation Standards

General Standards (apply to all modes of transport)
Medical Section
Medical Direction and Clinical Supervisor
    Medical Personnel
        Staffing
        Training
Commercial Escorts
Aircraft/Ambulance Section
    Medical Configuration
    Operational Issues
    Aircraft/Ambulance equipment
    Communications
Management and Administration Section
    Management/Policies
    Utilization Review
    Quality Management
    Infection Control

Rotor-Wing Standards
Certificate of the Aircraft Operator
Weather and Weather Minimums
Pilot Staffing and Training
Maintenance
Helipad and Refueling
Community Outreach

Fixed-Wing Standards
Certificate of the Aircraft Operator
Aircraft

Weather and Weather Minimums
Pilot Staffing and Training
Maintenance
Community Outreach

Ground Interfacility Standards
Vehicles
Driver Qualifications
Maintenance and Sanitation
Mechanic
Policies

---

ment, with a heavy emphasis on management experience. The first site surveyor training class was held in 1991 with classes repeated in 1995, 1997, and 1999 to keep up with attrition and site-visit demands.

ACCEPTING ACCREDITATION: BUYING INTO THE PROCESS

As mentioned earlier, most medical professionals understand accreditation because of exposure to the hospitals' accrediting agency—JCAHO. However, in developing an air medical accreditation process, aviation professionals had to be educated on the purpose and goals of accreditation. Although the aviation component was accustomed to regulations, they were not familiar with accreditation and did not understand the need for yet another process when most felt they were already overregulated by the FAA. The fixed-wing community was particularly baffled. Most fixed-wing transport services were owned and managed by private aviation operators who were totally unfamiliar with the term *accreditation*. CAAMS worked through the National EMS Pilots Association, as one of its member organizations, to try to gain wider acceptance and also developed a formal Aviation Advisory Committee to involve the fixed-wing community, managers from the major EMS Aviation Operators, and the FAA. The purpose of the Aviation Advisory Committee, which meets annually, is to provide updated information and to provide a forum for gathering input from the aviation professionals.

Another challenge facing CAAMS was the volatile health-care market of the 1990s. Hospitals were closing, merging, or buying up other hospitals, and if transport was part of hospital's system, it suddenly needed to demonstrate a positive financial outlook or cease to exist—quite a turnaround from the 1980s when hospitals did not worry about what the helicopter cost as long as it brought patients into the hospital and was available as a visible marketing tool. Therefore when the focus shifted to the bottom line of the budget, many hospital-based helicopter programs were fighting for survival and had difficulty justifying the cost of accreditation.

Justifying the costs of accreditation without financial incentives, such as reimbursement guarantees, were a constant source of criticism of CAAMS from its constituents. CAAMS began to

work with an aviation insurance broker in 1995 to develop an insurance incentive program. The broker would shop for underwriters willing to give premium discounts to a program based on the fact that the program was accredited. Some of the programs who were owned and operated under their own FAA Part 135 certificate did receive substantial savings in their premiums for hull and liability insurance.

The CAAMS Board of Directors also encouraged state EMS agencies to recognize accreditation in lieu of state licensure because CAAMS standards were usually more stringent that state licensing requirements. As states became familiar with the CAAMS standards, they started to change rules and regulations and to require CAAMS accreditation to uphold public confidence in the air medical transport services available to citizens of their state. Today Rhode Island, Washington, Utah, Arizona, Michigan, and certain counties in California and Nevada have rules that require CAAMS accreditation. Some of the federal programs, such as Indian Health Services, also require CAAMS accreditation for contractual purposes. And as managed care organizations become familiar with CAAMS, reimbursement is starting to be affected by a program's accreditation status. So by the late 1990s financial incentives were beginning to make a difference.

A survey was conducted in January 1998 to ask programs what motivated them to apply for accreditation. At the time there were 53 accredited services, and 47, or 89%, replied. Participants were asked to rate their reasons for applying for accreditation from the following listing.

- Benefits of an outside audit
- Competition
- Demonstrate a level of quality
- Federal transport contracts
- Indian Health Services contracts
- Lower aviation insurance premiums
- Managed care contracts
- Marketing tool
- State or county requirements
- Other

BOX 36-2 | **Frequently Cited Areas of Contingency**

Headstrike area in the aircraft is violated by equipment.

Equipment is not stored or secured appropriately.

Device for securing pediatric patients is not size appropriate.

There is no back-up source of oxygen.

There is no portable suction on board in addition to the on-board suction.

Fire extinguisher is only accessible only to the pilot.

The quality management or performance improvement program lacks follow-up and loop closure.

Medical director is not involved in the interviewing and hiring process for the medical personnel.

Skills maintenance program documentation is weak.

Initial orientation is not documented well.

Continuing clinical experiences are not documented.

Safety committee does not have representation from communications and maintenance.

There is no annual drill for the post incident/accident plan.

Despite all the complaints about costs and financial incentives, 77% of the participants chose "demonstrate a level of quality" as their highest priority for applying for accreditation. In order of highest to lowest priority, the survey showed: marketing tool, competition, managed care contracts, state or county requirements, lower aviation insurance premiums, Indian Health Services contracts, and federal transport contracts. This was a surprising result to the board because financial incentives were emphasized as a need by constituents but did not appear to be the most compelling reasons for applying for accreditation. The survey response was not only surprising but it was also inspiring. It appeared that medical transport services were still striving to create a better system and work toward a higher purpose despite the cutbacks, capitation, mergers, and reorganizations experienced by health-care providers in the 1990s.

Most medical transport services also find a number of intangible benefits as a result of going through the accreditation process, such as more cohesive working relationships, team building, a revitalized pride, and professionalism among personnel. Along with these benefits, the program receives a listing of the contingencies or areas that do not meet the intent of the accreditation standards or are not in compliance with the accreditation standards. The Commission tracks these areas of contingency and keeps a list of the most cited areas. Box 36-2 lists the most current frequently cited areas of contingency:

CAAMS changed its name in 1997 to the Commission on Accreditation of Medical Transport Systems (CAMTS) to capture a wider range of potential applicants and also to accommodate the need for standards and accreditation for the mobile intensive care ground services. Many of these ground MICU services consisted of pediatric and neonatal specialty teams, and many were part of an already existing air service. It was important for the service to be able to have its entire transport program accredited. Although the Commission on Accreditation of Ambulance Services (CAAS) exists for ground emergency services, CAAS does not have standards for critical care transport. Therefore CAMTS developed the ground standards—critical care standards were already in place—and began to fill this void in 1997 when it offered accreditation for ground critical care services as well as air medical services. In 2000 CAMTS also included basic life support (BLS) and advanced life support (ALS) ground standards to accommodate the transport services that either provided air or critical care ground services and also provided BLS and ALS ground transport.

Today there are 16 member organizations, each sending one representative to serve on the board of directors. Board members make all of the accreditation decisions, create and update policies, and revise the Accreditation Standards. In addition to the founding organizations listed earlier, CAMTS is proud to include the following member organizations:

Aerospace Medical Association (AsMA)

Air Medical Physicians Association (AMPA)

American Academy of Pediatrics (AAP)

American Association of Critical Care Nurses (AACN)

American Association of Respiratory Care (AARP)

Emergency Nurses Association (ENA)

National Air Transportation Association (NATA)

National Association of Neonatal Nurses (NANN)

National Association of State EMS Directors (NASEMSD)

It is the diversity and wealth of experience from the member organizations' board representatives that provide CAMTS with the strength and integrity to offer accreditation to medical transport services in North American and abroad and to continually improve medical transport services for patients now and in the future.

SUMMARY

Accreditation provides a framework for program evaluation and improvement. It also demonstrates to the public and the patients that we serve that a transport program complies with specific standards to ensure safe and competent patient transport.

REFERENCES

1. AIM/FAR: *91,105 flight crewmembers at stations,* New York, 1998, McGraw-Hill.
2. ASHBEAMS: *Air medical crew national standard curriculum,* Pasadena, Calif, 1988, US Department of Transportation.
3. Frazer R: Air medical accidents—20 year search for information, *AirMed* 5(5):34, 1999.
4. Helicopter Association International: *Helicopters 1948-1998—a contemporary history,* Alexandria, Va, 1998, HAI.
5. Joint Commission on Accreditation: *An introduction to the Joint Commission,* Chicago, 1988, The Commission.
6. McKenney S: Aeromedical evolution, *Aeromed* (May/June):22, 1986.
7. Richardson JG: *Health and longevity,* Philadelphia, 1914, Home Health Society.
8. Rhodes M et al: Field triage for on-scene helicopter transport, *J Trauma* 26(11):963, 1986.

37 CRITICAL CARE TRANSPORT: STRESS AND STRESS MANAGEMENT IN THE WORKPLACE

The world is becoming an increasingly volatile place in which to live. Violence and sudden death in the workplace are common occurrences, as evidenced daily on television and in the print media. Trauma, stressors, and stress sequelae are frequent topics on radio and television talk programs. This chapter discusses stress and stress symptomology pertinent to the health-care environment generally and the critical care transport industry specifically. In addition, cumulative stress or burnout is distinguished from traumatic or critical incident stress. Further, posttraumatic stress and posttraumatic stress disorder, or PTSD, are defined. Finally, stress management techniques for cumulative, traumatic stress, and PTSD are outlined.

STRESS IN THE WORKPLACE

Stress, its impact, and stress management are important research topics in the contemporary workplace. Adler[1] writes that the stress response, our "innate response to danger," once protected primitive humans from threats to their well-being; it

now may cause "nothing but trouble." Recent research shows the stress response affects the body, causing heart disease, ulcers, loss of memory, and lessened immune system response.

In 1929 Austrian endocrinologist Hans Selye identified "stressor" as any stimulus or demand placed on the organism. He used the term *stress* to describe the nonspecific response of the body to this demand or "stressor."[34] As designed, the human stress reaction serves to ensure survival of the individual. The brain perceives a threat and prepares the body to protect itself. In seconds after receiving the threat, multiple chemicals or hormones are secreted, including aldosterone, adrenaline, noradrenaline, and cortisol. These chemicals increase blood pressure, respiratory rate, and heart rate. The liver mobilizes sugar stores (gluconeogenesis), and fat reserves are processed into triglycerides for energy. Visual and hearing acuity are automatically sharpened. Blood is diverted from less-essential functions (i.e., digestion) to the brain and muscles. The body is prepared to survive a fight or flee to safety.[1,21,34]

However, modern civilization frequently stimulates the individual to "fight or flight," while withholding the opportunity to use the subsequent flood of chemicals. Rush hour commutes, project deadlines, proficiency certifications, oral presentations, and sales quotas act as psychologic stressors without immediate stress relief. Elevated blood pressure, increased heart rate, and excess sugars and fats in the system contribute to contemporary medical problems such as hypertension, coronary artery disease, and diabetes.[1]

Mitchell and Everly[34] indicate that excessive stress responses cause cognitive, physical, emotional and behavioral signs and symptoms. These responses can include the increased heart and respiratory rate and elevated blood pressure mentioned earlier. Additionally, symptoms can include fuzziness in thinking, difficulty making decisions, and memory dysfunction. Feelings of anger, depression, or being overwhelmed may result from excessive stress as can changes in eating, personal hygiene, or social interaction.

STRESS IN THE HEALTH-CARE ENVIRONMENT

Profound changes in the health-care environment in the 1990s have dramatically increased the types and amount of stress for health-care providers in general and nursing staff in particular. Rapid changes in insurance laws, revenue reimbursement, managed care, rightsizing, outsourcing, and streamlining the provision of medical care have created a climate of insecurity and uncertainty for caregivers. With the advent of the millennium, many health-care providers are closing their doors, whereas others are restructuring, downsizing, or even consolidating services. Health-care personnel, including nurses, find themselves with increasing responsibilities while continuing to be understaffed and already overworked.

Other factors contribute to health-care stress. Assaults to medical and nursing caregivers, irregular shift work, moral and ethical issues pertaining to patient care and treatment, and fear of contamination by bloodborne pathogens add to staff emotional stress, sense of victimization, and rate of turnover.[2,11,15,45] Burns and Harm[9] note that emergency department and pediatric intensive care staff find the unexpected death of a patient a profound source of stress. Marino[30] writes that nurses who

work with terminally ill patients and their bereaved survivors find cumulative grief an occupational hazard and source of burnout. Additionally, "horizontal violence," or anger, emotional violence, or aggressive behavior perpetrated by nurses on peers because of professional jealousy or a hostile work environment, can be destructive to involved personnel specifically and the profession as a whole.[48]

STRESS IN THE CRITICAL CARE TRANSPORT ENVIRONMENT

The last decade of the twentieth century was also a turbulent time for critical care transport. Coerced cooperation, consolidation, restructuring, and shutting down have been a constant as both air medical and ground-based transport programs struggle to survive monumental changes in referral patterns, reimbursements, executive vision, and configurations.* Rotorcraft providers have added fixed-wing capabilities. Air medical programs have added ground transport components. Transport personnel have found themselves either willingly evolving along with their programs or out of a job.

In addition to the sources of stress already noted, care providers in the critical care transport environment must deal with issues pertaining directly to the unique type of work they do. Ground and flight transport personnel "are expected to be proficient in performing advanced procedures, which may include endotracheal intubation, needle and surgical cricothyrotomy, chest needle decompression, tube thoracostomy . . . and assisting with emergency childbirth"[24] (Figure 37-1). Additionally, transport personnel are required to be proficient with complicated patient care issues for patients of all ages, as well as drugs, ventilators, and intra-aortic balloon pumps.[8,24] Furthermore, Isfort[24] notes, crew teamwork is absolutely essential for developing a realistic, workable plan of care for the patient.

There are physical requirements. Transport team members may need to walk great distances, lift heavy gurneys or Isolettes, and carry bulky

---

*References 3, 5, 6, 10, 16, 20, 22, 29, 33, 36, 38, 43.

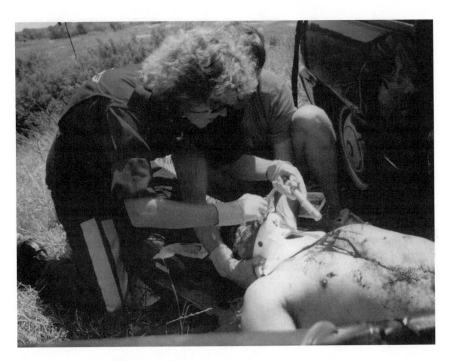

FIGURE 37-1   **Flight nurse intubating a critically injured patient.** (Photo courtesy of Margaret Watson Hopkins.)

equipment (Figure 37-2). There may also be personal weight restrictions, especially for air medical transport personnel, to stay in federal weight limit guidelines for each type of aircraft. Indeed, because of sometimes confining interior configurations of aircraft, there may be crew member size restrictions.

The working environment of the transport team can be stressful. In addition to potential lack of physical space in a vehicle or aircraft, a crew member must deal with irregular shifts, which often run into mandatory overtime because of end-of-shift transports. Meals may be irregular or even missed. Adequate hydration may be neglected.

Working outdoors in heat, rain, snow, wind, or ice may be a significant factor for transport personnel. Crew members may need to wade across flooded rice paddies in northern California or raft to a victim at a remote site in the mountains. The transport team may find themselves crawling under a vehicle in an attempt to reach a patient to establish an airway. Hypoxia at high altitudes can be a potentially fatal stressor for flight personnel.[7,8,23]

Bryan[8] writes that dealing with traumatized family members and often being the one who must deliver unpleasant information can be emotionally stressing: ". . . it is often the flight nurse who delivers the news that a loved one is seriously injured or deceased." Consequently excellent communication skills are essential. Transport personnel need to deal appropriately with caregivers at other facilities and family members. Additionally, team members are expected to facilitate conflict resolution in their own working groups. Finally, stressors in the form of required contributions to "outreach education, research, . . . safety, continuing quality improvement, public speaking and perhaps fund-raising" may occur.[24]

However, perhaps the most profound stressor that crew members must face is the personal potential for serious injury or death during a transport. The last 3 years of the 1990s and the opening of the twenty-first century have been somber years for the transport industry. Records gathered from the CONCERN Network of the Air and Surface Transport Nurses Association (ASTNA) indicate that from 14 December

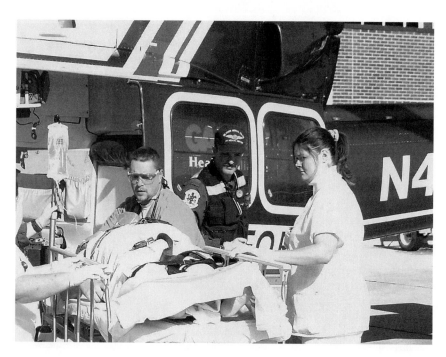

FIGURE 37-2   **Loading a patient into an aircraft.**

1997 until this writing, 14 American air medical programs and one program each from the United Kingdom and Australia have crashed, with the subsequent deaths of 41 flight personnel and serious or critical injuries to 10 others. Not since the early days of the air medical transport industry has such a loss of life occurred. The emotional impact on surviving crew peers can be devastating and lifelong.[23,34,39]

CUMULATIVE STRESS, CRITICAL INCIDENT STRESS, AND POSTTRAUMATIC STRESS DISORDER (PTSD)

CUMULATIVE STRESS OR BURNOUT

Stress is a complex relationship between a person and the environment, in which a person appraises a situation as taxing or exceeding one's resources and endangering one's well-being.[27]

Cumulative stress occurs after prolonged exposure to multiple stressors over a period of 1 to 10 years. These stressors are not necessarily severe. "Cumulative stress is usually caused by a combination of a wide range of work and nonwork stressors."[35] Cumulative stress develops slowly and subtly over a period of time. When the pressures of stress and life begin to overwhelm the transport worker's ability to cope, then the limits of wellness are being approached. If adequate stress management does not occur, burnout will be the inevitable result.[12] Burnout is very common in human services industries such as social services, mental health care, and medical care.

SIGNS OF BURNOUT

Dernocouer[12] indicates that affected individuals exhibit several common signs and symptoms of cumulative stress or burnout:

1. Negativity: Especially in persons who are generally positive or even tempered. Normally negative people may become even more negative.

2. Persistent feelings of lack of energy or fatigue: A good night's rest does not refresh.
3. Persistent cynicism: Usually noncynical individuals may puzzle their teammates with uncharacteristically sarcastic or cutting remarks. Cynical persons will become even more so.
4. Loss of motivation or enthusiasm for the job: Co-workers no longer seem to care about work or doing a good job.

PHASES OF BURNOUT

Mitchell and Bray[35] outline four phases of burnout. The "warning" phase of early cumulative stress or burnout occurs when the individual notes feelings of vague anxiety, depression, boredom, apathy, or emotional fatigue. The "mild symptoms" phase occurs in the team member who is beginning to show additional signs of distress. These symptoms include more frequent loss of emotional control; sleep disturbances; increased head, neck, back, or muscles aches; colds; increased physical or emotional fatigue; withdrawal from social contacts; irritability; and increasing depression.

During the third or "entrenched cumulative stress reaction" phase, individuals may find it difficult to make changes necessary to reverse this progression of stress. These persons will be in an increasingly emotionally painful condition. Their careers, personal happiness, and even family life may be in jeopardy. Such individuals may experience depression, increased self-medication with alcohol or nonprescription drugs, elevated blood pressure and/or cardiac problems, anorexia, profound sleep disturbances or restlessness, and more complete withdrawal from family, friends, and coworkers.

The fourth or "severe/debilitating cumulative stress reaction" phase is the most critical. At this phase, individuals may not or cannot pay attention to the many distress signals that are displayed. They may be self-destructive, and professional help will be necessary. If they do survive this phase without help, it is unlikely they will continue in the same vocation. Careers, and sometimes lives, end before they should. Victims may be both emotionally and physically sick with severe symptoms of cumulative stress and burnout: severe cardiac problems, diabetes, profound emotional depression, lowered self-confidence and esteem, inability to do the job or manage one's life, severe social withdrawal, or severely increased use of drugs or alcohol to numb the mind. They may overreact to events and have poor concentration and attention spans. They may be careless or forgetful or have frequent "accidents." They may have feelings of hostility or paranoia and moderate to severe thought disorders. They will be deeply impacted by their stress reaction.

It can take from 1 to 10 years for an individual to reach this fourth phase. Prevention of cumulative stress should be the goal in the contemporary, ever-evolving, medical transport industry. Transport program directors and concerned personnel who wish to reduce the potential for employee burnout and subsequent increased health insurance and disability costs will be wise to take proactive steps to provide ample stress management education and follow-up for staff.*

TRAUMATIC OR CRITICAL INCIDENT STRESS

Traumatic or critical incident stress differs from cumulative stress in that it is generally incident specific. It usually does not occur as a result of multiple, less-toxic stressors. Traumatic or critical incident stress occurs following a traumatic or critical incident. This type of incident is defined as ". . . a turning point event. A critical incident is *any* [italics added] event that has a stressful impact sufficient enough to overwhelm the usually effective coping skills of either an individual or a group."[34] Traumatic or critical incidents are generally unexpected, out-of-the-ordinary, and highly emotionally distressing events. Frequently they are also events with high media interest. They can have a strong emotional impact on even well-trained, experienced participants. Trauma research estimates that approximately 86% of individuals involved in a defined critical incident will have posttraumatic stress symptomology[34] (Figure 37-3).

---

*References 11, 12, 19, 27, 30, 34, 41, 45, 46.

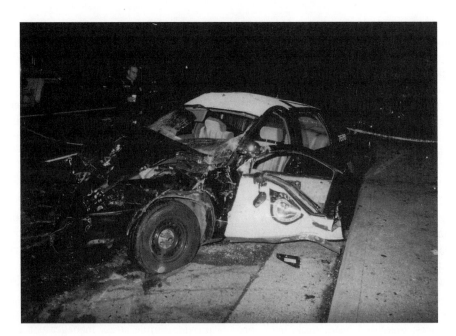

FIGURE 37-3   Police cruiser crash that involved the death of a police officer in the line of duty.

A traumatic or critical incident can happen to any individual. Citizens involved in a traffic crash in which loss of life occurs may suffer posttraumatic stress symptoms. The victim of rape, terrorism, a home invasion robbery at gunpoint involving threat of death, or torture during time of war is a candidate for posttraumatic stress symptomology.[14,17,47]

Traumatic incidents for emergency services and critical care transport personnel are frequently categorized into 10 areas (Box 37-1). Additional events that may trigger a critical incident stress response in a care provider can include (1) repetitive horrible events: alone, any single one might not be critical, but taken together, they overwhelm an individual's ability to cope with the impact; (2) symbolic events: events that remind a caregiver of the original incident—an anniversary memorial, for example, or a similar incident; and (3) multiple events: each event, like (1), in itself may not be horrible, but the events are simply cumulatively stressful until one finally occurs that is one too many. The provider is unable to use normal coping mechanisms to deal with subsequent emotions and symptoms.

Another potential critical incident trigger is (4) the event with personal meaning: the victim reminds the transporter of a family member or friend, or the incident is similar to one the worker has been involved in. Because of the personal nature of the event, coworkers may not be aware of the impact on the fellow employee. Consequently it is extremely important that critical care transport personnel be aware of their own backgrounds and "baggage" that can make a seemingly innocuous event a traumatic incident for them. Further, there are (5) threatening events: these can include being threatened by environmental dangers such as being injured in a hard landing or a traffic crash during transport. It can also include feeling in danger and threatened by a violent patient, a patient's family members, or possible bloodborne pathogens. Finally, (6) administrative abandonment of a caregiver can evoke emotions that are difficult to handle with normal coping mechanisms. Extreme anger, grief, depression,

---

| BOX 37-1 | **What Is a Critical Incident?** |

A critical incident is any event that has an impact stressful enough to overcome the usually effective coping skills of either an individual or a group. Critical incidents are usually sudden, powerful events that are outside of the range of ordinary human experience. The following are examples of such events.

1. Line-of-duty death.
2. Serious line-of-duty injury.
3. Co-worker suicide.
4. Multicasualty incidents (e.g., Oklahoma City, New York Trade Center, a multivehicle crash on the freeway, airplane crashes).
5. A police-involved shooting: either an officer is shot or an officer shoots another individual.
6. Injury or death to a civilian as a result of operational procedures (e.g., fire engine or ambulance vs. private vehicle; accidents as the result of high-speed chases).
7. Significant events involving children, especially injury or death to a child, especially if perpetrated by an adult. Ninety-five percent of the CISDs done in the United States have involved children.
8. Failed mission after extensive effort. Loss of the victim becomes very personal for the rescuer.
9. Excessive media interest: Continuous newspaper and TV coverage make it impossible to escape the event. Subsequent litigation adds to the memory.
10. Any other powerful event that strikes a chord in the transport provider. One individual's event may not be another's.

---

futility, anxiety, hopelessness, and fear for the future and one's livelihood are common reactions.[34]

POSTTRAUMATIC STRESS DISORDER (PTSD)

Transport personnel, by virtue of the jobs they perform, may find themselves exposed to trauma situations capable of jeopardizing their usually strong emotional and psychologic ability to respond appropriately. Untreated and frequently misunderstood, posttraumatic stress disorder can be a life-crippling problem.

Posttraumatic stress disorder was first officially recognized as a formal psychiatric disorder by the mental health community in 1980 following the Vietnam War. PTSD is one of the most widely used official diagnostic terms used to name psychologic sequelae that follow a traumatic event.

Posttraumatic syndromes date back in Western literature to 1666 as a result of the trauma of the Great Fire of London to the citizens of that city. But they are most commonly associated with problems encountered during wartimes. "Shell shock," "soldier's heart" (palpitations and chest pain), and "posttraumatic neurosis" are terms used to describe combat-related posttraumatic stress. However, it is important to note that "PTSD is now universally recognized as a potential response to any form of traumatic event, not just combat."[34]

Posttraumatic stress that lasts longer than 2 days but less than 30 days is termed acute stress disorder.[34] Posttraumatic stress that lasts longer than 30 days following the traumatic event is termed chronic posttraumatic stress disorder. *The Desk Reference to the Diagnostic Criteria from DSM-IV*[13] indicates that for both acute and chronic PTSD to be present:

- The person has been exposed to a traumatic event in which both of the following were present:
  - The person experienced, witnessed, or was confronted with an event or events that involved actual or threatened death or serious injury, or a threat to the physical integrity of self or others.
  - The person's response involved intense fear, helplessness, or horror.

ACUTE POSTTRAUMATIC STRESS DISORDER

Acute symptoms exist if the following factors are present:

- Either while experiencing or after experiencing the distressing event, the individual has three (or more) of the following dissociative symptoms:
  - A subjective sense of numbing, detachment, or absence of emotional responsiveness
  - A reduction in awareness of his or her surroundings (e.g., "being in a daze")
  - Derealization
  - Depersonalization
  - Dissociative amnesia (i.e., inability to recall an important aspect of the trauma)
- The traumatic event is persistently reexperienced in at least one of the following ways: recurrent images, thoughts, dreams, illusions, flashback episodes, or a sense of reliving the experience; or distress on exposure to reminders of the traumatic event.
- Marked avoidance of stimuli arouse recollections of the trauma (e.g., thoughts, feelings, conversations, activities, places, people).
- There are marked symptoms of anxiety or increased arousal (e.g., difficulty sleeping, irritability, poor concentration, hypervigilance, exaggerated startle response, motor restlessness).
- The disturbance causes clinically significant distress or impairment in social, occupational, or other important areas of functioning or impairs the individual's ability to pursue some necessary task, such as obtaining necessary assistance or mobilizing personal resources by telling family members about the traumatic experience.
- The disturbance lasts for a minimum of 2 days and a maximum of 4 weeks and occurs in 4 weeks of the traumatic event.
- The disturbance is not caused by the direct physiologic effects of a substance (e.g., a drug of abuse, a medication) or a general medical condition.

CHRONIC POSTTRAUMATIC STRESS DISORDER

Chronic posttraumatic stress disorder is a serious dysfunctional state that changes lives, ends careers, and destroys families (Box 37-2). Mitchell and Everly[34] write that the DSM-IV defines "a traumatic event as '. . . directly experiencing or witnessing actual or threatened death or serious injury or experiencing a threat to one's own physical integrity or the physical integrity of someone else.' " As noted earlier, "the response must be characterized by fear, helplessness, or horror."[34]

Mitchell and Everly[34] add that major factors predicting psychologic trauma include, among others:

1. Actual severe physical injury
2. Fear of severe physical injury
3. Fear of death
4. Torture or fear of torture
5. Sexual assault or fear of sexual assault
6. Watching someone else experience extreme pain, physical injury, or death
7. Death or injury to children
8. The violation or contradiction of a "core belief" or "critical expectation" (e.g., God, friendship, loyalty, fairness, justice, fidelity or competence)
9. Shame or guilt associated with factors other than those listed above

Further, Mitchell and Everly[34] mention that the 10th edition of *International Classification of Disease* defines a traumatic event as one that is "exceptionally threatening or catastrophic."[49] The ICD-10 notes that "PTSD may be so chronic as to transition into an enduring personality change as a direct result of the traumatic stressor, a 'trauma personality' of sorts." McCarty-Gould[31] writes that "PTSD can be an annoyance or it can be life-threatening."

Critical care transport personnel, particularly those who assist first responders with rescue, extrication, and immediate lifesaving strategies, may find themselves in situations in which they witness death or injury to a child or see someone slowly die at the scene of a traffic crash. They may be called on to do body recovery, make body identification, or give a death notification to grief-stricken family members. These obligations, which are a necessary part of the transport crew member's job, are, nonetheless, emotionally draining. Additionally, depending on the individual's psychologic hardiness and life stressors in action at a given time, a crew member may find

---

BOX 37-2 | **Chronic PTSD Symptoms**

A. The traumatic event is persistently reexperienced in one (or more) of the following ways:
   1. Recurrent and intrusive distressing recollections of the event, including images, thoughts, or perceptions
   2. Recurrent distressing dreams of the event
   3. Acting or feeling as if the traumatic event were recurring (includes a sense of reliving the experience, illusions, hallucinations, and dissociative flashback episodes, including those that occur on awakening or when intoxicated)
   4. Intense psychologic distress at exposure to internal or external cues that symbolize or resemble an aspect of the traumatic event
   5. Physiologic reactivity on exposure to internal or external cues that symbolize or resemble an aspect of the traumatic event
B. Persistent avoidance of stimuli associated with the trauma and numbing of general responsiveness (not present before the trauma), as indicated by three (or more) of the following:
   1. Efforts to avoid thoughts, feelings, or conversations associated with the trauma
   2. Efforts to avoid activities, places, or people that arouse recollections of the trauma
   3. Inability to recall an important aspect of the trauma
   4. Markedly diminished interest or participation in significant activities
   5. Feeling of detachment or estrangement from others
   6. Restricted range of affect (e.g., unable to have loving feelings)
   7. Sense of a foreshortened future (e.g., does not expect to have a career, marriage, children, or a normal life span)
C. Persistent symptoms of increased arousal (not present before the trauma), as indicated by two (or more) of the following:
   1. Difficulty falling or staying asleep
   2. Irritability or outbursts of anger
   3. Difficulty concentrating
   4. Hypervigilance
   5. Exaggerated startle response
D. Duration of the disturbance (symptoms in criteria A, B, and C) is more than 1 month
E. The disturbance causes clinically significant distress or impairment in social, occupational, or other important areas of functioning

Reprinted with permission from the *Diagnostic and statistical manual of mental disorders,* ed 4, text revision, Copyright 2000, American Psychiatric Association.

---

him- or herself suddenly stressed beyond what his or her normally vigorous coping strategies and emotional survival skills can handle.

Untreated PTSD can fester for a lifetime. In addition to a diagnosis of PTSD, the sufferer may also have other problems, such as alcoholism, panic disorder, and obsessive-compulsive disease. For example, an individual attempting to recompensate following a traumatic event may demonstrate obsessive and/or compulsive symptom patterns such as repetitive and persistent thoughts (obsessions) and/or repetitive behaviors or a rigid adherence to rules, rituals, and routines (compulsions).[17,28]

Not all transport personnel who experience a critical incident will develop PTSD. In fact, almost all who are involved in a critical or traumatic incident will begin to process and heal emotionally from the event in 3 weeks. However, some, because of their own personal stressors, may find that an event triggers something from their own background with which they are unable to deal. These are individuals who will benefit greatly from crisis-trained mental health professionals and an aggressive therapeutic approach to the problem. Some of these approaches will be discussed in following.

STRESS MANAGEMENT FOR THE TRANSPORT PROVIDER

Stress management techniques for cumulative stress (burnout), traumatic or critical incident stress, posttraumatic stress, and PTSD differ from one another. Although some techniques suggested to reduce cumulative stress symptoms may help alleviate the sequelae of a traumatic event, generally speaking, the strategies are different.

DEALING WITH CUMULATIVE STRESS

Dealing effectively with cumulative stress requires an individual to have some preexisting personality characteristics, the desire to learn new approaches, and some concrete techniques for reducing the impact of the stressors on both the mind and body.

Social support is extremely important for reducing the effects of burnout. This includes personal respect, empathy, genuineness, friendship, and opportunities for social interaction. This social support is essential from not only administrative superiors, but also co-workers and families.[19,27,41,42,46] Singh[41] advises transport organizations, which frequently have employees who rarely interact with co-workers because of shift scheduling, to proactively work on increasing social support "especially when 60% of stress occurring in paid occupations is due to relationships with colleagues."

Personal hardiness is also an excellent predictor of reduced chance of burnout. Simoni and Paterson[41] write that hardy personnel reduce stress through "reappraisal of stressors encountered and by using adaptive coping behaviors." They note that hardiness has three components or behaviors: (1) challenge, or openness to change and problem solving; (2) commitment, or a feeling of involvement; and (3) control, or a sense of personal influence. Transport personnel who experience less burnout are open to change, feel as if they are involved with change and problem solving, and finally, have a sense of control as it pertains to change. In other words, they feel their input makes a difference in their world. In an environment where change absolutely has become the norm, such attitudes and behaviors can literally be life and job savers.

Two types of coping behaviors identified are active or inactive and direct or indirect.[27,41] Active coping strategies, oriented toward the stress sources, are found to relate to low levels of burnout in nurses. Inactive coping strategies that involve avoidance or denial of the stressor have been shown to lead to higher levels of burnout and greater psychologic dysfunction under stress. Avoidance or denial of the stressor is emotionally exhausting. It leads to depersonalization of the crew member who denies the impact of the stressor. Finally, because the stressor continues to exert stress, the caregiver experiences lack of personal accomplishment. Nothing has changed except for a more negative emotional state for the crew member and an increased chance of burnout.

Direct and indirect coping behaviors also impact stress. Direct coping approaches are applied outwardly to the sources of stress. The objective is to either eliminate or reduce the size of the threat so the individual can better handle the situation (Box 37-3). Indirect coping approaches (Box 37-4) are those applied inwardly to one's own emotions, behaviors, and attitudes. The goal of indirect coping may include changing one's perception of the stressor or changing any of the components of the stress response.[27,41] These two coping approaches tend to diminish the impact of the stressors. Conversely, palliative coping measures, such as overeating, abuse of alcohol or nonprescription drugs, or overuse of unhelpful defense mechanisms, will produce higher levels of stress while potentiating burnout.

DEALING WITH TRAUMATIC OR CRITICAL INCIDENT STRESS

Crisis intervention is the approach used to alleviate the stress response experienced by individuals who have been involved in a critical incident. The crisis intervention approach is built on basic psychiatric principles that have proven effective over the years. These principles are used in current military stress relief operations and are essential in certain aspects of CISM crisis services. These principles are (1) immediacy, (2) proximity, and (3) expectancy.[34] A fourth principle frequently applied is brevity.

BOX 37-3 | **Direct Coping Strategies**

Direct coping strategies aim to eliminate or reduce the size of the threat so the person is better able to handle the situation.

1. Enhance health through exercise, adequate rest, and a balanced diet to produce a positive stressor-management effect.
2. Leave the stressful situation.
3. Change problematic aspects of the situation to reduce demand from the environment (e.g., interpersonal working conditions, short staffing, poor lighting, excessive noise).
4. Nurture social support. Social support is an important buffer against stressors. This can be done with selected friends or a self-help group.
5. Learn on one's own with books, tapes, and videos.
6. Increase one's knowledge base with a trained instructor.

From Kivisto J, Couture RT: Stress management for nurses controlling the whirlwind. *Nursing Forum*, 32:25-33, 1997.

Immediacy implies that support services for distressed personnel will take place as soon as possible after the traumatic incident. Proximity means that the intervention will take place as close to the scene as possible in a safe and controlled environment. In the civilian arena, this generally means at a predetermined meeting place such as a hospital or hall. Expectancy is defined as reassuring the participants in the intervention that they will be able to resume their normal duties and their usual activities when the stress reaction subsides. If they believe they will get better, they generally are motivated to work with the process. Brevity means that the interventions will be only as long as necessary to accomplish their goals.

Critical incident stress management (CISM) as promoted by the International Critical Incident Stress Foundation (ICISF) is a comprehensive program designed to mitigate the impact of critical incidents on the individuals who participate in them. CISM is based on sound crisis intervention techniques that have been practiced since World War I (Box 37-5). The process has been further perfected by research done concerning disaster responders, law enforcement issues, modern military involvement, and contributions from mental health and hospital services. It is becoming the standard of care in the emergency services, hospitals, industry, schools, the community, and the military internationally. The ICISF has been granted Special Consultive Status to the Economic and Social Policy Council of the United Nations.

CISM interventions accelerate the recovery of emergency services and critical care transport team members following a crisis event. The goals of CISM are to educate workers so they understand what has happened to them and to teach them appropriate crisis management coping skills. These coping skills will enable them stay on the job, decrease their stress responses to the incident, lessen the chance of emotional exhaustion, decrease turmoil in their lives and homes, minimize turnover in the workplace, and reduce employer expenses by reducing employee sick and stress leave.

CISM's comprehensive program involves seven components. These are (1) preincident education, (2) defusings, (3) demobilizations following disasters, (4) debriefings or CISDs, (5) support services for significant others, (6) individual consults or peer support, and (7) follow-up services.

One of the most important CISM components is preincident education. This is also called psychologic inoculation. The goals of preincident education are to (1) introduce workers to the potential stressors of the job in a realistic manner, including sights, sounds, and smells; (2) educate employees concerning stress responses that they may experience in potential crisis events as they perform their jobs; (3) teach appropriate coping skills and survival techniques; and (4) provide resources and referrals

BOX 37-4   Indirect Coping Strategies for Stress Management

Behavioral Interventions

The goal is to act differently so that new and effective coping patterns are acquired.

1. Slow down normal daily activities to enjoy the small pleasures in life.
2. Enjoy more humor in life by reading humorous books, watching humorous films. Allow yourself to laugh.
3. Spend time with positive people.
4. Decrease palliative coping behavior (overeating, abuse of alcohol or nonprescription drugs) and increase positive coping behavior (exercise, proper diet).
5. Take hardiness training (commitment, control, and challenge).
   a. Commitment: Tendency to involve oneself in activities with the environment.
   b. Control: Believing and acting as if one can influence events.
   c. Challenge: Individuals who feel appropriately challenged are more likely to demonstrate higher levels of confidence and have lower levels of disabling emotions and greater capabilities in using resources than individuals who feel threatened.
6. Reshape behaviors that are characteristic of type A personality traits (e.g., free-floating hostility, sense of time urgency and insecurity of status associated with a preoccupation with numbers). Like item1 above—slow down. It's OK.

Cognitive Interventions

The goal is to develop more realistic, positive, and self-supportive thinking patterns to positively enhance feelings and actions. These strategies are useful when one adds stress to life by exaggerating threat, catastrophizing, or putting self down.

1. Positive self-talk serves to defuse anxiety induced by exaggeration. The individual learns to use fewer self-critical remarks and to be more self-encouraging. This enables him or her to objectively assess the real risk in a situation and focus on personal strengths.
2. Mental imagery involves visualizing relaxing images and has the effect of calming the mind and inducing a more relaxed physiologic state.
3. Thought stopping is a two-step process: recognizing and stopping anxious thoughts, followed by a relaxation technique. The pleasant sensations of relaxation reinforce the thought-stopping process and decrease negative consequences.
4. Stress inoculation: The individual is educated about his or her stress reaction, trained in coping skills, and provided with opportunities to practice these skills.
5. Reframe the stressor. Is the event a threat or is it the individual's perception? For example, does a failing grade make the student a failure? Or can the issue be reframed by saying, "This problem can be fixed if I make some changes." The student must make the changes, but reframing the matter makes it less psychologically devastating.

Physiologic Interventions

The goal is to produce a physical state that is not compatible with the physiologic arousal that is generally associated with stress. This state is referred to as the relaxation response.

1. Learn diaphragmatic breathing. Sit quietly and take slow, deep breaths while expanding the abdomen rather than the chest. Relaxed breathing relaxes the person.
2. Practice progressive relaxation. Contract a muscle group for 20 seconds; relax it; progress from one muscle group to another throughout the body.
3. Practice yoga. Many have found it to be beneficial in acquiring a relaxed body and calm state of mind.

BOX 37-5	**Why Is CISM Effective?**

CISM defusing and debriefing interventions are effective because interventions:

1. Occur early—often within hours after the crisis event.
2. Offer the opportunity for catharsis or ventilation that can lower stress levels and help make sense of the trauma.
3. Allow co-workers to verbalize the trauma. Participants verbally reconstruct and express the specific traumas, fears, or regrets they experienced. Using words, they can make concrete the emotions, images, and memories that are keeping them off balance.
4. Provide a behavioral structure with a beginning and end, superimposed on the event that frequently represents chaos, suffering, and unanswerable questions. Research shows that this structured environment within which to "worry" reduces the tendency for worry to interfere with other activities.
5. Provide a psychologic structure for individuals to explore the critical incident from the cognitive or thinking level down through the emotional level and then back again to the everyday world.
6. Provide opportunity for group support. The sense of individual isolation is reduced, useful information is shared, and mutual comfort and help are given. The social network is restored.
7. Offer peer support. People who've been through the same experiences are there to reassure colleagues that life will be OK eventually.
8. Offer education on stress, and teach coping techniques for dealing with the physical and emotional effects of the critical incident on the body and mind.
9. Provide opportunity for follow-up. Additional peer support, mental health assistance, and chaplain involvement are built in for individuals who might like more assistance—even before they ask.
10. Are action oriented. People are not allowed to remain in a state of confusion. Participants in interventions feel their concerns are being taking seriously. They feel group leaders are in control and know what they are talking about.

for individuals who request further information. The concept of psychologic inoculation is rapidly gaining strength in many high-risk professions, including the emergency services (including fire service and law enforcement), social services, the government (including the FBI, BATF, Federal Marshals, and U.S. Federal Probation Department), schools, the military, hospitals, and business and industry. The increase in violence in the workplace along with the potential for line-of-duty death in high-risk professions has made such an emphasis on stress training imperative.[25,28,44,46]

Three other crisis interventions are commonly offered following a critical event. All of the interventions are completely confidential. It is emphasized that no one on the intervention team will ever discuss the meeting outside of the room. Participants are also encouraged to maintain confidentiality to foster a feeling of emotional security during the discussion.

The first intervention is one-on-one peer support or the individual consult. A CISM peer who has taken the Basic Critical Incident Stress Management training class can provide crisis intervention for one to three people following an incident. As noted earlier, a defined critical incident may affect only one worker involved in that incident. Because crisis interventions are response based rather than event based, interventions should be offered only when there is an indication that they are needed. When one to three people are affected, a single trained peer can intervene.

A defusing is the second crisis intervention offered. A defusing is an informal, educational discussion that takes place 8 to 12 hours following an incident. It is facilitated by coworker peers trained in Basic CISM. Depending on the size of the group, the discussion may last from 20 minutes to an hour. Participants share who they are, what their role was in the incident, and what happened from their point of view. They discuss any immediate stress responses they may have had. Peer team members then offer information on what they might possibly experience in the next few hours or days. Additionally, peers teach positive coping skills, including the need for proper diet and exercise to decrease the "fight or flight" chemicals in the body. The need to continue talking about the event to co-workers or family members, if necessary, is emphasized. Printed material is given out with additional information plus phone numbers of peer team members if participants would like to discuss the event privately.

The critical incident stress debriefing (CISD) is the third crisis intervention offered. This is a seven-phase, formal discussion that occurs between 24 and 72 hours following the event. It is facilitated by a mental health professional (e.g., social worker, therapist, or psychologist). However, it is emphasized that none of the crisis interventions, including the CISD, is psychotherapy. They are discussions of what happened from each individual's point of view and the impact that the event is having on the participants. They are educational and instructive. Support is given in a safe, secure environment, and individuals are encouraged to put into words the impact the event is having on them.[4]

Follow-up services are routinely offered after a crisis intervention. Follow-up includes a face-to-face conversation, a telephone call to each participant in the group, or a ride along in the case of a transport crew. It can also include referrals for additional help, if requested. This can mean referral to a crisis-trained therapist for in-depth treatment, a clergyperson for spiritual guidance, or even an attorney if legal advice is appropriate.

Another resource available to critical care transport teams is the Surface to Air Response Team for CISM (START for CISM). This CISM team is a national effort by CISM-trained air medical personnel to provide services to the national transport industry. It is composed of flight nurses, paramedics, pilots, and mechanics. Mental health professionals familiar with the unique culture of the transport industry are also on the team. The START team provides mutual aid to local CISM teams when

a transport provider requests help. The team also provides telephone consult services and assists with referrals as needed. The START team has responded members to work in tandem with local crisis teams following line-of-duty deaths, injuries, and other incidents that have affected individual crews and personnel. The START team is available without cost to requesting programs. The toll-free number for the START team is (877) 327-3737 (Figure 37-4).

CISM is a proven program that provides education and support for individuals who have been confronted with an incident that is so out of their ordinary realm of experience that they are unable to deal with it using normally strong coping skills. It provides an opportunity to put into words the most troublesome aspects of the event. It offers personnel the ability to understand the meaning of the incident and its impact on them. It promotes well-being, mental health, social support, insight, and perspective. It mitigates stress responses and accelerates recovery in normal people who are having normal responses to extraordinary events.[26,28,32,34]

DEALING WITH POSTTRAUMATIC STRESS DISORDER

Unmitigated stress following trauma can lead to PTSD. This disorder has the capability to destroy lives, marriages, and families. Although PTSD has been identified with Vietnam veterans and returning service personnel from other wars, it is not unique to combat survivors. Any individual who has had a traumatic event occur in his or her life that turned a world upside down is a potential candidate for PTSD. This includes civilian survivors of war, torture, rape, domestic violence, and sexual abuse. In addition, personnel in high-risk professions, including the critical care transport industry, can become victims of PTSD.

As noted earlier, PTSD is a posttraumatic stress syndrome that lasts longer than 4 weeks. Generally, the individual does not recover spontaneously but requires therapy. In the case of an entrenched disorder, intense therapy may last for years.[50]

Ochberg[37] suggests that three principles are fundamental to posttraumatic therapy. The first is the normalization principle; that is, "There is a general

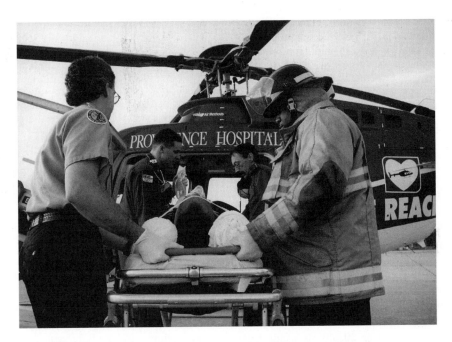

FIGURE 37-4   The air medical transport environment has its own unique types of stresses.

pattern of post-traumatic adjustment and the thought and feeling that make up this pattern are normal, although they may be painful and perplexing." Traumatized or victimized individuals are reacting normally to exceedingly abnormal events. However, they may confuse the abnormality of the event with abnormality in themselves. The crisis-trained therapist helps them see that they are having normal reactions to an event that is outside their life's norm. They are not crazy.

The second principle is the collaborative and empowering principle: "The therapeutic relationship must be collaborative, leading to empowerment of one who has been diminished in dignity and security.... The exposure to human cruelty, the feeling of dehumanization, and the experience of powerlessness creates a diminished sense of self."[37] Survivors of trauma, victimization, natural disasters and emergency services personnel who have participated in failed rescue or body recovery feel helpless, powerless, and diminished. They benefit from building a collegial and therapeutic alliance with a crisis-trained therapist who can assist them in empowering themselves.

The third principle is individuality. "Every individual has a unique pathway to recovery after traumatic stress."[37] The therapist and the client will explore this path together. They will be aware of the general direction they need to go, but will also be willing to discover new truths when it is necessary.

An adjunct to PTSD is a recent innovation called Eye Movement Desensitization and Reprocessing, or EMDR, developed by Francine Shapiro in the late 1980s. EMDR assists the individual who has incapacitating memories or intrusive images to reprocess those memories, remove their toxic elements, and put them into proper perspective. Shapiro and Forrest[40] write:

EMDR is a complex and powerful method of psychotherapy that integrates many of the most successful elements of a wide range of therapeutic approaches, even long-term Freudian analysis. In addition, it uses eye movements or other forms of rhythmical stimulation, such as hand taps or tones, in a way that seems to assist the brain's information-processing system to proceed at a rapid rate.[40]

Although EMDR appears radical and has its critics, it has been used with success since 1987. Well-documented research indicates that individuals have been helped and that a high success rate has been achieved by well-trained and competent practitioners of the therapy. Because it is so powerful, EMDR should never be used except with a licensed therapist. It is important for those interested in the process to understand that although there can be rapid results achieved and a dramatic lessening of intrusive images and memories, that it is not simple. It works only when it is used properly.

More published case reports and research support EMDR than any other method used in the treatment of trauma. Over 20,000 clinicians have been trained worldwide. Positive therapeutic results with the method have been reported with combat veterans, crime victims, police officers, sufferers of phobias and panic disorders, the bereaved, traumatized children, sexual assault victims, victims of accidents, and individuals with dissociative disorders. Additionally, there are more *controlled studies* of EMDR than of any other method used in the treatment of PTSD.[40]

CRITICAL CARE TRANSPORT: EVOLVING, DYNAMIC, AND LIFE CHANGING

The critical care transport environment, encompassing flight and ground personnel, is one of the most dynamic components of today's rapidly evolving medical care community. It is not surprising that it is also a high-risk profession. Change is a given. In addition to this unprecedented change, transport personnel also deal daily with the most critically ill patients. These practitioners are given the responsibility of receiving such patients, transporting, delivering appropriate care, and transferring care of those patients at the conclusion of their journey. Frequently these journeys begin inside a

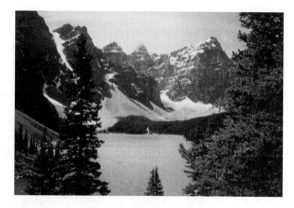

FIGURE 37-5   Hiking and taking photographs of that experience is one method of managing stress.

crushed vehicle on a freeway. Frequently they also end there.

Critical care transport personnel are proud of what they do. They are proud of their helicopters, fixed wings, and ambulances. They are proud of their skills. They are proud of their co-workers, their national associations, certifications, and uniforms. They are both proud and humbled when the family of one of their patients tells them, simply, "Thank you. You saved my child's life."

But these personnel also make some of the most difficult decisions any caregiver can make. Literally, their decisions can mean the difference between life and death for a patient. It is an awesome, stressful responsibility. It is not surprising that turnover in some programs is high and that burnout can mean the end of a career.

SUMMARY

Understanding stress in its various forms means understanding the impact that it has on the individual caregiver. It also means understanding the ways of gaining control over that impact. As transport personnel, we are controllers. We have to be. Learning about stress in its various forms and appropriate stress management strategies (Figure 37-5) gives us the opportunity to not only continue caring for our patients and our co-workers, but also to care for ourselves.[18]

REFERENCES

1. Adler J: Stress, *Newsweek* 58, June 14, 1999.
2. Appleton L: What's a critical incident? *The Canadian Nurse/L'Infirmiere Canadienne* 90(8):23, 1994.
3. Becknell J, Ostrow LS: Providers' primer on managed care, *J Emerg Med Serv* 81, 85, March 1996.
4. Blacklock E: Workplace stress: a hospital team approach, *Prof Nurse* 13:744, 1998.
5. Blumen I: Rising to the challenge: a UCAN tradition, *Air Med* 3(4):14, 16, 1997.
6. Bourn S: What's my line? *J Emerg Med Serv* 47, March 1995.
7. Boyko SM: Know your limitations: the hypoxic flight nurse, *J Emerg Nurs* 20:556, 1994.
8. Bryan S: Flight nursing, *J Emerg Nurs* 22:491, 1996.
9. Burns C, Harm NJ: Emergency nurses' perceptions of critical incidents and stress debriefing, *J Emerg Nurs* 19:431, 1993.
10. Cady G: Cooperation: an alternative to consolidation or bankruptcy, *J Emerg Med Serv* 34, 40, April 1994.
11. Caldwell MF: Incidence of PTSD among staff victims of patient violence, *Hosp and Comm Psych* 43:838, 1992.
12. Dernocoeur KB: *Streetsense: communication, safety, and control*, ed 3, Redmond Wash, 1996, Laing Research Services.
13. *Desk reference to the diagnostic criteria from DSM-IV*, Washington, DC, 1994, American Psychiatric Association.
14. De L Horne DJ: Traumatic stress reactions to motor vehicle accidents. In Wilson JP, Raphael, B, editors: *International handbook of traumatic stress syndromes*, New York, 1993, Plenum Press.
15. Dorevitch S, Forst L: The occupational hazards of emergency physicians, *Am J Emerg Med* 18:300, 2000.
16. Dries DJ: Positively influencing lives: Loyola Lifestar, *Air Med* 3(4):15, 20, 1997.
17. Everly GS Jr, Mitchell JT: *Critical incident stress management: a new era and standard of care in crisis intervention*, ed 2, Ellicott City, Md, 1999, Chevron.
18. Fenn J, Rega P, Stavros M, Buderer NF: Assessment of US helicopter emergency medical services' planning and preparedness for disaster response, *Air Med J* 18:12, 1999.
19. Firth H, McIntee J, McKeown P, Britton P: Interpersonal support amongst nurses at work, *J Adv Nurs* 11:273, 1986.
20. Garza MA: From mom and pop to big business: the ambulance industry consolidates, *J Emerg Med Serv* 44, April 1994.
21. Girdano DA, Everly JS Jr, Dusek DE: *Controlling stress and tension: a holistic approach*, Englewood Cliffs, NJ, 1993, Prentice Hall.
22. Herron H, Johnson R, Falcone RE: Grant LifeFlight: portrait of progressive expansion, *Air Med* 1(6):22, 1995.
23. High K, Vassar J: Flight crew safety: a compelling case example, *J Emerg Nurs* 22:52, 1996.
24. Isfort DA: So you want to be a flight nurse, *J Emerg Nurs* 25:531, 1999.
25. Kearns D: On a mission, *Air Med* 6(5):30, 2000.
26. Kalaine S: Critical incident stress management: taking care of our own, *Air Med* 5(6):34, 1999.
27. Kivisto J, Couture RT: Stress management for nurses: controlling the whirlwind, *Nurs Forum* 32:25, 1997.
28. Maggio M, Terenzi E: The impact of critical incident stress: is your office prepared to respond? *Federal Probation* 57(4):10, 1993.
29. Marasco ER., Bryant W: Baking the pie: will there be enough to go around? *Air Med* 6(5):28, 2000.
30. Marino PA: The effects of cumulative grief in the nurse, *J Intrav Nurs* 21:101, 1998.
31. McCarty-Gould C: *Crisis and chaos: life with the combat veteran*, Commack, NY, 1998, Kroshka Books.
32. McSkimming J: Training for life, *Air Ambulance* 4(2):18, 2000.
33. MedTrans President David White speaks out on high-performance EMS, expanded scope and his vision for the future, *J Emerg Med Serv* 7, 38, 40, December 1995.
34. Mitchell JT, Everly GS Jr: *Critical incident stress debriefing: an operations manual for the prevention of traumatic stress among emergency services and disaster workers*, ed 2, Ellicott City, Md, 1997, Chevron.
35. Mitchell JT, Bray G: *Emergency services stress: guidelines for preserving the health and careers of emergency services personnel*, Englewood Cliffs, NJ, 1990, Prentice Hall.
36. Morris M: A united effort, *Air Med* 1 (5):33, 1995.
37. Ochberg FM: Post-traumatic therapy. In Everly GS Jr, Lating JM, editors: *Pyschotraumatology: key papers and core concepts in post-traumatic stress*, New York, 1995, Plenum.
38. Reeder L: Bigger issues than the payers: the business of air medical transport, *Air Med* 1(1):42, 1995.
39. Robinson KS: Air medical crashes: a duty to serve or a duty to survive? *J Emerg Nurs* 25:351, 1999.
40. Shapiro F, Forrest MS: *EMDR: eye movement desensitization & reprocessing*, New York, 1997, Basic Books.

41. Simoni PS, Paterson JJ: Hardiness, coping and burnout in the nursing workplace, *J Prof Nurs* 13:178, 1997.

42. Singh RG: Relationship between occupational stress and social support in flight nurses, *Aviation Space and Environ Med* 61:349, 1990.

43. Smith BD: Healthy competition: is there always a better way? *Inter Air Ambulance Police Aviation: Millennium Issue* 28, 34, 2000.

44. Spitzer WJ, Burke L: A critical-incident debriefing program for hospital-based health care personnel, *Health and Social Work* 18:149, 1993.

45. Stanton T: Coping with stress on the job, *Kai Tiaki Nursing N Z* 17, Dec/Jan 1998-99.

46. Toscano R, Ponterdolph M: The personality to buffer burnout, *Nurs Manag* 29(8):32L, 32N, 32R, 1998.

47. Wardak AWH: The psychiatric affects of war stress on Afghanistan society. In Wilson JP, Raphael B, editors: *International handbook of traumatic stress syndromes,* New York, 1993, Plenum.

48. Wilson M: Horizontal violence: a challenge for nursing, *Kai Tiaki N Z* 24, Feb 2000.

49. World Health Organization: *International classification of diseases: classification of mental and behavioral disorders,* Geneva, Switzerland, 1992, Author.

50. Zaczek R: *Farewell darkness,* Annapolis, Md, 1994, Naval Institute.

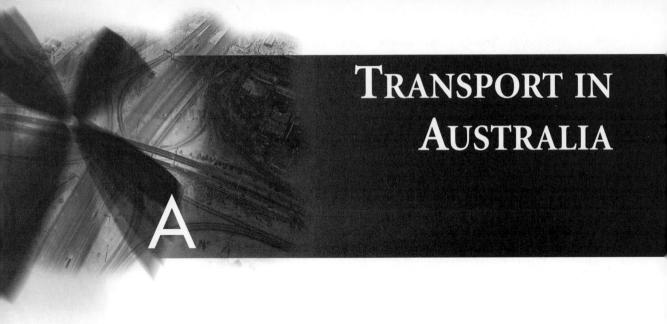

FLIGHT NURSING IN AUSTRALIA

INTRODUCTION

Flight Nurses Australia (FNA) has been an incorporated body since 1995 and was established by an interested, enthusiastic group of flight nurses who sought to promote their unique professional role.

It was challenging to represent the diversity of practice that exists across the vast distances of Australia in this specialty field.

1. **Aims**

    To promote flight nursing in the Australian region, representing the speciality of nursing in the aviation/transport environment, and to provide a professional identity and promote national recognition for flight nursing as a nursing specialty.

2. **Objectives**

    The objects for which the Association is established are:

    i. To provide a unified voice for flight nurses in the Australian region, promoting their general welfare, education standards, professional interests, and to uphold the status of flight nursing as a professional nursing specialty.

    ii. To uphold the role of the flight nurse as a valuable member of any aeromedical crew.

    iii. To facilitate and promote flight nursing knowledge through endorsement of Flight Nursing Courses, and continuing education via newsletters and conferences.

    iv. To provide a forum for communication and co-operation among flight nurses and other medical and non-medical personnel.

    v. To develop national standards for flight nursing practice and promote the delivery of quality care to our patients.

    vi. To promote research that relates to the impact of health delivery in the aviation/transport environment.

    vii. To act as an advisory body for aeromedical information relating to nursing practice in the aviation/transport environment.

HISTORY

The history of aeromedical services in Australia is analogous with that of the Royal Flying Doctor Service of Australia and along with the other two main fixed-wing aeromedical organizations—NT Aerial Medical Service and NSW Air Ambulance—employ the majority of flight nurses in Australia.

ROYAL FLYING DOCTOR SERVICE OF AUSTRALIA

The Royal Flying Doctor Service of Australia (RFDS) was the first aerial medical organization in the world and remains unique for its range of services. The RFDS was the vision of the Reverend John Flynn. He believed that the outback of Australia needed what he termed "a mantle of safety" for all those who lived, worked, and travelled through that unforgiving country.

The first record of flight nurses in Australia was recorded with the history of RFDS, although it has been a sadly forgotten history and not recorded to the extent that it has deserved. This history has been compiled by Jill Barclay while undertaking her PhD and is titled "The RFDS of Australia—The Nurses story." Much of the information obtained is courtesy of her research.

The first component of Flynn's "mantle of safety" consisted of a network of Australian Inland Mission hostels/hospitals staffed by nurses throughout the outback. The first hostel opened in 1912 at Oodnadatta. Within 14 years, 10 hostels/hospitals had been established, all staffed by registered nurses. The second component of his vision was an aeromedical service. The radical concept of combining airplane, radio, and medicine to outback Australia reached fruition in 1928 at Cloncurry, Queensland, in the form of an experiment.

In 1939 a young nurse, Meg McKay, wife of the Reverend Fred McKay, a boundary padre (later to be John Flynn's successor), flew from Cloncurry to Bulia to accompany the flying doctor and assist with immunization and surgery.

State Department of Health nurses also worked on RFDS aircraft for many years, usually being on call for flights, while working in the local hospitals.

However, the concept of a flying nurse was established in Flynn's mind, and in 1945 the Victorian, South Australian, and New South Wales sections of the Flying Doctor Service jointly funded an experiment of a flying nurse based at Broken Hill. Myra Blanch, a woman who had also worked for the Australian Inland Mission before serving in the second World War, was employed in the position. Her job description provides interesting reading.

1. *To engage in home nursing.*
2. *To relieve nursing staff in emergency cases in hospitals within the area of the Flying Doctor Service (FDS).*

3. *To give advice and help on matters of public health and prevention of disease; also medical advice when necessary. Also to dispense ante- and post-natal advice.*
4. *To broadcast talks over the Network on subjects of FDS interest in times to be arranged; also talks and visits to the schools.*
5. *To perform medical surveys and immunize children within the area.*
6. *It is intended that the nurse should, in the course of time, visit every homestead within the area, particularly those without radio or telephone communications.**

Myra Blanch carried out her duties with an incredible degree of excellence; her title, flying sister, was somewhat a misnomer. She did most of her traveling by any form of transport that was available. Additionally she did relieve the flying doctor during short absences and accompany him in the aircraft on request.* Despite the superb role model created by Myra Blanch, no other sections employed flight nurses at that point in time. However, the FDS did continue to use State Health Department nurses from local hospitals when required.

In 1947 the Western Australian Health Department appointed a Flying Infant Welfare Sister at Wyndham, a remote area town on the north of that state. While infant welfare was Lucy Garlick's prime role, she also relieved nursing staff at hospitals in the area, escorted patients to hospitals in the flying doctor aircraft, and when the doctor was unavailable, conducted the FDS clinics. During that time she reported that one of the doctors appointed to the flying doctor position had an extreme dislike of flying. So for 10 months she did all the aeromedical work herself.

However, it was not until the 1960s that other sections realized the value of assigned flight nurses. The Western Australian Health Department was first to appoint a registered nurse solely to

---

*Written radio reports prepared by the Honorary Secretary of the FDS Council for NSW Section and broadcast on a monthly basis to the NSW FDS Network, 1946–1954.

flying duties with the Victorian section of the RFDS.

The RFDS continued to employ flight nurses at all of their bases in the dual role of providing emergency care and basic health services to people living in isolated areas with no residential medical services.

The flight nurse population in the RFDS has increased from one in 1945 to around 80 in 2001. The service flies, on average, more than 8.8 million kilometers per year, sees over 155,000 clients in the outback, and evacuates approximately 14,500 clients to hospitals for further treatment.

NORTHERN TERRITORY AERIAL MEDICAL SERVICE (NTAMS)

Dr. Clyde Fenton founded the Northern Territory Aerial Medical Service (NTAMS), which commenced operations in Katherine in 1932 and was inaugurated as an official service in 1946. In the early formative years, 1932 to 1940, Department of Health nurses from Katherine Hospital flew with Dr. Clyde Fenton.

During World War II, NTAMS evacuations and medical advice was maintained by No. 6 Communication squadron of the RAAF. Post-war, when the service was inaugurated, flight nurses were provided by Alice Springs, Darwin, and Katherine hospitals for NTAMS flights. In 1948, the first full time Aerial Medical Service Flight Nurse, Ms. Meryl Nichols, was appointed.

The NTAMS provides similar functions as that of the RFDS but has its unique qualities.

Service provision includes:

- 24-hour emergency evacuation service to remote areas in the top end of the Northern Territory, oil rigs in the Timor Sea, ships at sea, and parts of Southeast Asia
- 24-hour medical consultation service to remote and isolated individuals in the top end, ships at sea, and oil rigs
- Interhospital transfers intrastate, interstate, and overseas
- Routine medical and nursing clinics to remote communities in the top end of the Northern Territory

There are three bases located in Darwin, Gove, and Katherine employing 15 flight nurses and one operations/flight nurse manager.

THE AIR AMBULANCE SERVICE OF NEW SOUTH WALES:

The Air Ambulance Service of New South Wales is based at Kingsford Smith Airport, Sydney, Australia.

The Service commenced operations on the 24 March 1967. The role of the Service is the interhospital transportation of patients throughout New South Wales including Lord Howe Island. The Service also transports New South Wales residents to and from Victoria, Queensland, and South Australia, covering an area of 800,000 square kilometers. Statistics over a 12-month period (2000-2001) show that they flew 2063 flights over 5408 hours and transported 4452 patients.

The four Super KingAir B200C aircraft are staffed by 16 flight nurses and 16 pilots. One flight nurse and one pilot per flight perform 93 percent of the work undertaken. Seven percent of the work is undertaken with the assistance of other medical personnel from retrieval services.

The flight nurses are employed by the Ambulance Service of New South Wales and are all Registered General Nurses and Registered Midwives with qualifications or extensive experience in critical care areas of nursing such as emergency and intensive care. After joining the service, additional training is given in aviation medicine, stabilization and transportation of differing medical conditions, and advanced life support protocols as per the Ambulance Service of New South Wales.

An external contractor employs the pilots and engineers. The coordination and planning of flights is managed 24 hours a day by Aeromedical and Retrieval Service Coordination Officers employed by the Ambulance Service of New South Wales. Each aircraft can carry two stretcher patients and two sitting patients.

THE SCOPE OF PRACTICE OF FLIGHT NURSING IN AUSTRALIA

Flight nurse practice is multidimensional with diverse characteristics that are defined by the operational scope and core business of the organization by whom they are employed.

The variation in aeromedical organizations includes the following:

- Aeromedical services that employ full-time flight nurses whose primary role is the preparation, stabilisation, and transport of patients across the lifespan and health specialities in the aeromedical environment. The transfer may be from either a primary, secondary, or tertiary level, and for some nurses it may also incorporate provision of primary health-care services.
- Specialist retrieval services who operate from a tertiary level facility and transport patients in their own speciality areas (i.e., adult, pediatric, or neonatal).
- International retrieval services who coordinate the repatriation of patients to and or from their country of origin and encompass the lifespan and health specialities.

FNA formulated their standards document in 2000. The intent of these standards is to ensure that all patients in Australia will be transported by expert flight nurses who have the knowledge and skills to provide the highest level of care during transport and at the hospital or scene.

The standards identify those elements that constitute the unique role of the flight nurse.

The implications for the flight nurse in complying with the standards is that they will be able to:

- Demonstrate the core competencies that are required for all registered nurses
- Practice at an advanced level in the unique context of flight nurse practice
- Frequently work in professional isolation
- Work as a sole practitioner or as a member of a team
- Provide care across the lifespan of diverse groups
- Provide health care across a diverse range of health specialities
- Work in consultation with a variety of health professionals

REFERENCES

Barclay J: The RFDS of Australia—the nurses story, *Oral History of Australia Journal.*

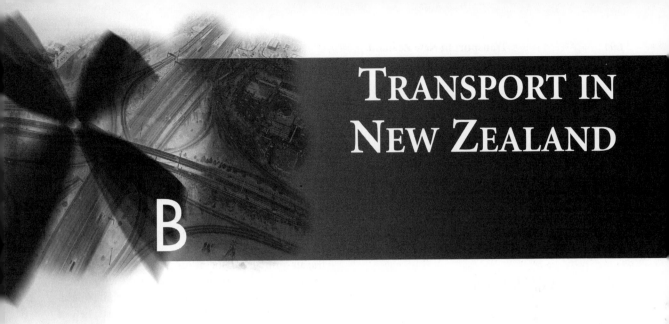

TRANSPORT IN NEW ZEALAND

B

HISTORY

In 1996 the New Zealand Flight Nurses Association (NZFNA) was formed as a national interest section of the New Zealand Nurses Organisation (NZNO). This association was formed to increase the knowledge of nurses who were caring for patients at higher altitudes and the effects that high altitude had on a patient, but also to promote networking amongst nurses working in this area.

Nurses were flying patients around New Zealand with minimal or no training in aviation nursing with retrospective stories being heard of patients deteriorating unexpectedly in flight. These nurses were generally taken from duty in hospital wards and being told to transfer a patient to another hospital.

In New Zealand there are a large number of air ambulance services per capita of population. This can be attributed to the terrain and the location of tertiary services.

TRAINING

The Aviation Industry Association Air Rescue/Air Ambulance Division (AIA/ARAA) had already developed recommended minimum training standards for medical attendants; however, these standards were largely unknown to many nurses working in the flight environment and were not generally being promoted by flight operators. This training was expected to be able to be completed in one day.

There was also no national training program specific for nurses in New Zealand. The NZFNA recognized the need for training nurses in aviation nursing and set about developing an introductory flight nurse's course with these needs in mind. This course focuses on physiology in the aviation environment and how those changes can affect a patient. The first course was held in April 1998 as a 3½-day course. A further seven courses have been held, with the course now extending 5 days.

Now many flight programs hold a training program specific to their own flight program requirements (in addition to nurses attending the introductory flight nurse's course) based on the minimum training standards from AIA and NZFNA Standards of Practice.

WORK REQUIREMENTS

Many of the flight programs in New Zealand are hospital based, being run through the hospital's critical care units. A smaller number of programs are run privately or through trust organizations.

Flight nurses in New Zealand are normally involved with the secondary interhospital transfer of patients. These patients are normally being transferred to a tertiary hospital for care not provided at regional and rural hospitals. Flight nurses do not practice primary response scene collection of patients.

Most nurses who are involved with flight nursing in New Zealand are critical care–trained nurses with a minimum of 5 years post-registration experience, who also have completed a post-registration critical care course, a New Zealand flight nurse's course, and advanced cardiac life support (ACLS) qualifications. Other qualifications the nurses may also possess include pediatric life support (PLS) and fundamentals of critical care support (FCCS).

PRACTICE CHALLENGES

Many of the programs are flying patients with unpressurized fixed-wing aircraft and helicopters. This obviously presents many challenges to flight nurses, needing to care for these patients who are being directly exposed to and affected by the reduced barometric pressure, reduced partial pressure of oxygen, and all the other associated stresses of flight.

New Zealand is divided into two main islands—the South Island and the North Island. Both of these islands have large mountain ranges dividing the east and west of the islands. This necessitates high altitude flights to climb over these ranges. The patient and crew are exposed to decreased pressures of gases (especially oxygen), cooler ambient temperatures, decreased humidity, and other associated stresses of flight.

The weather is also a major factor because it can vary greatly on each side of the mountain ranges. Flight nurses and crew members must maintain adequate temperature control for the patient and themselves by ensuring adequate layering of blankets and clothing.

Flight crews are required to take training in survival (especially mountain survival) because many fly over large areas of bush and forestry. Flight nurses are encouraged to have their own personal survival kit.

Because New Zealand is surrounded by water and has many rivers and lakes, additional training for flight crew includes sea survival and emergency underwater evacuation from aircraft.

Nurses in New Zealand do not hold patient clinics.

FLIGHT CREW PREPARATION/CONFIGURATION

Flight crew preparation and configuration varies greatly among programs. Nurses from within hospital programs are sourced either from being directly on shift in a unit to being the designated flight nurse on duty. Other programs have a nurse on duty from the air ambulance operation.

Doctors are normally sourced from within hospitals when required for missions, with some operations having doctors on duty for transports. Few of these doctors actually have aviation training and will often turn to the flight nurse for guidance and advice.

Respiratory therapists are not common in New Zealand; therefore they are not used in the transport scenario. Critical care flight nurses are responsible for managing ventilation and respiratory equipment during transports.

Paramedics are generally only involved with primary response helicopter work and do not work in the interhospital transfer environment. Paramedics in New Zealand do not have training in areas such as mechanical ventilation and inotrope management. Conversely, flight nurses do not have training in primary response aspects such as scene management, extrication, and mass casualty. Some programs in New Zealand may take a paramedic, but they act as crew members only, with a flight nurse/doctor being the primary caregiver.

The crew configuration is often related to the size of the aircraft being operated. Only a few operations in New Zealand have the ability to take an additional crew member. That crew member is generally responsible for the overall safety and loading of the aircraft.

PATIENT PREPARATION

As part of preparing the patient for transport, there first needs to be discussion from the referring doctor to the receiving doctor prior to a transfer request being initiated. Following acceptance of the patient at the receiving hospital, the flight medical team is notified. The flight doctor and flight nurse will then call the referring hospital for handover of the patient and to check that the receiving hospital has a bed available at the estimated time of arrival. A lot of this communication between flight crews and hospital/medical staff is done with mobile telephones.

Whenever possible, a relative is allowed to travel with the patient, but this is always subject to available space in the aircraft.

In regards to actual patient preparation, flight teams will always assess the patient prior to transport. This is to ensure that the patient's airway, breathing, circulation, and neurologic status are safe for transport.

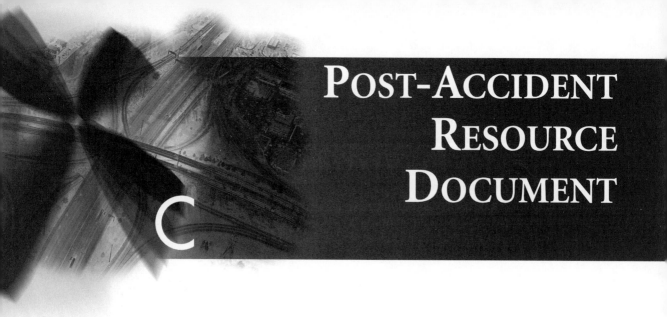

INTRODUCTION

Air medical transport services provide an essential life-saving function in the health-care and aviation systems. These services are generally high profile in nature, attracting positive attention from the media. Although air medical crashes are rare, when they occur, they instantly become an intensely emotional event.

This document describes the various phenomenon experienced by members of an air medical program following an aircraft incident. Its intended purposes are to assist air medical program leaders in progressing through the necessary critical functions required following a crash and to address the short- and long-term issues and decisions.

PHASE I: INTIAL SHOCK/REACTION (THE FIRST FEW HOURS)

When an air medical crash occurs, the timeliness and quality of information conveyed may vary depending on the circumstances. Notification of the crash may come to the communication center via scene witnesses (e.g., EMS, police, fire, and bystanders) or from the media. Rotor-wing crashes, which occur during takeoff or landing, usually are a witnessed event, whereas a fixed-wing crash may occur in a rural area far from the program's base of operation. With the advent of scanners, alpha-numeric paging systems, and media access to crash information, flight team members may receive information directly before official notification from a program representative.

POST-ACCIDENT INCIDENT PLAN

Your program's post-accident incident plan (PAIP) becomes the road map for your communications center staff to initiate the necessary critical steps which enhance crew survival and limit your program's liability. Priorities are:

- Verifying facts: crash location, other pertinent details
- Dispatching rescue crews: civil air patrol, air medical, or ambulance response to the crash site
- Activating notification list according to the PAIP
- Notifying security for crowd control at your base of operation/hospital

ROLE OF PROGRAM LEADERSHIP

The air medical program administrator's role will involve developing organization around the process, ensuring that the PAIP is being followed, and ensuring

Courtesy Association of Air Medical Services (AAMS). For more information contact the Association of Air Medical Services (AAMS), 526 King Street, Suite 415, Alexandria, Virginia 22314-3143; telephone: (703) 836-8732; fax: (703) 836-8920; Web page: www.aams.org.

that appropriate roles are assigned. Providing medical care to the victims of the crash—both air medical crew members and others involved in the crash—should be a high priority. The program leader should also ensure that the appropriate notifications are made to administration, the public relations director, the Part 135 operator (aviation site manager/lead pilot), and regulatory agencies such as the National Transportation Safety Board (NTSB), Federal Aviation Administration (FAA), and state health department. Flight team members must be notified of the event and directed to come to the program site where resources are available and factual information can be shared.

FAMILY MEMBER NOTIFICATION

As the person in charge, a program leader must ensure that family members of the on-board crew are notified. Ideally this notification should occur in person. Plan to send a responsible person to the location of the family members whenever feasible. Often the media will broadcast the information regarding the crash before notification of the family can occur. Minimally, this notification should occur by phone. Identify a private area at your facility, but away from the flight team, for the family members to gather. Assign an individual to provide factual information and to meet the needs of the family members. **Communicate facts only; do not speculate.**

In the first few hours, begin to organize a critical incident stress-diffusing session. Identify the agency of choice to conduct this, and plan to have as many crew members present as possible.

DEALING WITH THE MEDIA

Be sure that an appropriate individual is assigned to deal with the media. The media should have a place to convene away from the crash site or the flight team. A proactive approach to information sharing should help to limit speculation on the part of the media. When possible, one of the program leaders should be designated as a liaison for information sharing with the public relations official.

DECISION TO REMAIN IN SERVICE

A decision to remain in service may need to be addressed very quickly if you operate multiple aircraft.

The program administrator will need to quickly assess whether or not it would be appropriate depending on the flight team members' readiness to respond to a request for service. Such a decision should put safety first, keeping in mind that the profound effects on the air medical crew may minimize their effectiveness in providing patient care and in paying attention to safety principles for anywhere from hours to days following a crash. Flight team members will need time to seek information and process the events and results of the crash.

During this period, you should consider the availability of other air medical transport programs in your area. If this is a possibility, notify their communication center of your program's situation, and inform them that you may need to refer flight requests to their program.

You should also identify the scene coordinator, someone from your aviation team (pilot or mechanic) who should be assigned to coordinate activities at the crash site. The role of this individual is to coordinate the efforts of the various investigating agencies and to provide information to these agencies and the program administrator. This individual will also be the liaison to the Part 135 operator.

CRITICAL INCIDENT STRESS MANAGEMENT

An air medical crash will invoke a critical incident stress (CIS) response for many individuals both inside and outside of your program. Therefore the program leadership must recognize that psychologic assistance in dealing with the stress response and grieving process should be a required step for all members of the air medical team. The details about the assistance (who will be provide it, how it will be provided, and who will participate) should be identified in the post-accident incident planning process. Because individuals may not be able to adequately assess their own level of stress response, mandatory participation in the critical incident stress management (CISM) session is beneficial.

The mental health professionals involved in the CIS response can provide crucial assistance in assessing individual readiness for returning to flight. This assessment of all team members, including the program leader, is a crucial component of any PAIP and provides the information needed to determine the right time to return the program to service.

Despite CISM interventions and readiness assessments, air medical team members may experience a wide variety of post-stress phenomenon such as hypervigilence (e.g., obsession over the citing of wires in and around the landing zone) or flashbacks (e.g., triggered by a nighttime flight with circumstances similar to the crash). Such phenomenon may limit a team member's ability to perform his or her role. Strategies such as doubling up a flight team member or having additional flight team members on board as staffing and aircraft configurations allow can be helpful strategies as individuals start to perform their role on the aircraft following any critical incident.

Anger is an emotion commonly experienced by flight team members as a normal reaction to catastrophic loss and post-traumatic stress. Although individuals need to work through their anger, if misdirected this anger may be destructive to the rebuilding process. One-on-one counseling may be necessary to address individual stress reactions to an event.

Following a crash, team members are likely to continue in their role as members of the air medical team. This involvement provides an opportunity to experience regular acknowledgment and support from co-workers who can directly relate to their feelings. It is common for some staff to resign 6 to 12 months following a crash. The number resigning is based on numerous factors such as support both in and outside of work, and individual ability to cope with the work-related tragedy.

PHASE II: THE FIRST 24 HOURS— INITIAL DEVELOPMENT OF A PLAN

It is likely that the decision regarding the continuation of the air medical service will occur in the first 24 hours. It is often the ultimate test of your agency's support of the air medical program. If this decision was not addressed in the first few hours, this may become an essential decision to make and communicate to customers. The media can be a good source of getting this information out. Remember to notify emergency medical services

(EMS), public service groups, and communications centers when you return to service.

MANAGE THE MEDIA
Any positive relations developed with the media may pay off as the intense news coverage occurs. Plan to conduct regular news conferences and flight team interviews as appropriate. The public needs to know that your flight team can go on and that your program will continue. Providing the human side of this situation to the media may cause them to switch their focus from the negative aspects of the event. The local media (television and print) will likely cover this topic daily for several days to weeks. Flight program staff will need to expect this so that they will not be overwhelmed by the amount of media coverage.

INTERACTION WITH FAMILY MEMBERS
Plan interactions with family members of the crash victims. Program administration will need to contact family members to express concern for them and to determine if their needs are being met.

Family members of the air medical team may want to participate in a debriefing. The CISM team may be appropriate for this activity and the staff debriefing. In addition, family members may benefit from meeting with one of your program's pilots and representatives from administration. Their need for information will be heightened, especially with regard to program safety. Meeting the needs of team members' families will go a long way to gain the individual support necessary for return to work in the flight program.

KEEP LEADERSHIP INFORMED
Provide daily briefings to the CEO, the Board of Directors, and the line managers. It may be difficult for the program leadership to use objective decision-making skills during the crisis. Use the objectiveness of second-order people to assist with this and to validate decision making.

COMMUNICATE WITH THE AIR MEDICAL TEAM
Provide updated information from administration, planned CISM interventions, interaction with media, and successes (e.g., the positive encounters

and support from peers or customers). Regular staff meetings and on-going CISM interventions such as diffusing, debriefings, one-on-ones, and further individual counseling sessions may be needed on a daily basis for the first week or two. This is an opportunity to share information, common feelings, and experiences.

Contact neighboring air medical programs and the Concern Network if this has not already occurred. The industry recognition and support that results may be beneficial to the staff and program leadership.

LEGAL ISSUES

The legal consequences of a crash will quickly become apparent. Attorneys, risk managers, and your insurance carrier should be notified as early as possible. Be prepared to share your PAIP and steps taken to mitigate the event.

PHASE III: DAY 2 TO 5 IMPLEMENTATION/MODIFICATION

During this phase, many of the realities of the crash will become evident. The agencies that surround you will need to get back to business, whereas the air medical team members and leadership may continue to experience difficulty in coping with daily encounters and tasks.

CARING FOR THE INJURED VICTIMS

If there are survivors of the crash, caring for the injured crew members may require special attention to confidentiality issues, especially if it takes place at your base hospital/trauma center. It is common for flight team members to make regular visits to the injured flight team member(s). Their preoccupation with the injured team members' medical condition and concern for their family members may delay the individuals' return to flying.

HUMAN RESOURCES

Your human resources department staff will be essential in assisting with the processing of forms for the injured and deceased employees. They may be able to contact the hospital chaplain to coordi-

nate support for the rest of the hospital staff or agency employees.

REPLACING THE AIRCRAFT

Plans to replace the aircraft should be underway with a plan for return to service. It will be helpful to the flight team to know the plan for going back into service. All equipment on board the aircraft will need to be replaced. Using your equipment list should ease the process of identifying capital purchases required. When possible, designate an individual in your purchasing department to handle the process of timely equipment replacement. Equipment vendors may be able to provide loaner units to facilitate getting your aircraft back into service in a timely manner.

Identifying the tail number for the replacement aircraft may become a sensitive issue for flight team members. It is often wise to retire the tail number of the crash vehicle and start again. Flight teams may have a useful role in participating in tail number selection. There are several tasks appropriate to delegate to the flight team that are symbolic of the program moving forward, such as ordering and restocking the replacement aircraft. Opportunities to empower the staff with appropriate decisions may provide a mechanism to move beyond the immediate crisis.

PSYCHOLOGIC SUPPORT FOR STAFF

Ongoing assessment of team readiness to return to work and the available ongoing psychologic support are necessary for which to plan and communicate the need. Staff will need to understand the necessity of ongoing psychologic care, especially if individuals are not coping effectively with the stress. Inappropriate group dynamics may become evident as a coping mechanism, requiring an intervention for the entire group.

FUNERAL PLANNING

Death in the line of duty often translates to a public funeral; a ritual observed by firefighters, EMS personnel, and police officers. The EMS community will likely communicate this expectation early. Often there is no way to contain the outpouring of expected involvement, which may result in a public funeral. In many cases, the next of kin of the deceased may need to be convinced that a public funeral is in order. Identify a trusted member of the EMS community who has experience in planning a public funeral (member of a local fire department). This person may be invaluable in planning with the family and program leadership an otherwise overwhelming event. Religious officials will need to be involved in the planning along with the family so that the funeral plans are culturally sensitive to meet the needs of the family (e.g., Native-American burial practices) and those of the community at large.

Additionally, regular meetings with the designated individuals planning the public funeral will be necessary to ensure that the air medical program and staff needs are met. Municipal and state police involvement may be necessary to ensure that a processional of rescue vehicles can occur.

The air medical service leadership should consider taking the flight teams out of service to allow attendance at the funerals because participation in this ritual is an essential part of the healing process. Once again you have an opportunity to call on your neighboring flight program to cover your air medical transport requests. Several hours of down time following each funeral may be needed before team members can return to service.

MEMORIAL SERVICES

Memorial services may occur in addition to the public funeral. The CISM team and mental health workers can give advice regarding the appropriate timing for the memorial service. The service should provide an opportunity for team members to share personal remarks and eulogies. This can provide a sense of closure for some team members and an opportunity to move forward in the recovery process.

Participation in the funeral and memorial service is essential for all flight program staff. Consider taking your aircraft out of service for this time. Request coverage by other air medical services during this time. Ask a neighboring air medical service if they can reposition their aircraft to better cover your region. This will reduce the chance of air medical team mem-bers missing the service while conveying to the community your commitment to provide service.

REQUEST FOR MEMORIALS

Individuals or groups in the community may find a need to memorialize the aircraft crash site and deceased crew members. These issues may raise sensitivities with family members and the flight team, especially if suggestions are not consistent with the wishes of the family or flight team. Decisions about how to deal with these requests can be distracting and time consuming. Keep in mind that you do not have to deal with any of these issues right now. An urgent decision is rarely required. In many cases, it may be appropriate to delegate this responsibility to your public relations department.

DELAYED ISSUES

FORMAL INVESTIGATION

As the formal investigation continues, announcements of findings should be shared with key personnel in a timely manner. You may need to adopt a strategy to strive to inform air medical teams with information prior to learning this from the media. On-going regular meetings with the staff may be beneficial.

EVALUATE PROGRAM SAFETY

A plan to evaluate your program's safety program should include a review of:

- Safety and operational policies and procedures
- Safety education for staff
- Quality and effectiveness of crew resource management (CRM) training
- Community outreach safety education
- Quality of the program's safety culture

Reviewing these processes is a necessary step in providing reassurance for all members of the air medical team, administration, and risk management offices, with respect to the program's commitment to safety. A plan to evaluate safety will help to avoid the pitfall of reacting to requests based on stress and emotion rather than methodology. Involve the flight team, operator, and administration. Evaluate the effectiveness of your PAIP, and revise as necessary. An independent safety audit may be the choice to ensure objectivity. Develop a timetable for implementation of recommendations.

LEGAL ISSUES

We exist in a litigious society, and the number and nature of suits filed may surprise you. The news of such suits may become a significant distraction to the air medical teams as they work to re-enter the flight environment. Here are some issues to keep in mind:

- Insurance subrogation, the legal doctrine of substituting one creditor for another, can lead to litigation involving your customers. This could become an image problem for your program if the insurance provider sues your customer in the name of the operator or aircraft owner. Working closely with your legal department to support and reassure customers may be essential to preserve a positive working relationship.

- Anticipate filing deadlines and statue of limitations so that the flight team and public relations director can be prepared to manage the media. Often, announcements of lawsuit filings will appear in the press. Knowledge of lawsuits may generate a negative emotional response by air medical teams. Because your safety policy, procedures, and communications logs will likely be subpoenaed, consider archiving such documents as you update your manuals.

FINAL OUTCOME OF LAWSUITS

It often takes several years to settle lawsuits resulting from an air medical crash. It is possible that this will be reported in the media. Develop a relationship with your legal counsel regarding their commitment to communication with your program when legal activity is likely to attract the media's interest. Keeping your flight teams informed is essential.

EMOTIONAL SUPPORT FOR PROGRAM LEADERSHIP

To perform in the midst of an overwhelmingly emotional event, the leader probably will deny his or her own feelings of fear, grief, and anger to move the program forward. Although this may be necessary initially, if this process of denial goes on for too long, the program may be moving on and leaving the program leadership emotionally destitute and dysfunctional. Program managers must set aside some time to go through a formal grieving process and recognition of the intense impact the event has on them. Professional counseling is needed for all individuals involved. Without this assistance, inappropriate methods of dealing with the stress may eventually impair the long-term effectiveness of the manager. Seek the help of a professional counselor in a confidential setting, preferably away from the work environment. Plan time away from work with family and friends.

ANNIVERSARIES

The anniversary of a crash is a time of special recognition for the team and family members. Be prepared to deal with special requests for time off, and recognize that staff may need to be together. A meeting of the staff with an opportunity to talk about their feelings may be beneficial and should be offered to the flight team. Have your mental health workers available if team members need to speak in confidence about their feelings around the anniversary.

Each anniversary will be acknowledged in various ways by the staff. If the psychologic needs of the staff and program leadership are regarded as a high priority, it will be easier to deal with each anniversary.

REFERENCES

1. Hawkins M: Personal protective equipment in helicopter EMS, *Air Med J* 4(94):123-6, 1994.
2. Dodd R: Factors related to occupant crash survival in emergency medical services helicopters, *Aviation Science and Technology* 1992.
3. Low R, Sousa J, Dufresne D, et al: *IFR capability lowers accident rates of civilian helicopter ambulances: a multifactorial epidemiologic study*, Greenville, NC, 1997, East Carolina University School of Medicine.
4. Schneider C: Dollars and sense, *AirMed* Mar/Apr 18-19:21.4, 1997.
5. National Transportation Safety Board (NTSB): *Safety study, commercial emergency medical service*

helicopter operations, Report Number NTSB/SS-88/01, Washington, DC, 1988, NTSB.

6. Mitchell J, Everly G: *Critical incident stress debriefing: an operations manual for the prevention of traumatic stress among emergency services and disaster workers,* ed 2, Ellicott City, MD, 1996, Chevron Publishing Corp.

7. Mitchell J, Bray G: *Emergency services stress: guidelines for preserving the health and careers of emergency personnel,* Englewood Cliffs, NJ, 1990, Prentice Hall Publishers.

Post-Crash Resource Document
Association of Air Medical Services

POST-CRASH ADMINISTRATIVE CHECK LIST

Action Steps	Completion date/time	Comments
I. First 2 Hours		
A. Activate PAIP:		
1. Emergency/medical response to crash site.		
2. Complete notification list.		
3. Decide whether to remain in service (multiple aircraft).		
4. Identify and activate:		
a. Scene coordinator		
b. Base site coordinator		
c. Accident investigation team		
5. Identify a coordinator for the media.		
6. Convene flight team members.		
a. Provide updated information.		
b. Plan for initial CISM intervention.		
c. State expectation for ongoing CISM interventions.		
B. Notify family members, in person as applicable.		
C. Ensure that various coordinators have a checklist.		
II. First 24 Hours		
A. Liaison with public relations regarding managing the media.		
B. Interact with family members.		
C. Develop a plan to address flight team family member needs and CISM intervention.		
D. Inform leadership of your plan.		
E. Schedule a meeting with air medical team for information sharing and CISM.		
F. Notify attorneys, risk managers, and insurance carrier.		
III. First 2 to 5 Days		
A. Notify Human Resources, employee benefits, employment status, agency support		
B. Develop and communicate plan for aircraft replacement		
C. Develop and implement a plan for ongoing psychologic support for staff		
D. Designate an individual to plan a public funeral as indicated		
E. Designate individual to plan memorial service		
F. Identify a contact person to deal with requests for memorials		
IV. Delayed Issues 5 Days to 2 Weeks and Beyond		
A. Formal investigation: communicate initial findings.		
B. Evaluate program safety.		
C. Keep track of legal issues and communicate to staff:		
1. Insurance subrogation		
2. Filing deadlines/statute of limitations		
3. Final outcome of lawsuits		
D. Provide emotional support for program leadership. If you have not done this yet, it's time to make a plan.		
E. Anniversaries: plan meetings with staff and honor requests for time off.		

Add items to checklist as necessary.

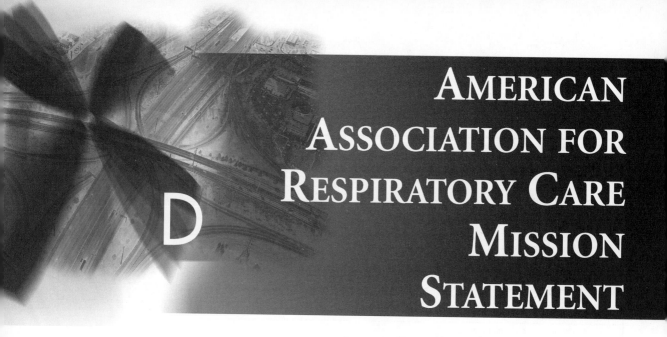

AMERICAN ASSOCIATION FOR RESPIRATORY CARE MISSION STATEMENT

The American Association for Respiratory Care (AARC) is formed to:

Encourage, develop, and provide educational programs for those persons interested in respiratory therapy and diagnostics

Advance the science, technology, ethics, and art of respiratory care through institutes, meetings, lectures, publications, and other materials

Facilitate cooperation and understanding among respiratory care personnel and the medical professions, allied health professions, hospitals service companies, industry, governmental organizations, and other agencies interested in respiratory care

Provide education to the general public in pulmonary health promotion and disease prevention

Courtesy American Association for Respiratory Care (AARC), Dallas, Texas.

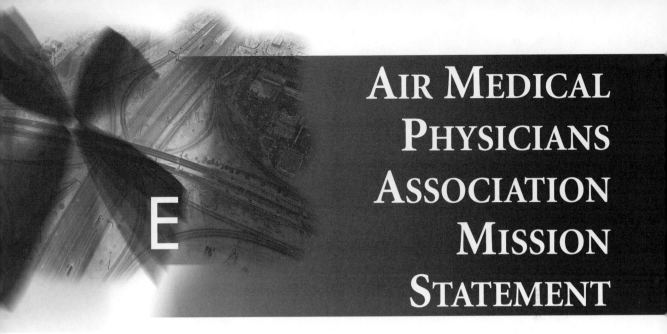

AIR MEDICAL PHYSICIANS ASSOCIATION MISSION STATEMENT

The Air Medical Physicians Association is a unique association comprised of physicians and professionals involved in medical transport who are committed to promoting safe and efficacious patient transportation through quality medical direction, research, education, leadership, and collaboration.

Courtesy Air Medical Physicians Association, Salt Lake City, Utah.

NATIONAL FLIGHT PARAMEDICS ASSOCIATION

F

MISSION STATEMENT

The National Flight Paramedics Association (NFPA) is dedicated to promoting the global development and growth of the paramedic profession.

VISION STATEMENT

The NFPA will evolve with the changing health-care environment and ensure that paramedics continue to perform a primary role in the critical care transport setting while maintaining the best interests of our patients.

MEDICAL CONDITION LIST AND APPROPRIATE USE OF AIR MEDICAL TRANSPORT

G

POSITION STATEMENT OF THE AIR MEDICAL PHYSICIAN ASSOCIATION

BACKGROUND

The Balanced Budget Act of 1997 initiated a process to convert all Medicare ambulance transport billing (including air) to a fee structure. Previous to this, ambulance reimbursement was done for the private ambulance industry under a fee structure reimbursement (commonly known as Part B) and, for hospital based ambulance service, under cost-based reimbursement (commonly known as Part A).

The new fee structure was developed in a process called Negotiated Rule Making (NRM). The NRM process established relative value units for each type of transport, rural modifiers, cost of living adjusters, and a phase-in schedule. As part of the NRM process, the Medical Conditions Work Group developed the Medical Condition List. This condition list was developed to simplify the issue of medical necessity for each level of transport and to reduce the importance of *ICD-9* codes to describe prehospital impressions. The Medical Condition List was developed because *ICD-9* codes are not designed to describe prehospital medical conditions. The standardization of medical necessity for different types of conditions created by the Medical Condition List will allow medical necessity to be aligned with appropriate use and will improve efficiency and simplify the billing and reimbursement process. The Medical Condition List was under consideration for possible inclusion in the final rule but was not included in the final rule published February 27, 2002. A commitment to develop the medical condition codes over the next 12 months was promised by the Center for Medcare and Medicaid Services (CMS) (formerly Health Care Finances Administration [HCFA]).

AMPA POSITION STATEMENT

AMPA supports the addition and adoption of the Medical Condition List, as submitted by the Medical Conditions Work Group, as a rational method of determining medically appropriate use of medical transport.

Furthermore, it is AMPA's position, as detailed in the Medical Condition List, that the determination of medical appropriateness for interfacility medical transport is determined by the a physician, as documented on a written Certification of Medical Necessity. Medical appropriateness of scene medical transport is determined by the requesting authorized prehospital provider, based on regional policy and their best medical judgment at the time of the request for transport. Further, AMPA supports that the Certificate of Medical Necessity for scene transport can be completed by the EMS control physician, receiving physician, or by the medical director of the transport program. AMPA supports that consultation with the transport provider medical direction is the optimal method of determining the appropriate mode of safe patient transport.

AMPA does not support the use of discharge ICD-9 codes to retrospectively determine medical appropriateness because this may adversely restrict access to appropriate care and negates the regional, environmental, and situational factors that are also important in determining medical appropriateness.

AMPA does not support a specification of a time needed for land transport as a general guideline. AMPA feels that when a time specification is made, it should be done regionally.

AIR MEDICAL TRANSPORT GUIDELINES DETAILED AS APPROPRIATE BY THE MEDICAL CONDITION LIST

AMPA supports the NRM workgroup recommendation to replace the list of conditions in section 2120.4 B (Medical Appropriateness) with:

- Acute neurologic emergencies requiring emergent/time sensitive interventions not available at the sending facility
- Acute vascular emergencies requiring urgent/time sensitive interventions not available at sending facilities

- Acute surgical emergencies requiring urgent/time sensitive interventions not available at the sending facility
- Critically ill patients with compromised hemodynamic/respiratory function who require intensive care during transport and whose time of transfer between critical care units must be minimized during transport
- Critically ill obstetric patients who require intensive care during transport and whose time of transfer between facilities must be minimized to prevent patient/fetal morbidity
- Acute cardiac emergencies requiring emergent/time-sensitive intervention not available at sending facility
- Critically ill neonatal/pediatric patients with potentially compromised hemodynamic/respiratory function, a metabolic acidosis greater than 2 hours post delivery, sepsis, or meningitis
- Patient with electrolyte disturbances and toxic exposure requiring immediate life-saving intervention
- Transplantation patients (fixed wing vs. helicopter)
- Patients requiring care in a specialty center not available at the sending facility
- Conditions requiring treatment in a Hyperbaric Oxygen Unit
- Burns requiring treatment in a burn treatment center
- Potentially life- or limb-threatening trauma requiring treatment at a trauma center, including penetrating eye injuries
- Emergency Medical Transport Active Labor Act (EMTALA) physician-certified inter-facility transfer (not a patient request)
- Emergency medical services (EMS) regional or state-approved protocol identifies need for on-scene air transport

Medical Condition List*
Draft—12/5/99

#	On-scene condition (general)	On-scene condition (specific)	Service level	Comments and examples (not all-inclusive)
Emergency conditions—non-traumatic				
1	Abdominal pain	With other signs or symptoms	ALS	Nausea, vomiting, fainting, pulsatile mass, distention, rigid, tenderness on exam, guarding
2	Abdominal pain	Without other signs or symptoms	BLS	
3	Abnormal cardiac rhythm/cardiac dysrhythmia	Potentially life-threatening	ALS	Bradycardia, junctional and ventricular blocks, non-sinus tachycardias, PVC's >6, bigeminy and trigeminy, vtach, vfib, atrial flutter, PEA, asystole
4	Abnormal skin signs		ALS	Diaphorhesis, cyanosis, delayed cap refill, poor turgor, mottled
5	Abnormal vital signs (includes abnormal pulse oximetry)	With symptoms	ALS	Other emergency conditions
6	Abnormal vital signs (includes abnormal pulse oximetry)	Without symptoms	BLS	
7	Allergic reaction	Potentially life-threatening	ALS	Other emergency conditions, rapid progression of symptoms, prior hx. of anaphylaxis, wheezing, difficulty swallowing
8	Allergic reaction	Other	BLS	Hives, itching, rash, slow onset, local swelling, redness, erythema
9	Animal bites/sting/envenomation	Potentially life- or limb-threatening	ALS	Symptoms of specific envenomation, significant face, neck, trunk, and extremity involvement; other emergency conditions
10	Animal bites/sting/envenomation	Other	BLS	Local pain and swelling, special handling considerations and patient monitoring required
11	Sexual assault	With injuries	ALS	
12	Sexual assault	With no injuries	BLS	
13	Blood glucose	Abnormal—<80 or >250, with symptoms	ALS	Altered mental status, vomiting, signs of dehydration, etc.
14	Respiratory arrest		ALS	Apnea, hypoventilation requiring ventilatory assistance and airway management
15	Difficulty breathing		ALS	

Continued

Medical Condition List*—cont'd
Draft—12/5/99

#	On-scene condition (general)	On-scene condition (specific)	Service level	Comments and examples (not all-inclusive)
Emergency conditions—non-traumatic—cont'd				
16	Cardiac arrest—resuscitation in progress		ALS	
17	Chest pain (non-traumatic)		ALS	Dull, severe, crushing, substernal, epigastric, left-sided chest pain associated with pain of the jaw, left arm, neck, back, and nausea, vomiting, palpitations, pallor, diaphoresis, decreased LOC
18	Choking episode		ALS	
19	Cold exposure	Potentially life- or limb-threatening	ALS	Temperature <95° F, deep frost bite, other emergency conditions
20	Cold exposure	With symptoms	BLS	Shivering, superficial frost bite, and other emergency conditions
21	Altered level of consciousness (non-traumatic)		ALS	Acute condition with Glascow Coma Scale <15
22	Convulsions/seizures	Seizing, immediate post-seizure, post-ictal, or at risk of seizure and requires medical monitoring/observation	ALS	
23	Eye symptoms, non-traumatic	Acute vision loss and/or severe pain	BLS	
24	Non-traumatic headache	With neurologic distress conditions	ALS	
25	Non-traumatic headache	Without neurologic symptoms	BLS	
26	Cardiac symptoms other than chest pain	Palpitations, skipped beats	ALS	
27	Cardiac symptoms other than chest pain	Atypical pain or other symptoms	ALS	Persistent nausea and vomiting, weakness, hiccups, pleuritic pain, feeling of impending doom, and other emergency conditions
28	Heat exposure	Potentially life-threatening	ALS	Hot and dry skin, temperature >105°F, neurologic distress, signs of heat stroke or heat exhaustion, orthostatic vitals, other emergency conditions
29	Heat exposure	With symptoms	BLS	Muscle cramps, perfuse sweating, fatigue
30	Hemorrhage	Severe (quantity)	ALS	Uncontrolled or significant signs of shock, other emergency conditions

*When using this chart, use all codes that apply.

Medical Condition List*—cont'd
Draft—12/5/99

#	On-scene condition (general)	On-scene condition (specific)	Service level	Comments and examples (not all-inclusive)
Emergency conditions—non-traumatic—cont'd				
31	Hemorrhage	Potentially life-threatening	ALS	Active vaginal, rectal bleeding, hematemesis, hemoptysis, epistaxis, active post-surgical bleeding
32	Infectious diseases requiring isolation procedures/ public health risk		BLS	
33	Hazmat exposure		ALS	Toxic fume or liquid exposure via inhalation, absorption, oral, radiation, smoke inhalation
34	Medical device failure	Life- or limb-threatening malfunction, failure, or complication	ALS	Malfunction of ventilator, internal pacemaker, internal defibrillator, implanted drug delivery device
35	Medical device failure	Health maintenance device failures	BLS	O_2 supply malfunction, orthopedic device failure
36	Neurologic distress	Facial drooping; loss of vision; aphasia; difficulty swallowing; numbness, tingling extremity; stupor, delirium, confusion, hallucinations; paralysis, paresis (focal weakness); abnormal movements; vertigo; unsteady gait/ balance; slurred speech, inability to speak	ALS	
37	Pain, acute and severe not otherwise specified in this list	Patient needs specialized handling to be moved: pain exacerbated by movement	BLS	
38	Pain, severe not otherwise specified in this list	Acute onset, unable to ambulate or sit	BLS	Pain is the reason for the transport
39	Pain, severe not otherwise specified in this list		ALS	Use severity scale (7-10 for severe pain), patit receiving pre-hospital pharmacologic intervention
40	Back pain—non-traumatic (T and/or LS)	Suspect cardiac or vascular etiology	ALS	Other emergency conditions, absence of or decreased leg pulses, pulsatile abdominal mass, severe tearing abdominal pain

Continued

Medical Condition List*—cont'd
Draft—12/5/99

#	On-scene condition (general)	On-scene condition (specific)	Service level	Comments and examples (not all-inclusive)
Emergency conditions—non-traumatic—cont'd				
41	Back pain—non-traumatic (T and/or LS)	New neurologic symptoms	ALS	Neurologic distress list
42	Poisons, ingested, injected, inhaled, absorbed	Adverse drug reaction, poison exposure by inhalation, injection or absorption	ALS	
43	Alcohol intoxication, drug overdose (suspected)	Unable to care for self; unable to ambulate; no risk to airway; no other symptoms	BLS	
44	Alcohol intoxication, drug overdose (suspected)	All others, including airway at risk, pharmacologic intervention, cardiac monitoring	ALS	
45	Post-operative procedure complications	Major wound dehiscence, evisceration, or requires special handling for transport	BLS	Orthopedic appliance; prolapse
46	Pregnancy complication/childbirth/labor		ALS	
47	Psychiatric/behavioral	Abnormal mental status; drug withdrawal	ALS	Suicidal, homicidal, hallucinations, violent, disoriented, DT's withdrawal symptoms, transport required by state law/court order
48	Psychiatric/behavioral	Threat to self or others, severe anxiety, acute episode or exacerbation of paranoia, or disruptive behavior	BLS	
49	Sick person	Fever with associated symptoms (headache, stiff neck, etc.)	ALS	
50	Sick person	Fever without associated symptoms	BLS	>102 in adults >104 in children
51	Sick person	No other symptoms	BLS	With other emergency conditions
52	Sick person	Nausea and vomiting, diarrhea, severe and incapacitating	ALS	
53	Unconscious, fainting, syncope	Transient unconscious episode or found unconscious	ALS	
54	Near syncope, weakness or dizziness	Acute episode or exacerbation	ALS	

*When using this chart, use all codes that apply.

Medical Condition List*—cont'd
Draft—12/5/99

#	On-scene condition (general)	On-scene condition (specific)	Service level	Comments and examples (not all-inclusive)
Emergency conditions—non-traumatic—cont'd				
55	Medical/legal	State or local ordinance requires ambulance transport under certain conditions	BLS	Minor with no guardian; During while intoxicated (DWI) arrest at MVA for evaluation; arrests and medical conditions (psych, drug overdose)
Emergency conditions—trauma				
56	Major trauma	As defined by ACS Field Triage Decision Scheme	ALS	Trauma with one of the following: Glascow <14; systolic BP <90; RR <10 or >29; all penetrating injuries to head, neck, torso, extremities proximal to elbow or knee; flail chest; combination of trauma and bums; pelvic fracture; two or more long bone fractures; open or depressed skull fracture; paralysis; severe mechanism of injury including: ejection, death of another passenger in same patient compartment, falls >20 feet, 20-inch deformity in vehicle or 12-inch deformity of patient compartment, auto pedestrian/bike, pedestrian thrown/run over, motorcycle accident at speeds >20 mph and rider separated from vehicle
57	Other trauma	Need to monitor or maintain airway	ALS	Decreased LOC; bleeding into airway; trauma to head, face, or neck
58	Other trauma	Major bleeding	ALS	Uncontrolled or significant bleeding
59	Other trauma	Suspected fracture/dislocation requiring splinting/ immobilization for transport	BLS	Spinal, long bones, and joints including shoulder elbow, wrist, hip, knee, and ankle; deformity of bone or joint
60	Other trauma	Penetrating extremity injuries	BLS	Isolated with bleeding stopped and good CSM
61	Other trauma	Amputation—digits	BLS	
62	Other trauma	Amputation—all other	ALS	
63	Other trauma	Suspected internal, head, chest, or abdominal injuries	ALS	Signs of closed head injury, open head injury, pneumothorax, hemothorax, abdominal bruising, positive abdominal signs on exam, internal bleeding criteria, evisceration
64	Other trauma	Severe pain requiring pharmacologic pain control	ALS	See severity scale

Continued

Medical Condition List*—cont'd
Draft—12/5/99

#	On-scene condition (general)	On-scene condition (specific)	Service level	Comments and examples (not all-inclusive)
Emergency conditions—trauma—cont'd				
65	Other trauma	Trauma NOS: it is up to the provider to provide sufficient documentation to support this claim	BLS	Ambulance required because injury is associated with other emergency conditions or other reasons for transport exist such as special patient handling or patient safety issues
66	Burns	Major—per ABA	ALS	Partial thickness burns >10% TBSA; involvement of face, hands, feet, genitalia, perineum, or major joints; third degree burns; electrical; chemical; inhalation; burns with preexisting medical disorders; burns and trauma
67	Burns	Minor—per ABA	BLS	Other burns than listed above
68	Lightning		ALS	
69	Electrocution		ALS	
70	Near drowning		ALS	
71	Eye injuries	Acute vision loss or blurring, severe pain or chemical exposure, penetrating, severe lid lacerations	BLS	

#	Reason for transport (general)	Reason for transport (specific)	Service level	Comments
Non-emergency				
72	Bed confined (at the time of transport)	Unable to get up without assistance; unable to ambulate; and unable to sit in a chair or wheelchair	BLS	Patient is going to a medical procedure, treatment, testing, or evaluation that is medically necessary
73	ALS monitoring required	Cardiac/hemodynamic monitoring en route	ALS	Expectation monitoring is needed before and after transport
74	ALS monitoring required	Advanced airway management	ALS	Ventilator dependent, apnea monitor, possible intubation needed, deep suctioning
75	ALS monitoring required	Intravenous (IV) meds required en route	ALS	Does not apply to self-administered IV medications
76	ALS monitoring required	Chemical restraint	ALS	
77	BLS monitoring required	Suctioning required en route	BLS	Per transfer instructions
78	BLS monitoring required	Airway control/positioning required en route	BLS	Per transfer instructions

*When using this chart, use all codes that apply.

Medical Condition List*—cont'd
Draft—12/5/99

#	Reason for transport (general)	Reason for transport (specific)	Service level	Comments
Non-emergency—cont'd				
79	BLS monitoring required	Third party assistance/ attendant required to apply, administer, or regulate or adjust oxygen en route	BLS	Does not apply to patient capable of self-administration of portable or home O_2; patient must require oxygen therapy and be so frail as to require assistance
80	Specialty care monitoring	A level of service provided to a critically injured or ill patient beyond the scope of the national paramedic curriculum.	SCT	
81	Medical conditions that contraindicate transport by other means	Patient Safety: Danger to self or others. In restraints	BLS	Refer to definition in the CFR—sec. 482.13(e).
82	Medical conditions that contraindicate transport by other means	Patient safety: Danger to self or others. Monitoring.	BLS	Behavioral or cognitive risk such that patient requires monitoring for safety.
83	Medical conditions that contraindicate transport by other means	Patient safety: Danger to self or others. Seclusion (Flight risk)	BLS	Behavioral or cognitive risk such that patient requires attendant to assure patient does not try to exit the ambulance prematurely. CFR sec. 482.13(f)(2) for definition.
84	Medical conditions that contraindicate transport by other means	Patient safety: risk of falling off wheelchair or stretcher while in motion	BLS	Patient's physical condition is such that patient risks injury during vehicle movement despite restraints. Indirect indicators include MDS criteria.
85	Medical conditions that contraindicate transport by other means	Special handling en route: isolation	BLS	Includes patients with communicable diseases or hazardous material exposure who must be isolated from public or whose medical condition must be protected from public exposure; surgical drainage complications
86	Medical conditions that contraindicate transport by other means	Special handling en route: patient size	BLS	Morbid obesity which requires additional personnel or equipment to transfer
87	Medical conditions that contraindicate transport by other means	Special handling en route: orthopedic device	BLS	Backboard, halotraction, use of pins and traction, etc.

Continued

Medical Condition List*—cont'd
Draft—12/5/99

#	Reason for transport (general)	Reason for transport (specific)	Service level	Comments
Non-emergency—cont'd				
88	Medical conditions that contraindicate transport by other means	Special handling en route: >1 person for physical assistance in transfers	BLS	
89	Medical conditions that contraindicate transport by other means	Special handling en route: severe pain	BLS	Pain must be aggravated by transfers or moving vehicle such that trained expertise of emergency medical technician (EMT) required (pain scale). Pain is present but is not sole reason for transport.
90	Medical conditions that contraindicate transport by other means	Special handling en route: positioning requires specialized handling	BLS	Requires special handling to avoid further injury (such as with >grade 2 decubiti on buttocks). Generally does not apply to shorter transfers < 1 hour. Positioning in wheelchair or standard car seat inappropriate due to contractures or recent extremity fractures—post-op hip as an example.
Inter-facility				
91	EMTALA-certified interfacility transfer to a higher level of care	Physician has made the determination that this transfer is needed—carrier only needs to know the level of care and mode of transport	BLS, ALS, SCT, Air	Excludes patient-requested EMTALA transfer. Specify what service is not available.
92	Service not available at originating facility, *and* must meet one or more emergency or non-emergency conditions		BLS, ALS, SCT, Air	
93	Service not covered	Indicates to carrier that claim should be automatically denied		

*When using this chart, use all codes that apply.

INDEX